D1498514

Breast Imaging

OTHER VOLUMES IN THE
EXPERT RADIOLOGY SERIES

Abdominal Imaging

Cardiovascular Imaging

Head and Neck Imaging

Imaging of the Chest

Imaging of the Musculoskeletal System

Imaging of the Spine

Image-Guided Interventions

FORTHCOMING VOLUMES IN THE
EXPERT RADIOLOGY SERIES

Imaging of the Brain

Gynecologic Imaging

Obstetric Imaging

Pediatric Neuroimaging

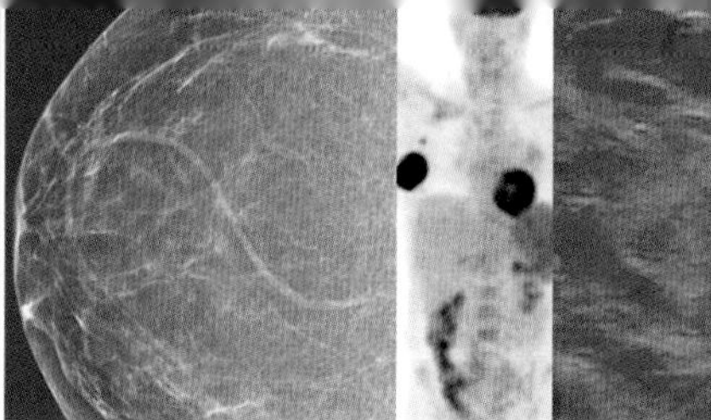

Breast Imaging

Lawrence W. Bassett, MD, FACR
Iris Cantor Professor of Breast Imaging
Vice Chair for Academic Affairs
Department of Radiological Sciences
David Geffen School of Medicine at UCLA
Los Angeles, California

Mary Catherine Mahoney, MD, FACR
Director of Breast Imaging
Barrett Cancer Center
Professor of Radiology
University of Cincinnati Medical Center
Cincinnati, Ohio

Sophia Kim Apple, MD
Director of Breast Pathology
Associate Professor
Department of Pathology and Laboratory Medicine
David Geffen School of Medicine at UCLA
Los Angeles, California

Carl J. D'Orsi, MD, FACR
Professor of Radiology, Oncology/Hematology
Director of Breast Imaging Research
Emory University Hospital
Atlanta, Georgia

ELSEVIER
SAUNDERS

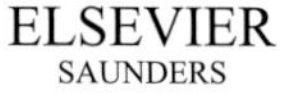

ELSEVIER
SAUNDERS

1600 John F. Kennedy Blvd.
Ste 1800
Philadelphia, PA 19103-2899

BREAST IMAGING
ISBN: 978-1-4160-5199-2
Copyright © 2011 by Saunders, an imprint of Elsevier Inc.

All rights reserved. No part of this publication may be reproduced or transmitted in any form or by any means, electronic or mechanical, including photocopying, recording, or any information storage and retrieval system, without permission in writing from the publisher. Details on how to seek permission, further information about the Publisher's permissions policies and our arrangements with organizations such as the Copyright Clearance Center and the Copyright Licensing Agency, can be found at our website: www.elsevier.com/permissions.

This book and the individual contributions contained in it are protected under copyright by the Publisher (other than as may be noted herein).

Notices

Knowledge and best practice in this field are constantly changing. As new research and experience broaden our understanding, changes in research methods, professional practices, or medical treatment may become necessary.

Practitioners and researchers must always rely on their own experience and knowledge in evaluating and using any information, methods, compounds, or experiments described herein. In using such information or methods they should be mindful of their own safety and the safety of others, including parties for whom they have a professional responsibility.

With respect to any drug or pharmaceutical products identified, readers are advised to check the most current information provided (i) on procedures featured or (ii) by the manufacturer of each product to be administered, to verify the recommended dose or formula, the method and duration of administration, and contraindications. It is the responsibility of practitioners, relying on their own experience and knowledge of their patients, to make diagnoses, to determine dosages and the best treatment for each individual patient, and to take all appropriate safety precautions.

To the fullest extent of the law, neither the Publisher nor the authors, contributors, or editors, assume any liability for any injury and/or damage to persons or property as a matter of products liability, negligence or otherwise, or from any use or operation of any methods, products, instructions, or ideas contained in the material herein.

Library of Congress Cataloging-in-Publication Data

Breast imaging / Lawrence W. Bassett ... [et al.]. - 1st ed.
p. ; cm.
Includes bibliographical references.
ISBN 978-1-4160-5199-2 1. Breast–Imaging–Textbooks. I. Bassett, Lawrence W. (Lawrence Wayne), 1942-
[DNLM: 1. Breast Neoplasms–diagnosis. 2. Diagnostic Imaging–methods. WP 870 B82847 2011]
RG493.5.D52B74 2011
618.1'90754–dc22

2010002588

Senior Acquisitions Editor: Rebecca Gaertner
Senior Developmental Editor: Jennifer Shreiner
Publishing Services Manager: Hemamalini Rajendrababu
Project Managers: Srikumar Narayanan and Bridget Healy
Designer: Steve Stave

Printed in China

Last digit is the print number: 9 8 7 6 5 4 3 2 1

Working together to grow
libraries in developing countries

www.elsevier.com | www.bookaid.org | www.sabre.org

ELSEVIER BOOK AID International Sabre Foundation

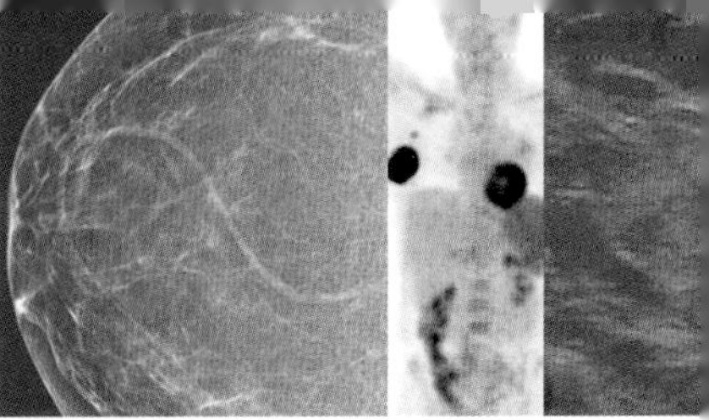

Contributors

Sophia Kim Apple, MD
Director of Breast Pathology
Associate Professor
Department of Pathology and Laboratory Medicine
David Geffen School of Medicine at UCLA
Los Angeles, California

Shida Banakar, PhD
Research Associate
Department of Radiological Sciences
David Geffen School of Medicine at UCLA
Los Angeles, California

Lawrence W. Bassett, MD, FACR
Iris Cantor Professor of Breast Imaging
Vice Chair for Academic Affairs
Department of Radiological Sciences
David Geffen School of Medicine at UCLA
Los Angeles, California

Eric A. Berns, PhD
Assistant Professor
Department of Radiology
Denver Health Medical Center
University of Colorado Denver School of Medicine
Denver, Colorado

Robyn L. Birdwell, MD, FACR
Section Head, Division of Breast Imaging
Brigham and Women's Hospital;
Associate Professor, Radiology
Harvard Medical School
Boston, Massachusetts

Adam Bracha, MD
David Geffen School of Medicine at UCLA
Los Angeles, California

Shireen L. Braner, PA, RT(R)(M)(QM), CBEC
Director of Breast Imaging
Imaging Department Magee-Womens Hospital
University of Pittsburgh Medical Center,
Pittsburgh, Pennsylvania

R. James Brenner, MD, JD
Director, Breast Imaging
Bay Imaging Consultants
Carol Ann Read Breast Health Center
Oakland, California;
Professor of Radiology
University of California, San Francisco
San Francisco, California

Louise A. Brinton, PhD
Chief, Hormonal and Reproductive Epidemiology Branch
National Cancer Institute
National Institutes of Health
Bethesda, Maryland

Priscilla F. Butler, MS, FACR, FAAPM
Senior Director, Breast Imaging Accreditation Programs
Department of Quality and Safety
American College of Radiology
Reston, Virginia;
Adjunct Professor
Department of Radiology
George Washington University Medical Center
Washington, DC

Ronald A. Castellino, MD
Professor Emeritus of Radiology
Stanford University School of Medicine
Stanford, California;
Member and Chairman Emeritus
Department of Radiology
Memorial Sloan-Kettering Cancer Center
New York, New York

Christopher Comstock, MD
Attending Radiologist
Director of Breast Imaging Education
Department of Radiology
Memorial Sloan-Kettering Cancer Center
New York, New York

Carl J. D'Orsi, MD, FACR
Professor of Radiology, Oncology/Hematology
Director of Breast Imaging Research
Emory University Hospital
Atlanta, Georgia

Jane M. Dascalos, MD
Radiology
Tower Imaging Medical Group
Los Angeles, California

Nanette D. DeBruhl, MD
Professor
Department of Radiological Sciences
David Geffen School of Medicine at UCLA
Los Angeles, California

D. David Dershaw, MD, FACR
Professor
Department of Radiology
Weill Cornell Medical College;
Director, Breast Imaging Section
Department of Radiology
Memorial Sloan-Kettering Cancer Center
New York, New York

Carol DeSantis, MPH
Epidemiologist
Department of Surveillance and Health Policy Research
American Cancer Society
Atlanta, Georgia

Laura Doepke, MD
Assistant Professor
Department of Radiological Sciences
David Geffen School of Medicine at UCLA
Los Angeles, California

Stephen W. Duffy, MSc, CStat
Professor
CR-UK Centre for EMS
Wolfson Institute of Preventive Medicine
Barts and The London School of Medicine and Dentistry
Queen Mary University of London
London, United Kingdom

Stephen A. Feig, MD, FACR
Professor of Radiological Sciences
University of California Irvine School of Medicine;
Director, Breast Imaging
Department of Radiology
UCI Medical Center
Orange, California

Richard H. Gold, MD
Professor Emeritus
Department of Radiological Sciences
David Geffen School of Medicine at UCLA
Los Angeles, California

David P. Gorczyca, MD
Staff Radiologist
Diagnostic Radiology, Breast Imaging, and MR Mammography
Red Rock Radiology
Las Vegas, Nevada

Jennifer A. Harvey, MD, FACR
Professor of Radiology
Chief, Division of Breast Imaging
University of Virginia School of Medicine
Charlottesville, Virginia

Anne C. Hoyt, MD
Associate Professor
Department of Radiological Sciences
David Geffen School of Medicine at UCLA
Los Angeles, California

Christopher P. Hsu, MD
Department of Radiological Sciences
David Geffen School of Medicine at UCLA
Los Angeles, California

Valerie P. Jackson, MD, FACR
Eugene C. Klatte Professor and Chair
Department of Radiology and Imaging Sciences
Indiana University School of Medicine
Indianapolis, Indiana

Ahmedin Jemal, DMV, PhD
Strategic Director, Cancer Surveillance
Department of Surveillance and Health Policy Research
American Cancer Society
Atlanta, Georgia

Joan Kramer, MD
American Cancer Society
Atlanta, Georgia

Gary M. Levine, MD
Director of Breast Imaging
Hoag Breast Care Center
Hoag Memorial Presbyterian Hospital
Newport Beach, California

Michael N. Linver, MD, FACR
Director of Mammography
Breast Imaging Center
X-Ray Associates of New Mexico, P.C.;
Clinical Professor
Department of Radiology
University of New Mexico School of Medicine
Albuquerque, New Mexico

Scott Lipnick, PhD
Biomedical Physics IDP
Department of Radiological Sciences
David Geffen School of Medicine at UCLA
Los Angeles, California

Jennifer Little, MD
Department of Radiological Sciences
David Geffen School of Medicine at UCLA
Los Angeles, California

Xiaoyu Liu, PhD
Graduate Student Researcher
Biomedical Physics IDP
Department of Radiological Sciences
David Geffen School of Medicine at UCLA
Los Angeles, California

January K. Lopez, MD
Department of Radiological Sciences
David Geffen School of Medicine at UCLA
Los Angeles, California

Mary Catherine Mahoney, MD, FACR
Director of Breast Imaging
Barrett Cancer Center;
Professor of Radiology
University of Cincinnati Medical Center
Cincinnati, Ohio

Ellen B. Mendelson, MD, FACR
Chief, Breast and Women's Imaging Section
Department of Radiology
Northwestern Memorial Hospital;
Professor of Radiology
Northwestern University Feinberg School of Medicine
Chicago, Illinois

Neda A. Moatamed, MD
Assistant Professor
Department of Pathology and Laboratory Medicine
David Geffen School of Medicine at UCLA
Los Angeles, California

Elizabeth A. Morris, MD, FACR
Attending Radiologist, Department of Radiology
Memorial Hospital for Cancer and Allied Diseases;
Associate Professor
Department of Radiology
Weill Cornell Medical College
New York, New York

Mary S. Newell, MD
Assistant Professor of Radiology
Assistant Director, Section of Breast Imaging
Director, Breast MRI
Director, Breast Imaging Fellowship Program
Department of Radiology
Emory University
Atlanta, Georgia

Dawn C. Nwamuo, MD
Breast Imaging Fellow
Department of Radiology
Stanford University
Palo Alto, California

Thomas Oshiro, PhD
Assistant Professor
Department of Radiological Sciences
David Geffen School of Medicine at UCLA
Los Angeles, California

Jennifer M.J. Overstreet, MD
Radiologist
Newport Harbor Radiology Associates
Newport Beach, California

Cheryce M. Poon, MD
Assistant Professor
Department of Radiological Sciences
David Geffen School of Medicine at UCLA
Los Angeles, California

Steven P. Poplack, MD, FSBI
Director, Breast Imaging
Department of Radiology
Dartmouth-Hitchcock Medical Center;
Associate Professor
Diagnostic Radiology
Dartmouth Medical School
Lebanon, New Hampshire

James W. Sayre, PhD
Professor
Department of Radiological Sciences
David Geffen School of Medicine at UCLA
Los Angeles, California

Helmuth Schultze-Haakh, PhD
MR Collaborations Manager
Siemens Medical Solutions USA, Inc.,
Malvern, Pennsylvania

Erum W. Sethi, MD
Department of Radiological Sciences
David Geffen School of Medicine at UCLA
Los Angeles, California

Edward A. Sickles, MD, FACR
Professor Emeritus of Radiology
Former Chief of Breast Imaging Service
Department of Radiology
University of California, San Francisco School of Medicine
San Francisco, California

Robert A. Smith, PhD
Director, Cancer Screening
Cancer Control Sciences
American Cancer Society
Atlanta, Georgia

A. Thomas Stavros, MD, FACR
Women's Imaging Radiologist
Sutter Pacific Women's Health Center
Santa Rosa, California

M. Albert Thomas, PhD
Professor
Departments of Radiological Sciences and Psychiatry
David Geffen School of Medicine at UCLA
Los Angeles, California

Katherine H. Walker, MD
Assistant Professor of Clinical Radiology
Indiana University School of Medicine
Indianapolis, Indiana

Colin J. Wells, MD
Assistant Professor of Radiology
Iris Cantor Center for Breast Imaging
Department of Radiological Sciences
David Geffen School of Medicine at UCLA
Los Angeles, California

Margarita L. Zuley, MD
Medical Director of Breast Imaging
Magee-Womens Hospital
University of Pittsburgh Medical Center;
Associate Professor
Department of Radiology
University of Pittsburgh School of Medicine
Pittsburgh, Pennsylvania

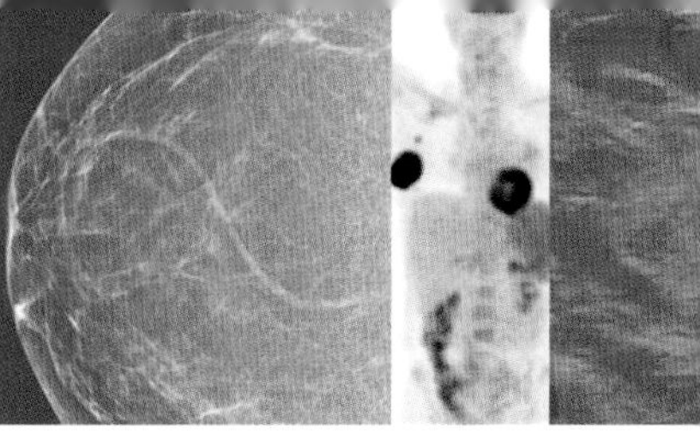

Preface

The editors of *Breast Imaging* are very excited about the introduction of this new and unique textbook for many reasons, including:

1. It has been designed to be the most up-to-date and comprehensive product for health care professionals who deal with breast diseases and especially physicians who interpret breast imaging exams.
2. It will provide an in-depth review on all aspects of breast imaging, including the newest technologies. The chapter authors are acknowledged as leading experts in the field.
3. It offers unique learning opportunities, including the ability to access the textbook for information on-line at a computer near the interpreting physician's workstation. For example, if the interpreting physician has questions about a breast imaging examination they are interpreting they can immediately access this textbook on-line for help.

Section 1 begins with a chapter on the history of the origins and development of the subspecialty of breast imaging. The next chapter, overseen by the lead author of the American Cancer Society Guidelines for Breast Cancer Screening, provides an opportunity to learn the newest information on the epidemiology of breast cancer and the impact of early detection on patient survival. The final chapter addresses controversies about breast cancer screening with mammography. The authors are acknowledged international experts in this arena. They provide evidence-based data that supports annual screening beginning at age 40, and this information will be important for interpreting physicians and other health care providers responding to questions from referring physicians and patients concerning screening mammography.

Section 2 encompasses comprehensive updates on breast imaging technologies. Leading experts in these technologies offer the current status of digital mammography, computer-aided detection, positioning, clinical image evaluation, and quality control in mammography. Experts in breast ultrasound and breast MRI have contributed additional chapters with thorough reviews and updates on these modalities. This section ends with a chapter that provides the most recent version of the American College of Radiology's Breast Imaging Reporting and Data System, authored by the overall Chair of the ACR BI-RADS Committee and Subcommittee Chairs for Mammography, Ultrasound, and MRI.

Sections 3, 4, and 5 are focused on imaging-pathology correlation. The authors of these chapters are pathologists and radiologists who specialize in breast diseases. Today the majority of breast biopsies are imaging guided, and the pathology results will determine subsequent patient management. We are confident that this publication provides the most comprehensive review of correlated imaging-pathology findings.

Section 3 presents the imaging and histology of the normal breast. We believe that this is fundamental to understand the imaging and histology of benign and malignant breast lesions.

Section 4 focuses on the Imaging of Benign Breast Diseases. The breast pathology and imaging authors worked together to provide a comprehensive review of the majority of benign lesions with histology and imaging correlates. There are chapters addressing both cystic and solid benign entities. In addition, proliferative lesions and benign calcifications are reviewed. Importantly, there is a review of high-risk benign breast lesions that may require excisional biopsy after an imaging-guided core needle biopsy.

Section 5 follows with a comprehensive review of the pathology and imaging of breast malignancies, ranging from ductal carcinoma-in-situ and invasive carcinomas to rare malignancies. There is also information about the role of imaging with neoadjuvant chemotherapy.

Section 6 introduces the current status of "Appropriateness Criteria" for the breast imaging workup. We are entering the era of "evidence-based medicine", which will require justification of our imaging protocols in the future health care system. The American College of Radiology Appropriateness Criteria were developed to identify appropriate workup protocols, justified by evidence in the scientific literature, for breast imaging findings associated with clinical findings or recalled from a screening mammogram. The authors of these chapters have been members of the ACR Appropriateness Criteria committee for breast imaging.

Section 7 presents the status of current imaging-guided interventional procedures. It also presents the pathologist's evaluation of the biopsy specimens and how they are processed. Finally, it addresses the breast imager's role in determining post-biopsy management.

Section 8 reviews the imaging findings in the surgically altered breast. Evaluating imaging studies after major surgery can be a challenge. However, the authors of these chapters are known experts in evaluating the post-surgical breast.

Section 9 is a comprehensive update on the current regulations in breast imaging. Like it or not, breast imaging is the most regulated field in radiology, and one of the most regulated in all of medicine. We are fortunate to have recruited the most authoritative contributors for each of these chapters that address MQSA and Accreditation Programs, The Medical Audit, Coding and Billing, and Medico-legal Issues.

Section 10 introduces Emerging Technologies in breast imaging. Each of the authors of these chapters is actively involved in research studies on these new and promising technologies of the future. It is an exciting venture.

We wish to thank our contributing authors for their excellent submissions to this book. We also want to thank our patients, families, friends, and coworkers for their help and patience in this endeavor. In summary, after our hard work we are proud to provide this new and unique textbook to you.

The Editors

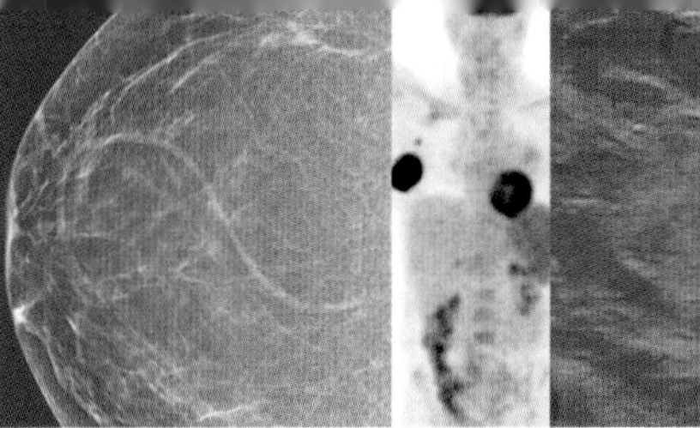

Contents

SECTION 1: INTRODUCTION

CHAPTER 1 **History of Breast Imaging** 3
Lawrence W. Bassett and Richard H. Gold

CHAPTER 2 **Epidemiology of Breast Cancer** 25
Robert A. Smith, Louise A. Brinton, Joan Kramer, Ahmedin Jemal, and Carol DeSantis

CHAPTER 3 **Screening Results, Controversies, and Guidelines** 56
Stephen A. Feig and Stephen W. Duffy

SECTION 2: IMAGING TECHNOLOGIES

CHAPTER 4 **Mammography and Digital Equipment** 79
Eric A. Berns

CHAPTER 5 **Computer-Aided Detection** 99
Robyn L. Birdwell and Ronald A. Castellino

CHAPTER 6 **Positioning in Mammography** 110
Margarita L. Zuley and Shireen L. Braner

CHAPTER 7 **Clinical Image Evaluation** 121
Lawrence W. Bassett and Laura Doepke

CHAPTER 8 **Mammography Quality Control: Digital and Screen-Film** 133
Priscilla F. Butler

CHAPTER 9 **Ultrasound Equipment** 146
Christopher Comstock

CHAPTER 10 **Ultrasound Indications and Interpretation** 153
A. Thomas Stavros

CHAPTER 11 **Magnetic Resonance Equipment and Techniques** 177
Thomas Oshiro, Helmuth Schultze-Haakh, and Jennifer Little

CHAPTER 12 **Magnetic Resonance Imaging: Indications and Interpretation** 195
Colin J. Wells and Nanette D. DeBruhl

CHAPTER 13 **BI-RADS, Reporting, and Communication** 213
Carl J. D'Orsi, Edward A. Sickles, Ellen B. Mendelson, and Elizabeth A. Morris

SECTION 3: IMAGING OF THE NORMAL BREAST

CHAPTER 14 **The Normal Breast** 223
Neda A. Moatamed, Lawrence W. Bassett, and Sophia Kim Apple

SECTION 4: IMAGING OF THE BENIGN BREAST DISEASE

CHAPTER 15 **Benign Cystic Lesions of the Breast** 239
Sophia Kim Apple, Laura Doepke, and Lawrence W. Bassett

CHAPTER 16 **Solid Benign Lesions of the Breast** 255
Sophia Kim Apple, Jane M. Dascalos, and Lawrence W. Bassett

CHAPTER 17 **Proliferative Lesions** 300
Sophia Kim Apple, Jennifer M.J. Overstreet, and Lawrence W. Bassett

CHAPTER 18 **Typical Benign Calcifications** 323
Sophia Kim Apple, Lawrence W. Bassett, and Erum W. Sethi

CHAPTER 19 **High-Risk Breast Diseases** 349
Sophia Kim Apple, Laura Doepke, and Lawrence W. Bassett

CHAPTER 20 **Infectious and Inflammatory Diseases of the Breast** 375
Sophia Kim Apple, Jane M. Dascalos, and Lawrence W. Bassett

SECTION 5: IMAGING OF THE BREAST MALIGNANCIES

CHAPTER 21 **Ductal Carcinoma in Situ and Paget's Disease** 391
Sophia Kim Apple, Jennifer M.J. Overstreet, and Lawrence W. Bassett

CHAPTER 22 **Invasive Ductal Carcinomas** 423
Sophia Kim Apple, Lawrence W. Bassett, and Cheryce M. Poon

CHAPTER 23 **Invasive Lobular Carcinoma** 483
Sophia Kim Apple, January K. Lopez, and Lawrence W. Bassett

CHAPTER 24 **Other Malignant Breast Diseases** 502
Sophia Kim Apple, Christopher P. Hsu, and Lawrence W. Bassett

CHAPTER 25 **The Effect of Neoadjuvant Chemotherapy and Radiation Therapy on Breast Tissue** 524
Sophia Kim Apple, Erum W. Sethi, and Lawrence W. Bassett

SECTION 6: **APPROPRIATENESS CRITERIA FOR BREAST IMAGING WORKUP**

CHAPTER 26 **American College of Radiology Appropriateness Criteria** 539
Lawrence W. Bassett

CHAPTER 27 **Appropriate Management of Masses** 542
Jennifer A. Harvey

CHAPTER 28 **Appropriate Management of Calcifications** 552
Jennifer A. Harvey

SECTION 7: **INTERVENTIONAL APPROACHES**

CHAPTER 29 **Image-Guided Percutaneous Biopsy** 563
Mary S. Newell and Mary Catherine Mahoney

CHAPTER 30 **Galactography** 597
Mary Catherine Mahoney, Valerie P. Jackson, and Lawrence W. Bassett

CHAPTER 31 **Presurgical Needle Localization** 605
Mary Catherine Mahoney and Valerie P. Jackson

CHAPTER 32 **Specimen Processing in Pathology** 611
Sophia Kim Apple

CHAPTER 33 **Post-Biopsy Management** 635
Anne C. Hoyt and Lawrence W. Bassett

SECTION 8: **THE SURGICALLY ALTERED BREAST**

CHAPTER 34 **The Conservatively Treated Breast** 649
D. David Dershaw and Adam Bracha

CHAPTER 35 **The Augmented Breast** 662
Nanette D. DeBruhl, Dawn C. Nwamuo, and David P. Gorczyca

CHAPTER 36 **Reduction Mammoplasty** 682
Valerie P. Jackson and Katherine H. Walker

SECTION 9: **REGULATIONS IN BREAST IMAGING**

CHAPTER 37 **The Mammography Quality Standards Act and Accreditation** 693
Priscilla F. Butler

CHAPTER 38 **The Medical Audit: Statistical Basis of Clinical Outcomes Analysis** 702
Michael N. Linver

CHAPTER 39 **Coding and Billing in Breast Imaging** 720
Michael N. Linver

CHAPTER 40 **Medical-Legal Aspects of Breast Imaging and Intervention** 728
R. James Brenner

SECTION 10: **EMERGING TECHNOLOGIES**

CHAPTER 41 **Emerging X-Ray-Based and Nuclear Technologies** 743
Carl J. D'Orsi

CHAPTER 42 **Ultrasound-Based Technologies Including Elastography and Automated Whole Breast Scanning** 751
Christopher Comstock

CHAPTER 43 **Recent Advances in Magnetic Resonance Spectroscopy in the Breast** 761
Xiaoyu Liu, Scott Lipnick, Shida Banakar, James W. Sayre, Nanette D. DeBruhl, Lawrence W. Bassett, and M. Albert Thomas

CHAPTER 44 **Minimally Invasive Percutaneous Breast Cancer Ablation** 772
Gary M. Levine and Steven P. Poplack

Index 777

SECTION

ONE

Introduction

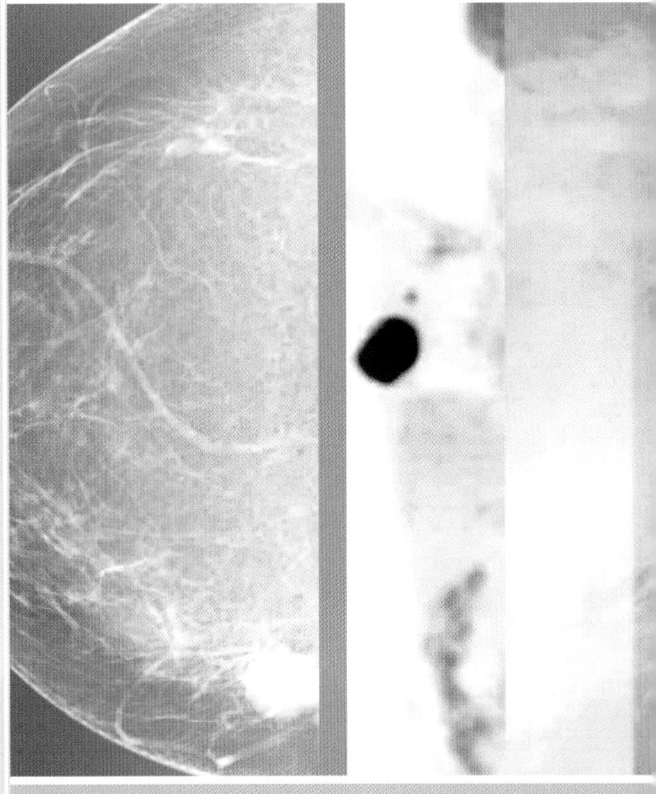

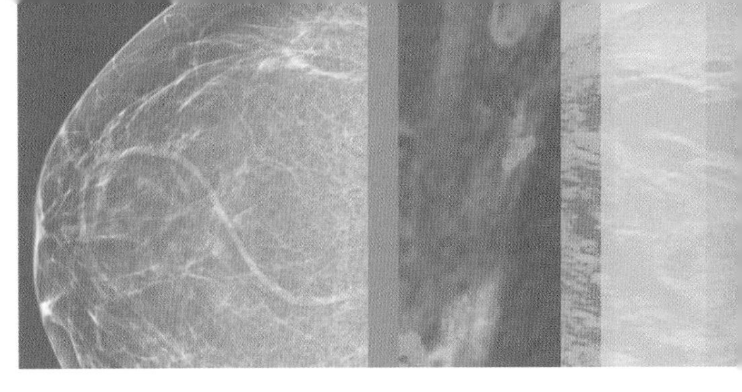

CHAPTER 1

History of Breast Imaging

Lawrence W. Bassett and Richard H. Gold

The relatively new subspecialty of breast imaging did not really play a major role until the 1980s when screening mammography became accepted. Breast imaging was not incorporated into the American Board of Radiology Certification Examination until 1990, when it became the 10th section and most recent addition to the examination. Nonetheless, the pioneers of mammography began their studies in the first decade of the 1900s. Later, new technologies were incorporated into breast imaging. In the 1990s breast imaging also encountered an awesome challenge as it became the most regulated subspecialty in radiology. Having achieved their goals in accommodating these strict regulations, radiologists practicing state-of-the-art breast imaging in their practices worked hard to have their subspecialty recognized for its importance to radiology. Their persistence and hard work led us to where we are today. In 2005, the American College of Radiology (ACR) established the Commission on Breast Imaging with a seat on the Board of Chancellors.

PIONEERS OF MAMMOGRAPHY

In 1895, Wilhelm Conrad Roentgen discovered the x-ray. In 1913, 18 years later, Albert Salomon[1] (Fig. 1-1), a surgeon at the Surgical Clinic of Berlin University, became the first to describe the usefulness of x-ray in the study of breast cancer. He performed radiography on more than 3000 mastectomy specimens and correlated the radiographic, gross, and microscopic findings (Figs. 1-2 and 1-3). Salomon found that radiographs were useful in demonstrating the spread of tumor to the axillary lymph nodes and to distinguish highly infiltrating carcinoma from circumscribed carcinoma. Additionally, he was the first person to observe on radiographs the microcalcifications associated with malignancy, although he did not appreciate their significance or the usefulness of his observation. After Salomon's paper on breast radiography, no related publications appeared until the late 1920s, when a number of articles on the use of radiography in the study of breast diseases were published independently in different parts of the world.

In Germany in 1927, surgeon Otto Kleinschmidt[2] reported the use of mammography as a diagnostic aid at the University of Leipzig Breast Clinic. In 1932, Walter Vogel,[3] also at the Leipzig clinic, published a paper on the mammographic differentiation of benign and malignant breast lesions.

In Spain in 1931, on the basis of examinations of 56 patients, J. Goyanes and colleagues[4] described the mammographic features of the normal breast and distinguished inflammatory from neoplastic lesions. Furthermore, they emphasized the importance of breast positioning in mammography.

In South America in 1929, Carlos Dominguez[5] of Uruguay described pneumomammography as a method to improve the delineation of lesions. The procedure required the injection of carbon dioxide into the retromammary and premammary spaces before radiography. It failed to become generally accepted.

In the United States great strides were made as well, as a result of the work of Stafford Warren (Fig. 1-4), a radiologist at Strong Memorial Hospital in Rochester, N.Y. In 1930, Warren[6] reported on the use of a stereoscopic technique for breast radiography, having performed it in 119 patients who subsequently underwent surgery (Fig. 1-5). In obtaining the mammograms, Warren used general-purpose radiographic equipment, "new" dual fine-grain calcium tungstate intensifying screens, a moving Potter-Bucky diaphragm (similar to today's reciprocating grids) to diminish scattered radiation, and the following technical factors: 50 to 60 kilovolt (peak) (kVp), 70 milliampere (mA), a target-to-film distance of 63 cm, and an exposure time of 2.5 seconds. He wrote, "In many of the cases,

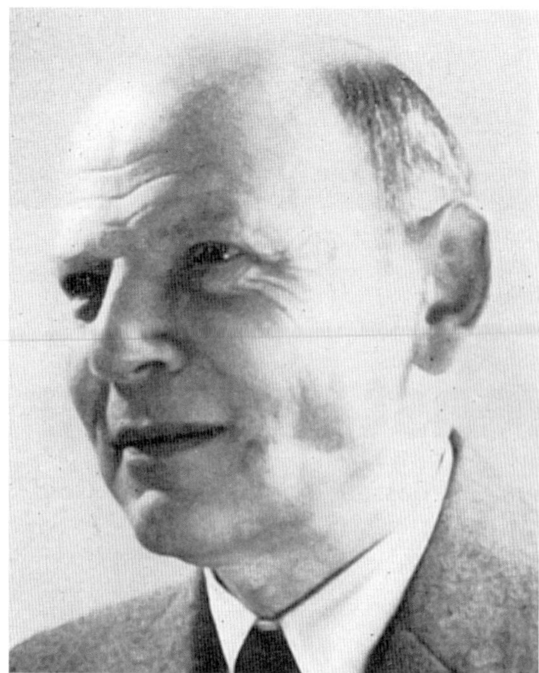

■ **FIGURE 1-1** Albert Salomon. *(Courtesy of Andre Bruwer, Tucson, Ariz.)*

there was no uniformity of opinion in the preoperative clinical diagnosis... The opinion from the mammogram on the other hand, was often very definite and most frequently correct." In fact, in the 119 cases, only eight interpretative errors were made, including four false-negative diagnoses in the 58 cases of cancer. Warren's accuracy in diagnosing breast cancer seemed to confirm the usefulness of mammography as a diagnostic tool. In addition, Warren described the mammographic appearance of normal breasts and the mammographic features associated with pregnancy and mastitis. In 1931, another American radiologist, Paul Seabold,[7] reported the mammographic appearance of normal breasts in various physiologic states ranging from puberty to post menopause, including changes seen during the menstrual cycle. Despite this surge of interest in mammography in the 1920s, progress in mammography had come to a halt in the United States by the mid 1930s. The most likely reasons were the unpredictable quality of the images and the inability to reproduce the high degree of accuracy reported by Warren. Thus, during the late 1930s, the majority of interested investigators were discouraged from pursuing mammography.

However, Jacob Gershon-Cohen (Fig. 1-6), a radiologist in Philadelphia, persisted in the study of mammography and made notable progress in diagnosing breast cancer. In 1938, he and his colleague, Albert Strickler, reported the range of normal radiographic appearances of the breast as a function of age and menstrual status, stressing the importance of understanding the appearance of the normal breast under all conditions of growth and physiologic activity before attempting the diagnosis of breast abnormalities.[8] In the 1950s, Gershon-Cohen and pathologist Helen Ingleby performed a roentgenologic-pathologic correlation of breast disease using whole-breast histologic sections, establishing mammographic criteria for the diagnosis of benign and malignant lesions. Gershon-Cohen emphasized the use of high-contrast images and breast compression and recommended the simultaneous exposure of two juxtaposed films for adequate exposure of both the thinner peripheral and thicker juxtathoracic tissues.

During the 1950s, interest in mammography also grew outside the United States. In France in 1951, Charles Gros and R. Sigrist[9] published many articles related to mammography, emphasizing mammographic criteria for benign and malignant lesions, and the indications for mammography. Later, Gros developed the prototypic dedicated mammography unit containing a molybdenum anode and a device to compress the breast.

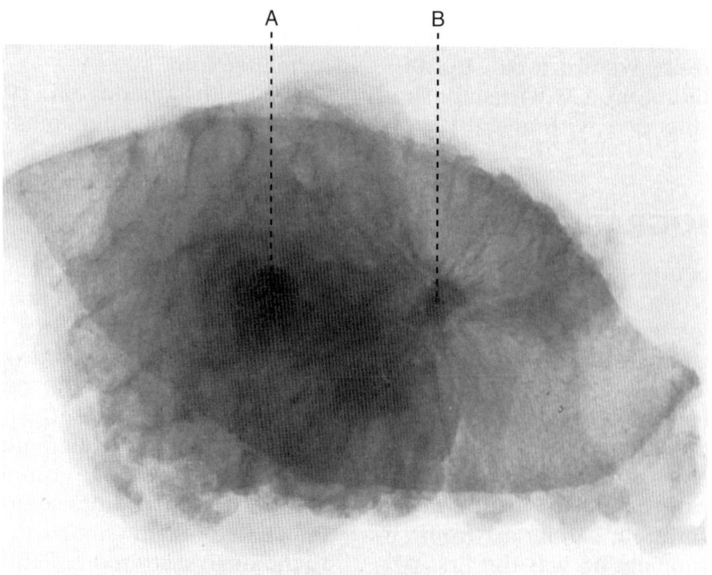

■ **FIGURE 1-2** Radiographs of breast tissue specimens obtained by Albert Salomon. Radiograph shows nipple (**A**) and carcinoma (**B**). *(From Salomon A: Beitrage zur Pathologie und Klinik der Mammacarcinome. Arch Klin Chir 1913;101:573-668.)*

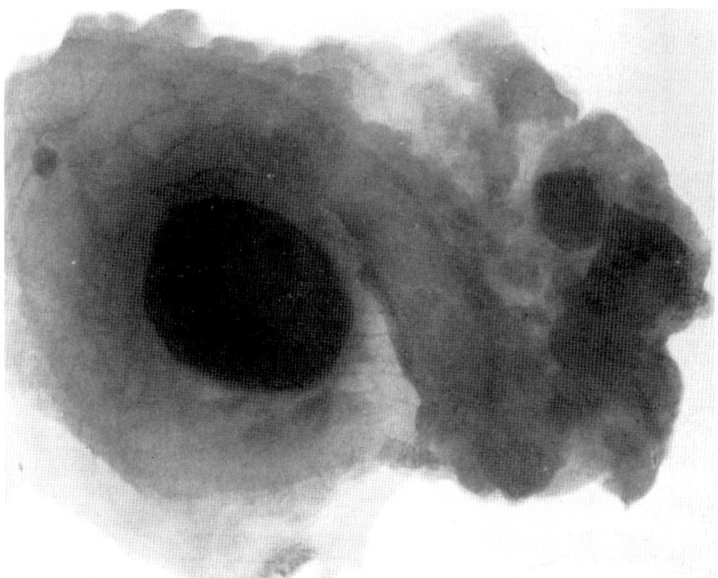

■ **FIGURE 1-3** Another case from the radiographs of breast tissue specimens obtained by Albert Salomon. The large mass (*left*) is an intracystic carcinoma, and the smaller masses (*right*) represent nodal metastases. *(From Salomon A: Beitrage zur Pathologie und Klinik der Mammacarcinome. Arch Klin Chir 1913;101:573-668.)*

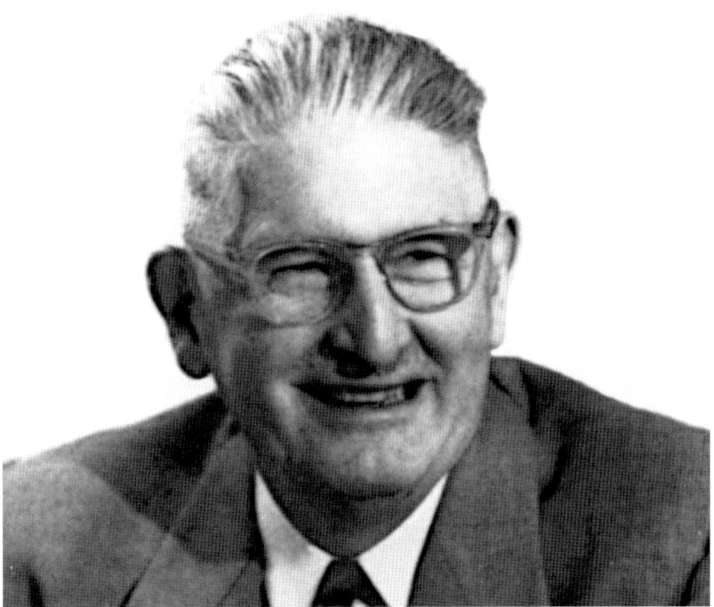

■ **FIGURE 1-4** Stafford L. Warren. *(Courtesy of Robert L. Egan, Atlanta, Ga.)*

In Uruguay, Raul Leborgne[10] (Fig. 1-7), a student of Dominguez, described the typical mammographic appearance of breast cancer and was the first person to emphasize the importance of microcalcifications in its diagnosis. He also stressed the usefulness of breast compression to immobilize the breast and diminish its thickness to enhance image quality (Fig. 1-8). To achieve compression, he used a long cone with a flat surface at its distal end. Furthermore, he used a low-kVp technique (20 to 30 kVp), nonscreen film, a 60-cm target-to-film distance, and 5 mA for each centimeter of compressed breast thickness. Leborgne also described the radiographic differences between benign and malignant calcifications and was the first person to report the significant association of microcalcifications with subclinical carcinoma, thus setting the stage for the use of mammography as a tool for cancer screening (Figs 1-9 to 1-12).

Despite these advances, mammography was rarely used in the United States in the 1950s because of its perceived lack of clinical usefulness and technical reproducibility. Then, in 1960, Robert Egan (Fig. 1-13), a radiologist at the M. D. Anderson Hospital in Houston, Texas, described a high-milliamperage/low-kilovoltage technique that resulted in dependable, reproducible, diagnostic-quality mammographic images. Egan modified general-purpose radiographic equipment to optimize soft tissue imaging

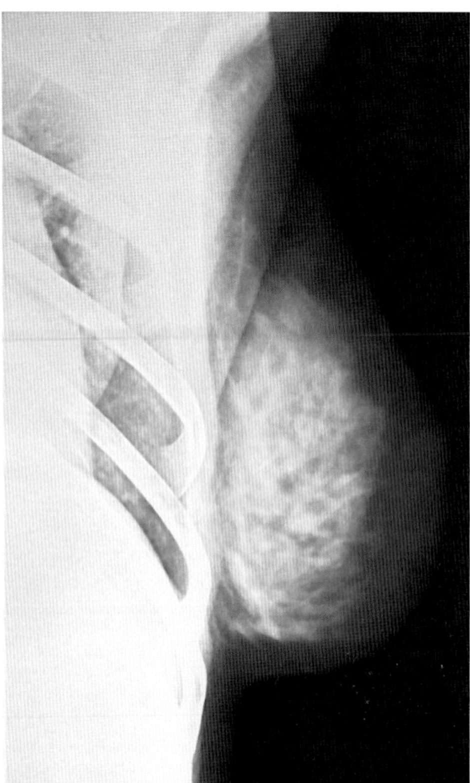

■ **FIGURE 1-5** Mammogram obtained by Stafford Warren (circa 1939) of a normal dense breast. *(Courtesy of Stafford L. Warren, Los Angeles, Calif.)*

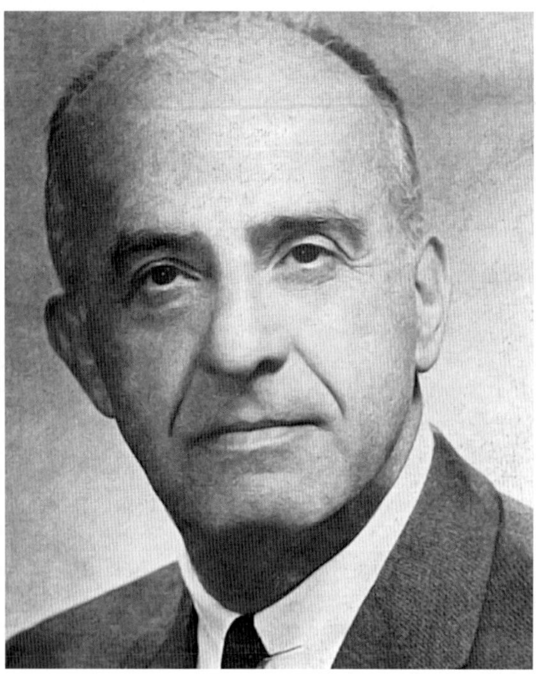

■ **FIGURE 1-6** Jacob Gershon-Cohen. *(From obituary: Jacob Gershon-Cohen. Radiology 1971;99:455.)*

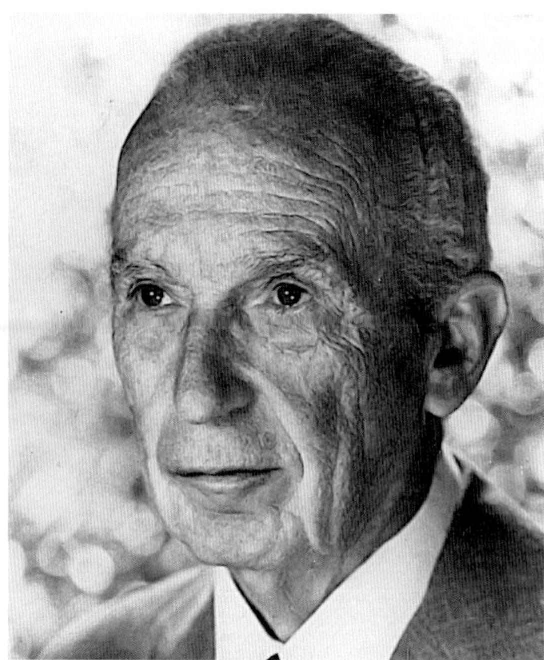

■ **FIGURE 1-7** Raul Leborgne. *(Courtesy of Felix Leborgne, Montevideo, Uruguay.)*

by limiting the filtration of the x-ray beam to the inherent filtration of a conventional glass-window x-ray tube, adjusting the control panel of the generator to produce accurate values below 30 kVp, using type M (industrial) Kodak film for high detail and high contrast, and employing a cylindrical cone to reduce scatter. He used the following technical factors: 26 to 28 kVp, 300 mA, a 90-cm target-to-film distance, and a 6-second exposure time (Fig. 1-14). At that time, mammography was performed at the M. D. Anderson Hospital in the "Section of Experimental Diagnostic Radiology."

Using this new technique, Egan reported excellent imaging results for the first 1000 breasts that he studied (634 patients).[11] In 1962, he described 53 cases of "occult carcinoma," which he defined as "one which remains totally unsuspected following examination by the usual methods used to diagnose breast cancer, including examination of the breast by an experienced and competent physician. To qualify for this definition, no symptoms or signs should be present." The success of mammography in detecting these clinically occult carcinomas provided further support for its use as a screening tool.

Egan's success in making reproducible images not only led to the widespread use of mammography to detect breast cancer but also elevated its status to national recognition. In 1963, the Cancer Control Program of the U.S. Public Health Service, the National Cancer Institute, and the M. D. Anderson Hospital jointly conducted a nationwide investigation involving 24 institutions to verify Egan's results and to determine the possible clinical applications of mammography (Fig. 1-15). The results of the study, presented in 1965, established the following: that (1) the Egan technique could be learned by other radiologists; (2) mammograms of acceptable quality could be reliably produced; (3) mammography could enable differentiation between benign and malignant lesions; and (4) mammography could be used as a screening tool in asymptomatic women.[12]

Those results led the ACR to establish a Mammography Committee, chaired by Wendell Scott, which initiated a nationwide training program for radiologists and technologists in the performance and interpretation of mammograms.[13]

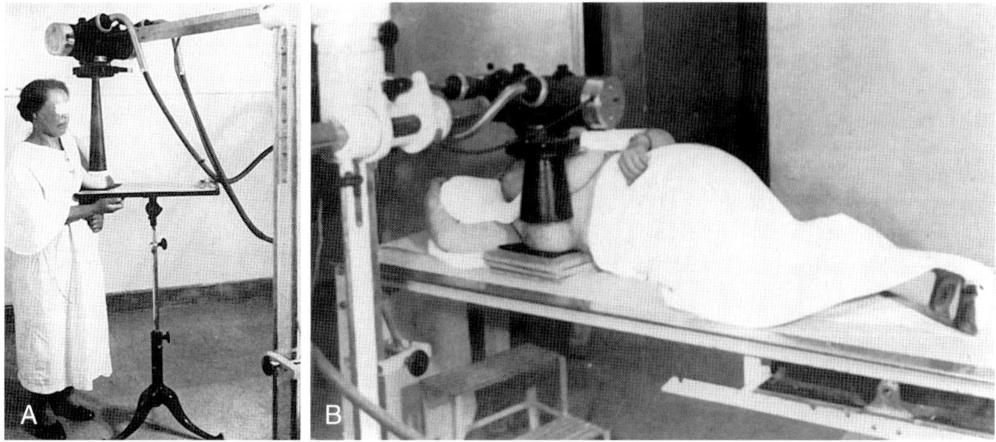

■ FIGURE 1-8 A, Raul Leborgne's positioning of the patient for a craniocaudal mammogram. Leborgne's caption reads, "Observe the characteristics of the cone and the compression pad interposed between it and the breast." **B,** Leborgne's positioning for the lateral view. *(**A,** From Leborgne R. Diagnosis of tumors of the breast by simple roentgenography. AJR Am J Roentgenol 1951;65:1-11; **B,** from Leborgne R. The breast in roentgen diagnosis. Montevideo, Uruguay, Impresora, 1953.)*

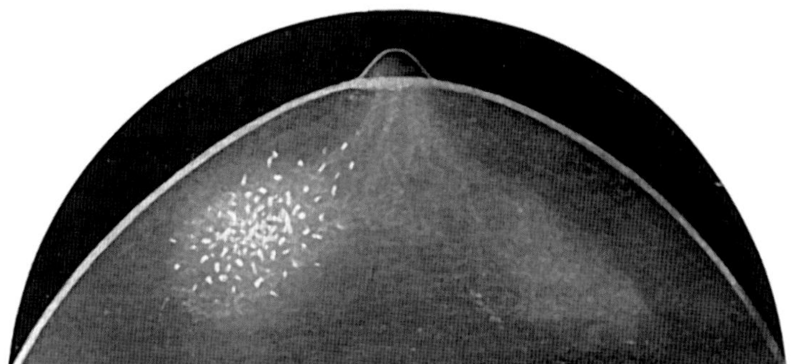

■ FIGURE 1-9 Raul Leborgne's diagram of calcifications in carcinoma. His caption reads, "Scattering of countless, punctiform or elongated calcifications, very closely grouped, particularly in center." *(From Leborgne R. The breast in roentgen diagnosis. Montevideo, Uruguay, Impresora, 1953.)*

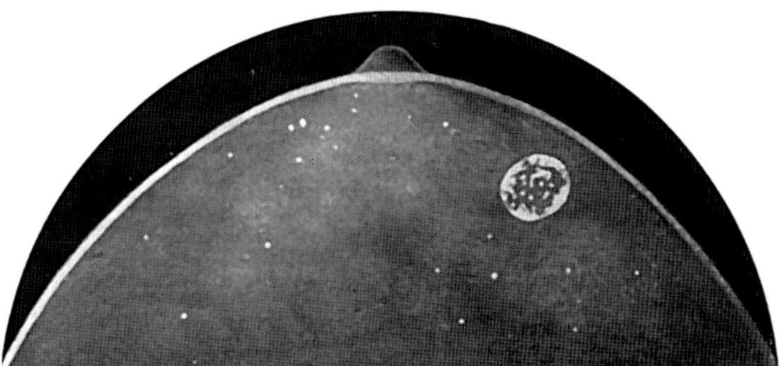

■ FIGURE 1-10 Raul Leborgne's diagram of calcifications in fibrocystic disease. His caption reads, "Small calcifications in a circumscribed area, predominating in the periphery (calcifications in cyst); and tiny, punctiform, rounded calcifications scattered throughout the breast in ductal desquamation." *(From Leborgne R. The breast in roentgen diagnosis. Montevideo, Uruguay, Impresora, 1953.)*

Those pioneers of mammography made three essential contributions to its evolution: They established a basis for future diagnostic criteria, they strove to improve image quality and reproducibility, and they stimulated widespread interest in mammography and its clinical uses. The wealth of insights and contributions of these physicians set the stage for an uninterrupted period of intense technologic progress.

THE ERA OF TECHNOLOGIC PROGRESS

Until the mid-1960s, mammography was performed with general-purpose radiographic equipment. The inability of this equipment to produce finely detailed, high-contrast images led Gros (Fig. 1-16) in France to develop the prototype of the first dedicated mammography unit (Fig. 1-17). This x-ray unit contained the following two innovations:

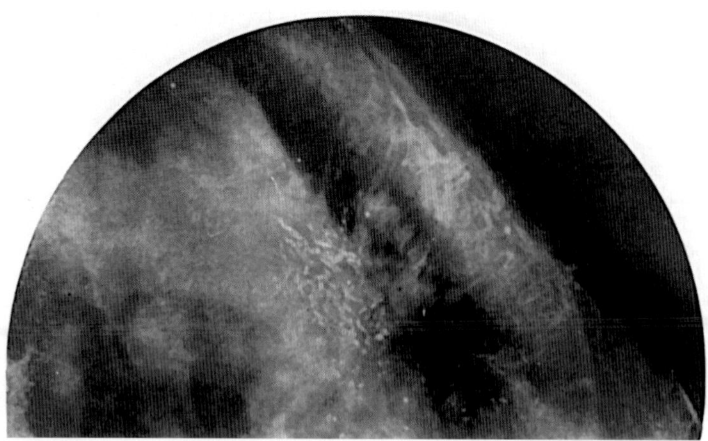

■ **FIGURE 1-11** Raul Leborgne's coned compression view shows calcifications in carcinoma. *(From Leborgne R. The breast in roentgen diagnosis. Montevideo, Uruguay, Impresora, 1953.)*

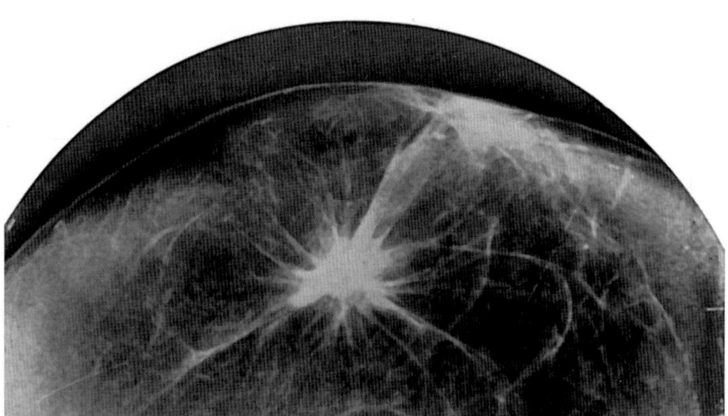

■ **FIGURE 1-12** Raul Leborgne's coned compression view reveals carcinoma with peripheral spicules. *(From Leborgne R. The Breast in roentgen diagnosis. Montevideo, Uruguay, Impresora, 1953.)*

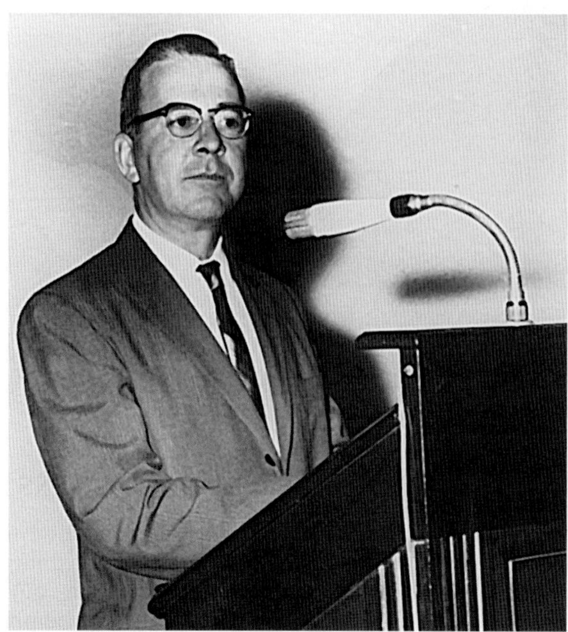

■ **FIGURE 1-13** Robert L. Egan, spreading the mammography gospel in 1967. *(Courtesy of Robert L. Egan, Atlanta, Ga.)*

(1) a molybdenum (rather than tungsten) target that provided high subject contrast because of the prominent photoelectric effect of the low-energy x-rays it produced; and (2) a built-in cone compression device that decreased the thickness of the breast and immobilized it during the exposure. In 1967, the Compagnie Generale de Radiologie (CGR), having developed the prototype with Gros, introduced the Senographe, the first commercially available dedicated mammography unit (Fig. 1-18). The molybdenum target, with its 0.7-mm focal spot, produced greater contrast among parenchyma, fat, and calcifications. The control panel, designed especially for mammography, offered exposure selections up to 40 mA and 40 kVp and exposure times up to 10 seconds. Built-in interchangeable compression cones decreased scattered radiation and motion unsharpness and separated overlapping breast structures. A rotating C-arm allowed patients to be examined in multiple projections while they sat upright. In the late 1960s, Gershon-Cohen tested the Senographe and reported that contrast, sharpness, and depiction of calcifications were significantly better in Senographe images than in images produced by modified general-purpose radiographic units. However, the improved image quality was achieved at the expense of higher radiation dose. Another disadvantage

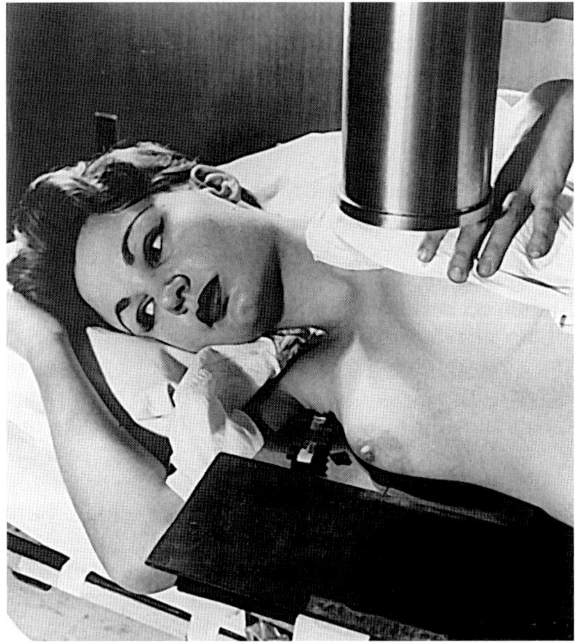

■ **FIGURE 1-14** Robert Egan's positioning for the mediolateral view. The patient lies on her side, her hand retracting her other breast. The cylindrical tube extending from the target was used to reduce scattered radiation. Technical factors used in obtaining the image included tungsten target, 2-mm focal spot, 28 kVp, 300 mA, 6-second exposure, approximately 90-cm source-to-image distance, Eastman Kodak Industrial Type M film, no screen, and no grid. *(Courtesy of Robert L. Egan, Atlanta, Ga.)*

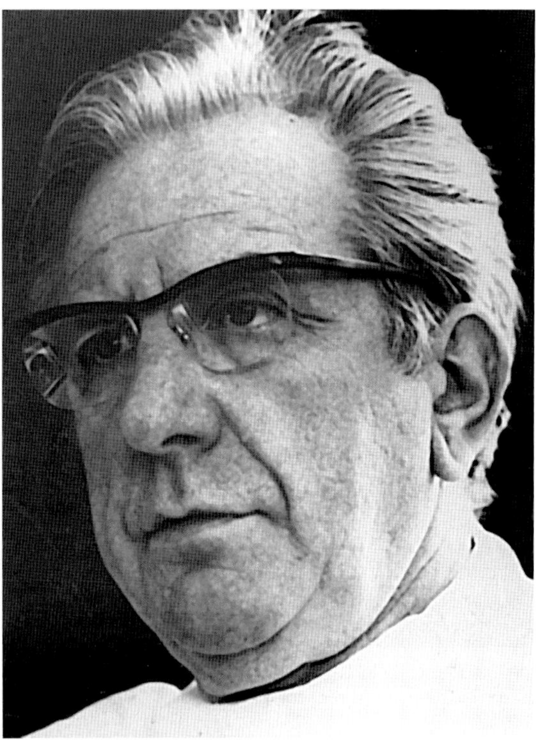

■ **FIGURE 1-16** Charles Gros. *(Courtesy of Dominique Gros, Strasbourg, France.)*

was the unit's relatively short source-to-skin distance, which resulted in mild magnification and occasional distortion of the image.

In the early 1970s, other dedicated mammography units were introduced, including the Mammomat (Siemens), MammoDiagnost (Philips), and Mammorex (Picker),, with each incorporating various technical improvements. The Diagnost-U (Philips), introduced in 1978 in the United States, was the first mammography unit with a built-in reciprocating grid. Stafford Warren used grids as early as 1930, but by the late 1970s practitioners had a renewed appreciation for their usefulness in overcoming image degradation due to scattered radiation.[14] Investigators in the mid-1980s confirmed the effectiveness of grids in improving image quality. Although they were effective in improving contrast and less expensive than reciprocating grids, stationary grids caused grid lines to appear in the image, a distraction to some radiologists. The better contrast resulting from the use of grids was achieved, nevertheless, at the expense of higher radiation dose. In 1986, Edward Sickles and William Weber[15] reported that grids were most effective in imaging dense breasts but offered little benefit for imaging fatty breasts.

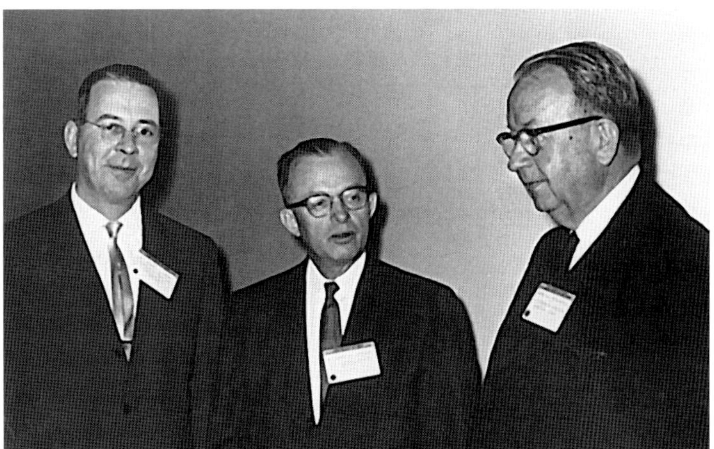

■ **FIGURE 1-15** The three men responsible for the 1963 Conference on the Reproducibility of Mammography (*from left to right*): Robert L. Egan, Lewis C. Robbins, (director of the U.S. Public Health Service Cancer Control Program), and Murray M. Copeland, (assistant director of M. D. Anderson Hospital). *(Courtesy of Gerald D. Dodd, Houston, Texas.)*

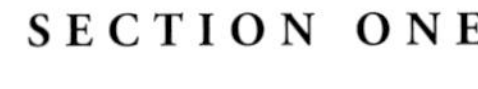

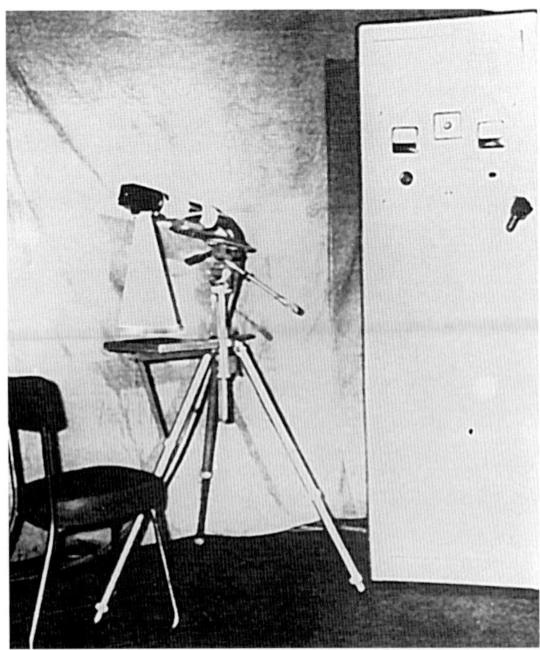

■ **FIGURE 1-17** Charles Gros' 1965 prototype of the Senographe, aptly called the Trepied ("three feet"). *(Courtesy of GE Medical Systems, Milwaukee, Wis.)*

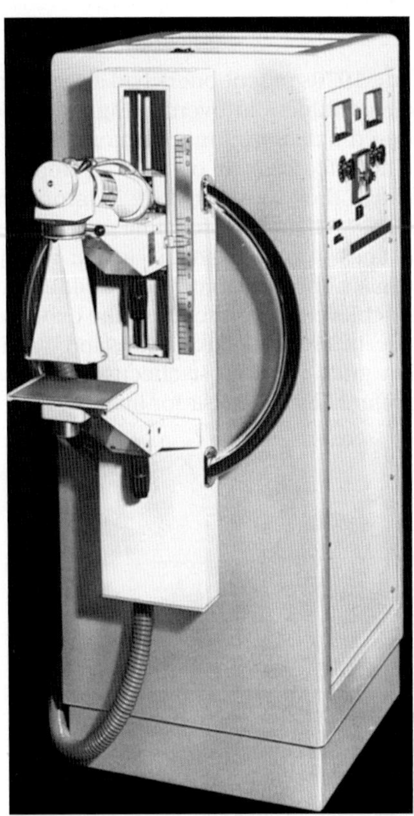

■ **FIGURE 1-18** First production model of the CGR Senographe in 1966. *(Courtesy of GE Medical Systems, Milwaukee, Wis.)*

During the late 1970s to early 1980s, mammography x-ray units underwent additional improvements. A foot pedal to control breast compression permitted the technologist to have both hands free to position the breast more accurately. The addition of an automatic exposure timer made image quality more consistent from one examination to the next. Photo timing also helped to make possible the screening of large populations because it allowed for the delayed batch processing of radiographs. In the late 1970s, a microfocal spot x-ray tube, which had already been used for magnified images of other organs, was placed into a mammography unit designed by Radiologic Sciences, Inc. Although magnification mammography provided highly detailed images of specific areas of interest, it required a higher radiation dose than standard mammography. Thus, the spot tube proved useful only as an adjunct to standard mammography.[16]

Higher image quality was achieved with the dedicated mammography unit but at the expense of a higher radiation doses. In 1970, in an effort to reduce both radiation dose and exposure time without sacrificing image quality, J. L. Price and P. D. Butler[17] of Great Britain first used a high-definition intensifying screen and film held in intimate contact in an air-evacuated polyethylene envelope. Bernard Ostrum and colleagues at the Albert Einstein Medical Center in Philadelphia, in association with the DuPont Co., conducted further experiments with screen-film combinations. In 1972, DuPont became the first manufacturer to market a dedicated screen-film system for mammography. A single-emulsion Cronex LoDose I film was placed in an air-evacuated, sealed polyethylene bag, with the film's emulsion side against a single Cronex LoDose calcium tungstate intensifying screen, thus reducing image blur by eliminating parallax unsharpness and image crossover. The new screen-film system allowed shorter exposures, thereby decreasing motion unsharpness and involving radiation doses 10 to 20 times lower than with direct film exposure. A variety of mammographic screen-film combinations were soon produced by various manufacturers with the aim of further reducing radiation dosage.

In 1974, the 3M Co. introduced rare-earth screens. Because such screens were more efficient than calcium tungstate screens in converting x-ray energy to light, they could be combined with faster-speed films. In 1975, the Eastman Kodak Co. introduced a complete mammographic image-recording system composed of a fast Min-R film and a rare-earth Min-R screen held tightly together in a special low-absorption Min-R cassette, thus eliminating the preparation time and vacuum-leakage problems associated with the polyethylene bag. In 1980, Eastman Kodak introduced the Min-R screen-Ortho-M film combination, which required half the radiation exposure required by the previous Min-R combination. In 1986, Eastman Kodak attempted to reduce the dose even further with the introduction of a two-screen dual-emulsion film system. Although this faster system did succeed in reducing radiation dosage, image resolution was decreased to an extent that many mammographers found unacceptable.

Film processing also played a crucial role in the evolution of mammography. Before 1942, all radiographs, including mammograms, were processed manually (Fig. 1-19).[18] Image quality and reproducibility depended on strict adherence to protocols regarding timing, solution formulation, freshness and temperature, and darkroom maintenance. In 1942, the Pako Co. introduced the first automated x-ray film processor, which processed films in approximately 40 minutes. In 1956, Eastman Kodak marketed the first roller transport processor (Fig. 1-20). This processor accommodated all

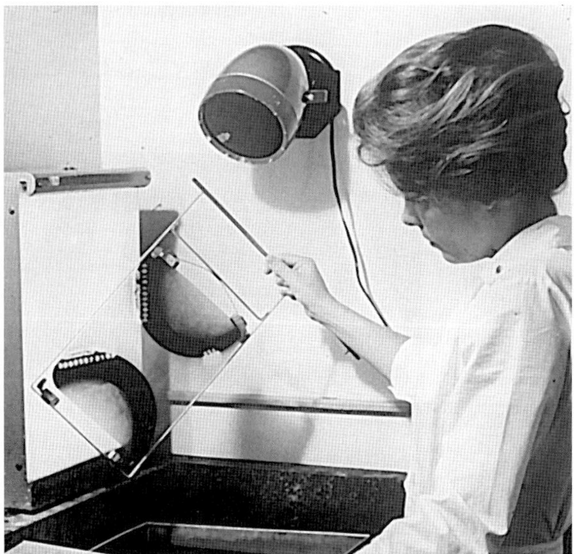

■ **FIGURE 1-19** One of Robert L. Egan's technologists hand-processing the nonscreen, industrial-grade mammography film used by Egan in the 1960s. *(Courtesy of Robert L. Egan, Atlanta, Ga.)*

types of films, processing them in about 6 minutes. In 1960, film handling was made easier and drying more rapid with the introduction of polyester film base. In 1965, Eastman Kodak introduced 90-second processing. These advances in film processing brought an end to the variability in image quality that had plagued manual processing.

While film mammography was continuing to evolve, xeromammography, an alternative method, emerged. In 1937, Chester Carlson developed the basic principles of xerography, which led to the commercial office copier in 1950.[19] In 1960, Howard Gould and associates reported that xeroradiography provided images of the breast with greater detail than those produced by conventional film mammography. In 1964, John Wolfe[20] (Fig. 1-21) began an investigation of xeromammography using a primitive Xerox radiographic unit consisting of five bulky components (Fig. 1-22). With the cooperation of the Xerox Corp., Wolfe made numerous modifications to the system, successfully condensing it into two components, a conditioner and a processor. In 1971, just before the introduction of the first dedicated screen-film system for mammography, the Xerox System 125 (Fig. 1-23) became commercially available.

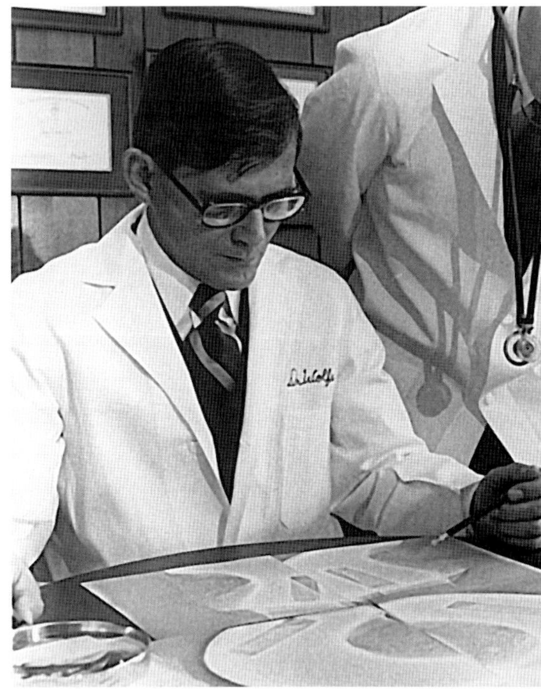

■ **FIGURE 1-21** John Wolfe in 1970. *(Courtesy of John N. Wolfe, Detroit, Mich.)*

When it was first introduced, positive-mode xeromammography produced high-contrast, high-resolution images at considerably lower radiation doses than were required for direct (nonscreen) film mammography. The superior image quality was attributed to a unique feature of xeroradiography, an edge enhancement phenomenon,

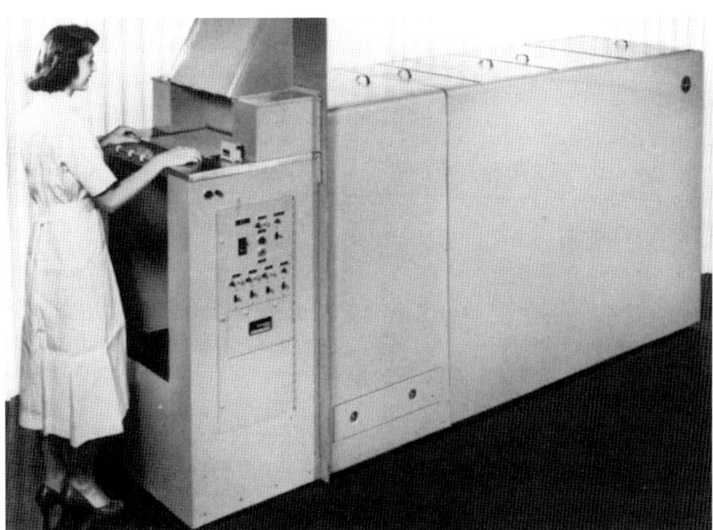

■ **FIGURE 1-20** First automatic roller transport processor, introduced in 1956, accommodated all radiographic films designed for exposure with intensifying screens. It was approximately 10 feet long and weighed nearly three quarters of a ton. *(Courtesy of Eastman Kodak Co., Rochester, N.Y.)*

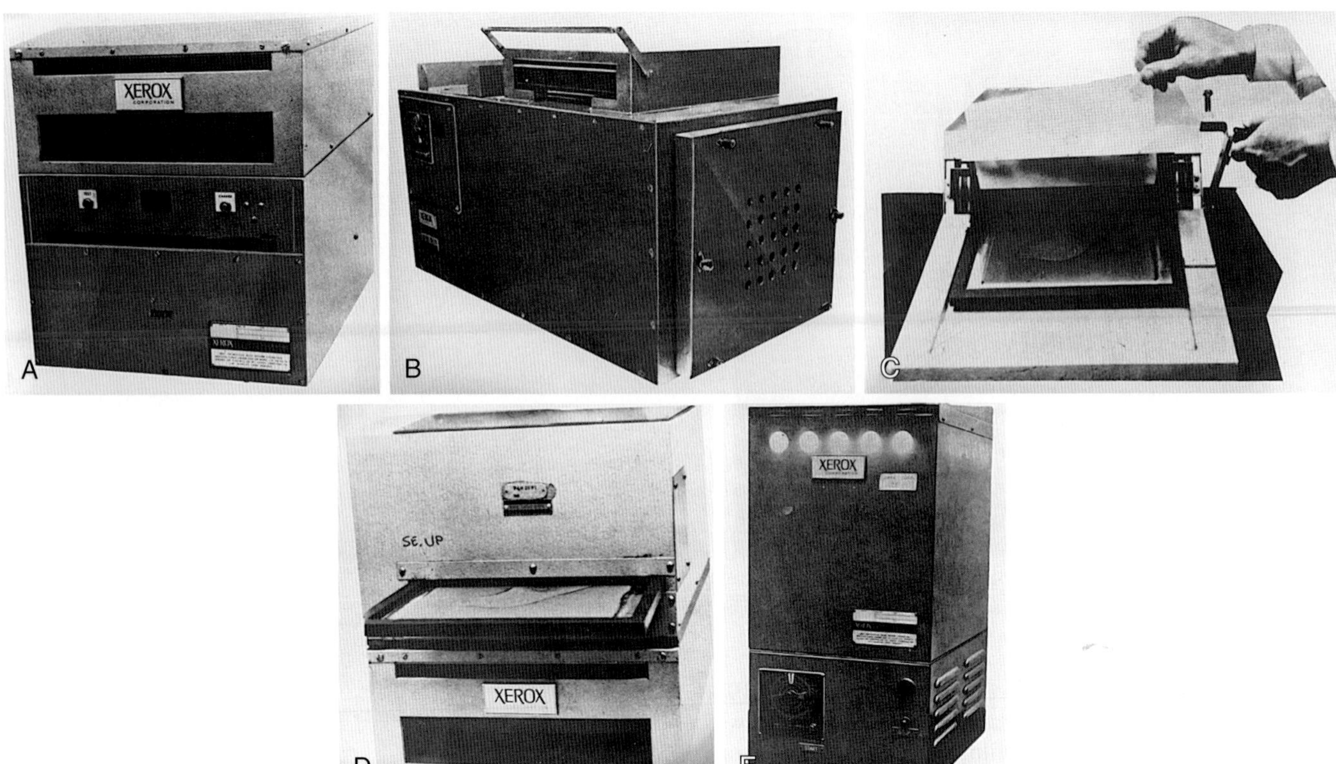

■ **FIGURE 1-22** Components of xeroradiography unit, circa 1953. **A,** Plate charger. **B,** Development chamber. **C,** Transfer unit. **D,** Plate cleaner. **E,** Relaxation unit. *(Courtesy of John N. Wolfe, Detroit, Mich.)*

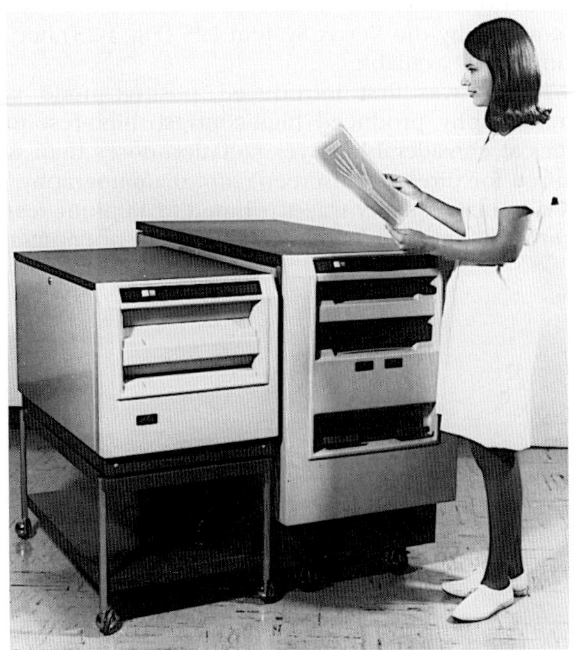

■ **FIGURE 1-23** The 125/6 system developed by Xerox was the first commercial xeromammography unit, marketed in 1971.

whereby the edges of high-density structures, especially spiculations and calcifications, were accentuated (Fig. 1-24A). By 1987, in an effort to further reduce radiation exposure, radiologists had been encouraged to switch to negative-mode imaging and to use additional filtration of the x-ray beam, factors that degraded xeromammographic image quality (see Fig. 1-24B). From the 1970s to the early 1980s, xeromammography and screen-film mammography were equally popular modes of breast imaging. However, by the 1980s, improvements in screen-film mammography led to better image quality and lower radiation dosage, resulting in its emergence as the dominant method of breast imaging. By 1988, the majority of facilities performing mammography in the United States were using screen-film systems, and 99% were using dedicated mammography equipment. By 1989, the growing popularity of screen-film mammography had resulted in the diminution of sales of xeromammographic systems to the point that the Xerox Corp., after introducing a black liquid toner for greater contrast (see Fig. 1-24C), stopped producing them.

The transition to digital mammography is now well under way in the United States, with more than 50% of mammography units being digital in 2009. An important step in the transition was the publication of the results of the ACR Imaging Network (ACRIN) Digital Mammography Imaging Screening Trial (DMIST), which validated the accuracy of digital mammography as equal to or better than screen-film mammography.[21]

OTHER MODALITIES FOR BREAST IMAGING

While x-ray mammography was evolving, other methods of breast imaging were also undergoing development. Ultrasonography, employing high-frequency ultrasonic waves, became particularly successful in differentiating cystic from solid masses. Transillumination, or light-

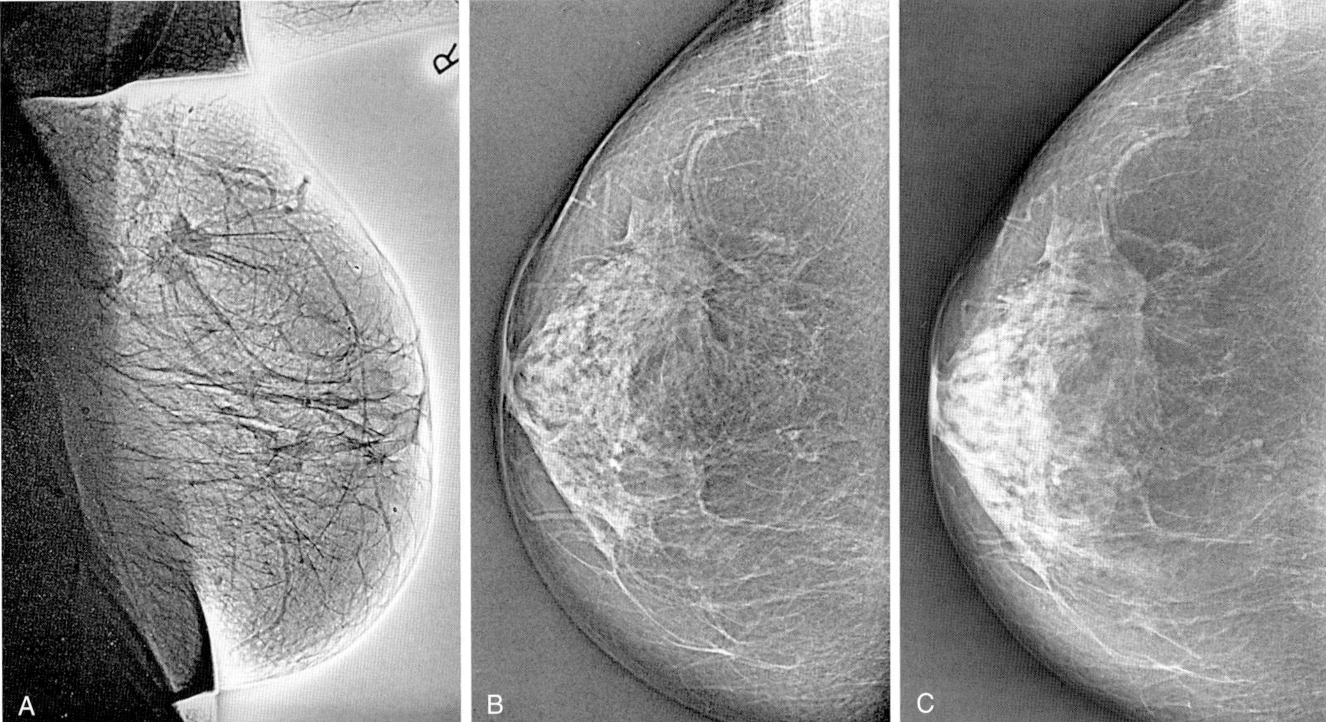

■ **FIGURE 1-24** Evolution of xeromammography. **A,** Positive-mode xeromammogram reveals a carcinoma in the upper hemisphere of the breast. Note the sharply defined spiculations. **B,** Negative-mode xeromammogram of another spiculated carcinoma. The image is "flatter" in contrast and less detailed than in **A. C,** Image from the same projection as in **B** but processed with liquid black toner.

scanning, was a technique based on imaging patterns of absorption of applied near-infrared and red electromagnetic radiation by the breast. Thermography used instruments to record abnormal patterns of infrared radiation emitted by the diseased breast.

Breast Ultrasonography

In 1880, the French physicists Pierre and Jacques Curie discovered the *piezoelectric effect*, whereby an electrical charge is produced in response to the application of mechanical pressure on certain crystals.[22] The first attempt to develop a practical application for this effect was that of Paul Langevin, who was commissioned by the French government during World War I to investigate the use of high-frequency ultrasonic waves to detect submarines, leading to the development of SONAR (an acronym derived from "sound navigation ranging") during World War II. Between the world wars, other applications of ultrasound were explored, including its role in medicine. During the 1920s and 1930s, ultrasound was used therapeutically for physical therapy and was evaluated for treatment of cancer. During the late 1940s and 1950s, the efficacy of ultrasonography as a diagnostic tool was explored. Karl Dussik of Austria ultrasonically depicted intracranial structures, becoming the first person to use this method for diagnosis. Other investigators, such as W. Guttner in Germany, Andres Denier in France, and Kenji Tanaka in Japan, joined in the effort to explore the diagnostic capabilities of ultrasound.

In the United States, George Ludwig[23] experimented with ultrasound, noting that the velocity of sound waves differed in various tissues, thus setting standards for later sonographic interpretation. In 1949, John Wild[24] used ultrasound to determine the thickness of the intestinal wall in various diseases. He determined that the echoes returning from tumors were different from those returning from normal tissues and suggested that these differences might make ultrasound useful for cancer detection. Later, Wild and John Reid constructed several "echoscopes," or hand-held, direct-contact ultrasound scanners, including vaginal and rectal scanners, and even an experimental system for breast cancer screening (Fig. 1-25).

These early investigators used A-mode ultrasound technology, whereby returning echoes were displayed on an oscilloscope. However, A-mode presentations were not anatomically based and difficult anatomic correlations were required of the investigators. Technologic advances were made in the late 1940s and early 1950s, primarily by Wild and Reid and by Douglas Howry and colleagues, leading to the development of B-mode scanning. This new mode of scanning allowed for more accurate anatomic images because the interfaces of tissue planes and the outlines of organs could be visualized. Wild and Reid employed B-mode contact scanning (Fig. 1-26), and Howry developed a water bath system, which necessitated placement of the patient in an immersion tank made from the gun turret of a B-29 bomber (Fig. 1-27). In the early 1960s, the use of B-mode scanning, with its better image quality, led to the commercial marketing of ultrasonographic equipment specifically intended for medical diagnosis. As a result, new applications of diagnostic ultrasonography were explored, including echocardiography, echoencephalography, Doppler ultrasonography, obstetric ultrasonography, ophthalmologic ultrasonography, abdominal ultrasonography, and breast ultrasonography.

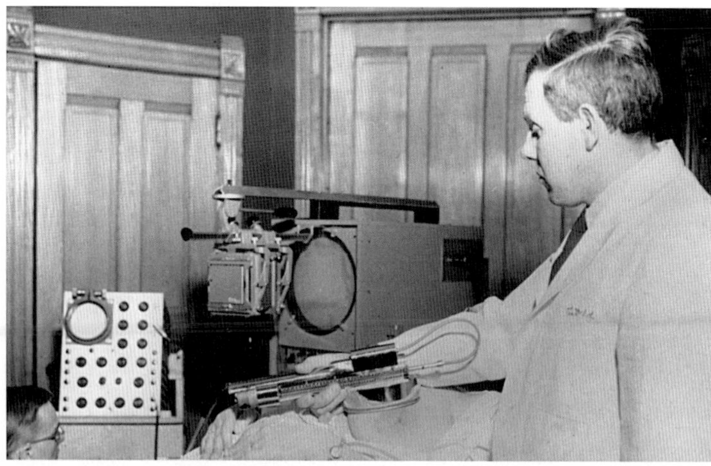

■ **FIGURE 1-25** John Wild (*right*) and John Reid (*lower left*) employing their B-mode contact scanner to image patients' breasts. *(Courtesy of Barry Goldberg, Philadelphia, Pa.)*

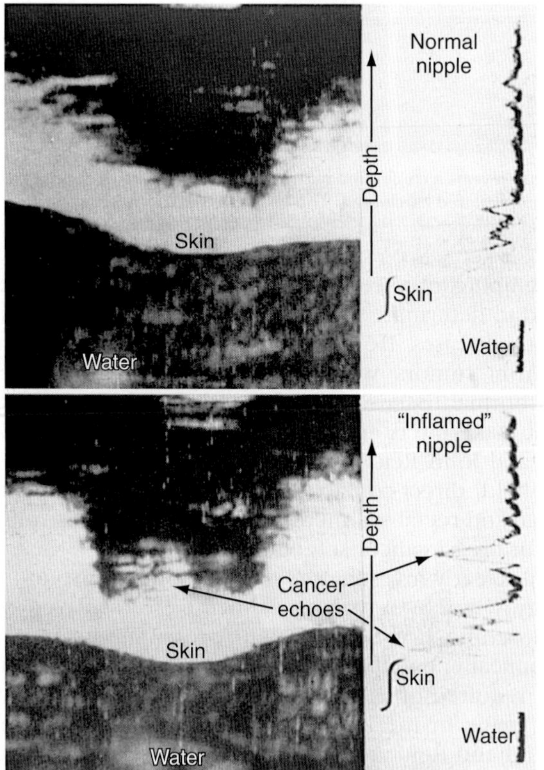

■ **FIGURE 1-26** Both A-mode (*at right*) and B-mode scans of an "inflamed" nipple and a normal nipple of the same patient, obtained by John Wild and John Reid in 1953. In the same breast with the "inflamed" nipple, Wild and Reid diagnosed a malignancy, which was later confirmed pathologically. This was the first B-mode scan ever produced of a carcinoma in the living human breast. *(Courtesy of Barry Goldberg, Philadelphia, Pa.)*

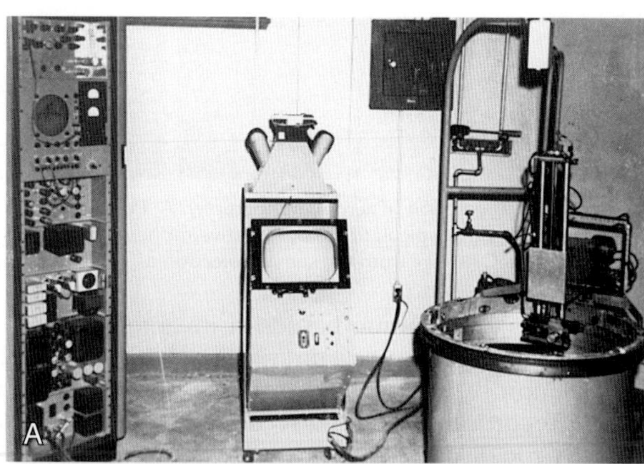

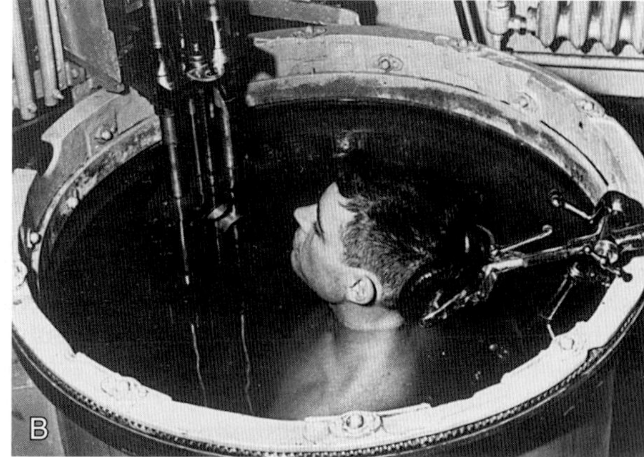

■ **FIGURE 1-27** B-29 gun turret scanner developed by Douglas Howry and his team. **A,** The water-bath system necessitated placement of the patient in an immersion tank, with lead weights on the patient's abdomen for consistent immersion level. **B,** Close-up view with experimental subject. *(Courtesy of Barry Goldberg, Philadelphia, Pa.)*

Breast ultrasonography began in 1951 when Wild and Reid in Minnesota and Toshio Wagai and his colleagues in Japan independently produced ultrasonographic images of breast tumors. Wild and Reid[25] were the first to develop equipment specifically designed for breast scanning, and they attempted to differentiate benign from malignant disease (see Fig. 1-26). They were able to detect some cancers as small as 2 to 3 mm and suggested that ultrasonography might prove beneficial in screening for early breast cancer. Furthermore, they were the first to differentiate between cystic and solid masses in the breast by means of ultrasonography.

Recognizing the potential advantages of ultrasonography in breast cancer detection, investigators around the world worked to develop better techniques and equipment to improve breast imaging. Japanese investigators persisted in their investigations of breast scanning, evaluating diagnostic criteria for various breast lesions. In 1968, British investigators P. N. T. Wells and K. T. Evans[26] reported their study of a large water-immersion breast scanner. Although they were able to obtain high-quality, high-resolution images, immersion scanners were clinically unsatisfactory. Also in 1968, Elizabeth Kelly-Fry and her colleagues[27] in Illinois initiated a study, supported by the Cancer Control Program of the U.S. Department of Health, Education, and Welfare, on the usefulness of ultrasonography in the detection of breast cancer. They found that the modality not only was useful for detecting small cystic and solid masses but also had potential for detecting breast cancer before it became palpable. In 1974, Jack Jellins, George Kossoff, and their associates[28] at the Australian Ultrasonics Institute, developed the Octoson (Fig. 1-28), a multipurpose water bath scanner with eight large-aperture transducers, and developed a gray scale to produce high-quality images. In fact, gray-scale echography was introduced as a direct result of the investigations conducted at the Ultrasonics Institute. Advances in echocardiography led to the development of real-time imaging equipment, which allowed for continuous viewing and recording of images.

Although the use of ultrasonography for breast cancer screening was first suggested by Wild in the 1950s, it was not until the late 1970s, as a result of nationwide concerns about the possibility of radiation-induced breast cancer from screening mammography, that this application was investigated on a large scale.[29] The resultant clinical studies showed that ultrasonographic screening was far less effective than screen-film mammographic screening of asymptomatic women. For example, in 1983, Sickles and coworkers[30] reported that in a prospective study of 1000 women, only 58% of 64 pathologically proven cancers were detected by ultrasonography, compared with 97% by mammography. The limitations of breast ultrasonography in screening included inability to depict microcalcifications, difficulty in imaging of fatty breasts, inability to differentiate benign from malignant solid masses, and unreliable depiction of solid masses smaller than 1 cm.

Nonetheless, the accuracy of differentiation of cystic versus solid masses showed an accuracy of 96% to 100%.[31,32] This alone made ultrasound an indispensible adjunct to mammography and reduced unnecessary biopsies by 30%. Continued technologic improvements have led to further investigations of the potential of ultrasound, resulting in a report on reliable ultrasound features for differentiation of benign and malignant solid masses.[33]

Continued technological advances have led to renewed interest in the potential of ultrasound as a screening tool for women with dense breasts. Published results of the ACRIN 6666 trial in 2008 indicated that additional cancers are detected with screening ultrasound.[34] However, this was at the expense of a considerable number of false-positive findings and unnecessary biopsies. The use of ultrasound for breast cancer screening continues to be controversial.

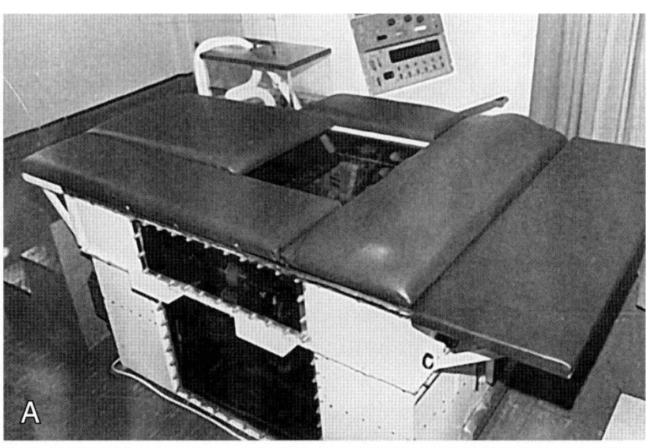

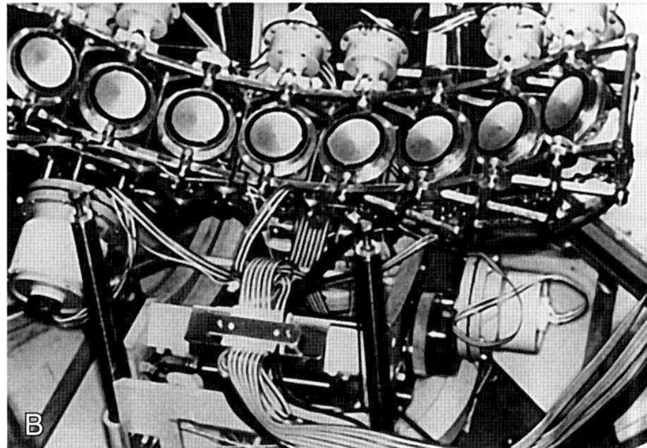

■ **FIGURE 1-28** Octoson prototype, developed by Jack Jellins, George Kossoff, and others at Australia's Ultrasonics Institute in 1974. **A,** The patient lay on a plastic membrane covering the water bath, and ultrasonic coupling was achieved by the application of oil between the skin and the plastic. **B,** Eight transducers were mounted within the water bath. *(Courtesy of Barry Goldberg, Philadelphia, Pa.)*

Light Scanning (Diaphanography)

In the late 1920s, Max Cutler investigated transillumination of the breast to access masses.[35] His work stimulated a more refined technique by Gros and his colleagues,[36] which they termed *diaphanography*. They used "cold" light that could penetrate even dense breast tissue and obtained a photographic image of the transilluminated breast. Advances by Ernest Carlsen combined cold light transillumination with an electronic system that analyzed light over a wide spectrum and stored the data for interpretation and retrieval.

Light scanning of the breast was based on the concept that cancer, because of its greater blood supply, absorbs more near-infrared and red electromagnetic radiation than benign tissue. As a consequence, instead of real-time viewing by the human eye, which is totally insensitive to near-infrared rays, the evaluation was made of an image on infrared-sensitive photographic film (Fig. 1-29).[37] Alternatively, a television camera sensitive to near-infrared radiation displayed the image on a television monitor. Electronic contrast enhancement of the video image increased the likelihood of visualizing subtle lesions. Although the technique was rapid, noninvasive, risk-free, and relatively inexpensive, prospective controlled feasibility studies showed light-scanning to be considerably less sensitive than mammography in the detection of nonpalpable cancer.[38] Nonetheless, research in this area continues to be more and more sophisticated.

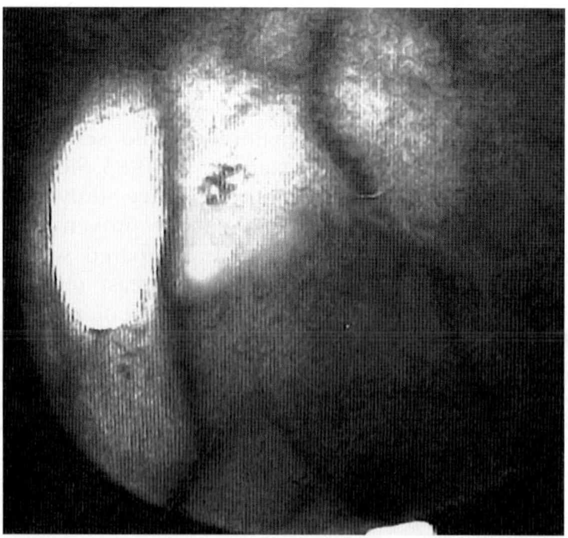

■ **FIGURE 1-29** Transillumination, or light-scanning. Photograph of a transilluminated breast reveals a large cyst. Images were obtained by using a "cold" light probe that could penetrate dense breast tissue. *(Courtesy of Christopher Merritt, New Orleans, La; reprinted from Merritt CRB, Sullivan MA, Segaloff A, McKinnon WP. Real-time transillumination lightscanning of the breast. Radiographics 1984;4:989-1009.)*

Thermography

Galileo constructed the first thermometer in 1595, but it was not until the 18th century that Herman Boerhaave first used thermometry in a clinical setting. In 1851, Carl Wunderlich began to periodically measure the temperature of his patients, thus giving thermometry a permanent role in clinical examination.

Thermography was first investigated for evaluating breast disease in 1956, when Ray Lawson,[39] having observed that breast cancer was associated with elevation of the temperature of the overlying skin, used modified military heat scanners for breast evaluation (Fig. 1-30). Although the mechanisms of tumor thermogenesis and heat transfer are not understood completely, increased blood perfusion at the site of the lesion is believed to be the primary factor responsible for the elevation in local skin temperature. Lawson's early experiments evolved into telethermography, in which infrared radiation emitted from the body was focused by an optical mirror and displayed on a cathode-ray tube. The image was photographed for a permanent record.

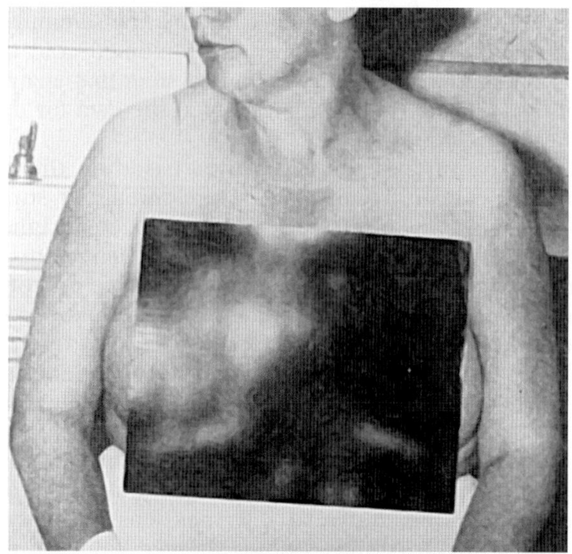

■ **FIGURE 1-30** Lawson's thermogram of a patient's breast superimposed on a photograph of the patient. The infrared display shows a white focus that corresponds to the site of increased skin temperature over a carcinoma in the right breast. *(From Lawson RN, Chughtai MS. Breast cancer and body temperature. Can Med Assoc J 1963;88:68-70.)*

A later method, contact liquid crystal thermography, involved placement of sheets of thin plastic containing heat-sensitive encapsulated liquid crystal cholesterol esters against the breast. Infrared radiation caused the black crystals to undergo changes in color, which varied with the infrared energies being emitted from the breast surface. Later, computed thermography employed multiple thermistors for infrared detection. The electronic signals were fed to a computer, which utilized various algorithms to determine whether the measurements were normal or abnormal without the necessity of imaging the breast.

However, numerous objective analyses have found that thermography is not reliable in detecting subclinical cancer.[40] Indeed, the poorest results were obtained in women whose cancers were most amenable to therapy. Also, thermography could not be used as a prescreening examination to identify patients requiring mammography or to reliably differentiate benign from malignant disease. In the Breast Cancer Detection Demonstration Project (BCDDP), the cancer detection rate for thermography was only 42%, a clinically unacceptable level, especially when compared with the rates of 57% for physical examination and 91% for mammography in that study. Furthermore, thermography had an unacceptably high number of false-positive results. Thus, thermography is not considered useful for breast cancer screening.

Radionuclide Imaging

In 1966, Whitley and coworkers[41] described a single case of breast carcinoma in which intravenously administered technetium 99m (^{99m}Tc) pertechnetate concentrated in the lesion. In a chapter contained in a 1969 textbook, Buchwald and colleagues[42] described the visualization of the tumor in 18 of 26 patients with breast carcinoma through the use of isotope Hg-197 mercuric chloride. Cancroft and Goldsmith[43] used ^{99m}Tc pertechnetate scintigraphy (Fig. 1-31) in six patients with palpable breast masses, of whom four had carcinoma (or "probable carcinoma" on the basis of physical examination or mammography), one had a biopsy-proven fibroadenoma, and the last had probable fibrocystic change that did not undergo biopsy. One of the four patients with presumed carcinoma refused biopsy and another, with bone metastases, was treated with radiotherapy to the primary lesion without biopsy. All of the biopsy-proven and presumed carcinomas showed increased radionuclide activity, and the benign lesions did not. However, any early enthusiasm generated for pertechnetate breast imaging was dissipated in 1974, when an investigation by Villarreal and associates[44] revealed significant numbers of false-negative and false-positive diagnoses of cancer with the modality. These investigators concluded that the procedure did not fulfill the requirements for a successful screening test.

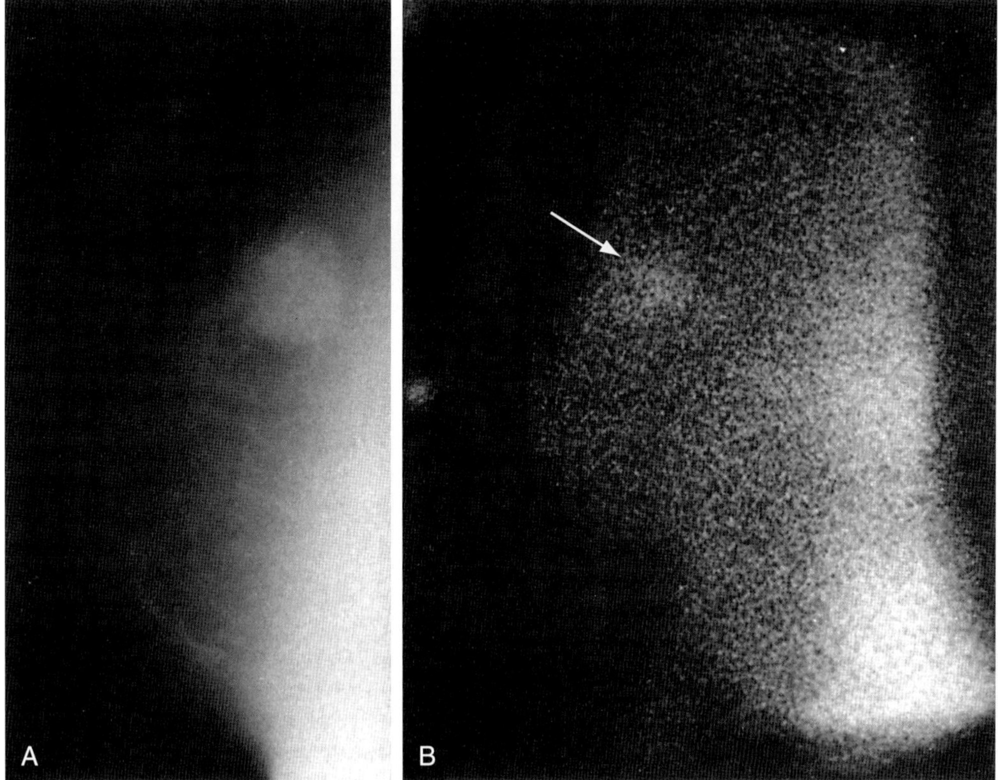

■ **FIGURE 1-31** Technetium-99m pertechnetate scintigraphy of breast carcinoma. **A,** Mediolateral mammogram demonstrates a mass with a spiculated margin. **B,** Gamma camera image shows focus of increased radionuclide activity (*arrow*). *(From Cancroft ET, Goldsmith SJ. ^{99m}Tc-pertechnetate scintigraphy as an aid to the diagnosis of breast masses. Radiology 1973;106:441-444.)*

In 1987, interest in radionuclide imaging of tumors was rekindled when ^{99m}Tc-methoxyisobutylisonitrile (MIBI), or sestamibi, was found to be taken up in a lung metastasis of a thyroid carcinoma.[45] The drug, originally designed as a myocardial perfusion tracer to assess coronary artery disease, has been investigated to determine its usefulness in the detection of breast cancer in patients scheduled to undergo breast biopsy. The results in these selected populations of women, most of whom had clinically suspicious lesions, have been variable; the modality shows good sensitivity for palpable lesions but more limited sensitivity for nonpalpable lesions.[46] The results of one preliminary investigation have suggested that scintimammography may be a valuable noninvasive complementary test in patients in whom mammography shows a low or indeterminate likelihood of cancer, especially when ACR Breast Imaging Reporting and Data System (BI-RADS) category 3 lesions–probably benign findings, have been found. Current investigations show promise for mammography-specific equipment that primarily images the breast, and there is potential for positron emission tomography (PET) when specifically designed for breast imaging.

Magnetic Resonance Imaging

The concept of cancer detection by magnetic resonance imaging (MRI) was first introduced by Raymond Damadian in 1971.[47] Investigations published between 1975 and 1978 showed that longitudinal relaxation time (T1) and transverse relaxation time (T2) differed between normal and malignant breast tissues in vitro.[48] In 1980, Mansfield and associates[49] reported the successful MRI localization of cancer in mastectomy specimens. Two years later, Ross and colleagues[50] reported the results of an in-vivo MRI investigation of the breasts of 65 women whose tissue varied from normal to dysplastic to cancerous. Seven of the women had carcinomas, two of which were clinically occult but mammographically suspicious. Using an early 0.045-tesla (T) FONAR QED 80 scanner, and imaging the patients in the supine position, these investigators found that the T1 relaxation times of dysplastic tissue and fibroadenomas overlapped those of malignant tissue.

In 1984, El Yousef and coworkers[51] published the results of an MRI study comparing the breasts of 10 normal volunteers with those of 45 patients with breast abnormalities (Fig. 1-32). These researchers used a 0.3-T system, scanning the volunteers and 25 patients in the supine position and without a surface coil, and scanning 20 patients in the prone position and with a dedicated breast surface coil. Using both spin-echo and inversion recovery pulse sequences, but obtaining only T1-weighted images, they compared their MR images with x-ray mammograms. Because they found considerable overlap in T1 relaxation times between cancer and benign breast lesions, El Yousef and coworkers determined that the contour and configuration of the abnormalities provided the best differential diagnostic criteria. This preliminary experience in breast MRI emphasized morphology as the most useful criterion to distinguish benign from malignant breast disease.

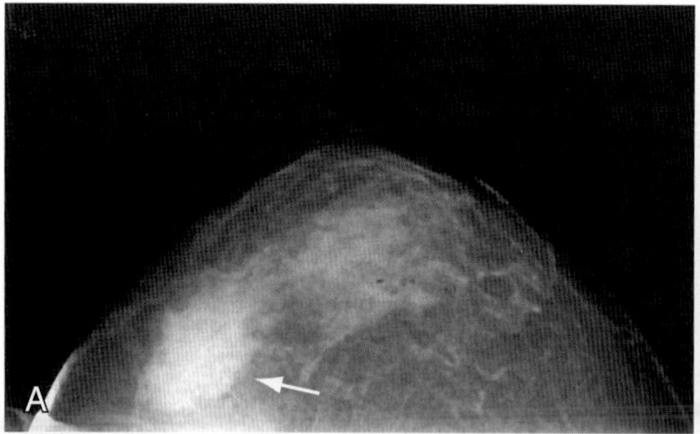

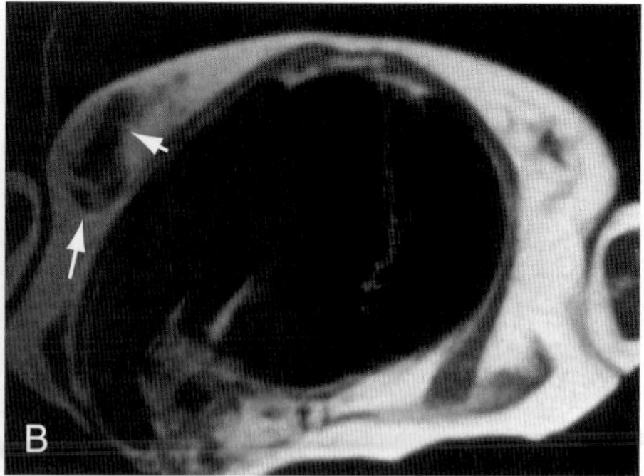

■ **FIGURE 1-32** Early magnetic resonance (MR) image of breast carcinoma. **A,** Craniocaudal mammogram shows an oval partially spiculated and partially indistinct mass (*arrow*). **B,** Axial spin-echo MR image (TR 500; TE, 30) of supine patient, obtained with cryogenic superconductive magnet (Teslacon) operating at 3.0 kilogauss. The cancer is marked by *arrows*. *(From El Yousef SJ, Duchesneau RH, Alfidi RJ. Nuclear magnetic resonance imaging of the human breast. Radiographics 1984;4:113-121.)*

In a scientific exhibit presented at the 1984 meeting of the Radiological Society of North America and an article published later, Alcorn and colleagues reported their experience with a 0.5-T magnet and a dedicated breast surface coil used to image breasts with varied pathology. These investigators blamed their necessarily imprecise calculations of T1 and T2 relaxation times for their lack of success in detecting breast cancer, and they were not optimistic about the value of morphology in detecting cancer that was surrounded by abundant parenchymal tissue. They ended their report with this prescient statement: "The future of MR imaging as an accurate modality for the detection of malignant breast neoplasms ... will probably depend upon the use of appropriate paramagnetic contrast substances as well as other technical improvements."

In 1986, Heywang and associates[52] evaluated the use of gadolinium enhancement (with intravenous gadolinium-labeled diethylenetriaminepentaacetic acid [Gd-DTPA]) to improve the differentiation between benign and malignant breast lesions. They found that most malignant tumors were enhanced but most benign lesions were not. The outgrowth of their work was the emergence of two different methods of contrast enhancement: dynamic, medium-resolution imaging *during* enhancement and three-dimensional high-resolution imaging *after* enhancement. The first method emphasized the value of information related to the time course of gadolinium enhancement, because malignant tumors theoretically enhance more rapidly than benign lesions. The proponents of this method maintained that clinically important enhancement was characterized by a 100% rise in signal intensity within the first 2 minutes after injection. The second method emphasized the value of whole-breast images for detecting unsuspected lesions. The investigators favoring this concept used ultimate signal intensity rather than dynamic information, with enhancement above 300 normalized units being considered clinically important.

Since these reports appeared, it has become clear that although cancers tend to enhance faster than benign lesions, there is overlap in their rates of enhancement. Another major limitation of breast MRI is its low specificity. The fact that most enhancing lesions are benign underscores the importance of lesion morphology as a diagnostic criterion. Continued advances in breast MRI, including the introduction of advanced computer-assisted design systems have overcome many of these limitations and improved the specificity of breast MRI. As a result, MRI for breast cancer detection and diagnosis is currently employed at the majority of breast imaging facilities in the United States and guidelines for breast MRI have been introduced by the American Cancer Society (ACS).[53] These issues will be covered in more detail in the chapters on breast MRI.

In 1993 and 1994, a large number of articles appeared describing the use of MRI to detect abnormalities of breast implants, such as silicone gel "bleed," leak, and rupture. When the effectiveness of MRI in this regard was compared with that of ultrasonography, mammography, and computed tomography (CT), MRI was generally found to be the most accurate method.[54,55] When a question of breast implant integrity cannot be answered through the use of conventional imaging methods, MRI is the most effective technology in detecting implant failure.

SCREENING MAMMOGRAPHY

Of the variety of modalities available for breast imaging, mammography has proven to be the most efficacious for breast cancer screening. The concept of using mammography as a screening tool was hypothesized by many of its pioneers; however, because their studies did not include controls, their work was largely ignored.

In an effort to determine the efficacy of screening mammography, several prospective large-scale clinical trials were performed. The first of these was conducted from 1963 to 1967 under the auspices of the Health Insurance Plan (HIP) of New York (Fig. 1-33).[56] Organized by Philip Strax, Louis Venet, and Sam Shapiro, the study was performed to determine whether periodic mammographic screening and physical examination could decrease mortality from breast cancer. The women in the study were equally divided into control and study groups. Those in the study group were requested to undergo annual physical examination and mammography for 4 consecutive years. The results of the study showed that the screened group had a 30% lower mortality overall than the control group of women; a 50% lower mortality was seen for those women who entered the study at 50 years or older. Although mortality was 23% lower among the screened women younger than 50 years, this finding lacked significance because of an inadequate number of women in this age group.

Radiographic Projections and Technical Factors

Craniocaudad

Ma—300
KvP—26
Time—6 seconds
Target-Film Distance—
22 to 40 inches

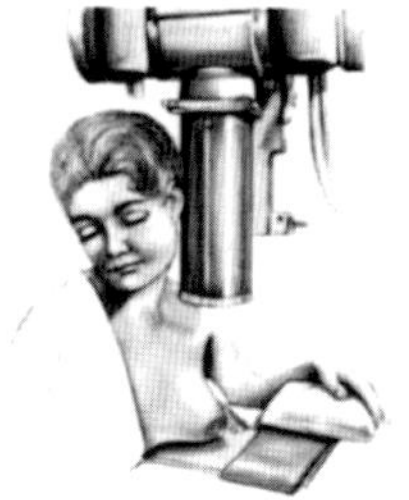

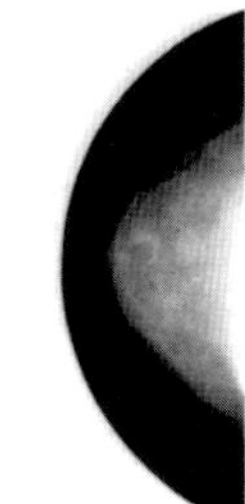

Mediolateral

Ma—300
KvP—28
Time—6 seconds
Target-Film Distance—
22 to 40 inches

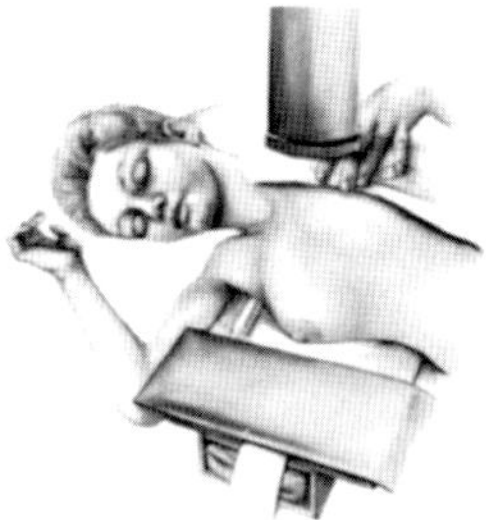

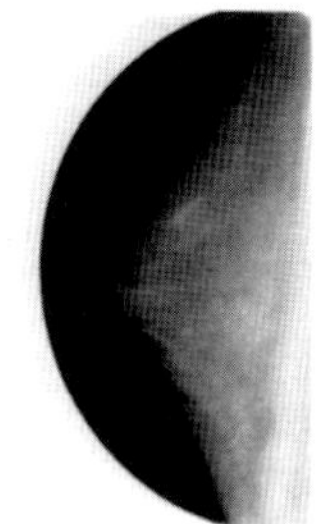

Axillary

Ma—300
KvP—54
Time—3½ seconds
Target-Film Distance—
Average Patient, 40 inches
Obese Patient, 30 inches

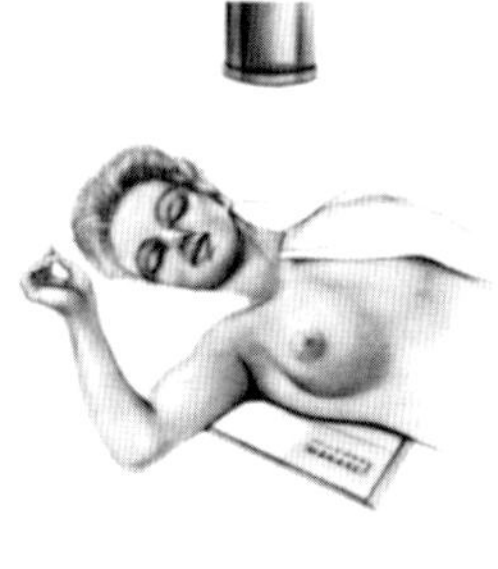

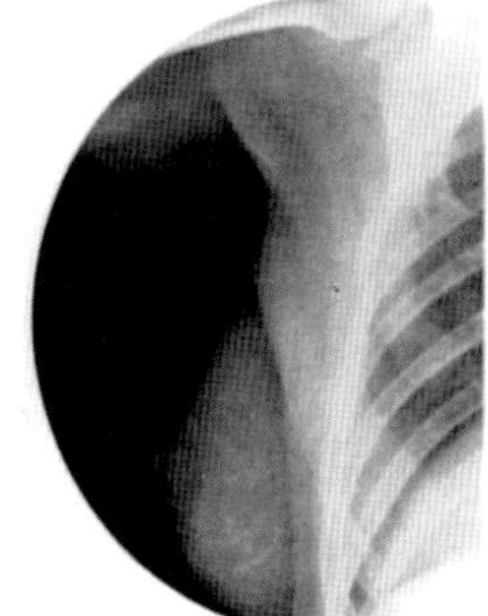

Film—Kodak Industrial X-ray Film, Type M (Estar Base), most satisfactory. Kodak Medical X-ray Film for Mammography (Estar Base) may be used.

Exposure Holder—Cardboard, with lead back.

Processing—Kodak Industrial X-ray Film, Type M. Process manually in fresh solutions. Development—5 to 8 minutes at 68 F, acid stop bath—30 seconds, fixation—12 to 15 minutes at 68 F, washing—20 minutes in running water.

Kodak Medical X-ray Film for Mammography. Designed to be processed in a Kodak X-Omat Processor for medical x-ray film using Kodak X-Omat chemicals.

Collimation—Extension cylinder, 4 by 12 inches.

Filtration—Inherent tube filtration only.

INDICATIONS FOR MAMMOGRAPHY

- Signs, Questionable Signs, or Symptoms of Disease of Breast
- Previous Radical Mastectomy
- High Familial Occurrence of Cancer of Breast
- Cancerophobia
- Previous Biopsy (Breast)
- Lumpy or Pendulous Breast
- Adenocarcinoma, Primary Site Undetermined
- Basis for Future Comparison

■ **FIGURE 1-33** Radiographic projections and technical factors for performing mammography were developed by Egan and taught to radiologists throughout the United States during the 1960s. Teaching aids such as this chart were often used. *(Courtesy of Eastman Kodak Co., Rochester, N.Y.)*

Subsequent studies in the United States and Europe have clearly shown the value of screening mammography of asymptomatic women. Responding to the results of these studies, various medical groups have established screening guidelines. In 1976, the ACR became the first group to adopt such guidelines. The ACR recommended that mammograms be performed at 1- to 2-year intervals for women younger than 50 years and annually for women age 50 or older. However, controversy surrounded the efficacy of screening women younger than 50 years. In 1980, the ACS recommended a baseline mammogram for all women 35 to 40 years of age. As a result of the BCDDP's findings, that significant numbers of cancers were detected by mammography in women age 40 to 49 years, the ACS recommended mammography at 1- to 2-year intervals for women in that age group. In 1989, the American College of Surgeons (ACS), National Cancer Institute (NCI), and nine other organizations joined in issuing a uniform set of guidelines: Screening should begin at age 40 years, followed by a mammogram every 1 to 2 years until age 50, after which a mammogram should be performed annually.[57] Important differences from previous guidelines were the deletion of a baseline mammogram and greater support for screening women between 40 and 49 years old.

The continuing controversies about the value of screening mammography will be the focus of Chapter 3: Screening Guidelines and Controversies. The authors, Stephen Feig and Stephen Duffy, are recognized experts who have analyzed international trials on the value of screening.

EDUCATION IN BREAST IMAGING

The usefulness of mammography significantly depends on the proper use of dedicated mammography equipment and the diagnostic skills of the interpreter, which can be achieved only through proper education. In 1965, it was determined that Egan's mammographic technique could be learned and used by other radiologists.[12] In 1967, the ACR established the Committee on Mammography, chaired by Wendell Scott, which undertook the responsibility of training radiologists and their technologists. With the assistance of Egan and with funding from the Cancer Control Program of the U.S. Public Health Service, 13 nationwide training centers using unique teaching aids were established. Radiologists and their technologists were encouraged to participate in a 1-week period of training at the center of their choice, with travel expenses paid by the program, and to return to the center after 2 or 3 months for a 3-day refresher course.[13] By 1969, when the program was discontinued, 1300 radiologists and 2300 technologists had been trained.

Despite growing interest and expanded training, the majority of radiologists remained unfamiliar with mammography. In an effort to increase its use, the ACR Committee on Mammography and Diseases of the Breast (formerly the Committee on Mammography) developed training tools that included a self-evaluation pretest, a continuing education text, and a detailed technical evaluation of available dedicated mammography equipment. Funded by the NCI, several new centers of training for radiologists and their technologists were active from 1975 through 1978.

In 1980, a survey found that radiology residency programs lacked adequate training in mammography. Some residents had no exposure to mammography, and only a few had rotations devoted exclusively to mammography.[58] During the early 1980s, as breast cancer detection by mammography increased, so did related medicolegal actions and recognition of the need for more effective mammography training of radiology residents. In 1983, the American Board of Radiology began to include questions related to breast disease and mammography in its written examinations, and beginning in 1990, a section on mammography was incorporated into its oral examinations. These actions reflected the growing importance of mammography and were major factors in improving mammography training.

These efforts to improve mammography training continue today. In 1997, the ACR developed the Committee on Mammography Interpretive Skills Assessment (ISA) under the leadership of Edward Sickles. The committee developed an interactive case-based tool that a radiologist could use on a computer to test and improve his or her mammography skills. The first edition (CD) of the mammography ISA was introduced in 2001, and three additional versions have since been produced. Another ACR Mammography Case Review has recently been released and another is currently under development.

History of the Society of Breast Imaging

In 1984, Marc Homer, Carl D'Orsi, Stephen Feig, Harold Moskowitz, Myron Moskowitz, and Edward Sickles initiated a plan to create a society of radiologists who were committed to advancing research, teaching, and clinical work in breast imaging and who would meet periodically with their peers to present new ideas and to seek advice on all aspects of breast imaging (M.J. Homer, personal communication, March 14, 2001). Thus was born the Society of Breast Imaging (SBI). The organizational meeting of the society was held in Boston on April 24, 1985, at which time the following objectives were established: (1) to improve and disseminate knowledge in the field of breast imaging; (2) to improve the quality of medical education in the field of breast imaging; (3) to foster research in all aspects of breast imaging; (4) to provide a medium for the exchange of ideas among professionals involved with breast imaging; (5) to provide meetings for presentation and discussion of papers, and for the dissemination of knowledge in the area of breast imaging; and (6) to establish a channel for publication of scientific reports in the field of breast imaging. In 1988, the SBI was welcomed as the newest member of the Intersociety Commission of the ACR. Although membership in the SBI was initially by invitation, a general membership category was established for radiologists in 1991 and an affiliate membership category was established for radiologic technologists in 1995. The first biennial meeting and postgraduate course of the national SBI occurred in 1993. The fourth postgraduate course, in 1999, played host to 860 registrants, exhibitors, and guests. The 2009 postgraduate course was held in May 2001. A program to fund worthy research in breast imaging was begun in 1998. For the fiscal year 2000-2001, the SBI awarded $35,487 in grant support to young investigators mentored by senior investigators with established records in breast imaging research. The SBI has also developed training curricula in breast imaging for residents and fellows.[59] By late 1999, the total membership of the SBI was more than 2000.

HISTORY OF THE REGULATION OF MAMMOGRAPHY

In 1975, Bicehouse[60] reported that surface radiation exposures delivered by mammography units in 70 medical facilities in eastern Pennsylvania ranged from 0.25 to 47 rad. Obviously, some facilities were using radiation doses too low to obtain diagnostic images while others were delivering excessive radiation. In 1975, the Bureau of Radiologic Health of the U.S. Food and Drug Administration (FDA), with the aid of state radiation control agencies, developed a mammography quality assurance program to minimize patient exposure while optimizing image quality. The purpose of the program, called Breast Exposure: Nationwide Trends (BENT), was to identify problems in dose and image quality and to help facilities improve mammography.[61] BENT consisted of four phases. During the first phase, mammography facilities were identified through a mailed questionnaire. During the second phase, facilities were sent survey cards for recording the technical factors used in mammography. The cards also contained thermoluminescent dosimeters (TLDs), which were used to measure entrance skin doses. The program performed analysis of the technical factors and TLD exposures before proceeding to the third phase, in which state surveyors visited facilities with problems in exposure and recommended corrective procedures. During the fourth and final phase, another TLD survey card was sent to assess changes in the performance of mammography. By 1977, 42 states were enrolled in BENT. Although only 7% of the facilities performing screen-film mammography were found to have unusually *high* radiation exposures, 29% were identified as having unusually *low* exposures, suggesting that films were being underexposed. Of the screen-film units selected for follow-up, 89% had tungsten anodes, indicating that general-purpose radiographic units were being used rather than dedicated mammography units.

Concern had been growing among some scientists that breast cancer might be induced through the exposure of healthy breast tissue to ionizing radiation. In September 1975, John C. Bailar III, editor of the Journal of the National Cancer Institute, met with the director of the NCI to discuss the possible radiation risks of mammography. Bailar expressed his concerns in an editorial, in which he concluded that "the overall benefits of mammography and screening of the general population have not been determined, and its hazards may be greater than are commonly understood .... There seems to be the possibility that the routine use of mammography in screening asymptomatic women may eventually take almost as many lives as it saves."[62] In October 1975, after a meeting among Bailar, NCI officials, and representatives of the ACS three experts were assigned to develop working groups to examine the pertinent issues. Lester Breslow was asked to determine the benefits of mammography in the HIP study, Arthur C. Upton to evaluate the possible radiation risks from mammography, and Louis B. Thomas to review the pathology of the cancers detected in the HIP study. The Breslow working group concluded that the entire benefit of screening in the HIP study was realized in women older than 50 years.[63] The report of the Upton group on radiation risks disclosed an excess of breast cancer in three populations previously exposed to radiation: young American and Canadian women treated with radiation for postpartum mastitis, young American and Canadian women with tuberculosis subjected to multiple chest fluoroscopy procedures, and Japanese women 10 years and older who had survived atomic bomb irradiation.[64] The group used a linear dose-response curve to determine that the annual risk of development of breast cancer secondary to mammography was 3.5 to 7.5 new cases per 1 million women (at least 35 years old) at risk per rad to both breasts. The concerns about the safety of mammography that were reported in the mass media in 1976 led to a "radiation scare" and a marked decline in the use of mammography. By the end of the 1970s, the future of mammography was uncertain!

The performance of mammography in the United States changed in the 1980s, when technologic advances allowed the reduction of radiation dose while simultaneously improving image quality. These advances resulted from the replacement of general-purpose radiographic equipment with tungsten anodes used for screen-film mammography and the introduction of dedicated mammography units that used molybdenum anodes. In 1979, 45% of all facilities performing mammography in the United States were using screen-film receptors, 45% were using xeromammography, and only 10% were using direct-exposure (nonscreen) film. By 1987, 54% of facilities used screen-film mammography, 30% xeromammography, 16% a combination of screen-film and xeromammography, and fewer than 1% direct film mammography.[65] By the end of the 1980s, screen-film mammography had become the predominant method and fewer than 1% of screen-film mammography examinations were performed with general-purpose radiographic equipment, leading to a striking reduction in radiation doses.

In 1986, specific guidelines for acceptable levels of radiation exposure in mammography were published by the National Council on Radiation Protection and Measurements.[66] The council recommended that the average glandular dose for a two-view examination not exceed 800 mrad per breast. By the end of the 1980s, the combination of decreased x-ray dosage and validation of the mortality reduction through mammography screening in European clinical trials had restored confidence in mammography.

Although concerns over radiation exposure from mammography had largely subsided, problems with image quality were resurfacing. In 1985 and 1988, the FDA and the Conference of Radiation Control Program Directors conducted nationwide assessments of phantom image quality and radiation doses under the National Evaluation of X-ray Trends (NEXT) program.[67] The NEXT-85 survey reported that a significant number of facilities had image quality problems. The NEXT-88 survey showed that there had been widespread replacement of general-purpose equipment by dedicated mammography units, a greater use of grids, and improvements in film processing; however, image quality was still variable, and 13% of facilities in the survey had unacceptable phantom image scores. In 1988, a report on screening sites participating in an ACS Breast Cancer Awareness Program in Philadelphia identified marked variations in the performance of film processors as a source of unreliable image quality. Forty-one percent of the mammography sites evaluated had unacceptably wide variations in processor performance over intervals as short as 2 weeks.[68] The ACR responded to the problems in image quality and the need to identify community-based sites that would perform quality mammography for the ACS screening projects by developing the Mammography Accreditation Program (MAP).[69] The ACR MAP began to accredit mammography facilities in August 1987. The accreditation program was voluntary and consisted of the following five parts: (1) a facility survey; (2) phantom image evaluation; (3) radiation dose measurement; (4) clinical image evaluation; and (5) processor performance. The program rapidly came to represent the standard for quality in mammography, and by the spring of 1991 a total of 4832 facilities had applied for ACR MAP accreditation.

One of the impediments to the use of screening mammography had been its relatively high cost, which was not reimbursed by all health insurance plans. In 1986, Maryland became the first state to pass legislation mandating screening mammography as a basic health insurance benefit. The first mammography quality assurance legislation was included in the Maryland reimbursement law. By 1994, 41 states and the District of Columbia had legislation or regulations concerning mammography, including quality assurance standards. However, the legislated requirements and mandated standards did not always apply uniformly to all mammography facilities from state to state or, for that matter, even within a state. A 1992 article in a law journal noted, "From a patient perspective, of course, practice guidelines or standards of care that differ from state to state merely heighten the confusion, fear, and risks surrounding mammography."[70]

Mammography regulations had reached the federal level in 1990, when the U.S. Congress passed the Omnibus Budget Reconciliation Act, creating the first budget to include federal funding for mammography screening. When the Health Care Financing Administration (HCFA) agreed to reimburse for screening mammography as a Medicare benefit for women 65 years and older and for disabled women between 35 and 64 years old, the administration also developed and imposed its own regulations and inspections as prerequisites for payment.[71] Although based largely on ACR MAP, the Medicare regulations included some controversial additional requirements, such as mandatory reports in lay language to examinees. The latter requirement was interpreted in varying ways by state inspectors. Some accepted a brief notification that the findings were normal or abnormal, whereas others demanded that a literal lay-language translation of the report that was sent to the referring health care provider to be sent to the patient after her examination. Some states applied the requirement for the lay-language report to all women undergoing mammography, whereas others restricted the requirement to self-referred women. When inspections began in December 1992, these inconsistencies made it difficult for facilities to comply with Medicare regulations. Furthermore, inspectors in the different states had a variable range of expertise and training and some Medicare inspectors were not employed by the Bureau of Radiologic Health. One report cited inspections by registered nurses whose experience came from inspecting long-term nursing care facilities. The practice of making unannounced inspections added to the friction that developed between the facilities and the Medicare inspectors.

By 1992, the differing quality assurance recommendations, guidelines, and regulations established by professional organizations, federal agencies, and state agencies had resulted in a disturbing variability in the quality of mammography across the United States.[72] In response to media exposés, public pressure, and the growing evidence of problems in mammography quality, the ACR-ACS Conference of Radiation Control Program Directors, American College of Obstetricians and Gynecologists (ACOG), and nearly 300 breast cancer support groups became united in their encouragement of federal standards and enforcement. With solid support from consumers and professional organizations, the Mammography Quality Standards Act (MQSA) was passed by Congress and signed into law by President George H. W. Bush in October 1992.[73]

The responsibility for implementing MQSA was delegated to the FDA in June 1993. According to MQSA, each of the approximately 10,000 facilities providing mammography would have to be certified by October 1, 1994, or cease performing mammography. The certificate would be issued for 3 years and would be renewable. The FDA was required to develop quality standards for accreditation bodies, personnel, equipment, record keeping, reporting, and dose limits. Among other mandates, the new law required that all facilities be evaluated annually by a certified medical physicist and inspected annually by approved inspectors. To accomplish this task within the time limit, the FDA established interim regulations that had to be met by October 1, 1994.[74]

The MQSA imposed a set of federal regulations on every facility and radiologist performing and interpreting mammograms. The interim regulations regarding accreditation were based on the original ACR Mammography Voluntary Accreditation Program. The final regulations were published on October 28, 1997, in the Federal Register.[75] When MQSA was re-authorized by Congress on October 9, 1998, a change was made in the final rule: A new requirement mandated that a report of the results of the screening procedure, prepared in lay language, be sent to each patient.

RECENT CHALLENGES AND ACCOMPLISHMENTS

The field of breast imaging has continued to face a number of challenges, but it has also dealt effectively with most of these and has made incredible progress. The challenges include continued controversies about the value of breast cancer screening, medicolegal issues, and a shortage of breast imagers. These issues will be addressed in several of the chapters in this textbook.

KEY POINTS

- The first mammogram was performed in 1927 in Germany.
- Stafford Warren performed the first mammograms in the United States.
- Robert Egan established a reproducible method for mammography.
- Mammography was not widely used in the United States until the 1980s.
- Breast imaging now includes mammography, ultrasonography, and MRI.
- Breast imaging has encountered many challenges and survived.
- Today breast imaging has finally been recognized as an essential component of radiology.

SUGGESTED READINGS

Bassett LW, Gold RH. The Evolution of Mammography. *AJR Am J Roentgenol* 1988;**150**:493-8.
Bassett LW. Breast imaging: current utilization, trends, and implications. *AJR Am J Roentgenol* 2007;**189**:612-3.
Gold RH, Bassett LW, Kimme-Smith C. Breast imaging: state-of-the-art. *Invest Radiol* 1986;**21**:298-304.
Sickles EA. Breast Imaging: from 1965 to the present. *Radiology* 2000;**215**:1-16.

REFERENCES

1. Salomon A. Beitrage zur Pathologie und Klinik der Mammacarcinome. *Arch Klin Chir* 1913;**101**:573-668.
2. Kleinschmidt O. Brustdruse. In: Zweife P, Payr E, editors. *Die Klinik der Bosartigen Geschwulste*. Leipzig: S. Hirzel; 1927. p. 5-90.
3. Vogel W. Die Roentgendarstellung der Mammatumoren. *Arch Klin Chir* 1932;**171**:618-26.
4. Goyanes J, Gentil F, Guedes B. Sobre la radiografiá de la glándula mamária y su valor diagnóstico. *Arch Espano de Oncol* 1931;**2**:111-42.
5. Dominguez CM. Estudio sistematizado del cancer del seno. *Bol Liga Uruguay Contr Cancer Genit Femen* 1929;**4**:145-54.
6. Warren SL. Roentgenologic study of the breast. *AJR Am J Roentgenol* 1930;**24**:113-24.
7. Seabold PS. Procedure in roentgen study of the breast. *Am J Roentgenol Radium Ther* 1933;**39**:850-1.
8. Gershon-Cohen J, Strickler A. Roentgenologic examination of the normal breast: its evaluation in demonstrating early neoplastic changes. *Am J Roentgenol Radium Ther* 1938;**40**:189-201.
9. Gros CM, Sigrist R. Radiography and transillumination of the breast. *Strasb Med* 1951;**2**:451-6.
10. Leborgne R. *The breast in roentgen diagnosis. Montevideo*. Uruguay: Impresora; 1953.
11. Egan RL. Experience with mammography in a tumor institution: evaluation of 1000 cases. *Radiology* 1960;**75**:894-900.
12. Clark RL, Copeland MM, Egan RL, Gallager HS, Geller H, Lindsay JP, et al. Reproducibility of the technic of mammography (Egan) for cancer of the breast. *Am J Surg* 1965;**109**:127-33.
13. Scott WG. Mammography and the training program of the American College of Radiology. *Am J Roentgenol Radium Ther Nucl Med* 1967;**99**:1002-8.
14. Barnes GT, Brezovich IA. The intensity of scattered radiation in mammography. *Radiology* 1978;**126**:243-7.
15. Sickles EA, Weber WN. High contrast mammography with a moving grid: Assessment of clinical utility. *AJR Am J Roentgenol* 1986;**146**:1137-9.
16. Haus AG, Paulus DD, Dodd GD, Cowart RW, Bencomo Jl. Magnification mammography: evaluation of screen film and xeroradiographic techniques. *Radiology* 1979;**133**:223-6.
17. Price JL, Butler PD. The reduction of radiation and exposure time in mammography. *Br J Radiol* 1970;**43**:251-5.
18. Haus AG, Cillinan JE. Screen film processing systems for medical radiography: a historical review. *Radiographics* 1989;**9**:1203-24.
19. Densdale A, Chester F. Carlson: Inventor of xerography. *Photogr Sci Eng* 1963;**7**:1.
20. Wolfe JN. History and recent developments in xeroradiography of the breast. *Radiol Clin North Am* 1987;**25**:929-37.
21. Pisano ED, Gatsonis C, Hendrick E, Yaffe M, Baum JK, Acharyya S, et al. Diagnostic performance of digital versus film mammography for breast-cancer screening. *N Engl J Med* 2005;**353**:1773-83.
22. Curie P. Dévelopment, par pression, de l'électricité polaire dans les cristaux hémièdres à faces inclinées. *C R Hébd Séances Acad Sci* 1880;**91**:294.
23. Ludwig GD. The velocity of sound through tissues and the acoustic impedance of tissues. *J Acoust Soc Am* 1950;**22**:862.
24. Wild JJ. The use of ultrasonic pulses for the measurement of biologic tissues and the detection of tissue density changes. *Surgery* 1950;**27**:183.
25. Wild JJ, Reid JM. Further pilot echographic studies on the histologic structure of tumors of the living intact human breast. *Am J Pathol* 1952;**28**:839-61.
26. Wells PN, Evans KT. An immersion scanner for two dimensional ultrasonic examination of the human breast. *Ultrasonics* 1968;**6**:220-8.
27. Kelly-Fry E, Kossoff G, Hindman HA. The potential of ultrasound visualization for detecting the presence of abnormal structures within the female breast. In: *Proceedings of the IEEE Sonics-Ultrasonics Symposium*. Boston: Mass; 1972. p. 25.
28. Jellins J, Kossoff G, Buddee FW, Reeve TS. Ultrasonic visualization of the breast. *Med J Aust* 1971;**1**:305-7.
29. Cole-Beuglet C, Goldberg BB, Kurtz AB, Patchefsky AS, Shaber GS, Rubin CS. Clinical experience with a prototype real-time dedicated breast scanner. *AJR Am J Roentgenol* 1982;**139**:905-11.
30. Sickles EA, Filly RA, Callen PW. Breast cancer detection with sonography and mammography: comparison using state-of-the-art equipment. *AJR Am J Roentgenol* 1983;**140**:843-5.
31. Hilton SW, Leopold GR, Olson LK, Wilson SA. Real-time breast sonography: Application in 300 consecutive patients. *AJR Am J Roentgenol* 1986;**147**:479-86.
32. Jellins J, Kossoff G, Reeve TS. Detection and classification of liquid-filled masses in the breast by gray scale echography. *Radiology* 1977;**125**:205-12.
33. Stavros AT, Thickman D, Rapp CL, Dennis MA, Parker SH, Sisney GA. Solid breast nodules: Use of sonography to distinguish between benign and malignant lesions. *Radiology* 1995;**196**:123-34.
34. Berg WA, Blume JD, Cormack JB, Mendelson EB, Lehrer D, Böhm-Vélez M, et al. Combined screening with ultrasound and mammography vs mammography alone in women at elevated risk of breast cancer. *JAMA* 2008;**299**:2151-63.
35. Cutler M. Transillumination as an aid in the diagnosis of breast lesions. *Surg Gynecol Obstet* 1929;**48**:721-9.
36. Gros CM, Quenneville Y, Hummel Y. Diaphanologie mammaire. *J Radiol Electrol Med Nucl* 1972;**53**:297-302.
37. Ohlsson B, Gundersen J, Nillsson DM. Diaphanography: a method for the evaluation of the female breast. *World J Surg* 1980;**4**:701-5.
38. Sickles EA. Breast cancer detection with transillumination and mammography. *AJR Am J Roentgenol* 1984;**142**:841-4.
39. Lawson R. Implications of surface temperatures in the diagnosis of breast cancer. *Can Med Assoc J* 1956;**75**:309-10.
40. Moskowitz M, Milbrath J, Gartside P, Zermeno A, Mandel D, et al. Lack of efficacy of thermography as a screening tool for minimal and stage I breast cancer. *N Engl J Med* 1976;**295**:249-52.
41. Whitley JE, Witcofski RL, Bolliger TT, Maynard CD. Tc99m in the visualization of neoplasms outside the brain. *Am J Roentgenol* 1966;**96**:706-10.
42. Buchwald W, Diethelm L, Wolf R. Scintigraphic delineation of carcinoma of the breast and parasternal lymph nodes. In: McCready VR, Taylor DM, Trott NG, et al., editors. *Radioactive isotopes in the localization of tumours*. New York: Grune & Stratton; 1969. p. 138-42.
43. Cancroft ET, Goldsmith SJ. ^{99m}Tc-pertechnetate scintigraphy as an aid to the diagnosis of breast masses. *Radiology* 1973;**106**:441-4.
44. Villarreal RL, Parkey RW, Bonte FJ. Experimental pertechnetate mammography. *Radiology* 1974;**111**:657-61.
45. Muller ST, Guth-Tougelides B, Crutzig H. Imaging of malignant tumors with MIBI-^{99m}Tc SPECT [abstract]. *J Nucl Med* 1987;**28**:562P.
46. Khalkhali I, Villanueva-Meyer J, Edell S, Connolly JL, Schnitt SJ, Baum JK, et al. Diagnostic accuracy of ^{99m}Tc-sestamibi breast imaging: multicenter trial results. *J Nucl Med* 2000;**41**:1973-9.
47. Damadian R. Tumor detection by nuclear magnetic resonance. *Science* 1971;**171**:1151-3.
48. Bouvee WMMJ, Getreuer KW, Smidt J, Lindeman J. Nuclear magnetic resonance and detection of human breast tumors. *J Natl Cancer Inst* 1978;**67**:53-5.
49. Mansfield P, Morris PG, Ordidge RJ, Pykett IL, Bangert V, Coupland RE. Human whole body imaging and detection of breast tumours by n.m.r. *Philos Trans R Soc Lond B Biol Sci* 1980;**289**:503-10.
50. Ross RJ, Thompson JS, Kim K, Bailey RA. Nuclear magnetic resonance imaging and evaluation of human breast tissue: preliminary clinical trials. *Radiology* 1982;**143**:195-205.

51. El Yousef SJ, Duchesneau RH, Alfidi RJ, Haaga JR, Bryan PJ, LiPuma JP. Magnetic imaging of the breast. Work in progress. *Radiology* 1984;**150**:761-6.
52. Heywang SH, Hahn D, Schmidt H, Krischke I, Eiermann W, Bassermann R, et al. MR imaging of the breast using gadolinium-DTPA. *J Comput Assist Tomogr* 1986;**10**:199-204.
53. Bassett LW, Dhaliwal SG, Eradat J, Khan O, Farria DF, Brenner RJ, et al. National trends and practices in breast MRI. *AJR Am J Roentgenol* 2008;**191**:332-9.
54. Mund DF, Farria DM, Gorczyca DP, deBruhl ND, Ahn CY, Shaw WW, et al. MR imaging of the breast in patients with silicone-gel implants: Spectrum of findings. *AJR Am J Roentgenol* 1993;**161**: 773-8.
55. Ahn CY, DeBruhl ND, Gorczyca DP, Shaw WW, Bassett LW. Comparative silicone breast implant evaluation using mammography, sonography, and magnetic resonance imaging: experience with 59 implants. *Plast Reconstruct Surg* 1994;**94**:620-7.
56. Shapiro S. Evidence on screening for breast cancer from a randomized trial. *Cancer* 1977;**39**(Suppl. 6):2772-82.
57. McIlrath S. Eleven medical groups endorse mammogram guidelines. *Am Med News* 1989;**32**:335.
58. Homer MJ. Mammography training in diagnostic radiology residency programs. *Radiology* 1980;**135**:529-31.
59. Feig SA, Hall FM, Ikeda DM, Mendelson EB, Rubin EC, Segel MC, et al. Society of Breast Imaging residency and fellowship training curriculum. *Radiol Clin North Am* 2000;**38**:915-20.
60. Bicehouse HJ. Survey of mammographic exposure levels and technique used in Eastern Pennsylvania. *Seventh Annual National Cancer Conference on Radiation Control;April 27 to May 2, 1975*. Hyannis, Mass: (DHEW Publication 76-8026). Bethesda, Md: DHEW; 1976.
61. Jans RG, Butler PF, McCrohan Jr JL, Thompson WE. Status of film/screen mammography: Results of the BENT study. *Radiology* 1979;**132**:197-200.
62. Bailar 3rd JC. Mammography: A contrary view. *Ann Intern Med* 1976;**84**:77-84.
63. Breslow L, Henderson BE, Massey FJ, et al. Report of NCI ad hoc working group on the gross and net benefits of mammography in mass screening for the detection of breast cancer. *J Natl Cancer Inst* 1977;**59**:473-8.
64. Upton AC, Beebe GW, Brown JM, et al. Report of NCI ad hoc working group on the risks associated with mammography in mass screening for detection of breast cancer. *J Natl Cancer Inst* 1977;**59**:579-93.
65. Bassett LW, Diamond JJ, Gold RH, McLelland R. Survey of mammography practices. *AJR Am J Roentgenol* 1987;**149**:1149-52.
66. National Council on Radiation Protection and Measurements. *Mammography: A user's guide*. (NCRP Report No. 85.) Bethesda, Md; 1986.
67. Reuter FG. *Preliminary report-NEXT-85*. National Conference on Radiation Control. Proceedings of the 18th Annual Conference of Radiation Control Program Directors: Charleston, W. Va: 1986. p. 111-20. CRCPD Publication 86-2.
68. Galkin BM, Feig SA, Muir HD. The technical quality of mammography in centers participating in a regional breast cancer awareness program. *Radiographics* 1988;**8**:133-45.
69. McLelland R, Hendrick RE, Zinninger MD, Wilcox PA. The American College of Radiology Mammography Accreditation Program. *AJR Am J Roentgenol* 1991;**157**:473-9.
70. Cocca SV. Who's monitoring the quality of mammograms? The Mammography Quality Standards Act of 1992 could finally provide the answer. *Am J Law Med* 1993;**19**:313-44.
71. U.S. Department of Health and Human Services. Interim final rules on conditions for Medicare coverage of screening mammography. *Fed Regist* 1990;**55**:53511-25.
72. U.S. General Accounting Office. *Screening mammography: Federal quality standards are needed*. Washington, DC: General Accounting Office; 1992. Publication No. GAO/T-HRD-92-39.
73. Mammography Quality Standards Act. *Public Law* 1992; p. 102-539.
74. U.S. Food and Drug Administration. Mammography facilities-requirements for accrediting bodies and quality standards and certification requirements; interim rules. *Fed Regist* 1993;**58**:67558-65.
75. MQSRA (Mammography Quality Standards Re-Authorization Act of 1998). Public Law 105-248.

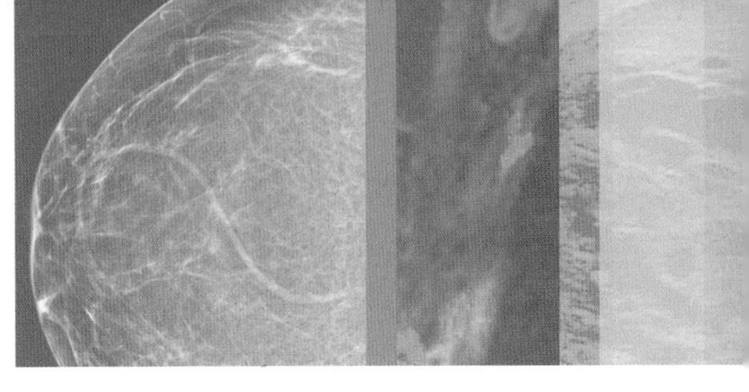

CHAPTER 2

Epidemiology of Breast Cancer

Robert A. Smith, Louise A. Brinton, Joan Kramer, Ahmedin Jemal, and Carol DeSantis

In the world, breast cancer is the most common cancer diagnosed in women, accounting for more than 1 in 10 new diagnoses each year and more than 1 million new cases annually. Breast cancer is the most common cause of death from cancer among women, with more than 400,000 deaths each year.[1] Among all cancers diagnosed in men and women, breast cancer is the most prevalent, with more than 4 million women in the world surviving breast cancer up to 5 years.[1]

In this chapter on the epidemiology of breast cancer, we focus on both the *descriptive epidemiology* of breast cancer, which principally relates to descriptive statistics and trends in risk, incidence, mortality and premature mortality, and *analytic epidemiology*, which goes beyond basic statistics and seeks to understand factors associated with risk of breast cancer occurrence and death. The statistics cited above speak to the global importance of breast cancer as a public health problem, but national statistics, specifically differences in the underlying risk of disease, also have provided important insights into the basic etiology of this disease. Moreover, patterns of risk are not static, as is evident by the increase in incidence in the developing world, and the decline in incidence in some developed nations.[2] Thus, incidence and mortality rates are affected not only by changes in behavior that affect disease risk, but also by secondary prevention measures, specifically use of mammography. Finally, insofar as assessment of absolute risk has been proposed as a basis for shared decision making about breast cancer interventions, it is important that clinicians be familiar with risk estimation tools and their strengths and limitations.

Through analytic epidemiological research we know a great deal about the underlying etiology of breast cancer, although few of the known risk factors, alone or in combination, offer a behavioral strategy that has proven or practical potential to measurably and confidently reduce risk. Risk reductions in women at elevated risk have been demonstrated through chemoprevention,[3,4] but the possibility of serious side effects in some women limits the potential of this strategy.[5-7] However, insofar as breast cancer is among women's greatest health concerns, it is important to look to the epidemiological research for strategies that may reduce risk, and help women make informed decisions regarding lifestyles and surveillance strategies.

BREAST CANCER STATISTICS: NUMBERS AND RATES

Each year, national and international agencies provide estimates of the number of newly diagnosed breast cancer cases and deaths, trends in rates, and survival.[8-10] In the United States, estimated numbers of cases and deaths are updated annually by the American Cancer Society (ACS),[9] while the National Cancer Institute (NCI) provides the most recent cancer statistics for the United States through the Surveillance, Epidemiology, and End Results Program (SEER).[8] An annual report on cancer statistics in the United States at the state and national level is produced by the Centers for Disease Control and Prevention (CDC) and NCI combining data from the CDC's National Program of Cancer Registries (NPCR) and NCI's SEER program.[11] Global cancer statistics are compiled by the International Agency for Research on Cancer (IARC)[10] and the World Health Organization (WHO) provides estimates of global cancer mortality.[12]

Worldwide estimates of the number of women diagnosed with breast cancer and the number of deaths from breast cancer are derived by applying age-specific cancer rates from a geographic region to the corresponding age specific population from the United Nations, which is provided in GLOBOCAN. U.S. estimates are projected using a spatio-temporal projection model based on high quality incidence data covering about 85% of the U.S. population.[13-15] Mortality data are collected in all industrialized countries and some developing countries, with available data estimated to cover approximately 30% of global deaths. Data from death certificates are abstracted and compiled in the WHO mortality database, covering about 30% of the world population.[12] The quality of mortality data as well as determination of the underlying cause of death is higher in high resource countries compared with low-resource countries.[15] In the United States, because deaths are enumerated by the Division of Vital Statistics of the National Center for Health Statistics (NCHS), the actual numbers of deaths from breast cancer usually are available within 3 to 4 years from the current calendar year.

Although the estimated annual numbers of new cases and deaths are important summary statistics, rates (events per population at risk) are better measures for comparisons over time and between population groups because the size of a population and its age composition influences the number of new cases and deaths from breast cancer. To remove the effect of different age distributions in populations, or trends in the same population over time, crude rates (number of cases per midyear unit of population) are standardized to a specific population distribution. An age-standardized rate, also referred to as an *age-adjusted* rate, is a weighted average of age-specific rates in a given population, where the weights are the proportions of persons in a standard population in the corresponding age groups.[16] Age-adjusted rates are only comparable when the same age standard is applied to each of the population being compared. Thus, apart from direct international comparisons (Figs. 2-1 through 2-5) age-adjusted international and U.S. breast cancer rates in this chapter are not directly comparable because the surveillance data are from different sources and use different standard populations. The international data presented in this publication are standardized to the 1960 world standard population, while incidence and mortality data in the United States and several European countries are standardized to the 2000 U.S. and European standard populations, respectively.[15]

The value of age standardization when comparing trends in breast cancer incidence and mortality rates is especially evident for U.S. trends because the average age of the population is increasing. Those women born in the first year of the postwar birth cohort reached 40 years of age in 1985, and each year a growing number of women enter age cohorts in which screening is recommended and age-specific breast cancer incidence and mortality are higher. Because breast cancer incidence and mortality rates increase with increasing age, crude rates increase over time in an aging population on that basis alone, whereas trends in age-adjusted incidence and mortality rates portray the underlying epidemiology of disease, as well as trends in breast cancer detection and treatment. Further, as a population's underlying age distribution and varying age distributions of sub-populations, such as may occur within different ethnic groups, grow increasingly different from the standardized distribution, the true (i.e., crude) rates and age-adjusted rates may become increasingly dissimilar. For example, in 1992, the crude incidence rate of female

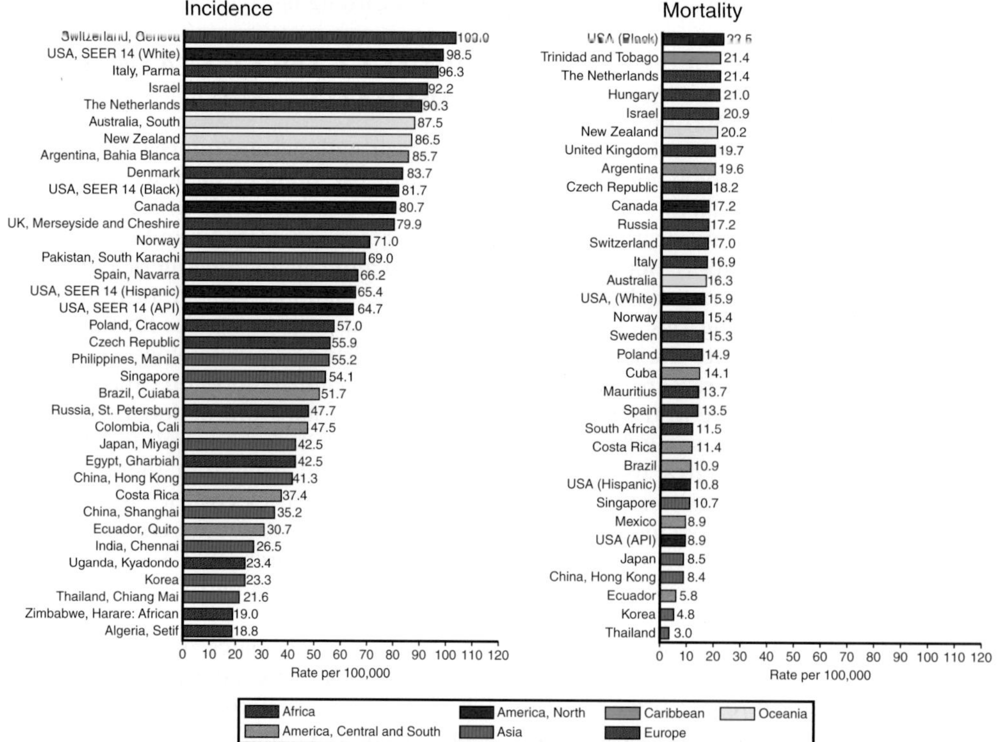

■ FIGURE 2-1 Female breast cancer incidence and mortality rates in select registries, 1998 to 2002. Rates are per 100,000 and age-standardized to the world population. *(Incidence data from Cancer Incidence in Five Continents, Volume IX, International Agency for Research on Cancer [IARC]. Mortality data from WHO Mortality Database. API: Asian/Pacific Islander.)*

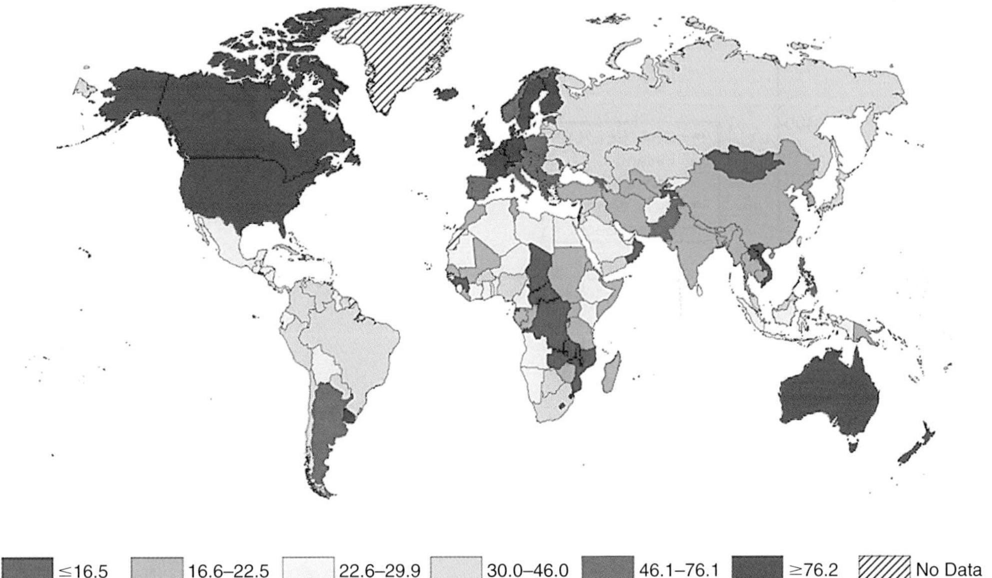

■ **FIGURE 2-2** International variation in age-standardized breast cancer incidence rates, 2002. Rates are per 100,000 and age-standardized to the world population. *(Data from GLOBOCAN 2002.)*

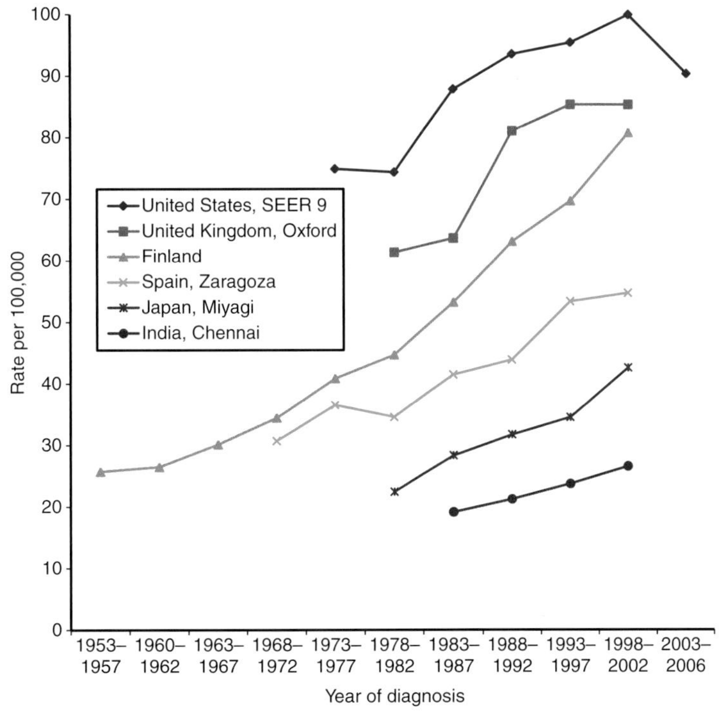

■ **FIGURE 2-3** Trends in breast cancer incidence rates in select registries. Rates are per 100,000 and age-standardized to the world population. *(Data from Cancer in Five Continents, Volumes I-IX, International Agency for Research on Cancer [IARC]. Data for United States from Surveillance, Epidemiology, and End Results [SEER] Program, 9 SEER Registries, 1973–2007, Division of Cancer Control and Population Sciences, National Cancer Institute, 2010.)*

breast cancer in the United States was 128.2 per 100,000, compared with an age-adjusted rate of 110.6 when standardized to the 1970 U.S. population, a difference of plus 16%.[17] As this example shows, apart from comparisons between different populations or a population over time, the adjusted rate for any one year has no inherent meaning as a stand-alone measure of disease burden.

Because of the aging of the U.S. population, there have been periods when clinicians and the public perceived rising breast cancer incidence rates in some subgroups of women when, in fact, rates have been quite stable or even declining.[18] Although age-adjusted breast cancer incidence rates in women younger than age 50 have changed very little between 1975 and 2007 (40.6 vs. 44.4 × 10^5), the

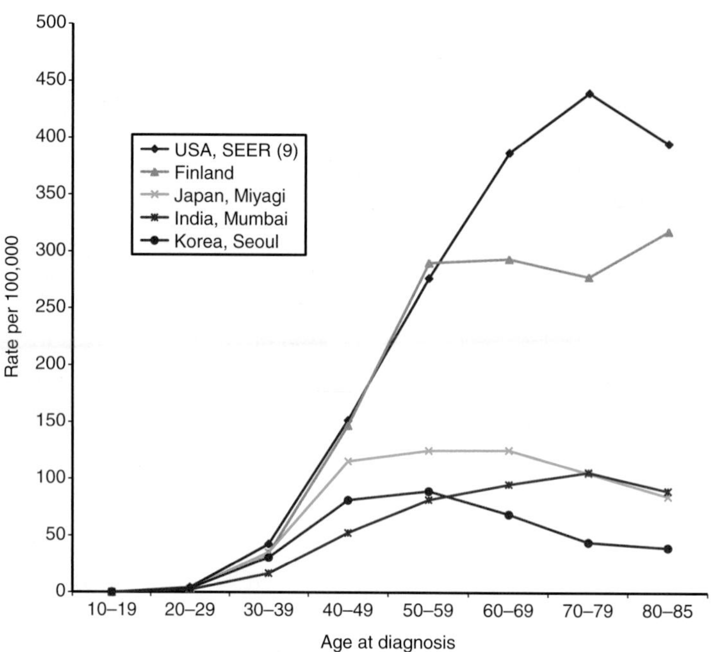

■ **FIGURE 2-4** Age-specific breast cancer incidence rates in select registries, 1998 to 2002. Rates are per 100,000 and age-standardized to the world population. *(Data from Cancer in Five Continents, Volumes IX, International Agency for Research on Cancer [IARC].)*

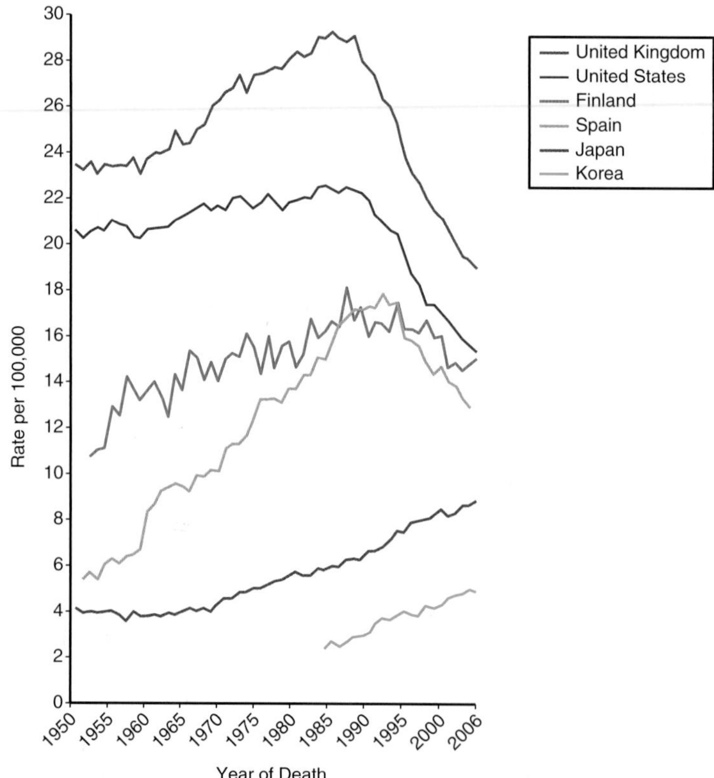

■ **FIGURE 2-5** Trends in breast cancer mortality rates in select countries, 1950 to 2006. Rates are per 100,000 and age-standardized to the world population. *(Data from WHO Mortality Database.)*

number of newly diagnosed cases has increased in these age groups, as increasingly larger numbers of women born since 1945 exceeded age 30 years. In 1970, approximately 11.6 million women were between the ages of 30 and 39 years, whereas in 1990, it is estimated that 21.1 million women were in that age group, roughly a doubling of the size of this age group over this 20-year period. Here, although age-adjusted breast cancer incidence rates for people younger than age 50 have been relatively stable, the growth in the size of the population at risk resulted in a near doubling of the annual number of cases in that age group over this period, and in successive age groups as well. As the baby boom cohort moved through into the age groups when breast cancer risk rises sharply, larger number of new cases diagnosed each year in younger women clearly made an impression in the clinical setting, despite the reassurance of epidemiologists that the United States was not experiencing an epidemic of breast cancer, at least not by classical definitions.

U.S. agencies elected to change the standard population from 1970 to 2000, to better reflect the current distribution of the U.S. population.[19] Beginning with the 1999 U.S. incidence and mortality data, incidence and mortality rates are adjusted to the 2000 U.S. population, and now more closely approximate true underlying rates. These new rates are not comparable to rates adjusted to the 1970 U.S. population, and thus comparisons between the new age-adjusted rates and rates in prior publications should be made with caution. For example, the 1998 age-adjusted incidence rate standardized to the 1970 U.S. population was 118.1 per 100,000 females,[20] whereas the 1998 incidence rate standardized to the 2000 U.S. population was 141.18 per 100,000 females,[8] a rate that more closely approximates the actual number of new cases per 100,000 females in that year. Unless otherwise specified (i.e., age-specific rates), rates for U.S. women in these discussions are expressed as the annual number of cases per 100,000 women, age-adjusted to the 2000 U.S. population, and derived from NCI's SEER*Stat database.[8,21]

INTERNATIONAL COMPARISONS

In the world, breast cancer incidence varies fivefold among nations.[1] These differences are due to variability in the population prevalence of known risk factors, but also the influence of screening programs on incidence, principally through the rate-inflating effect of advancing the time of diagnosis. In high resource countries, breast cancer is the most common malignancy diagnosed among women, and in middle and low resource countries, it typically ranks second to either cervical cancer or stomach cancer. Figure 2-1 shows 1998 to 2002 breast cancer incidence and mortality rates by country in seven global regions age-standardized to the World Standard Population, while Figure 2-2 shows a global map of the variation in 2002 age-adjusted breast cancer incidence rates in these same regions. Note that the highest incidence rates are in Western European countries and North America, whereas the lowest incidence rates included in this series are from Asia and Africa.

Breast cancer is also the leading cause of cancer mortality among women in the majority of industrialized nations.[1] Worldwide mortality rates reported in 2002 vary considerably and follow trends similar to those observed in the comparisons by incidence, although the rankings are not strictly parallel (see Fig. 2-1). For example, although white women in the United States have the second highest breast cancer incidence rates, mortality in U.S. white women ranks 15th in a comparison with mortality rates in the 33 countries shown in Figure 2-1. Because the mortality rate is a function of both the incidence rate and survival rates over time, differences in a country's comparative mortality ranking are influenced not only by the magnitude of breast cancer incidence but also by case fatality, which is influenced by patterns of detection and treatment. In addition, the comparative reliability of the medical diagnosis, reporting, and ascertainment of incident and mortality cases also influence these rates and rankings.[2] The highest breast cancer incidence rates occur in North American, Europe, Australia, New Zealand, and several Latin American countries. Incidence rates are considerably lower in Asia, Africa, and most of Central and South America.[22]

Global trends in breast cancer incidence and mortality are dynamic, principally because of changes in underlying risk factors as well as shifts in detection at more favorable stages and improvements in therapy. While industrialized nations experienced rising incidence rates in the last century, current trends show smaller increases in incidence or even a plateau or small declines in rates. Note in Figure 2-3 that age-adjusted incidence rates have declined in the United States and leveled off in the United Kingdom. In the United States, this downward trend in incidence is hypothesized to be in large part the result of a declining use of postmenopausal hormone treatment. In contrast, as low and middle resource countries have adopted modern lifestyles, here defined as postponement of childbirth, wider birth spacing, increased caloric consumption, exposures to exogenous estrogens, and declines in physical activity and increased weight gain, incidence rates have been rising. Whereas in the past, mammography screening would not have been considered in these regions because incidence and mortality rates were too low, rising incidence and mortality rates have led many countries to consider the implementation of screening programs.[23]

In all nations, the risk of breast cancer increases with age. While the pattern of rising age-specific rates in the premenopausal period is similar in most regions, age-specific postmenopausal rates are quite dissimilar (see Fig. 2-4). In Western countries age-specific incidence rates continue to rise, although at a slower rate than in the premenopausal period and with varying magnitude. In low-incidence countries, the slope of the age-specific incidence curve after menopause may be flat or even negative. This pattern in age-specific rates reflects a cohort effect—an increasing risk in successive generations of women rather than a true decline in risk with age. The younger age structure of many low-resource countries coupled with the flat age-specific incidence curve after menopause means that the average age at diagnosis is lower in low-resource countries compared with higher-resource countries, which often have older populations with a higher prevalence of breast cancer risk factors, such as early menarche and late menopause, late age at first live birth, lower parity, higher rates of postmenopausal obesity, and other risk factors associated with Western or modern lifestyles. In a comparison of trends in breast cancer incidence in Sweden and Singapore, Chia and colleagues[24] observed age-period and age-cohort effects on incidence in both populations, but the birth cohort effects were much greater among Singaporean women, which may be attributed to more rapid changes in reproduction and lifestyle patterns compared with Swedish women during the study period.

Figure 2-5 shows the trends in age-adjusted mortality rates in six countries. Breast cancer death rates have continued to decrease since 1990 in the United Kingdom, United States, and Spain largely due to early detection and improved treatment.[25-27] In contrast, death rates continue to increase in Japan because of increased incidence (decreasing age at menarche, increasing age at menopause, decreasing fertility, increasing age at first birth, and increasing height and weight).[28] An analysis of cancer mortality in 15 industrialized countries conducted in 1992 found that the breast cancer mortality rate was increasing in all regions and in most age-specific groups.[29] The average annual percent change between 1969 and 1986 ranged from 0.3% in two regions (the United States and the combined rate in New Zealand and Australia) to 1.2% in the combined average in three Eastern European countries (former German Democratic Republic, Czechoslovakia, and Hungary). More recently, for the periods 1985 to 1987 through 1995 to 1997, mortality has declined in some European countries (e.g., the United Kingdom, Wales, Sweden, Denmark, Spain), but in others, particularly Eastern Europe (Romania, Russian Federation, Estonia, etc.) mortality has been increasing. In Asia and Africa, breast cancer mortality rates also have been increasing, largely as a function of rising incidence. These trends are not uniform across all ages, since some countries have observed a decline in breast cancer mortality in women younger than age 50, but an increase in deaths in women older than age 50 (e.g., Israel, Kuwait, and Singapore).[22]

Comparisons of differences in international rates and trends over time have focused not only on known risk factors for breast cancer, but also on apparent lifestyle differences between cultures as a basis for hypothesis generation. However, what is most notable is that breast cancer incidence is increasing worldwide, with the most dramatic increases occurring in countries in which Western or modern lifestyles are becoming more prevalent. For example, while Japan still stands apart from other affluent countries in having a lower breast cancer incidence rate, the greater adoption of a Western lifestyle has resulted in a steady increase in breast cancer incidence and mortality.[30] Breast cancer incidence doubled between the 1960s and 1980s, with greater increases observed in urban versus rural areas and age-specific trends becoming more similar to North America and Europe.[31,32]

UNITED STATES TRENDS IN INCIDENCE, MORTALITY, AND SURVIVAL

In 2009, the ACS estimated that in the United States, 192,370 women would be diagnosed with invasive breast cancer, and an additional 62,280 women would be diagnosed with ductal or lobular carcinoma in situ.[9] Excluding cancers of the skin, invasive breast cancer is the most frequently diagnosed malignancy among women in the United States. In recent years, invasive and in situ breast cancer has accounted for nearly one in three newly diagnosed neoplasms in women. In the United States, breast cancer is the second leading cause of death from cancer among women, with an estimated 40,170 deaths in 2009, nearly 1 in 6 cancer deaths. Death from breast cancer is the leading cause of premature mortality from cancer among women. On average, a woman dying of breast cancer has lost nearly 19 years of life that she might have had if she had not died of this disease.[8] According to current incidence and mortality estimates, in a hypothetical cohort of women, approximately 1 in 7 will be diagnosed with invasive or in situ breast cancer in her lifetime, and 1 in 35 will die from this disease.[8] Breast cancer is far less common among men. In 2009, it was estimated that there would be 1300 newly diagnosed cases and 400 deaths among men, less than 1% of the annual incidence and mortality for both sexes.[9] Because the focus of this chapter principally is female breast cancer, numbers and rates relating to incidence and mortality are limited to women unless otherwise specified.

Trends in Incidence

The analysis of long-term trends in the incidence of breast cancer in the United States has relied on data from the few geographic areas that have supported cancer registries over a long period. Incidence data prior to 1973 are usually drawn from the Connecticut Tumor Registry or from five geographic areas (Atlanta, Connecticut, Detroit, Iowa, and Oakland, Calif).[8,33,34] Data from Connecticut (available since 1935), the five geographic regions (from 1950–1985), and data from 1973 to 1980 from SEER show a gradual annual increase over this period in the age-adjusted incidence rate of invasive breast cancer of less than 1% per year.[34] However, between 1980 and 1987, the age-adjusted incidence rate of breast cancer increased from 102.2 to 134.5 per 100,000, a relative increase in the incidence rate over the period of 27% or an average increase of approximately 4% per year (Fig. 2-6).[8] Between 1987 and 1998, incidence rates remained relatively stable, after which incidence rates have declined approximately 12% (see Fig. 2-6).

The long term trend in U.S. invasive and in situ breast cancer incidence rates shown in Figure 2-6 reveals several noteworthy historical events and periods when changes in patterns of detection or patterns of risk influenced rates. Although not shown in Figure 2-6, particularly noteworthy in the mid-1970s was the short-term increase in the incidence rate observed in 1974, believed to be primarily the result of an increase in the numbers of women who received breast examinations for screening or because of symptoms after two prominent women, former first lady Betty Ford and former second lady Happy Rockefeller, were diagnosed with breast cancer.[35] However, the 1974 to 1975 upturn in incidence rates was brief, as is clear from the subsequent decline in incidence rates after 1975 and then a return to the earlier trend. This phenomenon was a brief preview of what was to be experienced in the mid-1980s: a multi-year, significant increase in the annual breast cancer incidence rate due to advancing the time of detection with mammography, followed eventually by a decline in rates. A period of rising and declining incidence rates is consistent with a screening effect; that is, the observed

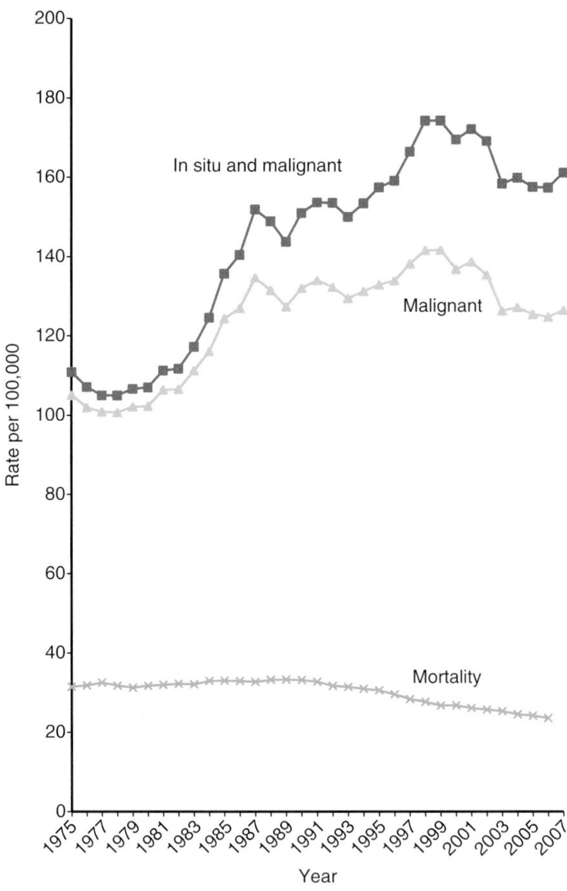

■ **FIGURE 2-6** Breast cancer incidence and mortality rates in U.S. women, 1975 to 2007. Rates are per 100,000, age-adjusted to the 2000 U.S. standard population. *(Incidence data from Surveillance, Epidemiology, and End Results [SEER] Program, 9 SEER Registries, 1973–2007, Division of Cancer Control and Population Sciences, National Cancer Institute, 2010, and have been adjusted for delayed reporting. Mortality data from National Center for Health Statistics, Centers for Disease Control and Prevention, 2009.)*

short-term increase in the incidence rate is not due to a change in the underlying epidemiology of disease but to a change in the rate of case detection. These cases having been detected prior to the time when they would have become clinically evident means a subsequent decline in the incidence rate can be anticipated.[36]

As seen in Figure 2-6, there was a dramatic increase in incidence during the period 1980 to 1987 that occurred during a period of rapid uptake of breast cancer screening with mammography.[37,38] According to Howard,[39] an evaluation of national surveys conducted between 1978 and 1983 indicated that only about 15% to 20% of American women had ever had a mammogram. In 1987, estimates from the National Health Interview Survey (NHIS) indicated that 39% of women aged 40 years and older had ever had a mammogram.[40] In 1992, according to estimates from the Mammography Attitudes and Usage Survey conducted by the Jacobs Institute of Women's Health, that number had increased to 74%.[41] During this time, a number of factors contributed to the increased use of mammography, including the growth of scientific support for the value of the procedure,[42-44] increasing acceptance by providers,[45,46] increasing acceptance by women,[41] and increasing access as measured by the growth in the number of installed dedicated mammography units.[47] Also during this period, an increasing number of women reported that they were screened on a regular basis according to recommended guidelines, or whenever their doctor recommended the test.[41] Thus, the evidence supports the interpretation that the magnitude of the increase in the incidence rates was associated with screening and represents the detection of occult cases that otherwise would have presented with symptoms in subsequent years. However, investigators also have concluded that the entirety of the recent increase in breast cancer incidence is not due solely to an increase in case detection. White and colleagues[48] concluded that an increase in screening accounts for the increase in incidence in women between the ages of 55 and 64 years but not entirely for women younger than 55 or older than 65 years. Likewise, Liff and associates[49] concluded that the increase in incidence was accounted for by both an increase in the use of mammography and a true increase in the rate of disease. As noted earlier, an average annual increase of slightly less than 1% per year has been observed with Connecticut tumor registry data long before the widespread availability and utilization of mammography. In addition, using Connecticut data, Holford and colleagues[50] showed higher age-specific incidence for successive cohorts of women born since 1970, again providing evidence that a true underlying increase in disease contributed in part to an increase in the incidence trend in the 1980s.

The fact that the age-adjusted incidence rate of in situ breast cancer (predominately ductal carcinoma in situ [DCIS]) also was increasing over this period is indicative of the influence of mammography on incidence rates, since most DCIS is detected with mammography and a diagnosis of DCIS is very uncommon before the age at which women begin mammography screening. Between 1975 and 2007, the age-adjusted incidence rate of in situ breast cancer increased from 5.8 to 34.8 per 100,000 women.[8] Age-specific incidence rates of in situ breast cancer also reveal the influence of mammography on detection. Between the ages of 35 and 39 when some women are advised to begin screening by their physician, despite the lack of endorsement from established guidelines, there is a greater difference in the rate of detection of in situ versus invasive breast cancer (10.0 vs. 58.9 per 100,000 women), whereas for women ages 55 to 59 the difference is much smaller (77.1 vs. 280.2 per 100,000 women).[8] Overall, detection of in situ breast cancer represents approximately 20% of all breast neoplasms diagnosed in the United States each year.[8]

The independent contributions of mammography and risk factors to breast cancer incidence trends also are evident in the period since the late 1990s, but in contrast to the earlier period, their influence has contributed to a decline in incidence rates.[51] In 2010, Edwards and colleagues[52] reported that the annual average percentage change in the age-adjusted incidence rate for the period 1996 to 2006 was a decrease of 2% per year. Two factors, declining use of postmenopausal hormones and declining mammography utilization, have been associated with this downturn in incidence rates. In July 2002, the National Heart, Lung, and Blood Institute announced the closing of the Trial of Estrogen Plus Progestin because of a lack of overall benefit and an observed increase in breast cancer risk.[53] According to Coombs and associates,[54] use of menopausal hormone therapy declined from 25% to 11.3% between 2000 and 2005, and incidence of breast cancer among women aged 40 to 79 years declined 8.8% over the same period, a decline that some observers have attributed almost entirely to reduced exposure to menopausal hormone therapy. However, just as breast cancer screening in asymptomatic women can result in an increase in the incidence rate due to advancing the time of diagnosis, a decline in mammography use also will result in fewer cases of breast cancer being detected in asymptomatic women. Breen and colleagues[55] analyzed data from the NHIS and reported a decline in mammography use between 2000 and 2005 (70% to 66%), findings that were corroborated by a CDC report using data from the Behavioral Risk Factor Surveillance System.[56] Jemal and colleagues[57] have suggested that the entirety of the decline in the breast cancer incidence rate is not attributable to a reduction in risk among women who stop or do not start using hormone therapy. They note that although sharp decreases in the incidence of estrogen-receptor positive tumors were observed in women aged 50 to 69 years between 2002 and 2003, age-specific rates of invasive breast cancer declined in all 5-year age groups from 45 years and older between 1999 and 2003, beginning 3 years before the announcement of the association between use of menopausal hormones and breast cancer risk. Analyses by tumor size and stage showed an average annual decrease in the incidence rate of tumors 2 cm or smaller in size of 4.1% from 2000 through 2003, while no decrease in incidence was observed for larger tumors or advanced disease over the same period. Thus, they concluded that the decline in incidence likely was due to a combination of reduced use of mammography as well as the benefit of reduced use of menopausal hormones.

Incidence and Age

The incidence of breast cancer increases with age (Fig. 2-7). The diagnosis of breast cancer is rare before age 25 years and begins to increase measurably afterwards. Between the ages of 20 and the mid-late 40s, the incidence rate of breast cancer increases rapidly, more than doubling in each successive 5-year age group. Near the age of menopause, and observable in the age-specific incidence rates after age 50, the increase in the age-specific incidence rate of breast cancer is slower compared with the pattern observed in premenopausal women. This pattern has been observed in other countries, although the increase in age-specific rates after the age of menopause is greater in Western countries than in Asian countries (see Fig. 2-4).[58]

Figure 2-7 shows average age-specific incidence rates during the periods 1975 to 1979, 1985 to 1989, and 2003 to 2007. Age specific rates during the 1975 to 1979 period are largely free of the influence of mammography screening, while age-specific rates shown for the periods 1985 to 1989 and 2003 to 2007 are influenced by the uptake of

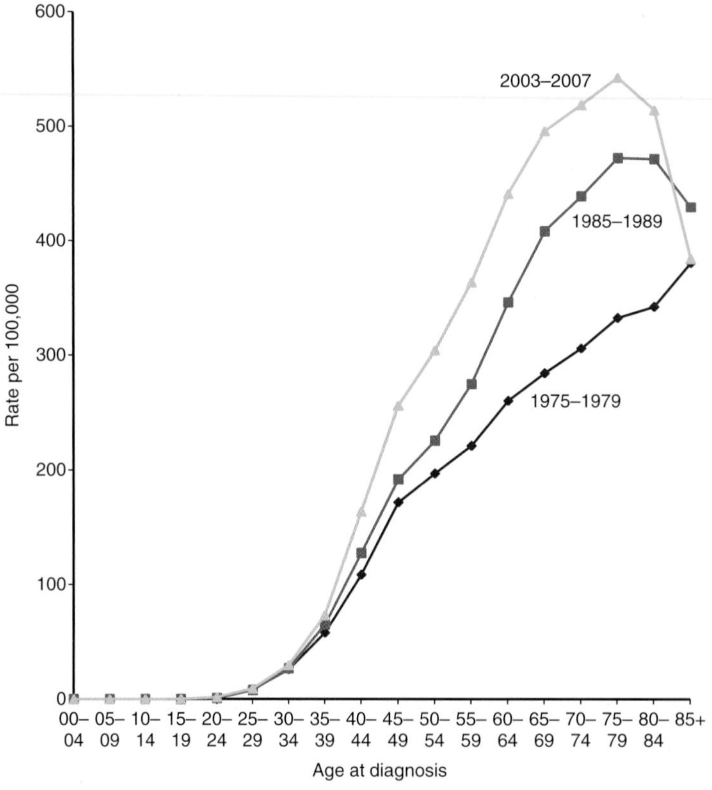

■ **FIGURE 2-7** Age-specific breast cancer incidence rates, U.S. women, 1975 to 2007. Rates are per 100,000 women within the specified age group. *(Data from Surveillance, Epidemiology, and End Results [SEER] Program, 9 SEER Registries, 1973–2007, Division of Cancer Control and Population Sciences, National Cancer Institute, 2010.)*

mammography. Before 1980, the breast cancer incidence rate was higher with each successive age group. This contrasts with data for the periods 1985 to 1989 and 2003 to 2007, which show a peak in incidence with the age group 75 to 79 years, followed by a decline in age-specific incidence. A decline in the age-specific incidence in older women was first observed in 1984 and has been evident ever since.[37]

The observed patterns of age-specific incidence over the three periods are mostly likely attributable to several underlying factors. Firstly, the shift in the age-specific pattern since the mid 1980s, specifically among older women, may be explained simply by different participation rates in screening and the interaction of age and lead time gained.[37] The introduction of screening should result in a visible increase in the incidence rate largely due to the increase in case finding in the pool of occult detectable cases. Because the average period of time that breast cancer is detectable with mammography prior to the onset of clinical symptoms—the *sojourn time*—is longer in postmenopausal women,[59,60] a more visible increase in the incidence rate should be observed in older compared with younger women due to the comparatively larger pool of detectable cases. This is evident in the age-specific trends in Figure 2-7. Furthermore, a higher rate of case findings in the initial years of a screening program also should lead to a more visible decline in the incidence rate in subsequent years. In contrast, a shorter sojourn time in younger women will contribute to a less visible increase in incidence and hence a smaller decline in the incidence rates in subsequent age cohorts following an increase in screening. Secondly, this change in the pattern of age-specific incidence rates among older women may also be influenced by the steady decline of screening rates as women get older.[61] Because age-specific incidence rates among women aged 80 years and older have not increased during the past decade at the same rate as those in women aged 60 to 79 years, the shift in the historical trend of higher incidence with higher age may be accounted for by higher rates of screening in women younger than 75. Thus, given the longer lead time in older women, a decline in age-specific incidence is consistent with a screening effect of advancing the time of detection, but the downward trend in age-specific incidence may also be influenced by declining screening rates after age 80.[62]

Although age-adjusted incidence rates have increased since the early 1970s, it is evident from the patterns visible in Figure 2-7 that change in age-specific rates has not been uniform. Among women younger than 40 years, the incidence of breast cancer has changed very little, while incidence rates among women aged 55 to 59 years have increased 54%. After age 85 years, age-specific incidence rates have fallen considerably, and for the 2003 to 2007 period they now are at the same average rate as 1975 to 1979.

INCIDENCE AND RACE OR ETHNICITY

White women have higher age-adjusted incidence rates for the 2003 to 2007 period compared with African American women (126.5 vs. 118.3 per 100,000), and these rates are higher than those for Asian and Pacific Islanders (90.0 per 100,000), American Indian/Alaskan natives (76.4 per 100,000) and Hispanics (86.0 per 100,000) albeit notable differences are evident in age-specific rates and trends over time (Fig. 2-8).[8] During the1998 to 2007 period, breast cancer incidence rates declined at an average rate of 1.6% per year among non-Hispanic white women, 1.0% per year among Hispanic women, and did not change significantly

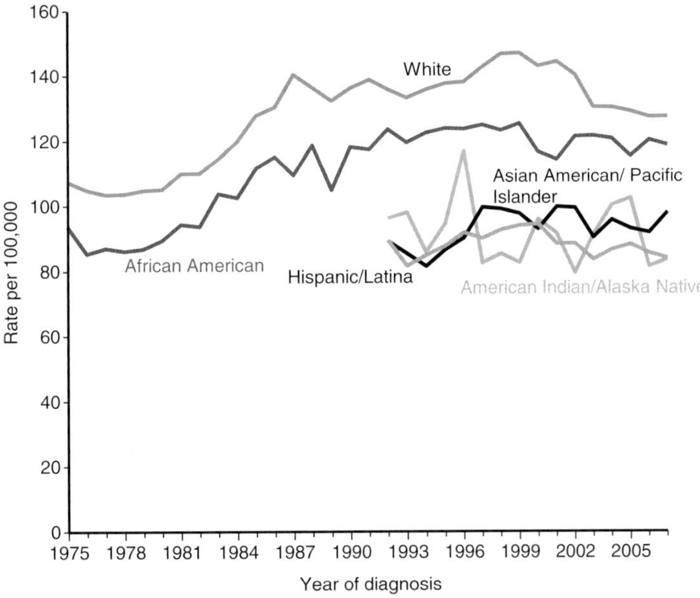

■ **FIGURE 2-8** Trends in breast cancer incidence rates by race and ethnicity, U.S. women, 1975 to 2007. Rates are per 100,000 and age-adjusted to the 2000 U.S. standard population. *(Data from Surveillance, Epidemiology, and End Results [SEER] Program, 1973–2007, Division of Cancer Control and Population Science, National Cancer Institute, 2010. Data for whites and African Americans are from the SEER 9 registries. Data for other races and ethnicities are from the 13 SEER registries.)*

among African Americans, Asians/Pacific Islanders or American Indians/Alaska natives.[8] The lack of a decline in incidence among African American women may be attributed to the lack of a significant recent decrease in mammography screening rates, as well as historically lower rates of menopausal hormone use.[55,63,64] Among women aged 35 years and younger, age-specific incidence rates are higher in African American women compared with white women, a difference that is especially evident among women aged 20 to 34 years. In comparison, among women aged 45 years and older, age-specific incidence rates are higher in white women compared with African American women.

TRENDS IN TUMOR SIZE, STAGE AT DIAGNOSIS, AND SURVIVAL

The trends in tumor size and stage at diagnosis since the early 1980s reflects growing participation rates in mammography, and likely to some degree improvements in breast imaging technology, use of problem solving imaging technology, and increased awareness of the importance of early detection resulting in women with palpable tumors reporting symptoms more promptly. Greater participation rates in mammography in the past two decades is reflected in trends in tumor size and stage at diagnosis over the same period. Figure 2-9 shows trends in the breast cancer incidence rates for the period 1988 to 2007 by tumor size for all race or ethnic groups combined, and then for white and African American women for tumors 2 cm or smaller, 2.1 to 5.0 cm, and larger than 5 cm. From 1988 to 2000, the incidence rate of smaller tumors (≤ 2.0 cm) among women of all races increased by 2.0% per year. Since 2000, the incidence rate of tumors 2.0 cm or smaller has declined by 3.3% per year. In contrast, the incidence rate of larger tumors (>5.0 cm) has increased since 1992 by 2.0% per year. The increase in prevalence of some underlying risk factors, such as postmenopausal obesity, menopausal hormone use, or both may have contributed to this pattern,[65] as well as factors that may be associated with reduced access to mammography screening. These trends also reveal that incidence rates of breast cancer by tumor size differed between white and African American women. African American women were less likely to be diagnosed with smaller tumors (≤ 2.0 cm) and more likely to be diagnosed with larger tumors (2.1 to 5.0 and >5.0 cm) than white women.

Figure 2-10 shows trends in breast cancer incidence by stage at diagnosis, expressed as extent of disease, for all race or ethnic groups and white and African American women. Among all women, localized breast cancer incidence rates increased through most of the 1980s and 1990s, but in 1999 began to decline by 2.3% per year. Incidence rates of regional-stage disease increased during the 1994 to 2001 period, after which rates declined at an average rate of 2.8% per year. Incidence rates of distant-stage disease have remained stable. African American women have higher rates of distant stage breast cancer compared with white women, and rates of distant-stage breast cancer among African American women have increased by 0.5% per year since 1975, whereas rates of distant stage breast cancer among white women have changed very little.

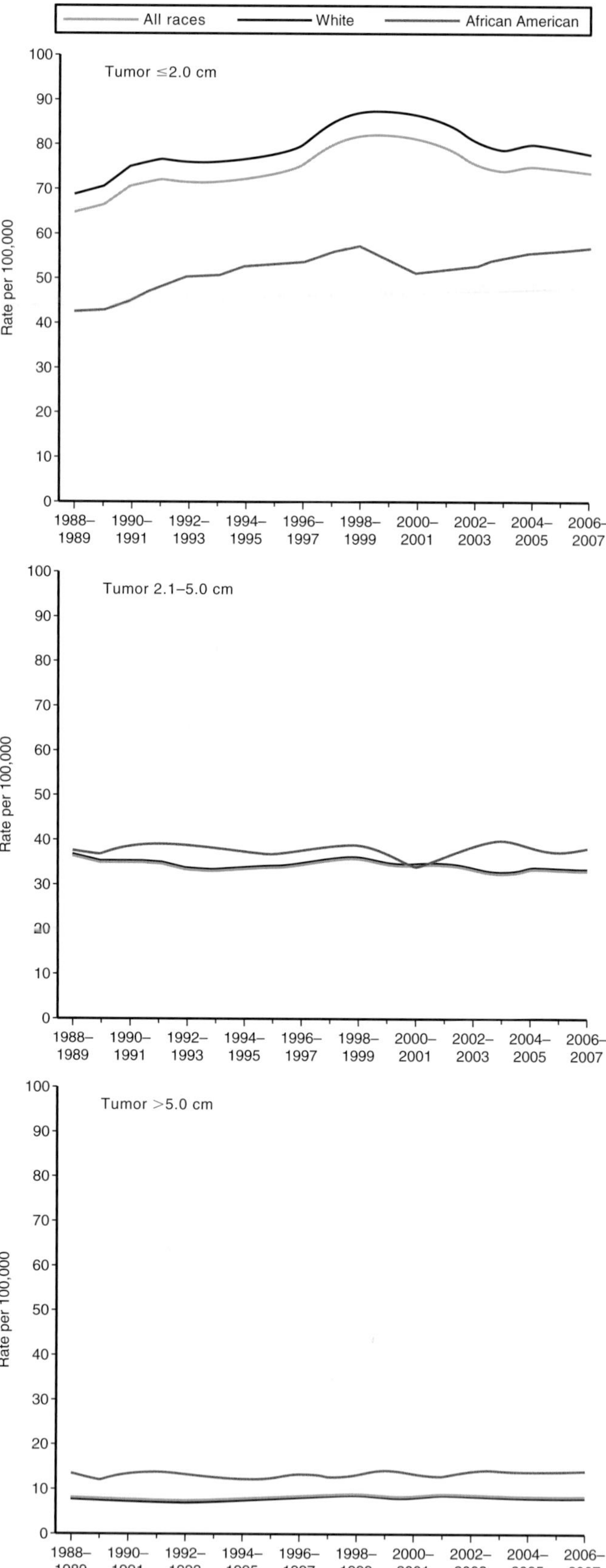

■ **FIGURE 2-9** Trends in breast cancer incidence rates by tumor size and race, U.S. women, 1988 to 1989 through 2006 to 2007. Rates are two-year moving averages and age-adjusted to the 2000 U.S. standard population. *(Data from Surveillance, Epidemiology, and End Results [SEER] Program, 9 SEER Registries, 1973–2007, Division of Cancer Control and Population Sciences, National Cancer Institute, 2010.)*

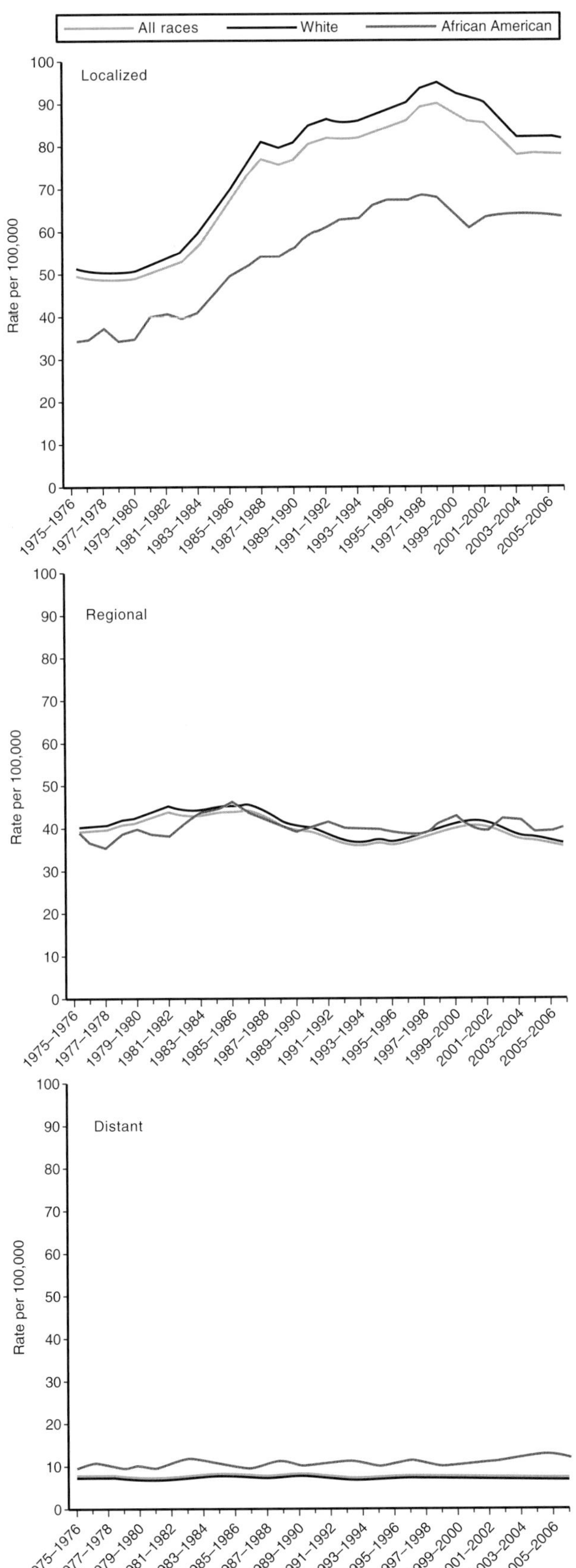

■ **FIGURE 2-10** Trends in breast cancer incidence rates by SEER historic stage and race, U.S. women, 1988 to 1989 through 2006 to 2007. Rates are two-year moving averages and age-adjusted to the 2000 U.S. standard population. *(Data from Surveillance, Epidemiology, and End Results [SEER] Program, 9 SEER Registries, 1973–2007, Division of Cancer Control and Population Sciences, National Cancer Institute, 2010.)*

The most recent national statistics show that about 60% of women diagnosed with breast cancer are diagnosed with localized disease, and approximately 33% are diagnosed with regional disease (Fig. 2-11). Only about 1 in 20 is diagnosed with distant disease. Figure 2-11 shows the proportion of all women diagnosed by stage, and the relative proportion of whites and African Americans diagnosed within each stage group. African Americans have lower rates of diagnosis of localized breast cancer compared with whites, and higher rates of regional and distant disease. Tumor size also is associated with survival, with smaller tumors having better survival compared with larger tumors. The influence of tumor size also is evident within stage groups. For example, among women diagnosed with regional disease, the 5-year relative survival is 95% for tumors 2.0 cm or smaller, 82% for tumors 2.1 to 5.0 cm, and 66% for tumors greater than 5.0 cm.[65]

The most recent 5-year period survival rate (i.e., for cases diagnosed from 1999 through 2006) for all stages of invasive disease is 89.9%.[8] When calculated by stage at detection, it is evident that survival is also much improved if breast cancer is diagnosed early. Figure 2-12 shows 5-year relative survival rates by stage at diagnosis and race for the period 1999 to 2006. For all races, the 5-year survival rate for invasive disease diagnosed at a localized stage is currently 98% for cases diagnosed in 1999 to 2006, whereas 5-year relative survival is poorer for women diagnosed with regional and distant stage disease. At each stage, survival is poorer in African American women compared with white women.[8]

The persistently worse average tumor characteristics in African American women, excess mortality compared with whites, and worsening disparity in breast cancer mortality rates is an ongoing source of concern and investigative effort to better understand differences in prognosis and outcomes in African American and white women. While there do appear to be some differences in tumor histologic features, such as a higher rate of receptor-negative tumors,[66,67] overall tumor characteristics when comparing African American and white women, these differences appear to account for a smaller fraction of the difference in outcomes compared with factors that affect access to the continuum of state-of-the-art care, specifically poverty and lack of health insurance. Lantz and colleagues[68] observed that African Americans were less likely than whites to have their breast cancer diagnosed early, and Smith-Bindman and colleagues[69] observed that African American women were more likely than white women to be diagnosed with large, advanced-stage, high-grade, and lymph node-positive tumors, a difference that was eliminated when adjusted for screening history. Gorey and associates[70] examined racial differences on breast cancer care and survival between 1975 and 2001 and observed that poorer survival and treatment increased over time, especially among younger African American women, who they observed were more likely to be uninsured, a difference among women with node positive disease that disappeared after adjustment for socioeconomic status. Investigations of disparities in breast cancer treatment using the NCI database found that African American women diagnosed with early stage tumors were 10% less likely to undergo lymph node biopsy (LNB) compared with whites[71] and were 24% less likely to undergo

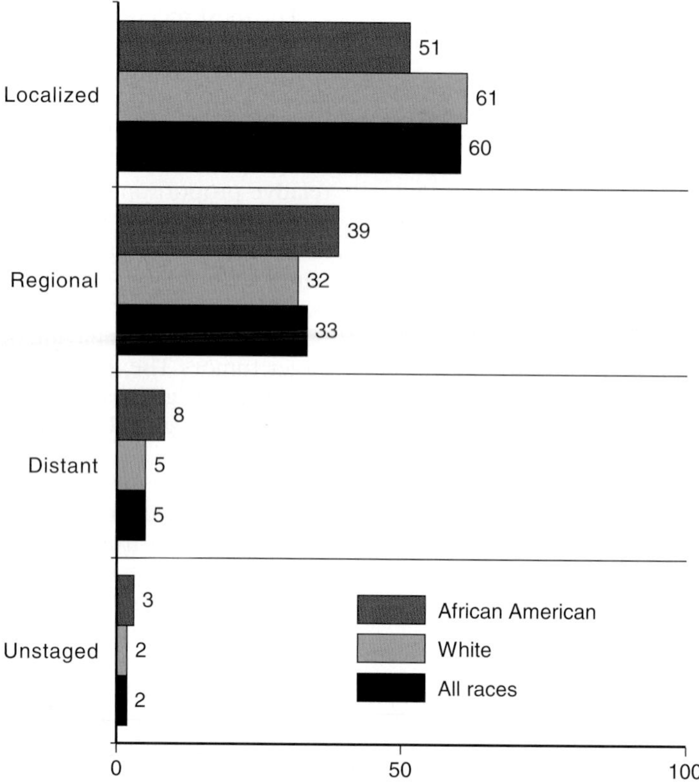

■ **FIGURE 2-11** Breast cancer stage distribution (%) by race, 1999 to 2006. *(Data from Surveillance, Epidemiology, and End Results [SEER] Program, 17 SEER Registries, 1973–2007, Division of Cancer Control and Population Sciences, National Cancer Institute, 2010.)*

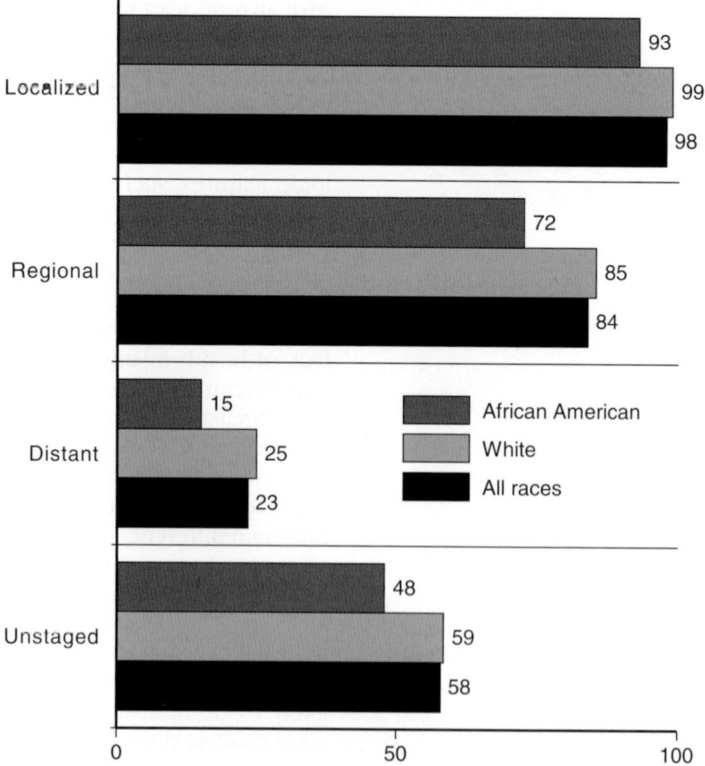

■ **FIGURE 2-12** Breast cancer five-year relative survival rates by SEER historic stage at diagnosis and race, 1999 to 2006. Survival rates are based on patients diagnosed between 1999 and 2006 and followed through 2007. *(Data from Surveillance, Epidemiology, and End Results [SEER] Program, 17 SEER Registries, 1973–2007, Division of Cancer Control and Population Sciences, National Cancer Institute, 2010.)*

sentinel lymph node biopsy compared with whites.[72] Others have observed disparities in receiving radiation therapy,[73] and tamoxifen and chemotherapy for regional disease.[74] Thus, the evidence indicates that, in addition to what appears to be some differences in worse histological tumor features in African American women, disparities that exist along the continuum of care in screening, diagnosis, and treatment account for the most of the disparities in breast cancer outcomes between African American and white women, differences that have their roots in lower socioeconomic status and access to care.

The most current survival data available for women diagnosed with breast cancer show a statistically significant improvement ($P < .05$) in 5-year survival for women with breast cancer diagnosed in the 1992 to 1999 period, compared with average survival for women diagnosed between 1975 and 1977 (89.9 % vs. 75.3%).[8] This improvement in the trend can be seen in the comparison of 5-year survival rates for women diagnosed with breast cancer in 1975 to 1979 with those diagnosed during the period 1985 to 1989, and women diagnosed in 2002, shown in Figure 2-13.

The historical trend in long-term survival should not be taken as the expected rate of survival for cases diagnosed today, and caution should be used in citing 5-, 10-, and 15-year survival data because each of those estimates is based on cases diagnosed that many years prior to the proportion surviving in 1991. Over this period, considerable improvements have been made in the overall stage at diagnosis, and treatment of breast cancer.

Mortality

Until 1987, breast cancer was the leading cause of cancer death among women, whereas it is now the second leading cause of death from cancer, following lung cancer.[9] It is the second leading cause of all premature mortality attributable to cancer, with an estimated 773,500 person-years of life lost in 2006, an average of 18.9 years per person dying of cancer.[75] The mortality rate from breast cancer was remarkably stable for several decades before 1990, ranging from 31.9 deaths per 100,000 women in 1950 to 33.3 in 1990.[75,76] Over the entire time period 1975 to 1990, the death rate for all races combined increased by 0.4% annually (see Fig. 2-6).[65] Beginning in 1990, the age-adjusted breast cancer mortality rate began to decline. Between 1990 and 1995, the mortality rate decreased annually by 1.8%, accelerating to an average annual decrease of 3.3% for the period 1995 to 1998. Between 1998 and 2006, the rate decreased by 1.9% annually.[75] Age-specific differences have been observed in declining breast cancer mortality rates (Fig. 2-14). From 1990 to 2006, death rates decreased by 3.2% per year among women younger than age 50 and by 2.0% per year among women ages 50 years and older. The decline in breast cancer mortality has been attributed to both improvements in early detection and therapy,[25]

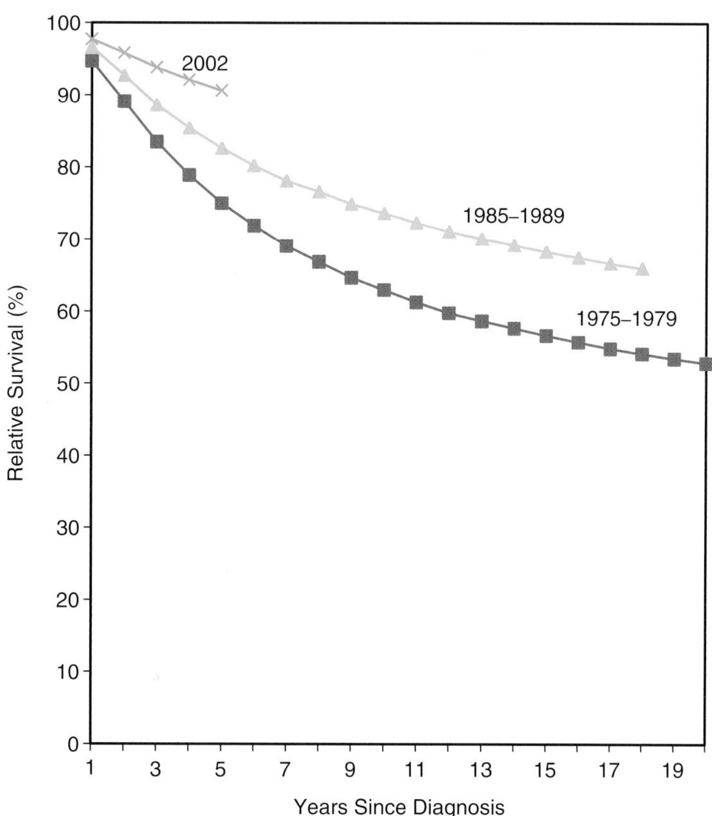

■ **FIGURE 2-13** Breast cancer relative survival rates (%) by years since diagnosis for U.S. women diagnosed during three time periods. *(Data from Surveillance, Epidemiology, and End Results [SEER] Program, 9 SEER Registries, 1973–2007, Division of Cancer Control and Population Sciences, National Cancer Institute, 2010.)*

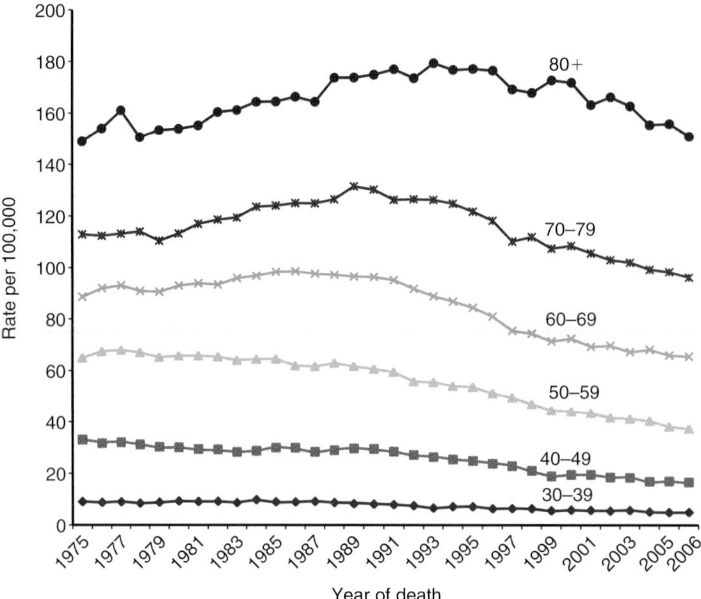

■ **FIGURE 2-14** Age-specific breast cancer mortality rates, U.S. white women, 1975 to 2006. Rates are per 100,000 women and age-adjusted to the 2000 U.S. standard population. *(Data from National Center for Health Statistics, Centers for Disease Control and Prevention, 2009.)*

although the relative contribution of each is a source of ongoing debate. In a report on the outcome of seven statistical models used to estimate the relative contributions of screening and therapy to declining breast cancer mortality, the estimated proportion of the total reduction in the rate of death from breast cancer attributable to screening ranged from 28% to 65% (median, 46%). The assumption would be that adjuvant treatment accounted for the remaining, and larger fraction, although it also is likely that in addition to benefits of adjuvant therapy, increased awareness resulting in faster response to breast cancer symptoms is also playing a role in detection of smaller tumors. In all likelihood, earlier detection through mammography screening and increased awareness has played a much greater role than adjuvant therapy in declining mortality because long-term survival has not dramatically improved within stage groups.[77] Moreover, Elkin and colleagues[78] demonstrated that a significant fraction of the improvement in survival within stage groups was attributable to the migration of tumor size between 1975 and 1990 to smaller tumors, which can be attributed to the use of mammography and improved awareness of the importance of reporting breast cancer symptoms immediately. Finally, in an evaluation of breast cancer mortality in Sweden in exposed and unexposed women during a prescreening and post screening epoch, Tabar and colleagues[79] estimated that screening accounted for more than two thirds of the observed difference in the death rate between women exposed and not exposed to mammography screening, with improvements in therapy and awareness accounting for the rest.

Racial or ethnic differences in mortality, and trends in mortality between 1975 and 2006 are noteworthy (Fig. 2-15). Overall, age-adjusted mortality rates for 2006 are higher in African American women (31.6 per 100,000) compared with white women (22.9 per 100,000). Age-specific rates increase steadily with age for both African American and white women, and unlike age-specific incidence rates, there is no peak in rates after which mortality rates decline. Age-specific mortality rates are considerably higher among women aged 80 to 84 years and 85 years and older, compared with women aged 70 to 79 years.[75] In every age category, African American females have higher age-specific breast cancer mortality compared with white women.

Prior to 1981, age-adjusted breast cancer mortality rates in African American women were similar to rates in white women. Between 1981 and 1990, rates were relatively stable in white women, but climbed steadily in African American women, peaking in 1998, and declining 8 years after breast cancer mortality began to decline in white women (see Fig. 2-15). In 2006, age-adjusted breast cancer mortality rates were 38% higher in African American women compared with white women.[75]

In general, trends in breast cancer mortality show that African American women and women of other racial or ethnic groups have not benefited to the same extent as white women from advances in early detection and therapy. From 1997 to 2006, female breast cancer death rates declined by 1.9% per year in non-Hispanic whites and Hispanics/Latinas, 1.6% in African Americans, 0.6% per year in Asian Americans/Pacific Islanders, and remained unchanged among African American women and Alaska natives.[75]

POPULATION TRENDS AND DISEASE CONTROL PROGRAMS

The introduction of early detection programs, new therapies, or changes in risk factors naturally leads observers to examine population trends in incidence, mortality, stage at diagnosis, and survival, and draw conclusions about the impact, or lack of impact of various factors on favorable,

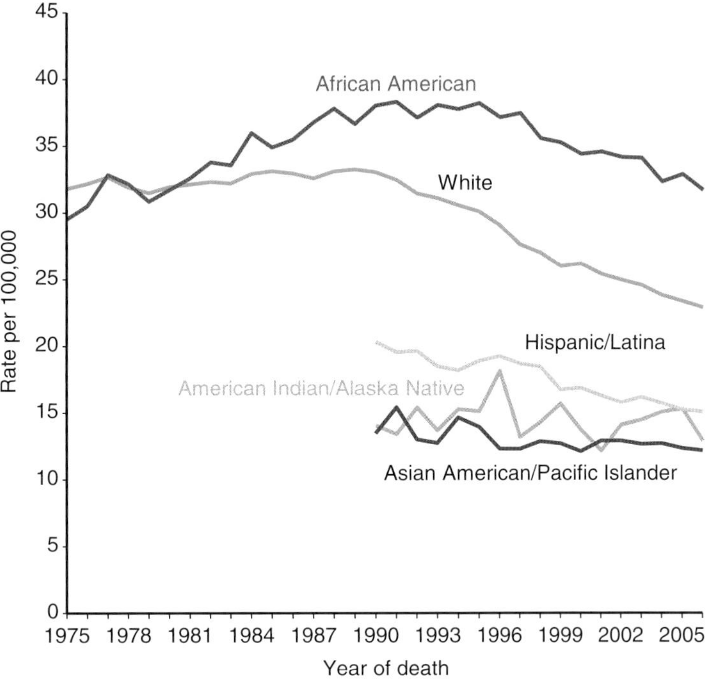

■ **FIGURE 2-15** Trends in breast cancer mortality rates by race and ethnicity, U.S. women, 1975 to 2006. Rates are per 100,000 and age-adjusted to the 2000 U.S. standard population. *(Data from National Center for Health Statistics, Centers for Disease Control and Prevention, 2009.)*

or unfavorable, end results. For example, some have questioned the value of breast cancer screening because trends in incidence and mortality weren't more favorable in the presence of significant rates of screening.[80] As the argument is commonly advanced, optimal screening should have produced a rise in incidence rates, followed by a fall in rates, and then a return to prescreening rates which now should have a more favorable distribution of tumor stages. This pattern would be due to the rise in incidence during the introduction of screening due to lead time, followed by the decline in incidence due to cancers that would have been detected in subsequent years if screening had not been introduced, and then a return to pre-screening incidence rates as early detection versus detection with symptoms becomes the common pathway to disease detection. Since breast cancer screening in the United States has not shown this pattern, but rather has been associated with an increase in localized disease without a commensurate decline in advanced disease, the conclusion is that modern screening is not very effective at altering the natural history of aggressive disease, and mostly detects less aggressive and indolent (i.e., overdiagnosed) cases.

It is unrealistic to observe this theoretical scenario of rising and falling incidence rates, with and rates then returning to equilibrium, for the simple reason that these commentators confuse the entire population with the potentially screened population, the *actually* screened population, and finally the *occasionally versus regularly* screened population. Thus, incidence rates include cancers detected in adults not eligible for screening, adults who have no access to screening, adults who are eligible, but refuse screening, adults who are irregularly screened, adults for whom screening has failed to detect early stage disease, and adults entering the screening cohort for the first time. Subsequent mortality rates also are affected by the detection rate in these different subgroups of the population, and the different opportunity structure for early detection.

Another common misinterpretation of trends in incidence data is to conclude that higher rates of breast cancer incidence following the introduction of screening are accompanied by a significant fraction of *overdiagnosis,* or the detection of a malignant breast cancer that would never have surfaced in the patient's lifetime in the absence of screening. The conclusion that much of the alleged excess of disease after the introduction of screening represents a significant level of overdiagnosis is readily discounted by the fact that the period of observation generally is too short. While overdiagnosis is likely to be a significant problem in prostate cancer screening,[81] it is most likely a small problem in breast cancer screening, and mostly limited to DCIS.[82,83] Short-term evaluation of population surveillance data is not a sound basis for judging the effectiveness of screening.[84]

CUMULATIVE AND RELATIVE RISK

Cumulative risk and relative risk (RR) are two fundamentally different measurements of the probability that a woman will be diagnosed with breast cancer. According to current estimates, approximately one in eight women, or 12.1% of a hypothetical cohort alive today, will be diagnosed with invasive breast cancer in her lifetime, and one in seven, or 14.5%, will be diagnosed with in situ or invasive breast cancer.[85] The reference to estimate has become customary as a symbolic expression of the magnitude of the risk women face. Lifetime risk is a measure of absolute risk, or cumulative risk, over a period defined as a lifetime for a population based on current estimates of incidence. RR is another measure of risk and is based on the occurrence of disease among women with a particular characteristic, that is, risk factor, compared with those without the characteristic. Measures of RR may also be adjusted for other known risk factors to eliminate the known or possible effects of confounding variables. The magnitude of the ratio is the RR, and it is expressed as a comparative likelihood of developing the disease or in terms of the protective effect associated with the risk factor. However, apart from the specific comparison, the measure and its magnitude have no inherent probabilistic meaning.

Each measurement, that is, cumulative risk and RR, has the potential to be misunderstood in the context of individual behaviors and individual risk. For example, the estimate of lifetime risk is an estimate of the proportion of a cohort that will have been diagnosed with breast cancer by a certain age. The proportion consists of women at less than a one in eight lifetime risk, as well as those with higher lifetime risk than one in eight. Further, the one in eight lifetime risk is cumulative, and because the incidence of breast cancer is lower when women are younger, the majority of the cumulative risk is delayed until later years of life. Thus, absolute risk over intervals of 10 and 20 years is considerably less, especially prior to the age of 65. With respect to RRs, risk approximations are done on the basis of RRs identified in the epidemiological literature. However, the use of RR as a basis of estimating individual risk can be misleading for the simple reason that it is a comparative measure, that is, it is a measure of risk for individuals with a known risk factor compared with the risk in individuals without the risk factor. Furthermore, the RR does not directly approximate the underlying probability of a diagnosis of breast cancer. Although relative odds may be greater by a factor of two or three times for a woman with a particular risk factor, the more important estimate is her absolute risk during particular time intervals, for example, within 1 year, during one or more decades, or during a lifetime. A rather large RR for breast cancer at an age when the absolute risk is very low will result in very few excess new cases, whereas a more modest RR applied to women at an age when the absolute risk is high will result in a significant number of excess cases. For example, Gail and Benichou[86,87] estimated the RR of breast cancer for a 40-year-old nulliparous woman whose mother developed breast cancer and who had no other risk factors to be 2.76 compared with women without that risk profile. Her absolute risk of developing breast cancer between age 40 and 70 years was estimated to be 11.6%. Over that 30-year period, the risk of developing breast cancer as estimated in the lifetime risk calculations (which are based on a hypothetical cohort of women representing all risk profiles) was 7.47%.[88] Although these two estimates are not directly comparable because they derive from different populations, they are useful to illustrate that RR estimates alone may inflate the perception of risk for women with a certain risk profile. On the other hand, risk between ages of 40 and 70 years for a woman with a family history of breast cancer in two first-degree relatives can be estimated to be 21% and will be higher if either or both had their disease diagnosed before menopause. In this instance, the use of this kind of counseling may serve to heighten both the woman's and her provider's attention to the importance of a program of routine screening at regular intervals.

Because women are concerned about breast cancer and their individual risk, it is important that clinicians and others understand these measurements and are equipped to appropriately counsel women.[89] It has been argued that this is especially true because risk perception typically is inaccurate, with few women correctly estimating risk, and most women either underestimating or overestimating risk.[90] Further, women with high perceived susceptibility to breast cancer not only significantly overestimate their risk of disease, but experience elevated distress and anxiety.[91] Conversely, women who underestimate risk may be less likely to understand the need for regular mammography.

Concerns about anxiety over breast cancer risk and the anxiety that occurs when mammography results are positive are well placed; the large majority of women will not develop breast cancer in their lifetime, and mammography offers proven benefits to women who attend regular screening. However, it is important to be realistic and not expect that risk perception and fear of breast cancer should correspond to actual risk or that the meaning women place on their risk should be proportional to their actual risk. The fact that women are more concerned about breast cancer than heart disease has more to do with the meaning they attach to each disease than perceptions of actuarial likelihood.

Lifetime Risk

In 1940, risk to age 85 years was 1 in 20, or 5%. By 1989, risk to age 85 years was estimated to be one in nine, or 11.1%.[92] Today risk to age 85 is estimated to be 12.1%.[85] The lifetime risk of breast cancer has changed during the last five decades, largely due to the long-term trend of increasing breast cancer incidence, parallel trends in increasing longevity, and the near-term influence of lead time on elevating age-specific rates. Life expectancy for cohorts of women born between 1900 and 1902 was 51 years, compared with 74 years for those born between 1959 and 1961.[93] Likewise, during this period, the age-specific incidence rate has increased in all age groups but most notably among women aged 40 years and older. The combination of increasing incidence and increasing longevity has meant a steadily increasing lifetime, or absolute, risk of developing breast cancer. Lifetime risk is a cumulative probability, and it is the function of two factors that vary at different ages, that is, the underlying incidence rate of disease and the rate of survival or withdrawal from the interval due to death from other causes.[88,92] Risk of being diagnosed with breast cancer can be estimated for an interval from birth (or any age) to some end point, such as one or more decades, or some age arbitrarily defined as a lifetime (i.e., 90 years) or for the combined lifetimes of the entire cohort. Lifetime risk represents the accumulated risk over successive intervals, each with a higher probability of a diagnosis of breast cancer than the previous interval, consistent with trends in age-specific rates. As noted previously, this observation highlights the problem of internalizing the lifetime risk as near-term risk.

TABLE 2-1. Probability of Developing Breast Cancer within the Next 10 Years by Age

If current age is ...	The probability of developing breast cancer in the next 10 years is:	Or 1 in:
20	0.06%	1760
30	0.44%	229
40	1.44%	69
50	2.39%	42
60	3.40%	29
70	3.73%	27
Lifetime risk	12.08%	8

Age-specific probabilities of developing invasive female breast cancer among those free of cancer at beginning of age interval. Based on cases diagnosed from 2004 to 2006. Percentages and "1 in" numbers may not be numerically equivalent due to rounding. Data from Surveillance, Epidemiology, and End Results (SEER) Program, 9 SEER Registries, 1973-2007, Division of Cancer Control and Population Sciences, National Cancer Institute, 2010. Probability derived using National Cancer Institute's DevCan Software, Version 6.4.0.

For example, as seen in Table 2-1 the average risk for a woman aged 30 years for the 10-year interval between age 30 and 40 years is estimated to be 0.44%, or 1 in 229, compared with a lifetime risk from 0 to "eventually" of 12.1%, or 1 in 8. However, between the ages of 60 and 70 years, a 60-year-old woman's risk is estimated to be 3.4%, or 1 in 29. It is important to appreciate that life-time risk is cumulative, i.e. the sum of successive age-specific probabilities as women increase in age. Thus, the cumulative probability to age 50 of being diagnosed with in situ or invasive breast cancer is 2.3% or 1 in 43. Risk to age 65 is 1 in 14, only half of the life time risk of being diagnosed with an in situ or invasive breast cancer. For women who are concerned about breast cancer risk, these estimates may provide a measure of reassurance that average risk over periods of 10 and 20 years is considerably less than the frequently expressed 1 in 8 (0 to age 85 years) estimates.

Risk Factors for Breast Cancer

Breast cancer has been the focus of wide-ranging epidemiological investigations, and yet it has been estimated that the established risk factors explain only slightly more than half of its occurrence.[94,95] The model by Bruzzi and colleagues[94] which incorporates the accepted risk factors of advancing age, family history of breast cancer in a first degree relative, early age at menarche, late age at menopause, nulliparity and late age at first full-term birth, and history of prior breast biopsies, does not account for some more recently recognized risk factors. These include fairly consistent increases in risk linked with lack of breastfeeding, obesity (for postmenopausal-onset disease only), and physical inactivity. Although dietary factors have received extensive attention (particularly dietary fat), few components have been definitely linked to breast cancer risk. The one exception is alcoholic beverage consumption, which has been consistently linked with elevations in risk. Exogenous hormones have also been intensively studied, with recent results indicating increases in risk with certain patterns of usage of both oral contraceptives and menopausal hormones, and beneficial effects of exposure to selective estrogen receptor modulators. Prediction models are currently being developed to incorporate additional risk factors and it is anticipated that these will allow a fuller understanding of the occurrence of breast cancer on a population basis.

Although we know a great deal about breast cancer risk factors, their interrelationships, and their interactions with host characteristics, risk prediction models perform poorly at the individual level and have questionable value for decision making, with the exception of identifying women at significant inherited risk. Unlike the population attributable fraction of lung cancer risk factors (i.e., smoking), the attributable fraction of individual breast cancer risk factors is low, population exposures are high, and many of the well-established breast cancer risk factors are not practically modifiable.[96] A further complication in understanding the occurrence of breast cancer relates to our limited understanding of biologic processes that leads to breast cancer. Although the important role of estrogens in the etiology of breast cancer has been recognized for some time,[97] it is clear that other biologic processes must also be taken into account. Increasing attention is being focused on other hormones, including androgens and progestogens, as well as a variety of proteins, such as insulin-like growth factors.[97-99] Additionally, it is increasingly being recognized that breast cancer is a heterogeneous disease, for which there may be subsets with distinct etiologies. Recent attention has attempted to assess etiologic variation by a variety of tumor markers, most notably by hormone receptor status.[100] New technologies, including tissue microarray,[101,102] may be particularly useful for expanding our knowledge of the etiology of this complex disease.

Most of the identified risk factors for breast cancer are associated with relatively low magnitudes of RR (Table 2-2). While many of the identified risk factors for breast cancer are not readily amenable to change, such as the age at menarche and menopause, height, or realistic (age at first live birth, parity, and birth spacing), it is nonetheless encouraging that some of the more recently identified risk factors are ones that are modifiable and offer clear opportunities for adoptive behaviors that are associated with lower breast cancer risk. Given this, it appears worthwhile to review some of the results relating to these factors.

Breastfeeding

The relationship of breastfeeding to breast cancer risk has long been debated, with it initially being assumed that any associations would merely reflect effects of other reproductive variables. However, of a large collaborative project involving data from 47 epidemiologic studies[103] showed that in addition to a 7% reduction in risk associated with each birth, a 4.3% reduction in risk was associated with every 12 months of breastfeeding. It was further estimated that the cumulative incidence of breast cancer in developed countries could be reduced by more than half, from 6.3 to 2.7 per 100 women by age 70, if women had the average number of births and lifetime duration of breastfeeding that occurs in many developing countries. While the estimated risk reduction is modest, more immediate

TABLE 2-2. Selected Risk Factors for Breast Cancer Incidence

Factors Influencing Risk	Approximate Relative Risks
Older ages (65-69 versus 30-34 yr)	17
Residency in North America or Europe versus Asia	4-5
Residency in urban areas	1.5
Higher education status or family income	1.5
Mother or sister with breast cancer	2-3
Nulliparity or late ages at first birth (≥30 yr versus <20 yr)	2-3
Absence of breastfeeding for long durations	1.5
Early ages at menarche (<12 yr versus ≥15 yr)	1.5
Late ages at menopause (≥55 yr versus natural menopause at <45 yr or removal of ovaries at a comparable age)	2
Biopsy-confirmed proliferative disease	2-4
Mammographically dense breasts	2-4
Obesity (postmenopausal only) (≥200 lbs versus <125 lbs)	2
Tallness (≥68 inches versus <62 inches)	1.5-2
Radiation to chest in moderate to high doses	2-4
History of breast cancer in one breast	2-4
History of primary cancer in endometrium, ovary	1.4-2

and certain advantages of breastfeeding accrue to the newborn infant, which may serve as the primary incentive to breastfeed. The American Academy of Pediatrics strong endorses breastfeeding during the first 6 to 12 months of life.[104]

Body Size

The relationship of body size to breast cancer risk has been extensively investigated, with differing associations having been observed for premenopausal and postmenopausal disease. For postmenopausal-onset disease, both weight and body mass index (BMI; defined as weight in kilograms divided by the square of height in meters) have been fairly consistently related to increases in risk. In a large case-control study, subjects in the upper quartile of BMI were at a 40% higher risk than those in the lower quartile.[105] This relationship is believed to be due to the ability of adipose tissue to convert precursor substrates to estrogens. Although particular attention has focused on obesity during adolescence, weight gain at older ages has more consistently been shown to be associated with breast cancer risk,[106] an encouraging finding from the perspective of prevention.

In contrast to relationships with postmenopausal breast cancer, body mass appears to be inversely related to premenopausal disease, with thin women being at highest risk.[107] In one meta-analysis, a BMI difference of 8 (i.e., the difference between a thin person and someone morbidly obese) resulted in a RR of 0.70 (95% confidence interval [CI], 0.5 to 0.9).[108] Although initially thought to be due to difficulties in detecting breast lesions in young, heavy women, this does not appear entirely to explain the relationship. Irregular anovulation, and consequently less exposure to endogenous hormones, has been proposed as an additional mechanism underlying the inverse association of body size to premenopausal breast cancer risk, although there remains a lack of full understanding of the increased breast cancer risk in overweight premenopausal women.

Among postmenopausal women, body fat distribution also appears to influence risk.[109,110] In a number of studies, women whose fat was distributed abdominally (i.e., around their waists) were at higher risk than those with peripheral fat distribution (including fat accumulation on the hips). This effect appeared to be independent of total body size. In the few studies in which body fat distribution has been examined for premenopausal women, inconsistent relationships have been observed

Physical Activity

There has been much enthusiasm regarding a potential beneficial effect of physical activity on breast cancer risk, especially given its modifiable nature. The relationship appears to be biologically plausible,[111] given that physical activity has been associated with changes in endogenous hormones, menstrual patterns, body fat distribution patterns, and other biologic repercussions that could benefit breast cancer risk (e.g., change in immunologic parameters).[112] The strongest support for physical activity as a potential preventive mechanism derives from a study of early-onset breast cancers, in which reductions in risk associated with regular physical activity were found to be independent of body size.[113] Although studies have produced conflicting results,[114-120] more recently the evidence for a protective effect of physical activity on risk of postmenopausal breast cancer is regarded as convincing, although the mechanisms are not clearly understood.[121] The need for more precision in the approach to measuring the influence of physical activity and associated and affected biomarkers has been stressed, including obtainment of objective measures of physical activity, collection of information on timing and intensity of activity levels, and consideration of all sources of activity (including physical activity resulting from household chores), and the influence on BMI, estrogens, androgens, sex hormone binding globulin, leptin, adiponectin, markers of insulin resistance, tumor necrosis factor-alpha, interleukin-6, and C-reactive protein.[121]

Alcohol Consumption

Although the relationship of breast cancer risk to most dietary factors remains unresolved, fairly consistent data have emerged regarding a potential adverse effect of consumption of alcoholic beverages. Longnecker,[122] in a meta-analysis of 38 case-control and cohort studies, showed a progressive increase in the risk of breast cancer with amount of alcohol consumed, with those consuming three or more drinks per day being at a 40% higher risk than non-drinkers. Typically a drink is equivalent to 10 grams of alcohol, which is found in the equivalent of a 12 oz.

can of beer, a 3 to 4 oz. glass of wine, or 1.0 oz. of spirits. Results were consistent across case-control and cohort studies. Adjustment for known breast cancer risk factors and dietary variables had little impact on observed relationships, and it appears it is consistent across different alcoholic beverages.[123] Lew and coworkers[124] examined the association between alcohol and breast cancer tumor characteristics in the National Institutes of Health (NIH)-AARP Diet and Health Study. Consistent with previous studies, alcohol was significantly positively associated with breast cancer risk, and specifically hormone receptor-positive tumors.

An important unanswered question is whether a reduction in alcohol consumption patterns can have a beneficial impact on breast cancer risk. One report showed that women who drank only early in life (prior to age 30) experienced a risk similar to those who continued to drink.[125] However, in another study, recent adult drinking appeared to be more important than drinking patterns earlier in life,[126] and Berstad and associates[127] also have observed increased breast cancer risk associated with recent alcohol consumption (≤ 5 years prior to diagnosis) in younger women, with average daily intake of 2 or more drinks per day being associated with an 82% excess risk compared with never drinkers. This would be consistent with the finding that alcohol is most strongly related to late stage tumors,[128] implying that it acts at a late stage in breast carcinogenesis.

Both intervention and cross sectional studies have shown alterations in endogenous estrogens associated with alcohol consumption,[129,130] providing a possible biologic explanation for the association of alcohol to breast cancer risk. There is also support for several other possible biologic mechanisms, including alcohol-induced changes in folate levels, increased cell permeability, and direct effects of contaminants such as nitrosamines in the alcoholic beverages. Further research is needed to clarify biologic mechanisms underlying the association of alcohol intake and breast cancer risk, particularly as related to periods and levels of consumption and types of alcoholic beverages. For example, although there has been little evidence of differential risk by type of alcoholic beverage, a recent study suggested that recent consumption of alcohol (≥ seven servings per week) versus lifetime consumption was associated with increased breast density.[131]

Despite enthusiasm for the possibility that cessation of alcohol consumption may be a means of reducing breast cancer risk, it appears that it would have only a minimal impact on overall disease burden. Because of the modest association between alcohol and breast cancer and the generally moderate level of alcohol intake among U.S. women, the proportion of breast cancer incidence attributable to alcohol intake appears relatively small, being only 2.1% in one analysis.[132]

Exogenous Hormone Use

Given the recognition of the importance of ovarian hormones in the etiology of breast cancer, much attention has focused on the relationship to risk of exogenous hormones, including oral contraceptives and menopausal hormones.

Oral Contraceptives

Oral contraceptives have been extensively studied in relation to breast cancer risk, with varying conclusions. Although the majority of studies have not confirmed an overall excess risk associated with oral contraceptive usage, a number of studies (including several meta-analyses) have suggested an increased risk associated with long-term usage for early onset cancers, usually defined as those occurring prior to age 45.[133-136] In the largest analysis, which involved pooling of data from 54 studies on 53,297 women with breast cancer and 100,239 without breast cancer, current and recent users were at increased risk (RR, 1.24; 95% CI, 1.15 to 1.33), with no evidence of an effect with duration of use.[137] The increased risk associated with recent use subsided within 10 years of cessation of oral contraceptive use. These findings suggest that the increased risk of breast cancer observed among young, long-term users may have been due primarily to recent usage, raising the possibility that oral contraceptives might act as late stage promoters. In contrast to the association between postmenopausal hormones and risk of lobular breast cancer, no association has been observed between ever use of oral contraceptives in young women and breast tumor histological subtypes.[138]

Given that an influence of oral contraceptives on the breast has been hypothesized to be greatest before the cellular differentiation that occurs with a first pregnancy, a number of investigations have evaluated effects of use of oral contraceptives prior to a first pregnancy. In the pooled analysis,[137] a significant trend of increasing risk with first use before age 20 years was observed. Among women diagnosed at ages 30 to 34 years, the RR associated with recent oral contraceptive use was 1.54 if use began before age 20 years and 1.13 if use began at older ages. However, in several studies not included in the meta-analysis, no such increase in risk was observed.[136,139]

Studies also have attempted to determine whether the effects of oral contraceptives are influenced by the presence of other breast cancer risk factors. Of particular interest has been whether effects are different in subjects with a family history of breast cancer. However, neither this factor, nor various other factors (including weight and alcohol use), appear to modify relationships with oral contraceptives. Several studies that have suggested that oral contraceptives may increase the risk of breast cancer more in subjects who are either *BRCA1* or *BRCA2* carriers require further confirmation with larger numbers.[140,141]

There has also been interest in whether specific formulations of oral contraceptives have unique influences on breast cancer risk. No consistent relationships have been seen with either dose of the progestin or estrogen considered, although methodologically it has been difficult to define this information and to consider it in a systematic fashion. Only limited data on the newer formulations of pills is available.[137] Also of interest is whether injectable progestogen contraceptives are associated with alterations in breast cancer risk. In a recent study in South Africa, no association was found with this exposure, in either older or younger women.[142]

Menopausal Hormones

The relationship of menopausal hormones to breast cancer risk was assessed in a re-analysis of data from 51 epidemiological studies, encompassing 52,705 women with breast cancer and 108,411 controls from 21 countries.[143] This showed a 2.3% (95% CI, 1.1% to 3.6%) increase in the RR of breast cancer for each year of hormone replacement therapy (HRT) use. This corresponded to a RR of 1.35 for users of 5 or more years and to a cumulative excess for women who began use of hormones at age 50 of approximately 2 cases per 1000 women for 5 years users, 6 cases per 1000 for 10 years users, and 12 cases per 1000 women for 15 year users. This increase was comparable with the effect on breast cancer risk of later menopause. The increased risk, however, was restricted to recent users, with no material excess observed 5 or more years after discontinuation.

Although it is accepted that recent long-term estrogen use is associated with some elevation in breast cancer risk, it was less resolved whether the addition of progestins to estrogens affects risk. Although this regimen had become increasingly common given the recognized advantages of progestins in terms of a reduction in endometrial cancer risk,[144] there was evidence that added progestins may adversely affect breast cancer risk. Notably, in vitro studies had shown that breast mitotic activity is higher during the luteal phase of the menstrual cycle, when progesterone levels are at their highest. A number of studies had provided support for the notion of a more deleterious effect of combined therapy. These included results from two large cohort studies, the Nurses Healthy Study[145] and the follow-up study of participants in the Breast Cancer Detection Demonstration Project (BCDDP).[146] Both studies showed a RR of 1.4 for combined therapy, as compared, respectively in the two studies, with RRs of 1.3 and 1.2 for estrogens alone. In the BCDDP study, the increased risk was limited to users within the prior 4 years and was largely confined to thin women, with the latter relationship possibly reflecting that heavier women may be less affected due to their higher levels of endogenous hormones. A potentially adverse effect for combined therapy had also been noted in two case-control studies, in Sweden[147] and Los Angeles County.[148] The Los Angeles study found a RR of 1.24 (95% CI, 1.1 to 1.4) for each 5 years of use of combined therapy, as compared with a RR of 1.06 (95% CI, 0.9 to 1.2) for each 5 years of estrogen use. The Swedish study also supported a notion of a duration effect, with the risk rising to 2.4 for users of 10 or more years.

In 1992, the NIH launched the Women's Health Initiative (WHI), which was the largest coordinated study of women's health ever undertaken. The objectives of the clinical trials were to evaluate the benefit and risk of HRT, dietary modification, and supplementation with calcium plus vitamin D on the overall health of post-menopausal women aged 50 to 79 years. In 2002, the National Heart, Lung, and Blood Institute (NHLBI) issued a press release announcing the closing of the trial to evaluate the risks and benefits of combined estrogen and progestin treatment in healthy menopausal women due to an increased risk of invasive breast cancer.[53] The trial also found increases in coronary heart disease, stroke, and pulmonary embolism in study participants on estrogen plus progestin compared with women taking placebo pills. The investigators observed a 26% excess incidence of breast cancer (hazard ratio [HR], 1.0 to 1.59), and an excess incidence of 8 cases of breast cancer per 10,000 women-years of observation among women randomized to receive conjugated equine estrogens, 0.625 mg/day, plus medroxyprogesterone acetate, 2.5 mg/day compared with the placebo group.[149] Following the announcement of the premature closing of the trial, the use of menopausal hormone therapy dropped dramatically and was followed by a decline in the incidence of breast cancer in the United States. Chlebowski and colleagues[150] examined temporal trends in the WHI observational study cohort to determine if the decline in the use of menopausal hormones was associated with a decline in breast cancer incidence. In the initial 2 years of the study, breast cancer incidence was lower in the group receiving estrogen plus progestin compared with the placebo group, but subsequently increased to a higher rated during the 5.6-year intervention period, then decreased rapidly after the trial was stopped. Frequency of mammography screening was similar in both groups, leading the investigators to conclude that differences in breast cancer incidence between the study group and the control group were associated with combination hormone therapy. Use of estrogen plus progestin was associated with increased breast density, even for short-term use,[151] a greater likelihood of a false positive mammogram and undergoing a breast biopsy,[152] and an increased risk of being diagnosed with lobular cancer.[153]

Selective Estrogen Receptor Modulators

Given the recognized adverse effects of HRT, much recent attention has focused on assessing alternative approaches to treating the menopause, including use of tamoxifen and other selective estrogen receptor modulators (SERMs). These agents are recognized as anti-estrogens, which presumably will offer many of the same advantages as HRT, while eliminating some of the disadvantages (i.e., no increase in breast cancer risk). Data indicate that these agents offer substantial advantages in terms of reducing breast cancer risk, with the most convincing data deriving from the National Surgical Adjuvant Breast and Bowel Project (NSABP).[3] This trial, which focused on women at an increased risk of breast cancer, found after 69 months of follow-up that those who had received tamoxifen had a 49% lower risk of invasive breast cancer than placebo-treated women. The beneficial effect pertained to women of all ages, but was most apparent among women with a history of lobular carcinoma in situ or atypical hyperplasia; in addition, the risk reduction was limited to estrogen receptor positive tumors. Two other trials, one in Britain[154] and the other in Italy,[155] however, did not find an effect of tamoxifen on breast cancer risk. This may have reflected limited sample sizes, high drop-out rates, or usage of other drugs (including HRT) among trial participants.

Studies are also beginning to evaluate the relationship of other SERMS to breast cancer risk. In the recently published Multiple Outcomes of Raloxifene Evaluation (MORE) trial of osteoporotic women, 120 mg of raloxifene daily decreased breast cancer risk by 76% (95% CI, 0.1 to 0.4).[156]

The results of the MORE trial led to the launch of the Study of Tamoxifen and Raloxifene (STAR) trial, a trial to evaluate the relative effectiveness of tamoxifen versus raloxifene in reducing breast cancer risk.[157] Given that tamoxifen had previously been linked with an increased risk of endometrial cancer,[3] while raloxifene was associated with an increased risk of thromboembolic disease,[156] the STAR trial was intended to also assess the relative adversity of both drugs. In 2006, Vogel and associates[4] reported that raloxifene is as effective as tamoxifen in reducing the risk of invasive breast cancer. Raloxifene was associated with a lower risk of thromboembolic events and cataracts, but was similar to tamoxifen with respect risk associated with other cancers, fractures, ischemic heart disease, and stroke.

Histologic and Mammographic Markers of Breast Cancer Risk

Noncancerous lesions of the breast have long been reported to be associated with an increased risk of breast cancer. Resolution of whether certain lesions are more predictive of risk than others has been complicated by the lack of uniformity of histologic classifications of benign breast disease. Dupont and Page[158] proposed diagnostic criteria that separate benign breast disease into the following three categories: (1) nonproliferative changes, including normal breast tissue, cysts, apocrine metaplasia, and mild ductal hyperplasia; (2) proliferative disease without atypia, including papillomas, sclerosing adenosis, fibroadenoma, and moderate to florid ductal hyperplasia of the usual type; and (3) atypical hyperplasia of either ductal or lobular type defined as epithelial proliferations with some features of ordinary hyperplasia and some features of carcinoma in situ. In a retrospective study of 3303 women with a breast biopsy showing benign breast disease, they found that 70% of women had nonproliferative lesions that were not associated with an increased risk of breast cancer.[158] The risk in women with proliferative disease without atypical hyperplasia was 1.9, and the risk in women with atypical hyperplasia was 5.3 compared with that of women without proliferative disease.

The appearance of the breast mammographically has also been found to be a predictor of subsequent breast cancer risk. A parenchymal pattern classification system, which takes into account the amount of the breast composed of ductal prominence, was initially proposed.[159] Direct measurements of dense areas of the breast have been found to be a less subjective and stronger indicator of risk. In one study,[160] breasts with areas of density of 75% or more were associated with nearly a fivefold elevation in risk, a magnitude of risk as great if not greater than most other established risk factors. Findings of a heritable component to mammographic density[161] suggest that a focus on identifying genes responsible for the phenotype could assist in furthering our understanding of etiologic processes. However, it is also clear that environmental factors can influence mammographic densities; notable recent findings in this regard relate to higher mammographic densities associated with combined estrogen and progestin therapy.[162] Boyd and colleagues[163] carried out three nested case-control studies to examine the association of proportion of density on an initial mammogram, breast cancer risk and mode of breast cancer detection. Women with less than 10% were the referent group. Compared with the low-density group, women with density in 75% or more were 4.7 times more likely to develop breast cancer (95% CI, 3.0 to 7.4). Women with at least 50% breast density accounted for half of all interval cancers. Thus, significant mammographic density was associated with both a high risk of breast cancer, and a high risk of failure to detect breast cancer on recent screening.

Family History and Risk Assessment

The proportion of women in the population with a family history of breast cancer in a first-degree relative (mother or sister) has been estimated to be approximately 8.4%. Further, the likelihood of having a family history of breast cancer in a first-degree relative increases with increasing age. Thus, among women aged 20 to 29 years, only 2.7% report a family history of breast cancer, while 11.6% of women aged 50 to 59 years report a family history of at least one first-degree relative with breast cancer. Of those who cite a family history of breast cancer in first-degree relatives, less than 10% have more than one relative affected, with only 1% having three or more first-degree relatives with breast cancer.[164] In series of breast cancer patients, a family history of breast cancer in a first-degree relative is more common, approaching 14%.[165,166] Even among breast cancer cases, however, having more than one family member affected is not common. In one large study, less than 2% of breast cancer cases reported having more than one first-degree relative affected by breast cancer.[165]

In general, only about 5% to 10% of all breast cancer can be accounted for on the basis of known hereditary breast cancer susceptibility disorders.[167-170] Thus, a true genetic predisposition to breast cancer is distinctly uncommon, and its presence generally is not signaled by the presence of only one affected family member. Because most women will not have had a family history to suggest increased breast cancer risk, clinicians must be cautious not to underestimate overall breast cancer risk among women without a family history, as other risk factors account for the majority of breast cancers in the general population and can be associated with a significantly elevated absolute risk.

Although the majority of women in the population do not have a family history of breast cancer, family history has long been recognized as a key risk factor for the development of this disease. The magnitude of risk has been shown to vary with the degree of relatedness, as the RR associated with having a first-degree relative with breast cancer is higher than that associated with having a second-degree relative with the same history (i.e., RR of 2.1 vs. 1.5).[171] Risk also increases as the number of affected family members increases, such that having three or more affected first-degree relatives is associated with a RR of 3.9.[165] Having a relative who was diagnosed with breast cancer at an earlier-than-usual age (which is typically defined as younger than age 50) also is associated with a higher risk.[171,172]

In order to accurately assess an individual's genetic risk of breast cancer, it is essential to collect a detailed history of cancer occurrence in relatives in both the maternal and paternal lineage, ideally for a minimum of three generations. This history should include cancers of all types, not only breast cancer, as the hereditary breast cancer syndromes often include an increased risk of other malignancies, such as ovarian cancer. Details regarding the breast cancer diagnosis, such as age at diagnosis, tumor characteristics, and bilaterality, should also be collected, and confirmed when possible with pathology reports[173] even though the accuracy of reported history of breast cancer actually is surprisingly high, often in the range of 90% or greater.[174,175]

Collecting detailed family history information can allow women with a family history of breast cancer to be stratified into those at moderate risk, and those at high risk, a distinction that is important for decisions about prophylactic measures and the appropriateness of high risk screening strategies.[173,176] Women from families with a history of breast cancer that is most often postmenopausal, unilateral, affecting one or two family members, and without a history of ovarian cancer or other genetically related malignancies are considered to be at moderate risk. These families make up a heterogeneous group, which includes families with breast cancer related to multiple susceptibility factors or environmental exposures including reproductive and lifestyle risk factors, families with several (coincidental) sporadic cancer cases, and some families that carry a mutation in a dominantly transmitted susceptibility factor with low penetrance. Models for individual risk assessment have been developed and may be useful in counseling moderate-risk families. These include the Gail model[177] and the Claus model.[172]

The Gail model incorporates personal risk factors such as age at menarche and history of previous breast biopsies, along with the history of breast cancer in first-degree relatives on the maternal side.[177] It is not suitable for estimating risk in cases where there is a possibility of carrying a mutation on a breast cancer susceptibility gene. The Claus model predicts breast cancer risk based on family history in first- and second-degree relatives, and thus is more sensitive to familial risks.[172] More recently, Tyrer and coworkers[178] published a model that incorporates both personal and familial risk factors.

High-risk women have families with a multi-generation history of breast cancer with early age at onset, bilateral or multifocal disease, and three or more first-degree relatives with breast or ovarian cancer, or both. The presence of both breast and ovarian cancer in the same person is a particularly strong clue to the possible presence of an inherited susceptibility. Women of Ashkenazi Jewish heritage with a significant family history are also at greater risk of carrying an altered breast cancer gene.[179,180] These histories indicate a substantial probability of having a mutation in a dominantly inherited breast cancer susceptibility gene with high penetrance.[172,181] The prevalence of dominant breast cancer-related mutations in the population is estimated to be 0.33%.[182] Women with a high-risk family history account for 5% to 7% of all breast cancer cases; they also account for 33% of women diagnosed with breast cancer before age 30.[174]

Individuals from high-risk families should be referred to multidisciplinary centers providing genetic counseling and access to genetic testing. Risk management strategies range from earlier and more intensive surveillance to chemoprevention and risk-reducing surgeries (such as bilateral mastectomy or oophorectomy).

MAJOR GENES AND SYNDROMES ASSOCIATED WITH AN INCREASED RISK OF BREAST CANCER

Germline mutations in a small number of genes seem to be responsible for most of the high risk of breast cancer seen in multiple-case families. These genes are inherited in an autosomal dominant manner and show high penetrance (i.e., most mutation carriers develop the phenotype and are affected by a syndromic cancer). Lifetime risk of developing a primary and secondary breast cancer, and developing breast cancer at an early age, is considerably higher than for average and moderate risk women. The importance of collecting a comprehensive family history in all women beginning in early adulthood cannot be overemphasized since possible mutation carriers are not easily identified without this information and, by virtue of their age, are presumed to be at the general, low background risk. If a family history of breast and other cancers on the maternal or paternal side is suggestive of the possibility of mutation carrier status, then careful evaluation can be done with specialized software that can estimate lifetime risk and risk of mutation carrier status.[178,183,184]

BRCA1 and *BRCA2*

Although breast cancer is associated with a number of family cancer syndromes, the majority of multiple case families (at least four cases of breast cancer) studied to date have demonstrated mutations in the *breast cancer 1, early onset* (*BRCA1*) or *breast cancer 2, early onset* (*BRCA2*) genes. Linkage to these two genes has been found in approximately 95% of the hereditary breast and ovarian cancer (HBOC) families studied by the Breast Cancer Linkage Consortium, with linkage to *BRCA1* more common than to *BRCA2*. The majority of those families with both male and female breast cancer could be linked to *BRCA2*.[185]

Studying family clusters of breast and ovarian cancer led to the discovery[186,187] and subsequent cloning[188] of the *BRCA1* gene, which is located on the long arm of chromosome 17. *BRCA1* is a large gene with 24 exons that encodes for a protein that is 1863 amino acids in length. It is important in the cellular response to DNA damage.[189] *BRCA1* acts as a tumor suppressor gene, and is inherited in an autosomal dominant pattern. Disease-associated mutations have been found scattered throughout the span of this large gene.[190] The initial estimates of the lifetime risk of breast cancer associated with *BRCA1* mutations approached 90%, because they were based on data from the multiple-case families that were used to map and clone the gene.[191] Subsequent estimates of breast cancer risk, obtained from less highly-selected populations, have generally been lower. A meta-analysis that combined data from 10 studies found an average cumulative risk of breast cancer by age 70 of 57% in carriers of a *BRCA1* mutation, and a 40% risk of ovarian cancer.[192] Female carriers of *BRCA1* mutations also have an increased risk of fallopian tube and primary peritoneal carcinoma,[193] while male mutation carriers have an increased risk of prostate cancer and male breast cancer.[194,195]

Studying HBOC kindreds with no evidence of linkage to the *BRCA1* gene led to the discovery of a second predisposition locus on chromosome 13, designated *BRCA2*.[196] Like *BRCA1*, *BRCA2* is a large gene with multiple documented disease-associated mutations scattered across its span.[190] Estimates of the cumulative risk of breast cancer in carriers of *BRCA2* mutations have also varied from a low of 28% to a high of 84%.[185,197] In the meta-analysis by Chen and colleagues,[192] the cumulative risk of breast cancer among women with a *BRCA2* mutation was 49% by age 70. This analysis found the average risk of ovarian cancer by age 70 in *BRCA2* carriers to be 18%.[192] Women with *BRCA2* mutations also have an increased risk of primary peritoneal carcinoma and fallopian tube carcinoma.[193] *BRCA2* is also associated with an increased risk of male breast cancer, as well as cancers of the pancreas and prostate.[185,198]

Although most HBOC families with germline mutations in *BRCA1 or BRCA2* have their own "private" mutations (i.e., nearly 1000 distinct mutations have been identified in each of these two genes),[190] in some populations one, or a small number of mutations account for the vast majority of the identified mutations. These are termed *founder* mutations; their high frequency is due to the presence of that *gene mutation* in a single ancestor or small number of ancestors. For example, in the Ashkenazi Jewish community, three specific mutations (*BRCA1* 185delAG and 5382insC, and *BRCA2* 6174delT) account for 85% to 90% of all *BRCA* mutations that occur.[199-201] Surveys in the general Ashkenazi population have suggested that 2% to 2.5% of all Ashkenazim carry one of these three mutations, regardless of their personal or family history of cancer.[180,202,203] By comparison, the prevalence of *BRCA* mutations in the general Caucasian population in the United States is estimated to be approximately 1 in 400.[204]

The term *founder mutation* is a general concept of which the Ashkenazi *BRCA* mutations are only a specific example. In fact, many other populations are known to have their own founder mutations in the *BRCA* genes. For example, specific French Canadian,[205] Icelandic,[206] Dutch,[207] and Japanese[208] founder mutations have been documented. The existence of one or several founder mutations that account for the majority of mutations in a given population allows for an altered testing strategy designed to efficiently rule out those specific *BRCA* mutations before moving on to more costly and labor intensive direct sequencing.

Li-Fraumeni Syndrome (*TP53*)

Li-Fraumeni syndrome (LFS) is a rare autosomal dominant cancer susceptibility syndrome that is characterized by sarcomas of the bone and soft tissue, brain tumors, adrenocortical carcinoma, and breast cancer.[209-211] Other cancers that are seen in this syndrome include those of the lung, stomach, colon, and ovary, as well as leukemia and malignant melanoma of the skin.[211] These malignancies occur at much younger ages than would be expected, often striking in childhood and early adulthood. In addition, many individuals are affected with multiple independent primary cancers.[212,213] Germline mutations in the *tumor protein p53 (TP53)* tumor suppressor gene have been documented in the majority of families with LFS.[211,212] In a large series, cancer risk among those with germline *TP53* mutations was estimated at 80% by age 50, with females at greater risk than males (93% in females by age 50 vs. 68% in males). The incidence of female breast cancer in this series was 100 times that of the general population.[214] In women diagnosed with breast cancer before age 40, the prevalence of germline mutations has been estimated to be approximately 1%.[215] In some of the families with LFS that do not show linkage to p53, a different gene, *CHK1 checkpoint homolog (S. pombe) (CHEK2)* (previously known as *hCHK2*), has been implicated.[216] However, this gene is not a common cause of this syndrome.[217]

Cowden Syndrome (*PTEN*)

Cowden syndrome (CS) is a rare autosomal dominant disorder associated with mutations in the *phosphatase and tensin homolog (PTEN)* gene, which is located on the long arm of chromosome 10.[218] Manifestations of CS include multiple benign hamartomas of the skin, mucous membranes (including the gastrointestinal tract), thyroid, and breast. Affected individuals also have an increased risk of cancers of the breast, gastrointestinal tract, thyroid, and uterus. The lifetime risk of breast cancer in women with CS has been estimated at 25% to 50%, with an average age at breast cancer diagnosis estimated to be in the range of 38 to 46 years of age.[219] Because the signs of CS can be subtle, the published prevalence for this syndrome, 1 in 200,000,[220] is thought by some investigators to be an underestimate.[219]

Peutz-Jeghers Syndrome (*STK11*)

Peutz-Jeghers syndrome (PJS) is an autosomal dominant disorder linked to mutations in the *serine/threonine kinase 11 (STK11)* gene, a tumor supressor gene on chromosome 19.[221,222] The cardinal features of PJS are pigmented oral lesions and multiple gastrointestinal polyps (both hamartomatous and adenomatous). The polyps seen in PJS can occur throughout the gastrointestinal (GI) tract, including the stomach, small intestine, and large intestine, and may lead to intussusception, bleeding, or even malignant transformation. Individuals with PJS have a markedly increased risk of cancer, with one study estimating a cumulative risk of 85% by age 70.[223] The most common cancers seen are gastrointestinal, including cancers of the colon, esophagus, stomach, small intestine, and pancreas. Women with PJS have an increased risk of breast cancer, with one series estimating a risk of more than 30% by age 60,[223] while another estimating a lifetime risk of 50%.[224]

E-Cadherin (*CDH1*)

Germline mutations in the gene *cadherin 1, type 1, E-cadherin (epithelial) (CDH1)*, which codes for the cell-cell adhesion molecule E-cadherin, have been linked to the hereditary diffuse gastric cancer syndrome. In this autosomal dominant disorder, individuals develop the diffuse form of gastric cancer at a young age (generally before the age of 50 years).[225] Female carriers of *CDH1* mutations also have an increased risk of lobular breast cancer, with a lifetime risk estimated at 20% to 40%.[225,226] In some families segregating *CDH1* mutations, breast cancer predominates to such an extent that evaluation for familial breast cancer syndromes is initiated.[227,228]

LOW PENETRANCE BREAST CANCER SUSCEPTIBILITY GENES

Inheritance of a major susceptibility gene accounts for up to 25% of the excess risk associated with a family history of breast cancer.[229] The remaining risk appears to arise from a number of lower risk gene mutations and variations. These gene changes may act alone or in combination to affect breast cancer risk.[230]

Ataxia Telangiectasia Mutated

Ataxia-telangiectasia (AT) is a rare autosomal recessive disorder caused by mutations in the *ataxia telangiectasia mutated* (*ATM*) gene, which is found on the long arm of chromosome 11.[231] This disorder is characterized by cerebellar degeneration, immunodeficiency, chromosome instability, increased sensitivity to ionizing radiation, and increased risk of cancer (particularly lymphoid malignancies). Affected individuals also display oculocutaneous telangiectasias.[232,233] Although AT itself is rare (requiring both copies of *ATM* to be mutated), with an estimated incidence of 3 per 1 million live births in Caucasians in the United States, heterozygote carriers for this disorder (i.e., those with only one altered copy of *ATM*) are thought to be relatively common. One estimate indicated that *ATM* carriers may comprise 1% of the U.S. population.[234] While *ATM* carriers are generally asymptomatic, investigators have found evidence of an increased in vitro sensitivity to ionizing radiation, at a level intermediate between that of individuals without the mutation and *ATM* homozygotes[235,236]

Family studies have revealed a twofold to threefold increased risk of developing[237] and dying[238] from cancer among *ATM* carriers. In particular, female carriers of *ATM* mutations have a modestly increased risk of breast cancer, with an estimated RR of 2.0.[239,240] Occasional studies have found an increased frequency of germline *ATM* mutations in familial breast cancer cases, although this gene does not appear to account for a significant proportion of familial breast cancer clusters.[241-244] However, the modest elevation in breast cancer risk in AT heterozygotes, when coupled with the relatively high frequency of *ATM* mutation carriers in the general population cited earlier, has produced estimates that 6% to 7% of U.S. breast cancer cases could be accounted for by AT heterozygosity,[245] a proportion rivaling that seen from *BRCA* mutations.

CHK2 Checkpoint Homolog

The CHK2 checkpoint homolog (S. pombe) (*CHEK2*) gene, located on the long arm of chromosome 22, is a gene that encodes a cell checkpoint kinase that has interactions with other gene products known to influence breast cancer risk, such as *TP53, ATM,* and *BRCA1*. An estimated 0.3% to 1.4% of the U.S. population carries a specific truncating mutation in *CHEK2*, known as 1100delC.[246] This mutation has been found at a higher frequency in individuals with bilateral breast cancer, and in cases with a positive family history of breast cancer.[247] Up to 5% of familial breast cancer cases which are *BRCA*-mutation negative were found to carry *CHEK2**1100delC.[247,248] Estimates for breast cancer risk associated with this mutation vary depending on family history. Although in unselected women this *CHEK2* mutation is associated with a twofold to threefold increase in breast cancer risk,[248,249] in women with a family history of the disease it seems to convey a higher risk compared with noncarriers (odds ratio [OR], 4.8; 95% CI, 3.3 to 7.2), with a cumulative risk to age 70 of 37%. Still, since the overall increase in risk seen with this mutation is modest, it is considered a low-penetrance breast cancer susceptibility allele. Other mutations in *CHEK2*, such as I157T, have been associated with breast cancer risk in other countries, including Israel, Poland, Latvia, and Finland.[250] As indicated previously, mutations in *CHEK2* have been implicated in some cases of Li-Fraumeni syndrome.[216,251,252]

BRIP1 and *PALB2*

BRCA1 interacting protein C-terminal helicase 1 (*BRIP1*) and *partner and localizer of BRCA2* (*PALB2*) genes encode for proteins that interact with the *BRCA* proteins: *BRIP1* with *BRCA1* and *PALB2* with *BRCA2*. Individuals with homozygous inactivating mutations of these genes develop Fanconi anemia, an inherited bone marrow failure syndrome.[253,254] Heterozygote carriers of these mutations have a twofold increased risk of breast cancer.[255,256] A founder mutation of *PALB2* seen in the Finnish population, 1592delT, appears to confer a much higher risk, and is associated with a lifetime risk of breast cancer of 40%.[257]

Polymorphisms Associated with Breast Cancer Risk

Polymorphisms are gene variants that are common in the general population. These often involve the change of a single nucleotide at a given position within a gene, and are thus often referred to as single nucleotide polymorphisms, or SNPs (pronounced *snips*). These variants may affect gene expression or protein function, but do not lead to gene inactivation. Genome wide association studies have uncovered a number of different polymorphisms, each of which has a modest effect on the risk of breast cancer. For example, the rs3803662 SNP in the *thymocyte selection-associated high mobility group box member 3* (*TOX3*) gene is associated with a 13% to 30% increased risk of breast cancer.[258] A recent paper estimated that the 18 breast cancer susceptibility loci identified to date account for approximately 8% of familial breast cancer risk.[258]

CONCLUSION

With the exception of family history and age, none of the identified risk factors is a particularly strong predictor of breast cancer, either alone or in combination. Further, any discussion of risk factors with patients should not be framed strictly in terms of RRs because they provide little information about probability of developing breast cancer over time, and also because some RRs are transitory over time. Genetic susceptibility results in highly elevated risk, but is rare.

Although a majority of women have at least one confirmed risk factor for breast cancer,[259] the majority of women diagnosed with breast cancer do not have a risk profile that readily distinguishes them from women who will not develop breast cancer. Thus, to date efforts to design screening programs based on risk factor profiles have not proved productive because estimates of the effectiveness of targeting women based on a handful of key risk factors, such as family history, age at menarche, and parity have shown that such a program would miss the majority of incident cases.[260] The majority of risk factors that influence a woman's risk of breast cancer, such as heredity, age, and onset of menarche and menopause, are beyond her control. Others, such as the timing of pregnancy, or her parity, are not easily or practically modifiable for obvious reasons. Lifestyle modifications (e.g., prudent diet, exercise, healthy BMI, and reducing alcohol intake) have not been convincingly associated with decreased breast cancer risk but can be advised based on inferential evidence of possible benefit, and because healthier lifestyles are consistent with good overall general health.

For women at average risk of breast cancer, *routine* screening according to recommended guidelines is the most important strategy to ensure early detection and reduce the risk of being diagnosed with an advanced breast cancer. For women at greater than average risk of breast cancer, intensified screening and chemoprevention have been proposed as protective methods. For women at exceptionally higher risk, heightened surveillance, chemoprevention, and prophylactic surgeries may be considered.[176] With increases in risk, clinicians face a greater responsibility to support shared decision making with their patients. Thus, from a public health standpoint, all women in appropriate age categories should be counseled about the importance of routine breast cancer screening, and providers need to recognize the important role they play in the achievement of a regular program of surveillance and helping women make informed decisions.

KEY POINTS

- Breast cancer is the most common cancer among women in the world, the leading cause of cancer mortality, and a leading cause of premature mortality.
- Global patterns show rising incidence, declining mortality in countries with early detection programs, and rising mortality in countries without early detection programs.
- Trends in incidence and mortality vary by race and ethnicity due to a combination of differential risk factors, and unequal access to care.
- Most risk factors for breast cancer are modest in influence and not easily modifiable.
- Some risk factors for breast cancer, such as avoiding postmenopausal hormones, moderate alcohol consumption, and avoiding weight gain do suggest strategies for risk reduction.
- Women who carry deleterious mutations on breast cancer susceptibility genes are at significantly elevated lifetime risk and should begin screening early, and make informed decisions about other preventive strategies.

SUGGESTED READINGS

Altekruse S, Kosary C, Krapcho M, Neyman N, Aminou R, Waldron W, et al. *SEER cancer statistics review, 1975-2007*. Bethesda, Md: National Cancer Institute; 2010.

Banks E, Canfell K. Invited commentary: hormone therapy risks and benefits–the Women's Health Initiative findings and the postmenopausal estrogen timing hypothesis. *Am J Epidemiol* 2009;**170**:24-8.

Coughlin SS, Ekwueme DU. Breast cancer as a global health concern. *Cancer Epidemiol* 2009;**33**:315-8.

Jemal A, Siegel R, Ward E, Hao Y, Xu J, Thun MJ. Cancer statistics, 2009. *CA Cancer J Clin* 2009;**59**:225-49.

Lund MJ, Trivers KF, Porter PL, Coates RJ, Leyland-Jones B, Brawley OW, et al. Race and triple negative threats to breast cancer survival: a population-based study in Atlanta, Ga. *Breast Cancer Res Treat* 2009;**113**:357-70.

Parkin DM, Fernandez LM. Use of statistics to assess the global burden of breast cancer. *Breast J* 2006;**12**(Suppl. 1):S70-80.

Parmigiani G, Chen S, Iversen ES, Friebel TM, Finkelstein DM, Anton-Culver H, et al. Validity of models for predicting BRCA1 and BRCA2 mutations. *Ann Intern Med* 2007;**147**:441-50.

Saslow D, Boates C, Burke W, Harms S, Leach MO, Lehman CD, et al. American Cancer Society guidelines for breast screening with MRI as an adjunct to mammography. *CA Cancer J Clin* 2007;**57**:75-89. Available at http://caonline.amcancersoc.org [Accessed June 6, 2010].

REFERENCES

1. Parkin DM, Bray F, Ferlay J, Pisani P. Global cancer statistics, 2002. *CA Cancer J Clin* 2005;**55**:74-108.
2. Parkin DM, Fernandez LM. Use of statistics to assess the global burden of breast cancer. *Breast J* 2006;**12**(Suppl. 1):S70-80.
3. Fisher B, Costantino JP, Wickerham DL, Redmond CK, Kavanah M, Cronin WM, et al. Tamoxifen for prevention of breast cancer: report of the National Surgical Adjuvant Breast and Bowel Project P-1 Study. *J Natl Cancer Inst* 1998;**90**:1371-88.
4. Vogel VG, Costantino JP, Wickerham DL, Cronin WM, Cecchini RS, Atkins JN, et al. Effects of tamoxifen vs raloxifene on the risk of developing invasive breast cancer and other disease outcomes: the NSABP Study of Tamoxifen and Raloxifene (STAR) P-2 trial. *JAMA* 2006;**295**:2727-41.
5. Gail MH, Costantino JP, Bryant J, Croyle R, Freedman L, Helzlsouer K, et al. Weighing the risks and benefits of tamoxifen treatment for preventing breast cancer [see comments]. published erratum appears in. *J Natl Cancer Inst* 2000 Feb 2;92:275. *J Natl Cancer Inst* 1999;**91**:1829-46.
6. Freedman AN, Graubard BI, Rao SR, McCaskill-Stevens W, Ballard-Barbash R, Gail MH. Estimates of the number of US women who could benefit from tamoxifen for breast cancer chemoprevention. *J Natl Cancer Inst* 2003;**95**:526-32.
7. Land SR, Wickerham DL, Costantino JP, Ritter MW, Vogel VG, Lee M, et al. Patient-reported symptoms and quality of life during treatment with tamoxifen or raloxifene for breast cancer prevention: the NSABP Study of Tamoxifen and Raloxifene (STAR) P-2 trial. *JAMA* 2006;**295**:2742-51.
8. Altekruse S, Kosary C, Krapcho M, Neyman N, Aminou R, Waldron W, et al. *SEER Cancer Statistics Review, 1975-2007*. Bethesda, Md: National Cancer Institute; 2010.
9. Jemal A, Siegel R, Ward E, Hao Y, Xu J, Thun MJ. Cancer statistics, 2009. *CA Cancer J Clin* 2009;**59**:225-49.

10. Ferlay J, Bray P, Pisani P, Parkin DM. *GLOBOCAN 2002: Cancer Incidence, Mortality, and Prevalence Worldwide*. Lyon: IARC Press; 2004.
11. U.S. Cancer Statistics Working Group. *United States Cancer Statistics: 1999-2006,1999-2006 Incidence and Mortality Web-based Report*. Atlanta: U.S. Department of Health and Human Services, Centers for Disease Control and Prevention and National Cancer Institute; 2010. Available at www.cdc.gov/cancer/npcr/uscs/2006/about.htm; [Accessed June 7, 2010].
12. *WHO Mortality Database*. WHO; 2010. Available at www.who.int/whosis/en/ [Accessed June 7, 2010].
13. Pickle LW, Hao Y, Jemal A, Zou Z, Tiwari RC, Ward E, et al. A new method of estimating United States and state-level cancer incidence counts for the current calendar year. *CA Cancer J Clin* 2007;**57**:30-42.
14. American Cancer Society. *American Cancer Society Facts & Figures 2009*. Atlanta: American Cancer Society; 2009.
15. American Cancer Society. *Global Cancer Facts & Figures 2007*. Atlanta: American Cancer Society; 2007.
16. Curtin L, Klein R. *Direct standardization (age-adjusted death rates). Healthy People 2000 Statistical Notes No. 6—Revised March 1995*. Department of Health and Human Services; 1995 DHHS Publication No. (PHS) 95-1237.
17. National Cancer Institute. *Personal communication*. 1995.
18. Swanson GM. Breast cancer risk estimation: a translational statistic for communication to the public. *J Natl Cancer Inst* 1993;**85**:848-9.
19. Edwards BK, Howe HL, Ries LA, Thun MJ, Rosenberg HM, Yancik R, et al. Annual report to the nation on the status of cancer, 1973-1999, featuring implications of age and aging on U.S. cancer burden. *Cancer* 2002;**94**:2766-92.
20. Ries L, Eisner M, Kosary C, Hankey BF, Miller BA, Clegg L, et al. *SEER Cancer Statistics Review, 1973-1998*. Bethesda, Md: National Cancer Institute; 2001.
21. *Surveillance, Epidemiology, and End Results (SEER) Program SEER*Stat Database: Incidence - SEER 9 Regs (1973-2007)*. Rockville, Md: National Cancer Institute, DCCPS, Surveillance Research Program, Cancer Statistics Branch; 2009 [computer program]. Version 6.6.2.
22. Bray F, McCarron P, Parkin DM. The changing global patterns of female breast cancer incidence and mortality. *Breast Cancer Res* 2004;**6**:229-39.
23. Anderson BO, Yip CH, Smith RA, Shyyan R, Sener SF, Eniu A, et al. Guideline implementation for breast healthcare in low-income and middle-income countries. *Cancer* 2008;**113**(Suppl. 8):2221-43.
24. Chia KS, Reilly M, Tan CS, Lee J, Pawitan Y, Adami HO, et al. Profound changes in breast cancer incidence may reflect changes into a Westernized lifestyle: a comparative population-based study in Singapore and Sweden. *Int J Cancer* 2005;**113**:302-6.
25. Berry DA, Cronin KA, Plevritis SK, Fryback DG, Clarke L, Zelen M, et al. Effect of screening and adjuvant therapy on mortality from breast cancer. *N Engl J Med* 2005;**353**:1784-92.
26. Duffy SW, Tabar L, Olsen AH, Vitak B, Allgood PC, Chen TH, et al. Absolute numbers of lives saved and overdiagnosis in breast cancer screening, from a randomized trial and from the Breast Screening Programme in England. *J Med Screen* 2010;**17**:25-30.
27. Cayuela A, Rodriguez-Dominguez S, Ruiz-Borrego M, Gili M. Age-period-cohort analysis of breast cancer mortality rates in Andalucia (Spain). *Ann Oncol* 2004;**15**:686-8.
28. Shin HR, Boniol M, Joubert C, Hery C, Haukka J, Autier P, et al. Secular trends in breast cancer mortality in five East Asian populations: Hong Kong, Japan, Korea, Singapore and Taiwan. *Cancer Sci* 2010;**101**:1241-6.
29. Hoel DG, Davis DL, Miller AB, Sondik EJ, Swerdlow AJ. Trends in cancer mortality in 15 industrialized countries, 1969-1986. *J Natl Cancer Inst* 1992;**84**:313-20.
30. Ferlay J, Bray P, Pisani P, Parkin DM. *GLOBOCAN 2000: Cancer Incidence, Mortality, and Prevalence Worldwide*. Lyon: IARC Press; 2001.
31. Wakai K, Suzuki S, Ohno Y, Kawamura T, Tamakoshi A, Aoki R. Epidemiology of breast cancer in Japan. *Int J Epidemiol* 1995;**24**:285-91.
32. Kawai M, Minami Y, Kuriyama S, Kakizaki M, Kakugawa Y, Nishino Y, et al. Reproductive factors, exogenous female hormone use and breast cancer risk in Japanese: the Miyagi Cohort Study. *Cancer Causes Control* 2010;**21**:135-45.
33. Devesa SS, Silverman DT, Young JL, Pollack ES, Brown CC, Horm JW, et al. Cancer incidence and mortality trends among whites in the United States, 1947-84. *J Natl Cancer Inst* 1987;**79**:701-70.
34. Kosary C, Hankey B, Brinton L, et al. *1995 Cancer Statistics Review*. Bethesda, Md: National Cancer Institute; 1995.
35. Hankey BF, Miller B, Curtis R, Kosary C. Trends in breast cancer in younger women in contrast to older women. *J Natl Cancer Inst Monogr* 1994;(16)7-14.
36. Morrison A. *Screening in Chronic Disease*. New York: Oxford University Press; 1992.
37. Kessler LG. The relationship between age and incidence of breast cancer. Population and screening program data. *Cancer* 1992;**69**(Suppl. 7):1896-903.
38. Smith RA, Haynes S. Barriers to screening for breast cancer. *Cancer* 1992;**69**(Suppl. 7):1968-78.
39. Howard J. Using mammography for cancer control: an unrealized potential. *CA Cancer J Clin* 1987;**37**:33-48.
40. Dawson DA, Thompson GB. Breast cancer risk factors and screening: United States, 1987. *Vital Health Stat* 1990;**10**:iii-iv, 1-60.
41. Horton JA, Romans MC, Cruess DF. Mammography attitudes and usage study, 1992. *Womens Health Issues* 1992;**2**:180-6; discussion 187-188.
42. American Cancer Society. *Mammography: Two statements of the American Cancer Society*. 1983 Atlanta.
43. Shapiro S. Evidence on screening for breast cancer from a randomized trial. *Cancer* 1977;**39**(Suppl. 6):2772-82.
44. Dodd GD. American Cancer Society guidelines on screening for breast cancer. An overview. *Cancer* 1992;**69**(Suppl. 7):1885-7.
45. American Cancer Society. Survey of physicians' attitudes and practices in early cancer detection. *CA Cancer J Clin* 1985;**35**:197-213.
46. American Cancer Society. 1989 survey of physicians' attitudes and practices in early cancer detection. *CA Cancer J Clin* 1990;**40**:77-101.
47. Brown ML, Kessler LG, Rueter FG. Is the supply of mammography machines outstripping need and demand? An economic analysis [see comments]. *Ann Intern Med* 1990;**113**:547-52.
48. White E, Lee CY, Kristal AR. Evaluation of the increase in breast cancer incidence in relation to mammography use. *J Natl Cancer Inst* 1990;**82**:1546-52.
49. Liff JM, Sung JF, Chow WH, Greenberg RS, Flanders WD. Does increased detection account for the rising incidence of breast cancer? *Am J Public Health* 1991;**81**:462-5.
50. Holford TR, Roush GC, McKay LA. Trends in female breast cancer in Connecticut and the United States. *J Clin Epidemiol* 1991;**44**:29-39.
51. Howe HL, Wu X, Ries LA, Cokkinides V, Ahmed F, Jemal A, et al. Annual report to the nation on the status of cancer, 1975-2003, featuring cancer among U.S. Hispanic/Latino populations. *Cancer* 2006;**107**:1711-42.
52. Edwards BK, Ward E, Kohler BA, Eheman C, Zauber AG, Anderson RN, et al. Annual report to the nation on the status of cancer, 1975-2006, featuring colorectal cancer trends and impact of interventions (risk factors, screening, and treatment) to reduce future rates. *Cancer* 2010;**116**:544-73.
53. National Institutes of Health. Press Release: NHLBI stops trial of estrogen plus progestin due to increased breast cancer risk, lack of overall benefit. In: *National Heart Lung, and Blood Institute*. Bethesda Md: National Institutes of Health; 2002.
54. Coombs NJ, Cronin KA, Taylor RJ, Freedman AN, Boyages J. The impact of changes in hormone therapy on breast cancer incidence in the US population. *Cancer Causes Control* 2010;**21**:83-90.
55. Breen N, A Cronin K, Meissner HI, Taplin SH, Tangka FK, Tiro JA, et al. Reported drop in mammography: is this cause for concern? *Cancer* 2007;**109**:2405-9.
56. Use of mammograms among women aged > or = 40 years-United States, 2000-2005. *MMWR Morb Mortal Wkly Rep* 2007;**56**:49-51.
57. Jemal A, Ward E, Thun MJ. Recent trends in breast cancer incidence rates by age and tumor characteristics among U.S. women. *Breast Cancer Res* 2007;**9**:R28.
58. Ursin G, Bernstein L, Pike M. *Breast cancer. Cancer Surveys Volume 19/20: Trends in Cancer Incidence and Mortality*. Imperial Cancer Research Fund; 1994.
59. Duffy SW, Chen HH, Tabar L, Day NE. Estimation of mean sojourn time in breast cancer screening using a Markov chain model of both

entry to and exit from the preclinical detectable phase. *Stat Med* 1995;**14**:1531-43.
60. Tabar L, Vitak B, Chen HH, Duffy SW, Yen MF, Chiang CF, et al. The Swedish Two-County Trial twenty years later. Updated mortality results and new insights from long-term follow-up. *Radiol Clin North Am* 2000;**38**:625-51.
61. Peek ME. Screening mammography in the elderly: a review of the issues. *J Am Med Womens Assoc* 2003;**58**:191-8.
62. Rao VM, Levin DC, Parker L, Frangos AJ. Recent trends in mammography utilization in the Medicare population: is there a cause for concern? *J Am Coll Radiol* 2008;**5**:652-6.
63. Hausauer AK, Keegan TH, Chang ET, Clarke CA. Recent breast cancer trends among Asian/Pacific Islander, Hispanic, and African-American women in the US: changes by tumor subtype. *Breast Cancer Res* 2007;**9**:R90.
64. Ravdin PM, Cronin KA, Howlader N, Berg CD, Chlebowski RT, Feuer EJ, et al. The decrease in breast-cancer incidence in 2003 in the United States. *N Engl J Med* 2007;**356**:1670-4.
65. American Cancer Society. *Breast Cancer Facts & Figures 2009-2010*. Atlanta: American Cancer Society; 2009.
66. Lund MJ, Trivers KF, Porter PL, Coates RJ, Leyland-Jones B, Brawley OW, et al. Race and triple negative threats to breast cancer survival: a population-based study in Atlanta, GA. *Breast Cancer Res Treat* 2009;**113**:357-70.
67. Cunningham JE, Montero AJ, Garrett-Mayer E, Berkel HJ, Ely B. Racial differences in the incidence of breast cancer subtypes defined by combined histologic grade and hormone receptor status. *Cancer Causes Control* 2010;**21**:399-409.
68. Lantz PM, Mujahid M, Schwartz K, Janz NK, Fagerlin A, Salem B, et al. The influence of race, ethnicity, and individual socioeconomic factors on breast cancer stage at diagnosis. *Am J Public Health* 2006;**96**:2173-8.
69. Smith-Bindman R, Miglioretti DL, Lurie N, Abraham L, Barbash RB, Strzelczyk J, et al. Does utilization of screening mammography explain racial and ethnic differences in breast cancer? *Ann Intern Med* 2006;**144**:541-53.
70. Gorey KM, Luginaah IN, Schwartz KL, Fung KY, Balagurusamy M, Bartfay E, et al. Increased racial differences on breast cancer care and survival in America: historical evidence consistent with a health insurance hypothesis, 1975-2001. *Breast Cancer Res Treat* 2009;**113**:595-600.
71. Halpern MT, Bian J, Ward EM, Schrag NM, Chen AY. Insurance status and stage of cancer at diagnosis among women with breast cancer. *Cancer* 2007;**110**:403-11.
72. Chen AY, Halpern MT, Schrag NM, Stewart A, Leitch M, Ward E. Disparities and trends in sentinel lymph node biopsy among early-stage breast cancer patients (1998-2005). *J Natl Cancer Inst* 2008;**100**:462-74.
73. Smith GL, Shih YC, Xu Y, Giordano SH, Smith BD, Perkins GH, et al. Racial disparities in the use of radiotherapy after breast-conserving surgery: a national Medicare study. *Cancer* 2010;**116**:734-41.
74. Banerjee M, George J, Yee C, Hryniuk W, Schwartz K. Disentangling the effects of race on breast cancer treatment. *Cancer* 2007;**110**:2169-77.
75. Horner M, Ries L, Krapcho M, Neyman N, Aminou R, Howlader N, et al. *SEER Cancer Statistics Review, 1975-2006*. Bethesda, Md: National Cancer Institute; 2009.
76. Ries L, Eisner M, Kosary C, Hankey B, Miller B, Clegg L, et al. *SEER Cancer Statistics Review, 1975-2000*. Bethesda, Md: National Cancer Institute; 2003.
77. Etzioni R, Urban N, Ramsey S, McIntosh M, Schwartz S, Reid B, et al. The case for early detection. *Nat Rev Cancer* 2003;**3**:243-52.
78. Elkin EB, Hudis C, Begg CB, Schrag D. The effect of changes in tumor size on breast carcinoma survival in the U.S.: 1975-1999. *Cancer* 2005;**104**:1149-57.
79. Tabar L, Vitak B, Chen HH, Yen MF, Duffy SW, Smith RA. Beyond randomized controlled trials: organized mammographic screening substantially reduces breast carcinoma mortality. *Cancer* 2001;**91**:1724-31.
80. Esserman L, Shieh Y, Thompson I. Rethinking screening for breast cancer and prostate cancer. *JAMA* 2009;**302**:1685-92.
81. Etzioni R, Penson DF, Legler JM, di Tommaso D, Boer R, Gann PH, et al. Overdiagnosis due to prostate-specific antigen screening: lessons from U.S. prostate cancer incidence trends. *J Natl Cancer Inst* 2002;**94**:981-90.
82. Duffy SW, Lynge E, Jonsson H, Ayyaz S, Olsen AH. Complexities in the estimation of overdiagnosis in breast cancer screening. *Br J Cancer* 2008;**99**:1176-8.
83. Yen MF, Tabar L, Vitak B, Smith RA, Chen HH, Duffy SW. Quantifying the potential problem of overdiagnosis of ductal carcinoma in situ in breast cancer screening. *Eur J Cancer* 2003;**39**:1746-54.
84. Etzioni R, Feuer E. Studies of prostate-cancer mortality: caution advised. *Lancet Oncol* 2008;**9**:407-9.
85. *DevCan: Probability of Developing or Dying of Cancer Software, Version 6.4.0*. Rockville Md: Statistical Research and Applications Branch, National Cancer; May 2009. [computer program].
86. Gail M, Benichou J. Assessing the risk of breast cancer in individuals. *Cancer Prevention* 1992;(June)1-15.
87. Gail M, Benichou J. Epidemiology and biostatistics program of the National Cancer Institute. *J Natl Cancer Inst* 1994;**86**:573-5.
88. Feuer E, Wun L, Boring C. Probability of developing cancer. In: Miller B, Gloeckler Ries, L, editors. *Cancer Statistics Review 1973-89*. National Cancer Institute; 1992 NIH Pub. No. 92-2789.
89. Vogel VG. Management of the high-risk patient. *Surg Clin North Am* 2003;**83**:733-51.
90. Crepeau AZ, Willoughby L, Pinsky B, Hinyard L, Shah M. Accuracy of personal breast cancer risk estimation in cancer-free women during primary care visits. *Women Health* 2008;**47**:113-30.
91. Absetz P, Aro AR, Sutton SR. Experience with breast cancer, pre-screening perceived susceptibility and the psychological impact of screening. *Psychooncology* 2003;**12**:305-18.
92. Seidman H, Mushinski MH, Gelb SK, Silverberg E. Probabilities of eventually developing or dying of cancer–United States, 1985. *CA Cancer J Clin* 1985;**35**:36-56.
93. National Center for Health Statistics. *Vital statistics of the United States, 1990*. Washington: U.S. Public Health Service; 1994.
94. Bruzzi P, Green SB, Byar DP, Brinton LA, Schairer C. Estimating the population attributable risk for multiple risk factors using case-control data. *Am J Epidemiol* 1985;**122**:904-14.
95. Madigan MP, Ziegler RG, Benichou J, Byrne C, Hoover RN. Proportion of breast cancer cases in the United States explained by well-established risk factors. *J Natl Cancer Inst* 1995;**87**:1681-5.
96. Rockhill B, Weinberg CR, Newman B. Population attributable fraction estimation for established breast cancer risk factors: considering the issues of high prevalence and unmodifiability. *Am J Epidemiol* 1998;**147**:826-33.
97. Key T, Appleby P, Barnes I, Reeves G; The Endogenous Hormones and Breast Cancer Collaborative Group. Endogenous sex hormones and breast cancer in postmenopausal women: reanalysis of nine prospective studies. *J Natl Cancer Inst* 2002;**94**:606-16.
98. Kaaks R, Lundin E, Rinaldi S, Manjer J, Biessy C, Söderberg S, et al. Prospective study of IGF-I, IGF-binding proteins, and breast cancer risk, in northern and southern Sweden. *Cancer Causes Control* 2002;**13**:307-16.
99. Hankinson SE, Willett WC, Colditz GA, Hunter DJ, Michaud DS, Deroo B, et al. Circulating concentrations of insulin-like growth factor-I and risk of breast cancer. *Lancet* 1998;**351**:1393-6.
100. Calle EE, Feigelson HS, Hildebrand JS, Teras LR, Thun MJ, Rodriguez C. Postmenopausal hormone use and breast cancer associations differ by hormone regimen and histologic subtype. *Cancer* 2009;**115**:936-45.
101. Hyman E, Kauraniemi P, Hautaniemi S, Wolf M, Mousses S, Rozenblum E, et al. Impact of DNA amplification on gene expression patterns in breast cancer. *Cancer Res* 2002;**62**:6240-5.
102. Gong Y, Yan K, Lin F, Anderson K, Sotiriou C, Andre F, et al. Determination of oestrogen-receptor status and ERBB2 status of breast carcinoma: a gene-expression profiling study. *Lancet Oncol* 2007;**8**:203-11.
103. Collaborative Group on Hormonal Factors in Breast Cancer. Breast cancer and breastfeeding: collaborative reanalysis of individual data from 47 epidemiological studies in 30 countries, including 50302 women with breast cancer and 96973 women without the disease. *Lancet* 2002;**360**:187-95.
104. Gartner LM, Morton J, Lawrence RA, Naylor AJ, O'Hare D, Schanler RJ, et al. Breastfeeding and the use of human milk. *Pediatrics* 2005;**115**:496-506.
105. Trentham-Dietz A, Newcomb PA, Storer BE, Longnecker MP, Baron J, Greenberg ER, et al. Body size and risk of breast cancer. *Am J Epidemiol* 1997;**145**:1011-9.

106. Trentham-Dietz A, Newcomb PA, Egan KM, Titus-Ernstoff L, Baron JA, Storer BE, et al. Weight change and risk of postmenopausal breast cancer (United States). *Cancer Causes Control* 2000;**11**:533–42.
107. van den Brandt PA, Spiegelman D, Yaun SS, Adami HO, Beeson L, Folsom AR, et al. Pooled analysis of prospective cohort studies on height, weight, and breast cancer risk. *Am J Epidemiol* 2000;**152**:514–27.
108. Ursin G, Longnecker MP, Haile RW, Greenland S. A meta-analysis of body mass index and risk of premenopausal breast cancer. *Epidemiology* 1995;**6**:137–41.
109. Ballard-Barbash R, Schatzkin A, Carter CL, Kannel WB, Kreger BE, D'Agostino RB, et al. Body fat distribution and breast cancer in the Framingham Study. *J Natl Cancer Inst* 1990;**82**:286–90.
110. Hall IJ, Newman B, Millikan RC, Moorman PG. Body size and breast cancer risk in black women and white women: the Carolina Breast Cancer Study. *Am J Epidemiol* 2000;**151**:754–64.
111. International Agency for Research on Cancer. *Weight control and physical activity*. Lyon: IARC Press; 2002.
112. Hoffman-Goetz L, Apter D, Demark-Wahnefried W, Goran MI, McTiernan A, Reichman ME. Possible mechanisms mediating an association between physical activity and breast cancer. *Cancer* 1998;**83**(Suppl. 3):621–8.
113. Bernstein L, Henderson BE, Hanisch R, Sullivan-Halley J, Ross RK. Physical exercise and reduced risk of breast cancer in young women. *J Natl Cancer Inst* 1994;**86**:1403–8.
114. Friedenreich CM, Thune I, Brinton LA, Albanes D. Epidemiologic issues related to the association between physical activity and breast cancer. *Cancer* 1998;**83**(Suppl. 3):600–10.
115. Moradi T, Nyren O, Zack M, Magnusson C, Persson I, Adami HO. Breast cancer risk and lifetime leisure-time and occupational physical activity (Sweden). *Cancer Causes Control* 2000;**11**:523–31.
116. Rockhill B, Willett WC, Hunter DJ, Manson JE, Hankinson SE, Colditz GA. A prospective study of recreational physical activity and breast cancer risk. *Arch Intern Med* 1999;**159**:2290–6.
117. Shoff SM, Newcomb PA, Trentham-Dietz A, Remington PL, Mittendorf R, Greenberg ER, et al. Early-life physical activity and postmenopausal breast cancer: effect of body size and weight change. *Cancer Epidemiol Biomarkers Prev* 2000;**9**:591–5.
118. Verloop J, Rookus MA, van der Kooy K, van Leeuwen FE. Physical activity and breast cancer risk in women aged 20–54 years. *J Natl Cancer Inst* 2000;**92**:128–35.
119. Wyshak G, Frisch RE. Breast cancer among former college athletes compared to non-athletes: a 15-year follow-up. *Br J Cancer* 2000;**82**:726–30.
120. Britton JA, Gammon MD, Schoenberg JB, Stanford JL, Coates RJ, Swanson CA, et al. Risk of breast cancer classified by joint estrogen receptor and progesterone receptor status among women 20–44 years of age. *Am J Epidemiol* 2002;**156**:507–16.
121. Neilson HK, Friedenreich CM, Brockton NT, Millikan RC. Physical activity and postmenopausal breast cancer: proposed biologic mechanisms and areas for future research. *Cancer Epidemiol Biomarkers Prev* 2009;**18**:11–27.
122. Longnecker MP. Alcoholic beverage consumption in relation to risk of breast cancer: meta-analysis and review. *Cancer Causes Control* 1994;**5**:73–82.
123. Tjonneland A, Christensen J, Olsen A, Stripp C, Thomsen BL, Overvad K, et al. Alcohol intake and breast cancer risk: the European Prospective Investigation into Cancer and Nutrition (EPIC). *Cancer Causes Control* 2007;**18**:361–73.
124. Lew JQ, Freedman ND, Leitzmann MF, Brinton LA, Hoover RN, Hollenbeck AR, et al. Alcohol and risk of breast cancer by histologic type and hormone receptor status in postmenopausal women: the NIH-AARP Diet and Health Study. *Am J Epidemiol* 2009;**170**:308–17.
125. Harvey EB, Schairer C, Brinton LA, Hoover RN, Fraumeni JF, et al. Alcohol consumption and breast cancer. *J Natl Cancer Inst* 1987;**78**:657–61.
126. Longnecker MP, Newcomb PA, Mittendorf R, Greenberg ER, Clapp RW, Bogdan GF, et al. Risk of breast cancer in relation to lifetime alcohol consumption. *J Natl Cancer Inst* 1995;**87**:923–9.
127. Berstad P, Ma H, Bernstein L, Ursin G. Alcohol intake and breast cancer risk among young women. *Breast Cancer Res Treat* 2008;**108**:113–20.
128. Swanson CA, Coates RJ, Malone KE, Gammon MD, Schoenberg JB, Brogan DJ, et al. Alcohol consumption and breast cancer risk among women under age 45 years. *Epidemiology* 1997;**8**:231–7.
129. Hankinson SE, Willett WC, Manson JE, Hunter DJ, Colditz GA, Stampfer MJ, et al. Alcohol, height, and adiposity in relation to estrogen and prolactin levels in postmenopausal women. *J Natl Cancer Inst* 1995;**87**:1297–302.
130. Reichman ME, Judd JT, Longcope C, Schatzkin A, Clevidence BA, Nair PP, et al. Effects of alcohol consumption on plasma and urinary hormone concentrations in premenopausal women. *J Natl Cancer Inst* 1993;**85**:722–7.
131. Flom JD, Ferris JS, Tehranifar P, Terry MB. Alcohol intake over the life course and mammographic density. *Breast Cancer Res Treat* 2009;**117**:643–51.
132. Tseng M, Weinberg CR, Umbach DM, Longnecker MP. Calculation of population attributable risk for alcohol and breast cancer (United States). *Cancer Causes Control* 1999;**10**:119–23.
133. Brinton LA, Daling JR, Liff JM, Schoenberg JB, Malone KE, Stanford JL, et al. Oral contraceptives and breast cancer risk among younger women. *J Natl Cancer Inst* 1995;**87**:827–35.
134. Hankinson SE, Colditz GA, Manson JE, Willett WC, Hunter DJ, Stampfer MJ, et al. A prospective study of oral contraceptive use and risk of breast cancer (Nurses' Health Study, United States). *Cancer Causes Control* 1997;**8**:65–72.
135. Romieu I, Berlin JA, Colditz G. Oral contraceptives and breast cancer. Review and meta-analysis. *Cancer* 1990;**66**:2253–63.
136. White E, Malone KE, Weiss NS, Daling JR. Breast cancer among young U.S. women in relation to oral contraceptive use. *J Natl Cancer Inst* 1994;**86**:505–14.
137. Collaborative Group on Hormonal Factors in Breast Cancer. Breast cancer and hormonal contraceptives: collaborative reanalysis of individual data on 53 297 women with breast cancer and 100 239 women without breast cancer from 54 epidemiological studies. Collaborative Group on Hormonal Factors in Breast Cancer. *Lancet* 1996;**347**:1713–27.
138. Nyante SJ, Gammon MD, Malone KE, Daling JR, Brinton LA. The association between oral contraceptive use and lobular and ductal breast cancer in young women. *Int J Cancer* 2008;**122**:936–41.
139. Wingo PA, Lee NC, Ory HW, Peterson HB, Rhodes P. Age-specific differences in the relationship between oral contraceptive use and breast cancer. *Obstet Gynecol* 1991;**78**:161–70.
140. Narod SA, Dube MP, Klijn J, Lubinski J, Lynch HT, Ghadirian P, et al. Oral contraceptives and the risk of breast cancer in BRCA1 and BRCA2 mutation carriers. *J Natl Cancer Inst* 2002;**94**:1773–9.
141. Ursin G, Henderson BE, Haile RW, Pike MC, Zhou N, Diep A, et al. Does oral contraceptive use increase the risk of breast cancer in women with BRCA1/BRCA2 mutations more than in other women? *Cancer Res* 1997;**57**:3678–81.
142. Shapiro S, Rosenberg L, Hoffman M, Truter H, Cooper D, Rao S, et al. Risk of breast cancer in relation to the use of injectable progestogen contraceptives and combined estrogen/progestogen contraceptives. *Am J Epidemiol* 2000;**151**:396–403.
143. Collaborative Group on Hormonal Factors in Breast Cancer. Breast cancer and hormone replacement therapy: collaborative reanalysis of data from 51 epidemiological studies of 52,705 women with breast cancer and 108,411 women without breast cancer. Collaborative Group on Hormonal Factors in Breast Cancer. *Lancet* 1997;**350**:1047–59.
144. The Writing Group for the PEPI Trial. Effects of hormone replacement therapy on endometrial histology in postmenopausal women. The Postmenopausal Estrogen/Progestin Interventions (PEPI) Trial. The Writing Group for the PEPI Trial. *JAMA* 1996;**275**:370–5.
145. Colditz GA, Hankinson SE, Hunter DJ, Willett WC, Manson JE, Stampfer MJ, et al. The use of estrogens and progestins and the risk of breast cancer in postmenopausal women. *N Engl J Med* 1995;**332**:1589–93.
146. Schairer C, Lubin J, Troisi R, Sturgeon S, Brinton L, Hoover R. Menopausal estrogen and estrogen-progestin replacement therapy and breast cancer risk. *JAMA* 2000;**283**:485–91.
147. Magnusson C, Baron JA, Correia N, Bergström R, Adami HO, Persson I. Breast-cancer risk following long-term oestrogen- and oestrogen-progestin-replacement therapy. *Int J Cancer* 1999;**81**:339–44.
148. Ross RK, Paganini-Hill A, Wan PC, Pike MC. Effect of hormone replacement therapy on breast cancer risk: estrogen versus estrogen plus progestin. *J Natl Cancer Inst* 2000;**92**:328–32.
149. Rossouw JE, Anderson GL, Prentice RL, LaCroix AZ, Kooperberg C, Stefanick ML, et al. Risks and benefits of estrogen plus progestin in healthy postmenopausal women: principal results from

the Women's Health Initiative randomized controlled trial. *JAMA* 2002;**288**:321-33.

150. Chlebowski RT, Kuller LH, Prentice RL, Stefanick ML, Manson JE, Gass M, et al. Breast cancer after use of estrogen plus progestin in postmenopausal women. *N Engl J Med* 2009;**360**:573-87.
151. McTiernan A, Martin CF, Peck JD, Aragaki AK, Chlebowski RT, Pisano ED, et al. Estrogen-plus-progestin use and mammographic density in postmenopausal women: Women's Health Initiative randomized trial. *J Natl Cancer Inst* 2005;**97**:1366-76.
152. Chlebowski RT, Anderson G, Pettinger M, Lane D, Langer RD, Gilligan MA, et al. Estrogen plus progestin and breast cancer detection by means of mammography and breast biopsy. *Arch Intern Med* 2008;**168**:370-7 quiz 345.
153. Ravdin PM. Hormone replacement therapy and the increase in the incidence of invasive lobular cancer. *Breast Dis* 2009;**30**:3-8.
154. Powles T, Eeles R, Ashley S, Easton D, Chang J, Dowsett M, et al. Interim analysis of the incidence of breast cancer in the Royal Marsden Hospital tamoxifen randomised chemoprevention trial. *Lancet* 1998;**352**:98-101.
155. Veronesi U, Maisonneuve P, Costa A, Sacchini V, Maltoni C, Robertson C, et al. Prevention of breast cancer with tamoxifen: preliminary findings from the Italian randomised trial among hysterectomised women. Italian Tamoxifen Prevention Study. *Lancet* 1998;**352**:93-7.
156. Cummings SR, Eckert S, Krueger KA, Grady D, Powles TJ, Cauley JA, et al. The effect of raloxifene on risk of breast cancer in postmenopausal women: results from the MORE randomized trial. Multiple Outcomes of Raloxifene Evaluation. *JAMA* 1999;**281**:2189-97.
157. Ford LG, Minasian LM, McCaskill-Stevens W, Pisano ED, Sullivan D, Smith RA. Prevention and early detection clinical trials: opportunities for primary care providers and their patients. *CA Cancer J Clin* 2003;**53**:82-101.
158. Dupont WD, Page DL. Risk factors for breast cancer in women with proliferative breast disease. *N Engl J Med* 1985;**312**:146-51.
159. Wolfe JN, Saftlas AF, Salane M. Mammographic parenchymal patterns and quantitative evaluation of mammographic densities: a case-control study. *AJR Am J Roentgenol* 1987;**148**:1087-92.
160. Byrne C, Schairer C, Wolfe J, Parekh N, Salane M, Brinton LA, et al. Mammographic features and breast cancer risk: effects with time, age, and menopause status. *J Natl Cancer Inst* 1995;**87**:1622-9.
161. Boyd NF, Dite GS, Stone J, Gunasekara A, English DR, McCredie MR, et al. Heritability of mammographic density, a risk factor for breast cancer. *N Engl J Med* 2002;**347**:886-94.
162. Greendale GA, Reboussin BA, Slone S, Wasilauskas C, Pike MC, Ursin G. Postmenopausal hormone therapy and change in mammographic density. *J Natl Cancer Inst* 2003;**95**:30-7.
163. Boyd NF, Guo H, Martin LJ, Sun L, Stone J, Fishell E, et al. Mammographic density and the risk and detection of breast cancer. *N Engl J Med* 2007;**356**:227-36.
164. Ramsey SD, Yoon P, Moonesinghe R, Khoury MJ. Population-based study of the prevalence of family history of cancer: implications for cancer screening and prevention. *Genet Med* 2006;**8**:571-5.
165. Collaborative Group on Hormonal Factors in Breast Cancer. Familial breast cancer: collaborative reanalysis of individual data from 52 epidemiological studies including 58,209 women with breast cancer and 101,986 women without the disease. *Lancet* 2001;**358**:1389-99.
166. Pharoah PD, Lipscombe JM, Redman KL, Day NE, Easton DF, Ponder BA. Familial predisposition to breast cancer in a British population: implications for prevention. *Eur J Cancer* 2000;**36**:773-9.
167. Anglian Breast Cancer Study Group. Prevalence and penetrance of BRCA1 and BRCA2 mutations in a population-based series of breast cancer cases. Anglian Breast Cancer Study Group. *Br J Cancer* 2000;**83**:1301-8.
168. Claus EB, Schildkraut JM, Thompson WD, Risch NJ. The genetic attributable risk of breast and ovarian cancer. *Cancer* 1996;**77**:2318-24.
169. Ford D, Easton DF, Peto J. Estimates of the gene frequency of BRCA1 and its contribution to breast and ovarian cancer incidence. *Am J Hum Genet* 1995;**57**:1457-62.
170. Wooster R, Weber BL. Breast and ovarian cancer. *N Engl J Med* 2003;**348**:2339-47.
171. Pharoah PD, Day NE, Duffy S, Easton DF, Ponder BA. Family history and the risk of breast cancer: a systematic review and meta-analysis. *Int J Cancer* 1997;**71**:800-9.
172. Claus EB, Risch N, Thompson WD. Autosomal dominant inheritance of early-onset breast cancer. Implications for risk prediction. *Cancer* 1994;**73**:643-51.
173. Hoskins KF, Stopfer JE, Calzone KA, Merajver SD, Rebbeck TR, Garber JE, et al. Assessment and counseling for women with a family history of breast cancer. A guide for clinicians. *JAMA* 1995;**273**:577-85.
174. Eerola H, Blomqvist C, Pukkala E, Pyrhönen S, Nevanlinna H. Familial breast cancer in southern Finland: how prevalent are breast cancer families and can we trust the family history reported by patients? *Eur J Cancer* 2000;**36**:1143-8.
175. Parent ME, Ghadirian P, Lacroix A, et al. The reliability of recollections of family history: implications for the medical provider. *J Cancer Educ* 1997;**12**:114-20.
176. Saslow D, Boates C, Burke W, Harms S, Leach MO, Lehman CD, et al; American Cancer Society Breast Cancer Advisory Group. American Cancer Society guidelines for breast screening with MRI as an adjunct to mammography. *CA Cancer J Clin* 2007;**57**:75-89. Available at http://caonline.amcancersoc.org [Accessed June 8, 2010].
177. Gail MH, Brinton LA, Byar DP, Corle DK, Green SB, Schairer C, et al. Projecting individualized probabilities of developing breast cancer for white females who are being examined annually. *J Natl Cancer Inst* 1989;**81**:1879-86.
178. Tyrer J, Duffy SW, Cuzick J. A breast cancer prediction model incorporating familial and personal risk factors. *Stat Med* 2004;**23**:1111-30.
179. Petrucelli N, Daly MB, Feldman GL. Hereditary breast and ovarian cancer due to mutations in BRCA1 and BRCA2. *Genet Med* 2010;**12**:245-59.
180. Struewing JP, Abeliovich D, Peretz T, Avishai N, Kaback MM, Collins FS, et al. The carrier frequency of the BRCA1 185delAG mutation is approximately 1 percent in Ashkenazi Jewish individuals. *Nat Genet* 1995;**11**:198-200.
181. Lynch HT, Watson P. Early age at breast cancer onset–a genetic and oncologic perspective. *Am J Epidemiol* 1990;**131**:984-6.
182. Claus EB, Risch N, Thompson WD. Genetic analysis of breast cancer in the cancer and steroid hormone study. *Am J Hum Genet* 1991;**48**:232-42.
183. Antoniou AC, Cunningham AP, Peto J, Evans DG, Lalloo F, Narod SA, et al. The BOADICEA model of genetic susceptibility to breast and ovarian cancers: updates and extensions. *Br J Cancer* 2008;**98**:1457-66.
184. Parmigiani G, Chen S, Iversen ES Jr, Friebel TM, Finkelstein DM, Anton-Culver H, et al. Validity of models for predicting BRCA1 and BRCA2 mutations. *Ann Intern Med* 2007;**147**:441-50.
185. Ford D, Easton DF, Stratton M, Narod S, Goldgar D, Devilee P, et al. Genetic heterogeneity and penetrance analysis of the BRCA1 and BRCA2 genes in breast cancer families. The Breast Cancer Linkage Consortium. *Am J Hum Genet* 1998;**62**:676-89.
186. Hall JM, Lee MK, Newman B, Morrow JE, Anderson LA, Huey B, et al. Linkage of early-onset familial breast cancer to chromosome 17q21. *Science* 1990;**250**:1684-9.
187. Narod SA, Feunteun J, Lynch HT, Watson P, Conway T, Lynch J, et al. Familial breast-ovarian cancer locus on chromosome 17q12-q23. *Lancet* 1991;**338**:82-3.
188. Miki Y, Swensen J, Shattuck-Eidens D, Futreal PA, Harshman K, Tavtigian S, et al. A strong candidate for the breast and ovarian cancer susceptibility gene BRCA1. *Science* 1994;**266**:66-71.
189. Gudmundsdottir K, Ashworth A. The roles of BRCA1 and BRCA2 and associated proteins in the maintenance of genomic stability. *Oncogene* 2006;**25**:5864-74.
190. Frank TS, Deffenbaugh AM, Reid JE, Hulick M, Ward BE, Lingenfelter B, et al. Clinical characteristics of individuals with germline mutations in BRCA1 and BRCA2: analysis of 10,000 individuals. *J Clin Oncol* 2002;**20**:1480-90.
191. Ford D, Easton DF, Bishop DT, Narod SA, Goldgar DE. Risks of cancer in BRCA1-mutation carriers. Breast Cancer Linkage Consortium. *Lancet* 1994;**343**:692-5.
192. Chen S, Parmigiani G. Meta-analysis of BRCA1 and BRCA2 penetrance. *J Clin Oncol* 2007;**25**:1329-33.
193. Levine DA, Argenta PA, Yee CJ, Marshall DS, Olvera N, Bogomolniy F, et al. Fallopian tube and primary peritoneal carcinomas associated with BRCA mutations. *J Clin Oncol* 2003;**21**:4222-7.
194. Liede A, Karlan BY, Narod SA. Cancer risks for male carriers of germline mutations in BRCA1 or BRCA2: a review of the literature. *J Clin Oncol* 2004;**22**:735-42.

195. Tai YC, Domchek S, Parmigiani G, Chen S. Breast cancer risk among male BRCA1 and BRCA2 mutation carriers. *J Natl Cancer Inst* 2007;**99**:1811-4.
196. Wooster R, Neuhausen SL, Mangion J, Quirk Y, Ford D, Collins N. Localization of a breast cancer susceptibility gene, BRCA2, to chromosome 13q12-13. *Science* 1994;**265**:2088-90.
197. Warner E, Foulkes W, Goodwin P, Meschino W, Blondal J, Paterson C, et al. Prevalence and penetrance of BRCA1 and BRCA2 gene mutations in unselected Ashkenazi Jewish women with breast cancer. *J Natl Cancer Inst* 1999;**91**:1241-7.
198. Giusti RM, Rutter JL, Duray PH, Freedman LS, Konichezky M, Fisher-Fischbein J, et al. A twofold increase in BRCA mutation related prostate cancer among Ashkenazi Israelis is not associated with distinctive histopathology. *J Med Genet* 2003;**40**:787-92.
199. Moslehi R, Chu W, Karlan B, Fishman D, Risch H, Fields A, et al. BRCA1 and BRCA2 mutation analysis of 208 Ashkenazi Jewish women with ovarian cancer. *Am J Hum Genet* 2000;**66**:1259-72.
200. Phelan CM, Kwan E, Jack E, Li S, Morgan C, Aubé J, et al. A low frequency of non-founder BRCA1 mutations in Ashkenazi Jewish breast-ovarian cancer families. *Hum Mutat* 2002;**20**:352-7.
201. Schubert EL, Mefford HC, Dann JL, Argonza RH, Hull J, King MC. BRCA1 and BRCA2 mutations in Ashkenazi Jewish families with breast and ovarian cancer. *Genet Test* 1997;**1**:41-6.
202. Oddoux C, Struewing JP, Clayton CM, Neuhausen S, Brody LC, Kaback M, et al. The carrier frequency of the BRCA2 6174delT mutation among Ashkenazi Jewish individuals is approximately 1%. *Nat Genet* 1996;**14**:188-90.
203. Roa BB, Boyd AA, Volcik K, Richards CS. Ashkenazi Jewish population frequencies for common mutations in BRCA1 and BRCA2. *Nat Genet* 1996;**14**:185-7.
204. Whittemore AS, Gong G, John EM, McGuire V, Li FP, Ostrow KL, et al. Prevalence of BRCA1 mutation carriers among U.S. non-Hispanic whites. *Cancer Epidemiol Biomarkers Prev* 2004;**13**:2078-83.
205. Tonin PN, Mes-Masson AM, Futreal PA, Morgan K, Mahon M, Foulkes WD, et al. Founder BRCA1 and BRCA2 mutations in French Canadian breast and ovarian cancer families. *Am J Hum Genet* 1998;**63**:1341-51.
206. Arason A, Jonasdottir A, Barkardottir RB, Bergthorsson JT, Teare MD, Easton DF, et al. A population study of mutations and LOH at breast cancer gene loci in tumours from sister pairs: two recurrent mutations seem to account for all BRCA1/BRCA2 linked breast cancer in Iceland. *J Med Genet* 1998;**35**:446-9.
207. Petrij-Bosch A, Peelen T, van Vliet M, van Eijk R, Olmer R, Drüsedau M, et al. BRCA1 genomic deletions are major founder mutations in Dutch breast cancer patients. *Nat Genet* 1997;**17**:341-5.
208. Sekine M, Nagata H, Tsuji S, Hirai Y, Fujimoto S, Hatae M, et al. Mutational analysis of BRCA1 and BRCA2 and clinicopathologic analysis of ovarian cancer in 82 ovarian cancer families: two common founder mutations of BRCA1 in Japanese population. *Clin Cancer Res* 2001;**7**:3144-50.
209. Li FP, Fraumeni JF. Soft-tissue sarcomas, breast cancer, and other neoplasms. A familial syndrome. *Ann Intern Med* 1969;**71**:747-52.
210. Li FP, Fraumeni JF, Mulvihill JJ, Blattner WA, Dreyfus MG, Tucker MA, et al. A cancer family syndrome in twenty-four kindreds. *Cancer Res* 1988;**48**:5358-62.
211. Olivier M, Goldgar DE, Sodha N, Ohgaki H, Kleihues P, Hainaut P, et al. Li-Fraumeni and related syndromes: correlation between tumor type, family structure, and TP53 genotype. *Cancer Res* 2003;**63**:6643-50.
212. Gonzalez KD, Noltner KA, Buzin CH, Gu D, Wen-Fong CY, Nguyen VQ, et al. Beyond Li Fraumeni Syndrome: clinical characteristics of families with p53 germline mutations. *J Clin Oncol* 2009;**27**:1250-6.
213. Hisada M, Garber JE, Fung CY, Fraumeni JF, Li FP. Multiple primary cancers in families with Li-Fraumeni syndrome. *J Natl Cancer Inst* 1998;**90**:606-11.
214. Hwang SJ, Lozano G, Amos CI, Strong LC. Germline p53 mutations in a cohort with childhood sarcoma: sex differences in cancer risk. *Am J Hum Genet* 2003;**72**:975-83.
215. Martin AM, Kanetsky PA, Amirimani B, Colligon TA, Athanasiadis G, Shih HA, et al. Germline TP53 mutations in breast cancer families with multiple primary cancers: is TP53 a modifier of BRCA1? *J Med Genet* 2003;**40**:e34.
216. Bell DW, Varley JM, Szydlo TE, Kang DH, Wahrer DC, Shannon KE, et al. Heterozygous germ line hCHK2 mutations in Li-Fraumeni syndrome. *Science* 1999;**286**:2528-31.
217. Siddiqui R, Onel K, Facio F, Nafa K, Diaz LR, Kauff N, et al. The TP53 mutational spectrum and frequency of CHEK2*1100delC in Li-Fraumeni-like kindreds. *Fam Cancer* 2005;**4**:177-81.
218. Nelen MR, Padberg GW, Peeters EA, Lin AY, van den Helm B, Frants RR, et al. Localization of the gene for Cowden disease to chromosome 10q22-23. *Nat Genet* 1996;**13**:114-6.
219. Pilarski R, Eng C. Will the real Cowden syndrome please stand up (again)? Expanding mutational and clinical spectra of the PTEN hamartoma tumour syndrome. *J Med Genet* 2004;**41**:323-6.
220. Nelen MR, Kremer H, Konings IB, Schoute F, van Essen AJ, Koch R, et al. Novel PTEN mutations in patients with Cowden disease: absence of clear genotype-phenotype correlations. *Eur J Hum Genet* 1999;**7**:267-73.
221. Hemminki A, Markie D, Tomlinson I, Avizienyte E, Roth S, Loukola A, et al. A serine/threonine kinase gene defective in Peutz-Jeghers syndrome. *Nature* 1998;**391**:184-7.
222. Jenne DE, Reimann H, Nezu J, Friedel W, Loff S, Jeschke R, et al. Peutz-Jeghers syndrome is caused by mutations in a novel serine threonine kinase. *Nat Genet* 1998;**18**:38-43.
223. Hearle N, Schumacher V, Menko FH, Olschwang S, Boardman LA, Gille JJ, et al. Frequency and spectrum of cancers in the Peutz-Jeghers syndrome. *Clin Cancer Res* 2006;**12**:3209-15.
224. Giardiello FM, Brensinger JD, Tersmette AC, Goodman SN, Petersen GM, Booker SV, et al. Very high risk of cancer in familial Peutz-Jeghers syndrome. *Gastroenterology* 2000;**119**:1447-53.
225. Cisco RM, Norton JA. Hereditary diffuse gastric cancer: surgery, surveillance and unanswered questions. *Future Oncol* 2008;**4**:553-9.
226. Pharoah PD, Guilford P, Caldas C. Incidence of gastric cancer and breast cancer in CDH1 (E-cadherin) mutation carriers from hereditary diffuse gastric cancer families. *Gastroenterology* 2001;**121**:1348-53.
227. Kaurah P, MacMillan A, Boyd N, Senz J, De Luca A, Chun N, et al. Founder and recurrent CDH1 mutations in families with hereditary diffuse gastric cancer. *JAMA* 2007;**297**:2360-72.
228. Suriano G, Yew S, Ferreira P, Senz J, Kaurah P, Ford JM, et al. Characterization of a recurrent germ line mutation of the E-cadherin gene: implications for genetic testing and clinical management. *Clin Cancer Res* 2005;**11**:5401-9.
229. Easton DF. How many more breast cancer predisposition genes are there? *Breast Cancer Res* 1999;**1**:14-7.
230. Pharoah PD, Antoniou A, Bobrow M, Zimmern RL, Easton DF, Ponder BA. Polygenic susceptibility to breast cancer and implications for prevention. *Nat Genet* 2002;**31**:33-6.
231. Savitsky K, Sfez S, Tagle DA, Ziv Y, Sartiel A, Collins FS, et al. The complete sequence of the coding region of the ATM gene reveals similarity to cell cycle regulators in different species. *Hum Mol Genet* 1995;**4**:2025-32.
232. Boder E. Ataxia-telangiectasia: some historic, clinical and pathologic observations. *Birth Defects Orig Artic Ser* 1975;**11**:255-70.
233. Epstein WL, Fudenberg HH, Reed WB, Boder E, Sedgwick RP. Immunologic studies in ataxia-telangiectasia. I. Delayed hypersensitivity and serum immune globulin levels in probands and first-degree relatives. *Int Arch Allergy Appl Immunol* 1966;**30**:15-29.
234. Swift M, Morrell D, Cromartie E, Chamberlin AR, Skolnick MH, Bishop DT. The incidence and gene frequency of ataxia-telangiectasia in the United States. *Am J Hum Genet* 1986;**39**:573-83.
235. Weeks DE, Paterson MC, Lange K, Andrais B, Davis RC, Yoder F, et al. Assessment of chronic gamma radiosensitivity as an in vitro assay for heterozygote identification of ataxia-telangiectasia. *Radiat Res* 1991;**128**:90-9.
236. Weil MM, Kittrell FS, Yu Y, McCarthy M, Zabriskie RC, Ullrich RL. Radiation induces genomic instability and mammary ductal dysplasia in Atm heterozygous mice. *Oncogene* 2001;**20**:4409-11.
237. Swift M, Sholman L, Perry M, Chase C. Malignant neoplasms in the families of patients with ataxia-telangiectasia. *Cancer Res* 1976;**36**:209-15.
238. Su Y, Swift M. Mortality rates among carriers of ataxia-telangiectasia mutant alleles. *Ann Intern Med* 2000;**133**:770-8.

239. Renwick A, Thompson D, Seal S, Kelly P, Chagtai T, Ahmed M, et al. ATM mutations that cause ataxia-telangiectasia are breast cancer susceptibility alleles. *Nat Genet* 2006;**38**:873-5.
240. Thompson D, Duedal S, Kirner J, McGuffog L, Last J, Reiman A, et al. Cancer risks and mortality in heterozygous ATM mutation carriers. *J Natl Cancer Inst* 2005;**97**:813-22.
241. Chenevix-Trench G, Spurdle AB, Gatei M, Kelly H, Marsh A, Chen X, et al. Dominant negative ATM mutations in breast cancer families. *J Natl Cancer Inst* 2002;**94**:205-15.
242. Larson GP, Zhang G, Ding S, Foldenauer K, Udar N, Gatti RA, et al. An allelic variant at the ATM locus is implicated in breast cancer susceptibility. *Genet Test* 1997;**1**:165-70.
243. Paglia LL, Lauge A, Weber J, Champ J, Cavaciuti E, Russo A, et al. ATM germline mutations in women with familial breast cancer and a relative with haematological malignancy. *Breast Cancer Res Treat* 2010;**119**:443-52.
244. Teraoka SN, Malone KE, Doody DR, Suter NM, Ostrander EA, Daling JR, et al. Increased frequency of ATM mutations in breast carcinoma patients with early onset disease and positive family history. *Cancer* 2001;**92**:479-87.
245. Athma P, Rappaport R, Swift M. Molecular genotyping shows that ataxia-telangiectasia heterozygotes are predisposed to breast cancer. *Cancer Genet Cytogenet* 1996;**92**:130-4.
246. Antoni L, Sodha N, Collins I, Garrett MD. CHK2 kinase: cancer susceptibility and cancer therapy - two sides of the same coin? *Nat Rev Cancer* 2007;**7**:925-36.
247. Vahteristo P, Bartkova J, Eerola H, Syrjäkoski K, Ojala S, Kilpivaara O, et al. A CHEK2 genetic variant contributing to a substantial fraction of familial breast cancer. *Am J Hum Genet* 2002;**71**:432-8.
248. Meijers-Heijboer H, van den Ouweland A, Klijn J, Wasielewski M, de Snoo A, Oldenburg R, et al. Low-penetrance susceptibility to breast cancer due to CHEK2(*)1100delC in noncarriers of BRCA1 or BRCA2 mutations. *Nat Genet* 2002;**31**:55-9.
249. Weischer M, Bojesen SE, Ellervik C, Tybjaerg-Hansen A, Nordestgaard BG. CHEK2*1100delC genotyping for clinical assessment of breast cancer risk: meta-analyses of 26,000 patient cases and 27,000 controls. *J Clin Oncol* 2008;**26**:542-8.
250. Kaufman B, Laitman Y, Gronwald J, Winqvist R, Irmejs A, Lubinski J, et al. Haplotypes of the I157T CHEK2 germline mutation in ethnically diverse populations. *Fam Cancer* 2009;**8**:473-8.
251. Lee SB, Kim SH, Bell DW, Wahrer DC, Schiripo TA, Jorczak MM, et al. Destabilization of CHK2 by a missense mutation associated with Li-Fraumeni syndrome. *Cancer Res* 2001;**61**:8062-7.
252. Vahteristo P, Tamminen A, Karvinen P, Eerola H, Eklund C, Aaltonen LA, et al. p53, CHK2, and CHK1 genes in Finnish families with Li-Fraumeni syndrome: further evidence of CHK2 in inherited cancer predisposition. *Cancer Res* 2001;**61**:5718-22.
253. Levitus M, Waisfisz Q, Godthelp BC, de Vries Y, Hussain S, Wiegant WW, et al. The DNA helicase BRIP1 is defective in Fanconi anemia complementation group. *J Nat Genet* 2005;**37**:934-5.
254. Reid S, Schindler D, Hanenberg H, Barker K, Hanks S, Kalb R, et al. Biallelic mutations in PALB2 cause Fanconi anemia subtype FA-N and predispose to childhood cancer. *Nat Genet* 2007;**39**:162-4.
255. Rahman N, Seal S, Thompson D, Kelly P, Renwick A, Elliott A, et al. PALB2, which encodes a BRCA2-interacting protein, is a breast cancer susceptibility gene. *Nat Genet* 2007;**39**:165-7.
256. Seal S, Thompson D, Renwick A, Elliott A, Kelly P, Barfoot R, et al. Truncating mutations in the Fanconi anemia J gene BRIP1 are low-penetrance breast cancer susceptibility alleles. *Nat Genet* 2006;**38**:1239-41.
257. Erkko H, Dowty JG, Nikkila J, Syrjäkoski K, Mannermaa A, Pylkäs K, et al. Penetrance analysis of the PALB2 c.1592delT founder mutation. *Clin Cancer Res* 2008;**14**:4667-71.
258. Turnbull C, Ahmed S, Morrison J, Pernet D, Renwick A, Maranian M, et al. Genome-wide association study identifies five new breast cancer susceptibility loci. *Nat Genet* 2010;**42**:504-7.
259. Seidman H, Stellman SD, Mushinski MH. A different perspective on breast cancer risk factors: some implications of the nonattributable risk. *CA Cancer J Clin* 1982;**32**:301-13.
260. Smith RA. Risk-based screening for breast cancer: Is there a practical strategy? *Semin Breast Dis* 1999;**2**:280-91.

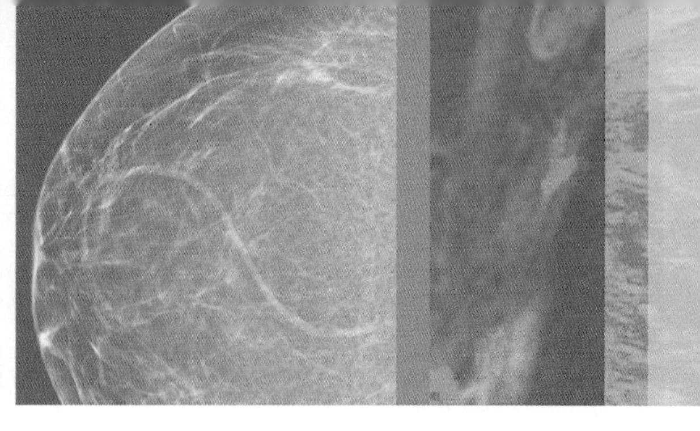

CHAPTER 3

Screening Results, Controversies, and Guidelines

Stephen A. Feig and Stephen W. Duffy

Screening is the periodic examination of a population to detect previously unrecognized disease. Breast cancer screening may be performed by means of mammography, clinical examination, and breast self-examination (BSE), alone or in combination. By definition, a breast cancer screening test is performed only on women who have no clinical abnormality to suggest breast cancer, although they may be at increased risk because of factors such as age, family history, and nulliparity. When the same test, such as mammography or clinical examination, is performed to evaluate a clinical sign or symptom or to evaluate an abnormality detected at screening, it is referred to as a *diagnostic (problem-solving) test*. Diagnostic testing is performed on an individual woman to answer a specific clinical question, such as the nature of her breast lump or nipple discharge, but screening is performed on large segments of the population as a public health measure.

Requirements for a screening test differ from those for a diagnostic test and include adequate sensitivity to detect early disease, acceptable specificity to minimize false-positive results, low risk, acceptable cost and cost-benefit ratio, availability of necessary equipment, and interpretive and performance expertise. Because the ultimate goal of screening is reduction in the number of deaths from breast cancer, of a statistically significant reduction in breast cancer mortality in a randomized controlled trial (RCT) is the 'gold standard' for proving benefit. Thus far, this result has been documented for mammography but not for physical examination or BSE alone.

SCREENING MODALITIES

Mammography, clinical examination, and BSE are complementary screening methods: Each modality should be capable of detecting cancers that are missed by one or both of the others. Detection by clinical examination or BSE depends on appreciation of tactile differences between a tumor and surrounding tissue. Presence of these tactile characteristics does not necessarily mean that a correspondingly visible mammographic finding will be present, especially in mammographically dense fibroglandular breasts. BSE may be advantageous in that it can be performed on a monthly basis and may detect interval cancers that surface between annual mammographic and clinical screenings. However, smaller tumors with higher survival rates are more likely to be detected by mammography than by clinical examination or BSE.[1]

The Breast Cancer Detection Demonstration Project (BCDDP), sponsored by the American Cancer Society (ACS) and National Cancer Institute (NCI), was a program that screened 280,000 women throughout the United States with both mammography and physical examination from 1973 to 1981. In this program, 39% (1375) of the 3548 cancers were found by mammography alone, 7% (257) by clinical examination alone, and 51% (1805) by both mammography and clinical examination. Moreover, the rate of detection at clinical examination was lowest for earlier-stage lesions. Of the 983 minimal cancers (invasive carcinoma measuring less than 1 cm and all ductal carcinoma in situ [DCIS]), 54% (484) were detected by mammography alone, 5% (42) by clinical examination alone, and 38% (340) by both mammography and clinical examination.[2]

Mammography is a more sensitive means of early detection than clinical examination or BSE. However, among women screened by both mammography and clinical examination, about 5% to 10% of detected cancers are found by clinical examination alone. BSE has been less efficient than mammography and clinical examination.[3] Breast cancer screening is most effective when all three modalities are used. The relative efficacy of any detection method depends on the quality of the examination being practiced. Major improvements in mammography since 1985, and especially since 1990, have enabled earlier detection of lesions than was possible in the BCDDP.[4]

Breast magnetic resonance imaging (MRI) can detect cancers missed by screening mammography and is recommended for supplementary screening of very high risk women. However, the high cost and need for intravenous contrast injection preclude the use of MRI for screening women at average risk.[5] Breast ultrasound can detect cancers missed by mammography in dense breasts. However high false positive biopsy rates are a current drawback to breast ultrasound screening.[6,7]

Digital mammography has proven to be useful for screening because its sensitivity and specificity have been shown to be comparable to those of conventional mammography among women aged 40 to 70 years. Additionally, digital mammography detects more cancers than film mammography in women with dense breasts and in those who are premenopausal or younger than age 50.[8]

Other modalities, such as thermography, which measures variation in breast temperature; light scanning (transillumination), which records transmission of light through the breast; and scanning with radionuclides, such as technetium Tc 99m sestamibi (^{99m}Tc-sestamibi), are still under investigation for screening.

HIGHER SURVIVAL RATES AMONG WOMEN WITH SCREENING-DETECTED CANCERS

Two related factors, tumor size and stage at time of diagnosis, represent the major determinants of survival rates among patients with breast cancer. Smaller cancers with no histologic evidence of spread to the regional lymph nodes have the best prognosis. The 20-year relative survival rates in the BCDDP were 80.5% (overall), 85% for cancers detected by mammography alone, 82% for cancers detected by physical examination alone, and 74% for cancers detected by both mammography and physical examination. Twenty-year relative survival rates were highly dependent on lesion size. The rate was 96% for in situ carcinomas. For invasive cancers, the rates were 88% for those measuring 0.1 to 0.9 cm, 78% for cancers 1.0 to 1.9 cm, 68% for cancers 2.0 to 4.9 cm, and 58% for cancers 5.0 to 9.9 cm.[9] These rates can be compared with survival data from the Surveillance Epidemiology and End Results (SEER) Program of the NCI, a population-based network of cancer registries that monitors cancer trends throughout the United States. Women with breast cancer entered into the SEER database during the BCDDP era (1973-1978), consisting largely of women who were not being screened, had a 20-year relative survival rate of 53%.[10]

Criteria for Benefit from Screening: Longer Survival versus Decreased Mortality

There are several reasons why "improved" survival rates among women who volunteer to be screened do not necessarily establish benefit from screening. They include selection bias, lead-time bias, length bias, and interval cancers.[11] Thus, differences in survival rates may be influenced by variables other than the screening process itself.

Selection bias refers to the possibility that women who volunteer for screening differ from those who do not volunteer in ways that may alter the outcome of their diseases, such as health status and behavioral factors. Therefore, survival rates in screened and nonscreened women may be influenced by variables other than the screening process itself.

Lead-time bias implies that screening may affect the date of detection but not necessarily the date of death from breast cancer. Let us suppose that a woman who has never been screened finds her breast cancer serendipitously in 2004. She dies from her disease five years later, in 2009. If this same woman had been screened, her cancer might have been detected by mammography in the year 2001. Although small, the cancer detected in this woman by mammography has microscopic dissemination beyond the breast. Despite screening, the woman will die from her disease in the year 2009. Because of screening, she is said to have survived for 8 years instead of 5 years. Therefore, the seemingly three-year improvement in survival is not real.

Length bias sampling postulates that cancers detected at screening contain a disproportionate number of less aggressive lesions. Their growth rates are so slow that in the absence of screening they might never reach sufficient size to surface clinically. Even if undetected, such cancers might never result in death.

Finally, more favorable survival rates for screen-detected cancers may be negated by lower survival rates for faster-growing *interval cancers* that are undetected by mammography and that surface clinically between screenings.

Considering these potential biases, benefit from screening cannot be proven by observation of improved survival rates. Rather, such proof requires prospective comparison of breast cancer death rates among a study group of women offered screening and a control group of women not offered screening in a RCT. Apart from the offer to be screened, these groups should not differ in any other substantial way. Therefore, a statistically significant difference in breast cancer deaths between the groups on follow-up may be considered proof of whether there is benefit from the screening. Observation of lower mortality for the screened group in a well-designed and well-conducted RCT is not affected by selection bias, lead-time bias, length bias, or interval cancers.

Results of Randomized Control Trials

Eight population-based trials of breast cancer screening by mammography alone or in combination with physical examination have been conducted. They are as follows: (1) the Health Insurance Plan of Greater New York (HIP) trial[12]; (2) the Swedish Two-County Trial consisting of Kopparberg and Östergötland counties[13]; (3) the Malmö (Sweden) Mammographic Screening Trial[14]; (4) the Stockholm (Sweden) trial[15,16]; (5) the Gothenburg (Sweden) Breast Screening Trial[17]; (6) the UK Age Trial[18]; and (7) the Edinburgh (Scotland) trial.[19] There has been one non-population-based RCT, the National Breast Screening Study (NBSS) of Canada.[20-22] In a population-based

RCT, study and control groups are randomly selected from a predefined population. In a non-population-based RCT, study and control groups are randomly selected from women who volunteer to participate.

Protocols and results for women of all ages at entry into RCT's are shown in Table 3-1. Mortality reduction is equal to 1 minus the relative risk (RR) of dying from breast cancer in the study group women versus the control group. The HIP trial, the first RCT ever conducted, found a 23% reduction in breast cancer deaths (RR = 0.77) among women aged 40 to 64 years who were offered screening mammography and physical examination.[12]

The Two-County Swedish Trial was the first to demonstrate a statistically significant benefit from screening by mammography alone. The latest 20-year follow-up for this trial found a 32% reduction in breast cancer deaths among women aged 40 to 74 years at entry.[13] In the Edinburgh trial, screening by annual physical examination and biennial mammography resulted in a statistically significant 29% decrease in breast cancer deaths among women aged 45 to 64 years at entry.[19] The Gothenburg Breast Screening Trial had a 23% reduction in deaths from breast cancer among women aged 40 to 59 years at entry into screening, a finding that had marginal statistical significance.[17]

Two Swedish screening mammography trials reported benefits that were not statistically significant. The Malmö Mammographic Screening Trial found a 19% reduction in breast cancer deaths among women who began screening between ages 45 and 69 years.[14] However, it should be noted that an extension of the Malmö trial found a significant reduction in breast cancer mortality in association with screening women aged younger than 50 years (see later discussion). The Stockholm trial described a 20% reduction in breast cancer deaths among women screened between 40 and 64 years of age.[16]

Combined results from a 15.8-year follow-up of women aged 38 to 75 years at entry into four Swedish trials (Malmö, Östergötland, Stockholm, and Gothenburg) showed a statistically significant 21% reduction in breast cancer mortality with screening.[23]

The Canadian NBSS failed to show any benefit for mammography screening in women aged 50 to 59 years. In that trial, women undergoing annual mammography and physical examination were compared with those being screening by physical examination alone.[20,21] Possible explanations for the variance between NBSS results and those of the seven other randomized trials include technical quality of mammography,[24-26] study design,[27-30] and control group contamination.[31]

In summary, of the eight randomized screening trials, seven showed evidence of benefit from screening. Breast cancer mortality reduction was statistically significant in each of three trials (HIP, Swedish Two-County, and Edinburgh) and in combined results from the Stockholm,

TABLE 3-1. Randomized Trials of Mammography Screening: Results for All Ages Combined

Trial (Years)*	Age at Entry (Years)	No. of Views	Frequency of Mammography (Months)	Rounds (No.)	CBE	Follow-up (Years)	RR (95% CI)	Mortality Reduction
Health Insurance Plan of Greater NY trial (1963-1969)[12]	40-64	2	12	4	Annual	18	0.77 (0.61-0.97)	23%†
Malmö Mammographic Screening Trial (1976-1986)[14]	45-69	1-2	18-24	5	None	12	0.81 (0.62-1.07)	19%
Swedish Two-County Trial, Kopparberg and Östergötland counties (1979-1988)[13]	40-74	1	23-33	4	None	20	0.68 (0.59-0.80)	32%†
Edinburgh trial (1979-1988)[19]	45-64	1-2	24	4	Annual	14	0.71 (0.53-0.95)	29%†
Canadian National Breast Screening Study (1980-1987)[21]	50-59	2+ CBE versus CBE	12	5	Annual	13	1.02 (0.78-1.33)	−2%
Stockholm trial (1981-1985)[15]	40-64	1	28	2	None	8	0.80 (0.53-1.22)	20%
Gothenburg Breast Screening Trial (1982-1988)[17]	40-59	2	18	4	None	14	0.77 (0.60-1.00)	23%
UK Age Trial (1991-2005)[18]	39-41	1-2	12	8	None	10	0.83 (0.66-1.04)	17%

CBE, Clinical breast examination; CI, confidence interval; RR, relative risk of death from breast cancer in study group/control group. Mortality reduction = 1 − RR.

*Superscript numbers indicate chapter references.

†Statistically significant.

Malmö, Östergötland, and Gothenburg trials, and marginally significant in the Gothenburg trial. Only one trial, the NBSS, found no evidence of benefit.

How the Controversy Regarding Screening Women 40 to 49 Years Old Began

Initial reports from the HIP trial found a difference in breast cancer death rates between study and control groups for women 50 years of age and older at entry that was apparent by year 4. However, a difference for women aged 40 to 49 years did not emerge until 7 to 8 years of follow-up. By 18 years of follow-up, the reduction in breast cancer deaths among study women aged 40 to 49 years at entry was 23%, the same as that for women aged 50 to 64 years at entry. Yet even by that time, benefit for younger women was still not statistically significant according to Shapiro and colleagues[12] who conducted and reported on the trial. This lack of statistical significance was a consequence of the relatively smaller number of younger women enrolled and the lower breast cancer incidence. Nevertheless, the apparent lack of statistically significant benefit led to controversy regarding screening of women in their 40s.[11,32,33]

However, the HIP trial was designed to determine the efficacy of screening a single group of all women aged 40 to 65 years rather than the efficacy of screening separate age groups. Attempts to subdivide the study group reduced statistical power. The observation that results for younger women lacked statistical significance has often been cited in the ongoing screening debate. The fact that the data for women aged 50 to 59 years and 60 years and older at entry, when analyzed separately, also lacked statistical significance was largely ignored.[12,34] Moreover, Chu and associates[35], using a different method of analysis, subsequently found statistically significant mortality reductions of 24% for women aged 40 to 49 years and 21% for those aged 50 to 64 years at entry into the HIP trial.

Despite the report by Chu and associates[35], some observers were still not convinced that screening would benefit women in their 40s for several reasons. Firstly, the reduction in the breast cancer death rates in the trials for younger women did not appear until several years after appearance of the reduction for women older than 50 years.[12] Secondly, results for younger women were not statistically significant for any other individual trial until 1997.

The controversy intensified in 1992 with publication of the 7-year follow-up report from the NBSS.[36] This study found no evidence of benefit among women aged 40 to 49 years who were offered five annual screenings by mammography and physical examination. There are several explanations for these disappointing results. Firstly, the technical quality of mammography was poor. During most of the trial, more than 50% of the mammograms were poor or completely unacceptable, even as assessed by the standards of the day.[25,26,37] Secondly, there are indications that the randomization process through which women were assigned to study and control groups was undermined.[28,37,38] All women were given a physical examination before randomization to the study trial. This protocol may have allowed preferential allocation of women with palpable masses (later stage breast cancers) to the study group. As a likely consequence, an excess of late-stage breast cancers and breast cancer deaths was found in the study group compared with the control group throughout the trial.[26,30]

Proof of Benefit for Screening Women Aged 40 to 49 Years

Beginning in 1993, several successive meta-analyses of combined data for multiple RCTs were performed in order to accrue a greater number of women-years of follow-up than possible from any one RCT alone. However, the earliest meta-analyses, published in 1993 and 1995, suggested little if any benefit from screening women younger than 50 years.[39-41]

Subsequent meta-analyses published by Smart and colleagues in 1995 and the Falun Meeting Committee in 1996 included later follow-up data.[42,43] These studies showed a statistically significant mortality reduction of 24%, for women aged 40 to 49 years at entry into the seven population-based RCTs (Table 3-2). They also found a 15% to 16% mortality reduction that barely missed statistical significance when the NBSS, a non-population-based RCT, was also included. A meta-analysis of these trials, published by Hendrick and colleagues in 1997, found statistically significant mortality reductions among women invited to undergo screening in their 40s: 18% for all eight RCTs and 29% for the five Swedish RCTs (see Table 3-2).[44] Thus, with increasing length of follow-up, successive meta-analyses have shown progressively greater and statistically significant mortality reductions for women who began screening between 40 and 49 years of age. Regardless of whether NBSS results are included or excluded, meta-analyses for screening women aged 40 to 49 years now show statistically significant benefit. Subsequently two other individual RCTs besides the HIP were each able to show statistically significant benefit for women aged 40 to 49 years (Table 3-3). Bjurstam and coworkers reported a statistically significant 45% mortality reduction for women aged 39 to 49 years at randomization in the Gothenburg trial.[45] Andersson and Janzon reported a statistically significant 35% breast cancer mortality reduction for women in the Malmö trial who began screening mammography at age 45 to 49 years.[46] A randomized trial of women aged 39 to 41 years at entry in the UK study showed a statistically nonsignificant 17% mortality reduction for those invited and a 24% mortality

TABLE 3-2. Meta-Analyses of Randomized Clinical Trials of Mammography Showing Statistically Significant Mortality Reduction for Women Aged 40 to 49 Years

Trials	Follow-up (yrs)	Mortality Reduction (%)
All eight trials*	10.5-18.0	15
Seven trials†	7.0-18.0	24
Five Swedish trials‡	11.4-15.2	29

*Health Insurance Plan of Greater New York (HIP), five Swedish trials, Edinburgh trial, UK Age Trial and National Breast Screening Study of Canada (NBSS-1).
†All trials except NBSS-1.
‡Malmö Mammographic Screening Trial; Swedish Two-County Trial, Kopparberg and Östergötland; Stockholm trial; and Gothenburg Breast Screening Trial.
Data from references 42-44.

TABLE 3-3. Follow-up of Randomized Clinical Trials of Mammography Showing Statistically Significant Breast Cancer Mortality Reduction for Women Aged 40 to 49 Years

Trial (years)*	Age at Entry (yrs)	No. of Views	Frequency of Mammography (mos)	Clinical Breast Exam	Follow-up (yrs)	Mortality Reduction (%)
Health Insurance Plan of Greater NY (1963-1969)[35]	40-49	2	12	Annual	18.0	24
Malmö Mammographic Screening Program (1976-1990)[46]	45-49	1-2	18-24	None	12.7	36
Gothenburg Breast Screening Trial (1982-1988)[45]	39-49	2	18	None	12.0	45

*Superscript numbers indicate chapter references.

reduction for those actually screened.[18] Deficiencies that restricted results in this study included use of one rather than two mammographic views on incidence screens, failure to biopsy many calcifications, low recall rates, insufficient women-years of follow-up, a low 68% compliance rate, considerable contamination of the 'unscreened' control population with private facilities offering mammograms, and mortality follow-up limited to 10 years. Later analysis likely to show much more benefits.

We also now have data from three "service screening" studies, each showing statistically significant mortality reduction from screening women aged 40 to 49 years, equal to that found for screening older women in these same studies. In Östergötland and Dalarma Counties in Sweden, Tabár and coworkers found breast cancer mortality reductions of 48% for women aged 40 to 49 years and 44% for all women aged 40 to 69 years. No such decline was seen in the 20-to 39-year age group, in which none were offered screening.[47] In British Columbia, Coldman and associates found that breast cancer deaths were reduced 39% among women aged 40 to 49 years versus 40% for all women aged 40 to 79 years.[48] In the two northern Swedish counties of Vasternorrland and Norrbotten, breast cancer deaths were reduced 36% to 38% for women aged 40 to 49 years versus 30% for all women aged 40 to 74 years.[49]

Should Women 75 Years of Age and Older Be Screened?

The question of mammographic screening for elderly women is clinically relevant, because there are almost 10 million women aged 75 years and older in the United States. The average life expectancy for a woman at age 75 is 13 years.[50] Women with good general health have a longer-than-average life expectancy. Thus, it is reasonable to expect that elderly women might benefit from screening. We know that reduction in breast cancer mortality among women aged 50 years and older becomes apparent within 4 years of entry into RCTs.[51] Therefore, for many older women with screening-detected breast cancer, death from another illness will not occur before they experience the benefit from screening.[52]

Strictly speaking, benefit from screening women 75 years and older has not been proven because this age group was not included in any RCT. Nevertheless, there is no biologic reason why early detection should not be effective for these women. Survival rates according to stage of disease are almost as high in older as in younger women.[53] The detection sensitivity of mammography is higher in elderly women because of their generally more fatty breast composition.[54,55] However, due to the lower life expectancy at future ages, there is a potential for diagnosis of tumors that would not have given rise to symptoms during the host's lifetime. Additionally, screening is only warranted if the woman is suitable for appropriate therapy in the event of a cancer diagnosis. Taking these considerations, especially comorbidity issues, it seems reasonable that screening mammography should be performed in women 75 years and older if their general health and life expectancy are good.[56,57]

Why Do Randomized Trials Underestimate the Benefit from Screening?

There are at least six reasons why results from all the early RCTs have underestimated the benefit to an individual woman undergoing screening with today's advanced mammography technology:

- Mammographic image quality below today's standards
- Use of only one mammographic view per breast in some RCT studies
- Noncompliance of some study group women
- Contamination of the control group
- Excessively long screening intervals (more than annual)
- Inadequate number of screening rounds

Firstly, there have been many technical improvements in mammographic technique since the early 1980s, when these trials were conducted. These innovations in mammographic equipment, screen-film systems, and processing as well as replacement of analog (film) mammography by digital mammography allow images to have better sharpness, exposure, and contrast.[58,59] Better image quality facilitates early detection of breast cancer.[4,60]

Secondly, women in the RCTs were mostly screened with one view per breast. Today's standard, two views per breast examination, has been shown to detect 3% to 11% (mean 7%) more cancers than found using a mediolateral oblique (MLO) view alone.[61-66] Of the seven population-based RCTs, only the HIP trial used two views on all examinations.[12,45] For example, The Gothenburg Trial used two-view mammography at the first screen and either single view or two views at subsequent screens, depending on breast density identified at the most recent prior mammogram. The Malmö trial used two views in the first two screenings but only a MLO view alone on all subsequent screenings, except in patients with dense breasts.[14] The Edinburgh trial used two-view screening on the initial screening but only one view on all subsequent screenings.[67] The Stockholm and Swedish Two-County trials used a single MLO view in all screenings.[13,15]

Two fundamental reasons why RCTs underestimate the benefit from screening are as follows: (1) Not all study group women accept the invitation to be screened *(noncompliance)*; and (2) some control group women obtained mammography screening outside the trial *(contamination)*. Yet, in order to avoid selection bias, an RCT must compare the breast cancer death rate among all study group women, both screened and nonscreened, with that among all control group women, including those who are screened on their own initiative. Thus, both noncompliance of some study women and contamination of control group women reduce the calculated benefit from RCTs.

Among the RCTs, the noncompliance rate ranged from 10% to 39%.[68] Studies performed on data from the individual trials have estimated that if all women in the study group had attended each screening round, there would have been at least an additional 10% reduction in breast cancer deaths.[63,64] Data from the Gothenburg, Malmö, and Swedish Two-County trials as well as the NBSS indicate that the rate of control group contamination ranged from 13% to 25%.[68]

Randomized trials might have also underestimated the potential benefit of screening because screening intervals were too long. Aside from the HIP trial, screening intervals in RCTs have been longer than the annual intervals now recommended.[69] For example, women in the Swedish Two-County Trial were screened every 24 to 33 months, and those in the Edinburgh trial every 24 months.[13,16,61] Numerous studies suggest that greater benefit should result from annual screening, especially for women aged 40 to 49 years, in whom breast cancer growth rates appear to be faster.[70-73] On the basis of a tumor growth rate model, Michaelson[74] calculated that annual screening would result in a 51% reduction in the rate of distant metastatic disease compared with a 22% reduction at a screening interval of 2 years.

It has been estimated that the use of annual screening in the Swedish Two-County Trial could have resulted in an additional 18% mortality reduction for women aged 40 to 49 years at entry, who were screened every 2 years, and an additional 12% mortality reduction for women aged 50 to 59 years at entry, who were screened every 33 months.[43] For women aged 39 to 49 at entry into the Gothenburg trial, who were screened every 18 months, it has been estimated that annual screening could have resulted in an additional 20% mortality reduction.[75]

Several investigators have used mathematical models of actual RCT data to calculate the benefit to an "average" woman who is screened every year and for whom results are not affected by noncompliance and contamination.[43,70,75,76] For example, on the basis of an observed 45% reduction in breast cancer mortality among women aged 39 to 49 years offered screening every 18 months in the Gothenburg trial, Feig calculated that the mortality reduction could have been as high as 65% with annual screening at the observed 80% compliance rate and as high as 75% at a 100% compliance rate.[75]

Finally, the fact that the results of some trials were based on a relatively short screening period and relatively small numbers of screening rounds represents a sixth reason why such trials may underestimate the potential benefits of screening. Such relatively short durations limit the mortality reduction estimates that can be made using standard methods of measurement. Screening frequency and length of follow-up should be sufficient to reach a "steady state" at which the greatest mortality reduction will be apparent. Put in rather cold terms, subjects in the control group have to have time to develop the disease, for it to become symptomatic and for it to cause death, while screening in the study group has to be sufficiently intensive to arrest this process. Using a new method of moving averages, Miettinen and colleagues showed that for women aged 55 to 69 years at entry into the Malmö Mammographic Screening Trial, mortality reduction was highest between 8 and 11 years of follow-up.[77] For that period, they calculated a 55% reduction in breast cancer deaths. This value was much higher than the 26% mortality reduction reported by Andersson and Nystrom, who had included data from before year 8, when benefit had not yet peaked, and from after year 11, when benefit was being diluted.[78]

SCREENING MAMMOGRAPHY GUIDELINES

Breast cancer incidence is decidedly lower for women in their thirties than among women aged 40 to 49, being 0.4 cases/1000 women/year versus 1.6 cases/1000 women/year, respectively. Less than 5% of all breast cancers occur before age 40 and less than 0.3% before age 30, compared with 19% for ages 40 to 49. Therefore, screening mammography is not advised for most women until age 40. Screening in their thirties may be considered only for those very few women who have extremely high risk for development of breast cancer at an early age.[69]

The time between screenings can affect the benefits. Because mortality rate reduction from screening is now well established, the goal should be to optimize the benefit by using the most appropriate screening intervals. Mounting evidence indicates that cancer in younger women has a shorter sojourn time and consequently a shorter lead time than cancer in older women.[71,73,79,80,81] *Sojourn time* is the maximum time between the earliest possible detection at screening and clinical finding in the absence of screening. *Lead time* is the average time between actual detection at screening and clinical finding in the absence of screening. If the interval between screenings is too long, many rapidly growing tumors will be detected by screening only shortly before they would have become clinically apparent, thereby reducing the benefit of screening.

Accordingly, many major medical organizations, including the ACS, the American College of Radiology (ACR), the American Medical Association (AMA), the American College of Surgeons (ACoS) and the Society for Breast Imaging (SBI), have recommended that women aged 40 to 49 years be screened annually.[69,81-83] This recommendation for annual mammography rather than mammography every 1 to 2 years for women aged 40 to 49 years is justified by the more rapid growth of breast tumors among younger women. These societies continue to recommend that women 50 years and older be screened annually. Breast cancer advocacy groups, such as the National Alliance of Breast Cancer Organizations (NABCO) and the Susan B. Komen Foundation, endorse the ACS recommendation. The American College of Obstetricians and Gynecologists (ACOG) recommends screening every 1 to 2 years between ages 40 and 49 and annually thereafter. Some authorities suggest that the interval between screenings can be lengthened as a woman ages. Nevertheless, it is likely that even in older women, some faster-growing cancerous tumors will become clinically apparent between biennial screenings, reducing the screening benefit. Women and their physicians should be aware that the major reason for accepting a longer screening interval at any age is a presumed reduction in screening costs, but that some consequent reduction in screening benefit will occur.

In November 2009, the U.S. Preventive Services Task Force (USPSTF) recommended that only very high risk women be screened between age 40 and 49 years, and that women aged 50 to 74 years be screened only every other year.[84] Shortly thereafter, the American Academy of Family Physicians (AAFP) and the American College of Preventive Medicine (ACPM) basically concurred by recommending that the conduct of screening for women aged 40 to 49 years be individualized and that women aged 50 to 74 years be screened every other year. The NCI deferred any change from its prior 2002 recommendation for screening every 1 to 2 years beginning at age 40 and continuing after age 50. The American College of Physicians (ACP) has thus far left unchanged its 2007 position, which is that women in their 40s should discuss screening with their physician in order to decide whether or not they should be screened.[85] The ACR, SBI, and ACoS have reaffirmed their recommendation for annual screening of all average risk women beginning at age 40. The ACR and SBI also advise that high-risk women start annual mammography before age 40.

Controversies Regarding Validity of Randomized Screening Trial Results

On the basis of results from RCTs conducted over the past quarter of a century and involving more than 500,000 women, consensus was reached in the medical community in favor of screening mammography.

In the face of such near-unanimous agreement about the value of screening mammography screening, two articles made the seemingly incredible claim that none of the trials provided any convincing evidence that screening prevents breast cancer deaths.[86,87] The authors of these articles, Gotzsche and Olsen, asserted that only two of the eight screening trials (the Malmö Mammographic Screening Trial and the NBSS) were valid, and that neither of these trials found evidence of benefit. The articles published in 2000 and 2001 received enormous publicity because of the sensational nature of their claim, which questioned the widely held belief in the efficacy of early detection through mammography screening.

The only two points on which Gotzsche and Olsen and all other observers agree are as follows: (1) that the NBSS failed to find benefit for screening in women aged 50 to 70 years with mammography and clinical examination versus clinical examination alone; and (2) the NBSS found no benefit for mammographic screening of women aged 40 to 49 years.[22,36] However, at this point advocates of screening part ways with Gotzsche and Olsen because their explanations for the negative NBSS results are vastly different. It is difficult to understand how Gotzsche and Olsen could view the NBSS as the paradigm of a well-conducted study for several reasons. Firstly, independent reviews found that the technical quality of mammography in the NBSS was poor even when measured by the standards of the 1980s, when the trial was conducted.[24-26] Secondly, performance of clinical breast examination before randomization of trial subjects may have allowed channeling of symptomatic women into the study group. The finding of an excess of advanced cancers in the study group aged 40 to 49 years suggests that randomization was not performed blindly.[26-29]

Thirdly, NBSS was not a population-based trial. Rather, participants were self-selected volunteers. Because self-selected women are more likely to be symptomatic, adequate randomization of such subjects is more problematic, especially when clinical examination has already been performed. Self-selected asymptomatic women may have higher survival rates than randomly selected asymptomatic women. Thus, benefit may be harder to demonstrate in a trial with such subjects than in a population-based trial. Contrary to the judgment of Gotzsche and Olsen, almost any of these problems in trial design and implementation could render the NBSS incapable of providing meaningful results.

The statement by Gotzsche and Olsen that the Malmö trial showed no evidence of benefit is even more difficult to understand. Gotzsche and Olsen considered only an early report of a small but insignificant 5% mortality reduction among women aged 45 to 70 years. They totally ignored later reports of breast cancer mortality reductions of 19% for women aged 45 to 70 years, 26% for women aged 55 to 70 years, and 36% for women aged 45 to 50 years at entry into the Malmö trial.[46] Moreover, several months after publication of the second Olsen and Gotzsche paper, Miettinen and associates reported using 3-year moving averages of RR estimates to estimate that the true mortality reduction from the Malmö trial was 55% for women aged 55 to 69 years and 60% for women aged 45 to 57 years at entry into screening.

Gotzsche and Olsen also claimed to have identified age differences of 1 to 5 months between study and control groups in the HIP and Edinburgh trials and all Swedish trials aside from the Malmö trial. The writers suggested that the observed reductions in breast cancer death rates were due to these age differences rather than to the screening process itself. Gotzsche and Olsen were unaware that when the screening trials used cluster randomization rather than individual randomization, such relatively small age differences were not unexpected, in some cases biased the studies against screening, and were in any case fully accounted for in analyses, leaving the conclusion of a significant mortality reduction unchanged.[88,89]

Screening trials and therapeutic trials are different in nature and may be different in design. In therapeutic trials, all participants have disease. The main variables are treatment versus no treatment and dose regimen. Study and control groups are small. Individual randomization is required, and small age differences are significant to the study. In screening mammography trials, there is low disease prevalence, so extremely large study and control groups are necessary. For this reason, individual randomization may not be practical, and cluster randomization is usually necessary.

The age difference between the two groups that Gotzsche and Olsen purported to have discovered in the Swedish Two-County Trial had been acknowledged by Tabár and colleagues in 1989.[90] In fact, after adjustment for age, mortality rates were only minimally different: 31% versus 30% for women aged 40 to 70 years in the Swedish Two-County Trial and 45% instead of 46% for women aged 39 to 49 years in the Gothenburg trial.[91] Thus, there was no way that these small differences in age could have altered the overall conclusion that mammography screening results in a substantial reduction in deaths from breast cancer.

In another criticism, Gotzsche and Olsen suggested that assignment of the cause of death among women in the Swedish screening trials might have been inaccurate. Accurate assignment of cause of death is critical to proper assessment of trial results. Death in a woman with breast cancer may be either causally related or unrelated to her malignancy. Because screening trials compare deaths due to breast cancer in women in study groups and control groups, attribution of the cause of death must be performed in a consistent and unbiased manner. However, the criticism by Gotzsche and Olsen was baseless. The methods for cause of death assignment in the Swedish trials had been previously described in detail by Nystrom and associates.[92] The process consisted of independent blind evaluation by four physicians and resulted in unanimous agreement in a remarkable 93% of cases.[23,92-94]

Gotzsche and Olsen also observed that no statistically significant decrease in death rates from all causes combined had yet been shown in any of the Swedish trials. They interpreted this observation to mean that any benefit from reduction in breast cancer deaths would be countered by increased deaths from other causes. This incorrect conclusion disregarded the fact that breast cancer accounts for only about 5% of total mortality. Thus, even the largest individual trial would be unlikely to demonstrate any statistically significant decrease in all-cause mortality. On this issue, Gotzsche and Olsen were proven wrong. Subsequent to publication of the second Olsen and Gotzsche paper, Nystrom and associates were, in fact, able to find a 2% decrease in all-cause mortality among study group women in five Swedish trials combined.[23,94] Additionally, Tabár and colleagues observed a significant 19% reduction in deaths from all causes among breast cancer cases in the group invited to screening in the Swedish Two-County Trial.[95] Thus, the Gotzsche and Olsen conjecture regarding all-cause mortality was incorrect.

To further their thesis that data from the Swedish Two-County trial was unreliable, Gotzsche and Olsen asserted that the reported study group size was different in the articles by Tabár and colleagues. In response to this criticism, Duffy and Tabár acknowledged that the study population size did in fact differ among their published reports.[96] In fact, Tabár and colleagues had previously noted that these differences were due to progressive identification and exclusion of women diagnosed with breast cancer before the trial began. [91] This is an acceptable and, in fact, commendable practice. The irony of this unjustified criticism is that Tabár and colleagues were faulted for practicing good science.

In their papers, Gotzsche and Olsen also reiterated the conclusion of a study by Sjonell and Stahle, which claimed that widespread screening in Sweden had not affected breast cancer mortality in the population.[97] The basic mistake by Sjonell and Stahle in this claim was that they had measured death rates too early after screening was started. Decreased mortality from screening should not be expected until 5 to 8 years after the start of screening. They had mistakenly begun to tally breast cancer deaths before the beginning of the service screening programs that they were attempting to assess.[95,98] Additionally, their calculations did not consider the increase in breast cancer incidence over time.

Although the report by Gotzsche and Olsen received considerable publicity in the U.S. media, no medical organization or government has changed its screening policy on the basis of their conclusions. After review of the Gotzsche and Olsen paper, eleven leading medical organizations (AAFP, ACS, ACOG, ACP, ACPM, AMA, American Society of Internal Medicine, Cancer Research Foundation of America, National Medical Association, Oncology Nursing Society, and the Society of Gynecologic Oncologists) reaffirmed their support of screening in a full-page advertisement published in the *New York Times* on January 31, 2002. Also, the NCI and the USPSTF concluded that despite Gotzsche and Olsen's contentions, the results from RCTs of screening were still valid.

Additionally, the Swedish National Board of Health and Welfare,[99] the Danish National Board of Health, the Health Council of the Netherlands,[100] the European Institute of Oncology, and the World Health Organization dismissed Gotzsche and Olsen's arguments and concluded that the evidence for benefit of screening for breast cancer was convincing.[98-102]

The "Over-Diagnosis" Controversy

Following the general acceptance of a substantial and significant reduction in mortality from breast cancer in association with mammographic screening, a new controversy has arisen on the subject of "over-diagnosis." This is defined as the diagnosis as a result of screening of histologically confirmed tumors which would not have given rise to symptoms in the patient's lifetime. This is essentially an epidemiological rather than pathological concept, although, if such tumors exist, one would expect them to be generally in-situ or minimally invasive cancers. For example a stage III breast cancer diagnosed by screening in a woman who dies in a road traffic accident the following day could be classified as a breast screening mammography "over-diagnosis"!

Analyses that rather crudely assess over-diagnosis on the basis of an increase in cancer incidence with the introduction of screening tend to estimate implausibly high rates of over-diagnosis, of the order of 30% to 50%.[103] These estimates are flawed, because they do not fully take account of numerous complicating factors in incidence of breast cancer and its interface with screening. Reasons for increased incidence observed with the introduction of screening include:

- Continuation of pre-existing trends of increasing breast cancer incidence in the late 20th century
- Acceleration of these trends by lead time—if screening confers an average lead time of two years, for example, we will observe 1994 incidence in 1992, 1995 incidence in 1993 and so on
- Lead time similarly accelerates age effects—we observe age 52 incidence at age 50, and so on
- A major surge of additional cancers, mostly due to lead time, is diagnosed with the prevalence screen when the program is introduced
- A similar surge of prevalence screen tumors occurring continuously at the minimum patient age of the screening program
- Over-diagnosis

Estimates that take account of the complexities listed above arrive at much smaller estimates, of the order of 10% or less,[104,105] consistent with estimates from long term follow-up of the Malmö trial.[106] It is intuitive that overdiagnosis of breast cancer is likely to be a minor phenomenon, since the populations subject to screening are generally middle aged women in the developed countries, who have excellent future life expectancy.

In another widely publicized article, Esserman and colleagues observed the following: (1) That following the widespread introduction of screening in the United States, breast cancer incidence has never returned to prescreening levels; and (2) that screening has not caused the relative incidence of regional cancer to decrease commensurate with the increased detection of early stage cancer.[107] Esserman acknowledged that breast cancer mortality has decreased during the screening era in our country but expresses uncertainty about the relative contributions of screening versus treatment to this accomplishment. She too is convinced that there is excessive diagnosis of slow-growing or biologically inert cancers. Our critique of her viewpoint is as follows: (1) That the increased incidence of breast cancer over the past 30 years is largely related to factors other than screening; and (2) that proof of mortality reduction through screening has been established in randomized trials and service screening studies and cannot be negated by distracting observations regarding the relative incidence of regional disease, which is influenced by factors such as overall breast cancer incidence, screening frequency, tumor growth rates, and screening compliance rates.

SERVICE SCREENING RESULTS

After the success of the Swedish randomized trials, organized service screening mammography became routine in nearly all Swedish counties by the 1990s. Unlike randomized trials, which are conducted primarily as clinical research studies, service screening is performed mainly as a public health initiative. Nevertheless, results from service screening projects have provided strong confirmation that screening mammography is effective in reducing mortality from breast cancer.[108]

Jonsson and coworkers[109] compared excess breast carcinoma mortality rates for the Swedish study group and control group counties. Study group counties were those in which screening was initiated between 1986 and 1987; control group counties were those in which screening was initiated in 1993 or later. Only women aged 50 to 69 years were evaluated because only half the counties began screening at age 40 years and some counties did not invite women to undergo screening after age 69 years. Women aged 50 to 69 years were thus invited to undergo screening in all counties. A 20% reduction in excess mortality from breast carcinoma was evident in the study group after a mean individual follow-up time of 8.4 years.[109]

A study by Tabár and colleagues[110] measured the effect of mammography in a population in which service screening is offered to all women 40 years and older. They compared breast cancer death rates in two Swedish counties over three periods: 1968 to 1977, when virtually no women were screened (prescreening era); 1978 to 1987, when half the population was offered screening in the RCT; and 1988 to 1996, after completion of the trial, when screening was offered to all women and 85% of the population was being screened. Compared with breast cancer death rates among women aged 40 to 69 years in the prescreening era, breast cancer death rates in 1988 to 1996 were 63% lower for screened women and 50% lower for the entire population (85% screened plus 15% not screened) (Table 3-4). During this time, reductions in death rates from breast cancer for screened women were similar to those for women screened during the trial (63% vs. 57%, respectively). However, during the RCT trial period (1978 to 1987), only half of the population was offered screening; for that era, breast cancer death rate reduction in the entire population was only 21%.

It seems probable that screening rather than advances in treatment was responsible for nearly all the benefit. The RRs of breast cancer death among nonscreened women aged 40 to 69 years were similar during the three

TABLE 3-4. Reduction in Population Death Rates from Breast Cancer in Women Diagnosed Between Ages 40 and 69 Years in Two Swedish Counties*

Screening Status	1978-1987 (Randomized Trial)	1988-1996 (Service Screening)
Screened	57%	63%
Invited to screening	43%	48%
Screened plus nonscreened	21%	50%

*Time of diagnosis either 1978-1987 or 1988-1996 compared with death rates from cancers diagnosed during 1969-1977 before screening began. All results were statistically significant at 95% confidence level.

Data from Tabar L, Vitak B, Chen HH, et al. Beyond randomized controlled trials: Organized mammographic screening substantially reduces breast cancer mortality. *Cancer* 2001;**91**:1724-1731.

consecutive periods (1.0, 1.7, and 1.19, respectively). Moreover, the breast cancer death rate for women aged 20 to 39 years, virtually none of whom were screened, showed no significant difference (1.0, 1.10 and 0.81, respectively) during these three consecutive periods.

Possibly, women who agree to be screened have selection bias factors that apart from the screening process improved their survival rates. Even assuming the maximum effect of selection bias, screening was shown to reduce breast cancer deaths by at least 50%.

A study by Duffy and coworkers assessed the effect of service screening in seven Swedish counties.[111] Among women aged 40 to 69 years, breast cancer mortality was 44% lower for screened women and 39% lower for women offered screening compared with the prescreening era. On the basis of breast cancer mortality trends, it was estimated that only 12% of the mortality reduction was due to improved therapy and patient management apart from the screening process. A further study of the 20-year experience in two Swedish counties found a significant 40% reduction in mortality with screening at ages 40 to 49 years.[47]

Garne and associates[112] found similar results for women in Malmö, Sweden. Between 1977 and 1992, breast cancer mortality among women 45 years and older in Malmö decreased 43%. During that same period, breast cancer deaths among women in this age group in the rest of Sweden diminished by only 12%. There was no change in mortality among women younger than 45 years. The decrease in mortality occurred in temporal relationship to the introduction of screening mammography and adjuvant therapy, consistent with a causal relationship. The Malmö trial (1976 to 1986) offered screening mammography to women aged 45 to 69 years. The screening compliance rate was estimated at 79%, and approximately 24% of control group women obtained screening outside the trial.[14]

In another service screening study, Jonsson and associates[109] found a 30% decrease in breast cancer mortality among women aged 40 to 74 years in two northern Swedish counties. Two adjacent counties where screening was not yet offered and that until that time had identical breast cancer mortality rates served as controls.

In Copenhagen, Denmark, Olsen observed a 25% reduction in breast cancer mortality among women aged 50 to 69 years invited to screening and a 37% mortality reduction among those actually participating.[113] Mortality comparisons were made to both historical and nonscreened national control groups.

In the Netherlands, Otto and coworkers[114] concluded that the 19.9% reduction in breast cancer mortality rates among women aged 50 to 75 years offered screening every other year was primarily attributed to the nationwide mammography screening program rather than to adjuvant chemotherapy. These trends persisted on longer term follow-up.[115]

In Finland, nationwide population-based breast cancer screening for women aged 50 to 59 years was introduced gradually between 1987 and 1991. Women born in even years began screening in 1987 or 1988. Women born in odd years, who began screening between 1989 and 1991, served as controls. An effect of screening emerged after 3 to 4 years of follow-up and rapidly diluted as controls were screened. For this narrow window of time, Hakama and colleagues[116] found that mortality from breast carcinoma was 24% lower among women who were offered screening and 33% lower among women who were actually screened.

In another service screening study in Finland, Parvinen and associates[117] found a 36% reduction in breast cancer deaths among women aged 55 to 69 years offered screening in the city of Turku compared with women in Helsinki where screening was not offered.

In Florence, Italy, Paci and colleagues[118] compared death rates from breast cancer among women aged 50 to 69 years in 1990 to 1996 with those in 1985 to 1986 when screening was not offered. In the 1990 to 1996 era, there was a 55% mortality reduction among those invited to screening and a 41% mortality reduction among those not yet invited. The authors concluded that about two thirds of the 55% reduction (37%) was due to therapeutic interventions and one third (18%) to screening.

A case-control study of women aged 50 to 74 years offered service screening mammography in five regions of Italy found a mortality reduction of 25% among those invited to screening and 50% among those actually screened.[119]

A service screening program in British Columbia, Canada, found a 40% reduction in breast cancer deaths among women having at least one mammographic screen. Correction for self-selection bias adjusted this estimate downwards to a 24% mortality reduction.[48]

Although there has not been any service screening study in the United States, screening mammography is regularly performed. Indeed, 70% of women age 40 and older report having had a mammogram in the past 2 years, and 55% in the past year.[120] As a consequence, the average woman with breast cancer is now 39% less likely to die from her disease than was her counterpart in the early 1980s when screening was much less common.[108] Screening has also resulted in a substantial down-staging of breast cancer[121] enabling more conservative treatment and allowing every current surgical, medical, and radiation treatment to be more effective.

Results from these many service screening studies indicate that the reductions in breast cancer mortality found in the RCTs can be obtained and exceeded in nonresearch, organized service screening settings. These programs effectively refute the claim by Gotzsche and Olsen that the benefits seen in the RCTs of screening were not real because of supposed flaws in randomization and ascertainment of cause of death.[122]

ADVERSE CONSEQUENCES AND COSTS OF SCREENING

A woman whose breast cancer is detected through screening is on average 50% less likely to die of that breast cancer than if she had not undergone screening.[108,111] However, only a tiny fraction of the population being screened each year benefits from mammographic examination, because the annual incidence of breast cancer is low and not all cases are detected by mammography. The major human cost of breast cancer screening is that it has to be applied to the population in order to benefit the small percentage of women who are destined to develop the disease. This is common to almost all primary and secondary prevention activities. Recent improvements in average life expectancy are the cumulative effects of mortality reductions of the order 1/1000 from one disease, 2/1000 from another, and so on. Breast cancer is a chronic disease, so the benefit from early detection may not be apparent for many years. In contradistinction, adverse consequences such as false-positive biopsy results occur sooner rather than later and affect more women. An even greater number of women may experience some anxiety that their examination may detect cancer. Moreover, the economic costs of screening are borne by nearly all members of society. All these benefits and risks must be carefully weighed in the determination of guidelines and policies for mammography screening.

That mammography produces benefit should no longer be subject to debate, because numerous randomized trials and service screening studies have produced unequivocal proof that screening can substantially lower the number of deaths due to breast cancer. Comparison of screening benefits with costs and adverse consequences, however, may reveal legitimate concerns. Such comparisons, like those discussed in the remainder of this chapter, can help determine when screening should begin and how often it should be performed. Analysis of risks from screening can lead to ways of reducing those risks without affecting cancer detection rates.

Breast Compression

The benefits of breast compression include the ability to obtain sharper images, with better exposure and more contrast, at lower radiation doses.[123] Improvements in breast compression devices and techniques over the past 30 years have allowed higher cancer detection rates and more comfortable examinations.[4]

When properly performed, mammography usually is not painful.[124] Some simple recommendations can minimize discomfort: First, "vigorous" compression is not necessary; rather, the breast should be compressed only until the skin is taut.[125] The patient should first be informed why compression is necessary and told that compression will be automatically released as soon as the exposure is taken. Also, pressure should be applied gradually, with manual fine-tuning for the final degree of compression. The patient should then let the technologist know of any excessive discomfort so that no further compression will be applied. Patients who experience tenderness just before their menstrual periods may want to schedule mammography at some other time, and taking a mild analgesic before mammography may be helpful. It is important to minimize any discomfort from mammography so that women will not be reluctant to undergo periodic screening.

Recall Rates

When screening mammograms are "batch-interpreted," the woman leaves the imaging center immediately after her standard two views per breast screening mammograms have been performed and checked for image quality by the technologist. The images are interpreted in batches by the radiologist at some later time, usually the same day. With batch-reading women receive their results from their referring health care provider or from the mammography facility, or from both, by mail. If screening mammography findings indicate that additional imaging is recommended, the patient must make an appointment to return for the diagnostic workup.

Because batch-reading is much more efficient and cost-effective than "on-line" interpretation (done before woman leaves the facility), it is the only practical way to perform screening mammography in the current environment of low reimbursement levels and high screening volume.[126] In contradistinction, on-line interpretation is necessary for diagnostic mammography because of the high percentage of abnormal study findings and the need to tailor each examination to the patient's clinical problem or findings on an abnormal screening mammograms.

Recall rate is defined as the percentage of patients asked to return for additional imaging evaluation after batch interpretation of screening mammography. Batch interpretation can be performed successfully only if recall rates are kept within acceptable limits. Recall rates that are too high cause patient inconvenience and anxiety, as well as increasing the cost and reducing the efficiency of the screening process. Unnecessarily high recall rates might also be a disincentive for women to undergo future screenings, for referring physicians to advise screening, and for medical care payers to support screening. On the other hand, if recall rates are too low, some subtle cancers may be missed, and some benign lesions may be subjected to an unnecessary biopsy because supplementary views or ultrasonography, or both, were not performed.

On the basis of published reports of recall rates for well-conducted screening programs, the ACR recommends that recall rates be maintained at 10% or less. [127] This upper limit value should probably be less for women in whom a previous mammogram that has been performed recently (e.g., within the last several years) is available for comparison. Hunt and colleagues found that recall rates for such women could be 30% lower than those for women having their initial mammogram.[128] These recommendations are supported from a study by Yankaskas and coworkers,[129] who found that a recall rate of 4.9% to 5.5% represents the best tradeoff between detection sensitivity (the percentage of cancers that are detected by screening mammography) and biopsy positive predictive value (PPV; the percentage of biopsies that reveal malignancy). Schell and colleagues[130] recommended recall rates of 10% for first and 6.7% for subsequent screening mammography. These recommendations are based on their observation of excessive increases in additional workups per additional cancers detected at recall rates higher than these values. The median recall rate at representative breast facilities in the United States has been measured at 9.8%, and about half of all facilities have recall rates higher than those recommended by the ACR.[131]

A study by Smith-Bindman and associates[132] found that recall rates at incidence screening at the Breast Cancer Surveillance Consortium (BCSC) in the United States were about twice as high as those at the National Health Service Breast Screening Programme (NHSBSP) in the United Kingdom (8.0% vs. 3.6%) yet cancer detection rates were the same in both countries. In another report, the authors concluded that radiologists in United States were interpreting too many screening exams as abnormal.[133] This conclusion differs from that of Moskowitz,[134] who evaluated recall rates and cancer detection rates at screening programs in North America and Europe. Among nine programs having recall rates of 2% to 10%, the higher recall rates were generally associated with higher cancer detection rates.[135]

It is well to remember that the purpose of breast cancer screening is to detect cancers earlier rather than just to detect more cancers. A critique of the study by Smith-Bindman and associates found that detection rates for DCIS as well as for early invasive cancers both 10 mm or less and 10 to 20 mm were higher at the BCSC in the United States than at the NHSBSP Program in the United Kingdom.[132]

These higher detection rates for minimal cancers in the United States may be partly related to higher recall rates. Excessively low recall rates may limit the benefits from screening. An expert panel of both academic and nonacademic breast radiologists in the United States advises that radiologists having recall rates of less than 5% or more than 12% should be considered for additional training.[136]

There are several common misconceptions regarding recall rates. Firstly, recall rates are not really false-positive rates, because most recalled patients do not undergo biopsy. However, we do use the term positive predictive value-1 (PPV1) to refer to the number of screening participants found to have cancer within one year after screening divided by the number of patients recalled from screening for additional imaging workup. A PPV1 of 5% to 10% is recommended by ACR.[127] Nevertheless, a "suspicious" category screening mammogram is not a positive diagnosis of any disorder: it is an indication for further investigation. In addition, recall rates for 10 subsequent screenings are not 10 times the rate for the initial screening, which has a higher recall rate than subsequent screenings because there are no previous exams with which to compare. Such misconceptions have appeared in the literature and need to be corrected.[137,138]

False-Positive Biopsy Results

An excessive rate of biopsies leads to anxiety, discomfort, and pain for the patient and also increases the cost and potentially decreases the use of screening mammography. The ACR recommends that the PPV when biopsy is *recommended* (PPV2; number of cancers detected per number of biopsies recommended) should be 25% to 40%.[127] PPV2 results are affected by patient age, risk factors, and presence of clinical signs and symptoms. Results from several centers have found that the PPV3 (number of cancers detected per number of biopsies actually *performed*) is about 22% for screening women aged 40 to 49 years, 35% for those aged 50 to 59 years, 45% for those aged 60 to 69 years, and 50% for those 70 years and older.[139-142] Although the PPV is lower for women aged 40 to 49 years, it is still acceptable. A complete imaging workup, including supplementary mammographic views and breast ultrasound, follow-up rather than biopsy for lesions that appear category 3—probably benign in the ACR's Breast Imaging Reporting and Data System (BI-RADS), and seeking second opinions for problematic cases can reduce unnecessarily high false-positive biopsy rates.

Ductal Carcinoma in Situ

The concept of over-diagnosis has been dealt with earlier. However, it is worth considering in more detail the detection of DCIS by screening. Coincident with the increasing use of mammography has been a marked increase in the detection of DCIS. Before the era of mammographic screening, DCIS represented less than 5% of all malignancies of the breast.[143] However, DCIS now accounts for between 20% and 40% of all nonpalpable cancers detected at screening and about 20% of all newly diagnosed cancers (screen-detected and non-screen detected) in the United States.[143] With appropriate treatment, the survival rate for patients with DCIS should be 99.5%. DCIS may be considered a frequent but nonobligate precursor of fatal breast cancer. In other words, all cases of invasive ductal carcinoma are believed to develop from DCIS, but not all cases of DCIS progress to invasive ductal carcinoma. Yet critics of screening have referred to DCIS as a *pseudocancer*, *false positive*, and *harm* from screening which leads to unnecessary biopsies and excessive surgery.

Justification for the use of DCIS as an index of the benefit of screening depends on how often and how rapidly DCIS evolves into invasive ductal carcinoma. As of yet, no direct method exists for determining the natural progression of DCIS. If patients with DCIS were never to undergo biopsy and the DCIS were left to develop into invasive carcinoma, there would be no way to establish that the initial lesion was DCIS. If DCIS is completely excised its natural history has been stopped, but there is no proof that it would have evolved into invasive ductal carcinoma.

Results from autopsy studies of women with no clinical evidence of breast cancer show a 6% to 14% prevalence of DCIS. These rates have been used to suggest that most cases of DCIS may never become clinically apparent. However, there are reasons why this conclusion is not justified. Firstly, most (45% to 56%) of the autopsy-detected cases of DCIS could not be identified by radiography performed on the surgical specimens.[143] Undoubtedly, an even higher percentage would not have been seen at mammography. If autopsy rates vary around 10% but mammography-detected rates are considerably lower than 1%, it is clear that mammographically detectable DCIS in living women is either a different entity from autopsy detectable DCIS in dead women, or a very special subgroup thereof. The DCIS found at autopsy is not representative of the type of DCIS detected by screening mammography, which would be larger, calcified, and, therefore, a faster-growing lesion. Secondly, detection rates for invasive ductal carcinoma at prevalence screening (a woman's first screening mammography) are two to three times higher than the expected incidence, consistent with a 2- to 3-year detection lead time. In the absence of screening, many cases of high-grade DCIS will not surface clinically as DCIS but rather as invasive carcinoma. Thus, it would not be surprising if the prevalence of mammographically visible DCIS at autopsy were even 10 to 20 times higher than the expected incidence of DCIS. Moreover, some cases classified as DCIS in the autopsy studies, which took place in the 1980s, would be reclassified as atypical hyperplasia according to current histology criteria.

Several follow-up studies of DCIS treated with biopsy alone also shed light on the invasive potential of DCIS. The lesions in these studies were categorized as benign at initial histologic review, and so wide excision was not performed. In one study, researchers found development of invasive ductal carcinoma at the biopsy site in 53% of cases within 9.7 years.[143] Another study showed development of invasive ductal carcinoma in 28% of cases by 10 years and 36% of cases within 24 years.[143] Recurrence rates for DCIS in series such as these have suggested to some observers that DCIS is unlikely to progress to invasive disease.

There are two reasons, however, why these studies should lead to just the opposite conclusion. Firstly, these studies underestimate the invasive potential of DCIS because they involved only cases of low-grade DCIS, that is, all histologic subtypes of DCIS except for comedocarcinoma, the most aggressive subtype. Comedocarcinoma typically accounts for 32% to 50% of all cases of DCIS detected at mammographic screening. Secondly, these studies included both cases in which the DCIS lesion was completely removed and cases in which some DCIS remained in the breast because biopsy margins were not sufficiently wide. Invasive ductal carcinoma would be expected only in this latter subgroup.

Based on a statistical model using the numbers of DCIS and invasive cancers detected at five different screening programs, Yen and colleagues[144] estimated that among cases of DCIS detected at prevalence (initial) screening, 63% were progressive and 37% were nonprogressive. At incidence (subsequent) screenings, 96% of detected cases of DCIS were progressive and only 4% were nonprogressive.

Among all cases of DCIS detected at the UK National Health Service Screening Programme, 60% were high grade, 20% intermediate grade, and 20% low grade.[145] It was estimated that 84% of high grade DCIS would, if undetected, progress to invasive disease in 5 years, most intermediate grade would progress to invasive disease in 10 years, and low grade could become invasive in 15 years or longer.

Because screening detects cancers years earlier than they would normally appear clinically, the incidence of invasive cancers will be lower than expected for several years after women cease participating in a screening program of limited duration. McCann and associates[146] estimated that 75% of this subsequent decreased incidence and lower mortality was due to screen-detected invasive cancers and 25% was from screen-detected DCIS. These investigators concluded that "Cancer for cancer, there is as much benefit from detection and treatment of DCIS as from detection and treatment of invasive cancer."

Screening Benefits versus Risks for Woman Aged 40 to 49 Years

Because the benefit of screening for women aged 40 to 49 years has now been established, the remaining screening issues for this age group are the smaller absolute reduction in breast cancer deaths and the higher relative rate of risks and procedures per cancer detected. However, differences in benefits between women aged 40 to 49 years and women aged 50 to 59 years are small. So are the differences in risks. Such changes occur gradually with age rather than abruptly at age 50.[139,140,147] Women aged 40 to 49 years have a lower incidence of breast cancer, a faster rate of breast cancer growth, and a tendency to have denser, more fibroglandular breast tissue, for which mammography is less sensitive. As a consequence, screening detection rates for women in their 40s are somewhat lower than those for women in succeeding decades. Biopsy PPV is also lower for women in their 40s. However, both detection rates and PPVs for women aged 40 to 49 years are well within acceptable limits (Table 3-5).

Some investigators have used inappropriate methods of comparison to suggest that detection rates are too low and false-positive rates are too high to support screening of women aged 40 to 49 years. Methods such as pooling data for women aged 40 to 49 years with data from younger women, pooling data for women aged 50 to 59 years with data from older women, and the exclusive use of data from the initial (prevalence) screening result in an inaccurate portrayal of screening outcomes for women in their 40s. Such improper assessment led Kerlikowske and associates[148] to make the misleading statement that screening of women younger than 50 years will detect only 20% as many cancers per 1000 women screened, will require 4 times as many diagnostic procedures per cancer detected, and will cause 2.5 times as many false-positive biopsy results for each cancer detected as screening of older women.

Proper assessment of the accuracy of screening mammography for women aged 40 to 49 years requires comparison of data for that age group only with data for women aged 50 to 59 years. The use of data from initial (prevalence) screening alone may be misleading. The use of data

TABLE 3-5. Detection Rates and Accuracy of Mammography at Three Screening Programs According to Age

	Age Range (yrs)				
Parameter	**30-39**	**40-49**	**50-59**	**60-69**	**70-79**
*Cancer detection rates:**					
MGH	NA	2.4	3.0	3.9	5.0
UCSF	2.9	3.4	5.4	7.5	9.5
NM	NA	3.5	4.8	7.0	9.5
Biopsy PPV:†					
MGH	NA	0.17	0.24	0.32	0.40
UCSF	0.16	0.26	0.35	0.43	0.55
NM	NA	0.25	0.32	0.41	0.60
Screening recall rates:‡					
MGH	NA	7.0	6.9	6.0	5.6
UCSF	2.3	2.0	1.9	2.0	1.4

*Cancers per 1000 women screened at first and subsequent screens combined.
†Cancers detected/biopsies performed at first and subsequent screens at MGH, subsequent screens only at UCSF.
‡Percentage of screening patients requiring supplemental imaging at first and subsequent screens at MGH, subsequent screens only at UCSF.
MGH, Massachusetts General Hospital; NA, not applicable; NM, X-ray Associates of New Mexico (private practice group); PPV, positive predictive value; UCSF, University of California at San Francisco.
Data from references 139-142, 147, 148.

from subsequent (incidence) screening alone is preferred, but combined data from prevalence and incidence screenings may also be used. Such an assessment indicates that screening of women aged 40 to 49 years detects at least 63% to 80% as many cancers, requires 1.7 times as many diagnostic imaging procedures, and results in 1.3 to 1.4 times as many false-positive biopsy results for cancers detected (Table 3-6).[147]

The increase in sensitivity and specificity from screening in women aged 50 to 59 years compared with screening in women aged 40 to 49 years is similar to that of screening in women aged 60 to 69 years compared with women aged 50 to 59 years and also to that of screening in women 70 years or older compared with women aged 60 to 69 years. Although mammography becomes more accurate as the age of the subject increases, there is no abrupt change in accuracy at the age of 50 years.[139,140,147]

Radiation Exposure

Misperceptions regarding radiation risk from mammography persist even though no woman has ever been shown to have experienced breast cancer as a result of mammography, not even from multiple examinations over many years' time at doses much higher than the current dose of 0.40 rad (0.004 Gy) for a two-view-per-breast examination. Such concern is based on the observation that some groups of women, such as Japanese atomic bomb survivors and North American women who were given radiation therapy for benign breast conditions such as postpartum mastitis or were monitored with multiple chest fluoroscopies during treatment for tuberculosis before 1940, were found to be at increased risk of breast cancer.[149-151] Among these women, excess risk was observed for doses from 100 to more than 1000 rad (1 to 10 Gy).

The hypothetical risk for mammography is based on a linear extrapolation from these high-dose studies. If there is any risk from mammography, it is extremely low and is lowest for those who are exposed when older than 35 years. The current mean breast dose of 0.4 rad (0.004 Gy) from mammography is markedly less than the mean glandular dose of 3.2 rad (0.032 Gy) from the mammography film systems that were used at most facilities until 1973.[152]

Screening benefits can be compared with radiation risks. On the basis of results from screening trials, we know that annual screening can reduce deaths from breast cancer detected among women aged 40 to 49 years by at least 35% and deaths from breast cancer detected among women 50 years and older by at least 46%.[149] Possible deaths from radiation exposure due to mammography can be estimated through the use of a linear RR extrapolation of risk found among populations that received extremely high doses. Calculations based on these assumptions indicate that 18,900 deaths from breast cancer can be averted when 1 million women are screened annually from age 40 years until age 74 years, and that at most, 21.6 excess deaths might be caused by radiation (Table 3-7). Thus, even if there is a risk from multiple mammographic examinations at a dose of 0.4 rad (0.004 Gy) each, the benefit from annual screening for women 40 years and older exceeds that theoretical risk by at least 875 to 1.[149]

Using similar assumptions, one can conclude that five biennial screenings between the ages of 40 to 50 years will result in 323.3 years of life expectancy gained per year of life lost; the corresponding benefit-to-risk ratio for 10 annual screenings is 243.3 years of life expectancy gained per year of life lost. Including benefits from earlier detection of cancers potentially caused by radiation, screening after age 50 would increase these respective benefit-to-risk ratios to 539.0, for biennial screening and 405.5 for annual screening.[150] Benefit-to-risk ratios for biennial screening are approximately 1.3 times higher than those for annual screening. However, the net benefits minus the risks are 1.5 times higher for annual screening than for biennial screening. These calculations favor annual over biennial screening. Regarding screening women aged 40 to 65 years at a total mean glandular dose of 4 mGy (0.4 rad), the National Council on Radiation Protection and Measurements has stated that "Even a reduction in breast cancer mortality rate of one percent confers more benefit than risk, in terms of reduced number of breast cancer deaths, and a reduction of 20-40 percent leads to a substantial decrease in the number of deaths."[152]

Cost -Effectiveness

Many investigators have calculated the cost-effectiveness of screening mammography. Their estimates have varied

TABLE 3-6. Relative Benefits and Risks of Screening According to Age Groups Being Compared

	Age Groups Being Compared (yrs)	
Parameter	**30-49 vs 50-69***	**40-49 vs 50-59†**
Detection rates	20%	63% to 80%
Diagnostic procedures per cancer detected	4×	1.7×
False-positive biopsy results per cancer detected	2.5×	1.3×-1.4×

*Prevalent screen data.
†Prevalent and incident screen data.
Data from Feig SA. Age-related accuracy of screening mammography: How should it be measured? *Radiology* 2000;**214**:633-640.

TABLE 3-7. Detection Benefits and Radiation Risks from Annual Screening Mammography of 1 Million Women from Age 40 to Age 74 years

Parameter	No. of women
Lives saved	18,900
Possible deaths caused	21.6
Benefit-risk ratio	875:1
Net benefit in lives	18,878

Data from Feig SA. Risk, benefit and controversies in mammographic screening. In: Haus AG, Yaffe MJ, editors. *Physical aspects of breast imaging—current and future considerations: 1999 syllabus, categorical courses in radiology physics.* Oak Brook, Il, Radiological Society of North America, 1999, p. 99-108.

TABLE 3-8. Median Cost Per Life-Year Saved for Annual Mammographic Screening of Women Aged 40 to 79 Years and Other Selected Types of Lifesaving Interventions

Intervention	Median Cost per Year of Life Saved ($)
Colorectal screening	3000
Cholesterol screening	6000
Cervical cancer screening	12,000
Antihypertensive drugs	15,000
Osteoporosis screening	18,000
Mammography screening	18,800
Coronary artery bypass surgery	26,000
Automobile seat belts and air bags	32,000
Hormone replacement therapy	42,000
Renal dialysis	46,000
Heart transplant	54,000
Cholesterol treatment	154,000

Data on nonmammographic interventions from Tengs TO, Adams M, Pliskin J, Safran DG, Siegel JE, Weinstein MC, et al. Five hundred life-saving interventions and their cost-effectiveness. *Risk Anal* 1995;**15**:369-390. Cost-effectiveness estimate for screening mammography from Rosenquist CJ, Lindfors KK: Screening mammography beginning at age 40 years: A reappraisal of cost-effectiveness. *Cancer* 1998;**82**:2235-2240.

because they have used different assumptions for benefits and costs and different methods of calculation. Many of these studies, such as one published by Salzmann and associates in 1997, are no longer valid because the benefits, particularly those for women aged 40 to 49 years, are now known to be much higher than previously believed.[153]

A later study by Rosenquist and Lindfors[154] estimated that annual screening mammography beginning at age 40 years and continuing until age 79 years would cost $18,800 per year of life expectancy saved. The assumption in this study was that annual screening would reduce breast cancer deaths by 36% for cancers detected in women aged 40 to 49 years and by 45% for cancers detected in women 50 to 79 years. The assumed costs included mammography at $64, core biopsy at $850, excisional biopsy of a nonpalpable lesion at $2400, and definitive treatment for breast cancer at $6100. Their final estimate for the cost-effectiveness of screening mammography is in the same general range as that for other commonly accepted interventions, such as screening for cervical cancer and osteoporosis (Table 3-8). The cost per year of life gained from annual screening mammography is higher than that for screening for colorectal cancer but is much lower than that for the use of seat belts and air bags in automobiles.[155]

THE 2009 U.S. PREVENTIVE SERVICES TASK FORCE CONTROVERSY

A controversy began in November 2009 when the USPSTF issued recommendations against routine screening of women aged 40 to 49 years (only very high risk women in this age group were advised to be screened), against annual screening of women age 50 to 74 (only screening every other year was recommended), against any screening at age 75 and older, against screening women with clinical examination at any age, and against teaching breast self-examination to women at any age.[156] The USPSTF is a government-appointed and government-supported group of health experts that reviews published research and makes recommendations about preventive health care issues such as screening for carcinoma of breast, cervix, prostate, and colon. Many members have earned PhDs and very few of the MD members are primarily involved in clinical care. There were no breast imagers or breast surgeons on the panel.

Public reaction to USPSTF was immediate and pronounced. Some women mistakenly thought that USPSTF supplanted older guidelines from the ACS, ACoS and ACR. Most women were either outraged or confused. A USA Today poll found that 47% strongly disagreed and 29% disagreed while only 5% agreed strongly and 17% agreed with the USPSTF advice.[157] The 2009 USPSTF recommendations were potentially more important than ones issued in 2002 because one provision in the proposed national healthcare legislation forbid Medicare and private insurers from paying for any medical care that did not conform to USPSTF policy. Kathleen Sebelius, the Secretary of Health and Human Services, was quick to deny that USPSTF recommendations were government policy. Several congressional representatives offered amendments to health care proposals exempting mammography screening from the USPSTF restrictions. Nevertheless, six states including California and New York soon stopped admitting new patients aged 40 to 49 years into state-supported mammography screening programs, ostensibly due to state budgetary programs but most certainly influenced by USPSTF recommendations. This current controversy is more dangerous than any prior controversies, because with expanding government constraints on the medical insurance companies, USPSTF recommendations could provide an excuse for third party payers to reduce their screening mammography coverage. Government, too, might seek to use "savings" from eliminated mammograms to help pay for proposed massive new health care initiatives.

The USPSTF argued that benefits from screening women aged 40 to 49 years were insufficient to justify screening the vast majority in that age group. Using results from randomized trials, they calculated that mortality reduction among women offered screening between ages 40 and 49, 50 and 59, 60 and 69, and 70 and 74 years was 15%, 14%, 32%, and 0 respectively.[156] The major mistake in this calculation was inclusion of results from the Canadian NBSS in the 40 to 49 and 50 to 59 age group. As discussed in the 40 to 49 year screening controversy section of this chapter, the NBSS had major problems in design and execution.[25,26] It appears that due to a fatal flaw in trial protocol, women with late stage breast cancers were preferentially enrolled in the NBSS study group resulting in excess breast cancer deaths in that arm. Additionally, all outside consultants confirmed that NBSS mammograms were technically poor, even by the standards of the 1980s when the trial was conducted. Excluding NBSS results from the USPSTF calculation would improve mortality reduction among 39-to-59-year-old women to 26% to 30% versus the 15% in the NBSS when included, thereby qualifying these women for screening according to USPSTF criteria.

USPSTF also ignored the facts that three separate randomized trials—HIP; Gothenburg, Sweden; and Malmö, Sweden—have shown statistically significant breast cancer mortality reductions of 25%, 45%, and 36% respectively for women offered screening between ages 39 and 49,[17,42,43,45,46] and that a meta-analyses of five Swedish trials found a statistically significant 29% mortality reduction in that age group.[11] USPSTF also ignored results from three service screening studies in Sweden and British Columbia that showed mortality reductions of 48%, 38%, 39% for women age 40 to 49 years.[47-49] USPSTF did include results of a randomized trial of women aged 39 to 41years at entry in the United Kingdom that showed a 17% mortality reduction for those invited.[18]

Besides the proven 30% to 48% mortality reduction for screening women in their 40s, there are other reasons why women in that age group need to be screened. Firstly, about 20% of women whose deaths are attributed to breast cancer, and about 40% of the years of life expectancy lost to breast cancer, are associated with cases diagnosed between ages 40 and 49.[12] Breast cancer incidence is lower in the 40s than in the 50s: 1.5/1000 versus 2.5/1000.[121] However, the U.S. female population age distribution is weighted towards younger women and they have longer normal life expectancies. Secondly, restricting screening in the 40s to only high risk women as advised by USPSTF would preclude detection of most breast cancers in that age group, because 70% of women with breast cancer have no known risk factors such as family history, clinical history, or prior biopsy results.[158]

At the other end of the age spectrum, USPSTF advised against screening women age 75 or older based on lack of data from randomized trials. Only one randomized trial included any women aged 70 to 74 years, and the number of women was too small for statistically meaningful results. The only possible reason that screening effectiveness might cease at older ages is the so called *over-diagnosis* phenomenon, where normal life expectancy is too short to allow improved survival to become manifest. We do know from randomized trials that benefit becomes apparent within 5 years after detection. Since the average older woman has a life expectancy of about 15 years, 9 years, and 5 years at ages 70, 80, and 90 respectively, there should be time for them to benefit from earlier detection. Women with no known co-morbid conditions have even longer life expectancies. Thus, the ACS recommends that screening continue regardless of age for women having a life expectancy of 5 years or longer. Moreover screening detection rates are greater above age 70 due to the higher breast cancer incidence and the improved sensitivity of mammography in fatty breasts.

The USPSTF recommendation for screening women age 50 to 74 every other year rather than annually is also seriously misguided. We know that annual screening[159] detects more early cancers than does screening at intervals of 2 or 3 years simply because breast cancers grow and become palpable over time. Annual screening is especially important for premenopausal women whose breast cancer growth rates are higher than those of older women. Although no randomized trial has been conducted to compare mortality reductions for comparable groups screened at different intervals, many indirect or inferential studies provide support for shorter screening intervals. Based on such studies, even the USPSTF agrees that annual screening should be more effective than biennial screening.[159] Its preference for biennial screening for women aged 50 to 74 years wa s based on mathematical modeling that showed that annual screening, while twice as frequent as biennial screening, may increase the number of averted deaths by 63%, rather than by 100%, while potentially doubling the false positive biopsy rate.[159] The use of the number of mammographic exams and biopsy rates implicitly represents a surrogate for cost. Thus, USPSTF acknowledges that annual screening saves more lives but infers that screening every other year is more cost-effective and therefore preferable.

Several investigators have estimated the increased benefits from annual screening from the observed benefits from screening every 24 months in the Swedish Two County trial and every 18 months in the Gothenburg, Sweden, trial along with the stage and expected death rates of interval cancers surfacing clinically between screens. In the Two County Trial, the observed mortality reduction was 24% for women aged 40 to 49 years and 39% for those aged 50 to 59 years. Using such data Tabár and coworkers, and Feig, in two separate reports, estimated mortality reductions of 35% and 46% for annual screening of these two respective age groups.[43,79] In Gothenburg, Bjurstam and associates found a 45% mortality reduction observed from screening women aged 39 to 49 years every 18 months (80% compliance).[45] Using data from that trial Feig estimated that annual screening of those women would have resulted in a mortality reduction between 65% (at 80% compliance) and 75% (at 100% compliance).[75] The USPSTF would seem to agree with the general conclusion of these studies that shorter screening intervals save more lives but was more concerned that the increase in benefit would be less than proportional to the increase in screening frequency, biopsy rates, and costs. However, the ACS believes that the extra cost and effort of annual screening is worth it; USPSTF does not.

USPSTF also ignored several computer simulations of breast cancer growth rates by Michelson and colleagues that estimated that annual screening would reduce breast cancer death rates for women aged 50 years by 52% compared with 27% for screening every second year and that the cost per year of life expectancy saved from annual screening at age 50 was $6756.00. [74] Lindfors and Rosenquist calculated that annual screening from age 40 to 79 would cost $18,800 per year of life gained.[154] Both of these cost estimates are within generally accepted costs for other medical preventive interventions.[155,163]

Three screening programs in the United States separately compared size and stage of cancers detected among women who had come for screening annually versus those who presented for screening every 2 years. White and colleagues[161] found that among women aged 40 to 49 years, those with a 2-year interval were more likely to have late stage disease at diagnosis than those with a 1-year interval. However, there was no increase in late stage disease for women 50 years of age or older with 2-year versus

1-year intervals. This result seems implausible unless one believes that breast cancers cease to grow after age 50. By contrast, Field and associates[162] found that among women age 65 and older, late stage cancers were substantially less frequent among those screened annually than among those screened biennially. Hunt and colleagues found that among women aged 40 to 79 years with previous normal mammography, those screened annually were more likely to have significantly smaller, lower stage cancer than those screened every other year.[128]

SUMMARY

Mortality reduction for women screened between ages 40 and 75 should be 40% to 50%. Annual screening should begin at age 40 and should be more effective than less frequent screening. The main risks and other adverse consequences from screening include discomfort or pain from breast compression, the need to recall patients for additional imaging, and false-positive biopsy results. Although these risks affect a larger number of women than the number who benefit from screening, the risks are far less consequential than the life-sparing benefits from early detection. Detection of DCIS is a benefit rather than a risk from screening. Radiation risk, even for multiple screenings, is negligible at current mammography doses. Most of the confusion among women, controversy in the media, and misunderstanding among supposed experts could be prevented by simply reading and understanding the screening literature.

KEY POINTS

- Randomized trials, the gold standard for establishing benefit, have proven that screening women aged 40 to 70 years can reduce breast cancer mortality by at least 30%. Service screening studies indicate that this benefit may be as high as 45% to 50%
- The ACS, ACR, and the SBI recommend annual screening beginning at age 40 and continuing as long as a woman's life expectancy is at least 5 years. Annual screening is probably more effective than screening at longer intervals. Limiting screening to only high risk women will miss at least 70% of all cancers.
- Very high risk women may begin screening mammography before age 40. In some patients, supplementary screening with ultrasound or breast MRI may be appropriate.
- Adverse consequences of screening such as callbacks for additional imaging, false positive biopsies, potential over-diagnosis, and any hypothetical radiation risk do not outweigh the benefits from early detection

SUGGESTED READINGS

Feig SA. Adverse effects of screening mammography. *Radiol Clin North Am* 2004;**42**:807-20.

Feig SA. Methods to identify benefit from mammographic screening. *Radiology* 1996;**201**:309-16.

Smith RA. Breast cancer screening among women younger than age 50: A current assessment of the issues. *CA Cancer J Clin* 2000;**50**:312-36.

Smith RA. Risk based screening for breast cancer: is there a practical strategy? *Semin Breast Disease* 1999;**2**:280-91.

Tabár L, Vitak B, Chen HH, Duffy SW, Yen MF, Chiang CF, et al. The Swedish Two-County Trial twenty years later. *Radiol Clin North Am* 2000;**38**:625-52.

REFERENCES

1. Senie RT, Lesser M, Kinne DW, Rosen PP. Method of tumor detection influences disease-free survival of women with breast carcinoma. *Cancer* 1994;**73**:1666-72.
2. Seidman H, Gelb SK, Stilverberg E, LaVerda N, Lubera JA. Survival experience in the breast cancer detection demonstration project. *CA Cancer J Clin* 1987;**37**:258-90.
3. Feig SA. Should breast self-examination be included in a mammographic screening program? *Recent Results Cancer Res* 1990;**119**:151-64.
4. Feig SA. Screening mammography: Effect of image quality on clinical outcome. *AJR Am J Roentgenol* 2002;**178**:805-7.
5. Saslow D, Boetes C, Burke W, Harms S, Leach MO, Lehman CD. American Cancer Society guidelines for breast screening with MRI as an adjunct to mammography. *CA Cancer J Clin* 2007;**57**:75-89.
6. Berg WA, Blume JD, Cormack JB, Mendelson EB, Lehrer D, Böhm-Vélez M. Combined screening with ultrasound and mammography vs mammography alone in women at elevated risk of breast cancer. *JAMA* 2008;**299**:2151-63.
7. Berg W. Tailored supplementary screening for breast cancer. What now and what next? *AJR Am J Roentgenol* 2009;**192**:390-9.
8. Pisano ED, Gatsons C, Hendrick E, Yaffe M, Baum JK, Acharyya S, et al. Diagnostic performance digital versus film mammography for breast cancer screening. *N Engl J Med* 2005;**353**:1773-83.
9. Smart CR, Bryne C, Smith RA, Garfinkel L, Letton AH, Dodd GD, et al. Twenty-year follow-up of the breast cancers diagnosed during the Breast Cancer Detection Demonstration Project. *CA Cancer J Clin* 1997;**47**:134-49.
10. Ries L, Eisner MP, Kosary CL, Hankey BF, Miller BA, Clegg L, et al. *SEER Cancer Statistics Review, 1973-1998*. Bethesda Md: National Cancer Institute; 2001.
11. Feig SA. Methods to identify benefit from mammographic screening. *Radiology* 1996;**201**:309-16.
12. Shapiro S, Venet W, Strax P, Venet L. *Periodic Screening for breast cancer, the Health Insurance Plan Project and its sequelae 1963-1986*. Baltimore: Johns Hopkins University Press; 1988.

13. Tabár L, Vitak B, Chen HH, Duffy SW, Yen MF, Chiang CF, et al. The Swedish Two-County Trial twenty years later. *Radiol Clin North Am* 2000;**38**:625-52.
14. Andersson I, Aspegren K, Janzon L, Landberg T, Lindholm K, Linell F, et al. Mammographic screening and mortality from breast cancer: The Malmö Mammographic Screening Trial. *BMJ* 1988;**297**:943-8.
15. Frisell J, Eklund G, Hellstrom L, Lidbrink E, Rutqvist LE, Somell A. Randomized study of mammography screening: preliminary report on mortality in the Stockholm trial. *Breast Cancer Res Treat* 1991;**18**:49-56.
16. Frisell J, Lidbrink E, Hellstrom L, Rutqvist LE. Followup after 11 years: update of mortality results in the Stockholm mammographic screening trial. *Breast Cancer Res Treat* 1997;**45**:263-70.
17. Bjurstam N, Bjorneld L, Warwick J, Sala E, Duffy SW, Nyström L, et al. The Gothenburg Breast Screening Trial. *Cancer* 2001;**97**:2387-96.
18. Moss SM, Cuckle H, Evans A, Johns L, Waller M, Bobrow L. Effect of mammographic screening from age 40 years on breast cancer mortality at 10 years' follow-up: a randomised controlled trial. *Lancet* 2006;**368**:2053-80.
19. Alexander FE, Anderson TJ, Brown HK, Forrest AP, Hepburn W, Kirkpatrick AE, et al. 14 years of follow-up from Edinburgh randomised trial of breast cancer screening. *Lancet* 1999;**353**: 1903-8.
20. Miller AB, Baines CJ, To T, Wall C. Canadian National Breast Screening Study: 2. Breast cancer detection and death rates among women aged 50 to 59 years. *CMAJ* 1992;**147**:1477-88.
21. Miller AB, To T, Baines CJ, Wall C. Canadian National Breast Screening Study-2: 13-year results of a randomized trial in women aged 50-59 years. *J Natl Cancer Inst* 2000;**92**:1490-9.
22. Miller AB, To T, Baines CJ, Wall C. The Canadian National Breast Screening Study-1: breast cancer mortality after 11 to 16 years of follow-up: A randomized screening trial of mammography in women age 40 to 49 years. *Ann Intern Med* 2002;**137**:305-12.
23. Nystrom L, Andersson I, Bjurstam N, Frisell J, Nordenskjöld B, Rutqvist LE. Long-term effects of mammography screening: Updated overview of the Swedish randomised trials. *Lancet* 2002;**359**:909-19.
24. Baines CJ, Miller AB, Kopans DB, Moskowitz M, Sanders DE, Sickles EA, et al. Canadian National Breast Screening Study: Assessment of tech nical quality by external review. *AJR Am J Roentgenol* 1990;**155**:743-7.
25. Kopans DB. The Canadian Screening Program: A different perspective. *AJR Am J Roentgenol* 1990;**155**:748-9.
26. Kopans DB, Feig SA. The Canadian National Breast Screening Study: A critical review. *AJR Am J Roentgenol* 1993;**161**:755-60.
27. Bailar JC, MacMahon B. Randomization in the Canadian National Breast Screening Study: A review of evidence for subversion. *Can Med Assoc J* 1997;**156**:193-9.
28. Boyd NF. The review of randomization in the Canadian National Breast Screening Study: Is the debate over? *Can Med Assoc J* 1997;**156**:207-9.
29. Boyd NF, Jong RA, Yaffe MJ, Tritchler D, Lockwood G, Zylak CJ. A critical appraisal of the Canadian National Breast Screening Study. *Radiology* 1993;**189**:661-3.
30. Tarone RE. The excess of patients with advanced breast cancer in young women screened with mammography in the Canadian National Breast Screening Study. *Cancer* 1995;**75**:997-1003.
31. Sun J, Chapman J, Gordon R. Survival from primary breast cancer after routine clinical use of mammography. *Breast J* 2002;**8**:199-208.
32. Fletcher SW, Black W, Harris R, Rimer BK, Shapiro S. Report of the International Workshop on Screening for Breast Cancer. *J Natl Cancer Inst* 1993;**85**:1644-56.
33. Smith RA. Breast cancer screening among women younger than age 50: A current assessment of the issues. *CA Cancer J Clin* 2000;**50**:312-36.
34. Hurley SF, Kaldor JM. The benefits and risks of mammographic screening for breast cancer. *Epidemiol Rev* 1992;**14**:101-30.
35. Chu KC, Smart CR, Tarone RE. Analysis of breast cancer mortality and stage distribution by age for the Health Insurance Plan clinical trial. *J Natl Cancer Inst* 1998;**80**:1125-32.
36. Miller AB, Baines CJ, To T, Wall C. Canadian National Breast Screening Study: 1. Breast cancer detection and death rates among women aged 40 to 49 years. *CMAJ* 1992;**147**:1459-76.
37. Warren-Burhenne LJ, Burhenne HJ. The Canadian National Breast Screening Study: a Canadian critique. *AJR Am J Roentgenol* 1993;**161**:761-3.
38. Mettlin CJ, Smart CR. The Canadian National Breast Screening Study: an appraisal and implications for early detection policy. *Cancer* 1993;**72**:1461-5.
39. Elwood JM, Cox B, Richardson AK. The effectiveness of breast cancer screening in younger women. *Online J Curr Clin Trials* 1993; Feb 25: Doc 32.
40. Glasziou PP, Woodward AJ, Mahon CM. Mammographic screening trials for women aged under 50: a quality assessment and meta-analysis. *Med J Aust* 1995;**162**:625-9.
41. Kerlikowske K, Grady D, Rubin SM, Sandrock C, Ernster VL. Efficacy of screening mammography: a meta-analysis. *JAMA* 1995;**273**:149-54.
42. Smart CR, Hendrick RE, Rutledge JH, et al. Benefit of mammography screening in women ages 40 to 49 years. Current evidence from randomized controlled trials. [erratum appears in *Cancer* **75**: 2788]. *Cancer* 1995;**75**:1619-26.
43. Falun Meeting Committee and Collaborators. Breast-cancer screening with mammography in women aged 40-49 years. Swedish Cancer Society and the Swedish National Board of Health and Welfare. *Int J Cancer* 1996;**68**:693-9.
44. Hendrick RE, Smith RA, Rutledge JH, Smart CR. Benefit of screening mammography in women aged 40-49: a new meta-analysis of randomized controlled trials. *Natl Cancer Inst Monogr* 1997;**33**:87-92.
45. Bjurstam N, Bjorneld L, Duffy SW, Smith TC, Cahlin E, Eriksson O. The Gothenburg Breast Screening Trial: First results on mortality, incidence, and mode of detection for women ages 39-49 years at randomization. *Cancer* 1997;**80**:2091-9.
46. Andersson I, Janzon L. Reduced breast cancer mortality in women under 50: updated results from the Malmö Mammographic Screening Program. *J Natl Cancer Inst Monogr* 1997;(22): 63-8.
47. Tabár L, Yen MF, Vitak B, Chen HH, Smith RA, Duffy SW. Mammography service screening and mortality in breast cancer patients: 20-year follow-up before and after introduction of screening. *Lancet* 2003;**361**:1405-10.
48. Coldman A, Phillips N, Warren L, Kan L. Breast cancer mortality after screening mammography in British Columbia women. *Int J Cancer* 2007;**120**:1076-80.
49. Jonsson H, Bordas P, Wallin H, Nyström L, Lenner P. Service screening with mammography in Northern Sweden: effects on breast cancer mortality - an update. *J Med Screen* 2007;**14**:87-93.
50. U.S. Bureau of the Census. *Statistical Abstract of the United States*. 209th ed. Washington, DC: U.S. Government Printing Office; 2009.
51. Feig SA. Mammographic screening of elderly women. *JAMA* 1996;**276**:446.
52. Mandelblatt JS, Wheat ME, Monane M, Moshief RD, Hollenberg JP, Tang J. Breast cancer screening for elderly women with and without comorbid conditions. *Ann Intern Med* 1992;**116**:722-30.
53. Yancik R, Reis LG, Yates JW. Breast cancer in women: A population based study of contrasts in stage, survival, and surgery. *Cancer* 1989;**163**:976-81.
54. Faulk RM, Sickles EA, Sollitto RA, Ominsky SH, Galvin HB, Frankel SD. Clinical efficacy of mammographic screening in the elderly. *Radiology* 1995;**194**:193-7.
55. Wilson TE, Helvie MA, August DA. Breast cancer in the elderly patient: early detection with mammography. *Radiology* 1994;**190**:203-7.
56. Costanza ME. Issues in breast cancer screening in older women. *Cancer* 1994;**74**:2009-15.
57. Walter LC, Covinsky KE. Cancer screening in elderly patients: A framework for individual decision making. *JAMA* 2001;**285**:2750-6.
58. Conway BJ, Suleiman OH, Reuter FG, Antonsen RG, Slayton RJ. National survey of mammographic facilities in 1985, 1988, and 1992. *Radiology* 1994;**191**:323-30.
59. Haus AG. Dedicated mammography x-ray equipment, screen-film processing-systems, and viewing conditions for mammography. *Semin Breast Dis* 1999;**2**:30-54.
60. Young K, Wallis MG, Ramsdale ML. Mammographic film density and detection of small breast cancers. *Clin Radiol* 1994;**49**:461-5.
61. Andersson I, Hildell J, Muhlow A, Pettersson H. Number of projections in mammography: Influence on detection of breast disease. *AJR Am J Roentgenol* 1978;**130**:349-51.
62. Anttinen I, Pamilo M, Roiha M, Soiva M, Suramo I. Baseline screening mammography with one versus two views. *Eur J Radiol* 1989;**9**:241-3.
63. Bassett LW, Bunnell DH, Jahanshahi R, Gold RH, Arndt RD, Linsman J. Breast cancer detection: One versus two views. *Radiology* 1987;**165**:95-7.

64. Muir BB, Kirkpatrick AE, Roberts MM, Duffy SW. Oblique-view mammography: adequacy for screening. *Radiology* 1984;**151**:39-41.
65. Sickles EA, Weber WN, Galvin HB, Ominsky SH, Sollitto RA. Baseline screening mammography: One vs two views per breast. *AJR Am J Roentgenol* 1986;**147**:1149-53.
66. Thurfjell G, Taube A, Tabár L. One-versus two-view mammography screening: a prospective population based study. *Acta Radiol* 1994;**35**:340-4.
67. Roberts MM, Alexander FE, Anderson TJ, Chetty U, Donnan PT, Forrest P, et al. Edinburgh trial of screening for breast cancer: mortality at seven years. *Lancet* 1990;**335**:241-6.
68. Humphrey LL, Helfant M, Chan BK, Woolf SH. Breast cancer screening: A summary of the evidence for the U S Preventive Services Task Force. *Ann Intern Med* 2002;**137**:347-60.
69. Smith RA, Saslow D, Sawyer KA, Burke W, Costanza ME, Evans 3rd WP, et al, American Cancer Society High-Risk Work Group; American Cancer Society Screening Older Women Work Group; American Cancer Society Mammography Work Group; American Cancer Society Physical Examination Work Group; American Cancer Society New Technologies Work Group; American Cancer Society Breast Cancer Advisory Group. American Cancer Society Guidelines for Breast Cancer Screening: Update 2003. *CA Cancer J Clin* 2003;**53**:141-69.
70. Feig SA. Determination of mammographic screening intervals with surrogate measures for women aged 40-49 years. *Radiology* 1994;**193**:311-4.
71. Moskowitz M. Breast cancer: Age specific growth rates and screening strategies. *Radiology* 1986;**161**:37-41.
72. Pelikan S, Moskowitz M. Effects of lead-time, length bias, and false-negative reassurance on screening for breast cancer. *Cancer* 1993;**71**:1998-2005.
73. Tabár L, Fagerberg G, Day NE, Holmberg L. What is the optimum interval between screening examinations? An analysis based on the latest results of the Swedish Two-County Breast Cancer Screening trial. *Br J Cancer* 1987;**55**:547-51.
74. Michaelson JS, Halpern E, Kopans DB. Breast cancer computer simulation method for estimation of optimal intervals for screening. *Radiology* 1999;**212**:551-60.
75. Feig SA. Increased benefit from shorter screening mammography intervals for women ages 40-49 years. *Cancer* 1997;**80**:2035-9.
76. Tabár L, Fagerberg G, Chen HH. Efficacy of breast cancer screening by age: new results from the Swedish Two-County Trial. *Cancer* 1995;**75**:2507-17.
77. Miettinen OS, Henschke CI, Pasmantier MW, Smith JP, Libby DM, Yankelevitz DF. Mammographic screening: no reliable supporting evidence? *Lancet* 2002;**359**:404-6.
78. Andersson I, Nystrom L. Mammography screening. *J Natl Cancer Inst* 1995;**87**:1263-4.
79. Feig SA. Estimation of currently attainable benefit from mammographic screening of women aged 40-49 years. *Cancer* 1995;**75**: 2412-9.
80. Duffy SW, Day NE, Tabár L, Chen HH, Smith TC. Markov models of breast tumor progression: some age-specific results. *Natl Cancer Inst Monogr* 1997;(22)93-7.
81. Feig SA, D'Orsi CJ, Hendrick RE, Jackson VP, Kopans DB, Monsees B, et al. American College of Radiology Guidelines for Breast Cancer Screening. *AJR Am J Roentgenol* 1998;**171**:29-33.
82. Council on Scientific Affairs. *Mammography screening for asymptomatic women*. Report No. 16. Chicago: American Medical Association; 1999.
83. Lee CH, Dershaw DD, Kopans DB, Evans P, Monsees B, Monticciolo D, et al. Breast cancer screening with imaging: recommendations from the Society of Breast Imaging and the ACR on the use of mammography, breast MRI, breast ultrasound, and other technologies for the detection of clinically occult breast cancer. *J Am Coll Radiol* 2010;**7**:18-27.
84. Calonge N, Petitti DB, DeWitt TG, et al. US Preventive Services Task Force: Screening for breast cancer: U.S. Preventive Services Task Force recommendation statement. *Ann Intern Med* 2009; **151**:716-26.
85. Elmore JG, Choe JH. Breast cancer screening for women in their 40s: moving from controversy about data to helping individual women. *Ann Intern Med* 2007;**146**:529-31.
86. Gotzsche PC, Olsen O. Is screening for breast cancer with mammography justifiable? *Lancet* 2000;**355**:129-34.
87. Olsen O, Gotzsche PC. Cochrane review on screening for breast cancer with mammography. *Lancet* 2001;**358**:1340-2.
88. De Koning HJ. Assessment of nationwide cancer-screening programmes. *Lancet* 2000;**355**:80-1.
89. Duffy SW. Interpretation of the breast screening trials: a commentary on the recent paper by Gotzsche and Olsen. *Breast* 2001;**10**:209-12.
90. Tabár L, Fagerberg G, Duffy SW, Day NE. The Swedish Two County trial of mammographic screening for breast cancer: recent results and calculation of benefit. *J Epidemiol Community Health* 1989;**43**:107-14.
91. Bjurstam N, Bjorneld L, Duffy SW, Prevost TC. The Gothenburg Breast Screening Trial [authors' reply]. *Cancer* 1998;**83**:188-90.
92. Nystrom L, Larsson LG, Rutqvist LE, Lindgren A, Lindqvist M, Rydén S, et al. Determination of cause of death among breast cancer cases in the Swedish randomized mammography screening trials. A comparison between official statistics and validation by an endpoint committee. *Acta Oncol* 1995;**34**:145-52.
93. Nystrom L, Rutqvist LE, Wall S, Lindgren A, Lindqvist M, Rydén S, et al. Breast cancer screening with mammography: Overview of Swedish randomised trials. [published erratum appears in *Lancet* 1993;**342**:1372]. *Lancet* 1993;**342**:973-8.
94. Nystrom L. Screening mammography re-evaluated [letter to the editor]. *Lancet* 2002;**355**:748-9.
95. Tabár L, Duffy SW, Yen MF, Warwick J, Vitak B, Chen HH, et al. All cause mortality among breast cancer patients in a screening trial: support for breast cancer mortality as an end point. *J Med Screen* 2002;**9**:159-62.
96. Duffy SW, Tabár L. Screening mammography re-evaluated [letter to the editor]. *Lancet* 2000;**355**:747-8.
97. Sjonell G, Stahle L. [Mammography screening does not reduce breast cancer mortality.]. *Lakartidningen* 1999;**96**:904-13.
98. Rosen M, Rehnqvist N. No need to reconsider breast screening programme on basis of results from defective study [letter to the editor]. *BMJ* 1999;**318**:809-10.
99. Swedish Board of Health and Welfare. *Vilka Effekter Har Mammografic screening?*. Referat av ett expertmote anordnat av Socialstyrelsen och ancerfonden i; Stockholm den 15 February 2002.
100. *The Benefit of Population Screening for Breast Cancer with Mammography*. The Hague: Health Council of the Netherlands; 2002.
101. Veronisi U, Forrest P, Wood W. *Statement from the chair: Global Summit on Mammographic Screening*. Milan: European Institute of Oncology; June 3-5, 2002.
102. International Agency for Research on Cancer: *Mammography screening can reduce deaths from breast cancer*. Lyon, France: IARC Press; 2002.
103. Zahl PH, Strand BH, Maehlen J. Incidence of breast cancer in Norway and Sweden during introduction of nationwide screening: prospective cohort study. *BMJ* 2004;**328**:921-4.
104. Olsen AH, Agbaje OF, Myles JP, Lynge E, Duffy SW. Overdiagnosis, sojourn time and sensitivity in the Copenhagen mammography screening program. *Breast J* 2006;**12**:338-42.
105. Duffy SW, Agbaje OF, Tabár L, Vitak B, Bjurstam N, Björneld L, et al. Overdiagnosis and overtreatment of breast cancer: estimates of overdiagnosis from two trials of mammographic screening for breast cancer. *Breast Cancer Res* 2005;**7**:258-65.
106. Zackrisson S, Andersson I, Janzon L, Manjer J, Garne JP. Rate of overdiagnosis of breast cancer 15 years after end of Malmo mammographic screening trial: follow-up study. *BMJ* 2006;**332**:689-92.
107. Esserman L, Shieh Y, Thompson I. Rethinking screening for breast cancer and prostate cancer. *JAMA* 2009;**302**:1685-92.
108. Feig SA. Effect of service screening mammography on population mortality from breast carcinoma. *Cancer* 2002;**95**:451-7.
109. Jonsson H, Nystrom L, Tornberg S, Lenner P. Service screening with mammography of women aged 50-69 years in Sweden: Effects on mortality from breast cancer. *J Med Screen* 2001;**8**:152-60.
110. Tabár L, Vitak B, Chen HH, et al. Beyond randomized controlled trials: Organized mammographic screening substantially reduces breast carcinoma mortality. *Cancer* 2001;**91**:1724-31.
111. Duffy SW, Tabár L, Chen HH, et al. The impact of organized mammography service screening on breast cancer mortality in seven Swedish counties: A collaborative evaluation. *Cancer* 2002;**95**:458-69.
112. Garne JP, Aspegren K, Balldin G, Ranstam J. Increasing incidence of and declining mortality from breast carcinoma: trends in Malmö, Sweden, 1961-1992. *Cancer* 1997;**79**:69-74.
113. Olsen AH, Njor SH, Vejborg I, Schwartz W, Dalgaard P, Jensen MB, et al. Breast cancer mortality in Copenhagen after introduction of mammography screening: cohort study. *BMJ* 2005;**330**:220.

114. Otto SJ, Fracheboud J, Looman CW, Broeders MJ, Boer R, Hendriks JH, et al. Initiation of population-based mammography screening in Dutch municipalities and effect on breast-cancer mortality: a systematic review. *Lancet* 2003;**361**:1411-7.
115. Otten JD, Broeders MJ, Fracheboud J, Otto SJ, de Koning HJ, Verbeek AL. Impressive time-related influence of the Dutch screening programme on breast cancer incidence and mortality, 1975-2006. *Int J Cancer* 2008;**123**:1929-34.
116. Hakama M, Pukkala E, Heikkila M, Kallio M. Effectiveness of the public health policy for breast cancer screening in Finland: a population based cohort study. *BMJ* 1997;**314**:864-7.
117. Parvinen I, Helenius H, Pylkkanen L, Anttila A, Immonen-Räihä P, Kauhava L, et al. Service screening mammography reduces breast cancer mortality among elderly women in Turku. *J Med Screen* 2006;**13**:34-40.
118. Paci E, Duffy SW, Giorgi D, et al. Quantification of the effect of mammographic screening on fatal breast cancers: The Florence Programme 1990-96. *Br J Cancer* 2002;**87**:65-9.
119. Puliti D, Miccinesi G, Collina N, De Lisi V, Federico M, Ferretti S, et al. Effectiveness of service screening: a case-control study to assess breast cancer mortality reduction. *Br J Cancer* 2008;**99**:423-7.
120. American Cancer Society. *Cancer prevention and early detection facts and figures, 2009*. Atlanta Ga: American Cancer Society; 2009.
121. http://seer.cancer.gov/statfacts/html/breast.html Accessed March 10, 2010.
122. Feig SA. How reliable is the evidence for screening mammography? *Recent Results Cancer Res* 2003;**163**:129-39.
123. Feig SA. Mammography equipment: Principles, features, selection. *Radiol Clin North Am* 1987;**15**:897-911.
124. Stomper PC, Kopans DB, Sadowsky NL, Sonnenfeld MR, Swann CA, Gelman RS, et al. Is mammography painful? A multicenter patient study. *Arch Intern Med* 1988;**148**:521-4.
125. American College of Radiology. *Mammography quality control manual*. Reston, Va: American College of Radiology; 1999.
126. Feig SA. Economic challenges in breast imaging: A survivor's guide to success. *Radiol Clin North Am* 2000;**38**:843-52.
127. D'Orsi CJ, Bassett LW, Berg WA, et al. *Illustrated breast Imaging Reporting and Data System-Mammography*. 4th ed. Reston, Va: American College of Radiology; 2003. p. 234.
128. Hunt KA, Rosen EL, Sickles EA. Outcome analysis for women undergoing annual versus biennial screening mammography: a review of 24,211 examinations. *AJR Am J Roentgenol* 1999;**173**:285-9.
129. Yankaskas BC, Cleveland RJ, Schell MJ, Kozar R. Association of recall rates with sensitivity and positive predictive values of screening mammography. *AJR Am J Roentgenol* 2001;**177**:543-9.
130. Schell MJ, Yankaskas BC, Ballard-Barbash R, Qaqish BF, Barlow WE, Rosenberg RD. Evidence based target recall rates for screening mammography. *Radiology* 2007;**243**:681-9.
131. Rosenberg RD, Yankaskas BC, Abraham LA, Sickles EA, Lehman CD, Geller BM, et al. Performance benchmarks for screening mammography. *Radiology* 2006;**241**:55-66.
132. Smith-Bindman R, Chu PW, Miglioretti DL, Sickles EA, Blanks R, Ballard-Barbash R, et al. Comparison of screening mammography in the United States and the United Kingdom. *JAMA* 2003;**290**:2129-37.
133. Smith-Bindman R, Kerlikowske K. Optimal recall rates following mammography [letter to the editor]. *JAMA* 2004;**291**:821-2.
134. Moskowitz M. Retrospective reviews of breast cancer screening: What do we really learn from them? *Radiology* 1996;**199**:615-20.
135. Feig SA. Adverse effects of screening mammography. *Radiol Clin North Am* 2004;**42**:807-20.
136. Carney PA, Sickles EA, Monsees B, Bassett LW, Brenner RJ, Feig SA, et al. Identifying minimally acceptable interpretive performance criteria for screening mammography. *Radiology* 2010;**255**:354-61.
137. Elmore JG, Barton MB, Moceri VM, Polk S, Arena PJ, Fletcher SW. Ten-year risk of false positive screening mammograms and clinical breast examinations. *New Engl J Med* 1998;**338**:1089-96.
138. Feig SA. A perspective on false positive screening mammograms. *ACR Bulletin* 1998;**54**:8-13.
139. Kopans DB, Moore RH, McCarthy KA, Hall DA, Hulka CA, Whitman GJ, et al. Positive predictive value of breast biopsy performed as a result of mammography: there is no abrupt change at age 50 years. *Radiology* 1996;**200**:357-60.
140. Kopans DB, Moore RH, McCathy KA, et al. Biasing the interpretation of mammography screening data by age grouping: Nothing changes abruptly at age 50. *Breast J* 1998;**4**:139-45.
141. Linver MN, Paster SB. Mammography outcomes in a practice setting by age: prognostic factors, sensitivity, and positive biopsy rate. *Natl Cancer Inst Monogr* 1997;**33**:113-7.
142. Sickles EA. Auditing your practice. In: Kopans DB, Mendelson EB, editors. *Syllabus: a categorical course in breast imaging*. Oak Brook, Ill: Radiological Society of North America; 1995. p. 81-91.
143. Feig SA. Ductal carcinoma in situ: implications for screening mammography. *Radiol Clin North Am* 2000;**38**:653-68.
144. Yen MF, Tabár L, Smith RA, Smith RA, Chen HH, Duffy SW. Quantifying the potential problem of overdiagnosis of ductal carcinoma in situ in breast cancer screening. *Eur J Cancer* 2003;**39**:1746-54.
145. United Kingdom National Health Service. *NHS Breast Screening Programme & Association of Breast Surgery at BASO: an audit of screen detected breast cancers for the year of screening April 2007 to March 2008*. UK West Midlands Cancer Intelligence Unit; 2009.
146. McCann J, Treasure P, Duffy SW. Modeling the impact of detecting and treating ductal carcinoma in situ in a breast screening programme. *J Med Screen* 2004;**11**:117-25.
147. Feig SA. Age-related accuracy of screening mammography: How should it be measured? *Radiology* 2000;**214**:633-40.
148. Kerlikowske K, Grady D, Barclay J, Sickles EA, Eaton A, Ernster V. Positive predictive value of screening mammography by age and family history of breast cancer. *JAMA* 1993;**270**:2444-50.
149. Feig SA. Risk, benefit and controversies in mammographic screening. In: Haus AG, Yaffe MJ, editors. *Physical aspects of breast imaging-current and future considerations: 1999 syllabus, categorical courses in radiology physics*. Oak Brook, Ill: Radiological Society of North America; 1999. p. 99-108.
150. Feig SA, Hendrick RE. Radiation risk from screening mammography of women aged 40-49 years. *Natl Cancer Inst Monogr* 1997;**22**:119-24.
151. Feig SA. Mammographic screening of women aged 40-49 years. Benefit, risk, and cost considerations. *Cancer* 1995;**76**:2097-106.
152. National Council on Radiation Protection and Measurements. *NCRP Report No. 149, a guide to mammography and other breast imaging procedures*. Bethesda Md: National Council on Radiation Protection & Measurements; 2004.
153. Salzmann P, Kerlikowske K, Phillips K. Cost-effectiveness of screening mammography of women aged 40-49 years of age. *Ann Intern Med* 1997;**127**:955-65.
154. Rosenquist CJ, Lindfors KK. Screening mammography beginning at age 40 years: a reappraisal of cost-effectiveness. *Cancer* 1998;**82**:2235-40.
155. Tengs TO, Adams ME, Pliskin JS, Safran DG, Siegel JE, Weinstein MC, et al. Five hundred life saving interventions and their cost-effectiveness. *Risk Anal* 1995;**15**:369-90.
156. Nelson HD, Tyne K, Naik A, Bougatsos C, Chan BK, Humphrey L, U.S. Preventive Services Task Force. Screening for breast cancer: an update for the U.S. Preventive Services Task Force. *Ann Intern Med* 2009;**151**:727-37.
157. Szabo L. Women are insistent on mammograms, poll shows. *USA Today* November 24, 2009.
158. Smith RA. Risk based screening for breast cancer: is there a practical strategy? *Semin Breast Disease* 1999;**2**:280-91.
159. Mandelblatt JS, Cronin KA, Bailey S, Berry DA, de Koning HJ, Draisma G, et al. Effects of mammography screening under different screening schedules: model estimates of potential benefits and harms. *Ann Intern Med* 2009;**151**:738-47.
160. Wallberg B, Michelson H, Nystedt M, Bolund C, Degner L, Wilking N. The meaning of breast cancer. *Acta Oncol* 2003;**42**:30-5.
161. White E, Miglioretti DL, Yankaskas BC, Geller BM, Rosenberg RD, Kerlikowske K, et al. Biennial versus annual mammography and the risk of late-stage breast cancer. *J Natl Cancer Inst* 2004;**96**:1832-9.
162. Field LR, Wilson TE, Strawderman M, Gabriel H, Helvie MA. Mammographic screening in women more than 64 years old: a comparison of 1- and 2-year intervals. *AJR Am J Roentgenol* 1998;**170**:961-5.
163. Gold M, Siegel J, Russell L, Weinstein M. *Cost-effectiveness in health and medicine*. New York: Oxford University Press; 1996.

SECTION

TWO

Imaging Technologies

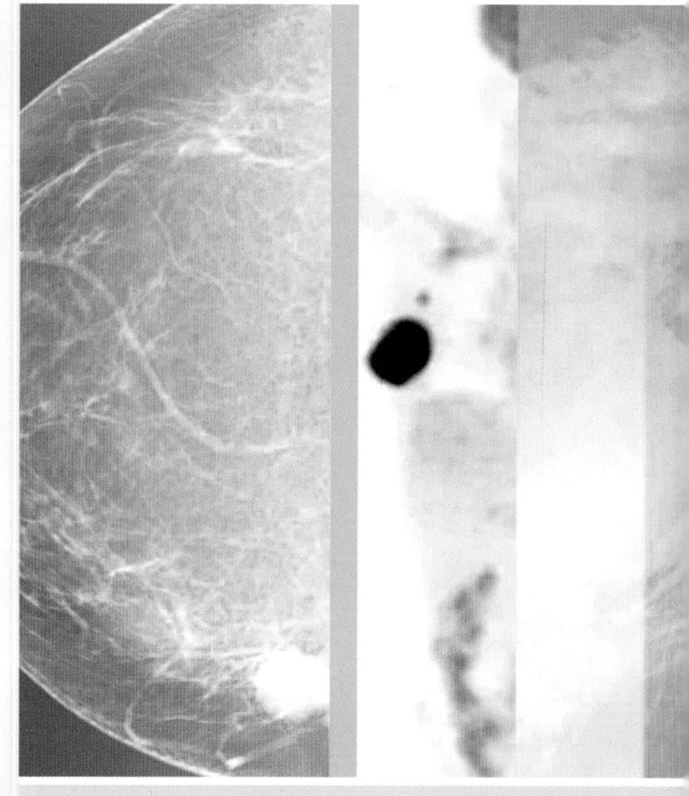

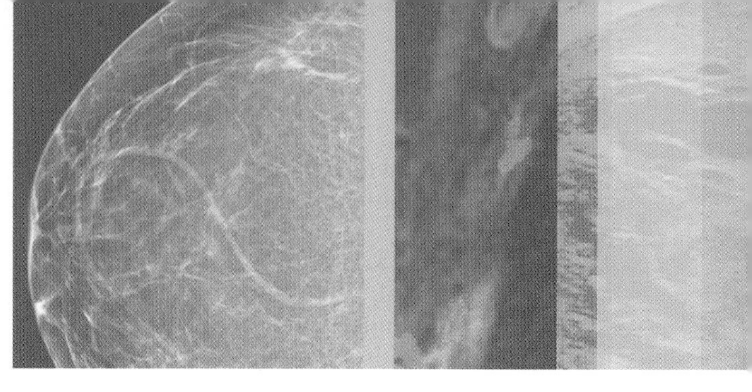

CHAPTER 4

Mammography and Digital Equipment

Eric A. Berns

In 1913, German surgeon Albert Salomon was the first to use x-ray imaging to view the gross anatomy of mastectomy specimens and was the first to demonstrate successful visualization of microcalcifications.[1] In 1949, Raoul Leborgne introduced imaging techniques for mammography that included the use of low kVps (20-30 kilovolts peak per second [kVps]) and light compression during exposure.[2] These ideas resulted in improved image contrast, better patient positioning, and reduced patient motion. Leborgne eventually wrote a classic textbook on breast radiography and ductography.[3] In 1960, Robert L. Egan described a high milliamperage, low kilovoltage technique using a conventional x-ray unit and high-resolution industrial film that resulted in easily reproducible techniques and positioning.[4]

Through the middle of the 1960s, mammography had been performed using general purpose x-ray units with no compression and using industrial grade film. These x-ray units typically had tungsten targets that produced insufficient subject contrast in soft-tissues. In 1965, Charles Gros in cooperation with Compagnie Generale de Radiologie (CGR) developed the first x-ray unit dedicated to mammography, called the Senographe.[5] The Senographe had two significant improvements over general purpose x-ray units. The first was a molybdenum target material (0.7 millimeter nominal focal spot size) that provided higher subject contrast when operated in the 22 to 30 kVp range. The second was a built-in compression device that provided uniformly decreased breast thickness and breast immobilization. This compression device was important because it reduced scatter, reduced patient motion, and spread out overlapping tissues, resulting in improved image quality.

In 1967, the first production Senographe mammography unit became commercially available. In the early 1970s, other dedicated mammography units were designed and made available by various manufacturers. Siemens Corp. introduced the Mammomat, Royal Philips Electronics introduced the MammoDiagnost, and Picker Corp. introduced the Mammorex. All of these units employed a molybdenum target, had similar designs of separate compression devices, and had fixed source to image receptor distances. In 1978, Philips introduced the Diagnost-U mammography unit that was the first to employ a reciprocating grid designed specifically for mammography.

Mammography image receptors evolved over the decades with the introduction of screen-film systems and xeroradiography systems in the early 1970s. In 1971, Xerox Corp. introduced xeroradiography as an alternative method for recording the x-ray image. It quickly became the predominant medium for mammography. Xeroradiography used a selenium-coated aluminum plate inside a cassette. An electrostatic charge was applied to the plate immediately before exposure to blank the plate. The plate was then exposed to x-rays forming a latent electrostatic image. The plate was developed in a reading device similar to a Xerox copy machine. Initially, xeroradiography produced high-contrast, high-resolution images at doses lower than film mammography. With continuing improvements in screen-film mammography through the 1980s, including lower doses due to the use of faster screen-film cassettes and higher contrast due to improved film and film processing, xeromammography slowly was replaced by screen-film mammography. Production of xeromammography units was discontinued in 1989.

In 1972, DuPont was the first company to introduce a dedicated screen-film system for mammography. In 1974, a new screen made of gadolinium oxysulfide coupled with orthochromatic film was introduced by 3M. This screen had higher efficiency in converting x-rays to green light, allowing the use of faster films that provided even lower patient doses without sacrificing image quality.[6,7]

In 1975, Eastman Kodak Co. introduced the first systems housed in a special, rigid, low-absorption cassette. The Kodak Min-R film and Min-R screen system held the film firmly in contact with the screen and allowed for elimination of problems associated with the darkroom and vacuum-bag systems of other manufacturers. In 1980, Eastman Kodak introduced the Min-R screen—Ortho M film combination that reduced patient dose by half that of Min-R film. In 1996, Eastman Kodak introduced Min-R 2000 film and Min-R 2000 cassettes that again improved subject contrast.

By 1988, most facilities in the United States were using screen-film systems and 99% were using dedicated mammography equipment.[8]

Film processors also have evolved over time. Until 1942, all medical x-ray film was developed by hand and image quality depended strongly on the skill and accuracy of personnel following guidelines from the manufacturer. The first automatic film processor was introduced in 1942 by the Pako Co. with processing times of 40 minutes. In 1956, Eastman Kodak introduced the first automatic film processor with a roller transport mechanism that allowed for processing of film of different sizes.[9] This automatic film processor could process films in 6 minutes. In 1965, Eastman Kodak improved processing time to 90 seconds, which is still the standard today for screen-film mammography systems.

In late 1996 and early 1997, the first prototype full-field digital mammography units were installed in the United States for clinical evaluation for U.S. Food and Drug Administration (FDA) approval. The first study to comparing screen-film and full-field digital mammography in a clinical study group was published in March 2001.[10]

On January 28, 2000, the GE Senographe 2000D was the first full-field digital mammography unit to be approved by the FDA for commercial use. Its initial approval was for image interpretation from printed films (hardcopy). On November 13, 2000, the GE Senographe 2000D received approval by the FDA for softcopy interpretation of digital mammograms. Table 4-1 shows the FDA approval months and years for commercial use for each full-field digital mammography manufacturer and model with each corresponding detector type.

For a more detailed account of the history of mammography there are four papers by Gold,[11] Bassett,[12] Houn,[13] and Hendrick,[14] that are particularly helpful.

TABLE 4-1. FDA Approval Months and Years For Full-Field Digital Mammography Manufacturers, Models and Detector Type

Full-Field Digital Mammography Detector Types		
Manufacturer and Model	**FDA Approval Months and Years**	**Detector Type**
GE Senographe 2000D	January, 2000	Cesium iodide
Fischer Senoscan	September, 2001	Slot-scanning CCD array
Lorad Digital Breast Imager	March, 2002	Tiled CCD array
Lorad/Hologic Selenia	October, 2002	Selenium
GE Senographe DS	February, 2004	Cesium iodide
Siemens Mammomat Novation DR	August, 2004	Selenium
GE Essential	April, 2006	Cesium iodide
Fuji FCRMS	July, 2006	Computed radiography
Hologic Selenia with Tungsten Target	November, 2007	Selenium
Siemens Mammomat Novation S	February, 2009	Selenium
Hologic Selenia S	February, 2009	Selenium
Hologic Selenia Dimensions 2D	February, 2009	Selenium

CCD, charge-coupled device; FCRMS, Fuji Computed Radiography Mammography Suite; FDA, U.S. Food and Drug Administration.

EQUIPMENT

Mammography Equipment Overview

The formation of the screen-film (SFM) and full-field digital (FFDM) mammographic images is depicted in Figure 4-1. Photons from the x-ray source are incident on the breast. Variations in tissue composition give rise to differences in attenuation, which in turn spatially modulates the transmitted x-ray beam (the x-ray image). The exiting x-rays are then captured by an intensifying screen or digital image receptor. Spatial variations in the x-ray energy absorbed in the intensifying screen for SFM and absorbed in the digital detector for FFDM and give rise to differences in screen or detector response and light output. These differences, in turn, result in differences in film density or digital signal to produce the mammographic image (see Fig. 4-1). Breast disease is manifested as small differences in subject contrast between lesions and their surroundings and by microcalcifications.

Visualization of these subtle subject contrast variations requires a high-contrast imaging system, in terms of both the x-ray spectrum incident on the breast and the image receptor. It is important not only to see the subtle lesions and microcalcifications but also to be able to delineate their borders to distinguish benign from malignant. This requires a sharp or high-resolution imaging system. Such borders also are easier to see if their sharpness is not degraded by graininess or artifacts. Image quality in mammography, and in medical imaging in general, depends on contrast, spatial resolution, noise, and artifacts.

Mammography is the most technically demanding radiographic examination. In clinical practice, the technical quality of the image depends on the adequate control of the following factors: (1) patient positioning and compression; (2) equipment selection; (3) technique; (4) exposure factors; and (5) image processing. Controlling and optimizing these factors in turn depend on equipment design and performance, image processing, technologists' training, and the assistance given to a site by the medical physicist. The objectives of this chapter are to review equipment design and performance considerations.

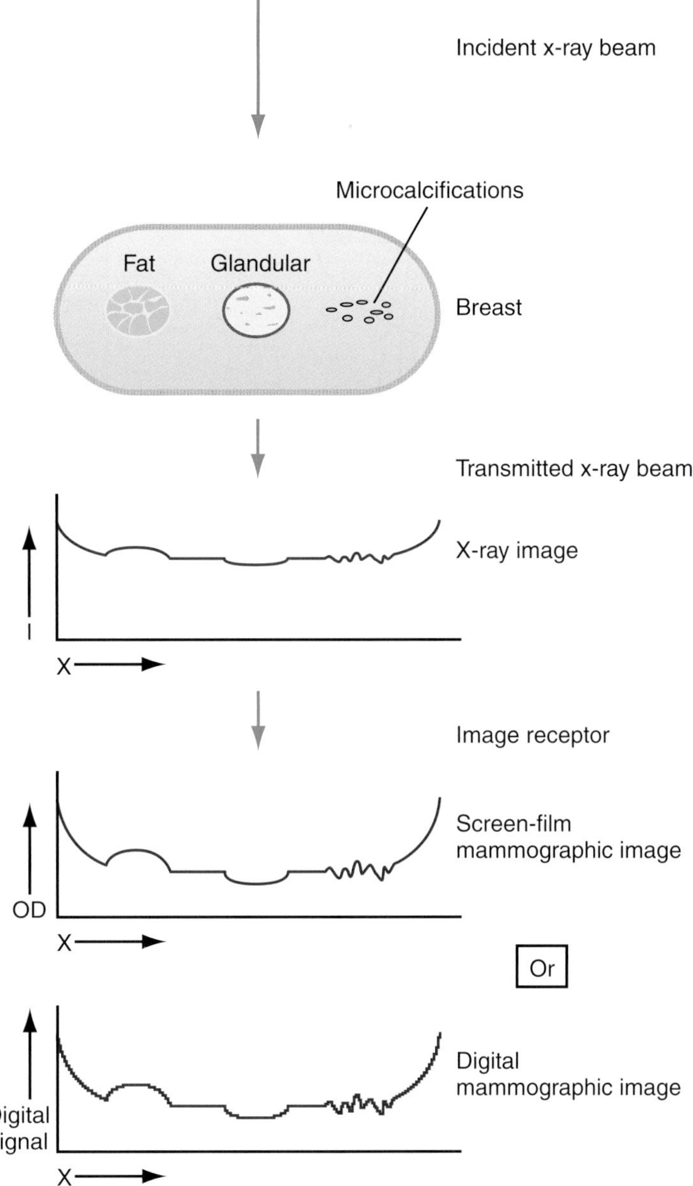

■ **FIGURE 4-1** Formation of the screen-film and digital mammography image. The incident x-ray beam, spatially modulated by the attenuation differences in the breast, forms the x-ray image. The x-ray image is, in turn, converted to a radiographic image by the source-film or digital processing system.

THE MAMMOGRAPHY UNIT

A mammography unit consists of an x-ray generator and control, U-arm, x-ray source assembly, collimator, compression device, breast support and grid assemblies, an image receptor— either screen-film or digital—and automatic exposure control (AEC) subsystem. A detailed diagram can be seen in Figure 4-2. Mammography Quality Standard Act (MQSA) regulations require that mammography units be operated with both 18 × 24 cm and 24 × 30 cm image receptors and be equipped with moving grids matched to the image receptor sizes.[15] In addition, diagnostic units have a magnification stand. The MQSA requires that in diagnostic units, the grid between the source and image receptor is removed for magnification procedures.[15]

The U-arm can be raised or lowered via a motor drive and can be rotated clockwise and counterclockwise. The x-ray source assembly (x-ray tube, tube housing, and filters) is mounted to the top of the U-arm and covered with a shroud. The collimator is mounted directly below the source assembly and is also covered by the source assembly shroud. The compression device is built into the vertical section of the U-arm. A horizontal mounting plate for attaching the grid assemblies and magnification stand is located at the bottom. The AEC subsystem consists of an AEC sensor and associated electronics for SFM systems while for FFDM systems, the AEC system is built into the detector itself. Figure 4-2 shows the geometry of a mammography unit and the relative locations of the x-ray tube, x-ray target, the tube housing, tube port, x-ray tube filtration, collimator, compression paddle, patient breast, grid, and image receptor.

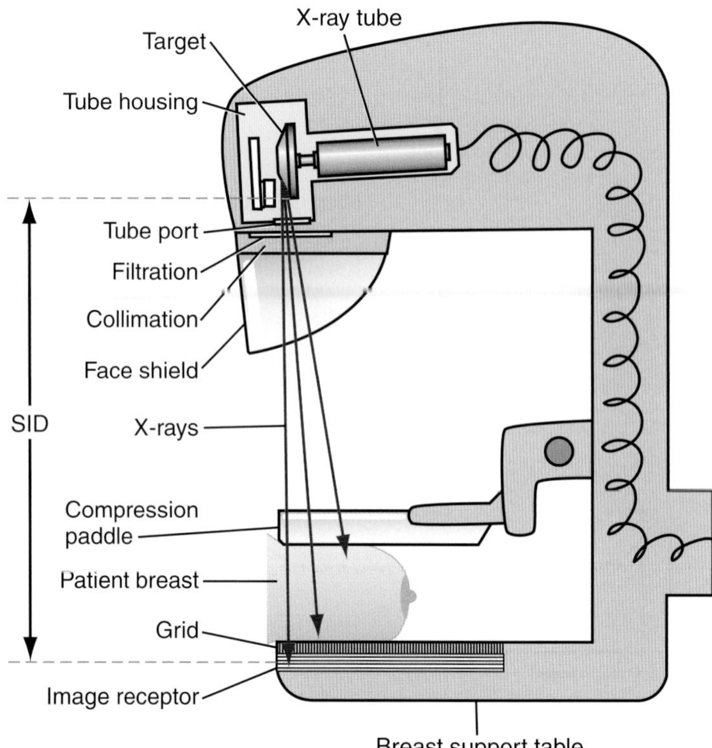

■ **FIGURE 4-2** The geometry of a mammography unit and the relative locations of the x-ray tube, x-ray target, the tube housing, tube port, x-ray tube filtration, collimator, compression paddle, patient breast, grid, and image receptor. The control and shield are not separate and are attached to the column. SID, source-to-image distance.

Generator

All mammography units currently being manufactured use high-frequency x-ray generator technology. The input is typically single phase, which in turn is rectified and capacitor smoothed to achieve a direct current (DC) voltage waveform. The DC output is fed to an inverter circuit, which converts DC to pulses of high-frequency alternating current (AC). The output of the inverter is capacitor coupled to the primary winding of the high-tension transformer, where the voltage is stepped up, is rectified, and charges a high-voltage capacitor that is in parallel with the x-ray tube. Often, a voltage doubling circuit is employed at this stage to reduce transformer cost. Typically, the cathode is grounded. On a few units, the anode is grounded. This latter arrangement is claimed to reduce off-focus radiation and improve image quality.

A voltage divider is placed across the x-ray tube and used to obtain a kilovolt (kV) feedback signal. The feedback signal is compared with the reference signal selected by the operator. If the feedback signal is less than the reference signal, the inverter pulsing rate is increased. Likewise, if the feedback signal is greater than the reference signal, the inverter pulsing rate is decreased. The inverter is pulsed at the maximum rate when an exposure is initiated and decreases as the high-voltage capacitor across the x-ray tube approaches the selected value. The inverter pulsing rate during an exposure stabilizes at a value that depends on the x-ray tube potential and milliamperage (mA) selected and is greater at higher x-ray tube potentials and currents. A typical pulsing rate is 5000 to 10,000 hertz (Hz). In an alternative design, pulsing occurs at a constant frequency but the pulse width is modulated.

Closed-loop control, or kV and mA feedback, is inherent to high-frequency x-ray generator design. Its use results in a high degree of reproducibility that is independent of commonly experienced line voltage fluctuations. The on-off switching time of high-frequency mammographic generators is on the order of a millisecond, and the kV waveforms typically have very little ripple (<4%) and are essentially constant potential. Modern mammographic high-frequency x-ray generator designs are compact and offer exquisite exposure reproducibility.

X-ray Tube and Filter

Mammography x-ray tubes typically have a large focal spot (0.3 mm) that is employed for grid work and a small focal spot (0.1 mm) that is used for magnification work. Most mammography systems require a beryllium window tube port to minimize beam hardening. X-ray target materials used by SFM and FFDM manufacturers typically include molybdenum (Mo), rhodium, (Rh), and tungsten (W). Each target typically has one or two user selectable options that can include Mo, Rh, aluminum (Al), or silver (Ag) for added filtration. Filters are used primarily to optimize the x-ray spectra reaching the image receptor for the characteristics of a given patient.

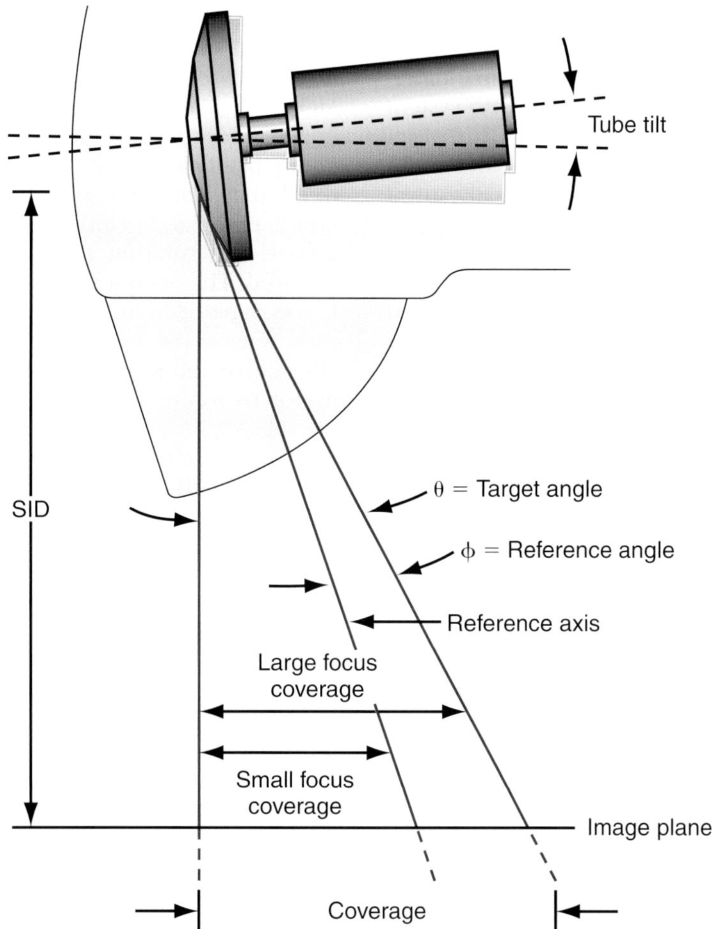

■ **FIGURE 4-3** Geometry of a mammography x-ray tube. Illustrated are the rotor and target, focal spot, target angle, reference angle and axis, source-to-image distance (SID), and coverage, or field of view (FOV). The size of the focal spot is specified by the mammography unit manufacturer as the projected dimensions (width and length) at the reference angle in a plane perpendicular to the reference axis.

As illustrated in Figure 4-2, the x-ray tube focal spot or source is located directly above the chest wall edge of the image receptor. The geometry of the x-ray tube target is illustrated in Figure 4-3. A number of factors depend on the x-ray tube target angle: Heel effect (less radiation intensity on the anode side than on the cathode side along the x-ray tube axis); coverage (the cathode-anode field-of-view dimension before the radiation falls off to an unusable degree in the anode direction); and the effective or projected focal spot being smaller (in the tube axis direction) than the area of the target struck by high-speed electrons or line focus principle. These result in a number of practical tradeoffs. The smaller the target angle, (1) the smaller the coverage and the more pronounced the heel effect; (2) the greater the area struck by electrons; and (3) the greater the loadability (permissible kV × mA product). Loadability also increases with increasing focal spot size, anode disk diameter, and anode rotation speed.

To use the heel effect to best advantage and also to minimize equipment bulk in the vicinity of the patient's head, the cathode is positioned toward the chest wall and the anode toward the U-arm. Radiation coverage depends on and increases with x-ray tube effective target angle. The effective target angle is equal to mechanical target angle plus the tube tilt angle.

According to MQSA regulations, the site's medical physicist must measure system resolution on installation of a mammography unit and annually thereafter.[15] For SFM systems the limiting system resolution is measured at 28 kVp for grid technique, and also for magnification technique on diagnostic units. The resolution patterns are positioned 4.5 cm above the grid or magnification stand cover and 2 cm from the chest wall edge and are measured for all screen-film combinations employed with a given technique. For both grid and magnification techniques, the limiting spatial resolution associated with the focal spot should be about 11 line pair per mm (lp/mm) for the length and about 13 lp/mm for the width. (The focal spot length is the projected focal spot dimension associated with the x-ray tube's cathode-anode axis, and the width is the projected dimension transverse to the tube's axis.) For FFDM, the limiting spatial resolution is typically measured using line-pair bar patterns and scoring them on a digital display. Each manufacturer has different requirements for its spatial resolution. The primary factors determining the system resolution is the dimensions of the focal spot. Mammography units with smaller focal spots have better performance. It is not uncommon for focal spot system resolution to exceed 15 lp/mm (length and width) for both large and small focal spots. There is a noticeable difference between mammography images obtained with system resolution of 11 lp/mm and 15 lp/mm.

To minimize patient motion, the large focal spot should be capable of 100 mA or more over the clinically used range of tube potentials. Similarly, the small focal spot should be capable of 30 mA or more. There are marked differences between the x-ray tube loadability of different mammography units. A large focal spot limit of 100 mA over the useful range of tube potentials is common. In some units, the mA falls from 100 mA to 70 mA as the tube potential is increased above 28 kVp. This undesirable feature compromises one's ability to obtain high-quality images on thick, dense breasts. For one manufacturer's unit, the x-ray tube current remains relatively constant in the 140-mA range as the tube potential increases from 25 to 30 kVp. As a result, one is able to use a lower kVp and obtain higher-contrast images for a woman with thick, dense breasts than is possible with other units. The higher mA values are achieved when high-speed anode rotation is employed. With high-speed anode rotation, 140 mA and 45 mA are achievable on the large and small focal spots, respectively, on widely used x-ray tubes over the clinical range of tube potentials.

U-Arm and Imaging Geometry

The x-ray source assembly (x-ray tube, tube housing, and filter) and collimator are mounted at the top of the U-arm, and the image receptor is mounted at the opposite end or bottom. The U-arm can be raised or lowered via a motor drive and can be rotated 180 degrees from the vertical in both clockwise and counterclockwise directions. The MQSA regulations require that the motion of the tube-image receptor U-arm assembly be capable of being fixed in any position where it is designed to operate and, once fixed, that it not undergo unintended motion when the unit is energized or in the event of power interruption.[15] Two U-arm rotation designs are currently being manufactured. The simplest design is to counterbalance the U-arm, have it held in place with electromagnetic locks, then release the locks to manually rotate the U-arm. The alternative and more complex design is to use an electric motor to rotate the U-arm. Both designs work well and are reliable.

The source-to-image distance (SID) on mammography units currently being manufactured is between about 65 and 66 cm. This distance permits good patient access and flexibility in positioning. Longer SIDs increase tube loading, whereas shorter SIDs limit patient access and can compromise image quality, particularly when magnification is employed. The ray orthogonal to the image receptor should project along the chest wall and should be aligned with the chest wall edge of the compression paddle (see Fig. 4-2). This geometry maximizes the chest wall breast tissue imaged.

Both SFM and FFDM units have a face shield that does several things. The first is to keep the patient from leaning into the x-ray beam during exposure. This keeps unwanted tissue from creating artifacts on the image and secondly prevents the patient from unnecessary x-ray exposure (Fig. 4-4).

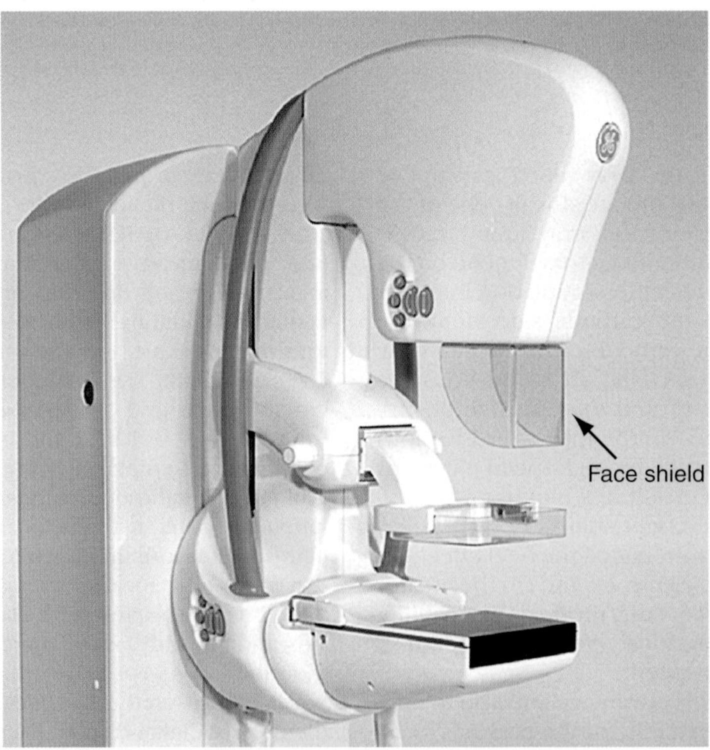

■ **FIGURE 4-4** A typical face shield for mammography that keeps the patient from leaning into the x-ray beam during exposure, getting unnecessary exposure, and keeps unwanted tissue from creating artifacts. *(Image courtesy of GE Medical Systems.)*

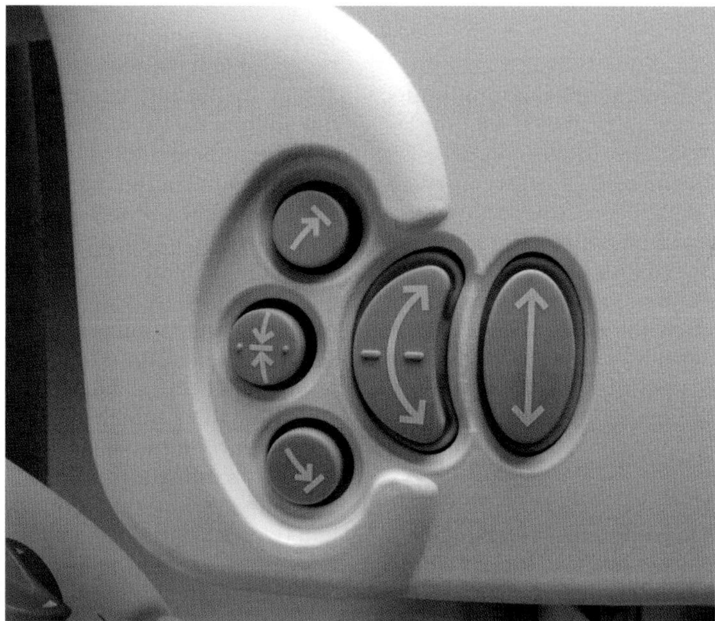

■ **FIGURE 4-5** Control buttons on a digital mammography gantry that operates the movement of the U-arm.

On all SFM and FFDM units there are control buttons on the gantry that operate the movement of the U-arm (Figs. 4-4 and 4-5). These controls are used by the technologist to raise and lower the U-arm, to rotate the U-arm for oblique imaging, to turn on and off the light-field, and to operate the compression devices. There are typically several sets of these control buttons positioned in convenient locations for the technologist.

Collimator

The collimator determines the x-ray FOV. Two general approaches are employed. In high-end units, the collimator blades are automatically motor driven to the size of the image receptor, and for a given image receptor size, the operator can reduce (cone down) the FOV to two or more smaller sizes by pushing a button (Fig. 4-6). In less expensive units, the collimator automatically switches between the small size (typically 18 × 24 cm) and the large size (24 × 30 cm) FOVs, and different diaphragms are manually switched out for the small focal spot and magnification as well as for coned-down views. On a number of less expensive units, the diaphragms are also manually switched between the small and large FOVs. From the technologists' perspective, because the grid and magnification stands are changed, there is little difference in terms of convenience, particularly for units on which the collimator automatically switches between the small and large size FOVs.

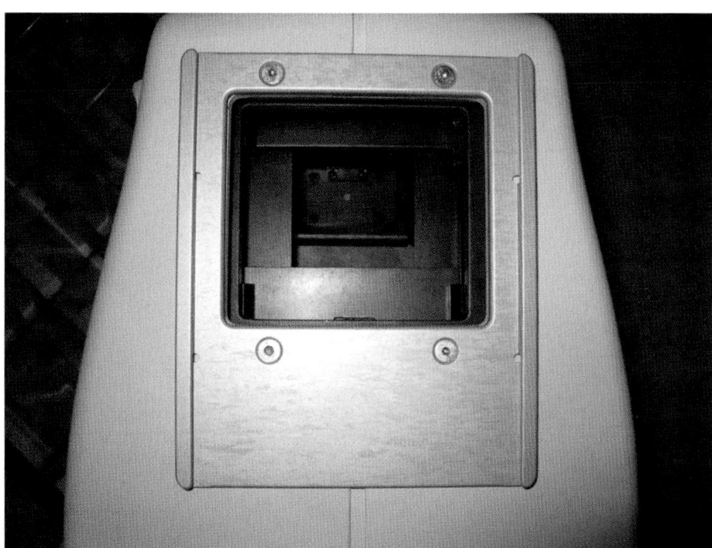

■ **FIGURE 4-6** Collimator blades on a digital mammography unit. The collimator adjusts the x-ray field to match the desired field of view.

Compression Devices

All mammography units are equipped with a compression device consisting of mechanical drive components located within the vertical section of the U-arm and a selection of paddles (Fig. 4-7). The MQSA regulations require that the compression initially be power driven and operable by hands-free controls on either side of the patient and that it have manual fine-adjustment controls that are also operable from both sides of the patient.[15] Also, a system must be equipped with different-sized compression paddles that match the sizes of all full-field image receptors provided with the system, the chest wall edge of the compression paddles must be straight and parallel to the edge of the image receptor, and paddles for special purposes (i.e., spot compression) may be provided.

A diagnostic SFM or FFDM mammography unit is typically equipped with five or more compression paddles: small, large, and spot grid technique paddles, and small and spot magnification technique paddles. Only small and large grid technique paddles are needed on a screening unit. As illustrated in Figure 4-2, the central ray (the ray orthogonal to the image receptor) should project parallel to the chest wall, and the chest wall edge or lip of the paddle should be aligned with the central ray. According to MQSA regulations, the projection of the paddle lip must not be projected on the film and must not extend beyond the chest wall of the film by more than 6 mm (1% of the SID).[15] In practice, the paddle lip should not extend beyond the film's edge by more than 3 mm. If the paddle lip extends much beyond the chest wall edge of the film, tissue close to the chest wall will not be imaged. Also, the chest wall lip of the paddle should be about 3 cm high. If the lip is too short, the superimposition of tissue above the breast can be a problem on obese women.

The MQSA regulations specify that the paddle must be flat and parallel to the breast support cover and must not deflect from parallel by more than 1 cm when compression is applied.[15] The compression force at which the deflection is checked is not specified. However, the maximum compression force for the initial power drive must be between 25 and 45 pounds; presumably, if the paddle deflects 1 cm or less under 25 pounds of compression force, the regulation is satisfied. It should be noted that the regulations permit paddles that are not designed to be flat and parallel to the breast support cover during compression, and these paddles do not need to meet the deflection requirement but do need to meet the manufacturer's design specifications and maintenance requirements.[15] In clinical practice, a deflection of about 2 cm is not a problem because of the following: (1) a decrease of tissue thickness as one goes from the chest wall to the nipple tends to compensate for the heel effect and for the increasing x-ray beam path length through the breast due to beam angulation; and (2) a compression paddle that deflects 1 to 2 cm results in a more comfortable experience for women undergoing the examination than a rigid paddle (i.e., one that does not deflect). Also important for comfort are the radius measurements of the compression paddle and grid cover chest wall edges. The radii of these edges should be about 4 mm. Smaller radii result in a more abrupt edge and greater patient discomfort. Larger radii, particularly for the grid cover, result in increased bulk and wasted space between the grid and grid cover. Recently, new "flex" paddles have been introduced into clinical practice to allow for improved tissue visualization due to reduced patient

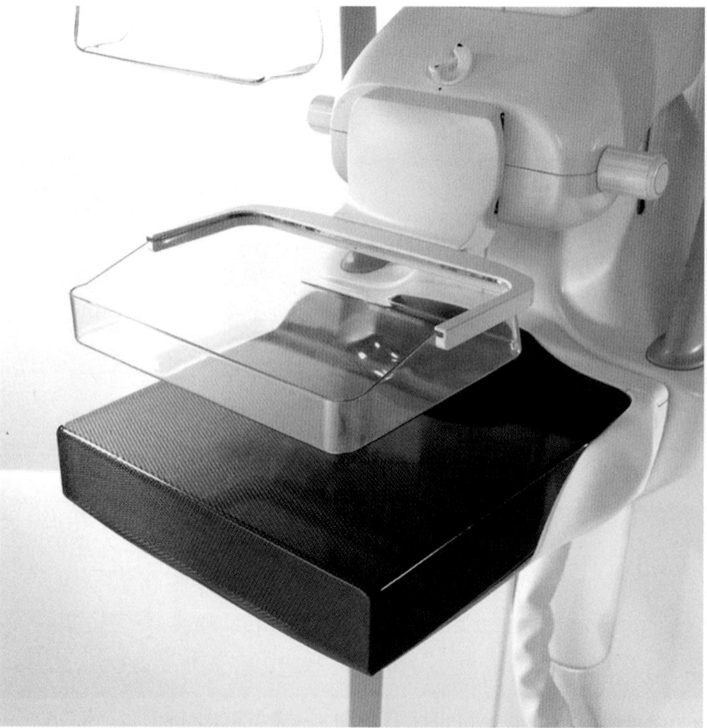

■ FIGURE 4-7 Compression paddle consisting of mechanical drive components located within the vertical section of the U-arm. *(Image courtesy of GE Medical Systems.)*

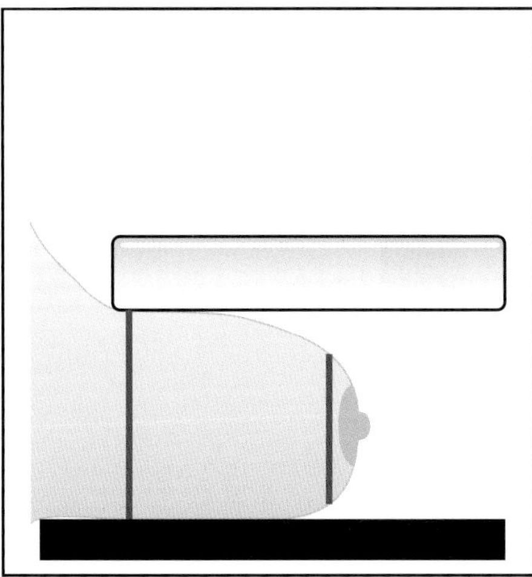

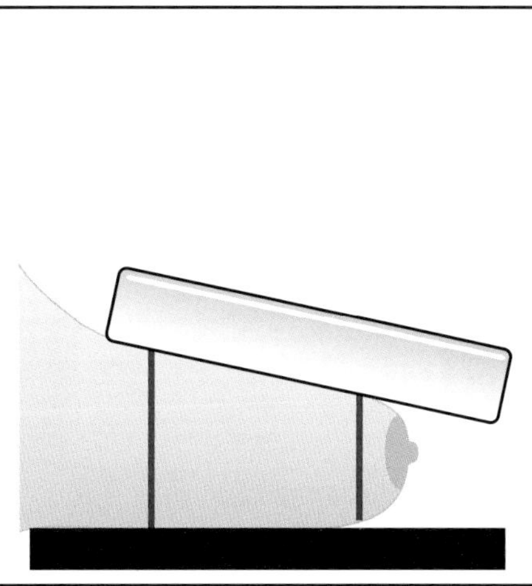

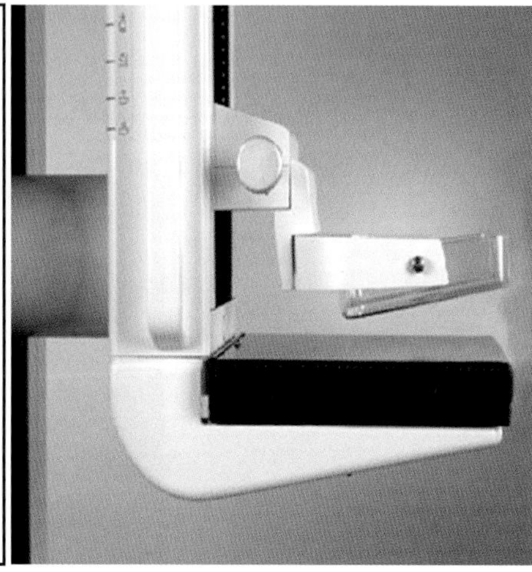

■ **FIGURE 4-8** Illustration of a conventional paddle providing compression parallel to the image receptor. Illustration of a flex paddle providing compression aligned with the top of the breast. Photograph of a flex paddle illustrating the flex capability of the device. *(Courtesy of Hologic, Inc.)*

motion. Additionally, these flex paddles can provide a small improvement in patient comfort (Fig. 4-8).

Compression improves image contrast and reduces the radiation dose to the breast. Image contrast is increased because the thickness of the breast is reduced and there is less attenuation of the x-ray beam (less beam hardening), the relative intensity of scatter is less,[16] and a lower-kVp technique can be employed. An additional advantage is that breast tissue is spread out over a larger area, reducing the superimposition of overlying structures and increasing the number of x-rays employed to image the breast.[17] Breast thickness is more uniform, permitting the use of high-contrast films. Patient motion is reduced because the breast is constrained and, with decreased breast thickness, exposure time and radiation dose are reduced.

Foot Pedals and Digital Display for Compression

Both SFM and FFDM units have two ways to provide compression to the compression paddle. The first uses a set of foot pedals located on the floor on either side of the U-arm. These foot pedals provide compression to a specified maximum force of 45 pounds.[15] The foot pedals are used for initial compression and aid the technician during positioning of the patient (Fig. 4-9). The second type of compression uses the manual knob at the compression paddle itself. This method is typically used to fine-tune the amount of compression applied after the initial compression is applied.

At the base of the U-arm, near the floor, or, at the top of the U-arm stand, there is a small digital display that presents the compression force, compression thickness, and the angle of the U-arm (Fig. 4-10). This is important because it reports to technologists information that helps them optimize patient positioning. Proper positioning and compression are among the most important aspects of providing good image quality.

Radiation Output

The MQSA regulations require that mammography units be capable of producing a minimum radiation output rate of 800 milliroentgens per second (mRs) measured 4.5 cm

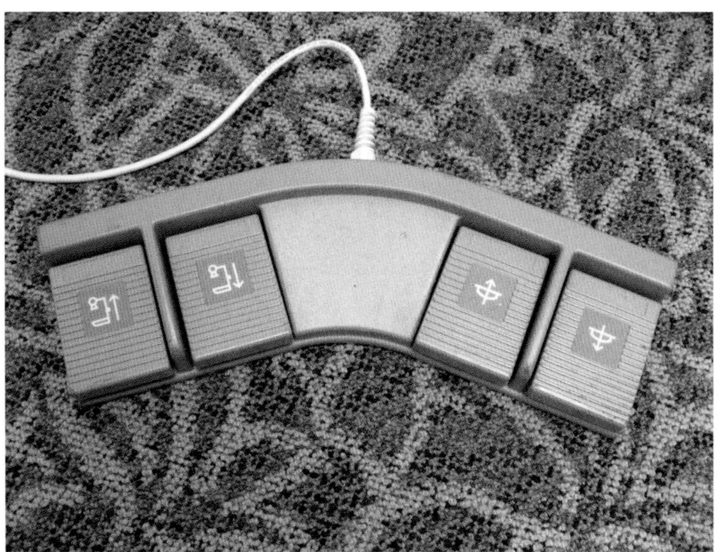

■ **FIGURE 4-9** Foot pedals used for initial compression.

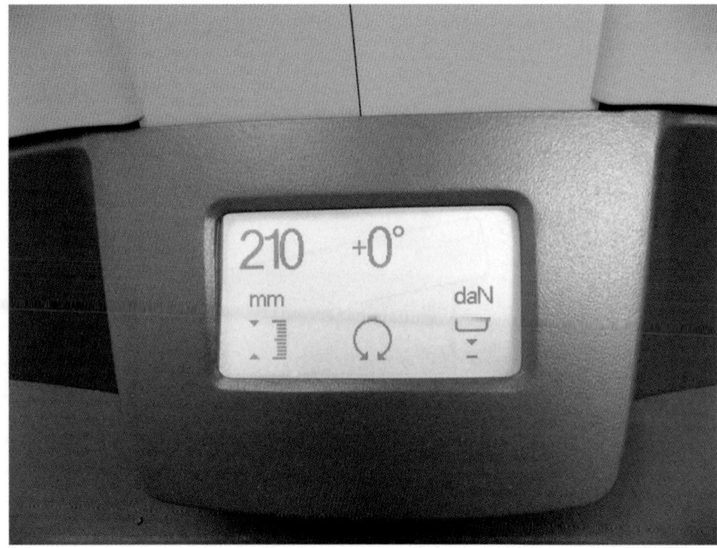

■ **FIGURE 4-10** Digital display presenting the compression force, compression thickness, and the angle of the U-arm.

above the grid breast support surface when operated at 28 kVp in the standard Mo/Mo target-filter mode. All mammography units currently being manufactured meet this requirement. However, measured radiation output rates vary from manufacturer to manufacturer, from 1000 to 2000 mR per second. The main reason for this factor of two in output rate is the loadability of the x-ray tube or the maximum mA the x-ray tube can achieve. Other factors, such as filter thickness, play a role. Obviously, a unit with a higher radiation output rate will allow shorter exposure times on small and medium breasts and will have greater capability to penetrate thick, dense breasts without employing excessively high kVp values.

Antiscatter Grid Assembly

All SFM and FFDM mammography units must have grid assemblies and moving grids.[15] However, several FFDM manufacturers have designed their systems without grids and some may only have one image receptor size. The assemblies, which mount on the U-arm's mounting plate, consist of a grid, grid drive motor and associated electronics, and image receptor. From top to bottom, a grid assembly comprises a breast support plate or grid cover, grid, image receptor, and bottom plate. Mammography Quality Standards Act (MQSA) regulations also require that the grid assemblies fit snugly on the mounting.

In clinical practice, the ratio of scatter to primary radiation emerging from the breast ranges from 0.3 to 1.5.[10] As a result, only 40% (thick, dense breast) to 75% (thin breast) of the possible contrast is imaged unless scatter is controlled.

A typical grid consists of lead lamellae separated by radiolucent spacers (Fig. 4-11). The height of the lead lamellae divided by the interspace thickness defines the grid ratio. In mammography, typical ratios are 4:1 or 5:1, and lamellae

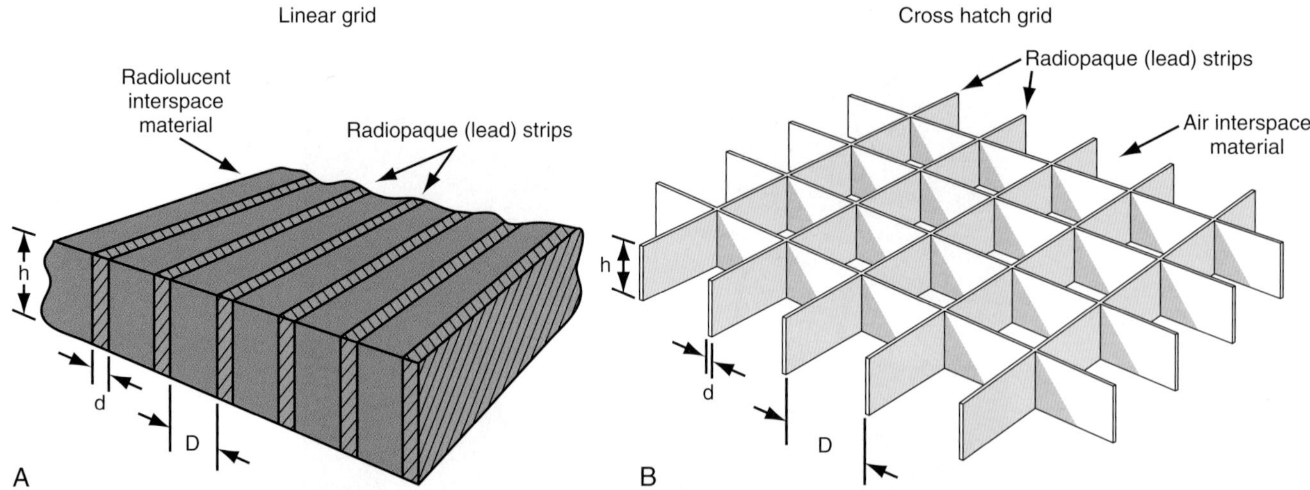

■ **FIGURE 4-11** **A,** Conventional mammography grid, width of lead lamellae. D, width of radiolucent interspace material; d, width of radiopaque strips; h, height of grid. Not shown are the top and bottom carbon fiber covers. *Black lines* represent radiopaque lead strips that make up the grid. The lead strips are focused on the focal spot so that the primary and information-carrying x-rays "see" only the edges of the strips. **B,** Principle of Lorad high-transmission cellular (HTC) grid. The grid controls scatter in two directions. A conventional linear grid controls scatter in only one direction.

strip densities are 30 to 50 lines/cm. The grid is positioned as shown in Figure 4-2, so that the primary or information-carrying x-rays strike only the edges of the lead lamellae and only a small percentage are absorbed. Scattered x-rays do not travel in a straight line from the focal spot to the image receptor. As a result, they strike a much greater area of lead and, compared with primary x-rays, are preferentially absorbed. The lamellae are projected by the primary beams as lines, and during an exposure, the grid is moved through a distance of 20 or more grid line spacings to blur out the lines. Ideally, a grid would transmit all the primary x-ray beam and absorb all the scatter. In practice, however, mammography grids transmit 60% to 75% of the primary x-rays and absorb 75% to 85% of the scatter.[18]

The performance of a grid depends on two factors: the improvement in contrast and the increase in dose that results when it is used. The factors are known as the contrast improvement factor (CIF) and the Bucky factor. When one compares two grids, the grid that has the higher CIF and lower Bucky factor is better. Both the CIF and Bucky factor of mammography grids vary with the ratio of scatter to primary x-rays emerging from the breast and, thus, with breast thickness. It has long been realized that conventional mammography grids are limited in performance. Although improved efficiency has been demonstrated, the majority of systems achieving it have not been capable of conventional positioning flexibility or of accommodating both small and large FOVs. One approach that does not have these limitations is the cellular, air-interspace grid introduced by Lorad (Hologic, Inc., Bedford, Mass.) in the mid-1990s. The grid, referred to as the HTC (high-transmission cellular) grid, is schematically shown in Figure 4-11. A linear grid controls scatter in one direction, and the cellular grid controls scatter in two directions. The HTC grid exhibits superior contrast improvement for all phantom thicknesses and tube potentials studied. It also has a lower (superior) Bucky factor for 2- and 4-cm phantom thicknesses and slightly higher Bucky factor (2.6% higher) for the 8-cm phantom thickness. In clinical practice, the HTC grid results in better contrast than a linear grid.

Automatic Exposure Control (AEC) System

A fundamental requirement in mammography is that the image receptor, either film or digital, be properly exposed. If the image receptor is not correctly exposed, breast structures will not be displayed with maximum contrast, information will be lost, and cancers will be missed. Proper exposure depends on the AEC system performance. The AEC on a mammography unit should provide consistent film density or signal intensity as breast thickness is varied for the range of x-ray tube potentials employed clinically.

In screen-film mammography, the AEC sensor is located in the U-arm mounting plate behind the image receptor (Fig. 4-12). The sensor detects x-rays that penetrate the breast and screen-film cassette and then generates a current proportional to the detected x-ray energy fluence. The current is amplified and charges a capacitor. The voltage across the capacitor is compared with a reference value, and when the two are equal, the exposure is terminated. Mammography units manufactured before 1990 did not achieved consistent film density because breast thickness and x-ray tube potential were varied.[7,19] Factors contributing to this unacceptable performance were greater beam hardening with increasing breast thickness, film reciprocity law failure, and AEC sensor dark current.[17]

Modern SFM AECs apply corrections for these effects and, if set up correctly, generally achieve acceptable performance. The MQSA regulations require that the AEC track to within ±0.15 OD (optical density) of the average OD as breast phantom thickness is varied from 2.0 to 6.0 cm over the clinically used range of tube potentials, filters, and x-ray tube target materials.[9]

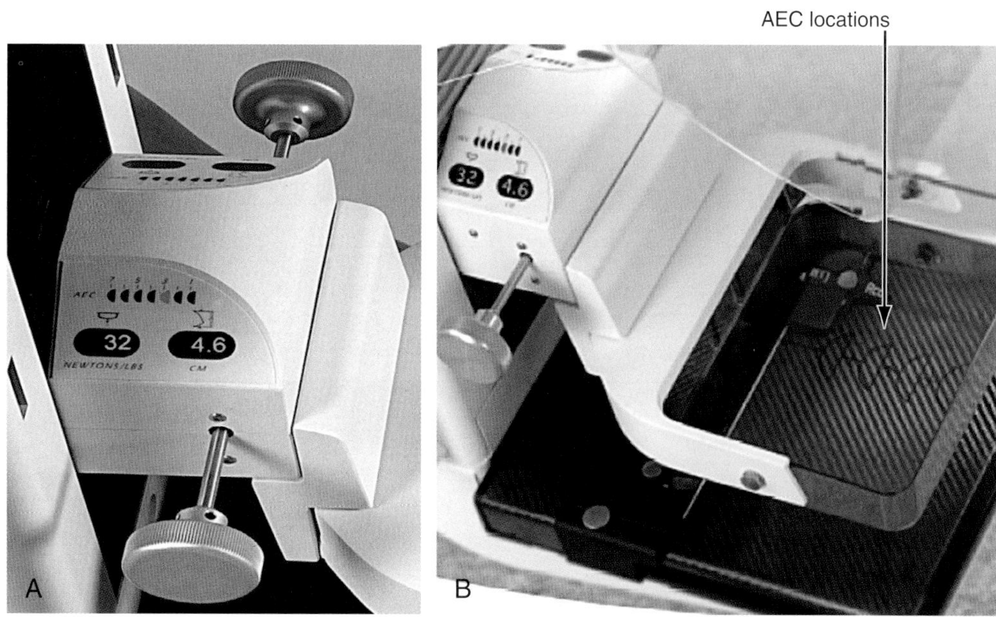

FIGURE 4-12 **A,** Display of automatic exposure control (AEC) sensor locations. **B,** Automatic exposure control sensor locations displayed on paddle. *(Courtesy of Hologic, Inc.)*

In FFDM, the AEC sensor is typically all, or part of, the digital detector itself. There is no separate AEC sensor as in SFM. The AEC function typically works by taking a short "pre-exposure" to determine the correct technique factors by evaluating breast thickness, breast density, and so on, and then continuing with a longer exposure that is determined by the pre-exposure. The FFDM manufacturer establishes the parameters for determining exposure parameters and often recommends to facilities what AEC mode to use.

For SFM, a mammography AEC should meet a number of other specifications. The sensor should have a range of movement (~8 cm) from close to the chest wall to out toward the nipple, so that it can be placed under the dense glandular tissue. A number of discrete positions are preferred, with the positions shown on the compression paddle (an MQSA regulation). A feature appreciated by technologists on one manufacturer's units is the additional ability to shift the sensor laterally about 2 centimeters on either side of the center line of the mounting plate. To assist the technologist, the lateral as well as the chest wall-to-nipple sensor positions are shown on the paddle.

For SFM, the AEC sensor should sample an adequate region of the breast. If it is too small (i.e., 1 cm^2), only a small area of the breast will determine the screen-film exposure, and because breast tissue is highly variable, greater exposure (and density) variations will occur than with a larger sensor. Two solutions to this problem that work well in practice are the following: (1) employing a D-shaped pickup with a sensitive area of 5 cm^2 or more; and (2) using an array of three 1-cm^2 sensitive sensors and summing the results of the three. Two of the sensors are positioned 4 cm apart, and the third is located in the middle of the other two and 2 cm anteriorly. In either approach, a larger area of breast tissue is sampled, but not so large that it extends beyond the boundaries of small breasts encountered. Sampling a larger area of breast tissue results in greater consistency in clinical film OD.

For SFM, the AEC should have a separate density calibration for grid and magnification techniques and two screen-film combination selections for each technique. (Several units also have a small and large grid assembly adjustment.) The unit should automatically select a default screen-film combination (programmable) for each technique—that is, a standard-speed screen-film system for grid technique and a faster screen-film system for magnification technique. It should also have 11 exposure steps (i.e., -5 to +5) with an exposure change of about 10% per increment. (The exposure change per increment should be programmable.) An exposure change of 10% corresponds to a film OD change of 0.15 to 0.20 for a typical mammography screen-film system. This is a desirable degree of film OD control for the technologist. An OD change of 0.10 or less per increment is too fine, and a change of 0.30 or more is too great.

The operator should be able to select between two manual techniques: Auto time and an optimized auto mode that selects the kVp or the kVp and filter. In the auto time AEC mode, the operator selects the kVp (and filter) and the unit determines the exposure time to achieve the correct film OD. In the optimized auto AEC mode, the unit selects the kVp and filter and determines the exposure time. On units that have dual targets, this latter mode also selects the target. Some manufacturers also offer an auto kVp AEC mode, in which the Mo/Mo target-filter is selected by the operator and the unit selects the kVp and determines the exposure time.

Magnification Stand

The MQSA regulations require that mammography systems used to perform noninterventional problem-solving procedures have radiographic magnification capability available for use by the operator.[15] For magnification work, the grid is removed and replaced on the U-arm's mounting plate by the magnification stand (Fig. 4-13). The regulations further require that at least one magnification value

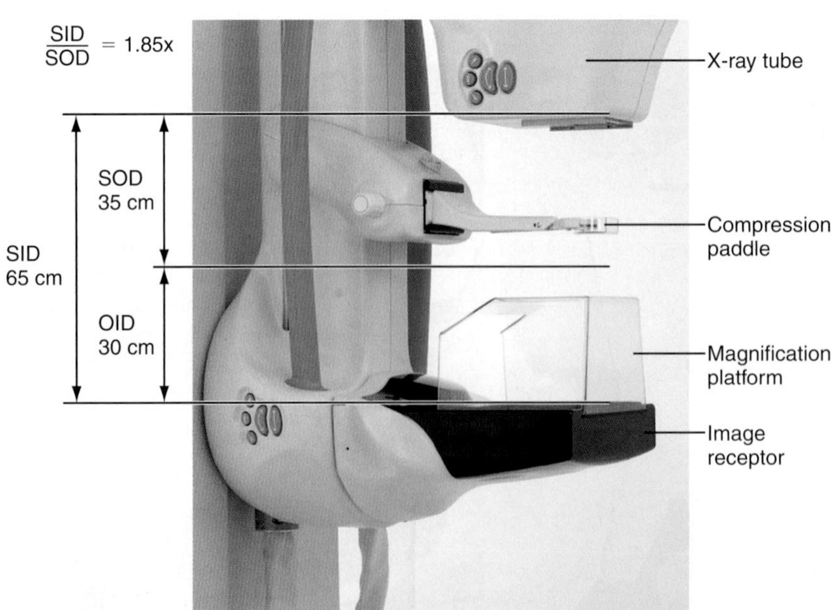

■ **FIGURE 4-13** Magnification stand used in mammography with associated smaller compression paddle. Geometry figures illustrate the magnification factor of 1.85. OID, object-to-image; SID, source-to-image; SOD, source-to object. *(Image courtesy of GE Medical Systems.)*

within the range of 1.4 to 2.0 be provided.[15] Implicit in this requirement and to meet the MQSA regulations system resolution, the unit must also have a small focal spot. For a 65-cm SID, space constraints limit the maximum magnification (2 cm above the breast support) to less than × 2.0. Although one or more manufacturers offer two magnification values (i.e., × 1.5 and × 2.0), the majority offer one value in the × 1.5 to × 2.0 range.

Magnification is employed to better delineate a region of interest of the breast. Image quality is improved because of the following: (1) system spatial resolution is better; and (2) more x-ray photons are used to image the structure of interest, and there is a 30% to 40 % decrease in effective noise.[19] Two important points of practical importance are to be pointed out: Firstly, magnification system resolution (0.1-mm focal spot) is better than grid technique, and secondly, the size of the small focal spot critically affects magnification system resolution. For example, at × 1.7, the system modulation transfer function (MTF) response with a 0.2-mm focus is degraded compared with the 0.1-mm focal spot response. The MQSA regulations are not overly stringent in this regard, requiring that the limiting spatial resolution associated with the width and length of the small focal spot be 13 lp/mm or more and 11 lp/mm or more, respectively.[15] Compared with a system with limiting resolutions of 13 lp/mm (width) and 11 lp/mm (length), images obtained with a system with limiting resolutions of 15 lp/mm appear sharper and microcalcification borders are better delineated. The measured system resolutions of a mammography unit are important parameters that have a direct impact on image quality, particularly the magnification system resolutions.

Additional factors affecting magnification image quality are kVp, exposure time, and FOV. If the small focal spot has sufficient loadability (i.e., ≥30 mA at 25 kVp), lower kVp and shorter exposure time techniques can be employed. Lowering the kVp increases subject contrast, and there is less chance of patient motion problems with shorter exposure times. Scatter depends on the FOV. Data for the dependence on the relative intensity of scatter on FOV in magnification mammography are limited, but fundamental imaging physics principles suggest that the smaller the FOV, the smaller the relative intensity of scatter imaged. The problem with decreasing the FOV too much is that it makes positioning difficult and also decreases the surround and the ability of the reader to orient himself or herself. A reasonable compromise is a 12 ×18-cm FOV at the image plane (~7 cm × 10.5 cm at the object plane). A problem with a 12 × 18-cm FOV is that a significant region of the image receptor is not exposed and must be masked for optimal viewing. However, the improvement in perceived image contrast more than compensates for this minor inconvenience.

Acquisition Workstation

Digital mammography (FFDM) has an acquisition workstation (AW) which is the first place the mammography technologist will experience the difference between SFM and FFDM. The AW is where the technologist will interact with the FFDM unit to acquire and manage images (Fig. 4-14). The AW consists of a computer, computer monitor, keyboard, mouse or trackball, and software specific to the FFDM manufacturer. The technologist will use the AW to perform patient acquisitions starting with entering patient data manually or obtaining patient data from a radiology information system. Once the patient data is entered, the technologist will adjust technique parameters using the acquisition console (Fig. 4-15). These parameter typically include selecting the automatic mode, tube target/tube filter combination, kVp, and mAs. The technologist can also select things such as image view, image laterality, and technologist ID.

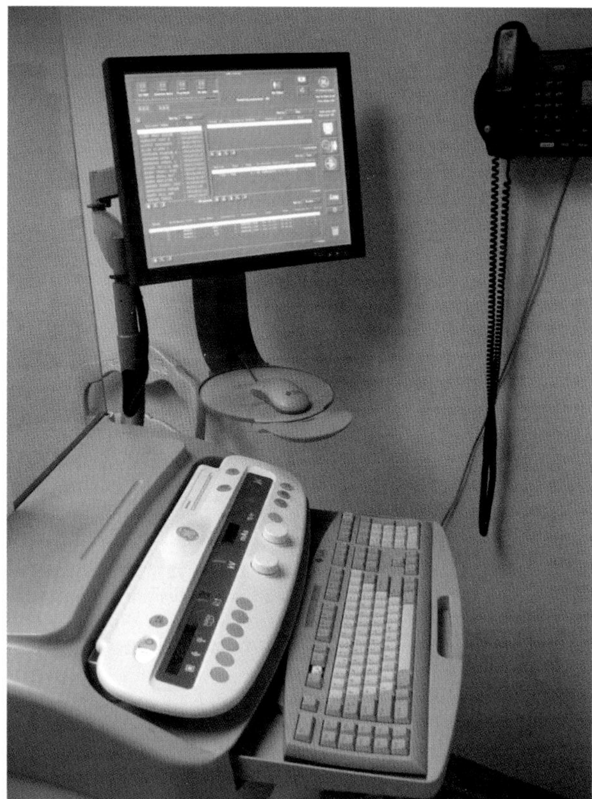

■ FIGURE 4-14 The acquisition workstation (AW) consisting of a computer, computer monitor, keyboard, mouse or trackball, and software specific to the full-field digital mammography (FFDM) manufacturer. The technologist uses the AW to perform patient acquisitions starting with entering patient data manually or obtaining patient data from a radiology information system.

Once the image is acquired, the technologist can use the AW to review the image and evaluate for quality. He or she can either accept the image and send it on for interpretation or reject and repeat the image. The AW is where the technologist performs all the tasks related to imaging of the patient and it allows technologists to view and interact with the digital image.

Radiologist Review Workstation

At the end of the FFDM imaging chain the radiologist has a review workstation (RW) which usually houses a pair of high-resolution monitors where the digital mammography images are interpreted. A typical radiologist RW consists of two high-resolution 5-megapixel (MP) monitors

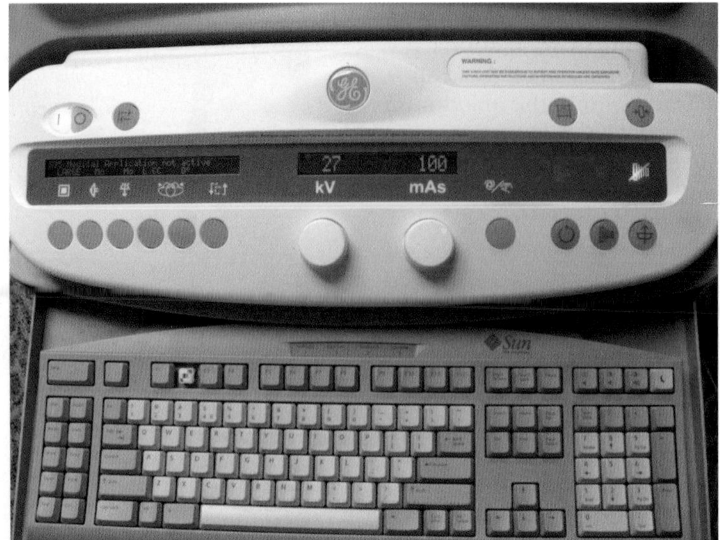

■ **FIGURE 4-15** The acquisition console shown here is where the technologist will adjust acquisition parameters such as automatic mode, tube target/tube filter combination, kVp, and mAs. The technologist can also select things like image view, image laterality, and technologist ID.

and a single lower resolution 2-MP monitor (Fig. 4-16). The 5-MP monitors are used for interpretation of digital mammograms while the single 2-MP monitor is often used for reading images from other modalities such as ultrasound, magnetic resonance (MR), or computed tomography (CT). The 2 MP monitor is also used for viewing the browser software for finding and reading patient lists.

Another important component of a RW that is designed for digital mammography is the dedicated keypad. This keypad has an array of single-stroke keys that are designed to navigate through mammography images and cases. Each manufacturer has its own version of a keypad while some use the keyboard with programmable "hotkeys."

Two important characteristics of display monitors are brightness and contrast. Brightness can be described by luminance (L) levels that are measured in candela per meter squared (cd/m^2). The Lmin and Lmax of a monitor can be measured and it is usually recommended that the Lmin be less than 1.0 cd/m^2 and the Lmax be at least 450 cd/m^2 or higher. Contrast should comply with the American Association of Physicists in Medicine (AAPM) Task Group 18 recommendations and should not deviate from the Digital Imaging and Communications in Medicine grayscale standard display function (DICOM GSDF) contrast values by more than 10%.[20]

Laser Printers

Dry laser printers in medical imaging have come to replace most, and at some point all, wet-chemistry film processors. These printers can be as small as a desktop printer to as

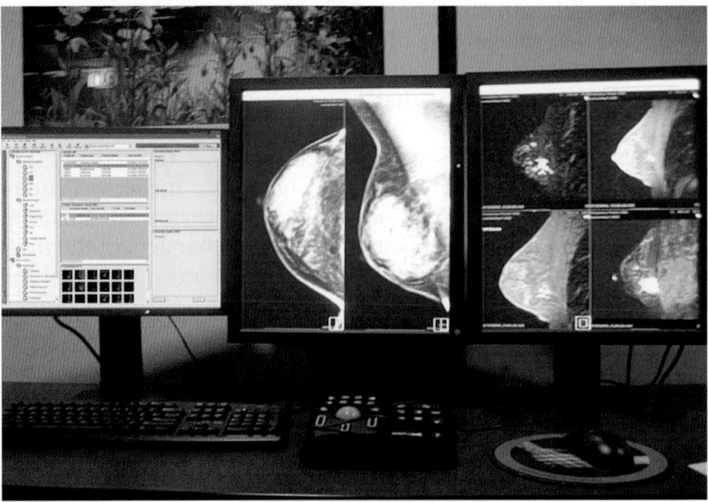

■ **FIGURE 4-16** Radiologist review workstation (RW), which is usually a pair of high-resolution monitors where the digital mammography images are interpreted. A typical radiologist RW consists of two high-resolution 5-megapixel (MP) monitors and a single lower resolution 2-MP monitor.

large as a floor-standing printer much the same size as the old wet-chemistry multi-loaders. The main advantage of the dry laser printers is their reliability and consistency. No longer do you see the dramatic fluctuations in optical densities that you would with the wet processors.

There is an MQSA requirement that all mammography facilities be able to provide final interpretation quality hard-copy images. So, a facility must have a laser printer somewhere within its imaging network. Currently the FDA only recommends that printers be cleared for FFDM by the Office of Device Evaluation (ODE) and does not require FDA approval. The American College of Radiology (ACR) has published several recommendations for printers and two of these consist of the printer being able to produce spatial sampling to match the detector element size of the FFDM detector, and printers conforming to the DICOM GSDF[21]. Finally, it is required by the FDA that all printers used with FFDM systems comply with a quality assurance program that is substantially the same as that recommended by the FFDM manufacturer.

Storage

The advent of FFDM has introduced the new challenge of storage and transmission of digital images. Digital images are relatively large images and require a lot of memory to store and display. There is the added complication that previous studies are needed for comparison. Therefore, a robust storage and retrieval system has become one of the most important features of a digital mammography system.

Digital image files of uncompressed images range from 8 megabytes (MB) for 18 cm × 23 cm FOV at 100 microns up to 50 MB for 24 cm × 30 cm FOV at 50 microns. Therefore a standard screening exam of 4 views can require from 32 to 200 MB. If you add prior studies from multiple years this number can grow exponentially and can easily outpace other modality storage needs in radiology.

An additional complication in digital mammography is the use of computer aided detection (CAD) which uses a *for-processing* image. This image is also known as a *raw* image and has no image processing applied to the image. A *for-presentation* image is used for diagnosis on the digital display and is different from the for-processing image. Therefore, for each image there are actually two images that may need to be stored, a for-processing and a for-presentation.

It is important to recognize that digital mammography needs a large storage device and high-speed data transmission to handle such large files.

Image Receptors: Film versus Digital

Film

Currently, several manufacturers supply intensifying screen cassettes and film designed for mammography. To maximize spatial resolution, these are all single screen, single emulsion film systems. The film consists of silver bromide grains in a gelatin matrix (emulsion) coated onto a polyester base. The emulsion layer is typically 10 μm, and the polyester base 180 μm in thickness. The intensifying screen consists of terbium-activated gadolinium oxysulfide (Gd_2O_2S:Tb) phosphor particles and binder layer coated on a polyester base. The phosphor particles are about 10 μm in size, the thickness of the layer is about 75 μm, and the thickness of the (polyester) base is about 225 μm. The coating weight of Gd_2O_2S:Tb phosphor is about 33 mg/cm^2. Gd_2O_2S:Tb is a bright phosphor that emits green light to which mammography film is sensitized (i.e., mammography film is orthochromatic).

The film is designed to have high contrast. This is accomplished with emulsions using a narrow silver bromide grain-size distribution of small cubic grains measuring approximately 1 μm. As illustrated in Figure 4-17, the x-ray beam is incident on the cassette and sequentially passes through the top of the cassette, the film base, and the film emulsion, and then strikes the intensifying screen. Although a (very) small percentage of x-rays are absorbed by the emulsion's silver halide grains, the majority are absorbed in the intensifying screen and are converted to light, which in turn exposes the film. A small percentage penetrate the screen and strike the AEC sensor. The percentage of the x-rays absorbed per unit thickness in the phosphor layer is greatest close to the film and decreases with increasing depth in the screen. Less light diffusion and blur are associated with x-rays absorbed close to the film, and greater diffusion occurs for x-rays absorbed farther away from the film. For this reason, the film, screen, and cassette geometry shown in Figure 4-18 is employed rather than the reverse; this geometry maximizes screen-film spatial resolution.

Mammography screen-film manufacturers typically offer one film and two screen speeds—standard and medium. The medium-speed system has slightly less spatial

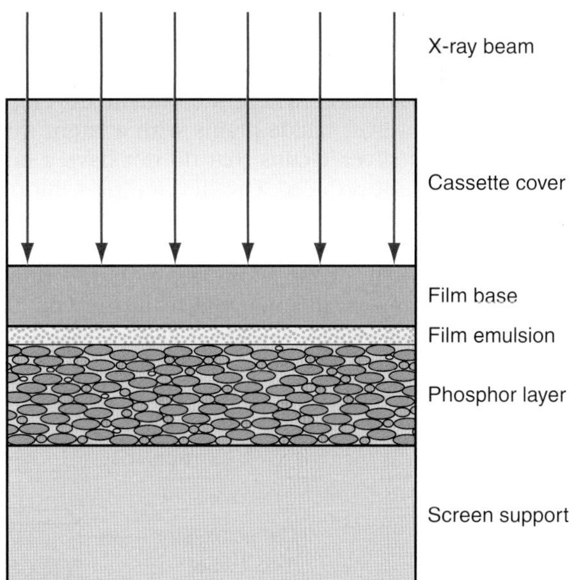

■ **FIGURE 4-17** Screen-film system geometry. The x-rays transmitted by the patient (and grid) are incident on the cassette. They sequentially pass through the top (polycarbonate) cover of the cassette, the film base, and the film emulsion layer and are incident on the phosphor layer of the intensifying screen. Most are absorbed by the phosphor layer, and only a few pass through the cassette and strike the automatic exposure control (AEC) sensor positioned below the screen-film cassette. The x-rays absorbed by the screen's phosphor layer are converted to light, exposing the film.

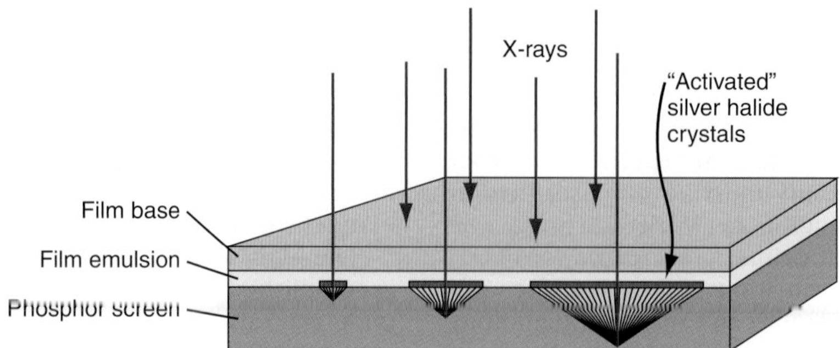

■ **FIGURE 4-18** A cross-section view of the film, screen, and cassette geometry. This geometry is employed rather than the reverse to maximize screen-film spatial resolution.

resolution and slightly more noise than the standard-speed system. However, the differences are subtle. The standard-speed screen is commonly employed for the majority of work at most mammography centers. The medium-speed screen, however, can be employed to advantage in two areas, magnification techniques and grid work for imaging of thick, dense breasts. In these cases, one must increase the kVp and exposure time to obtain a properly exposed image with the standard-speed system. With the medium-speed system, the subtle decrease in spatial resolution and subtle increase in image noise are more than compensated for by the reduced exposure time and lower kVp techniques that can be employed.

Film Processing Overview

The exposure of film to light results in the formation of latent image centers on grains that have received a sufficient amount of light. A latent image center consists of 4 to 10 silver atoms clustered at a surface sensitivity speck on a grain. Film development consists of first immersing the film in the developing solution, where the organic developing agents reduce the silver halide grains with a latent image center to metallic silver. Grains that do not have a latent image center are not reduced. The developing solution is basic (pH ~10.2). The fixing solution is acidic (pH ~ 4.2), and development is stopped when the film is immersed in the fixing solution. In the fixing solution, the remaining undeveloped grains are removed from the emulsion. Fixation is followed by washing and drying the film. Film processing is important and has a significant impact on mammography image quality. If the processing is subpar, film speed and film contrast are compromised.

Digital Detectors

There are several different types of digital detectors being used in digital mammography. These include slot scanning with a scintillator and a charge-coupled device (CCD) array, a flat-panel scintillator and an amorphous silicon diode array, a flat-panel amorphous selenium array, and photostimulable phosphor plates (computed radiography or CR). These different detectors are described in the following section.

Slot-Scan Charge-Coupled Device System

The Slot-Scan CCD system used by Fischer Medical Imaging uses a long, narrow, rectangular detector that is approximately 1 cm × 24 cm. The detector is made from thallium activated cesium iodide (CsI) phosphor with fiber optic coupling to a CCD. The CsI phosphor is deposited on a coupling plate that consists of millions of optical fibers that conduct light from the phosphor to the CCD array that converts the light into an electronic signal which is then digitized (Fig. 4-19). The x-ray beam is collimated to match the detector dimensions in the shape of a narrow fan beam.

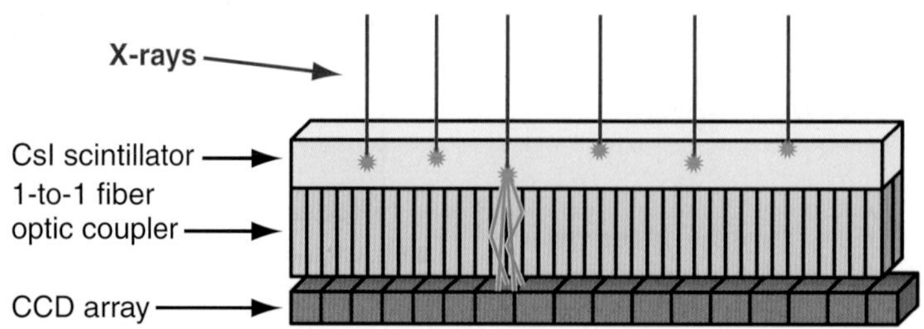

■ **FIGURE 4-19** Cross sectional view of a cesium iodide (CsI) with charge-coupled device (CCD) slot-scan detector. X-rays pass through the CsI scintillator producing visible light. The visible light is transmitted through the one-to-one fiber-optic coupler until it reaches the CCD array where the digital signal is formed.

To acquire an image the detector and x-ray fan beam scan laterally across the breast in synchrony. The detectors fixed matrix size is 400 × 2028 pixels with a total FOV of 21 × 29 cm resulting in an image matrix of 4096 × 5625 pixels. The total scan time is approximately 5.2 seconds with an effective exposure time of 200 milliseconds (msec). The detector element size is approximately 54 microns in standard resolution and 27 microns in high resolution. This type of system is no longer in commercial production since Fischer Medical Imaging was bought by Hologic in the mid 2000s.

Flat-Panel Phosphor System

The flat-panel phosphor system uses a large area glass plate onto which a large two dimensional matrix of light sensitive diodes and thin film transistors (TFTs) have been deposited. On top of this, a layer of linear columns of CsI crystals are deposited (Fig. 4-20). As x-ray photons are absorbed in the CsI crystals they are converted to visible light. The visible light travels down the columnar CsI crystals and is detected by the photodiodes. Each light sensitive diode is connected by TFT to a control and data line and read out as a digital signal. The CsI crystals are grown in long, tubular, structures that work to contain the light as it travels down the crystal (Fig. 4-21). This property works to reduce lateral spread and allows the detector to be made thicker to provide high quantum efficiency.

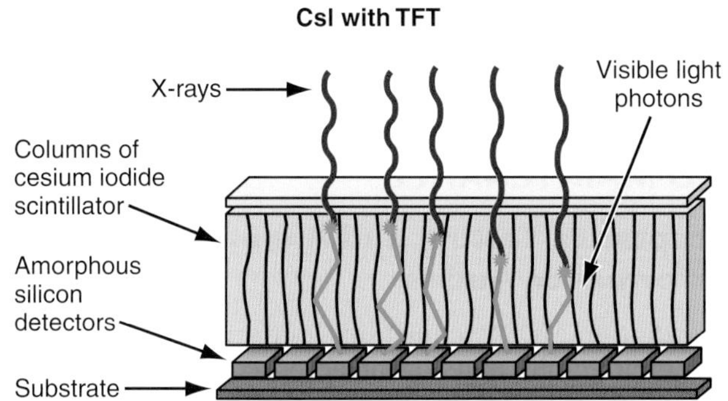

■ **FIGURE 4-20** Cross-sectional view of a cesium iodide (CsI) with thin film transistors (TFT) detector. X-rays are absorbed by the CsI scintillator producing visible light. The visible light is transmitted through the columnar CsI structures until it reaches the amorphous silicon detectors and the digital signal is formed. *(Image courtesy of GE Medical Systems.)*

The a-SI CsI detector system is used by GE Medical Systems in its Senographe 2000D, DS, and Essential systems. The 2000D and DS employ a 1920 × 2304 pixel matrix on a 19.2 × 23 cm detector with a 100 micron pixel size. The Essential uses a 2400 × 3100 matrix on a 24 × 31 cm detector with the same 100 micron pixel size.

Selenium Flat-Panel System

The Selenium flat-panel system is currently employed by both Hologic and Siemens Medical Systems for their FFDM systems. This detector design utilizes an x-ray absorber made of amorphous selenium. When the amorphous selenium absorbs x-rays and electric charge is liberated an electron-hole pair is formed. When an electric field is placed between the electrodes via electrodes on the upper and lower surface of the selenium, the charge from the electron-hole pair can be collected onto a readout surface (Fig. 4-22). The charge on the readout surface is then converted to a digital signal. Amorphous selenium is a good photoconductor with a high x-ray absorption characteristic (>95%) in the mammography energy ranges. Another advantageous characteristic is its narrow line-spread function that helps improve spatial resolution.

The selenium systems typically have FOVs of 24 × 29 cm and a pixel size of 70 microns. Matrix size is fixed at 3328 × 4096 pixels.

Computed Radiography System

Computed radiography (CR) systems in digital mammography are similar to those used in conventional radiography. These detectors employ a plastic sheet coated with a

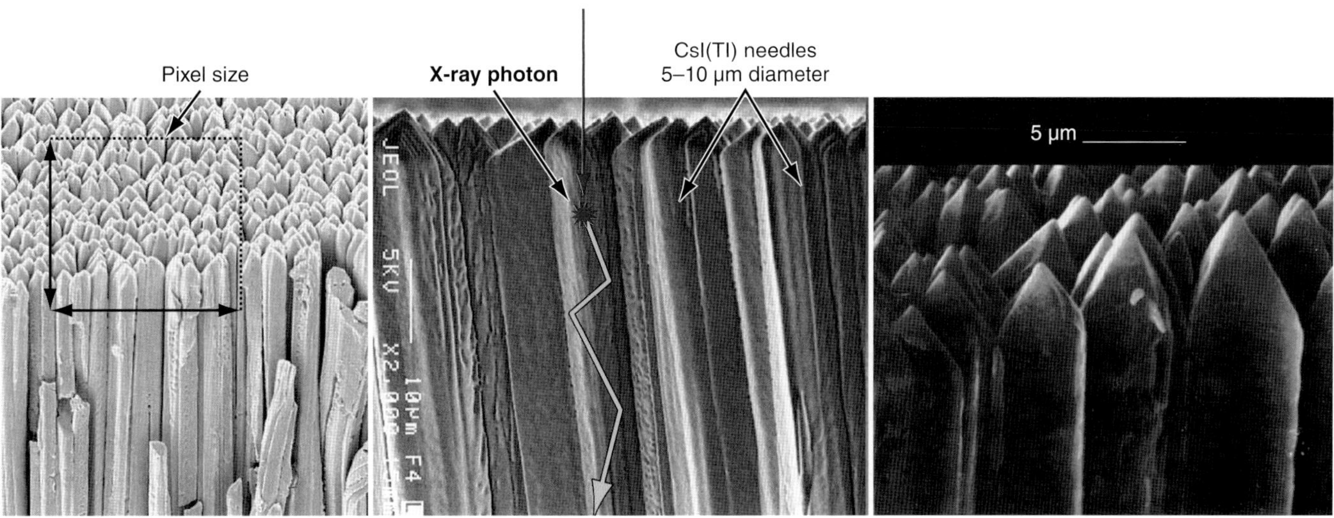

■ **FIGURE 4-21** The cesium iodide (CsI) crystals are grown in long, tubular, structures that work to contain the light as it travels down the crystal. Here are a set of high-resolution images showing magnified CsI crystals. *(Images courtesy of GE Medical Systems.)*

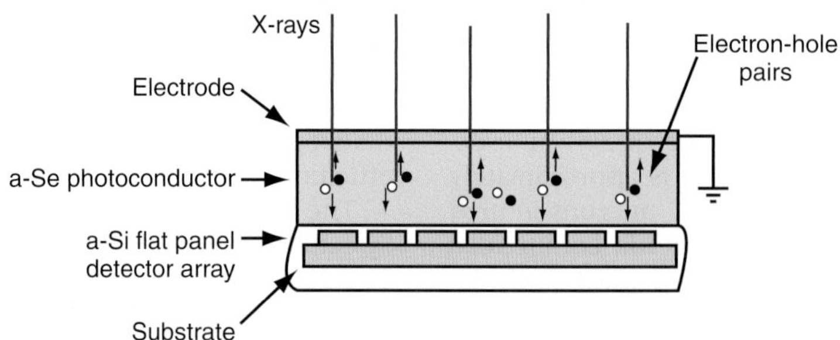

■ **FIGURE 4-22** Cross-sectional view of an amorphous selenium with thin film transistors (TFT) detector. When the amorphous selenium absorbs x-rays and an electric charge is liberated, an electron-hole pair is formed. When an electric field is placed between the electrodes via electrodes on the upper and lower surface of the selenium, the charge from the electron-hole pair can be collected onto a readout surface. The charge on the readout surface is then converted to a digital signal.

photostimulable phosphor material as the x-ray absorber. These are typically made from $BaFBR:Eu^{2+}$. The phosphor plates are exposed to x-rays and an electronic charge is stored at the location of the absorbed x-ray. The charges are stored in "traps" and are proportional to the amount of incident x-rays. The image is read in a CR reader by a precision laser beam. During the scanning process a red laser beam discharges the traps causing stimulated emission of blue light that is collected by light guides that funnel the light into photo-multiplier tubes (Fig. 4-23). The resulting signal from the photomultiplier tubes is logarithmically amplified, digitized, and processed for display.

Many manufacturers use CR in FFDM but only Fuji Medical Systems has an FDA approved device for use in the United States as of February 2010. Its system provides two CR cassette sizes that match the traditional screen-film mammography cassette sizes of 18 × 24 cm and 24 × 30 cm. Image matrix sizes are 1770 × 2370 pixels and 2364 × 2964 pixels. Spatial resolution for this system utilizes a 50 micron pixel size.

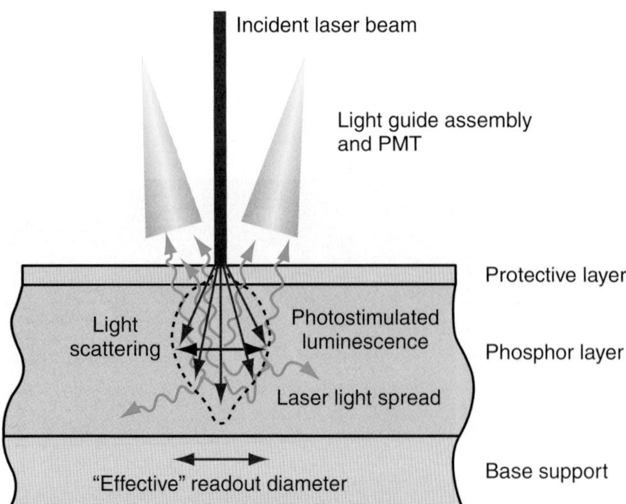

■ **FIGURE 4-23** Cross sectional view of a computed radiography imaging plate and readout schematic. During the scanning process, a red laser beam discharges the traps causing stimulated emission of blue light that is collected by light guides that funnel the light into photo-multiplier tubes. The resulting signal from the photomultiplier tubes (PMTs) is logarithmically amplified, digitized, and processed for display. *(Image courtesy of Fuji Medical Systems.)*

EQUIPMENT PERFORMANCE AUDITS AND MAINTENANCE

Acceptance Testing and Annual Performance Audits

According to MQSA regulations, performance evaluations of mammography units or image processors must be performed by (or under the direct supervision of) a qualified medical physicist whenever a new unit or processor is installed or whenever a unit or processor is dissembled and reassembled at either the same or at a new facility.[15] All problems found that do not satisfy MQSA regulations must be corrected, the correction documented, and the documentation reviewed by the medical physicist before the unit is put into clinical use. The MQSA regulations also require that each facility undergo an annual equipment performance audit by a medical physicist. As with the initial or acceptance testing of a unit, problems found in meeting MQSA regulations must be corrected, the correction documented, and the documentation reviewed by the medical physicist.

With an annual audit, however, there are requirements depending on the test for either SFM or FFDM that either the facility can continue to use the unit and has 30 days from the date of the audit (not the date of the report) to correct the problems, or, must fix the problem before further clinical use of the unit. It is beyond the scope of this chapter to detail these, but it is important for a facility to know which tests have to be repaired immediately and which tests have 30 days to be repaired. Two important quality control tests with have to be corrected immediately are: accreditation (ACR) phantom image quality and dose. If the phantom image made at the time of an annual audit does not satisfy the minimum standards of the accreditation body or if the average glandular phantom dose exceeds 300 mrad, the unit cannot be used for mammography until the problem is corrected.

Additional Medical Physics Equipment Evaluations

The MQSA regulations require that evaluations be performed by a qualified medical physicist (or by an individual under the direct supervision of a qualified medical physicist) whenever major components of a mammography unit or processor are changed or repaired.[15] These evaluations are used to determine whether the new or repaired component meets MQSA performance standards. All problems are to be corrected before the new or repaired component is put into service. Examples of major equipment component replacement that require medical physics testing are the x-ray tube, digital detector replacement, collimation subassembly, compression subassembly, AEC sensor and associated circuitry, and grid assemblies. Examples of processor major components that require medical physics testing are replacement or rebuilding of processor racks (as opposed to routine cleaning and preventive maintenance).

Equipment Maintenance and Repair

The warranty on a new mammography unit is typically a year, during which the vendor maintains the unit and corrects problems. The quality and reputation of a vendor's service organization are an important consideration in purchasing a unit. After the warranty period, the five service options for a facility are a full service contract, partial service contract, no service contract, in-house service, and risk insurance with a third party. With no service contract, the facility pays time and materials for each repair and replaced component. Partial service contracts are variable but typically have most of the features of a full service contract, excluding glassware (x-ray tubes). It is highly recommended that digital mammography units maintain a service contract that covers the entire detector and related parts. These are extremely expensive to replace.

When one is purchasing a new unit, it is a good idea to require documentation of the costs of full service and the type of partial service contracts in which the facility is interested for a period of 5 years beyond the warranty period. This provides the purchaser a degree of price protection. Service contracts are an important cost consideration, and adding a 5-year full-service cost to the initial cost of the unit is known as its life cycle cost. If the service contract price for a mammography unit seems too high, either the equipment is not well engineered and requires an excessive amount of service or the service contract price is inflated. Either of these reasons detracts from the unit's desirability. Some equipment manufacturers sell new units at a relatively small profit margin with the intent of making a substantial profit on parts and service. Response time during regular working hours, evenings, and occasionally on weekends is also important; this issue should be documented before a unit or a service contract is purchased.

In-house service can be cost effective and provide timely response.[22] However, it is feasible only for larger facilities and must be well managed. Smaller facilities are limited to vendor or third-party equipment maintenance, either with or without a service contract. With in-house service replacement, parts can be a problem. Obtaining a purchase order for a part can take considerable time and effort at larger institutions. The process can be expedited with a parts contract, whereby the in-house service person need not obtain a purchase order before ordering a needed part.

There are at least two service risk insurance options. For one, the facility directly calls the service vender of choice to arrange for problems to be fixed, and the insurance company pays the service bill. For the other, the facility calls the third party risk insurer, which in turn arranges for the unit to be fixed with either the vendor or another service organization. Insurance options add a layer of bureaucracy, slow down repairs, and involve an additional party that is making money from the service. In the author's experience, risk insurance offers little or no advantage for mammography.

A cost-effective approach for a smaller facility is to expect to pay for time and materials, or to have no contract. To avoid a budget crisis, a service account should be set up and money added each year or each quarter equal to the cost of a full service contract, so as to pay for time and materials or repairs as needed. When the money in the account exceeds the cost of replacing the x-ray tube, the amount added the next year need only be equal to a service contract excluding glassware, and so on. With this approach, the facility is self-insured and, provided that there is not a catastrophic equipment failure, saves money. Also, if a site is planning to not have a full service contract, it is advantageous on a new unit to schedule the medical physicist's annual performance audit a month or more before the end of the warranty period and request that the physicist send the report in immediately after completing the survey. The problems that are identified by the medical physicist and must be corrected are then covered by the warranty.

With any of the preceding service options, the original equipment manufacturer's preventive maintenance recommendations should be reviewed and the key points followed. For example, on some manufacturers' units, the automated AEC algorithms depend on the compressed breast thickness reading. If the reading is off by a centimeter or more, the wrong kVp and filter can be selected and image quality compromised. This is one of the many settings on a unit that must be checked and calibrated periodically. Preventive maintenance can minimize unnecessary and unexpected downtime.

Acknowledgment

The author is grateful for Dr Gary Barnes, whose treatment of this topic in the last incarnation of this book greatly informed the present chapter.

KEY POINTS

- Modern mammography equipment utilize screen-film or full-field digital technologies. Both contain very sophisticated technologies which continue to evolve.
- Full-field digital mammography systems use very different detector technologies that have different components with different specifications. As a result, these detectors have different pixel sizes, image matrix sizes, and spatial resolution.
- Both screen-film and full-field digital mammography are governed by the laws written in the MQSA regulations. These regulations detail requirements both for personnel (Radiologists, Technologists, and Medical Physicisits) and for mammography equipment including quality control.

REFERENCES

1. Salomon A. Beitrage zur pathologie und klinik der mammacarcinome. *Arch Klin Chir* 1913;**101**:573-668.
2. Leborgne RA. Diagnosis of Tumors of the Breast by Simple Roentgenology. *Am J Roentgenol Radium Ther* 1951;**65**:1-11.
3. Leborgne RA. *The Breast in Roentgen Diagnosis. Montevideo*. Uruguay: Impresora Uruguaya; 1953.
4. Egan RL. Experience with mammography in a tumor institution: evaluation of 1000 cases. *Radiology* 1960;**75**:894-900.
5. Gros CM. Methodologie: Symposium Sur Le Sein. *J Radiol Electrol Med Nucl* 1967;**48**:638-55.
6. Buchanan RA, Finkelstein SI, Wickersheim KA. X-ray exposure reduction using rare earth oxysulfide intensifying screens. *Radiology* 1976;**118**:183-8.
7. Haus AG. Technologic improvements in screen-film mammography. *Radiology* 1990;**174**:628-37.
8. Conway BJ, McCrohan JL, Reuter FG, Suleiman OH. Mammography in the 80s. *Radiology* 1990;**177**:335-9.
9. Russell HD. Rapid processing of x-ray film. *Photographic Science and Engineering* 1959;**3**:32-4.
10. Lewin JM, Hendrick RE, D'Orsi CJ, Isaacs PK, Moss LJ, Karellas A, et al. Comparison of full-field digital mammography with screen-film mammography for cancer detection: Results of 4,945 paired examinations. *Radiology* 2001;**218**:873-80.
11. Gold HR. The evolution of mammography. In: Bassett LW, editor. *Radiologic Clinics of North America: Breast Imaging*, vol. 30. Philadelphia: WB Saunders; 1992. p. 1-19.
12. Bassett LW, Gold RH, Kimme-Smith C. *History of the technical development of mammography. RSNA AAPM Syllabus on Technical Aspects of Breast Imaging*. 3rd ed. 1994.
13. Houn F, Elliott ML, McCrohan JL. The Mammography Quality Standards Act of 1992. In: *Radiologic Clinics of North America: Breast Imaging*. vol. 33. Philadelphia: WB Saunders; 1995. p. 1059-65.
14. Hendrick RE. Quality assurance in mammography. In: Bassett LW, editor. *Radiologic Clinics of North America: Breast Imaging*, vol. 30. Philadelphia: WB Saunders; 1992. p. 243-55.
15. Department of Health and Human Services. FOA 21 CFR Part 900: April 28, 1999.
16. Barnes GT, Brezovich IA. Contrast: effect of scattered radiation. In: Logan WW, editor. *Breast Carcinoma: The Radiologist's Expanded Role*. New York: John Wiley & Sons; 1977. p. 73-81.
17. LaFrance R, Gelskey DE, Barnes GT. A circuit modification that improves mammographic phototimer performance. *Radiology* 1988;**166**:773-6.
18. Barnes GT. Contrast and scatter in x-ray imaging. *Radiographics* 1991;**11**:307-23.
19. Barnes GT. Tube potential, focal spot, radiation output and HVL measurements on screen-film mammography units. In: Barnes GT, Frey GD, editors. *Screen-Film Mammography: Imaging Considerations and Medical Physics Responsibilities*. Madison, WI: Medical Physics; 1991. p. 67-113.
20. Samei E, Bodano A, Chakraborty D, Compton K, Cornelius C, Corrigan K, et al. Assessment of display performance for medical imaging systems: Executive summary of AAPM TG 18 Report. *Med Phys* 2005;**32**:1205-25.
21. ACR Practice Guideline. *Practice guideline for determinants of image quality in digital mammography*. 2007 (Res. 35).
22. Barnes GT, McDanal W. When is inhouse service cost effective? *Proc SPIE* 1980;**233**:286-90.

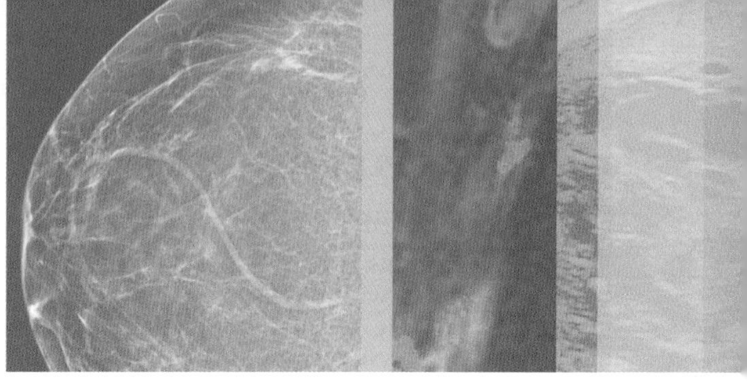

Computer-Aided Detection

Robyn L. Birdwell and Ronald A. Castellino

The terms *computer-aided detection* and *computer-aided diagnosis* are often used to describe the same process and, to confound the problem, they share the same acronym, CAD. In this chapter, the term *CADe* will be used to indicate those computer systems designed to aid the radiologist *detect* features worrisome for breast cancer. The term *CADx* will refer to those computer systems designed to aid the radiologist *classify* detected (either by the radiologist alone or with CADe input) features worrisome for breast cancer as being benign or malignant. Although to our knowledge such a system does not yet exist, the term *CADr* might refer to a computer system that independently both detects and then classifies candidate lesions and then issues the final report.

Research on CADe systems began several decades ago to address the known false-negative rate in screening mammography, which was generally accepted as being around 20%. The reasons for this error rate are varied but can be conveniently considered to be errors of visual perception or of cognition.[1] In an error of perception, the unreported cancer is completely overlooked by the observer or is looked at but not long enough to allow detection or recognition. In an error of cognition, the unreported cancer is looked at long enough (perceived) but erroneously judged to not represent an actionable finding warranting further investigation.[2] Bird and colleagues reported that some 43% of missed breast cancers were due to cancers being overlooked (perception errors), 52% to misinterpretation (cognitive errors), and 5% to suboptimal technique.[3]

A CADe system addresses perception errors. (A CADx system would address cognitive errors.) It is important to note that a CADe system is *not* equivalent to a "second reader" as occurs with double-reading protocols that use two radiologists. The CADe system marks (detects) features that require assessment (interpretation) by the same radiologist who first read the examination unaided by CAD. Thus, a CADe system is really a "second detector/perceiver." Depending on the protocol used, double reading with two radiologists may be independent with all abnormal findings recalled for additional evaluation or may be achieved via consensus, limiting the number of recalls after some degree of arbitration. Regardless of the double-reading method used, interpretation of a mammogram by two (or more) humans differs from adding CADe "look again" marks to the interpretation by one radiologist.

Even though a CADe system (correctly) marks a subsequently proven cancer (a true-positive CADe mark), the assessment of this lesion as to whether further investigation is warranted is done by the radiologist. And, at times, a true-positive CADe mark will be dismissed by the radiologist. When this occurs, the radiographic appearance of the marked cancer falls into two overlapping and subjective categories. The first is when the mammographic features of the cancer are sufficiently nonspecific that recalling all such similar findings in a screening population for further imaging would result in an unacceptably high recall rate (low positive predictive value for cancer). In this instance, the radiologist is correct in dismissing such nonspecific findings, even though the cancer is not diagnosed. The second category is when the mammographic features of the cancer are sufficiently compelling such that most radiologists would recall the woman for further investigation. In this instance, this undiagnosed cancer would be considered an error of cognition.

In 1998, the U.S. Food and Drug Administration (FDA) approved the first commercially available CADe system for mammography, and within several years FDA approval for CADe systems from other vendors followed. Initial modest adoption of CADe technology by American mammography practices steadily increased after publication of early studies supporting its impact on increasing the cancer detection rate[4,5] and approval of reimbursement to support the purchase and maintenance of the CADe systems. However, a few recent published studies have challenged the reported value of CADe, and the residual controversy on the impact of CADe in clinical practice will be addressed here.

BASIC PRINCIPLES

The Mammographic Image

The CADe algorithms require a digital image to analyze for features associated with the mammographic appearances of breast cancer (Fig. 5-1). For screen-film mammography (SFM) acquisition systems, the analog information on the processed films is converted to digital information, such as with a laser scanner, at resolutions typically in the 50-μm and 12-bit gray scale range. This digitization process inherently introduces noise into the digital dataset, which, if significant, can affect the reproducibility of the true-positive and false-positive CADe marks on the same image when serially digitized. Fortunately, with current scanners the reproducibility of the true-positive marks is very high.

For digital mammography acquisition systems, the image is already in a digital format, which addresses the reproducibility issue. However, potential differences in CADe output (true- and false-positive marks) might arise if the CADe system processed the raw data obtained by the digital mammography unit versus the processed image used for image interpretation.

The CADe Algorithms

CADe systems use varying proprietary strategies such as segmentation, filters, pattern recognition, neural networks, and others to analyze the mammographic images. The algorithms are designed to search for features that are associated with the mammographic appearances of breast cancer, which can be divided into two broad categories: microcalcifications and masses (which include spiculated and nonspiculated margins and areas of architectural distortion). These findings can at times coexist as masses containing microcalcifications. The CADe systems produce different marks for indication of microcalcifications and masses.

Because the CADe algorithms identify numerous candidate lesions on the mammographic image, those that possess "stronger" morphologic features such as densities with spiculated margins are selected to be displayed for the radiologist. This hierarchical selection/exclusion process is used to decrease the number of false-positive CADe marks. The center of a CADe mark of the correct category (microcalcification or mass) placed within the confines of a biopsy-proven cancer is considered a true-positive mark, and the center of a CADe mark not placed within a cancer is a false-positive CADe mark.

CADe Sensitivity and Specificity

CADe "stand-alone" sensitivity refers to the fraction of cancers correctly marked by a CADe system. The false marker rate serves as a surrogate for CADe specificity.

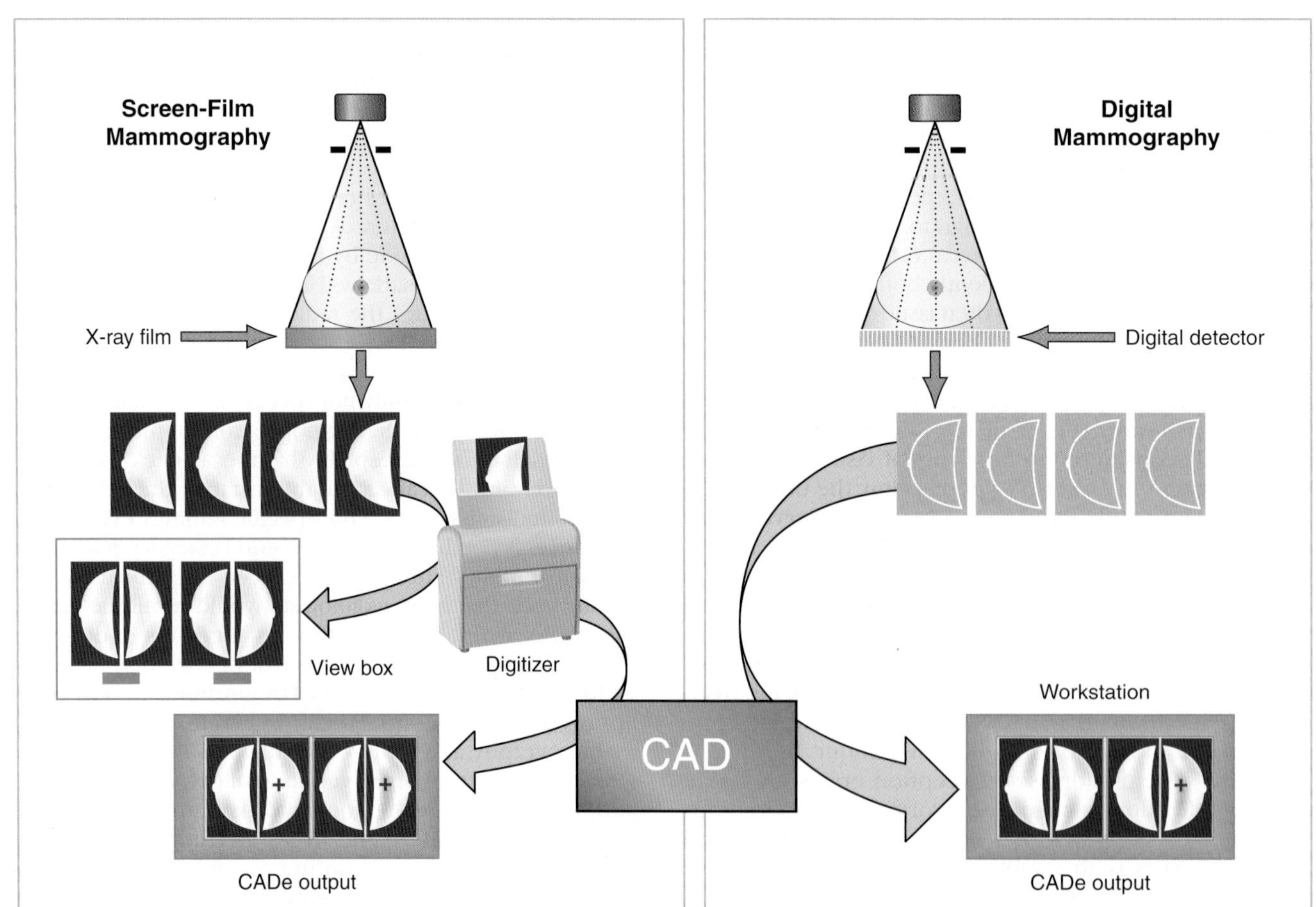

■ **FIGURE 5-1** Schematic illustrates differences in steps required to produce CADe output. *Left*, The analog film image must be digitized to enable analysis by the CAD algorithms. The analog films are reviewed on a viewbox in the standard fashion. CAD input is provided on adjacent CRT or flat panel display, or paper printout. *Right*, The CAD algorithms analyze the digitally acquired image that is transferred to the radiologist's workstation. The CAD results are available on the readout workstation.

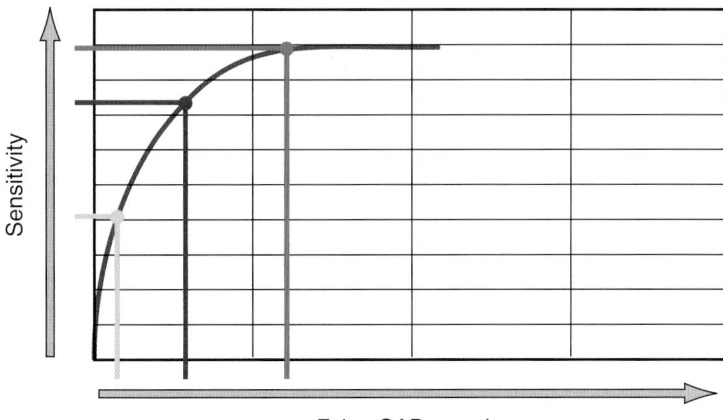

■ **FIGURE 5-2** Schematic of an fROC plot for a CADe algorithm. Three different points (orange, red, and green) are selected on the fROC curve. As sensitivity is increased (moving higher along the x-axis) there is an increase in the false marker rate (moving toward the right on the y-axis).

As with human observers, CADe system performance can be described on receiver operating characteristic (ROC) curves (Fig. 5-2). An increase in sensitivity is accompanied by an increase in the false marker rate. Conversely, an increase in specificity (i.e., a decrease in the false marker rate) is accompanied by a decrease in sensitivity.[6] Most FDA-approved CADe systems are set to work at a false marker rate of around two false marks per four-view normal case. More recently, vendors have provided more than one operating point on the fROC curve to accommodate reader preference (i.e., opting for the higher sensitivity versus the lower false marker rate).

Reading Protocol

According to the FDA current guidelines for case review with CADe systems, the case is first reviewed in the usual fashion without CADe input and a decision is reached as to whether the case is normal or if a perceived lesion(s) is interpreted as requiring further workup. The marks from the CADe system are then reviewed to determine if any overlooked features warrant further workup. In this scenario there are two important rules to follow:

1. Always evaluate a finding of concern noted on the initial review without CADe input even if not marked by the CADe system. This is because the CADe algorithms are not 100% sensitive and some visible and actionable cancers will not be marked by the CADe system (a false-negative CADe case).
2. Never evaluate a finding simply because it is marked by the CADe system unless that finding (which was presumably overlooked on the initial review) is judged to warrant recall. This is because the CADe algorithms provide many false-positive CADe marks.

The purpose of a CADe system is to alert the radiologist to findings that may represent cancer and that may have been overlooked on the initial, unaided review. The radiologist must then decide (interpret) which of these CADe prompts warrant patient recall.

Of note, there has been recent interest in using CADe input as a concurrent detector, or even as the initial, and only, detector. Paquerault and coworkers[7] reported a reader study that compared observer performance when a CADe system was used as a second reader to concurrent-use CADe. They concluded that "readers may benefit as much or more when using CAD in a concurrent mode than with CAD as a second reader when detecting mass-like objects in mammographic backgrounds." Yaffe and associates[8] reported that if CADe was used as a prescreening tool with digital mammography, and if only cases with one or more CADe marks were referred for review by the radiologist, only 1 of 71 cancers would not have been referred. This one cancer was missed by a panel of 10 readers without CADe input. At this threshold, there would have been a reduction in workload of 14% without a loss of sensitivity.

Learning Curve

The introduction of new technologies is accompanied by a period during which the practitioner gains increased skills in the most effective implementation to enhance patient care. With increasing experience, outcomes are improved and complications are diminished. The adoption of CADe in a clinical practice is no exception, and radiologists will experience a learning curve on the optimal use of this technology. More specifically, most users will find that their recall rate will increase as they learn how to best manage the false-positive CADe marks, that is, that the marked features require the same interpretive rigor as features that they perceive and evaluate unaided by CADe input.

During the first 2 months of CADe use, Dean and Ilvento[9] experienced a doubling of their recall rate (from 6.2% before CADe implementation to 13.4%). Over the study period, however, the recall rate declined to 6.75%. Their experience suggests that the learning curve, as judged by a decrease in the inflated recall rate associated with initial use of CADe, may take as long as 1 year. Of importance, an increase in recall rate should also result in a comparable increase in the cancer detection rate. As was shown in this study, although the impact of CADe on radiologist performance resulted in an increase in the recall rate of 8.9% (from 6.2% to 6.75%), the cancer detection rate increased by 11.4%.

EVALUATION OF CADE SYSTEMS

Initial evaluations of a CADe algorithm are generally done in a laboratory-type setting. These include determination of stand-alone sensitivity on cancer cases and false marker rates (a surrogate for specificity) on normal cases. Subsequent evaluations investigate the impact of a CADe system on radiologist performance in a real-life clinical practice setting. CADe system input should initially lead to an increase in the cancer detection rate by decreasing the number of overlooked, or missed, cancers. In order to diagnose more cancers, the recall and biopsy rates will increase as well. Importantly, the increase in the recall and biopsy rates due to CADe input should be concordant with (i.e., similar to or less than) the increase in the cancer detection rate. After some time during which the CADe system has increased the detection rate by detecting cancers that ordinarily would have been diagnosed as interval cancers or at the next screening round, the detection rate will likely drift down to a baseline level based on the number of visible and actionable cancers that the radiologist will diagnose unaided and then aided by CADe input. However, one would expect an increase in the proportion of more favorable cancers (smaller in size and lower grade and stage) than before installation of a CADe program.

CAD Stand-Alone Performance Studies

In CAD stand-alone performance studies, mammograms of biopsy-proven cancers and of normal cases (usually defined as mammograms read as normal with one or more years of subsequent normal examinations) are collected and analyzed by a CADe system. For cancer cases, a true positive CADe mark is defined as follows: A CADe mark (1) whose center lies within the confines of the known cancer on the mammogram; and (2) is of the correct classification (microcalcification or mass). CADe stand-alone *case sensitivity* is defined as the percentage of cancers correctly marked on at least one of the standard four-view screening examinations. CADe stand-alone *image sensitivity* is defined as the percentage of cancers correctly marked on the number of views (one or both) on which the cancer is visible. For practical purposes (in a clinical setting), a CADe mark on only one of the two views that both have a visible cancer is of little importance, because the view with the marked cancer should be sufficient to alert the radiologist to a feature that warrants further consideration. Once prompted, if the lesion is also visible on the other (nonmarked) view, the radiologist should identify it independently.

A *false-positive CADe mark* is one whose center lies outside the confines of a cancer (if a cancer is present on the image). Because (by definition) the normal cases collected for stand-lone performance studies have no visible cancers, any CADe mark present is a false-positive mark. This is generally reported as the average number of false marks per four-view normal case and serves as a surrogate for specificity.

Stand-alone performance studies are useful to determine the robustness of a CADe system, in that they provide data on the sensitivity of the algorithms for correctly marking the broad categories of breast cancer features (microcalcifications and masses) and, importantly, the false CADe marker rate. This is particularly useful for developers of CADe systems because they evaluate the impact of new versions of algorithm performance on the same test set for improvements in CADe sensitivity and false marker rates.

A note of caution: stand-alone performance results reported by researchers in academic and private settings, and by CADe vendors, are almost always done on their own case sets of cancer and normal cases. These case sets are dissimilar and will vary in the composition and complexity of both cancer and normal cases. Therefore, to compare the performance of two different CADe systems (or different versions of the same CADe system), comparative standalone performance studies must use the same test set of cancer and normal cases. Several investigators have compared the performance of different CADe systems on the same test case set (known cancers and normal cases) for cancers manifesting as architectural distortions,[10] masses,[11] and small (<16 mm), noncalcified invasive cancers.[12] In this way, and for those particular cases sets, one can determine which CADe system has the superior performance, as measured by the sensitivity (true-positive CADe marks) and false marker rate (the average false-positive CADe marks per four-view normal case) (Figs 5-3 and 5-4).

In all fairness, it should be noted that stand-alone performance studies that use cancers detected by radiologists in clinical practice as the gold standard do not present a complete measure of CADe sensitivity. In such studies, CADe sensitivity essentially will always be less than 100%, that is, CADe will appear less sensitive than radiologists. However, we know that 15% to 20% of visible and actionable cancers are *not* diagnosed in clinical practice and that some of these missed cancers will be correctly marked by CADe.[13] Therefore, a more complete measure of CADe standalone sensitivity would be to also include CADe performance on the baseline mammograms on which there is, in retrospect, visible and actionable evidence of interval cancers and cancers diagnosed at the next screening round. A few studies have taken this approach.[14]

Potential Impact of CADe on Missed Cancers Studies

Missed cancers studies consist of screening mammograms that were originally read as normal in clinical practice but in retrospect (and with knowledge of the location of a subsequently diagnosed cancer) are judged to have visible evidence of the missed cancer. These cases are analyzed by a CADe system, and the number of correctly marked retrospectively visible cancers is determined. If one assumed that all correct CADe marks would be acted upon, the potential impact of CADe on radiologist sensitivity could be calculated.[4,5] This, however, is

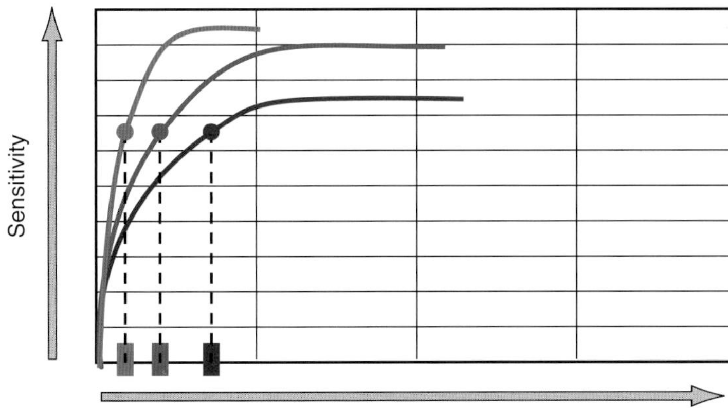

■ **FIGURE 5-3** Schematic of three fROC curves (green, blue, and red) for three different CADe algorithms. Although each algorithm has the same sensitivity at the location of the colored dots, the corresponding false marker rates increase with the poorer performing algorithms.

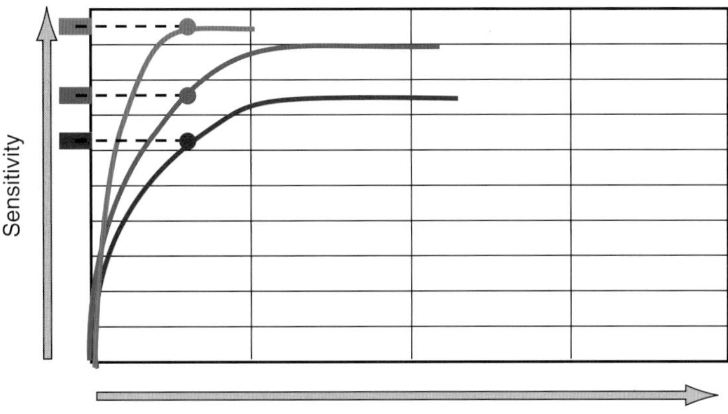

■ **FIGURE 5-4** Schematic of three fROC curves (green, blue, and red) for three different CADe algorithms. Although each algorithm has the same false marker rate at the location of the colored dots, their corresponding sensitivity decreases with the poorer performing algorithms.

unrealistic in that many of these cancers, although retrospectively visible, are so nonspecific in appearance that even when marked by CADe would likely be interpreted (and correctly so) as nonactionable (not warranting recall).[15] Therefore, a subset of the these missed cancers is developed by further characterizing the "visible in retrospect" cancers as being "actionable," that is, ones that most radiologists would both perceive and interpret as warranting recall.

Two large retrospective studies reporting on the potential impact of CADe on radiologist performance were reported in 2000 and 2003.[4,5] Although using somewhat different methodology, the two studies had similar conclusions. Radiologist sensitivity without CADe was 79% and 75%, respectively. These results mirrored the findings of numerous prior reports. The estimated potential reduction in false-negative rates in the detection of breast cancer with CADe input was calculated as 77% and 65%, respectively.

More recently, Skaane and colleagues[14] evaluated the results of 3683 women who had both film and digital screening mammograms with prospective independent double reading of each technique. All of the women were followed for 2 years to include cancers diagnosed in the interval between screening rounds and detected at the next screening round. The analysis focused on the cancers diagnosed at baseline screening and the subsequent cancers (interval and next screening round) that were judged to be visible and actionable in retrospect. Radiologist's sensitivity for double reading film mammograms was 77% compared with 85% for CADe stand-alone performance ($P = .57$). For digital mammograms, the sensitivity for double reading was 64% compared with 95% for CADe stand-alone performance ($P = .006$). Again, assuming that all true-positive CADe marks would be acted upon, the calculated potential sensitivity of independent double reading with CADe input on this case material could be as high as 90% for film mammograms and 100% for digital mammograms.

The previous studies assume that all true-positive CADe marks would be acted upon, which does not occur in clinical practice. Although the potential of CADe was shown to be very encouraging, it is the studies performed in a real clinical practice setting that have demonstrated the real world impact of CADe on radiologist performance. In these studies, various metrics, such as CADe-prompted changes in recall rates, biopsy rates, cancer detection rates, are tracked to determine the impact of CADe on radiologist performance.

Historical Controlled Studies

Historical controlled studies are usually retrospective in design and conducted in a clinical practice setting. They compare the performance of radiologists before (the historical control) and after the introduction of CADe into their clinical practice. Because the study compares data from two different time periods, changes in patient demographics (e.g., prevalent vs. incident screens, age of the women), the number and experience of the interpreting radiologists, and the imaging technology employed in the different time periods could bias the results.

As summarized in Table 5-1, most large historical controlled studies have reported an increase in cancer detection, accompanied by a concordant increase in the workup rate, with CADe input compared with the pre-CADe period. Gur and colleagues[16] reported only a modest (1.72%) increase in the cancer detection rate with CADe input for the 24 radiologists who read 115,571 screening mammograms, 56,432 before and 59,139 after implementation of CADe in their clinical practice. However, Feig and associates[17] pointed out that the low-volume radiologists in this study (17 of the 24 readers) had a 19.7% increase in the cancer detection rate with CADe input, accompanied by a lower 14.1% increase in the recall rate. They note, "Thus, the use of computer-aided detection allowed the low volume radiologists to increase their collective detection rates to a rate equal to that of the high-volume radiologists."

In 2004, Cupples and coworkers[18] reported a 16.3% increase in the cancer detection rate with CADe input, accompanied by a 7.8% and 6.6% increase in the recall and biopsy rates, respectively, for radiologists who read 27,274 screening mammograms, 7,872 before and 19,402 after implementation of CADe in their clinical practice. There was a 164% increase in the detection of small (=10 mm) invasive cancers and the mean age at screening detection of cancer was 5.3 years younger in the CADe group.

In 2007, Fenton and colleagues[19] published a historical control study that concluded that CADe input was detrimental to radiologist performance. On the basis of data retrospectively collected by mailed questionnaires, they reported that the cancer detection rate increased only 1.2%, accompanied by an alarming increase in the recall (30.1%) and biopsy (19.7%) rates. They also reported a 4.5% increase in radiologist sensitivity and a 33.1% increase in detection of ductal carcinoma in situ (DCIS) with CADe input. Numerous flaws in study design and analysis[20] have been pointed out, including the survey method versus prospective data collection and the study time period (1998-2002), ignoring interval improvements in the CADe algorithm performance. But perhaps the most important flaw is the almost complete lack of clinical experience with CADe. A total of 31,186 mammograms were read with CADe by 38 radiologists, for an averaged CADe experience of 821 cases per radiologist. The results ignored the expected learning curve related to stabilization of the recall rates over time. Furthermore, their reported decreased accuracy was due to increased false-positive findings and not fewer detected cancers; there was a statistically significant increase in detection of DCIS.[19]

In 2008, Gromet[21] published a historical controlled study comparing the performance of the single (first) radiologists who double read 112,413 screening mammograms (the historical control) to that of single radiologists who read 118,808 mammograms after the implementation of their CADe program. There were nine radiologists who read an average of 13,201 mammograms with CADe (as compared with 38 radiologists who averaged 821 examinations in the study by Fenton and coworkers).[19] The performance of the single radiologists with CADe input as compared with the first reader (without CADe) in the double-reader historic control arm showed an increase in sensitivity of 11.1% (from 81.4% to 90.4%; $P < .0001$), accompanied by a 3.9% increase in the recall rate (from 10.2% to 10.6%).

Prospective, Sequential Read Studies

Prospective, sequential read studies, also performed in a real clinical practice setting, are prospectively designed as follows. The radiologists read the mammogram in the standard fashion without CADe input and record their interpretations. The CADe marks are then displayed in the radiologist's record if the CADe prompts resulted in a change in interpretation. In this study design, bias can occur when, for example, the radiologist competes with the CADe system and reviews all studies with heightened awareness or the radiologist is less observant, knowing that the CADe system is a useful second reader/observer, especially in the detection of suspicious microcalcifications.

As detailed in Table 5-2, five such studies have been published.[9,22-25] All studies reported an increase in the cancer detection rate (average 9.8%, range 4.7%-19.5%). In those studies providing such data there was a similar wide range in recall rates (9.2%-18.1%) and biopsy rates (5.2%-19.6%). A possible explanation for this divergence is that the academic practices in general had a lower increase in both cancer detection and workup rates.

On balance, well-designed and carefully performed prospective clinical studies are considered to be the preferred methodology to evaluate the impact of a new intervention (in this case CADe) in clinical practice (screening mammography).

Double Reading versus a Single Reader with CADe

Because double reading of screening mammograms is performed in some U.S. practices and is mandated in certain countries (e.g., the United Kingdom and Northern Europe), some studies have addressed whether practices using human-human double reading could replace their second human reader with a CADe system. In the historical controlled study reported by Gromet,[21] sensitivity increased 2.7% (from 88.0% to 90.4%) and the recall

TABLE 5-1. Historical Control Clinical Studies on Screening Mammograms Read with Computer Aided Diagnosis (CADe) Assistance

		Recall rate			Biopsy rate			Detection rate/1000					
Study	***N* =**	**pre CAD**	**with CAD**	**% change***	**pre CAD**	**with CAD**	**% change**	**control**	**with CAD**	**% change**			
Gur et al (2004) [16]													
All readers (*n*=24)													
historical control	56,432	11.39			n/a			3.49					
read with CAD	59,139		11.40	0.09%		n/a			3.55	1.72%			
High volume readers (*n*=7)													
historical control	44,629	11.62			n/a			3.61					
read with CAD	37,500		11.05	-4.91%		n/a			3.49	-3.32%			
Low volume readers [17] (*n*=17)													
historical control	11,803	10.52			n/a			3.05					
read with CAD	21,639		12	14.07%		n/a			3.65	19.67%			
Cupples et al (2005) [18]													
historical control	27,274	7.7			1.37			3.68					
read with CAD	19,402		8.3	7.79%		1.46	6.57%		4.28	16.30%			
Fenton et al (2007) [19]											Sensitivity		
historical control	84,900	10.1			1.47			4.15			80.4		
read with CAD	31,186		13.2	30.69%		1.76	19.73%		4.20	1.20%		84.0	4.48%
Gromet (2008) [(21)]											Sensitivity		
** historical control	112,413	10.2			1.26			4.12			81.4		
read with CAD	118,808		10.6	3.92%		1.44	14.29%		4.20	1.94%		90.4	11.06%

n/a, not available.
* Change in radiologist performance (read with CADe / historical control) × 100
** First reader in the pre-CADe double reading program – see text.

TABLE 5-2. Five Prospective, Sequential Read Clinical Studies on Computer Aided Diagnosis (CAD) with Mammography

Publication (practice type)	Number of Exams	Number of Recalls				Number of Biopsies				Number of Cancers			
		pre CADe	with CADe	Total	Change*	pre CADe	with CADe	Total	Change*	pre CADe	with CADe	Total	Change*
Freer[22] (community)	12,860	830	150	980	**18.07%**	107	21	128	**19.63%**	41	8	49	**19.51%**
Birdwell [23] (Stanford University)	8,682	790	73	863	**9.24%**	172	9	181	**5.23%**	27	2	29	**7.41%**
Morton [24] (Mayo Clinic)	21,349	2,101	199	2,300	**9.47%**	256	21	277	**8.20%**	105	8	113	**7.62%**
Dean [9] (community)	5,631	n/a	n/a	n/a		n/a	n/a	n/a		30	4	34	**13.33%**
Ko [25] (community/ Tufts)	5,016	607	89	696	**14.66%**	101	6	107	**5.94%**	43	2	45	**4.65%**
TOTAL	**53,538**	4,328	511	4,839	**11.81%**	636	57	693	**8.96%**	246	24	270	**9.76%**

n/a, not available.
*Change in radiologist performance with CADe / historical control × 100

rate decreased 10.9% (from 11.9% to 10.6%) for the single reader with CADe input compared with the double-reading program. Georgian-Smith and associates[26] found no statistical difference between cancer detection by a human second reader versus CADe.

Gilbert and colleagues[27] published a prospective study of 28,723 film screening mammograms independently read by both double reading and single reading with CADe input. The reported estimated sensitivity was similar for single reading with CADe and double reading (87.2% vs. 87.7%, respectively). However, the recall rate was higher for single reading with CADe than double reading (3.9% vs. 3.4%, respectively). The authors concluded, "Single reading with computer-aided detection could be an alternative to double reading..." which primarily is of interest to practices that perform double reading. Of more pertinence to most U.S. practices that perform single reading, they stated, "Where single reading is standard practice, computer-aided detection has the potential to improve cancer detection rates to the level achieved by double reading."

COMMENTS

CADe and Digital Mammography

The ACRIN multi-institutional study group comparing film and digital mammography reported radiologist sensitivities of 0.66 and 0.70 (not statistically significant) for reading the film and digital mammograms, respectively.[28] Clearly, cancers were (and are) missed by interpreting radiologists on both analog and digital images. The investigators also found that radiologists' performance reading digital compared with film mammograms was superior in women who were younger, premenopausal, and/or had dense breast tissue. If indeed radiologists reading digital mammograms find additional cancers, then is there a need for CADe with this modality?

CADe stand-alone performance studies have reported sensitivities for known cancers manifesting as microcalcifications and masses on digital mammograms to be comparable to reported stand-alone CADe sensitivities on film mammograms. Furthermore, the CADe false marker rates on digital and film mammograms are similar as well.[29,30] If digital acquisition and display systems actually display more features due to cancer, then detection assistance becomes of even greater importance. As discussed earlier, Skaane and associates reported a 64% sensitivity for radiologists for independent, double-reading digital screening mammograms and, assuming all correct CADe marks were acted upon, a calculated potential for CADe input to increase sensitivity to 100%.

Brancato and colleagues[31] have to date the only prospective, sequential-read clinical study of radiologist performance with CADe input on consecutive screening digital mammograms (n = 2596). They reported a 14.3% increase (two additional cancers) detected due to CADe input. Of interest, there was a 3.3% increase (three additional cancers) detected with CADe input on mammograms in 829 symptomatic women at sites other than that of the complaint (i.e., at asymptomatic regions of the breast). Data on the impact of CADe on recall rates was not provided separately for the screening and symptomatic mammograms. For the combined group, CADe input increased the recall rate by 9.8%.

False-Positive CADe Marks

The vast majority of CADe marks do not mark cancers, and these false CADe marks are often cited as a severe drawback to the use of CADe systems. To some extent this is correct, in that an excessive number of false CADe marks can lead some readers to the following: (1) an increase in the number of unnecessary recalls; (2) a disregard of a true-positive CADe mark due to the presence of numerous nuisance prompts, leading to a lost opportunity to diagnose cancer, or (3) both. Zheng and associates[6] showed that more than two false CADe marks per four-view examination had such deleterious effects, and vendors have generally set their operating points at two false CADe marks per four-view mammogram or lower levels.

Visual search studies have shown that radiologists detect many features and findings on a radiographic image that elicit a longer visual fixation (dwell time) or result in a second look—or both—before interpreting the finding.[32] In many ways, this is analogous to the false CADe marks, that is, much like radiologists, CADe systems search the image for worrisome features; however, CADe systems do not provide an interpretation as to the likelihood (probability) of malignancy versus benignancy, which the radiologist provides with an American College of Radiology Breast Imaging and Reporting Data System (BI-RADS) score.

In clinical practice, most false CADe marks are readily dismissed as marking nonsuspicious entities (e.g., vascular and other benign calcifications, summation shadows of normal glandular tissue, tissue projecting over the pectoralis muscle). These marks primarily represent a nuisance factor to the radiologist. A much smaller number have features of concern and require a more studied evaluation before (correctly) dismissing the finding. In this instance, the radiologist may well have independently noted this finding before displaying the CADe marks and will have already interpreted it as not warranting recall. In either case, the radiologist must decide if the finding of concern warrants further evaluation, regardless of whether it was first detected by the radiologist or only after subsequent review of the CADe marks.

CADe Impact on Recall Rates

There are legitimate concerns that the numerous false CADe prompts could result in an unacceptable increase in recalls for women who do not have breast cancer. Clinical studies (both historical control and prospective, sequential read) (see Tables 5-1 and 5-2) have shown that CADe input, not surprisingly, increases radiologists' recall rate. Almost all such studies, however, have also documented an increase in the cancer detection rate. What is important is whether the increase in recalls for further evaluation (usually imaging studies) is consistent with the increase in cancers detected. After all, additional cancers cannot be diagnosed without additional recalls and, in a subset of recalls, biopsies. Most of these studies have shown just that—the increase in recalls is accompanied by a comparable increase in cancer detection. Furthermore, when tracked, the cancers diagnosed with CADe input have generally been smaller in size and at an earlier stage than those diagnosed before CADe.[9,18,22]

CONCLUSIONS

CADe is designed as an adjunct to the radiologist in the interpretation of mammograms. Prospective data support the incremental benefits of increased cancer detection in the clinical setting of CADe use. Training and experience are very important not only in the use of the system as it is designed and FDA approved but also in recognizing the strengths and weaknesses of the present systems. Radiologists initiating the use of CADe should expect an increase in their call-back rate and should audit their practice closely. After as long as 1 year, there should be a return to about the same recall rate as was present before CADe use as the radiologist becomes more experienced in the dismissal of the many false-positive CADe marks. The audit should also be expected to demonstrate an increase in cancer detection.

DISCLOSURE: Dr. Castellino was the **Chief Medical Officer,** R2 Technology **(1999-2006)** and subsequently **Chief Medical Officer,** Hologic, Inc **(2006-2009)** manufacturers of computer aided detection **(CAD)** systems for mammography; **and, occassionally consults for Hologic, Inc.**

KEY POINTS

- CADe systems are designed to decrease observational oversights (missed cancers) and increase the proportion of more favorable (smaller, earlier stage) cancers.
- Training and experience are very important, not only in the use of the system as it is designed and FDA approved but also in recognizing the strengths and weaknesses of the present systems.
- When using a CADe system, always evaluate a finding of concern noted on the initial review without CADe input, even if not marked by the CADe system, and never evaluate a finding simply because it is marked by the CADe system.
- The preponderance of literature shows that CADe used in the clinical practice setting increases cancer detection, accompanied by a comparable increase in the recall rate.

SUGGESTED READINGS

Giger ML, Chan HP, Boone J. Anniversary paper: history and status of CAD and quantitative image analysis: the role of *Medical Physics* and AAPM. *Med Phys* 2008;**35**:5799-820.

Helvie M. Improving mammographic interpretation: double-reading and computer-aided diagnosis. *Radiol Clin North Am* 2007;**45**:801-11.

Nishikawa RM. Current status and future directions of computer-aided diagnosis in mammography. *Comp Med Imaging Graph* 2007;**31**:224-35.

Nishikawa RM, Pesce LL. Computer-aided detection evaluation methods are not created equal. *Radiology* 2009;**251**:634-6.

REFERENCES

1. Krupinski EA. The future of image perception in radiology: synergy between humans and computers. *Acad Radiol* 2003;**10**:1-3.
2. Kundel HL, Nodine CF, Carmody DP. Visual scanning, pattern recognition and decision-making in pulmonary nodule detection. *Invest Radiol* 1978;**13**:175-81.
3. Bird RE, Wallace TW, Yankaskas BC. Analysis of cancers missed at screening mammography. *Radiology* 1992;**184**:613-7.
4. Warren-Burhenne LJ, Wood SA, D'Orsi CJ, Feig SA, Kopans DB, O'Shaughnessy KF, et al. Potential contribution of computer-aided detection to the sensitivity of screening mammography. *Radiology* 2000;**215**:554-62.
5. Brem RF, Baum J, Lechner M, et al. Improvement in sensitivity of screening mammography with computer-aided detection: a multiinstitutional trial. *AJR Am J Roentgenol* 2003;**181**:687-93.
6. Zheng B, Leader JK, Abrams G, Shindel B, Catullo V, Good WF, et al. Computer-aided detection schemes: the effect of limiting the number of cued regions in each case. *AJR Am J Roentgenol* 2004;**182**:579-83.
7. Paquerault S, Wade DI, Petrick N, et al. Observer evaluation of computer-aided detection: second reader versus concurrent reader scenario. *Proc SPIE* 2007;**6515**.
8. Yaffe M, Jong R, Wolrman J, et al. Performance of CAD for pre-screening with digital mammography. *RSNA* 2005.
9. Dean JC, Ilvento CC. Improved cancer detection using computer-aided detection with diagnostic and screening mammography: prospective study of 104 cancers. *AJR Am J Roentgenol* 2006;**187**:20-8.
10. Baker JA, Rosen EL, Lo JY, Gimenez EI, Walsh R, Soo MS. Computer-aided detection (CAD) in screening mammography: sensitivity of commercial CAD systems for detecting architectural distortion. *AJR Am J Roentgenol* 2003;**181**:1083-8.
11. Gur D, Stalder JS, Hardesty LA, Zheng B, Sumkin JH, Chough DM, et al. Computer-aided detection performance in mammographic examination of masses: assessment. *Radiology* 2004;**233**:418-23.
12. Ellis RL, Meade AA, Mathiason MA, Willison KM, Logan-Young W. Evaluation of computer-aided detection systems in the detection of small invasive breast carcinoma. *Radiology* 2007;**245**:88-94.
13. Birdwell RL, Ikeda DM, O'Shaughnessy KF, Sickles EA. Mammographic characteristics of 115 missed cancers later detected with screening mammography and the potential utility of computer-aided detection. *Radiology* 2001;**219**:192-202.
14. Skaane P, Kshirsagar A, Stapleton S, Young K, Castellino RA. Effect of computer-aided detection on independent double reading of paired screen-film and full-field digital screening mammograms. *AJR Am J Roentgenol* 2007;**188**:377-84.
15. Ikeda DM, Birdwell RL, O'Shaughnessy KF, Sickles EA, Brenner RJ. Computer-aided detection output on 172 subtle findings on normal mammograms previously obtained in women with breast cancer detected at follow-up screening mammography. *Radiology* 2004;**230**:811-9.
16. Gur D, Sumkin JH, Rocketed HE, Ganott M, Hakim C, Hardesty L, et al. Changes in breast cancer detection and mammography recall rates after the introduction of a computer-aided detection system. *J Natl Cancer Inst* 2004;**96**:185-90.

17. Feig SA, Sickles EA, Evans WP, Liner MN. Letter to the Editor: Re: Changes in breast cancer detection and mammography recall rates after the introduction of a computer-aided detection system. *J Natl Cancer Inst* 2004;**96**:1260-1.
18. Cupples TE, Cunningham JE, Reynolds JC. Impact of computer-aided detection in a regional screening mammography program. *AJR Am J Roentgenol* 2005;**185**:944-50.
19. Fenton JJ, Taplin SH, Carney PA, Abraham L, Sickles EA, D'Orsi C, et al. Influence of computer aided detection on performance of screening mammography. *N Engl J Med* 2007;**356**:1399-409.
20. Letters to the Editor. *N Engl J Med* 2007;**357**:83-5.
21. Gromet M. Comparison of computer-aided detection to double reading of screening mammograms: review of 231,221 mammograms. *AJR Am J Roentgenol* 2008;**190**:854-9.
22. Freer TW, Ulissey MJ. Screening mammography with computer-aided detection: prospective study of 12,860 patients in a community breast center. *Radiology* 2001;**220**:781-6.
23. Birdwell RL, Bandodkar P, Ikeda DM. Computer aided detection with screening mammography in a university hospital setting. *Radiology* 2005;**236**:451-7.
24. Morton MJ, Whaley DH, Brandt KR, Amrami KK. Screening mammograms: interpretation with computer-aided detection–prospective evaluation. *Radiology* 2006;**239**:375-83.
25. Ko JM, Nicholas MJ, Mendel JB, Slanetz PJ. Prospective assessment of computer-aided detection in interpretation of screening mammography. *AJR Am J Roentgenol* 2006;**187**:1483-91.
26. Georgian-Smith D, Moore RH, Halpern E, Yeh ED, Rafferty EA, D'Alessandro HA, et al. Blinded comparison of computer-aided detection with human second reading in screening mammography. *AJR Am J Roentgenol* 2007;**189**:1135-41.
27. Gilbert FJ, Astley SM, Gillan MG, Agbaje OF, Wallis MG, James J, et al; for the CADET II Group. Single reading with computer-aided detection for screening mammography. *N Engl J Med* 2008;**359**:1675-84.
28. Pisano ED, Gatsonis C, Hendrick E, Yaffe M, Baum JK, Acharyya S, et al. Diagnostic performance of digital versus film mammography for breast- cancer screening. *N Engl J Med* 2005;**353**:1773-83.
29. Kim SF, Moon WK, Cho N, Cha JH, Kim SM, Im JG. Computer-aided detection in full-field digital mammography: sensitivity and reproducibility in serial examinations. *Radiology* 2008;**246**:71-80.
30. The JS, Schilling KJ, Hoffmeister JW, Friedmann E, McGinnis R, Holcomb RG. Detection of breast cancer with full-field digital mammography and computer-aided detection. *AJR Am J Roentgenol* 2009;**192**:337-40.
31. Brancato B, Houssami N, Francesca D, et al. Does computer-aided detection (CAD) contribute to the performance of digital mammography in a self-referred population? *Breast Cancer Res Treat* 2008;**111**:373-6.
32. Nodine CF, Mello-Thomas C, Weinstein SP, Kundel HL, Conant EF, Heller-Savoy RE, et al. Blinded review of retrospectively visible unreported breast cancers: an eye-position analysis. *Radiology* 2001;**221**:122-9.

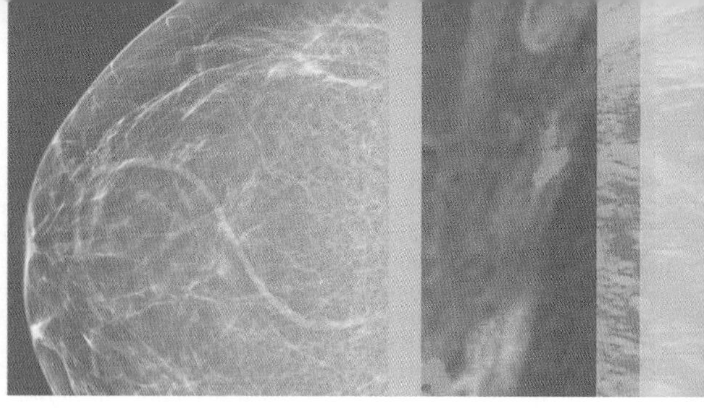

CHAPTER 6

Positioning in Mammography

Margarita L. Zuley and Shireen L. Braner

For digital mammography, many parameters in the image acquisition and display are new or different from what existed for screen-film mammography. The imaging chain includes more variables that can influence the final quality of the images and, thus, quality of interpretation. For example, processing algorithms and the application of various window width and window level look-up tables for the display of the dynamic range is notably different across vendors and highly influential on the image for display. Radiologists are faced with new terminology such as analog to digital units (ADU) and detective quantum efficiency (DQE) that are important to both image quality and dose. Still, one of the most important components of a high-quality mammogram is appropriate positioning. In this chapter we discuss positioning from both the radiologist's and technologist's standpoints. We will review all the standard and optional views, their purposes and review how to judge the quality of positioning of any image. For in the end, the radiologist is responsible for overseeing that each patient receives a quality evaluation from acquisition to interpretation.

Quality mammography in large part is dependent on excellent technique in positioning and acquisition of images. The current guidelines that we have in place for virtually all aspects of mammography are, in large part, a result of the cooperation and foresight of several well-known organizations and governmental agencies. In the beginning, the process of quality oversight was managed by multiple different entities. In the 1980s the American Cancer Society (ACS) determined that there was an unacceptable amount of variability in the quality of mammography as well as the radiation dose per study. The ACS approached the American College of Radiology (ACR) and requested that the ACR begin an accreditation process in order to help to improve the situation. The ACR formed the Breast Task Force as a result and began the Mammography Accreditation Program (MAP) in 1987 as a voluntary program that now has become required.[1,2] Coincident with this, in 1990, the U.S. Congress passed a law permitting Medicare reimbursement of mammography and required that facilities seeking Medicare reimbursement register and follow guidelines that were similar to those of the ACR. In addition, several states required that facilities follow their regulations to perform mammography. Then, in the 1990s, the ACR partnered with the Centers for Disease Control and Prevention (CDC) to form the Cooperative Agreement for Quality Assurance Activities in Mammography.[3,4] This partnership brought together radiologists and technologists to further define standard mammographic positioning and also to disseminate that information to facilities. In 1992, the Mammography Quality Standards Act (MQSA) was signed into law. The act defined minimum federal standards that facilities had to meet in order to provide mammography services.[5,6] This law was intended to eliminate all of the variability in requirements that had grown from the early days of mammography quality control. The U.S. Food and Drug Administration (FDA), a branch of the Department of Health and Human Services, was charged with approving accrediting bodies as well as certifying facilities. In turn, by request from the FDA, the ACR became the primary accrediting body for the standards and regulations that evolved from this history. Several states (Iowa, Arkansas and Texas) also are currently approved by the FDA as accrediting bodies.[7] The first ACR Mammography Quality Control Manual was published in 1990 with subsequent editions published in 1992, 1994 and, most recently, in 1999.[8] Currently, a digital mammography quality control manual is being developed and will be published in the very near term. In order to be accredited through the ACR's MAP, appropriate positioning of images is vital. In fact, the single largest reason for a facility not passing the accreditation process is unsatisfactory clinical images, and the single largest reason for that failure has historically been inadequate positioning.[9] Positioning failures have also been blamed for higher false negative rates after screening and lower sensitivity of mammography.[10] This chapter is meant to review standard positioning and especially to discuss changes and challenges related to the use of digital mammography.

EQUIPMENT

In 1999 the FDA determined that full-field digital mammography (FFDM) would be classified as a class III device. This meant that all FFDM systems had to pass strict criteria by the FDA to be used on patients in the United States. The first such system passed in 2000 and currently, there are multiple direct ray (DR) and computed ray (CR) systems on the market. The first product to market had a relatively small surface area for imaging, which resulted in a significant number of patients requiring more than two views of each breast to include all of the tissue. This is called tiling. Not only does tiling lead to higher radiation exposure for each breast, but also is more of a challenge to interpret. Therefore, newer systems have evolved with larger surface area detectors. Each of these systems has slightly different detector sizes and thicknesses; thus, they each pose a learning situation for positioning. In addition, several of the vendors have the ability to change the active part of the detector, or essentially its imaging size, with the use of different sized paddles and variable positioning of the paddles over the detector surface. The use of curved detectors in conjunction with slit and slot scanning is also new and may require adjustments by the technologists to optimize patient positioning. Having said all of this, the basics of positioning that have been created and disseminated to us through the efforts of the ACR and many dedicated radiologists and technologists through the last 20 and more years still holds true and are the foundation from which these minor positioning accommodations are made.

ANATOMY

In order to understand the rationale for the required positioning, an understanding of the regional anatomy and anatomy of the breast is useful. The breast is a modified sweat gland positioned between the second and sixth rib from superior to inferior and between the layers of the superficial and deep pectoral fascia anteriorly and posteriorly. Posterior to the deep pectoral fascia sit the pectoralis major and pectoralis minor muscles. The lateral margin of the breast is located at the mid axillary line and the medial margin is the sternum. The tail of the breast, also called the tail of Spence, extends into the axilla. Regional lymph node drainage is typically to the ipsilateral axillary chain, and to a lesser extent to the ipsilateral internal mammary chain. Ductal anatomy includes lactiferous sinuses that are immediately below the nipple surface. These arborize into ducts throughout the breast, which can be divided into lobules based on the ductal anatomy. The ducts then lead to terminal duct lobular units. It is in these terminal duct lobular units that the majority of breast abnormalities arise. Frequently there are anastomoses between these ductal segments. Intervening between these ducts is a mixture of fibroglandular and adipose tissue as well as thin suspensory ligaments, called Cooper ligaments. These suspend the breast from the nipple to the chest wall.

BASIC CONCEPTS OF POSITIONING

In order to view the anatomy of the breast, and hence any potential pathology, proper positioning requires as complete a visualization of the entire organ as is possible in any given patient. The lateral and inferior portions of the breast are far more mobile than the superior and medial portions. Therefore standard views have been developed to maximize this mobility and pull as much breast tissue toward the more fixed borders and onto the imaging device as is possible.[11,12] Of note, all mammographic views are defined by the direction of the x-ray beam from the tube toward the detector. The mediolateral oblique view (MLO) is the single best view to image the majority of the breast tissue.[13-15] The upper inner portion of the breast is the least successfully included portion, and so the other standard mammographic view, the craniocaudal (CC), should include as much medial tissue as is possible without excluding lateral tissue.

Special Circumstances

The two standard views, the MLO and the CC are used for the majority of patients, but occasionally in patients with impaired mobility such as the wheelchair-bound patient, and patients with special circumstances such as patients with kyphosis or severe scoliosis, or even pacemakers, use of other views is more appropriate. Tailoring the exam to accommodate these limitations in mobility and different body habitus allows quality mammography still to be performed.

Considerations for women who have physical limitations or mobility would include: consider using a mammography positioning chair with locking wheels; use cushions to raise the patient into position; use pillows or soft positioning foam to provide support to the patient in maintaining an upright position; remove the face shield and lean the patient's head forward along the side of the detector; tilt the tower so the detector is parallel to the breast line, realizing the plane of the breast tissue of the patient with physical limitations may not sit perpendicular to the chest wall; remove wheelchair arms if possible and remember to lock wheelchair wheels and turn off electric wheelchairs after positioning the patient (Fig. 6-1A and 6-1B).[16]

Breast Compression

Even with the excellent imaging characteristics of the digital detectors and advances in processing algorithms, breast compression during positioning is still one of the most important factors for a high quality, low dose image.[17] The majority of digital systems work by recording the compression thickness. The systems use a very low dose initial exposure to generate a limited ADU map of the compressed breast. Based on that test exposure and thickness, most systems have an automatic exposure control (AEC) that then selects the appropriate kilovolt peak (kVp), milliampere seconds (mAs) and target/filter combination for the image. So, in digital imaging not only

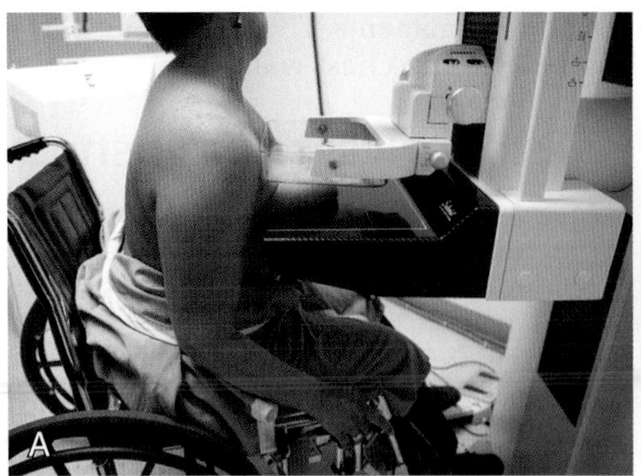

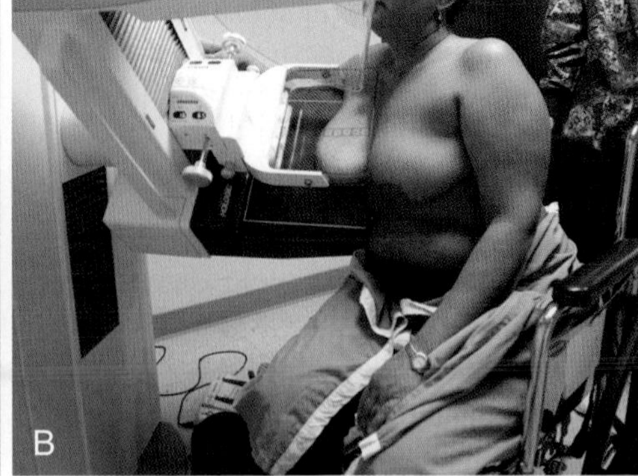

■ **FIGURE 6-1** A and B, These images demonstrate positioning of a patient in a wheelchair.

is compression important for tissue immobilization and separation of structures, but it is also important for image dose and quality. Figures 6-2A and 6-2B show how an image is degraded by insufficient compression. Most digital systems are made with two types of paddles. The first is a rigid paddle, the inferior surface of which stays entirely parallel to the breast support. With this paddle design, the breast is compressed to a uniform thickness so that equal penetration of the x-ray beam is possible throughout the entire organ. The second design is a flexible paddle that has springs on the chest wall side. These flexible paddles are meant to allow equal compressive force in the thicker posterior aspects of the breast and the thinner anterior portion simultaneously. The processing algorithms compensate for the variable compression thickness and create an image for display that has a homogeneous appearance. With either paddle, compression should be firm enough to compress the breast as much as possible such that the exposure is as minimal and fast as possible, both to limit dose and to limit motion unsharpness. A major part of quality positioning is adequate breast compression. The technologist must master the art of firm compression that includes as much tissue as is possible for each view and compresses as much as the patient can tolerate without causing undo discomfort that may dissuade the patient from returning for yearly screening.

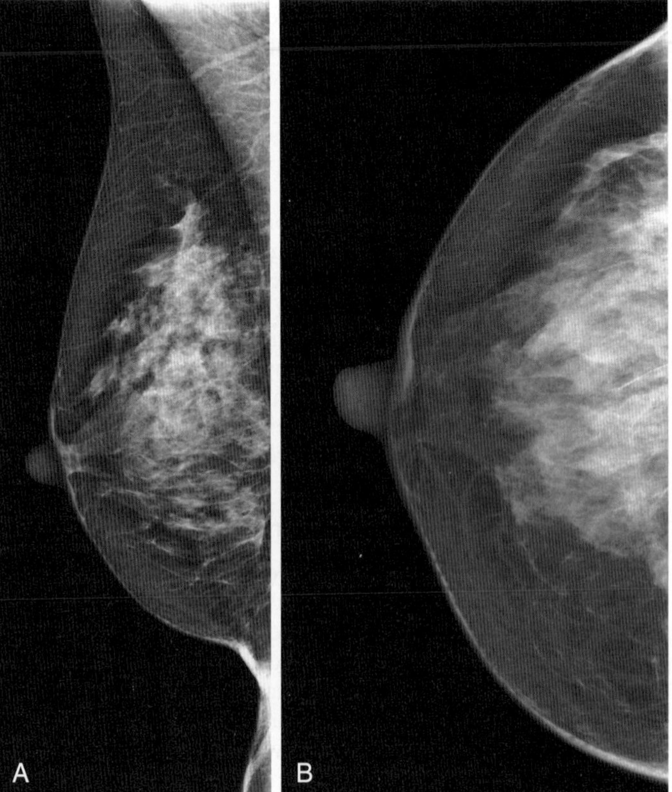

■ **FIGURE 6-2** A and B, craniocaudal (CC) and mediolateral oblique (MLO) views from the same patient. **A,** The MLO is well compressed with good image quality. **B,** The CC is poorly compressed, which resulted in a flat, gray image with little detail.

Labeling and Soft Copy Display

With the advent of soft copy review, several new considerations are necessary with respect to labeling and display. Most diagnostic workstations can be configured such that each reader, or at least each facility, can choose what information is routinely seen during soft-copy interpretation, and that information can be toggled on and off during reading. This is to reduce distractions from the displayed image. For digital imaging, view descriptors are not only important for image recognition, but on many workstations, they drive hanging protocols. Therefore, several new views and view modifiers have been added to the standardized labeling codes. The order of the terminology for views is now also standardized. First, an "R" or "L" will be displayed to indicate laterality. Then prefix modifiers such as "S" for spot compression will be displayed, then the view name such as MLO will be listed, and finally any suffix modifiers, such as "ID" for Implant Displaced will be listed. Table 6-1 lists the views and accepted abbreviations. Along with kVp, mAs, compression thickness, view angle and other acquisition parameters that we are accustomed to reviewing on images, ADU is a new digital parameter that is useful. (Currently, one vendor calls this Exposure Index, or EI.) This is one of the best ways to check the signal-to-noise ratio of the image. Each vendor has a target range of ADUs. If an image does not have enough dose, the image will appear noisy and the ADU value will be low. Conversely, when the ADU values are too high, too much dose was given for the view.

TABLE 6-1. Imaging Views and Abbreviations in Mammography

Abbreviations	View Names
Standard Views	
MLO	Mediolateral oblique
CC	Craniocaudal
Additional Views	
LMO	Lateromedial oblique
SIO	Superoinferior oblique
ISO	Inferosuperior oblique
FB	From below
XLCC	Exaggerated lateral craniocaudal
AT	Axillary tail
CV	Cleavage
TAN	Tangenital
Modifiers	
Prefixes (before the view name)	
M	Magnification
S	Spot
RM	Rolled medial
RL	Rolled lateral
Suffixes (after the view name)	
ID	Implant displacement

In addition to the acquisition parameters and patient and view identifiers that radiologists are used to seeing on screen-film images, soft copy interpretation requires that the reader understand if the displayed image is being viewed at full resolution, true size, or fit to viewport mode.[18] The term *full resolution*, also known as *view actual pixels* means that each pixel acquired on the detector at acquisition is viewed by one pixel on the display monitor.[19] *True size* means that the breast is being viewed at real, physical size. This mode is important for surgical or stereotactic biopsy planning. *Fit to viewport* is the most common mode of display and is used to simultaneously display more than one view on a monitor. In this mode, adjacent pixel values are averaged together so that the entire image can be displayed smaller and of lower resolution. This mode is very good for comparing current and prior as well as symmetry as an initial step in a display protocol. However, it does not show the radiologist all of the information in the image; that is only done at full resolution. Labeling of the images with this display resolution so that the radiologist understands if all the detail in the image is present or not is a new aspect of interpretation with digital mammography. At soft-copy display, it is also important that the chest wall side of the breast is justified to the chest wall side of the display monitor in every step of a hanging protocol, no matter the resolution of display. Excellent positioning by the technologist to include posterior tissue is not very helpful if the radiologist never sees it due to faulty workstation functionality. This discussion has a correlate in printed digital images. The mammograms can be printed in a *fit to film* mode, full resolution mode or true size mode, and the images should be justified to the edge of the film so that all of the acquired posterior tissue is printed onto the film. In addition, when any image is printed to film, standard MQSA required labeling should still be used with all information printed on the side of the film opposite the chest wall, not overlying breast tissue and the view label should be in the axillary portion of the image, opposite the chest wall. The resolution of the printed image should be on the image as well as a ruler for accurate measurement.

STANDARD MAMMOGRAPHIC VIEWS

Mediolateral Oblique View

The MLO and CC views are the two primary images obtained in both screening and diagnostic mammography. For the radiologist, assessment of image positioning and compression is an integral part of interpretation of any mammogram. The MLO view includes the maximal amount of axillary and posterior tissue, because it is obtained at an angle that is parallel to the fibers of the underlying pectoral muscle. This angle varies with body habitus, and is steeper for taller patients and less steep for shorter women. It is best achieved by utilizing the mobility of the lateral tissue toward the medial fixed tissue. Encouraging the patient to relax her upper body muscles will allow for more mobility thereby visualizing more tissue. The digital detector has more depth than the film-screen cassette and requires the patient to be placed more forward on the detector to access the most breast tissue. For the MLO, the pectoral

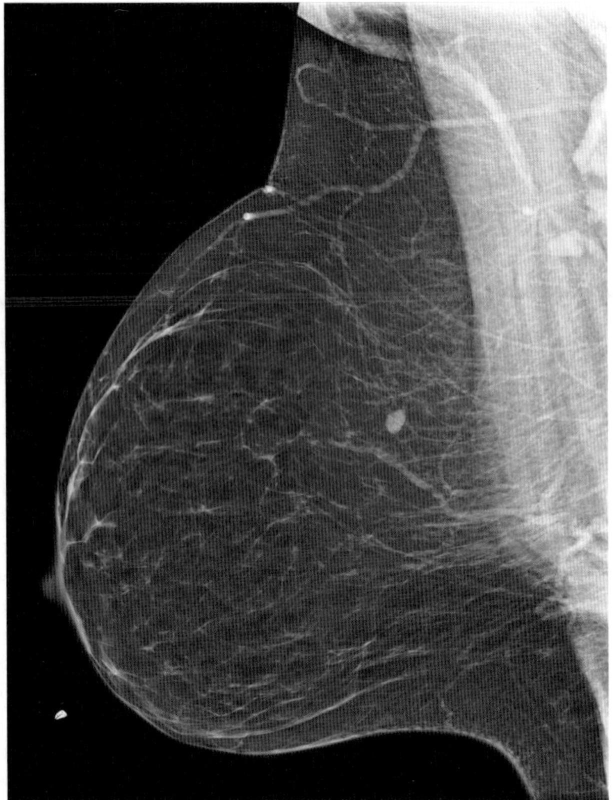

■ **FIGURE 6-3** An example of a well positioned mediolateral oblique (MLO) view.

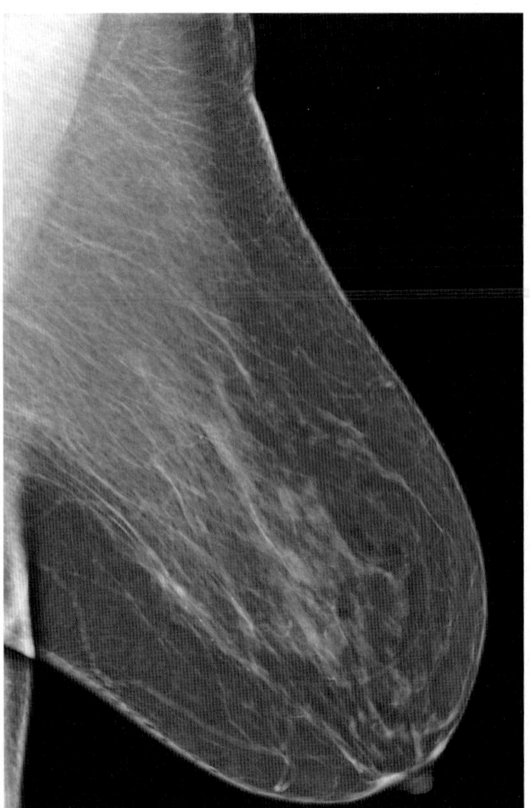

■ **FIGURE 6-4** For this mediolateral oblique (MLO) view, the breast was not adequately compressed, which resulted in drooping of the tissue, motion and insufficient inclusion of posterior tissue.

muscle should be seen to the level of the nipple and should have a convex anterior boarder, because it is relaxed. Also, the inframammary fold should be present and the nipple should be in profile on most images (Fig. 6-3). Insufficient compression leads to motion unsharpness, which can obscure subtle findings such as spiculated masses and fine calcifications. Most frequently, motion on the MLO is present in the inferior part of the breast because of lack of compression. This is often associated with a drooping breast (Fig. 6-4). The technologist must use a sweeping *up and out* motion of the inferior portion of the breast to avoid the drooping breast image and overlapping tissue (Fig. 6-5). Some patients will require more than one MLO view. For example, in some patients, in order to include sufficient posterior tissue, the anterior breast tissue is not adequately compressed. In this situation, an anterior compression MLO should be performed. Also, in some women, the breast is too large for the image detector and so multiple tiled images are necessary in order to include all of the breast tissue. Computed ray (CR) technology allows the ability to use one of two standard cassette sizes, much like screen-film. Some

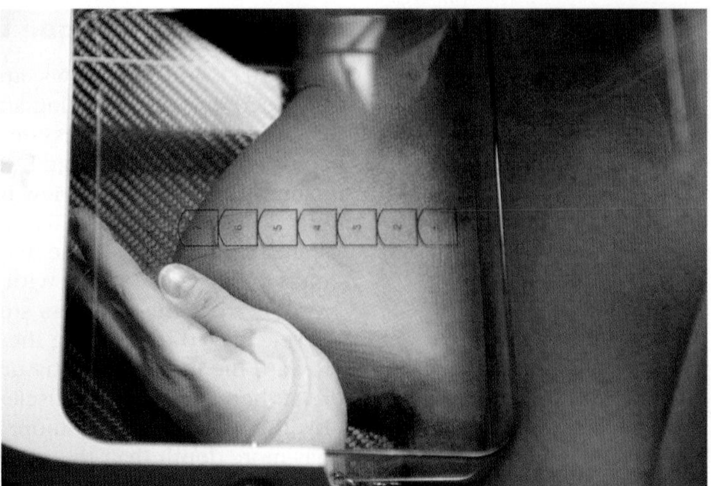

■ **FIGURE 6-5** Proper positioning for the mediolateral oblique (MLO) view.

DR companies have allowed either the entire detector surface, or a portion thereof to be used for imaging to accommodate these different sizes, in order to minimize the need for tiling.

Craniocaudal View

The other standard view, the CC view, should include some pectoral muscle in at least 25 % of images and should include as much posterior medial tissue as possible, because the one area that the MLO does not image completely is the upper inner quadrant. The radiologist should look for a small amount of included skin at the most medial aspect of the image to indicate that sufficient medial breast tissue has been included. Care should be taken, however, not to cut off too much lateral tissue. In order to avoid this, the technologist will pull on lateral tissue just before final positioning of the compression paddle. If some lateral tissue trails off of the posterolateral edge of the CC view, an exaggerated lateral CC view can be done. The distance from the nipple to the chest wall edge of the image should be within 1cm of the distance on the MLO from the nipple to pectoral muscle. Again, the nipple should be in profile as often as possible, but not at the expense of adequate compression or posterior tissue (Fig. 6-6). Technically this view is accomplished by using the natural mobility of the inferior aspect of the breast and raising the breast at the inframammary fold, placing the breast support at this level and then bringing down the compression paddle onto the tissue (Figs. 6-7A and 6-7B). This allows the less mobile posterior medial tissues to be more completely imaged and is less uncomfortable for the patient. Encouraging the patient to maintain a relaxed shoulder and moving her head forward around the tube assembly will allow the technologist to pull in the maximum amount of tissue. If the technologist will drape her arm over the patient's shoulder of the breast being imaged, this will allow for more relaxation and decrease the pulling sensation the patient may feel during compression. It is important that attention be made toward eliminating skin folds while smoothing breast tissue into the position to be imaged.

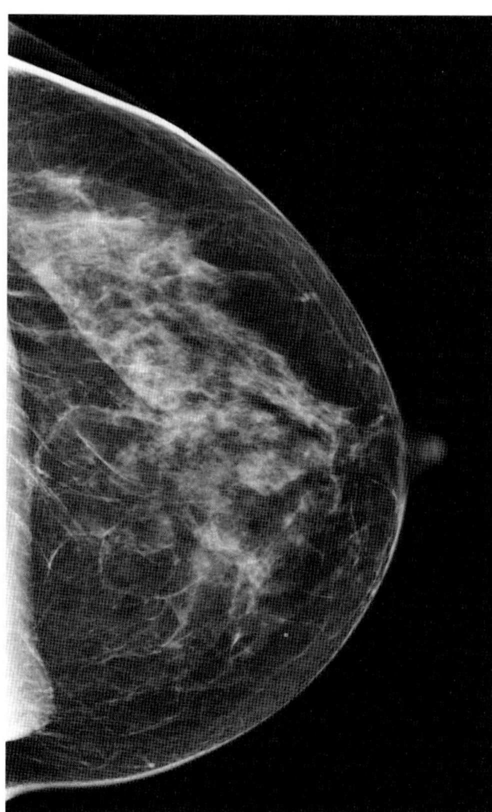

■ **FIGURE 6-6** An example of a well positioned craniocaudal (CC) view.

Additional Views

After a potential finding is identified on the standard views, the radiologist must determine if the finding is real or just superimposition of adjacent structures in the case of a possible mass or architectural distortion. Additional views are also used to evaluate the precise location of a real finding and to evaluate its character and extent further. Several techniques have been used to accomplish these goals. The first technique is angulation of the x ray tube to change the orientation of the breast tissue slightly so as to move normal superimposed adjacent structures apart. The second technique is to roll the breast tissue and repeat a view, with the concept the same as for tube angulation. The third is to apply spot compression to maximize local compression and separate tissues, and the final technique is to use geometric magnification. Magnification can be added to any of other techniques as well. It is important the technologist have the ability to spatially visualize the area of concern when employing the additional views. The radiologist and technologist act as a team when discussing how to pinpoint the lesion for the view requested.

Mediolateral and Lateromedial Views

The most commonly performed angled view is the 90-degree view. This can be performed as a mediolateral (ML) or a lateromedial (LM). The correct beam direction is the one that places the area of interest closest to the image detector, in order to minimize geometric blur. Frequently this view is used to solve problems in findings seen on the MLO and to triangulate the precise location of a finding. Lesions medial to the nipple will move superiorly on the 90-degree view from their location on the MLO and lesions that are lateral will move inferiorly. Also the more peripherally positioned the lesion on the CC, the more the lesion will move on the 90-degree view as compared with its location on the MLO view. As in the MLO view, the 90-degree view requires lifting and using an *up and out* positioning technique to obtain the most breast tissue possible within the image (Fig. 6-8). One note with digital imaging is that any view that has a beam direction opposite of a standard view could hang backwards at soft-copy display.[19] This occurs because all digital images carry orientation tags in the Digital Imaging and Communications in Medicine (DICOM) header that follow the predominate beam direction. By convention, the standard beam directions are from either medial to lateral as for the MLO or from head to foot, as for the CC. So a ML 90-degree view will hang appropriately but a LM view may not because

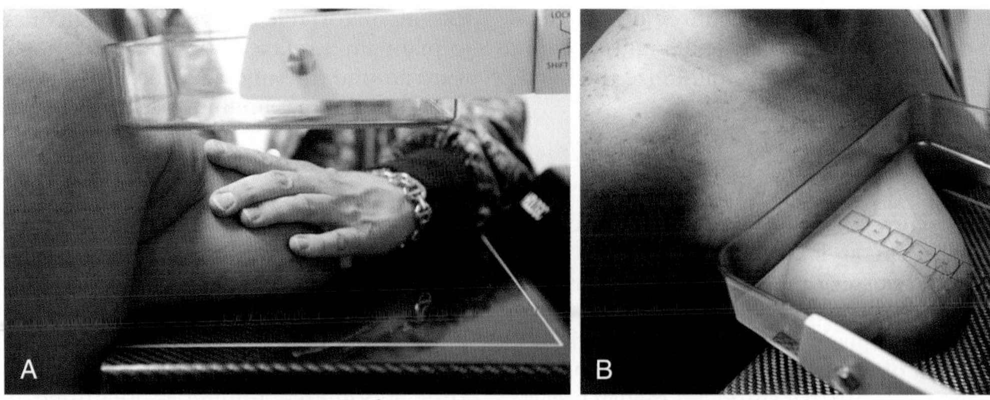

■ **FIGURE 6-7** A and B, Proper positioning for the craniocaudal (CC) view.

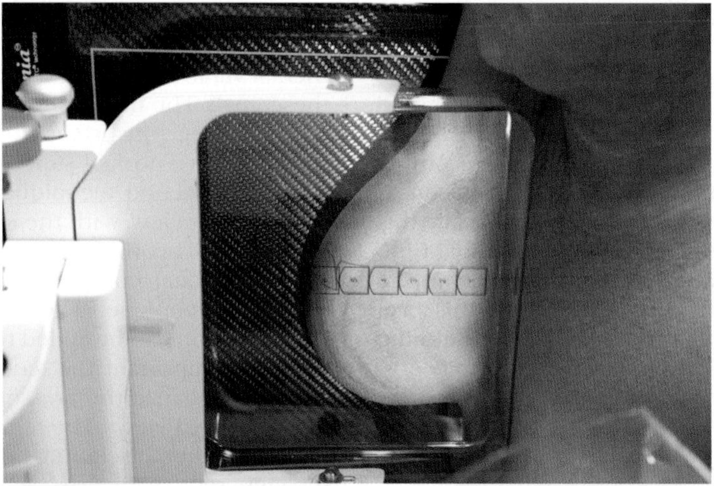

■ **FIGURE 6-8** The 90-degree mediolateral (ML) view.

it has reverse beam orientation. This is especially important for facilities that interpret digital mammography on soft-copy workstations because most workstations have the ability to toggle all display annotations on and off, as described earlier. Potentially, therefore, a radiologist could interpret an incorrectly hanging left 90-degree LM view (Fig. 6-9). It is the radiologist's responsibility to be aware of every additional view that has been taken on any patient and to ensure that each of those views is displayed correctly. Having the technologist judge that the image will hang correctly on the diagnostic workstation based on how the image is displayed at the acquisition workstation in the x-ray room is a mistake, because often times the acquisition unit is made by a different vendor from the diagnostic workstation and so the display functionality may be different. The incorrect display could be the fault of insufficient use of the DICOM orientation tags by the acquisition vendor, or incorrect implementation of those tags by the display vendor.

Lateromedial Oblique View

The lateromedial oblique (LMO) view is an infrequently used view that can be used for problem solving, especially in patients with pacemakers or a difficult to image body habitus. For this view, the beam moves from the lower outer quadrant to the upper inner quadrant toward the detector. As in the MLO view, the breast tissue must be supported by the technologist's hand in an *up and out* sweep to decrease a drooping breast image. Care must also be taken that the upper arm tissue does not overhang the breast tissue before or after compression. If the upper arm tissue overhangs the breast tissue during compression, it may become trapped between the breast and the compression paddle, causing the patient unnecessary discomfort and pinching. If the upper arm tissue overhangs the breast tissue after compression, it will obscure breast tissue. This is a reverse orientation view, like the 90-degree LM, and so care must be taken to ensure that this view hangs correctly at display.

Superoinferior Oblique View

The superoinferior oblique (SIO) view is another angled problem-solving view where the beam travels from the superolateral breast to the inferomedial breast. If this view is done at a relatively shallow angle so that the predominant beam direction is head to foot, this view will display correctly, but if the angle is steeper than 45 degrees, the predominant tube angle becomes lateral to medial and the

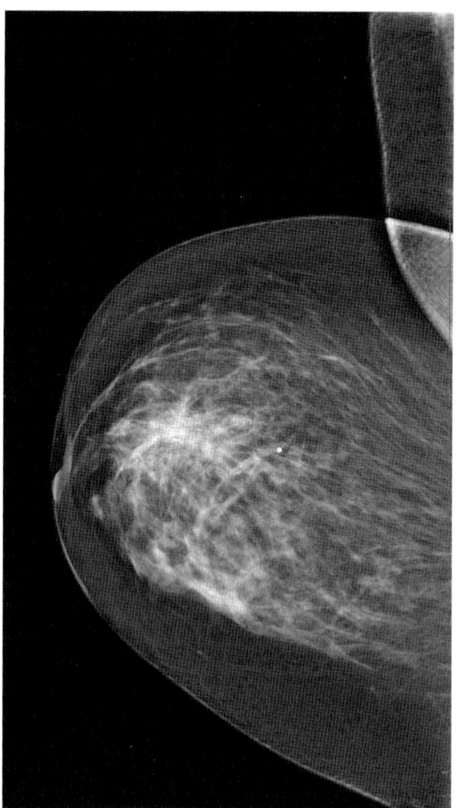

■ **FIGURE 6-9** This lateromedial view is displayed upside down at the diagnostic workstation because the orientation tags are not appropriately applied.

same reverse orientation discussion as for the LM view applies.

Inferosuperior Oblique View

Exactly opposite of the SIO view is the ISO, or inferosuperior oblique. This is a rarely used view for problem solving and again, care must be taken with reverse orientation issues if the predominant beam angle is foot to head.

From Below View

Imaging far posterior superior lesions is well done with the CC view from below (FB) because the object-to-source distance is reduced and the compression paddle does not displace this tissue since it comes up from the bottom (Fig. 6-10). This view is also used for hard to position patients such as patients with kyphosis or male patients and for needle localizations when the closest skin surface to the area being localized is the inferior surface. Once again, this is a reverse orientation view and so potentially it may hang for the radiologist as the opposite breast CC if the workstation does not use the orientation tags correctly.

Rolled Views

Instead of changing the tube angle to reorient tissues that are adjacent to each other, some prefer to perform rolled views. These are usually done to determine if a density that is seen on the CC view is due to superimposition of structures or real. The rolled views can be done either medially (...RM) or laterally (...RL).

Exaggerated Lateral Craniocaudal View and Axillary Tail View

The most common additional view used to include more tissue is the exaggerated lateral CC view (XLCC). This view is used when tissue trails off of the lateral margin of the breast on the original CC view or to image far posterior lateral lesions or axillary tail lesions. Figures 6-11A and 6-11B illustrate this. The technologist will position the patient as she would during the routine CC view but then rotate the patient until the lateral aspect of the breast is positioned on the detector (Fig. 6-12). Another view, the axillary tail (AT) view, is also used to image the axilla. This view is specifically meant to display the entire axillary tail. The angle is less steep than that of an MLO but will be dictated by the patient's body habitus by placing the detector parallel to the axillary tail. As in the MLO, the

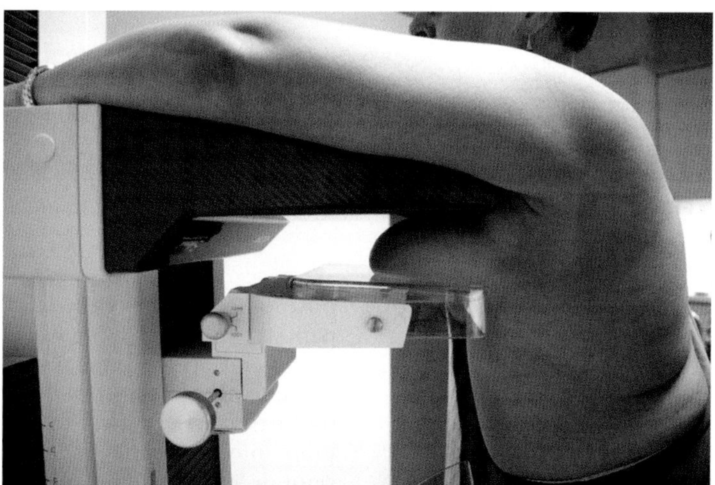

■ **FIGURE 6-10** Proper positioning for the craniocaudal or from below (FB) view.

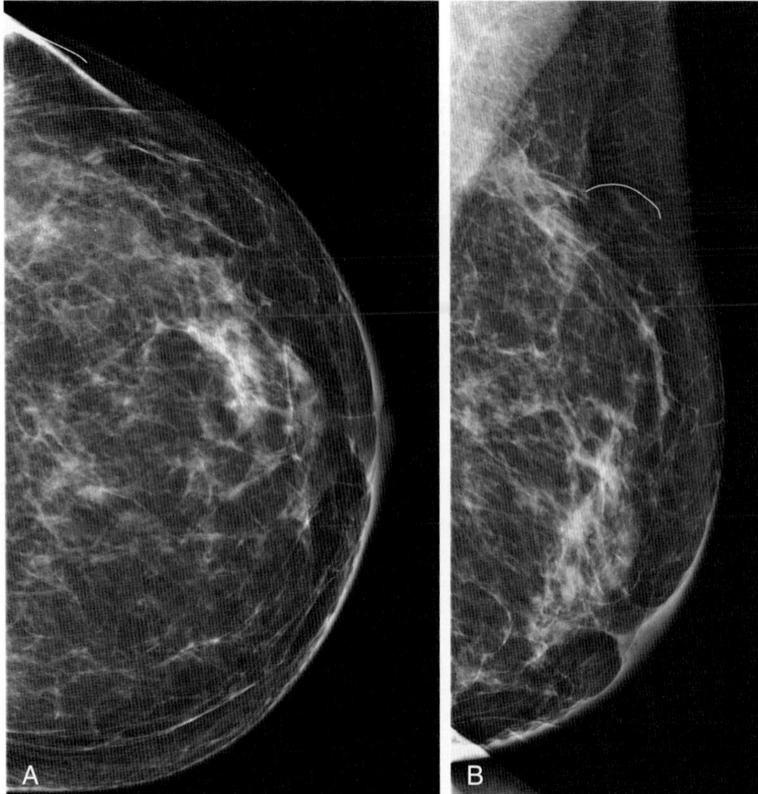

■ **FIGURE 6-11** The craniocaudal (CC) view (**A**) does not include the most posterior lateral tissue. An exaggerated lateral CC view (XLCC) taken on the same patient (**B**) shows how the XLCC view better demonstrates the posterior lateral tissue.

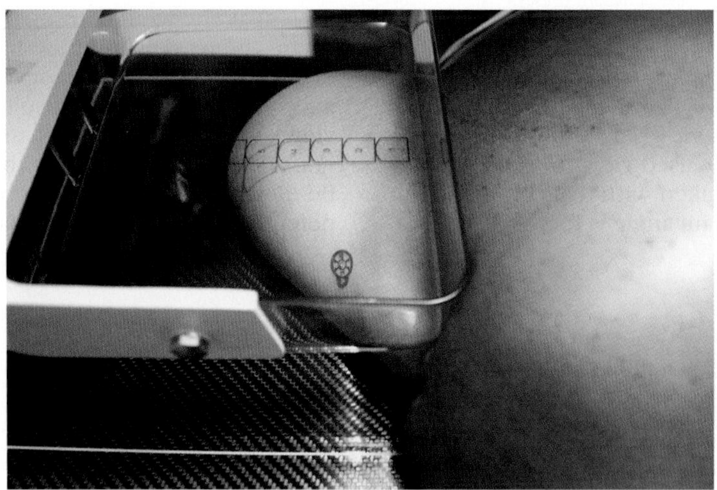

■ **FIGURE 6-12** The properly positioned exaggerated lateral CC (XLCC) view.

arm of the side being imaged is draped over the top of the detector (Fig. 6-13).

Cleavage View

The cleavage view (CV) is used to evaluate far posterior medial lesions. The medial aspects of both breasts are imaged with this view and so display can be confusing. The technologist stands behind the patient during the positioning of this view and wraps her arms around the patient, pulling both breasts into position. The technologist may stand on the medial side of the breast being imaged if she is unable to properly position from behind. Turning the patient's head away from the side of interest will allow more medial tissue to be accessed. During acquisition, right or left should be chosen so that the breast of interest is displayed on the top of the radiologist's monitor and is oriented in the same direction as the original CC view.[19]

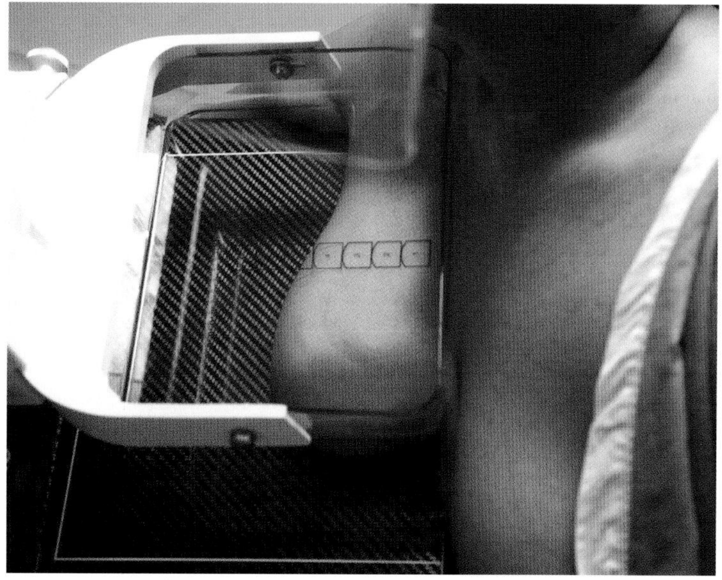

■ FIGURE 6-13 Positioning for the axillary tail view (AT).

Tangential View

Palpable lesions are frequently well demonstrated with the tangential view (TAN). For this view, a lead maker is placed on the skin directly over the palpable area, and the image is acquired so that the beam is in tangent to the marker. This maneuver moves the lesion as close to the subcutaneous fat as possible so that the margins of the area can be assessed more thoroughly.[20] The TAN is also used to evaluate if calcifications are in the skin.[21,22] This is done by deciding which skin surface is closest to the calcifications on the initial two-view mammogram. The technologist then uses either the fenestrated paddle or open paddle with cross hairs that are meant for needle localizations and acquires an image with this paddle on the closest skin surface, over the area of calcium. The skin is then marked with a lead marker directly over the calcium and a TAN is obtained to that marker.

Implant Views

For patients with implants, eight views are typically performed, including each of the two standard views for each breast with and without the implant in the field. In order to see as much posterior tissue as possible, the implants are included in the field of view, but compression is limited with this and so the implants are then displaced toward the chest wall and as much breast tissue as possible is then compressed and imaged.[23] The displacement of the implant is achieved by pushing the implant posterior and superiorly while gently pulling the breast tissue forward and holding the displaced implant and anterior tissue in place with the compression paddle. This technique is performed in both the CC and MLO views. The implant displaced (ID) views (e.g., MLOID, CCID) may display as a second CC view for the radiologist or as an extra view depending on the functionality of the diagnostic workstation.

Magnification

Geometric magnification can be added to any of the above additional views and can be used with or without coning of the beam. Just as in screen-film mammography, a microfocal spot is used to reduce some of the geometric unsharpness inherently created with this technique. Unlike screen-film mammography, however, with digital mammography, the spatial resolution increases with magnification. This occurs because more pixels are used to sample a small area with magnification. Mass margins and calcifications are well demonstrated with this technique. Just as with screen-film, the dose to the patient is higher and the exposure time longer than with contact imaging and so appropriate positioning and compression are important to minimize motion blurring and repeating of images.

In conclusion, though positioning is one of the topics that radiologists leave to the radiologic technologists to master, a basic understanding of each view, how it used and how it should be judged from a quality perspective is critical to interpretation and good patient care.

KEY POINTS

- Positioning is important in interpretation.
- Each additional view has specific uses.

SUGGESTED READINGS

Eklund GW, Cardenosa G.The art of mammographic position. *Radiol Clin North Am* 1992;**30**:21-53.

Siegel E, Krupinski E, Samei E, Flynn M, Andriole K, Erickson B, et al. Digital mammography image quality: image display. *J Am Coll Radiol* 2006;**3**:615-27.

REFERENCES

1. Hendrick RE. Quality assurance in mammography. *Radiol Clin North Am* 1992;**30**:243-55.
2. Destouet JD, Bassett LW, Yaffe MJ, Butler PF, Wilcox PA. The ACR's Mammography Accreditation Program: ten years of experience since MQSA. *J Am Coll Radiol* 2005;**2**:585-92.
3. Heinlein RW, Bassett LW. *Diagnosis of diseases of the breast*. 2nd ed. 1992; Philadelphia: Elsevier; 2005; p. 102-539.
4. Yaffe MJ, Hendrick RW. Recommended specifications for new mammography equipment: report of the ACR-CDC focus group on mammography equipment. *Radiology* 1995;**197**:19-26.
5. The Mammography Quality Standards Act. *Public Law* 1992; 102-539.
6. MQSA. Mammography Quality Standards Act regulations 21 CFR part 900. *Mammography* 2002.
7. Federal Register: Rules and Regulations. February 6, 2002;**67**(25).
8. *Mammography Quality Control Manual*. Restin, Va: American College of Radiology; 1999.
9. Bassett LW, Farria DM, Bansal S, Farquhar MA, Wilcox PA, Feig SA. Reasons for failure of a mammography unit at clinical image review in the American College of Radiology Mammography Accreditation Program. *Radiology* 2000;**215**:698-702.
10. Taplin SH, Rutter CM, Finder C, Mandelson MT, Houn F, White E. Screening mammography: clinical image quality and the risk of interval breast cancer. *Am J Roentgenol* 2002;**178**:797-803.
11. Eklund GW, Cardenosa G. The art of mammographic positioning. *Radiol Clin North Am* 1992;**30**:21-53.
12. Bassett LW, Hirbawi IA, DeBruhl N, Hayes MK. Mammographic positioning: evaluation from the view box. *Radiology* 1993;**188**:803-6.
13. Bassett LW, Gold RH. Breast radiography using the oblique projection. *Radiology* 1983;**149**:585-7.
14. Lundgren B, Jakobsson S. Single view mammography. a single and efficient approach to breast cancer screening. *Cancer* 1976;**38**:1124-9.
15. Sickles EA, Weber WN, Galvin HB. Baseline screening mammography: one vs two views per breast. *AJR Am J Roentgenol* 1986;**147**:1149-53.
16. Maiki F, Cardoso K. *Breast health access for women with disabilities: training for the mammography technologist*. Alta Bates Summit Medical Center, Rehabilitation Services Department. *www.bhawd.org*; January 2006.
17. Berkowitz JE, Gatewood OMB, Donovan GB, Gayler BW. Dermal breast calcifications: localization with template-guided placement of skin marker. *Radiology* 1987;**163**:282.
18. Pisano ED, Zuley M, Baum JK, Marques HS. Issues to consider in converting to digital mammography. *Radiol Clin North Am* 2007;**45**:813-30.
19. IHE technical Framework. Available at. *www.ihe.net/technicalframework/* [accessed 3/18/2010].
20. Faulk RM, Sickles EA. Efficacy of spot compression - magnification and tangential views in mammographic evaluation of palpable breast masses. *Radiology* 1992;**185**:87-90.
21. Berkowitz JE, Gatewood OM, Gayler BW. Equivocal mammographic findings: evaluation with spot compression. *Radiology* 1989;**171**:369-71.
22. Kopan DB, Meyer JE, Homer MJ, Grabbe J. Dermal deposits mistaken for breast calcifications. *Radiology* 1983;**149**:592-4.
23. Eklund GW, Busby RC, Miller SH, Job JS. Improved imaging of the augmented breast. *AJR Am J Roentgenol* 1988;**151**:469-73.

CHAPTER 7

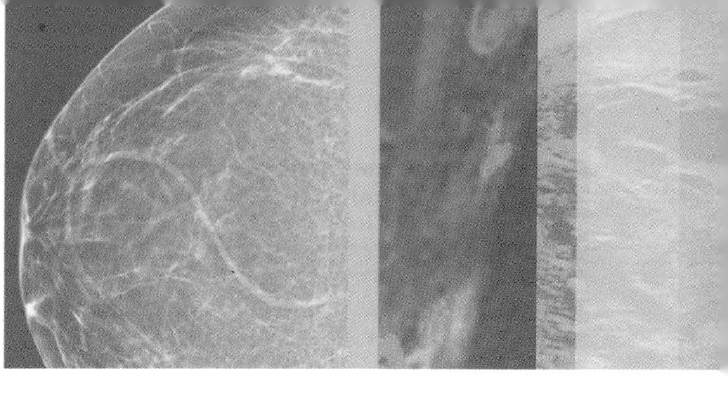

Clinical Image Evaluation

Lawrence W. Bassett and Laura Doepke

Maintaining high-quality clinical images is one of the most important goals of a quality assurance program for mammography. Learning to recognize specific deficiencies in the clinical images and their possible causes allows the interpreting physician and radiologic technologist to correct image deficiencies as soon as possible. In addition to the ongoing daily assessment of clinical images by the interpreting physician and radiologic technologist, an external review of selected clinical images is mandated by the Mammography Quality Standards Act (MQSA).[1,2] The external clinical image evaluation is performed at least every 3 years and is done by specially trained radiologists under the auspices of U.S. Food and Drug Administration (FDA)-approved accrediting bodies.[3]

CLINICAL IMAGE REVIEW

The clinical image review of the American College of Radiology Mammography Accreditation Program (ACR MAP) requires that a screening examination of each breast of a woman with fatty breasts (ACR Breast Imaging Reporting and Data System [BI-RADS] type 1 or 2) and of a woman with dense breasts (BI-RADS type 3 or 4) be submitted for each mammography unit.[4] If a facility submits mammograms identified as a fatty breast that is actually dense (> 50% dense), or mammograms of a dense breast that is actually fatty (< 50% dense), the submitted mammograms will be returned with a request to submit a case with appropriate density criteria. Because of variations in body habitus and the ability of the patient to cooperate, it is not possible to attain ideal breast positioning and compression in all women. Therefore, facilities are requested to submit what they consider to be representative images of their best work.

The clinical image evaluation includes an assessment of these following eight categories: (1) positioning; (2) compression; (3) exposure; (4) contrast; (5) sharpness; (6) noise; (7) artifacts; and (8) labeling. Each of these categories for image quality assessment are reviewed in detail in this chapter.

In 1997, 1034 units failed their initial clinical image evaluation submission.[5] In these failed initial applications, 6128 categories were cited by reviewers as deficient. These deficiencies included 1250 (20%) with deficiencies in positioning, 944 (15%) in exposure, 887 (14%) in compression, 806 (13%) in sharpness, 785 (13%) in contrast; 703 (11%) in labeling, 465 (8%) in artifacts, and 288 (5%) in noise. A significantly higher proportion of failures were attributed to positioning deficiencies for fatty breasts than for dense breasts ($P = .028$). Higher proportions of failures in dense breasts were related to compression ($P < .001$) and exposure ($P < .001$) deficiencies. Table 7-1 summarizes the most common deficiencies of the eight clinical image evaluation categories reported in that study.

A follow-up study in 2005 showed a considerable improvement in images submitted for accreditation in 2003.[6] From 1987 (the inception of the ACR accreditation program) to 1991, only 70% of the mammography units facilities applied for accreditation passed on their first attempt. In 2003, 88.3% of the units passed on their first submission of images, indicating a marked improvement in the quality of mammography since MQSA went into effect and the accreditation program was mandated.

The following focuses on the eight categories of the clinical image evaluation.

Positioning

Breast positioning has improved dramatically over the years. This is due to a better understanding of the anatomy and mobility of the breast and improved capabilities of modern dedicated mammography equipment.[7] The standard screening views are the mediolateral oblique (MLO) and the craniocaudal (CC). Because these are the

TABLE 7-1. Clinical Image Evaluation Categories and Potential Deficiencies

Category	Potential Deficiencies
Positioning	Poor visualization of posterior tissues Sagging breast on MLO Inadequate amount of pectoralis major muscle on MLO Nonstandard angulation of MLO Breast positioned too high on image receptor on MLO Posterior nipple line on CC not within 1 cm of MLO Excessive exaggeration on CC view: Portion of breast image cut off Skin folds Other body parts projected over breast
Compression	Poor separation of parenchymal densities Nonuniform exposure levels Patient motion
Exposure	Generalized underexposure Inadequate penetration of dense areas Generalized overexposure
Contrast	Inadequate contrast Excessive contrast
Sharpness	Poor delineation of linear structures Poor delineation of feature margins Poor delineation of microcalcifications Poor film-screen contact
Noise	Visually striking mottle pattern Noise-limited visualization of detail
Artifacts	Punctate or lint Scratches or pickoff Roller marks Equipment related artifacts; e.g., grid lines Hair, deodorant, etc. Image handling Image fogging
Labeling	Failure to properly identify: patient, facility, exam date, view at axillary side, radiologic technologists, number of cassette and screen

CC, craniocaudal view; MLO mediolateral oblique view.

only views employed for screening mammography, the goal should be to image as much breast tissue as possible on these views.[8]

Before beginning the actual positioning maneuvers, the radiologic technologist performing screen-film mammography (SFM) or computed radiography mammography (CRM) determines which size image receptor is most appropriate for the woman being examined. Both 18 × 24 cm and 24 × 30 cm image receptors are usually available. For full field digital mammography (FFDM) units there is usually only one image receptor size, which varies with manufacturers.

Positioning for the Mediolateral Oblique View

The MLO is the view that provides the best opportunity to show all of the breast tissue in a single image (Fig. 7-1). Because the breast lies primarily on the pectoralis muscle, a generous amount of pectoralis muscle should be included to ensure that far posterior breast tissues are shown. It is desirable for the muscle to extend inferiorly to the posterior nipple line (PNL) or below; this can be achieved in greater than 80% of women.[8] On the MLO, the PNL is drawn at an angle approximately perpendicular to the muscle (usually about 45 degrees), extending from the nipple to the pectoralis muscle or to the edge of the film, whichever comes first (Fig. 7-2). Whenever possible, the fibroglandular tissue should not extend to the edge of the film, because this would imply that additional posterior tissue was excluded from the image. Thus, it is desirable to see fat posterior to all the fibroglandular tissue when possible.

Skin folds on the image should be avoided because they can obscure a lesion or mimic an abnormality (Fig. 7-3). Occasionally, skin folds in the axilla cannot be avoided, but these should not pose problems in interpretation. If proper positioning methods have been used during the initiation and application of compression, the breast should not sag.

Positioning for the Craniocaudal View

The overriding goal for positioning the CC view should be to include all of the posteromedial tissue, because this

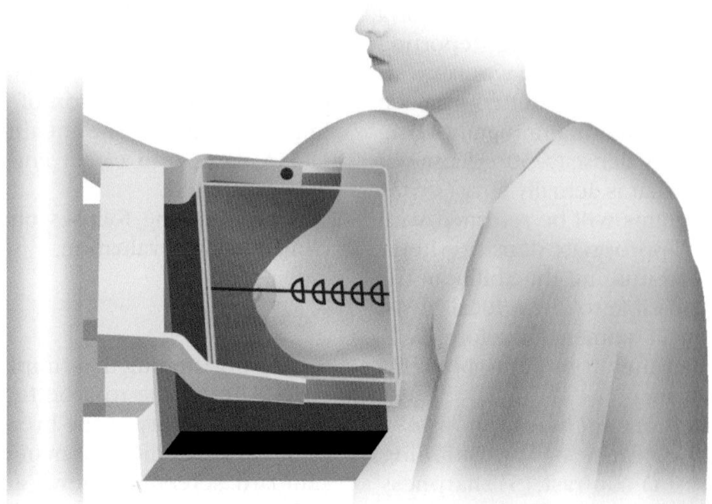

■ **FIGURE 7-1** Woman properly positioned for mediolateral oblique (MLO) view.

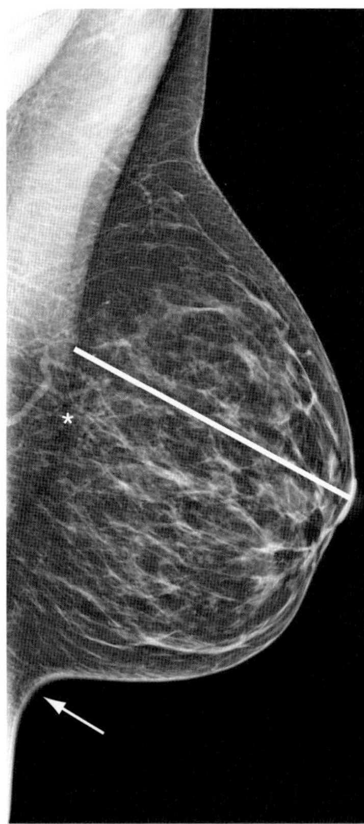

■ **FIGURE 7-2** Proper positioning for the mediolateral oblique (MLO) mammography view: Note inclusion of a generous amount of pectoralis muscle, extension of the muscle below the posterior nipple line (a line drawn at a 45 degree angle from the nipple extending to the anterior edge of the pectoralis muscle), visualization of retromammary fat (*asterisk*) posterior to the fibroglandular tissues, and open inframammary fold (*arrow*).

is the area of the breast most likely to be excluded in an MLO (Figs. 7-4 and 7-5). If proper methods are used, the radiologic technologist can include all of the posteromedial fibroglandular tissue without resorting to exaggerated medial positioning of the CC. Exaggerated medial positioning may result in unnecessary exclusion of posterolateral tissue (Fig. 7-6). However, while as much lateral tissue as possible should be included on the CC, lateral tissue should never be included at the expense of medial tissue.

Visualization of the pectoralis muscle is evidence that sufficient posterior breast tissue has been included on the CC. However, the pectoralis muscle is seen in only about 30% of properly positioned CC views.[8] The measurement of the PNL is a reliable index as to whether the CC includes sufficient posterior tissue when the muscle is not visualized. On the CC, the PNL is drawn directly posterior from the nipple to the edge of the film. A good general rule is that the measurement of the PNL on the CC should be within 1 cm of its length on the MLO. Although the length of the PNL is usually greater on the MLO, in approximately 10% of correctly positioned cases, the PNL is longer on the CC.[8]

Compression

Compression decreases breast thickness and makes it more uniform.[9] Decreased thickness reduces dose, scatter radiation, and object unsharpness. Uniform thickness means that film optical densities are more likely to correspond to subtle attenuation differences in the tissue rather than to thickness differences. Adequate compression also prevents motion unsharpness.

Inadequate compression is manifested by overlapping breast structures, nonuniform tissue exposure and motion unsharpness (also called *blur*). Motion due to inadequate compression is more commonly seen on the MLO than on the CC view, because the breast is supported by the image receptor or "bucky" on the CC view (Fig. 7-7).

Contrast

Radiographic contrast can be described as the degree of variation in optical density between different areas of the image. The different shades of gray on the film allow us to perceive attenuation differences in the breast tissues. Contrast in mammography image receptor systems has improved markedly over the years.

The ability to obtain unlimited contrast is one of the greatest advantages of soft copy reading with FFDM. In addition, the capacity for postprocessing at the workstation allows for contrast adjustments. But when digital films are printed out as hard copy it is important to achieve the best contrast settings prior to printing the image. If the printer contrast range settings are too wide, contrast will be inadequate. However, if the printer contrast range settings are too narrow, the contrast will be excessive.

For SFM, film processing is one of the most important determinants of image contrast.[10] Films should be developed according to the manufacturer's specifications. Longer processing times increase image contrast, although they also increase image noise because of the accompanying lower radiation exposure. Processor temperature is also crucial, and the processor thermometer should be checked regularly for accuracy. Although high contrast is desirable, if the contrast is too high, it may be impossible to see both thick and thin parts on the same image. Thus, a balance must be reached between contrast and latitude when selecting the type of film to use for mammography.

Exposure

The high-contrast and low kilovolt (peak) (kVp)-techniques used in mammography result in a small exposure latitude.[11] In other words, even small differences in kVp or milliampere-seconds (mAs) result in large variations in optical density. Therefore, kVp and mAs must be carefully selected, and phototimer performance must be precise over the range of kVp, breast thickness, and density values encountered in clinical practice. Proper functioning of the phototimer should be evaluated using varying thicknesses of breast-equivalent phantom material during initial calibration of the mammography unit, during the annual survey by the medical physicist, and at least monthly during the phantom image evaluation by the radiologic technologist. The mammography generator should have sufficient output to adequately image large breasts and dense breasts with reasonably short exposure times (less than 2 seconds). The radiologic technologist can monitor exposures for each clinical image based on the length of time of the audible exposure.

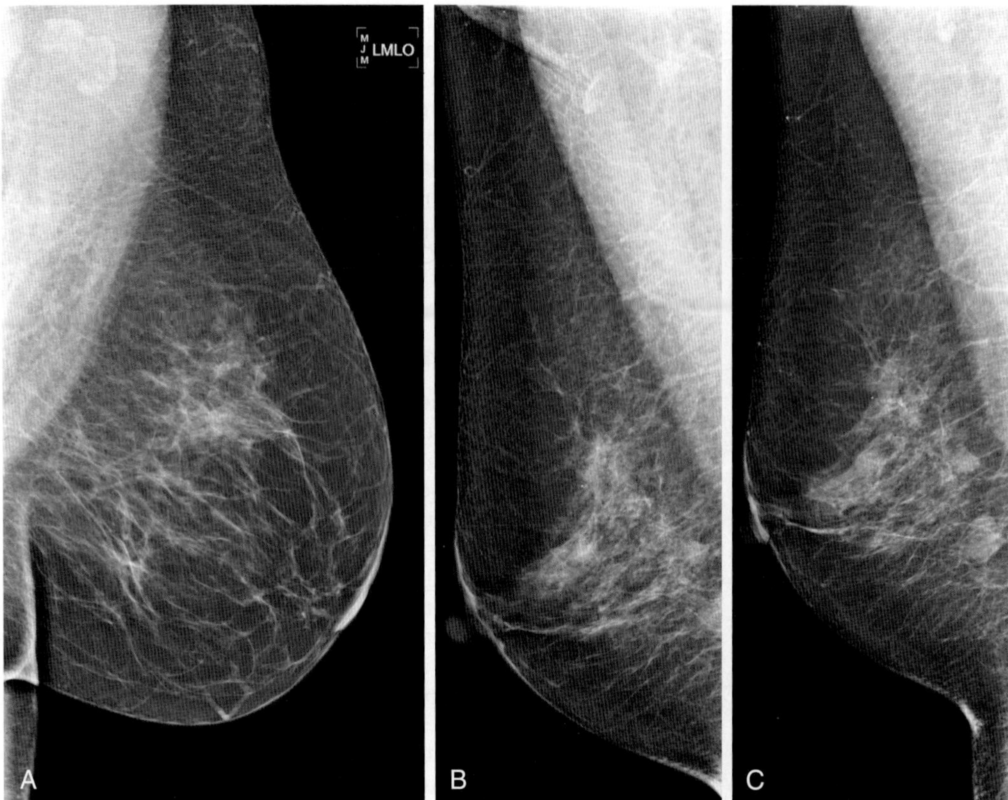

■ **FIGURE 7-3** A, Deficiencies in positioning for mediolateral oblique (MLO) mammography view: Sagging breast. The technologist did not hold the breast up and out as compression was applied. Note the low position of the nipple and prominent inferior skin fold near the chest wall. **B-C,** Deficiencies in positioning for mediolateral oblique (MLO) mammography view: absence of the inframammary fold. The value in seeing an open inframammary fold is demonstrated in images (**B**) (without the inframammary fold) and (**C**) (open inframammary fold) where a mass in the inferior hemisphere is partially obscured in the image without the inframammary fold.

Proper mammographic exposure must be evaluated under correct viewing conditions. These viewing conditions are reviewed in the ACR Mammography Quality Control Manuals and include adequate workstation or viewbox light (luminance), low ambient room light (illuminance) to minimize light reflected off the workstation monitor or surface of the film, and masking of films to eliminate extraneous viewbox light that has passed through the unexposed area of the film from reaching the eye. For FFDM ambient room light should be about equivalent to the workstation monitor's luminance, and for SFM ambient light should be as minimal as possible. In particular, there should not be viewboxes or other strong light sources directly across the room as they may reflect on the monitor or film. It may be necessary to rearrange a room to achieve optimal reading conditions.

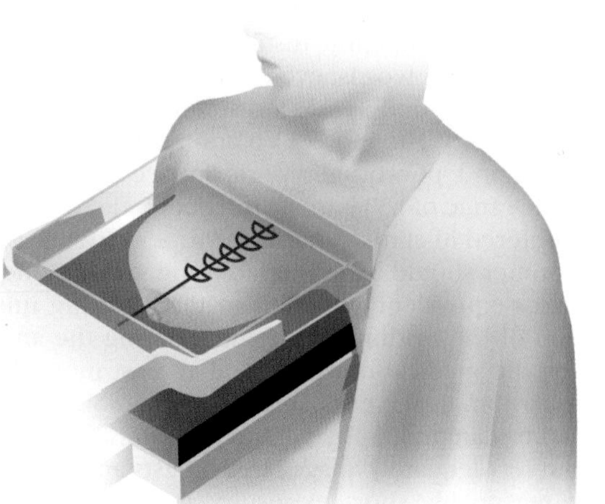

■ **FIGURE 7-4** Woman properly positioned for the craniocaudal (CC) mammography view.

Underexposure has been shown to be a more frequent image deficiency than overexposure. Underexposure is manifested by inability to see details in dense fibroglandular tissue. Because lesions can be obscured within underexposed dense tissue, underexposure is a potentially more serious error since it can lead to false-negative examinations. The pectoralis muscle is one of the densest structures on the MLO, and it is important that the muscle be exposed sufficiently to show underlying breast tissue (Fig. 7-8). Overexposure results in loss of details in the thin or fatty parts of the breast. However, overexposure is frequently a recoverable error that can be compensated for with FFDM by adjusting the image and with SFM by using high luminance view boxes combined with masking of extraneous light, or by *hot lighting* overexposed areas of the film. Underexposure, on the other hand, is an unrecoverable error that requires repeat imaging.

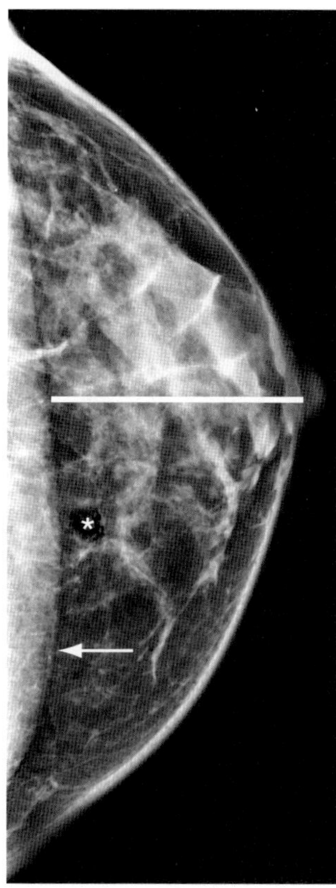

■ **FIGURE 7-5** Evidence of proper positioning for the craniocaudal (CC) view includes the presence of the pectoralis muscle (*arrow*) on the image, posterior nipple line (line from nipple to chest wall) within 1 cm of its length on the mediolateral oblique (MLO) view, inclusion of retromammary fat (*asterisk*) posterior to all medial fibroglandular tissue, and location of the nipple in the midline of the image. Note that some posterior lateral tissue extends beyond the edge of the film.

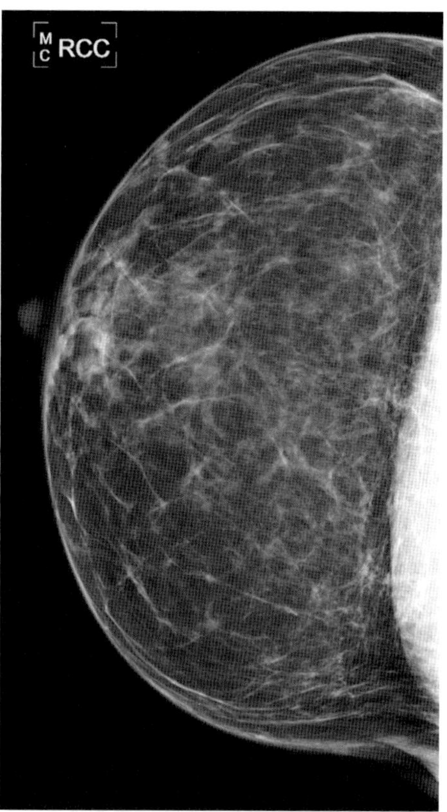

■ **FIGURE 7-6** Exaggerated craniocaudal (CC) mammography view positioning. The nipple is rotated toward the lateral aspects of the breast rather than located at the midline, as in Figure 7-5. This exaggerated positioning might have been intentional to ensure that all of the posteromedial tissue was included but is unnecessary and results in the exclusion of posterolateral tissue.

Noise

Noise, or radiographic mottle, compromises the ability to discern small details, such as calcifications, in mammography images. Quantum mottle is the major source of noise in mammography. It is caused by a statistical fluctuation in the number of x-ray photons absorbed at individual locations in the image receptor.[11] The fewer the total number of photons (for indirect exposure receptors) or x-rays (for direct exposure receptors) that produce the image, the greater the amount of quantum mottle that will be observed. Thus, image recording systems that are faster, underexposed, or processed too aggressively have the potential for more noise. Noise is more likely to be a problem in high-contrast images because high contrast makes the mottle more evident.

The recent increasing focus on reducing radiation doses creates a real challenge for research to decrease radiation without increasing noise.

Sharpness

Sharpness is the ability of the imaging system to define an edge or margin against the surrounding tissue. Unsharpness, often referred to as *blur*, is manifested by blurring of the edges of fine linear structures (Fig. 7-9), tissue borders, and calcifications. Types of unsharpness that may be encountered include geometric, motion, parallax and screen unsharpness, and blurring due to poor film-screen contact.[11]

An increase in focal spot size, a longer object-to-film distance, and a shorter source-to-image distance increase geometric unsharpness. Over the last decade, the focal spot sizes of dedicated mammography units have been reduced for both contact and magnification mammography.

For SFM, a loss of intimate contact between the screen and film results in the further spread of light from the screen before it reaches the film. Poor film-screen contact can result from poorly designed or damaged cassettes, improper placement of the film in the cassette (Fig. 7-10), dirt lying between the film and the screen, or air trapped between the film and the screen at the time the film is loaded. Complete elimination of the air after the cassette is loaded may take up to 15 minutes. Thus, it is recommended that the radiologic technologist wait at least 15 minutes before exposing cassettes after they are loaded.

Artifacts

An artifact can be defined as any density variation on an image that does not reflect true attenuation differences in the subject. Full-field digital mammography (FFDM) artifacts can result from problems with the x-ray equipment (Fig. 7-11).

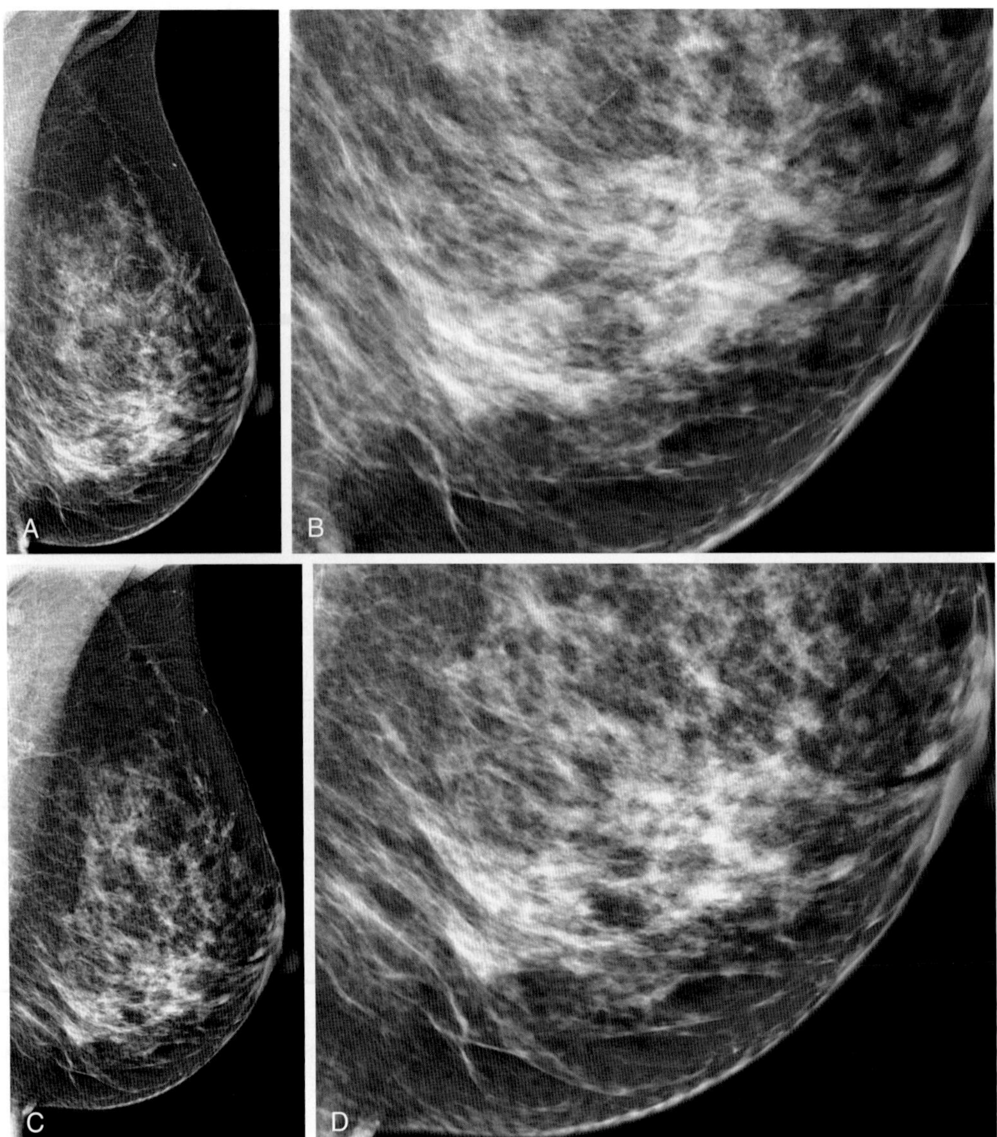

■ **FIGURE 7-7** **A,** Motion unsharpness due to inadequate compression. Linear structures are blurred throughout the lower half of the breast on this mediolateral oblique (MLO) mammography view. **B,** A closer view of the area of unsharpness. **C,** Same patient as in A and B without motion unsharpness. **D,** A closer view of the lower half of the breast where motion unsharpness was previously seen and is now resolved due to improved compression.

For SFM, artifacts are usually due to darkroom cleanliness, film handling, screen maintenance, or processing. The presence of multiple artifacts on images suggests problems with quality control at a facility. The processor can be the source of many different types of artifacts, including roller marks, loader marks, and chemical residues (Fig. 7-12). Routine processor maintenance, replenishment of chemicals, cleaning of rollers, and daily quality assurance activities are essential.

Equipment-related artifacts include grid lines and equipment parts superimposed on the image. When a moving grid is used, the grid lines should not be visible on the image. If grid lines are observed regularly, the drive mechanism should be repaired or replaced. Occasionally, it may be difficult to determine whether parallel linear artifacts are related to improper function of the grid or processor rollers. Two images of a uniform phantom, such as the ACR mammography phantom, acquired with the same technical factors but introduced at right angles to each other can be used to determine whether linear artifacts are due to a faulty grid (the lines do not change direction relative to the properly positioned phantom) or to the processor (the lines do change orientation relative to the phantom).

Improper size, design, or alignment of the compression device can result in inadequate visualization of deep tissues. If the device is improperly aligned with the image receptor, the posterior lip of the compression device may appear on the image.

Labeling

Radiologists are frequently called on to review mammograms from other facilities. A review of mammograms from facilities across the country submitted for clinical image evaluation to ACR MAP in 1993 revealed that

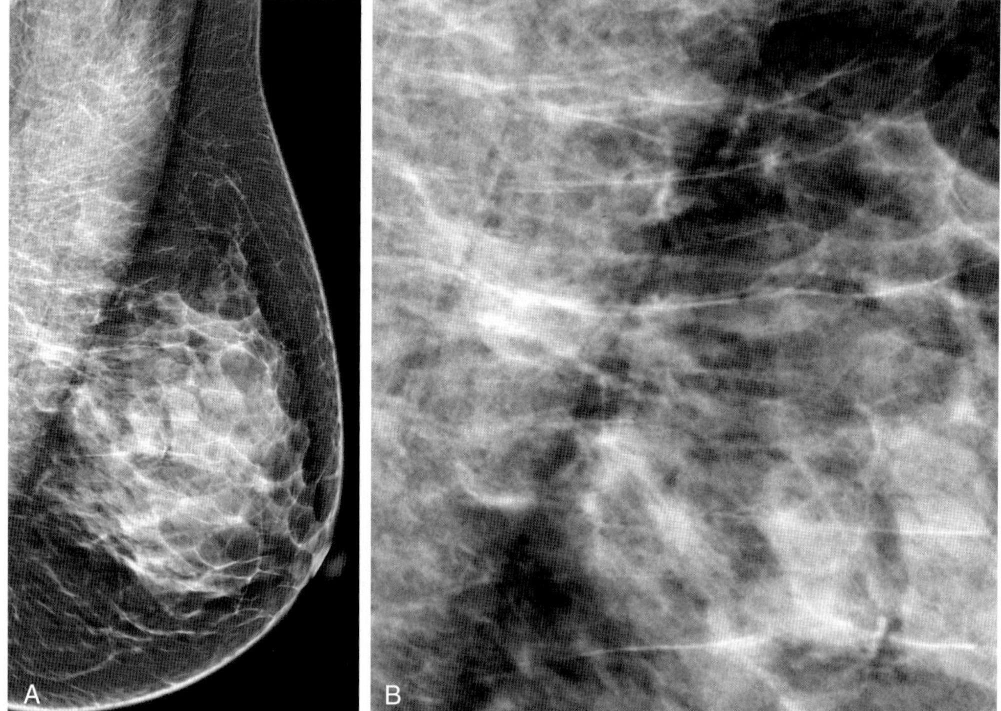

■ **FIGURE 7-8** A and B, Mediolateral oblique (MLO) mammography view showing adequate exposure of the pectoralis muscle in order to show underlying breast tissue.

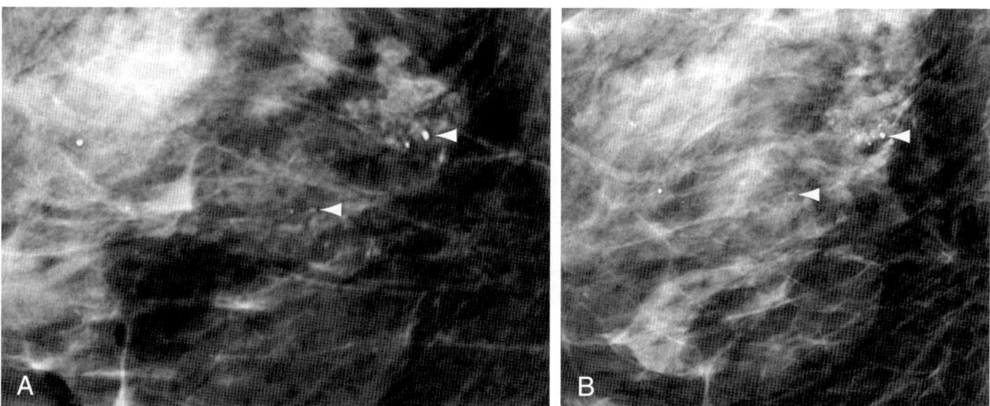

■ **FIGURE 7-9** Blurring of calcifications on the mediolateral oblique (MLO) mammography view due to motion secondary to inadequate compression. **A,** On the initial mediolateral oblique view the image appears blurry with some of the calcifications poorly visualized (*arrows*) secondary to motion. **B,** On the repeat MLO view without motion the calcifications (*arrows*) are better seen.

nonstandardized labeling practices were prevalent.[12] In addition to nonstandardized formats, films often did not contain enough information to adequately identify the facility or the patient (Figs 7-13 and 7-14). In many cases, eccentric methods for designation of view and laterality resulted in confusion or incorrect information (Fig. 7-15).

Standardized methods for labeling films have been developed to ensure correct identification of facilities, patients, laterality, and view (Fig. 7-16). These labeling guidelines for mammography films can be divided into those that are considered essential or required, highly recommended, or just recommended. Required items include identification label, view and laterality, cassette number (Arabic numeral), and initials of the radiologic technologist who performed the examination. The identification label should include facility name and address (at least city, state and ZIP code), examinee's first and last name, and a unique additional identifier (e.g., medical record number or date of birth). It is strongly recommended that the identification label be "flashed" on the image to make it as permanent as possible and so that it can be transferred onto copy films. Paper identification labels are discouraged. The laterality and view marker should be placed at the location on the image near the axilla to facilitate proper orientation of the image.

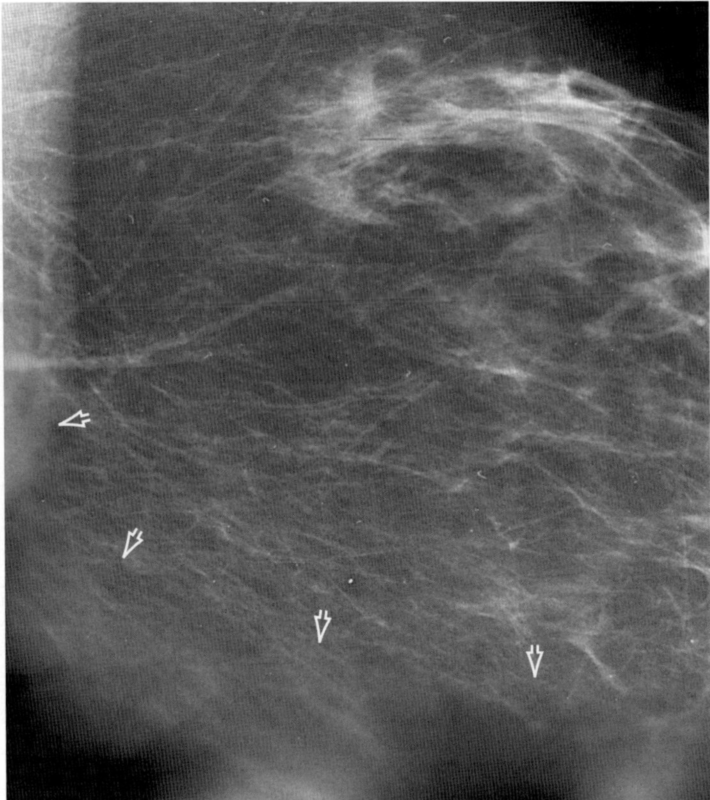

■ **FIGURE 7-10** Loss of film-screen contact. Much of the detail is blurred (*arrows*) in the lower part of the image, a result of improper loading of the film into the cassette.

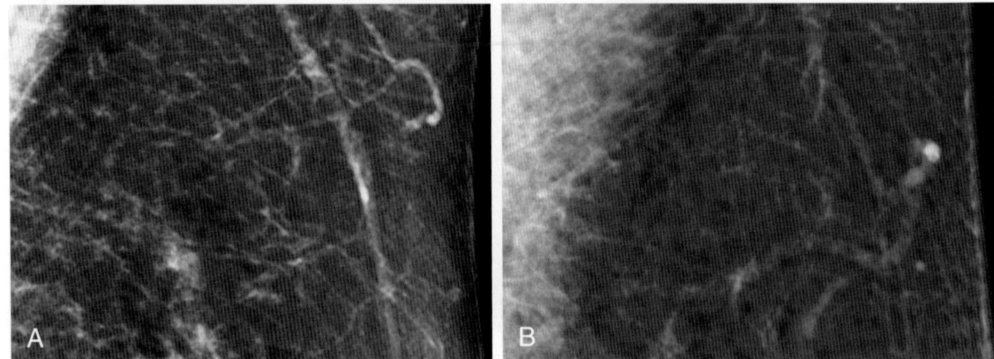

■ **FIGURE 7-11** Two close-up images of mammograms on the same patient with (**A**) and without (**B**) grid artifact. Notice on the image with the grid artifact there is a superimposed crosshatch pattern. On the image without the grid artifact, this pattern is absent.

SUMMARY

Clinical image evaluation is an important quality control activity that should be performed on a daily basis by every physician who interprets mammograms. The interpreting physician's evaluation of the clinical images complements other quality assurance activities, such as phantom image evaluation. Ongoing feedback to the radiologic technologists about good quality or image deficiencies is recommended. Learning to recognize the most likely causes of image deficiencies expedites the rapid correction of problems and maintenance of a high quality breast imaging practice.

KEY POINTS

- Clinical image evaluation is an essential component of the ACR Mammography Accreditation Program.
- Clinical image evaluation should be conducted on a daily basis.
- There are eight essential components of clinical image evaluation.

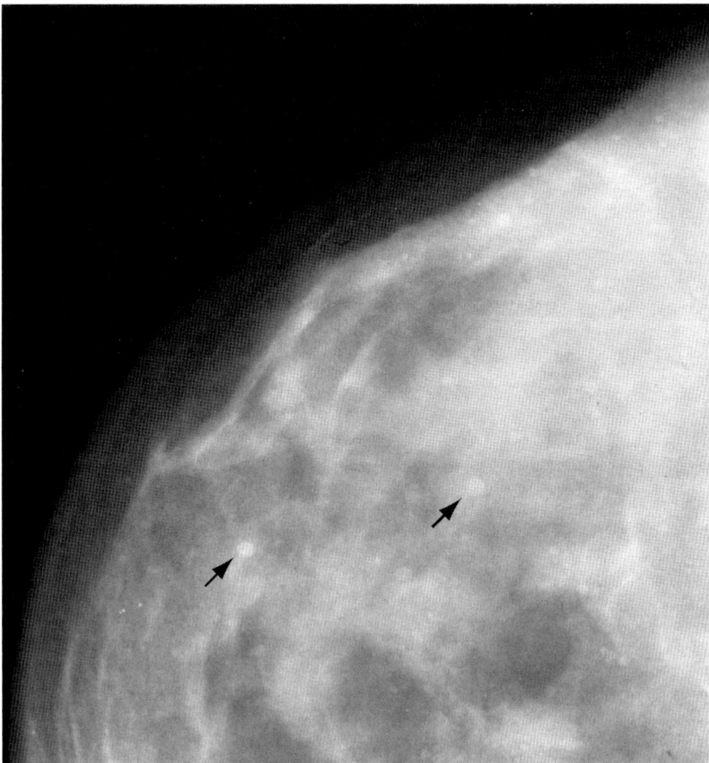

■ **FIGURE 7-12** Multiple artifacts (*arrows*) visible on all of the mammography films of this patient were due to residue of chemicals on the processor rollers, secondary to poor maintenance.

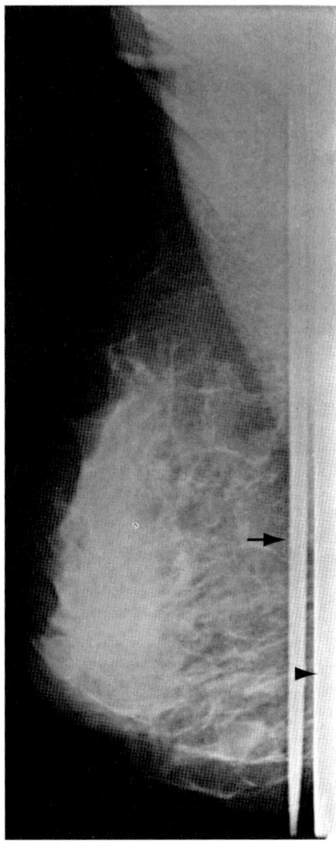

■ **FIGURE 7-13** Improper alignment of compression device. The posterior lip of the compression device (*arrow*) is superimposed on the posterior aspect mammography of the breast. Additional posterior breast tissue is excluded by excessive collimation (*arrowhead*). The following essential information was not provided in the film labeling: location of facility, patient's full name, ID number or birth date for patient, screen identification, and technologist's initials. View should be labeled "RMLO." Compression and exposure are also inadequate. (*From Bassett LW. Clinical Image Evaluation. Radiol Clin North Am 1995;33:1027-1039.*)

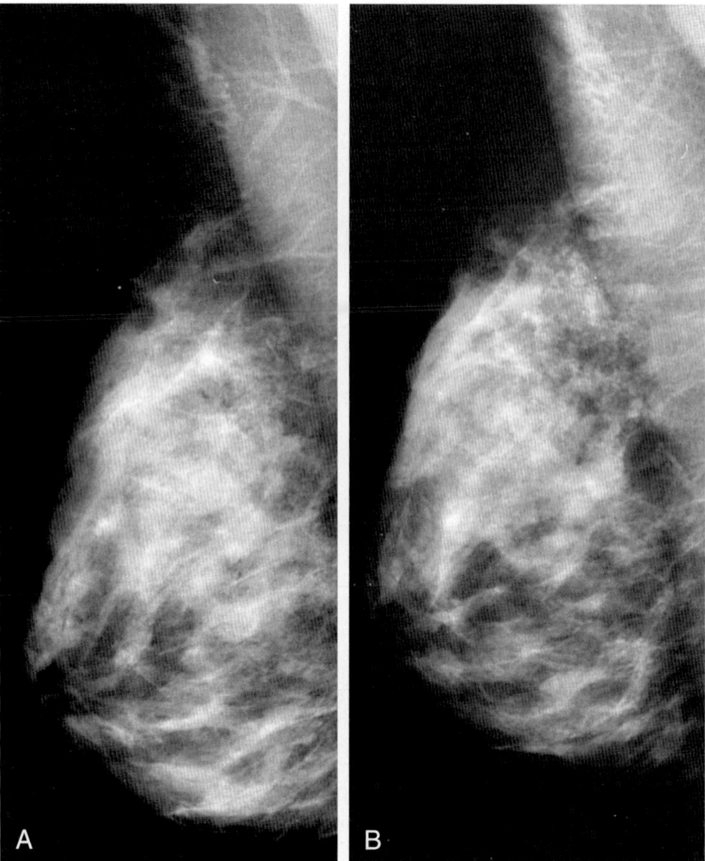

■ **FIGURE 7-14** Different labeling of films for same patient. **A,** Mediolateral (MLO) view with nonstandardized labeling. Facility name (partially masked) is provided but no address. The patient's last name (partially masked) but no first name is given, and no unique ID number is provided. Designation for view incorrect (should be "MLO," not "Axillary") and radiologic technologist is not identified. **B,** MLO view of same patient obtained 2 years later with standardized labeling (facility address partially masked, examinee name masked). Note improved positioning.

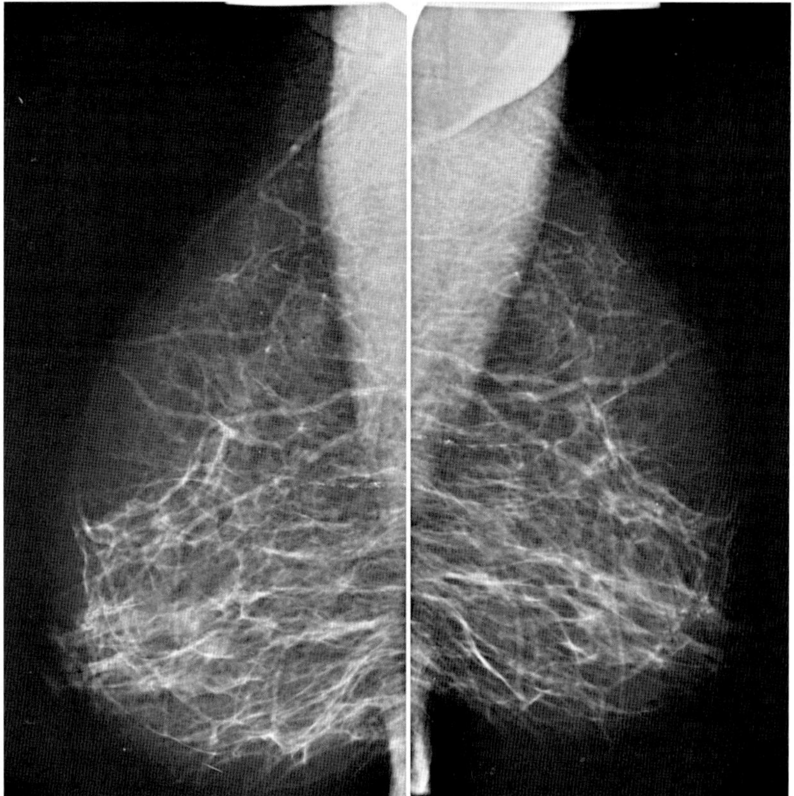

■ **FIGURE 7-15** Confusion can result when facilities use eccentric labeling methods. In the system shown here, the laterality marker (L-R) and view marker (MLO-CC-AX) wheels were supposed to be rotated until the correct view and laterality were in direct opposition. The device results in the presence of both right and left laterality designations and three different view selections on every film. This was confusing to radiologists comparing these films with new mammograms. The system was apparently also confusing to the radiologic technologist spinning the wheels: The RMLO was incorrectly identified "LCC." One of the craniocaudal (CC) views was also labeled incorrectly.

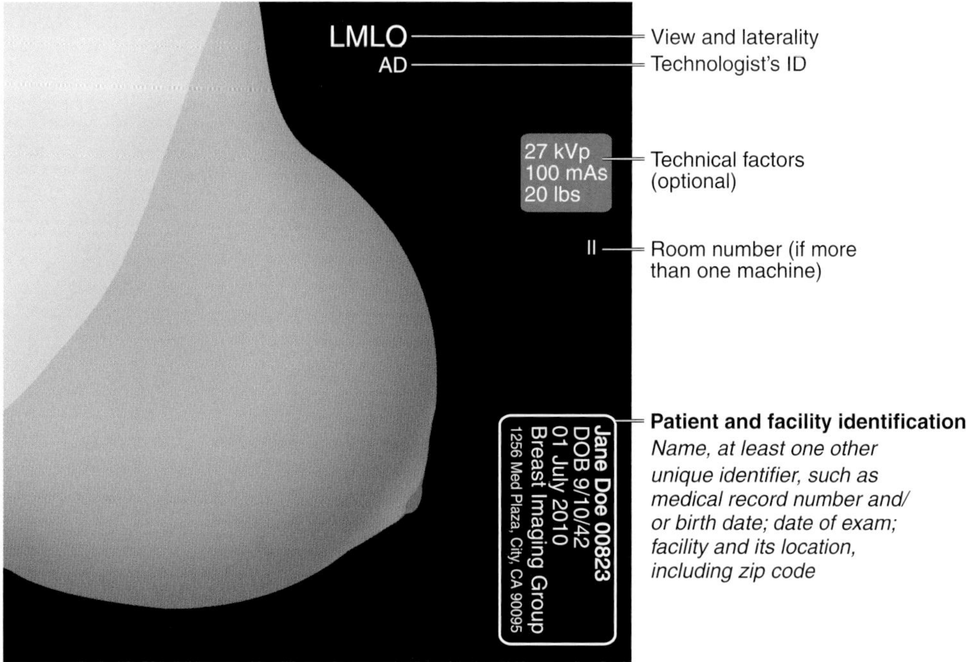

■ **FIGURE 7-16** Recommendations for labeling of mammograms.

SUGGESTED READINGS

Bassett LW, Hirbawi IA, DeBruhl N, Hayes MK. Mammographic positioning: evaluation from the view box. *Radiology* 1993;**188**:803-6.

Hendrick RE. Quality assurance in mammography: accreditation, legislation, and compliance with quality assurance standards. *Radiol Clin North Am* 1992;**30**:243-55.

www.acr.org/accreditation/mammography.aspx.

REFERENCES

1. The Mammography Quality Standards Act. *Public Law* 1992;102-539.
2. Food and Drug Administration. Mammography facilities-requirements for accrediting bodies and quality standards and certification requirements; interim rules. *Fed Regist* 1993;**58**:67558-65.
3. Hendrick RE. Quality assurance in mammography: accreditation, legislation, and compliance with quality assurance standards. *Radiol Clin North Am* 1992;**30**:243-55.
4. McLelland R, Hendrick RE, Zinninger MD, Wilcox PA. The American College of Radiology Mammography Accreditation Program. *AJR Am J Roentgenol* 1991;**157**:473-9.
5. Bassett LW, Farria DM, Bansal S, Farquhar MA, Wilcox PA, Feig SA. Reasons for failure of a mammography unit at clinical image review in the American College of Radiology Mammography Accreditation Program. *Radiology* 2000;**215**:698-702.
6. Destouet JM, Bassett LW, Yaffe MJ, Butler PF, Wilcox PA. The ACR's Mammography Accreditation Program: 10 years of experience since MQSA. *J Am Coll Radiol* 2005;**2**:585-94.
7. Eklund GW, Cardenosa G. The art of mammographic positioning. *Radiol Clin North Am* 1992;**30**:21-53.
8. Bassett LW, Hirbawi IA, DeBruhl N, Hayes MK. Mammographic positioning: evaluation from the view box. *Radiology* 1993;**188**:803-6.
9. Helvie MA, Chan HP, Adler DD, Boyd PG. Breast thickness in routine mammograms: effect on image quality and radiation dose. *AJR Am J Roentgenol* 1994;**163**:1371-4.
10. Kimme-Smith C, Rothschild PA, Bassett LW, Gold RH, Moler C. Mammographic film-processor temperature, development time, and chemistry: effect on dose, contrast and noise. *AJR Am J Roentgenol* 1989;**152**:35-40.
11. Curry TS, Dowdey JE, Murry RC. The radiographic image. In: Curry TS, Dowdey JE, Murry RC, editors. *Christensen's Physics of Diagnostic Radiology*. 4th ed Philadelphia: Lea & Febiger; 1990. p. 196-218.
12. Bassett LW, Jessop NW, Wilcox PA. Mammography film-labeling practices. *Radiology* 1993;**187**:773-5.

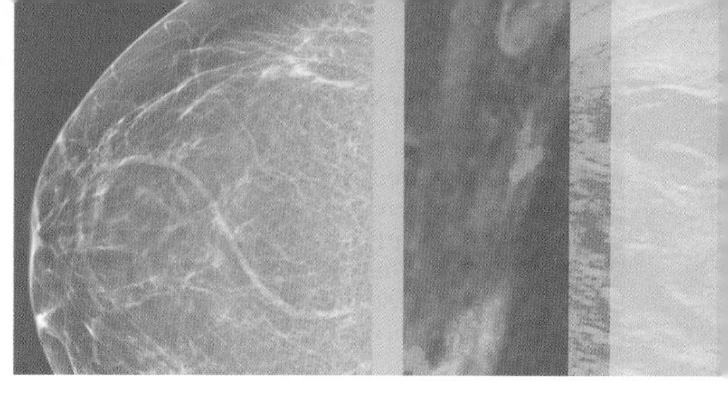

CHAPTER 8

Mammography Quality Control: Digital and Screen-Film

Priscilla F. Butler

Quality control (QC) is defined as "the overall system of activities whose purpose is to provide a quality of product or service that meets the needs of the users; also, the use of such a system. The aim of quality control is to provide quality that is satisfactory, adequate, dependable, and economic."[1] Although the term quality assurance (QA) is often used interchangeably with QC, it has a broader meaning; quality assurance is "a system of activities whose purpose is to provide assurance that the overall quality control job is in fact being done effectively. The system involves a continuing evaluation of the adequacy and effectiveness of the overall quality control program with a view to having corrective measures initiated where necessary."[1] Quality control is an integral part of quality assurance. The definition of quality control for mammography that is used by the Agency for Health Care Policy and Research (AHCPR) is "The routine monitoring of performance and functioning of x-ray imaging and processing equipment."[2] That definition is the focus of this chapter.

Although the concepts of quality assurance and quality control were used by industry for some time, they were first applied to diagnostic radiology in the mid-1970s. A number of scientific papers were published then examining the benefits of implementing QC programs in terms of reduced radiation dose for the patient, improved image quality, and decreased facility costs.[3-6] Several film manufacturers introduced training programs in QC for their customers to ensure that they would obtain the best possible results. As far back as 1973, the Council of the American College of Radiology (ACR) approved resolutions encouraging quality imaging, QA, and QC by their membership.[7] In 1979, the U.S. Food and Drug Administration (FDA) published a recommendation that all diagnostic facilities implement QA programs.[8] Several individuals and organizations published books and reports to serve as resources for diagnostic facilities implementing this new concept.[9-15]

In 1987, the ACR established the first voluntary, national program to accredit mammography facilities that demonstrated high-quality mammography. Gerald Dodd, former chairman of the ACR's Breast Task Force, recognized the need for a detailed instructional manual on quality control to aid facilities in achieving the necessary high quality for good patient care as well as accreditation. The ACR formed the Committee on Mammography Quality Assurance, chaired by R. Edward Hendrick, to develop the ACR's Mammography Quality Control Manual. The first version was published in 1990[16] as three separate manuals: one for the radiologic technologist, one for the medical physicist, and one for the radiologist. The ACR published an updated, single-manual version in 1992.[17] The 1992 Mammography Quality Standards Act (MQSA) significantly enlarged the impact of the ACR's QC manual. In 1993, the FDA's newly published interim rules for mammography facilities required them to conduct substantially the same QC tests and meet the performance criteria outlined in the 1992 manual.[18] The ACR revised the manual in 1994 to fit its new role as a regulatory document,[19] and the FDA adopted the 1994 manual by reference in a subsequent rule.[20] In 1997, the FDA published its final rule for mammography facilities, with specific details on required QC and performance criteria.[21] The ACR manuals were no longer referenced in the regulations. Consequently, in 1999,[22] the ACR's Committee on Mammography Quality Assurance modified the manual again to be consistent with the FDA's final rule requirements. Also, to encourage further improvements in image quality beyond the baseline standards set by the FDA, the manual recommends several additional tests and tighter performance criteria in some areas.

RESPONSIBLE INDIVIDUALS

Teamwork

Mammography QC takes a team approach. Officially, this team consists of radiologists (interpreting physicians), mammography technologists, and medical physicists. The team is often supplemented with the expertise of representatives and service personnel from x-ray equipment, film, and processor manufacturers. Under the FDA's final rule,[21] the facility must assign specific individuals to perform QA and QC activities who are qualified for their assignments and who will be allowed adequate time to perform these duties. The FDA's final rule spells out the regulated role of each official team member (Table 8-1), but in the hectic pace of health care today, many individuals do not realize the extent of their responsibilities.

All radiologists, medical physicists, and radiologic technologists working in mammography must meet the FDA-required minimum criteria for qualification.[21] These requirements are summarized in Table 8-2. They apply to part-time or locum tenens staff as well. Mammography personnel should also be aware of the FDA's requirements for reestablishing qualifications if they no longer meet continuing education or continuing experience requirements.

Supervising Radiologist

The facility's supervising radiologist (or lead interpreting physician, as described in the FDA's final rule) has the responsibility for ensuring that all QA requirements are met. He or she is ultimately responsible for the clinical image quality produced at the facility and the level of patient care provided. In addition, the supervising radiologist must ensure that the individuals he or she has assigned to conduct QA tasks are qualified to perform these tasks, have sufficient time to carry out these duties, and perform them adequately.

A single individual, who is an interpreting physician at the facility, must be designated as the supervising radiologist or lead interpreting physician; designating multiple lead interpreting physicians is not allowed and may lead to confusion. Although the supervising radiologist need not be on site, the ACR recommends that this individual review the QC technologist's results at least quarterly and the medical physicist's survey report annually to ensure that all required tests are being performed and that they meet minimum standards. The lead interpreting physician can easily document this by initialing the QC charts or report at the time of review.

Radiologist

The facility's radiologists (interpreting physicians) are an essential component of a strong QC program because they have an opportunity to evaluate the current clinical image quality with each film they interpret. In addition, by comparing current patient images with those done at the same facility the prior year (or with previous films taken at other facilities), radiologists can detect changes in quality over time.

The FDA's final rule requires that all radiologists interpreting mammograms for the facility follow the facility's procedures for taking corrective action when they are asked to interpret images of poor quality. An example of an appropriate procedure would be to provide written or verbal feedback to technologists on image quality parameters such as positioning, compression, optical density, contrast, patient motion, and technique factors. Radiologists typically have no problem providing timely feedback to technologists when they interpret the mammograms at the same site where the patients are imaged. However, this important feedback is often neglected when radiologists

TABLE 8-1. Quality Assurance (QA) Responsibilities of Mammography Personnel Required by U.S. Food and Drug Administration (FDA)

Individual	Responsibilities
Lead interpreting physician	Has general responsibility to ensure that the QA program meets all FDA requirements Must ensure that individuals assigned to QA tasks are qualified to perform these tasks and that their performance is adequate
Reviewing (audit) interpreting physician	Must review and discuss the medical audit results with the other interpreting physicians (this may be the lead interpreting physician)
Interpreting physician	Follow the facility procedures for corrective action when asked to interpret images of poor quality Participate in the facility's medical outcomes audit program
Medical physicist	Must perform the facility's annual survey Must provide the facility with an annual survey report Is responsible for mammography equipment evaluations (when applicable)
Quality control technologist	Must be a qualified mammography technologist Responsible for all QA duties not assigned to the lead interpreting physician or the medical physicist. Normally, he or she is expected to perform these duties May assign other qualified personnel or may train and qualify others to do some or all of the tests. Retains the responsibility to ensure that assigned duties are performed according to the regulations
Other personnel qualified to perform the QA tasks	Must have technical training appropriate for the assigned task(s) Training must be documented

TABLE 8-2. Summary of Mammography Personnel Qualifications as Required by the U.S. Food and Drug Administration (FDA)

Requirement	Interpreting Physicians	Medical Physicist	Radiologic Technologist
Initial credentialing	Medical license *and* certification by ABR, AOBR, or RCPS *or* appropriate training (see text)	Certification by ABR or ABMP *or* state licensure *or* state approval	ARRT or ARCRT registered *or* state licensure
Initial training	60 hours Category I CME (40 hours if qualified before 4/28/99) 8 hours in each modality	Master's degree in physical science with 20 hours of physics and 20 hours of conducting surveys *or* If qualified before 4/28/99, B.S. in physical science with 10 hours of physics and 40 hours of conducting surveys 8 hours in each modality	If qualified after 4/28/99, 40 hours of training 8 hours in each modality
Initial experience	240 exams within 6 months of qualifying date *or* If board certified at first opportunity, 240 exams in any 6 months within last 2 years of residency	One facility and 10 mammography units *or* If qualified before 4/28/99 with B.S. in physical science, one facility and 20 units	If qualified after 4/28/99, 25 exams under direct supervision
Continuing experience	960 exams in 24 months	Two facilities and 6 mammography units in 24 months	200 exams in 24 months
Continuing education	15 hours Category I CME in 36 months	15 CEUs in 36 months	15 CEUs in 36 months

ABMP, American Board of Medical Physics; ABR, American Board of Radiology; AOBR, American Osteopathic Board of Radiology; ARCRT, American Registry of Clinical Radiologic Technologists; ARRT, American Registry of Radiologic Technology; B.S., bachelor of science degree; CEU, Continuing Education Units; CME, Continuing Medical Education in mammography; FDA, U.S. Food and Drug Administration; RCPS, Royal College of Physicians and Surgeons of Canada.

interpret images off-site. Off-site radiologists should make special efforts to ensure that technologists receive appropriate and timely image quality critique to help improve their performance.

All radiologists interpreting mammograms must meet the following FDA requirements.[21]

Initial Qualifications

Every radiologist interpreting mammograms must:

- Be licensed to practice medicine.
- Be certified in diagnostic radiology by the American Board of Radiology (ABR), the American Osteopathic Board of Radiology (AOBR), or the Royal College of Physicians and Surgeons (RCPS) of Canada or have at least 3 months (2 months if initially qualified before April 28, 1999) of documented training in mammography interpretation, radiation physics, radiation effects, and radiation protection.
- Have 60 hours of documented Category I continuing medical education (CME) in mammography (40 hours if initially qualified before April 28, 1999), at least 15 of which must have been acquired in the 3 years immediately before the physician met his or her initial requirements.
- Have interpreted mammograms from examinations of 240 patients within the 6 months immediately prior to his or her qualifying date or in any 6 months within the last 2 years of residency if the physician becomes board certified at his or her first possible opportunity.
- Receive at least 8 hours of training in any mammographic modality (e.g., digital) for which he or she was not previously trained before beginning to use that modality.

Continuing Experience

Every radiologist interpreting mammograms must continue to interpret or multi-read at least 960 mammographic examinations over a 24-month period.

Continuing Education

Every radiologist interpreting mammograms must earn at least 15 hours of category I CME credit in a 36-month period.

Reestablishing Qualifications

Any radiologist who does not maintain the required continuing qualifications must reestablish his or her qualifications before resuming the independent interpretation of mammograms. A radiologist who does not meet the continuing experience requirements must either (1) interpret or multi-read at least 240 examinations under the direct supervision of an interpreting physician or (2) interpret or multi-read a sufficient number of examinations, under the direct supervision of an interpreting physician, to bring the total up to 960 examinations for the prior 24 months. These interpretations must be done within the 6 months immediately before the radiologist resumes independent interpretation. A radiologist who does not meet the continuing education requirements must obtain additional category I CME hours in mammography to bring the total up to the required 15 credits in the previous 36 months before resuming independent interpretation.

Medical Physicist

The medical physicist is responsible for performing the facility's annual survey. This includes evaluating the QC conducted by the facility's QC technologist as well as conducting the annual tests. Furthermore, the medical physicist must conduct a mammography equipment evaluation of the x-ray unit or film processors whenever a new unit or processor is installed, a unit or processor is disassembled and reassembled at the same or a new location, or major components of the unit or processor are changed or repaired. Although the medical physicist may not delegate these tests to unqualified individuals, he or she may directly supervise tests conducted by trainees.

Communicating survey and equipment evaluation results in a timely manner is an essential part of the medical physicist's responsibilities. The reports must eventually be in written form, but the physicist should either leave the facility a preliminary written report summary or provide a verbal summary immediately after completing the survey to reassure the facility that there are no problems or to allow the facility to quickly take corrective action.

Additionally, "the medical physicist should be available to answer questions for the QC technologist carrying out the QC measurements listed in the ACR Mammography QC Manual whenever problems are encountered. Radiologists and QC technologists should rely on the medical physicist as a resource for questions and problems regarding mammography image quality and QC.

All medical physicists surveying mammography equipment must meet the following FDA requirements.[21]

Initial Qualifications

Every medical physicist who surveys medical equipment must:

- Either be licensed or approved by a state or be certified in Diagnostic Radiological or Imaging Physics by the ABR or the American Board of Medical Physics.
- Have a master's degree or higher in a physical science, 20 semester hours of physics, 20 contact hours of training in conducting surveys of mammography facilities, and experience in conducting mammography surveys of at least 10 units and at least one facility; or, if qualified before April 28, 1999, have qualified as a medical physicist under the interim regulations, and have a bachelor's degree or higher in a physical science, 10 semester hours of physics, 40 contact hours of training in conducting surveys of mammography facilities, and experience in conducting mammography surveys of at least 20 units and at least one facility.
- Have at least 8 hours of training with any mammographic modality (e.g., digital) before surveying units with that modality.

Continuing Experience

Every medical physicist who surveys medical equipment must survey at least two mammography facilities and a total of at least six mammography units within a 24-month period.

Continuing Education

Every medical physicist who surveys medical equipment must earn at least 15 CME hours or continuing education units (CEUs) in a 36-month period.

Reestablishing Qualifications

Any medical physicist who does not maintain the required continuing qualifications may not perform the surveys without the supervision of a qualified medical physicist. Before independently surveying another facility, the medical physicist must reestablish qualifications. Any medical physicist who does not meet the continuing experience requirement must complete a sufficient number of surveys under the direct supervision of a qualified medical physicist to bring the total surveys up to the required 2 facilities and 6 units in the previous 24 months. No more than one survey of a specific unit within a period of 60 days can be counted towards the total mammography unit survey requirement. Any medical physicist who does not meet the continuing educational requirements must obtain a sufficient number of continuing education units to bring the total units up to the required 15 in the previous 3 years.

Quality Control Technologist

The facility-designated QC technologist must be a qualified mammography technologist. She or he is responsible for conducting the daily, weekly, monthly, and semiannual QC tests. It is essential that this individual be given sufficient time to conduct these tests and take (or arrange for) appropriate corrective actions to address identified problems. Although a single designated QC technologist who has overall responsibility for routine QC generally allows for better management of the system, it is sometimes helpful to assign a backup QC technologist to cover the absence of the primary QC technologist. However, this backup person must be adequately trained to conduct and evaluate the tests in precisely the same way as the primary QC technologist in order to minimize artificial variations in results.

Normally, the QC technologist is expected to personally conduct each of the required QC tests. However, the FDA final rule allows the flexibility of assigning some QC tasks to other qualified individuals. For example, many hospitals designate a non-mammography technologist to conduct the processor QC testing and evaluation on each processor in the facility (both within and outside mammography). This practice is acceptable as long as (1) the individual is appropriately qualified and trained and (2) appropriate documentation of those qualifications and training are available. It is important to note, however, that the designated mammography QC technologist is responsible for ensuring that the tasks are done properly by standardizing test methodology, reviewing all data, overseeing repeat testing before calling the medical physicist or service personnel, and conferring with the radiologist and medical physicist.

All mammography technologists, including the quality control technologist, must meet the following FDA requirements.[21]

Initial Qualifications

Every mammography technologist must:

- Have general certification from the American Registry of Radiologic Technology or the American Registry of Clinical Radiologic Technologists or be licensed to perform general radiographic procedures in a state.

- Meet the mammography-specific training requirements by having at least 40 hours of documented training in mammography, including the following: (1) training in breast anatomy and physiology, positioning, and compression, QA/QC techniques, and imaging of patients with breast implants; (2) performance of a minimum of 25 mammography examinations under direct supervision of an appropriate MQSA-qualified individual; and (3) at least 8 hours of training in the use of any mammographic modality (e.g., digital) before beginning to use that modality independently.

Continuing Experience

Every mammography technologist must perform at least 200 mammography examinations in a 24-month period.

Continuing Education

Every mammography technologist must earn at least 15 CEUs in a 36-month period.

Reestablishing Qualifications

Any mammography technologist who does not maintain the required continuing qualifications must reestablish her or his qualifications before performing unsupervised mammography examinations. A technologist who does not meet the continuing experience requirements must perform a minimum of 25 mammography examinations under the direct supervision of a qualified mammography technologist. Any technologist who does not meet the continuing education requirements must obtain a sufficient number of continuing education units in mammography to bring the total up to at least 15 in the previous 3 years, at least 6 of which must be related to each modality used by the technologist in mammography.

QUALITY CONTROL TESTS

The FDA clearly specifies the QC tests that must be performed on mammography equipment.[21] In the 1999 ACR Mammography Quality Control Manual,[22] several additional tests are recommended to further address common image quality problems. These requirements and recommendations are summarized in Tables 8-3 and 8-4. Although performance of the recommended tests are not required for ACR accreditation, the ACR recommends that facilities follow the procedures and performance criteria outlined in the 1999 manual.

TABLE 8-3. Screen-Film Mammographic Quality Control Tests for Technologists

Test	FDA Required	Minimum Frequency	Required and Recommended Performance Criteria*	Time Frame for Corrective Action
Darkroom cleanliness		Daily	Few dust artifacts *should* appear on images.	
Processor QC	✓	Daily	Base + fog *must* be within ± 0.03 of operating level. Mid-density and density difference *must* be within ± 0.15 of operating level.	Immediately
Mobile unit QC	✓	Daily	Test *must* be passed each time unit is moved to a different location and before the unit is used on patients.	Immediately
Screen cleanliness		Weekly	Few dust artifacts *should* appear on images.	
Viewboxes and viewing conditions		Weekly	Marks on viewbox surfaces should be removed. Multiple-viewbox light *should* be uniform in color and intensity.	
Phantom images	✓	Weekly	Background optical density *must* be ≥ 1.20; the operating level should be ≥ 1.40. The density difference operating level *should* be ≥ 0.40. The 4 largest fibers, 3 largest speck groups, and 3 largest masses *must* be visible.	Immediately
Visual checklist		Monthly	Each item *should* function as appropriate.	
Repeat analysis	✓	Quarterly	Repeat rate *should* be < 2% (or < 5% if approved by radiologist and medical physicist). A change in rate of ± 2% *must* be investigated.	Within 30 days of the test date
Analysis of fixer retention	✓	Quarterly	Residual fixer *must* be ≤ 0.05g/m^2 (5 μg/cm^2).	Within 30 days of the test date
Darkroom fog	✓	Semi-annually	Fog *must* be ≤ 0.05.	Immediately
Screen-film contact	✓	Semi-annually	Large areas (> 1 cm) of poor contact are unacceptable; cassettes with such areas *must* be repaired or removed from service.	Immediately
Compression	✓	Semi-annually	For initial power drive, maximum compression *must* be between 25 and 45 pounds.	Immediately

*Required by the U.S. Food and Drug Administration, recommended by the American College of Radiology. Required criteria are designated by the use of *must*, and recommended criteria by the use of *should*.
ACR, American College of Radiology; FDA, U.S. Food and Drug Administration; QC, quality control.

TABLE 8-4. Screen-Film Mammographic Annual Quality Control Tests for Medical Physicists

Test	FDA Required	Required and Recommended Performance Criteria*	Time Frame for Corrective Action
Mammographic unit assembly evaluation	✓	Systems with automatic decompression *must* have (1) override capability to allow maintenance of compression and (2) continuous display of the override status. Items that are hazardous or inoperative or that operate improperly *should* be repaired.	Within 30 days of the test date
Collimation assessment	✓	Both left + right and anterior + chest edge x-ray field-light field deviations *must* be ≤ 2% SID. X-ray field *must* not exceed any side of image receptor by > 2% SID. X-ray field *must* not fall within chest wall side of image receptor. X-ray field *should* not fall within image receptor by > 2% on the right and left sides or by > 4% on the anterior side. Compression paddle edge *must* not extend beyond image receptor by > 1% SID or appear on the image.	Within 30 days of the test date
Evaluation of system resolution	✓	For all focal spot sizes and anode materials: With the bars parallel to the anode-cathode axis, the system resolution *must* be ≥ 13 lp/mm With the bars perpendicular to the anode-cathode axis, the system resolution *must* be ≥ 11 lp/mm.	Within 30 days of the test date
AEC system performance	✓	Over 2 to 6 cm, optical density *must* be maintained within ±0.15 of the mean. Over 2 to 8 cm and various modes, *should* maintain optical density within ±0.30 of the mean. Each density control step *should* result in a 12% to 15% change in mA or an approximate 0.15 increase in optical density.	Within 30 days of the test date
Uniformity of screen speed	✓	Density range (for same size cassette) *must* be ≤ 0.3.	Within 30 days of the test date
Artifact evaluation	✓	Artifacts *must* not be significant.	Within 30 days of the test date
Image quality evaluation	✓	Background optical density *must* be ≥ 1.20; the operating level should be ≥ 1.40. The density difference operating level *should* be ≥ 0.40. The 4 largest fibers, 3 largest speck groups, and 3 largest masses *must* be visible.	Immediately
kVp accuracy and reproducibility	✓	Measured kVp *must* be within ± 5% of the indicated. Coefficient of variation *must* be ≤ 0.02 or ≤ 2%.	Within 30 days of the test date
Beam quality assessment (HVL)	✓	HVL (in mm Al) *must* be ≥ kVp/100. HVL (in mm Al) should be ≥ kVp/100 + 0.03. HVL (in mm Al) should be < kVp/100 + C (where *C* is 0.12 for Mo/Mo, 0.19 for Mo/Rh, 0.22 for Rh/Rh, and 0.30 for W/Rh).	Within 30 days of the test date
Breast exposure and AEC reproducibility	✓	Coefficient of variation for AEC reproducibility *must* be ≤ 0.05 or ≤ 5%.	Within 30 days of the test date
Average glandular dose	✓	Average glandular dose *must* be ≤ 0.3 rad (3.0 milligray) for a standard breast.	Immediately
Radiation output rate	✓	The radiation output rate at 28 kVp with Mo/Mo *must* be ≥ 800mR/sec at any SID at which the system is designed to operate. System *must* be able to maintain this rate when averaged over 3 sec.	Within 30 days of the test date
Viewbox luminance and room illuminance		Viewbox luminance *should* be ≥ 3000 cd/m^2. Room illuminance *should* be ≤ 50 lux or preferably less.	

*Required by the U.S. Food and Drug Administration and recommended by the American College of Radiology. Required criteria are designated by the use of *must*, and recommended criteria by the use of *should*.

ACR, American College of Radiology; AEC, automatic exposure control; cd, candela; FDA, U.S. Food and Drug Administration; HVL, half-value layer; kVp, kilovolt (peak); lp/mm, line pairs per millimeter; mm A1, millimeters of aluminum; Mo, molybdenum; QC, quality control; Rh, rhodium; SID, source-image distance; W, tungsten.

Although only minimum testing frequencies are specified in Tables 8-3 and 8-4, these tests should be performed whenever problems occur so that the causes may be identified before they affect clinical image quality or patient safety. In addition, if the QC program has just begun, the tests should be conducted more frequently for the first few months; this approach will give the QC technologist more experience in a shorter time and also provide better baseline data regarding the reliability of imaging equipment. Tests also should be conducted after service or preventive maintenance has been performed. It is particularly important that the processor QC test be performed any time the processor is serviced.

The phantom image test should also be carried out at these times to test for processing artifacts.

The mammography facility must ensure that a medical physicist performs an equipment evaluation of the mammography unit and film processor at installation and conducts a complete survey at least annually. Under the FDA's final rule, the medical physicist is required to perform an equipment evaluation whenever a new unit or processor is installed, a unit or processor is disassembled and reassembled in the same or a new location, or major components of a mammography unit or processor equipment are changed or repaired (Box 8-1). The equipment evaluation must determine whether the new or changed equipment meets the applicable MQSA requirements for mammography equipment (Table 8-5) in addition to the applicable QC requirements for equipment (see Tables 8-3 and 8-4). All problems must be corrected before the new or

BOX 8-1 Equipment Changes for Which Mammography Equipment Evaluations Are Required by the U.S. Food and Drug Administration*

Automatic exposure control replacement
Collimator replacement
Filter replacement
Newly installed x-ray unit (even if used)
Newly installed processor (even if used)
X-ray unit or processor disassembled and reassembled at the same or new location
X-ray tube replacement

**All problems must be corrected before the new or changed equipment is put into service for examinations or film processing.*

TABLE 8-5. Mammography Quality Standards Act Requirements for Mammography Equipment

Feature	Requirement(s)	Rule Section	Effective Date
Motion of tube-image receptor assembly	The assembly shall be capable of being fixed in any position where it is designed to operate. Once fixed in any such position, it shall not undergo unintended motion.	3(i)	4/28/99
	This mechanism shall not fail in the event of power interruption.	3(ii)	4/28/99
Image receptor sizes	Systems using screen-film image receptors shall provide, at a minimum, for operation with image receptors of 18 ∞ 24 cm and 24 ∞ 30 cm.	4(i)	4/28/99
	Systems using screen-film image receptors shall be equipped with moving grids matched to all image receptor sizes provided.	4(ii)	4/28/99
	Systems used for magnification procedures shall be capable of operation with the grid removed from between the source and image receptor.	4(iii)	4/28/99
Beam limitation and light fields	All systems shall have beam-limiting devices that allow the useful beam to extend to or beyond the chest wall edge of the image receptor.	5(i)	4/28/99
	For any mammography system with a light beam that passes through the x-ray beam-limiting device, the light shall provide an average illumination of not less than 160 lux (15 ft-candles) at the maximum SID.	5(ii)	4/28/99
Magnification	Systems used to perform non-interventional problem-solving procedures shall have radiographic magnification capability available for use by the operator.	6(i)	4/28/99
	Systems used for magnification procedures shall provide, at a minimum, at least 1 magnification value within the range of 1.4 to 2.0.	6(ii)	4/28/99
Focal spot selection	When more than one focal spot is provided, the system shall indicate, prior to exposure, which focal spot is selected.	7(i)	4/28/99
	When more than one target material is provided, the system shall indicate, prior to exposure, the preselected target material.	7(ii)	4/28/99
	When the target material and/or focal spot is selected by a system algorithm that is based on the exposure or on a test exposure, the system shall display, after the exposure, the target material and/or focal spot actually used during the exposure.	7(iii)	4/28/99
Application of compression	Each system shall provide an initial power-driven compression activated by hands-free controls operable from both sides of the patient.	8(i)(A)	10/28/02
	Each system shall provide fine adjustment compression controls operable from both sides of the patient.	8(i)(B)	10/28/02

Continued

TABLE 8-5. Mammography Quality Standards Act Requirements for Mammography Equipment—Cont'd

Feature	Requirement(s)	Rule Section	Effective Date
Compression paddle	Systems shall be equipped with different-sized compression paddles that match the sizes of all full-field image receptors provided for the system.	8(ii)(A)	4/28/99
	The compression paddle shall be flat and parallel to the breast support table and shall not deflect from parallel by more than 1.0 cm at any point on the surface of the compression paddle when compression is applied.	8(ii)(B)	4/28/99
	Paddles intended by the manufacturer's design to not be flat and parallel to the breast support table during compression shall meet the manufacturer's design specifications and maintenance requirements.	8(ii)(C)	4/28/99
	The chest wall edge of the compression paddle shall be straight and parallel to the edge of the image receptor.	8(ii)(D)	4/28/99
	The chest wall edge may be bent upward to allow for patient comfort but shall not appear on the image.	8(ii)(E)	4/28/99
Technique factor	Manual selection of mAs or at least one of its component parts (mA and/or selection and display time) shall be available.	9(i)	4/28/99
	The technique factors (kVp and either mAs or mA and seconds) to be used during an exposure shall be indicated before the exposure begins, except when AEC is used, in which case the technique factors that are set prior to the exposure shall be indicated.	9(ii)	4/28/99
	Following AEC mode use, the system shall indicate the actual kVp, and mAs (or mA and time) used during the exposure.	9(iii)	4/28/99
Automatic exposure	Each screen-film system shall provide an AEC mode that is operable in all control combinations of equipment configuration provided, e.g., grid, non-grid; magnification, non-magnification; and various target-filter combinations.	10(i)	4/28/99
	The positioning or selection of the detector shall permit flexibility in the placement of the detector under the target tissue. The size and the available positions of the detector shall be clearly indicated at the x-ray input surface of the breast compression paddle. (Note: This applies *only* to systems using screen-film image receptors.) The selected position of the detector shall be clearly indicated.	10(ii)	4/28/99
	The system shall provide means for the operator to vary the selected optical density from the normal (zero) setting.	10(iii)	4/28/99
X-ray film	The facility shall use x-ray film for mammography that has been designated by the film manufacturer as appropriate for mammography.	11	4/28/99
Intensifying screens	The facility shall use intensifying screens for mammography that have been designated by the screen manufacturer as appropriate for mammography and shall use film that is matched to the screen's spectral output as specified by the manufacturer.	12	4/28/99
Film processing solutions	For processing mammography films, the facility shall use chemical solutions that are capable of developing the film in a manner equivalent to the minimum requirements specified by the film manufacturer.	13	4/28/99
Lighting	The facility shall make special lights for film illumination, i.e., hotlights, capable of producing light levels greater than that provided by the viewbox, available to the interpreting physician.	14	4/28/99
Film masking devices	Facilities shall ensure that film masking devices that can limit the illuminated area to a region equal to or smaller than the exposed portion of the film are available to all interpreting physicians interpreting for the facility.	15	4/28/99

AEC, automatic exposure control; kVp, kilovolt (peak); mA, milliamperes; mAs, milliamperes per second; SID, source-image distance.

changed equipment is put into service for examinations or film processing and before the facility may apply for accreditation of a mammography unit. In order to prevent scheduling delays, the facility should notify the medical physicist as soon as possible of upcoming equipment additions and changes so that an equipment evaluation may be scheduled immediately after installation or modification and before the equipment is used for mammography.

Full-field digital mammography (FFDM) is different from screen-film mammography in a number of ways. The detector is different, the image processing is different, and so is the QC. The FDA requires that the facility's QC technologist and medical physicist follow the QC procedures specified by the manufacturer of an FFDM unit. Although some of the tests specified by the various manufacturers are similar for different FFDM units, most are considerably different. Also different manufacturers specify different frequencies and performance criteria. The FDA final rule requires that facilities with FFDM units follow their manufacturer's current QA requirements.[23-25] The ACR is currently developing a quality control manual for digital mammography that should harmonize the existing manufacturer-specified tests and reduce the complexity of this important testing for both medical physicists and radiologic technologists. Consequently, the following tests primarily apply to screen-film mammography.

TABLE 8-6. Time Required for Radiologic Technologist Quality Control Tests

Nature of Procedure/Task and Minimum Performance Frequency	Time Required*
Daily	
Darkroom cleanliness	5 min
Processor QC	20 min
Weekly	
Screen cleanliness	10 min
Viewbox cleanliness	5 min
Monthly	
Phantom images	30 min
Visual checklist	10 min
Quarterly	
Repeat analysis	60 min
Analysis of fixer retention	5 min
Meetings with radiologist	45 min
Semiannually	
Darkroom fog	10 min
Screen-film contact	80 min
Compression	10 min
Total time for QC per year	160 hours

*Estimated times include setup, testing, and recording of results for a facility with two mammography units, one processor and 16 cassettes.
Adapted from Farria DM, Bassett LW, Kimme-Smith C, DeBruhl N. Mammography quality assurance from A to Z. Radiographics 1994;14:371-385.

Tests Performed by the Radiologic Technologist

Reaping the benefits of QC requires an investment of time. The mammography facility's supervising radiologist and management must give the QC technologist sufficient time each day to perform these important tests and evaluate their results. The approximate times needed to perform the QC tests are listed in Table 8-6.[26] Some of the technologist's QC tasks can be carried out simultaneously with other tests. For example, while waiting for the processor to warm up, the QC technologist can clean the darkroom and screens, check the viewbox and viewing conditions, review the visual checklist, or test the mammography unit's compression. Consequently, once an efficient routine is established, only a modest amount of time is required for a successful mammographic QC program.

Darkroom Cleanliness (Screen-Film)

For the production of high-quality clinical images, it is critical that artifacts on film images be minimized through maintenance of the cleanest possible conditions in the darkroom. The single-emulsion films that are currently in use for screen-film mammography are particularly sensitive to dust and dirt between the screen and film. Although the cause of the resulting prominent artifacts is obvious, the dust may degrade screen-film contact and produce image blurring, and the artifacts may mimic microcalcifications, leading to misdiagnosis. The QC technologist should minimize dust and dirt as much as possible.

Processor Quality Control (Screen-Film)

Processor QC procedures are designed to confirm and verify that the film processor and processor chemistry system are working in a consistent manner. Before conducting processor QC, the QC technologist should verify that the processor is performing consistently with the film manufacturer's specifications and then should establish baseline operating levels. This procedure should be carried out with new processors or whenever a significant change is made in imaging procedures (e.g., different film, a change in brand or type of chemicals, a change in processing workload). Once baseline operating levels are established, processor QC must be performed daily, at the beginning of the workday, before any patient films are processed but after the processor has warmed up. All levels falling outside the established performance criteria (described in Table 8-3) must be corrected before the processor is used to develop patient films.

Screen Cleanliness (Screen-Film)

The screen cleanliness procedure is similar to the darkroom cleanliness check, in that it ensures that mammographic cassettes and screens are free of dust and dirt particles that might degrade image quality or mimic microcalcifications.

Phantom Image

Routinely exposing a breast-simulating phantom and evaluating the image permits a facility to evaluate changes in image quality without exposing a patient to radiation. The phantom image test ensures that the film optical density, digital image noise level, contrast, uniformity, and image quality due to the entire imaging chain are maintained at optimum levels.

Darkroom Fog (Screen-Film)

Inappropriate darkroom safe lights and other light sources inside and outside the darkroom can fog mammographic films. Fog reduces contrast. The darkroom fog test allows a facility to detect, identify, and eliminate the sources of fog that cannot be seen with the human eye.

Screen-Film Contact (Screen-Film)

Screen-film contact has a significant influence on image sharpness. Sharpness is essential in mammography for the detection of microcalcifications. The screen-film contact test ensures that optimum contact is maintained between the intensifying screen and film in each mammography cassette.

Compression

Appropriate compression is essential for high-quality mammography. Compression diminishes the thickness of tissue that must be penetrated by radiation, thereby reducing scattered radiation and increasing contrast, while limiting radiation exposure of the breast. Compression improves image sharpness by reducing the breast thickness, thereby minimizing focal spot blurring of structures in the image, and by minimizing patient motion. In addition, compression makes the thickness of the breast more uniform, resulting in more uniform image densities with film. The compression test determines whether the mammography system can provide adequate compression in both the manual and powered modes and ensures that the equipment does not allow too much compression to be applied.

Repeat Analysis

Repeating mammograms raises cost, decreases efficiency, and increases patient exposure. The repeat analysis allows the facility to determine the number and causes of repeated mammograms so that problems may be identified and corrected.

Viewboxes and Viewing Conditions

Poor viewboxes and viewing conditions may impair the visibility of breast structures on even the highest-quality screen-film image. Although most interpretations of digital images are performed on monitors, attention should also be paid to the quality of the viewboxes if previous images are reviewed on hard copy. High ambient lighting and low viewbox brightness coupled with dirty viewbox surfaces can reduce the apparent contrast of films and obscure clinical information. Testing ensures that the viewboxes and viewing conditions are optimized and then maintained at an optimum level. If mammography technologists use a separate viewbox to check the density and quality of the screen-film mammograms and QC films, this viewbox should be similar to the reading viewbox in luminance and light color. In addition, the ambient lighting conditions should be similar to those used in the reading room.

Analysis of Fixer Retention in Film (Screen-Film)

Excessive residual fixer (thiosulfate, hyposulfite, or "hypo") can turn films brown and reduce their archival stability. This analysis determines the quantity of residual fixer in processed film.

Visual Checklist

The visual check ensures that the mammographic x-ray system's indicator lights, displays, mechanical locks, and detents are working properly and that the mechanical rigidity and stability of the equipment is appropriate.

Tests Performed by the Medical Physicist

Mammographic Unit Assembly Evaluation

The mammographic unit assembly evaluation ensures that all locks, detents, angulation indicators, displays, mechanisms, and mechanical support devices for the x-ray tube, compression device, and image receptor holder assembly are operating properly.

Collimation Assessment

If the x-ray field extends too far beyond the edges of the image receptor, the patient may be exposed to unnecessary radiation. If the x-ray field falls too far within the image receptor, breast tissue may be missed on the image, and the unattenuated light passing through large, unexposed portions of the film may degrade visibility of low-contrast structures. Collimation assessment ensures that that the x-ray field aligns with the light field, the collimator allows for full coverage of the image receptor by the x-ray field (but does not allow significant radiation beyond its edges), and the chest wall edge of the compression paddle aligns with the chest wall edge of the film.

Evaluation of System Resolution

The visualization of microcalcifications significantly depends on the resolving capability of a mammographic system. Therefore, the medical physicist evaluates the limiting resolution of the entire mammography system, including effects from geometric (focal spot) blurring and the detector.

Automatic Exposure Control System Performance Assessment

A properly functioning automatic exposure control (AEC) system will allow the technologist to produce an appropriate and consistent film optical density (or digital image noise level) for breasts of varying densities and thicknesses and with the use of various imaging modes. The performance of the mammography unit's AEC system should be assessed so that consistent image optical density (or digital image noise level) can be maintained and modified with the density control function.

Uniformity of Screen Speed (Screen-Film)

Variations among the speeds of intensifying screens can result in variations in image optical densities from cassette to cassette. The uniformity of the radiographic speed of image receptors routinely used for mammographic imaging therefore is assessed.

Artifact Evaluation

This is one of the most important tests conducted by the medical physicist. Excessive artifacts have the potential to obscure or mimic important clinical detail. Artifact evaluation assesses the severity and source of artifacts visualized on mammograms or phantom images so that they may be eliminated or minimized.

Image Quality Evaluation

Although the QC technologist performs an image quality evaluation weekly, the medical physicist is in the unique position to offer suggestions for image quality improvement on the basis of his or her experience evaluating phantom images from other units and facilities. In addition, the medical physicist can note changes that may have occurred from year to year. This evaluation allows the medical physicist to assess mammographic image quality and to detect temporal changes in image quality.

Accuracy and Reproducibility of Kilovolt (Peak)

Image contrast, exposure time, and patient exposure can be impacted by the selection and accuracy of the kilovolt (peak) (kVp). The medical physicist therefore ensures that the actual kVp is accurate (within ± 5% of the indicated kVp) and that the kVp is reproducible, having a coefficient of variation equal to or less than 0.02. The stability of modern x-ray generators has decreased the necessity of conducting this test on a yearly basis.

Beam Quality Assessment (Half-Value Layer Measurement)

A low beam quality could be a cause for excessive radiation exposure; a high beam quality could be a cause of poor image contrast. Quality beam assessment ensures that the half-value layer of the x-ray beam is adequate and also provides data to enable the estimate of average glandular dose.

Breast Entrance Exposure, Reproducibility of Automatic Exposure Control, Average Glandular Dose, and Radiation Output Rate

The medical physicist must also measure the typical entrance exposure for an average patient (approximately 4.2-cm compressed breast thickness; 50% adipose, 50% glandular composition), estimate the associated average glandular dose, assess short-term AEC reproducibility, and measure the air kerma (radiation output) rate.

Viewbox Luminance and Room Illuminance

The luminance of the viewboxes for interpretation or QC of mammography images should be evaluated to ensure that they meet or exceed minimum levels, that the room illuminance levels are below prescribed levels, and that viewing conditions have been optimized.

WHERE TO GO FOR HELP

High-quality mammography takes routine attention to producing quality mammograms, constant awareness of the performance of mammography equipment and chemistry, organizational skills, and, especially, knowing where to go for information and guidance. Currently a number of sources are available for help, whether one prefers reading information on paper, cruising the Internet, or talking with an expert. This section summarizes some of the best sources:

Table 8-7 lists some of the governmental and organization contacts and has blanks for filling in contact information for specific mammography equipment and units. The QC technologist can photocopy the table, fill in contact names, addresses, and so on, and store it by the phone or computer so as to keep all essential QC contact information in one place.

Medical Physicists

The QC technologist should contact her or his medical physicist first when there are questions about how to perform or evaluate QC, if problems cannot be solved, or if they frequently reoccur. The medical physicist should serve as the facility's primary consultant on image quality.

Manufacturers' Representatives

Manufacturers' representatives or service personnel for the mammography unit, the film processor, the film, or the screen are typically specially trained to evaluate and

TABLE 8-7. Contact Information for Quality Control Questions*

Source	Name	Phone Number	Web Site
Medical Physicist			
Mammography Unit Manufacturer			
Film and Screen Manufacturer			
Processor Unit Manufacturer			
Processor Service/Chemistry Company			
Consultant			
American College of Radiology	Mammography Accreditation Program Information Line	1-800-227-6440	www.acr.org
U.S. Food and Drug Administration	Mammography Quality Standards Act (MQSA) Hotline	1-800-838-7715	www.fda.gov/cdrh/mammography

*This table may be photocopied and the relevant information filled in for each unit; the copy may be kept by the telephone or computer for reference when questions arise.

address problems related to their products. Because it is sometimes difficult to identify the specific cause of a problem in a system that consists of many components, it may be useful to obtain the assistance of all the representatives at the same time. Many manufacturers maintain telephone "help" lines and Web sites to further assist customers.

Independent Consultants

Independent consultants in mammography may bring special expertise to the facility when researching specific issues such as problems with performance of QC or patient positioning.

The American College of Radiology's Mammography Accreditation Program

The ACR offers three sources of information and assistance with QC problems in mammography:

- 1999 ACR Mammography Quality Control Manual: This "cookbook"-style manual[22] is the best source of information on how to perform and evaluate the QC tests required by the FDA and recommended by the ACR.
- The ACR Web Site (www.acr.org): This information-packed Web site is not for members only. The site contains frequently asked questions, downloadable QC forms from the ACR's 1999 QC manual, information on stereotactic breast biopsy accreditation and breast ultrasound accreditation, the Breast Imaging Reporting and Data System (BI-RADS) lexicon, and the ACR's Breast Guidelines.
- The Breast Imaging Accreditation Information Line (800-227-6440): The phone line is staffed by experienced mammography technologists who can help with questions on accreditation, the FDA regulations, or other general mammography or QC issues.

U.S Food and Drug Administration

The FDA also offers several resources for mammography QC.

- MQSA Web Site (www.fda.gov/cdrh/mammography): The FDA has developed an extremely useful and user-friendly Web site to help mammography facilities understand the current regulations and implement their requirements. Both the text of the MQSA and the Final Rule are available.
- The FDA's Policy Guidance Help System:This question-and-answer guidance document, updated several times a year, reflects the FDA's current thoughts on the regulations implementing the MQSA. It can be accessed directly though the FDA's Web site (www.fda.gov/cdrh/mammography).The system is organized as a series of books or main topics.

SUMMARY

The radiologist, medical physicist, and mammography technologist, working together as a team, are the keys to providing optimum quality mammography images, which will ultimately give patients the best medical care possible.

KEY POINTS

- **Under MQSA, the lead interpreting physician has the responsibility to ensure that all quality assurance requirements are met.**
- **The facility's quality control technologist is responsible for conducting most routine QC; a qualified medical physicist must conduct certain in-depth QC tests annually.**
- **Under MQSA, if certain designated tests fail, the facility may not perform mammography with the unit or component until the problem is corrected.**
- **The FDA's final regulations outline the specific screen-film QC tests that must be performed at all mammography facilities.**
- **The FDA's final regulations specify that facilities performing digital mammography must follow their digital equipment manufacturer's QC tests.**

SUGGEST READINGS

American College of Radiology, Committee on Quality Assurance in Mammography: *Mammography quality control manual.* Reston, VA: American College of Radiology; in press.

www.acr.org.

REFERENCES

1. Thomas Jr W. *SPSE Handbook of photographic science and engineering*. New York: John Wiley & Sons; 1973.
2. Bassett LW, Hendrick RE, Bassford TL, et al., Quality Determinants of Mammography. *Clinical practice guideline*. No. 13. Rockville, MD: Agency for Health Care Policy and Research, Public Health Service, U.S. Department of Health and Human Services; October 1994. AHCPR Publication No. 95-0632.
3. Trout ED, Jacobson G, Moore RT, Shoub EP. Analysis of the rejection rate of chest radiographs obtained during the coal mine "black lung" program. *Radiology* 1973;**109**:25-7.
4. Hall CL. Economic analysis of a quality control program. In: Application of optical instrumentation in medicine VI. *Proc Soc Proceedings of SPIE* 1977;**127**:271-5.
5. Patrylak J. Counting x-ray retakes reduces cost. *Applied Radiology* 1978;7:35-6.
6. Goldman L, Vucich JJ, Beech S, Murphy WL. Automatic processing quality assurance program: impact on a radiology department. *Radiology* 1977;**125**:591-5.
7. American College of Radiology. *Digest of council actions*. Reston, Va: American College of Radiology; 2001.

8. U.S. Department of Health and Human Services, Food and Drug Administration. Quality assurance programs for diagnostic radiology facilities: final recommendation. *Fed Regist* 1979;**44**:71728–40.
9. Gray JE. Photographic quality assurance in diagnostic radiology, nuclear medicine and radiation therapy. Vol I, *The basic principles of daily photographic quality assurance*. Washington, DC: DHEW; 1976. HEW Publication (FDA) 76-8043.
10. Hendee WR, Rossi RP. *Quality assurance for radiographic x-ray units and associated equipment*. Washington, DC: DHEW; 1979. HEW Publication (FDA) 79-8094.
11. Hendee WR, Rossi RP. *Quality assurance for fluoroscopic x-ray units and associated equipment*. Washington, DC: DHEW; 1980 HEW Publication (FDA) 80-8095.
12. Gray JE, Winkler NT, Stears J, Frank ED. *Quality control in diagnostic radiology*. Rockville, MD: Aspen Publishers; 1983.
13. National Council on Radiation Protection. *Mammography-a user's guide*. Bethesda, Md: National Council on Radiation Protection and Measurements; 1986. NCRP Report #85.
14. National Council on Radiation Protection. *Quality assurance in diagnostic imaging*. Bethesda, Md: National Council on Radiation Protection and Measurements; 1988. NCRP Report #99.
15. American Association of Physicists in Medicine (AAPM). *Equipment requirements and quality control for mammography*. College Park, Md: AAPM Diagnostic X-Ray Imaging Committee Task Group # 7; 1990. Report No. 29.
16. American College of Radiology. *Mammography quality control manual*. Reston, Va: American College of Radiology; 1990.
17. American College of Radiology. *Mammography quality control manual*. Reston, VA: American College of Radiology; 1992.
18. U.S. Department of Health and Human Services, Food and Drug Administration. Mammography facilities-requirements for accrediting bodies and quality standards and certification requirements: Interim rules. *Fed Regist* 1993;**58**(243).
19 American College of Radiology. *Mammography quality control manual*. Reston, VA: American College of Radiology; 1994.
20. U.S. Department of Health and Human Services, Food and Drug Administration. Quality standards and certification requirements for mammography facilities. *Fed Regist* 1994;**59**(189).
21. American College of Radiology. *Mammography quality control manual*. Reston, Va: American College of Radiology; 1999.
22. U.S. Department of Health and Human Services, Food and Drug Administration. Quality mammography standards: correction, final rule. *Fed Regist* 1997;**62**(217).
23. GE Medical Systems Senographe 2000D QAP. *Quality control tests for MQSA facilities*. Milwaukee, Wis: 2001. QC Manual 2277390-100, Revision 3.
24. Fischer Imaging SenoScan Full Field Digital Mammography System Operator Manual. Denver: Aug. 2001. P-55933-OM Revision.
25. Lorad Selenia Full-Field Digital Mammography System Quality Control Manual. Danbury, Conn: Dec. 2001.
26. Farria DM, Bassett LW, Kimme-Smith C, DeBruhl N. Mammography quality assurance from A to Z. *Radiographics* 1994;**14**:371–85.

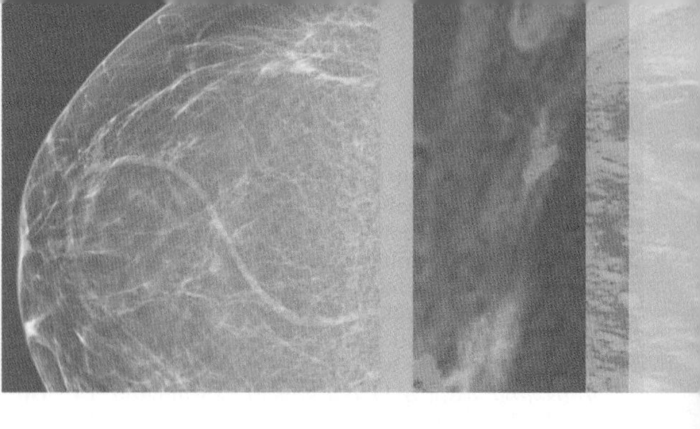

CHAPTER 9

Ultrasound Equipment

Christopher Comstock

Despite the best scanning techniques and interpretive skill, breast ultrasound quality is ultimately limited by the equipment being used. This chapter will present the basic elements of ultrasound equipment necessary to ensure high-quality breast ultrasound. The technical requirements to produce high-quality breast ultrasound images are greater than that for most other tissues in the body. Breast ultrasound requires both high spatial and high contrast resolution. Additionally, resolution must be maintained throughout the image and in particular, near the skin surface (near field). The American College of Radiology (ACR) accreditation program and the ACR Practice Guideline for the Performance of a Breast Ultrasound Examination require an electronically focused, linear array transducer with a minimum center frequency of 10 megahertz (MHz).[1] Additional tools such as spatial compounding, coded harmonics and three-dimensional (3D) methods may also help to improve breast ultrasound quality.

TRANSDUCERS

Breast ultrasound imaging requires transducers that can provide high-resolution near-field imaging. To accomplish this, most current breast ultrasound systems employ a 10 to 15 MHz linear array transducer with electronic focusing. Arrays can contain up to 512 elements spaced over several centimeters along the long axis. B-mode ultrasound images are created when the transducer elements generate (transmit) pulses of sound and then listen (receive) for returning echoes over a certain period of time. Through the process of continuous dynamic electronic focusing, during both transmit and receive, the returning echoes can be focused on one or more depth settings. By concentrating the narrowest part of the ultrasound beam (focal zone) at the area of interest, lesion detail can be improved and the effects of volume averaging (slice thickness artifact) can be diminished (Fig. 9-1). Lateral resolution is best within the focal zone of the beam. However, adding too many focal zones can ultimately slow the frame rate. In addition to long-axis electronic focusing, manufacturers use unique methods to further improve quality by improving short-axis focusing, axial resolution and contrast resolution.

SPATIAL RESOLUTION

Resolution is the ability of a transducer to separate signals produced by two reflectors when they are close together either perpendicular to the beam or parallel to the beam. High-resolution breast ultrasound requires good spatial resolution in three planes. The spatial resolution is determined by both lateral (X and Y) and axial (Z depth) resolution. In a linear array, the piezoelectric elements are aligned along the long-axis (Y) of the transducer (Fig. 9-2). If just the single elements were used to transmit and receive, the beam produced by such a narrow element would diverge rapidly after traveling only a few millimeters and result in poor lateral resolution due to beam divergence. In order to overcome this, adjacent elements—typically 8 to 16—are pulsed simultaneously.[2] By delaying the timing of the firing of the elements in the group (from inner to outer), the focal zone can be adjusted (beam narrowed along the long-axis plane); this is called long-axis focusing (Fig. 9-3). The time delays determine the depth of focus for the transmitted beam. The same delay factors can also be applied to the group of elements during the receiving phase resulting in dynamic focusing of the returning echoes. If multiple focal zones are selected, multiple pulses are performed by the same group of element with varied time delays for each focal zone depth (Fig. 9-4). In this manner, a single scan line in the ultrasound image is acquired. To generate the next adjacent scan line, another group of elements is created by shifting one element position over along the transducer array from the previous group. The process is repeated until the entire image is formed.

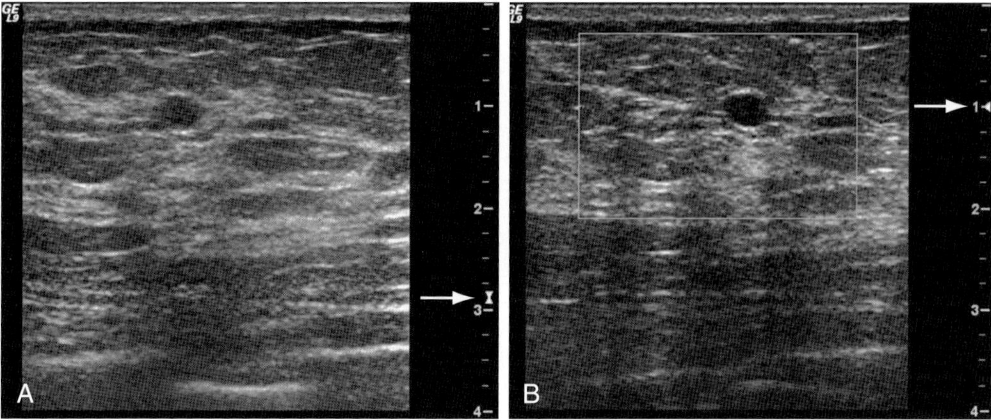

■ **FIGURE 9-1** The importance of focal zone setting. **A,** A small oval indistinct hypoechoic lesion in the near-field. The focal zone is positioned deep in the field of view (*arrow*). **B,** With the focal zone set appropriately (*arrow*), it is clear that the lesion is a cyst. By centering the focal zone (narrowest part of the beam) on the lesion, the effects of volume averaging (slice thickness artifact) can be reduced and lesion detail improved.

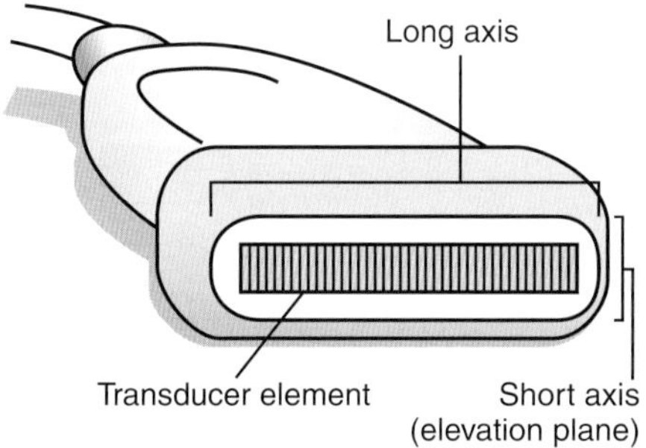

■ **FIGURE 9-2** Linear array transducer. In a linear or 1D array, the individual piezoelectric elements are aligned along the long-axis (Y) of the transducer. The short axis X (elevation plane) of a single element wide linear array cannot be electronically focused and is therefore fixed. The short-axis resolution is determined by the manufacturer's acoustic lens that is built into the particular transducer. The short-axis focus of breast imaging transducers is optimized for the near field imaging.

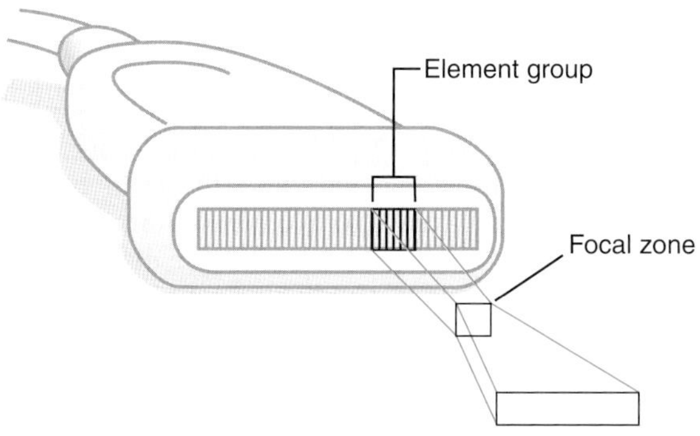

■ **FIGURE 9-3** Long axis focusing. By firing a group of elements—typically 8 to 16—rather than a single element, lateral resolution can be improved. By delaying the timing of the firing of the elements in the group (from inner to outer), the focal zone can be adjusted (beam narrowed along the long-axis plane) and is called long-axis focusing. The time delays determine the depth of focus for the transmitted beam. To generate the next adjacent scan line, another group of elements is created by shifting one element position over, along the transducer array from the previous group. The process is repeated until the entire image is formed.

The short axis (X elevation plane) of a single element wide linear array cannot be electronically focused and is therefore fixed. The short-axis resolution is determined by the manufacturer's acoustic lens that is built into the particular transducer. The short-axis focus of breast imaging transducers is optimized for the near-field imaging. Rectangular or matrix array transducers with unequal rows of transducer elements are two-dimensional (2D), but are termed 1.5D, because the number of rows is much less than the number of columns. These transducers provide dynamic, electronic focusing in both the long and short axes (Fig. 9-5).

Axial resolution (Z depth) is related to transducer frequency, bandwidth and pulse length. Because axial resolution is inversely proportional to frequency, quality breast ultrasound requires high-frequency transducers, typically between 7 and 15 MHz. They also employ composite backing materials to highly dampen the transducer elements in order to shorten the reflected pulse, allowing closely spaced reflectors along the Z-plane to be resolved.

HARMONIC IMAGING

The pulsed ultrasound beams used to form images are composed of a spectrum of frequencies rather than a single frequency. The bandwidth is the range of frequencies in the ultrasound beam and the center frequency is the middle frequency in the range. Much of the artifact within an image that degrades the contrast resolution is generated by side lobes and/or backscatter from lower frequency components within the sound beam. Because axial resolution is better with wider bandwidth ultrasound beams, simply filtering out the lower frequencies, thereby narrowing the beam, will also reduce resolution. Use of coded harmonics is a technique that transmits coded ultrasound pulse sequences and decodes them on receipt to improve image resolution and reduce artifacts.[3,4] With coded harmonics, a digitally encoded pulse is transmitted at one frequency and received at a multiple of the transmitted frequency and decoded (Fig. 9-6). By receiving only

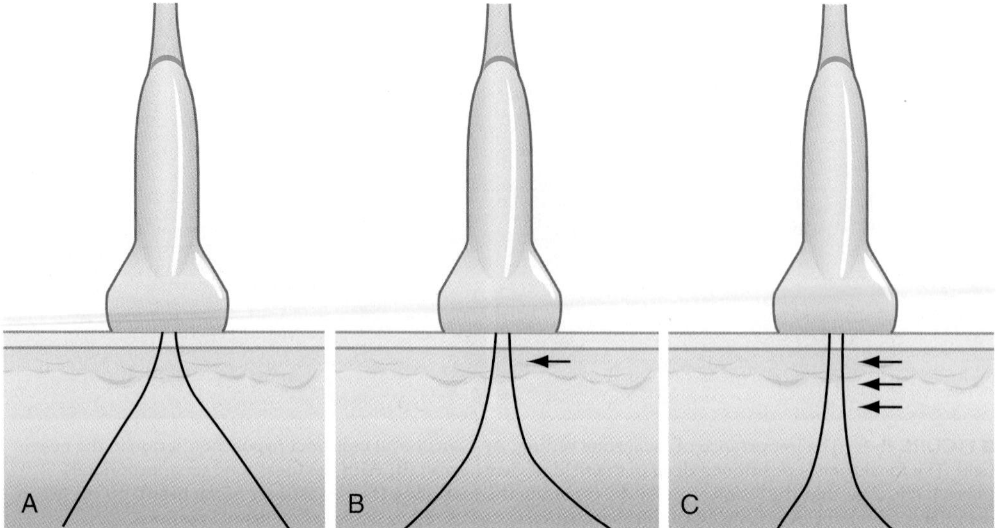

■ **FIGURE 9-4** Multiple focal zones. Without long axis focusing, the sound beam would diverge rapidly, reducing resolution **(A)**. By adding a single near-field focal zone (*arrow*), beam divergence can be reduced **(B)**. With the addition of multiple focal zones (*arrows*), beam divergence can be reduced throughout the field of view **(C)**. The addition of too many focal zones could, however, affect image frame rate.

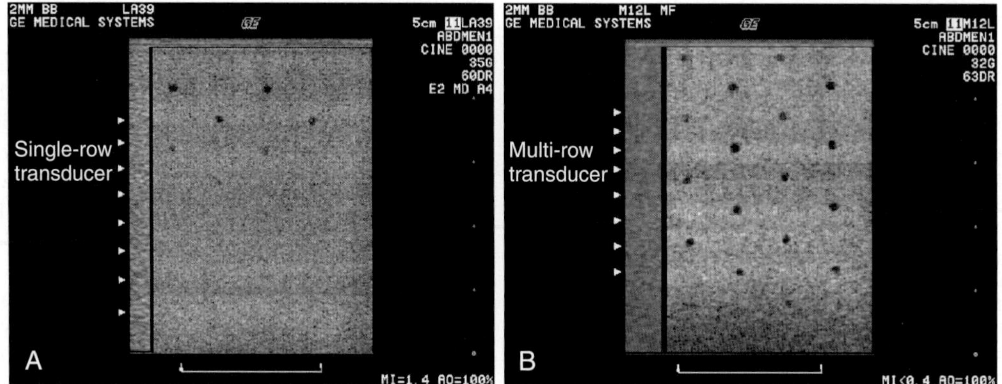

■ **FIGURE 9-5** Short axis focusing. **A,** Demonstrates a linear array image with multiple long axis focal zones but fixed near-field short axis focusing. **B,** In addition to long axis focusing, matrix array transducers (1.5D arrays) can also focus in the short axis. With the ability to focus in the short axis and create multiple short axis focal zones (in addition to the long axis focal zones), the matrix array transducer is seen to have better lateral resolution throughout the entire field of view. *(Courtesy of GE Medical Systems.)*

the higher frequency signals and excluding the lower frequency signals of the returning echoes, image artifact can be diminished (Fig. 9-7). In addition, coded harmonic imaging can improve penetration and reduce unwanted signals such as reverberation, speckle artifact and clutter, particularly in the mid and far-field.

SPATIAL COMPOUND IMAGING

Another method to improve ultrasound image contrast and resolution is called spatial compounding.[5] Standard ultrasound images, using a linear array, are generated by ultrasound beams that propagate perpendicular to the long axis of the transducer. In spatial compounding, by the use of electronic beam steering, multiple images (3 to 9) are obtained at different angles and combined to form a single image in real time (Fig. 9-8). By compounding multiple images together, real echoes will stand out while artifactual echoes will tend to average out. In addition, by imaging a lesion from different angles, the margins as well as the internal features of the lesion may be better interrogated (Fig. 9-9). It should be noted that for very small cancers that are detected primarily due to their posterior acoustic shadowing, spatial compounding may make the posterior shadowing less apparent (Fig. 9-10). In those situations, it may be better to apply spatial compound imaging for analysis, once the lesion has been detected using standard ultrasound imaging.

In addition to image acquisition techniques, postprocessing algorithms such as speckle reduction may help to further improve image quality. Speckle is an artifact created by reflections of an ultrasound pulse that degrades

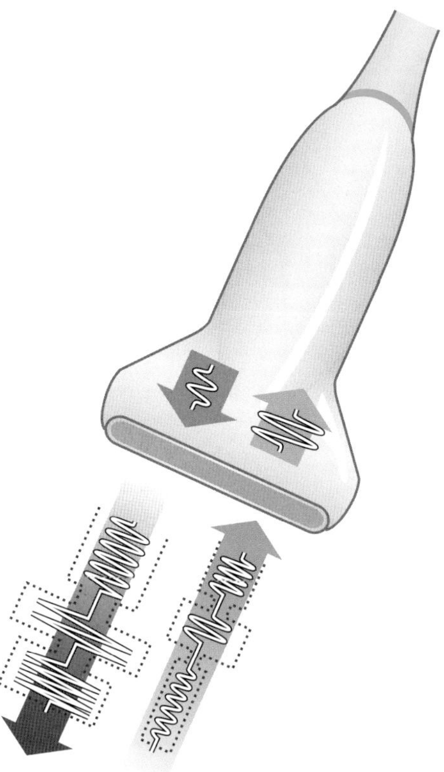

■ **FIGURE 9-6** Harmonic imaging. With coded harmonics, a digitally encoded pulse is transmitted at one frequency and received at a multiple of the transmitted frequency and decoded. By receiving only the higher frequency signals and excluding the lower frequency signals of the returning echoes, image artifact can be diminished. *(Courtesy of GE Medical Systems.)*

spatial and contrast resolution. In speckle reduction imaging, a real-time adaptive algorithm is applied to the ultrasound image to smooth regions where no feature, or edges, appear and maintain or enhance edges and borders (Fig. 9-11).

FIELD OF VIEW

Standard imaging from most linear arrays provides a rectangular field of view. Certain manufacturers provide options to create a larger field of view to allow measurement of large lesions or to show the relationship between two separate lesions. One method, commonly called *virtual convex* generates a wider field of view by steering (phasing) the ends of the transducer to create a trapezoidal shaped beam (Fig. 9-12). However, due to beam divergence, the resolution in the triangular ends of the beam may be lower than in the field of view directly below the transducer. Another method used to create a large static field of view is achieved by capturing a large single image across a region of the breast. This landscape or panoramic view is recorded while the transducer is manually moved along its long axis over the breast (Fig. 9-13).

THREE-DIMENSIONAL AND FOUR-DIMENSIONAL ULTRASOUND

In addition to enhancing lesion evaluation, the ability to perform 3D or volumetric ultrasound analysis of breast lesions may be advantageous for certain clinical applications such as comparing serial studies, and evaluating response to therapy, as well as for computer-aided

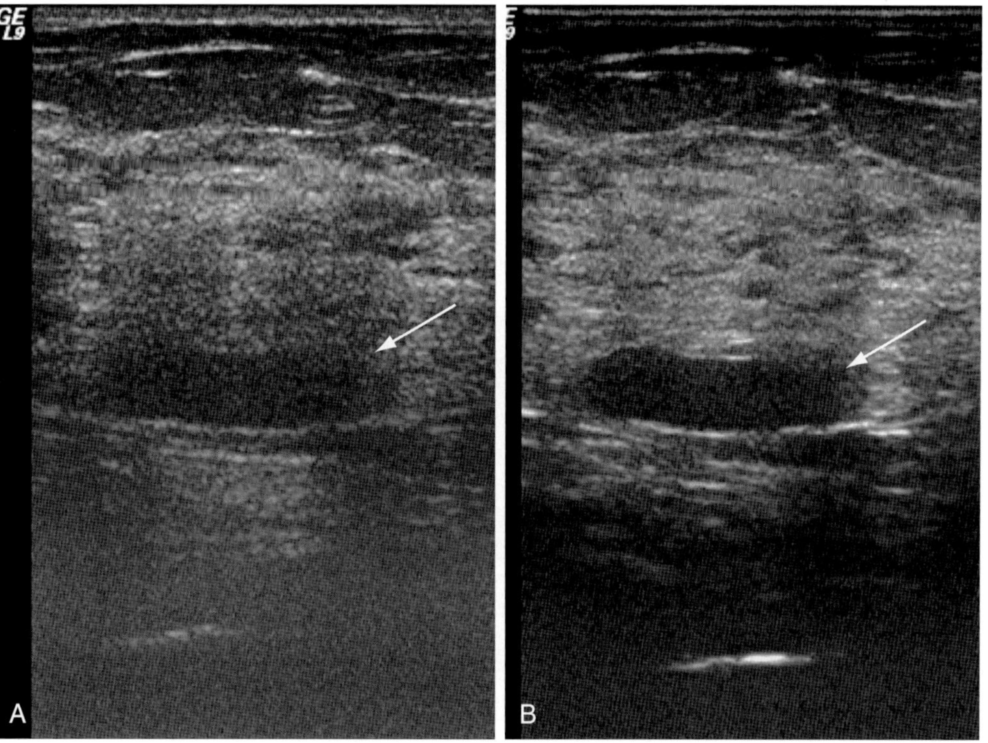

■ **FIGURE 9-7** Coded harmonic imaging. **A,** An oval hypoechoic lesion is seen deep within the breast (*arrow*). **B,** With the use of coded harmonic imaging, lesion detail is improved and noise is reduced.

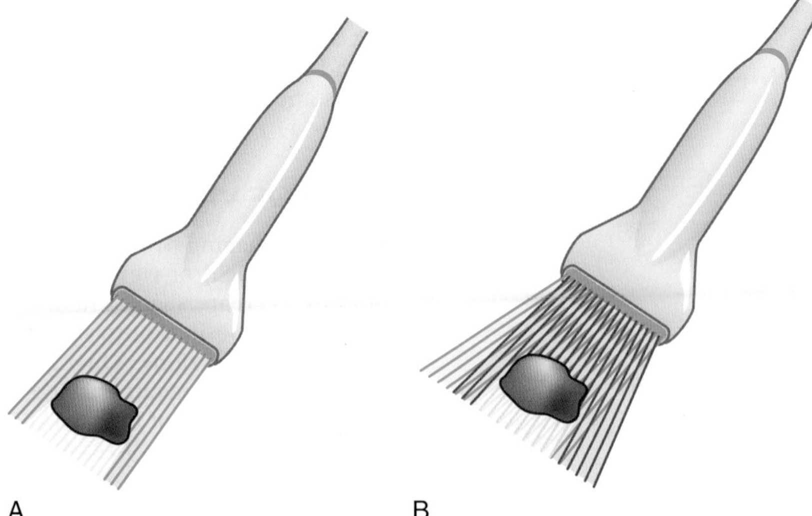

■ **FIGURE 9-8** Spatial compound imaging. **A,** With standard ultrasound imaging, the sound beams propagate perpendicular to the long-axis of the transducer. **B,** In spatial compounding, by the use of electronic beam steering, multiple images (3 to 9) are obtained at different angles and combined to form a single image in real time.

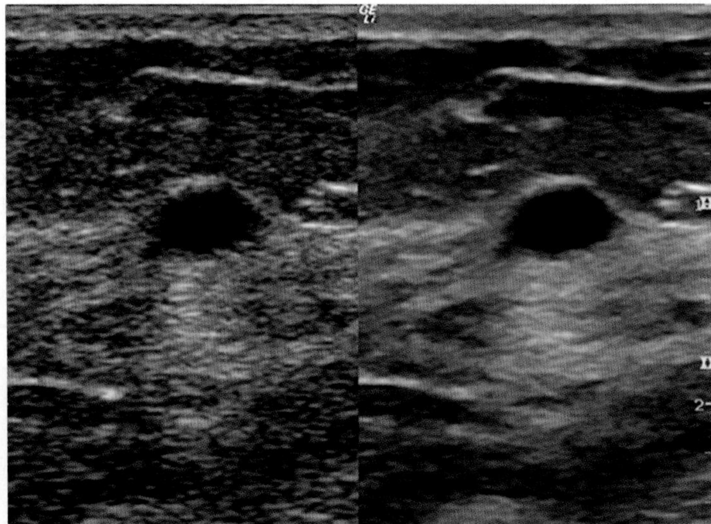

■ **FIGURE 9-9** Spatial compound imaging and lesion detail. The left-hand image demonstrates standard ultrasound imaging of a cyst. By compounding multiple images together (*right-hand image*), artifactual echoes are reduced. In addition, because the lesion is imaged from multiple angles during spatial compounding, the margins as well as the internal features of the cyst are seen in better detail. *(Courtesy of GE Medical Systems.)*

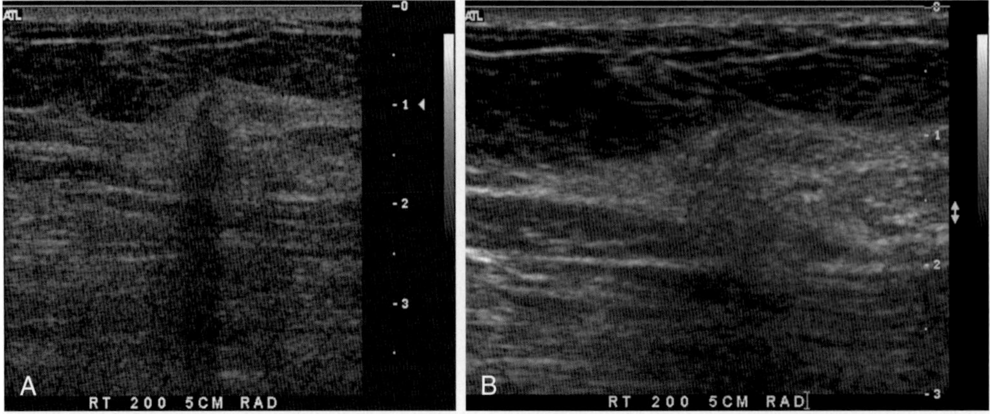

■ **FIGURE 9-10** Spatial compound imaging and posterior acoustic shadowing. **A,** Standard ultrasound demonstrates a small hypoechoic irregular breast cancer in the center of the image that demonstrates posterior acoustic shadowing. **B,** The same area is imaged using spatial compounding. The lesion is less evident due to the diminished posterior acoustic shadowing of the spatially compounded image.

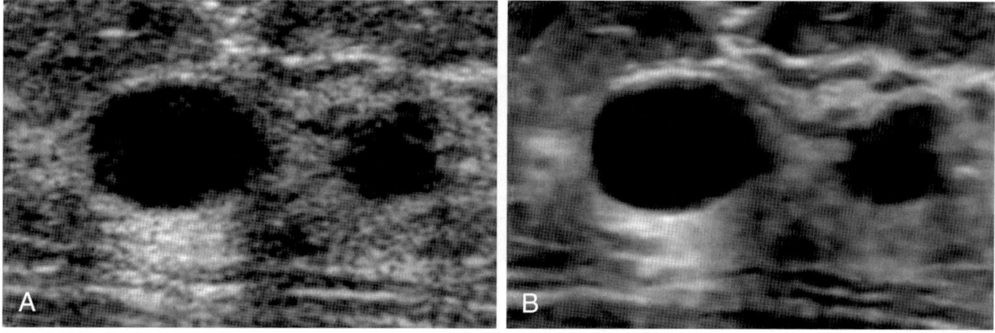

■ **FIGURE 9-11** Speckle reduction imaging. **A,** Standard ultrasound image of breast cysts. **B,** Same area imaged using speckle reduction imaging. In speckle reduction imaging, a real-time adaptive algorithm is applied to the ultrasound image to smooth regions where no feature, or edges, appear and maintain or enhance edges and borders. *(Courtesy of GE Medical Systems.)*

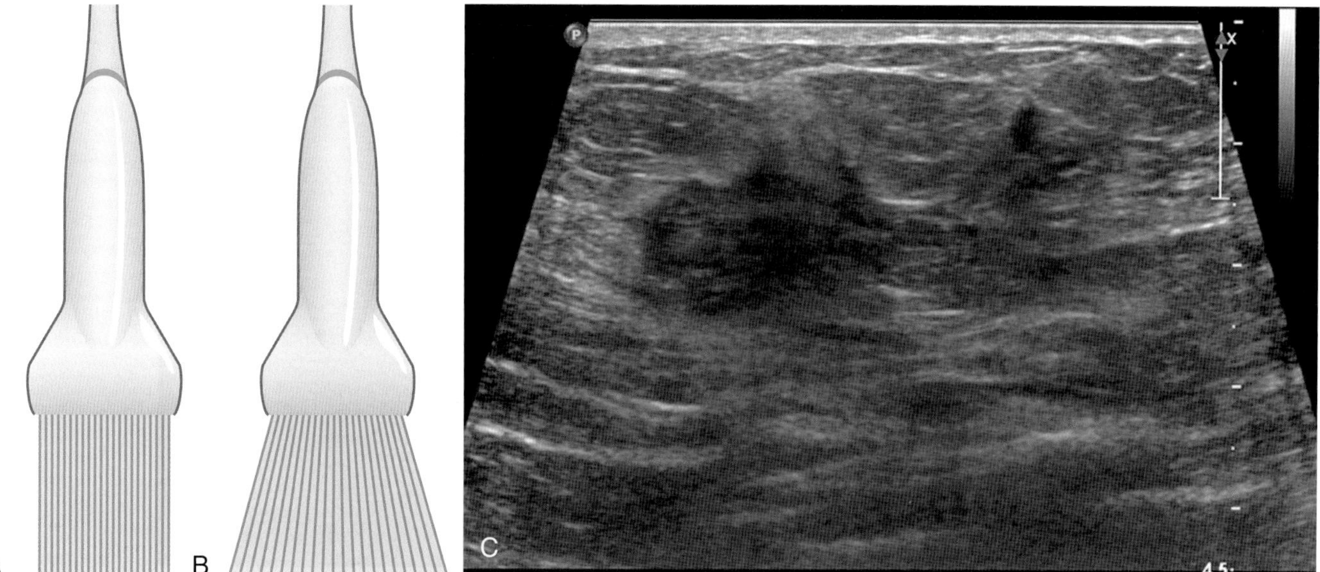

■ **FIGURE 9-12** Enhanced field of view. **A,** Standard imaging from a linear array transducer generates a rectangular field of view. **B,** By electronically steering the ends of the transducer, a wider field of view is generated (commonly called "virtual convex"). However, due to beam divergence, the resolution in the triangular ends of the beam may be lower than in the field of view directly below the transducer. **C,** A wider field of view may be useful when measuring larger lesions or in showing the relationship between two or more separate lesions.

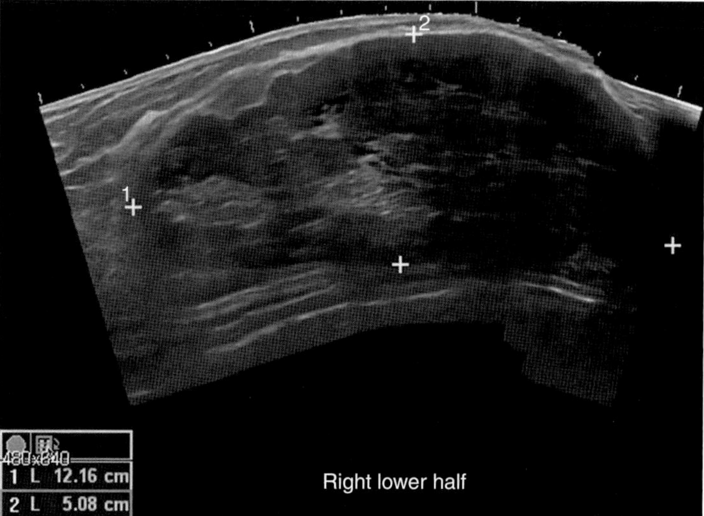

■ **FIGURE 9-13** Panoramic imaging. Another method used to create a large static field of view is achieved by capturing a large single image across a region of the breast. This landscape or panoramic view is recorded while the transducer is manually moved along its long axis over the breast. *(Courtesy of Dr. Al Tehan.)*

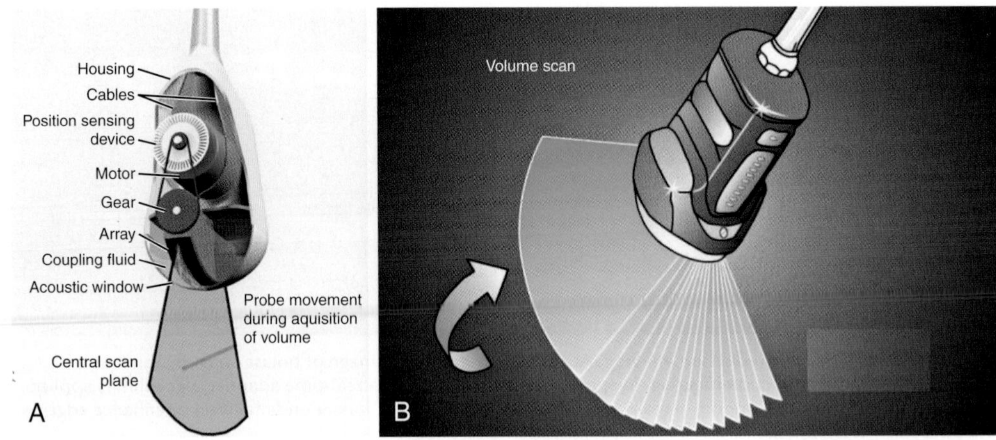

■ **FIGURE 9-14** 3D Imaging. Breast ultrasound systems perform 3D imaging by mechanically sweeping a liner array, which is coupled to a position sensing mechanism **(A)**, to obtain a large number of 2D planes that are used to create a 3D image block or volume **(B)**. *(Courtesy of GE Medical Systems.)*

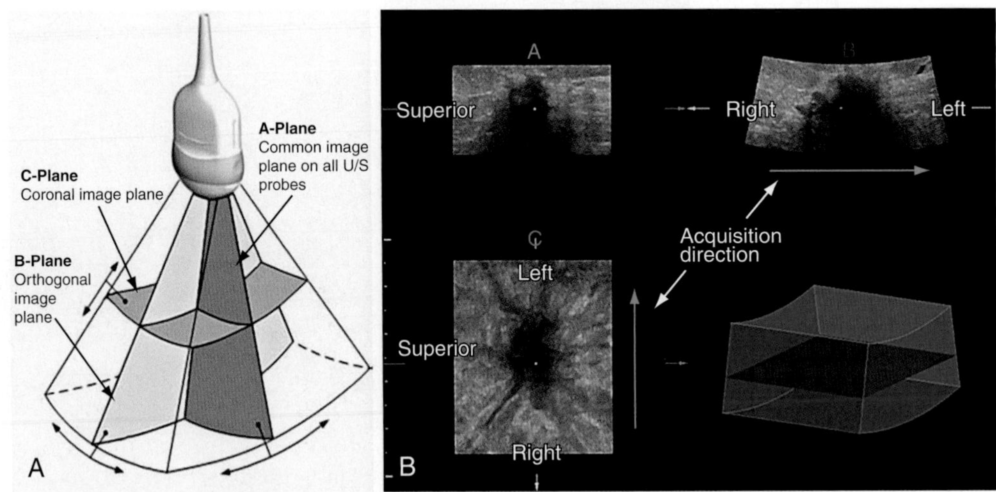

■ **FIGURE 9-15** Viewing 3D breast ultrasound. The 3D image volume can be described by three orthogonal planes along the direction of the beam **(A)**. It can be viewed by scrolling through the individual 2D images or viewed in multiplanar displays **(B)** and by various volume rendering algorithms. This allows a breast lesion to be reconstructed and analyzed in any projection. *(Courtesy of GE Medical Systems.)*

diagnosis (CAD) applications. There are currently no commercially available transducers that utilize a 2D array of elements to perform 3D imaging. 3D breast ultrasound systems perform 3D imaging by mechanically sweeping a liner array, which is coupled to a position sensing mechanism, to obtain a large number of 2D planes that are used to create a 3D image block or volume (Fig. 9-14).[6] Once the 3D image volume is obtained, it can be viewed by scrolling through the individual 2D images or viewed in multiplanar displays and by various volume rendering algorithms (Fig. 9-15). This allows a breast lesion to be reconstructed and analyzed in any projection and aids in demonstrating its relationship to other breast structures or lesions. When sequential 3D volumes are obtained of the same area over time, a 4D image data set can be created. This may be useful in observing physiologic changes of a breast lesion in three dimensions.

Understanding the basic technical aspects of ultrasound equipment will help to ensure the highest possible breast ultrasound image quality. Further advances in ultrasound technology will continue to improve the accuracy of breast ultrasound. In addition, improvements in transducer materials, efficiency and ergonomics have made scanning by technologists and physicians easier.

REFERENCES

1. ACR practice guideline for the performance of a breast ultrasound examination. *American College of Radiology* Revised 2007 (Res. 34).
2. Woo J. *A short history of the development of ultrasound in obstetrics and gynecology. Obstetric ultrasound. Linear arrays.* Available at www.ob-ultrasound.net/lineararrays.html. Accessed June 9, 2010.
3. Sehgal CM, Weinstein SP, Arger PH, Conant EF. A review of breast ultrasound. *J Mammary Gland Biol Neoplasia* 2006;**11**:113-23.
4. Desser TS, Jeffrey RB. Tissue harmonic imaging techniques: physical principles and clinical applications. *Semin Ultrasound CT MR* 2001;**22**:1-10.
5. Entrekin R, Jackson P, Jago JR, Porter BA. Real time spatial compound imaging in breast ultrasound: technology and early clinical experience. *Medicamundi* **43**: 1999; 31-4.
6. Weismann CF, Datz L. Diagnostic algorithm: How to make use of new 2D, 3D and 4D ultrasound technologies in breast imaging. *Eur J Radiol* 2007;**64**:250-7.

CHAPTER 10

Ultrasound Indications and Interpretation

A. Thomas Stavros

A BRIEF HISTORY OF BREAST ULTRASOUND

The indications for breast ultrasound continue to evolve. Screening breast ultrasound as a possible replacement for mammography was tried unsuccessfully in the early 1970s. Following this failed attempt, breast ultrasound fell into some degree of disrepute. In overreaction, many breast imagers in the United States loss confidence in breast ultrasound for most of a decade for any purpose other than distinguishing cyst from solid. Gradually, through the 1990s and 2000s, breast ultrasound has re-emerged as the key and first diagnostic breast modality that is used after mammography. Its diagnostic and guidance roles continue to expand and evolve, and recently we have begun the process of reevaluating ultrasound as an ancillary screening tool that is used after mammography in women with high risk, dense breast tissue, or both, on mammography. Both hand-held and automated approaches are being evaluated. Additionally, new technical developments have occurred within ultrasound, such as static and shear-wave elastography, three-dimensional (3-D) ultrasound, assessment of the entire radiofrequency spectrum, and computer-aided diagnosis (CAD).

A LEXICON FOR ULTRASOUND

Diagnostic breast ultrasound is quite operator dependent. Additionally, reporting of breast sonography and the recommendations generated by the reporting have varied greatly—too greatly. Referring physicians were too often confused by the reports and uncertain how to proceed based upon the sonographic findings that radiologists reported.

To help standardize the examination, reporting, and recommendations, the American College of Radiology (ACR) added a Breast Imaging, Reporting, and Data System (BI-RADS) lexicon for ultrasound to the BI-RADS lexicon that already existed for mammography. Adherence to the ultrasound BI-RADS lexicon helps us standardize descriptors and facilitates characterization of cystic and solid lesions and assignment of a BI-RADS category helps us make more consistent recommendations for further imaging or management.

All findings (whether a lesion or normal tissues) must be described within the BI-RADS lexicon and the examination must be assigned an overall BI-RADS category. When there are multiple findings, the overall BI-RADS category chosen will generally be that of the finding with the highest suspicion. The BI-RADS category given after the ultrasound examination is meant to be based upon the combined mammographic and ultrasound findings if, as in most cases, mammography was done first, not just upon the sonography findings alone. The individual BI-RADS descriptors are too numerous to discuss in detail here, but are clearly defined and illustrated at the ACR Web site, *www.acr.org*.

For each final BI-RADS category, a recommendation about management should be given.

The BI-RADS categories are not written in stone, but general definitions and recommendations for each are similar to those for mammography and are listed in Table 10-1.

The recommendations only rarely vary from those above. Note that the BI-RADS 5 category indicates a risk of malignancy of 95% or higher. In reality, this is difficult to achieve with ultrasound alone. However, the category assigned after ultrasound should be based upon the combined mammographic and sonographic findings, which

TABLE 10-1. General Definitions and Recommendations for Each of the Breast Imaging Reporting and Data System (BI-RADS) Categories for Ultrasound

BI-RADS Category	Descriptor	% Risk of Malignancy	Common Recommendations
0	Incomplete, needs additional workup		Additional imaging workup
1	Normal	0%	Depending upon indication, clinical follow-up and/or annual mammography
2	Benign	About 0%	Depending upon indication, clinical follow up and/or annual mammography
3	Probably benign	≤ 2%	Short interval follow-up versus biopsy
4	Suspicious	> 2% and < 95%	Biopsy
4a	Mildly suspicious	> 2% and < 10%	Biopsy
4b	Moderately suspicious	> 10% and < 50%	Biopsy
4c	Highly suspicious	≥ 50% and < 95%	Biopsy
5	Malignant	≥ 95%	Biopsy
6	Proven malignant		Treatment

together are expected to have a 95% or greater risk of malignancy. Note also that the BI-RADS 4 category spans from greater than 2% risk to less than 95% risk. This is a huge category for which optional 4a, 4b, and 4c subcategories have been created. Unfortunately, neither the ranges of malignant risk for each subcategory nor the rules for assigning lesions to subcategories have been defined.

As a practical rule, all three of BI-RADS 4 subcategories must undergo biopsy. However, there are other reasons that subcategorizing BI-RADS 4 lesions may be of benefit.

First, if new imaging examinations are to be used most efficiently, (i.e., examinations such as shear-wave elastography) their benefit would most likely accrue for lesions that lie within the BI-RADS 3 and 4a categories, where positive predictive value is low. For example, future studies may show that a "normal" shear-wave elastogram in a BI-RADS 4a lesion would reduce its risk from more than 2% to less than 2%, allowing it to be downgraded to BI-RADS 3. Alternatively, data may show that an "abnormal" elastogram in BI-RADS 3 lesions raises their risk from less than 2% to more than 2%, forcing an upgrade from BI-RADS 3 to BI-RADS 4a, suggesting the need for biopsy. It is highly unlikely that a "normal" elastogram in a patient with a BI-RADS 4b, 4c, or 5 lesion would ever reduce the risk of malignancy to less than 2%. Thus, a normal elastogram in such patients would be considered "discordant" and biopsy would be performed regardless of elastography results. Furthermore, if elastography results changed risks between the BI-RADS 4 subcategories or between BI-RADS 4 and BI-RADS 5, it would have much less clinical benefit. All would need biopsy anyway. Sub-categorization of the BI-RADS categories may also help assess the concordance of histologic and imaging findings in patients who undergo minimally invasive biopsy. A non-specific benign diagnosis such as benign fibrocystic change might be considered concordant if the biopsied lesion was BI-RADS 4a, but discordant if the lesion was 4b or higher. Thus, the benefit of BI-RADS 4 subcategories would be in defining a subgroup that might benefit from additional testing and in better adjudicating imaging and histologic results.

The BI-RADS Breast Ultrasound Lexicon is, of course, far from perfect. It was developed by consensus among experts whose opinions varied, and thus, it was a compromise that could only partially satisfy any one expert. Nevertheless, I feel quite sure that its use has decreased variability in reporting and management of breast pathology. It is currently undergoing its first revision and the second edition will be available soon. While breast ultrasound is not included in the Mammography Quality Standards Act (MQSA) at this time, it will likely be incorporated at some time in the future. It is also likely that accreditation, "pay-for-performance," and continuous quality improvement will mandate its use. However, its terminology is based largely upon pattern recognition rather than anatomic or histopathologic descriptions, a limitation, in my view. BI-RADS descriptors, categories, and management recommendations will likely be necessary as a minimum, but descriptors beyond BI-RADS might be helpful and necessary. BI-RADS is intended to be a living and evolving system, and additional descriptors or subcategories beyond BI-RADS that are found helpful may be incorporated into later versions of the lexicon.

INDICATIONS

Current indications for breast ultrasound include:

1. Palpable abnormalities
2. Mammographic abnormalities
3. Pain
4. Nipple discharge
5. Follow-up of lesions not biopsied (Mostly BI-RADS 3 lesions)
6. Determination of extent of lesion in patients with suspicious or malignant nodules
7. Assessment of regional lymph nodes in patients with suspicious or malignant lesions
8. Second look after magnetic resonance imaging (MRI)
9. Guiding interventional procedures
10. Screening

Palpable Abnormalities

Palpable abnormalities comprise the most common indication for targeted diagnostic breast ultrasound. Every palpable abnormality should be evaluated sonographically, regardless of the mammographic findings. This is especially true when the mammogram is negative, but shows dense tissue in the vicinity of the palpable abnormality on the mammogram. A negative mammogram should never dissuade one from aggressively evaluating the palpable abnormality sonographically. Many palpable lesions that are not visible mammographically can be beautifully demonstrated sonographically.

In our department, the sonographic examination is usually targeted to the palpable abnormality and the remainder of the ipsilateral breast. However, protocols do vary from department to department and range from targeted exams to bilateral whole breast ultrasound. In most instances, evaluation of a palpable abnormality requires only a very quick, targeted, and definitive exam. Sonography commonly demonstrates a collection of normal breast tissue or a definitively benign simple or complicated cyst to be the cause of the palpable abnormality. The negative predictive value of such an examination is more than 99%, allowing us to avoid unnecessary biopsy in almost all cases. In some cases, sonography will show that a complex mass or solid nodule causes the palpable abnormality. Such lesions can be characterized into BI-RADS 3, 4, or 5 categories, facilitating management decisions. Management of palpable lesions that are characterized BI-RADS 3 is still controversial. Some insist that all palpable lesions, regardless of their BI-RADS classification, undergo biopsy. We do not concur. We believe that patients with palpable BI-RADS 3 lesions can be offered the option of follow-up rather than biopsy. In some cases, a suspicious or malignant lesion (BI-RADS 4 or 5) causes the palpable abnormality. In such cases, we always extend the exam to include the regional lymph nodes (discussed later in this chapter).

It is important to palpate while scanning before deciding that normal tissue or a benign lesion such as a simple cyst causes the palpable abnormality. Every patient has normal breast tissue and a fairly large percentage of patients also have benign breast cysts. However, simply showing that normal tissue or a benign cyst exists in the general vicinity does not prove that it causes the palpable abnormality. To do so requires palpating while scanning. There are a variety of ways of simultaneously palpating while scanning (Fig. 10-1). Which method works best will vary, depending upon lesion size, lesion tension, lesion depth, and firmness or softness of tissues surrounding the palpable abnormality. Discussion of each of these techniques is beyond the scope of this chapter.

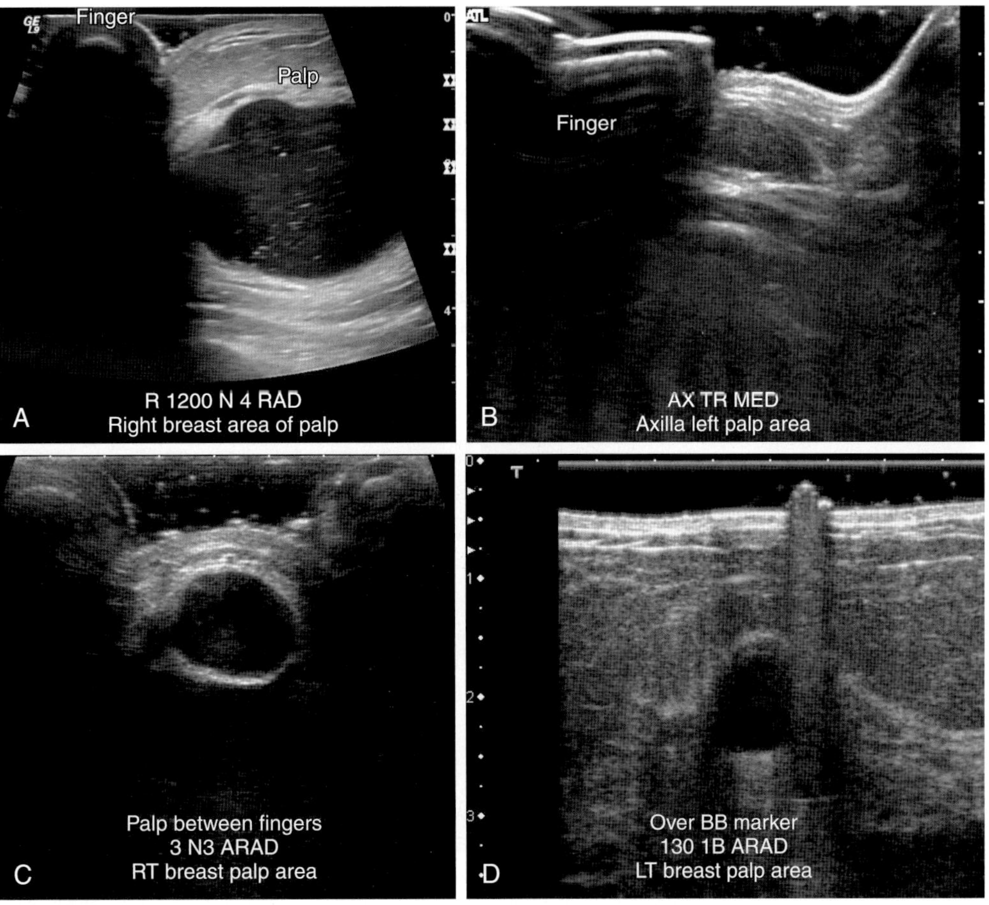

■ **FIGURE 10-1** Examples of images that document sonographic-clinical correlation, simultaneous scanning and palpation: with the side of the index finger (**A**), with the tip of the index finger (**B**), between the index and middle fingers (**C**), and with a paper clip (**D**).

Mammographic Abnormalities

Mammographic abnormalities constitute a growing indication and the second most common indication for diagnostic breast ultrasound. These mammographic abnormalities range from small vague focal asymmetries, to architectural distortions, nodules and masses. Even calcifications can benefit greatly from sonographic assessment in some patients. Mammographic abnormalities, of course, may also be palpable.

Like palpable abnormalities, mammographic abnormalities can be caused by normal tissue, benign cysts and clusters of cysts, benign complicated cysts, and solid nodules or masses that cause various degrees of suspicion. To prove that normal tissue or a definitively benign lesion causes the mammographic abnormality we must make sure that there are not two separate lesions, one that is visible mammographically and a second one that is visible sonographically. To do this we must carefully correlate size, shape, location, and surrounding tissue density between the mammogram and the sonogram. This is generally best accomplished by comparing the craniocaudal (CC) mammographic view with the transverse ultrasound plane. The mediolateral oblique (MLO) view is obtained at an unknown angle of between 30 and 60 degrees off vertical, making it difficult to reproduce the exact oblique plane sonographically. If a lesion is visible only on an MLO view, it is best to obtain a true mediolateral or lateromedial view with which to correlate a true longitudinal ultrasound plane. In correlating size between the mammogram and sonogram, maximum diameter works better than mean diameter. (Mean diameter, however, may be better for assessing size change on short interval follow-up examinations.) In correlating location, remember that mammographic compression pulls lesions away from the chest wall, while sonographic compression pushes lesions towards the chest wall. Thus, lesions often appear to be much closer to the chest wall on ultrasound than they appear to be on mammography. In correlating location, remember that the mammographic screening pair of MLO and CC are not obtained at 90 degrees to each other. The MLO is angled from high medial to low lateral, causing lateral lesions to project superior to their true locations and medial lesions to project inferior to their true locations in most, but not all, patients. Furthermore, the farther peripheral the lesion is located, the more pronounced is this effect. Finally, when doing shape correlation, remember that mammography cannot show the compressed diameter of partially compressible lesions, while ultrasound can. This means that lesions that appear elliptical on ultrasound (their true shape) will appear falsely round or spherical on mammography. This same phenomenon may result in mean diameters of lesions appearing larger on mammography than on sonography. For this reason, we prefer maximum diameter to mean diameter when correlating sonographic findings with mammographic findings. Finally, we correlate with surrounding tissue densities to obtain a higher degree of certainty about the correlation.

We note whether the lesion has a border silhouetted by dense tissue on the mammogram and try to find fibrous or glandular tissue abutting the lesion on ultrasound. We note whether dense tissue lies superficial or deep to the lesion. (Fig. 10-2) We note the relationship to definite nearby structures such as a vessel, an intramammary lymph node, or a Cooper ligament.

In most cases, the correlation of size, shape, location, and surrounding tissue density will enable us to be sure that we have identified the correct lesion sonographically. However, there will be a few cases the correlation is less certain. The most common cases that are difficult are those in which there are multiple mammographic lesions of similar size, where it is difficult to be certain which lesion on the MLO view correlates with which lesion on the CC view. Correlation can also be difficult when mammographic abnormalities are visible only on one view. Finally, it can be difficult when there are small architectural distortions without mass effect, such as in cases of radial scars and in cases where there is a small solid nodule that is isoechoic with surrounding fat. In such cases, harmonics can make the lesion relatively

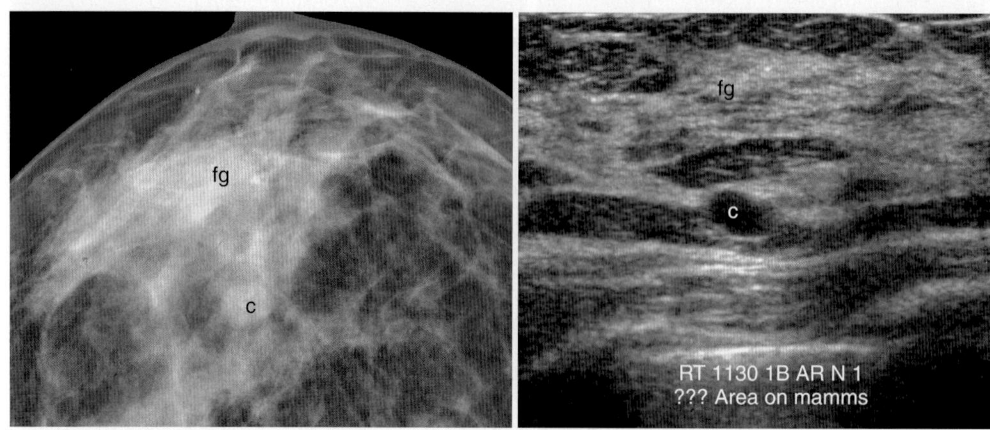

■ FIGURE 10-2 Example of mammographic-sonographic correlation. **A,** The oval, circumscribed mass on the craniocaudal (CC) view of the mammogram lies at 11:30 o'clock. It is deep to fibroglandular tissue (fg) and bulges into the retromammary fat. **B,** On sonography its size, shape, and location correlate perfectly with the ultrasound. The surrounding tissues also match those on the mammogram. The cyst lies deep to fibrous tissue and bulges into the retromammary fat.

more hypoechoic, and the surrounding fat relatively more hypoechoic, improving the conspicuity of the lesion. It can also be helpful to change the search algorithm from the usual one of looking for hypoechoic lesions to one of looking for the hyperechoic capsule or pseudo-capsule that surrounds most lesions.

While mammography can show smaller and more numerous calcifications than can sonography, it can still be very useful to assess suspicious mammographic calcifications with ultrasound for several reasons. Firstly, sonography may show the calcifications well enough to enable ultrasound-guided vacuum biopsy, which is quicker and cheaper than stereotactic biopsy. Ultrasound guidance is also truly real-time, while stereotactic biopsy is not. It will always be important to perform a specimen radiograph and a postmarker deployment mammogram, regardless of whether the biopsy was performed with sonographic or mammographic guidance. Secondly, ultrasound may show a mass or nodule that represents the invasive part of the lesion that is not visible mammographically (Fig. 10-3). Such lesions should be biopsied sonographically in addition to stereotactic biopsy of the calcifications. Calcifications usually lie within the in situ components of the lesion. Stereotactic biopsy of the calcifications often leads to underdiagnosis of associated invasion. Thirdly, the lesion may have non-calcified in situ components that ultrasound can show, which are not visible mammographically. Thus, ultrasound can show the lesion to be significantly larger than suspected from mammographic findings. In such cases, ultrasound-guided biopsies can be used to map the extent of the lesion and to guide preoperative multi-wire bracketing localization. Fourthly, sonography can be used to assess lymph nodes for metastasis and to guide biopsy of suspicious lymph nodes in patients with suspicious calcifications. And finally, the use of color or power Doppler together with gray scale ultrasound in planning and performing the biopsy can enable us to identify large vessels in the area of the suspicious lesion and can enable us to avoid them during biopsy, minimizing the chances of large postbiopsy hematomas. Generally, this cannot be accomplished with stereotactically guided biopsies. In our department, large hematomas are more likely to occur with stereotactically guided biopsies than with ultrasound-guided biopsies.

Breast Pain

Focal breast pain can be a valid, but low-yield, indication for diagnostic breast ultrasound. Some effort should be made to distinguish bilaterally symmetric (particularly upper outer quadrant pain) and cyclical pain from focal unilateral pain that is not cyclical. It is probably not justified to perform targeted diagnostic bilateral breast ultrasound in patients with symmetrical cyclical pain, although such patients may well remain candidates for bilateral whole breast supplementary screening ultrasound if they have dense tissue on mammography.

Focal pain is most often caused by benign fibrocystic change with or without associated acute inflammation that is sonographically demonstrable. Sonographically normal appearing breast is the most common cause of focal breast pain. Less frequently, an acutely inflamed breast cyst or duct causes the pain (Fig. 10-4). Inflamed sebaceous cysts also cause pain and inflammation. Other benign causes, such as abscess, trauma, or superficial, venous thrombosis are much less common. In all patients with focal pain, such as those with lumps, simultaneous palpation and scanning should be used to make sure that the structure being image is, in fact, tender.

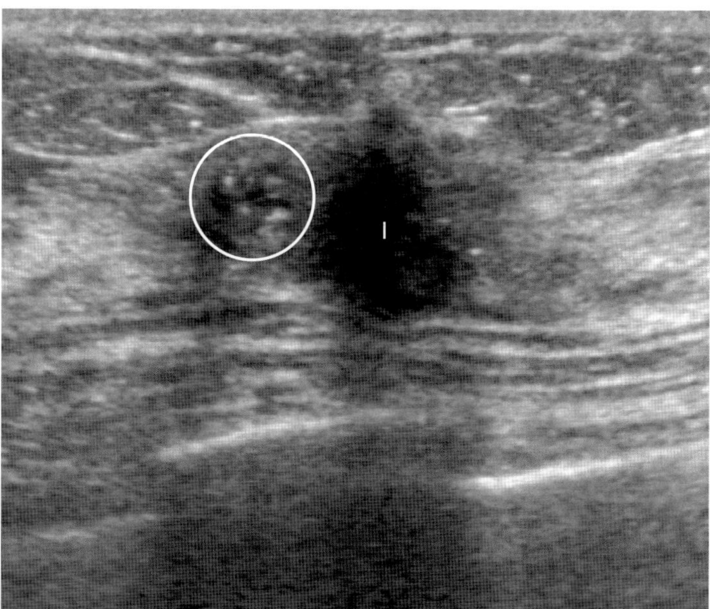

■ **FIGURE 10-3** Sonography of mammographically detected suspicious clustered coarse, heterogeneous calcifications shows the calcifications (*circle*), but also shows a nearby non parallel, oval, hypoechoic shadowing invasive carcinoma (I). Stereotactically-guided biopsy of calcifications often leads to a diagnosis of carcinoma in situ, but underdiagnoses invasion. Ultrasound enables us to identify and appropriately guide biopsy of it.

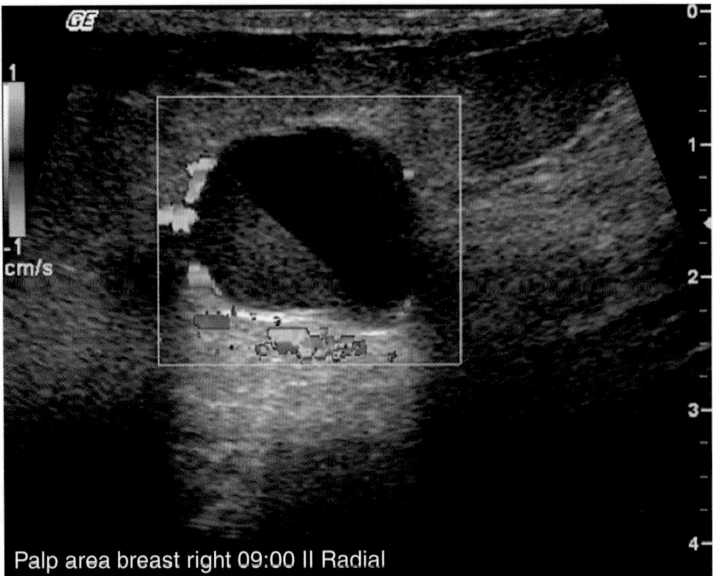

■ **FIGURE 10-4** Ultrasound of an inflammatory cyst. The triad of findings that indicate acute inflammation of a breast cyst include uniform isoechoic wall thickening, fluid-debris level, and hyperemia in the pericystic tissues. The inflammatory vessel has a course that lies parallel to the cyst wall.

Malignant lesions are an uncommon, but real, cause of pain. This most often occurs in grade 3 invasive malignant lesions that invade perineurally or in lesions such as medullary carcinoma that have a significant immune response associated with them.

Nipple Discharge

Assessing nipple discharge is a niche application for breast ultrasound, but its importance has grown since the advent of ultrasound-guided directional vacuum-assisted biopsy (DVAB). Mammography alone is not very useful for assessing nipple discharge. Galactography is the procedure of choice. However, ultrasound can also be very useful. Ultrasound-guided DVAB of intraductal papillary lesions (IPLs) is far more practical than is stereotactically guided biopsy using galactographic contrast within the ducts as guide. Of course surgical excision remains a viable option, but this too, might require sonographically guided localization.

While galactography is the procedure of choice for assessing nipple discharge, most believe that it should be reserved for high-risk nipple discharge. High risk discharge is defined as the following: (1) spontaneous; (2) unilateral; (3) from a single duct orifice; and (4) clear, serous, serosanguineous, or frankly bloody. Such discharge indicates an increased risk of an underlying papilloma or malignancy. Low risk secretions more typically exhibit the following characteristics: (1) expressible only; (2) bilateral; (3) from multiple duct orifices; and (4) milky or greenish. Low risk secretions are more typical of benign duct ectasia or benign fibrocystic change. While we agree that galactography should be reserved for high-risk secretions, sonography, because it is so cheap and non-interventional, can be justified even in patients with low risk secretions. Intraductal papillary lesions (IPLs) do occur in patients with benign duct ectasia, so merely demonstrating duct ectasia does not exclude an IPL. The lumen of each ectatic duct should be interrogated for IPLs.

We routinely schedule patients with high-risk nipple discharge for both galactography and ultrasound. We generally obtain the galactogram first. We follow the galactogram with sonography, whether or not the galactogram is successful, positive, or negative. The ultrasound can be useful regardless of the galactographic results. When the galactogram is technically unsuccessful, the ultrasound may be our only way to find the lesion. When the galactogram is positive, ultrasound may show the extent of the lesion more accurately than does the galactogram, particularly when there is *duct cut-off* sign (Fig. 10-5). Additionally, IPLs are far more commonly multiple than the galactographic literature suggests. This makes sense, since only a single lobar duct is injected during galactography, while sonography can show IPLs in other ducts as well. Thus, it is important to evaluate all the ducts with ultrasound, in patients with nipple discharge, even if the galactogram shows an IPL in one duct only. Finally, when the galactogram is negative, it may be falsely so because the wrong duct may have been cannulated or because inspissated secretions within the duct have diluted the contrast or prevented adequate filling. Ultrasound may be able to show the lesion better than galactography in such cases.

Ultrasound-guided DVAB has become our procedure of choice for biopsy of IPLs. We try to remove the lesion and some of the surrounding tissue when the lesion is small, as it usually is, and we always deploy a marker (Fig. 10-6). If the biopsied lesion has malignant or atypical histology, ultrasound guided needle localization of the marker will be necessary to guide surgical excision. Performance of DVAB of IPLs is controversial primarily because some pathologists are reticent to evaluate papillary lesions from any sort of minimally invasive biopsy specimen. Our pathologists, on

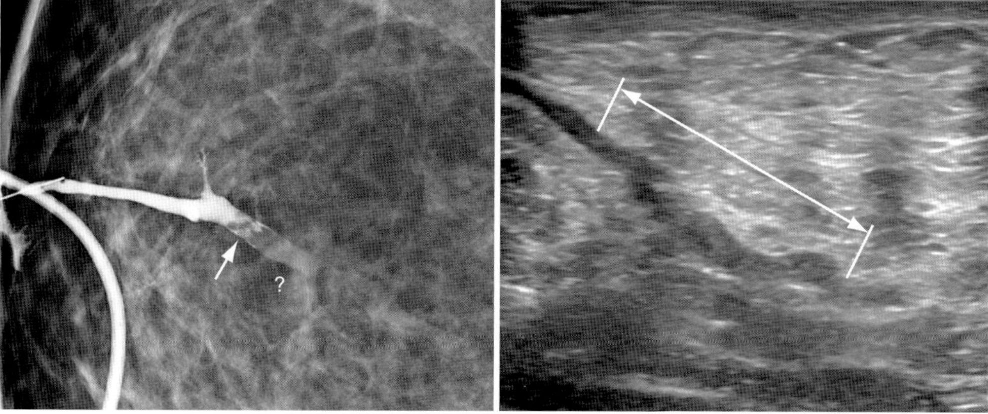

■ **FIGURE 10-5** A, The ductogram shows a *duct cut-off* sign, indicating the presence of an intraductal papillary lesion (IPL), but does not show the length of the lesion. **B,** Sonography, on the other hand, shows the exact length of the IPL. (Histology indicates a benign large duct papilloma.)

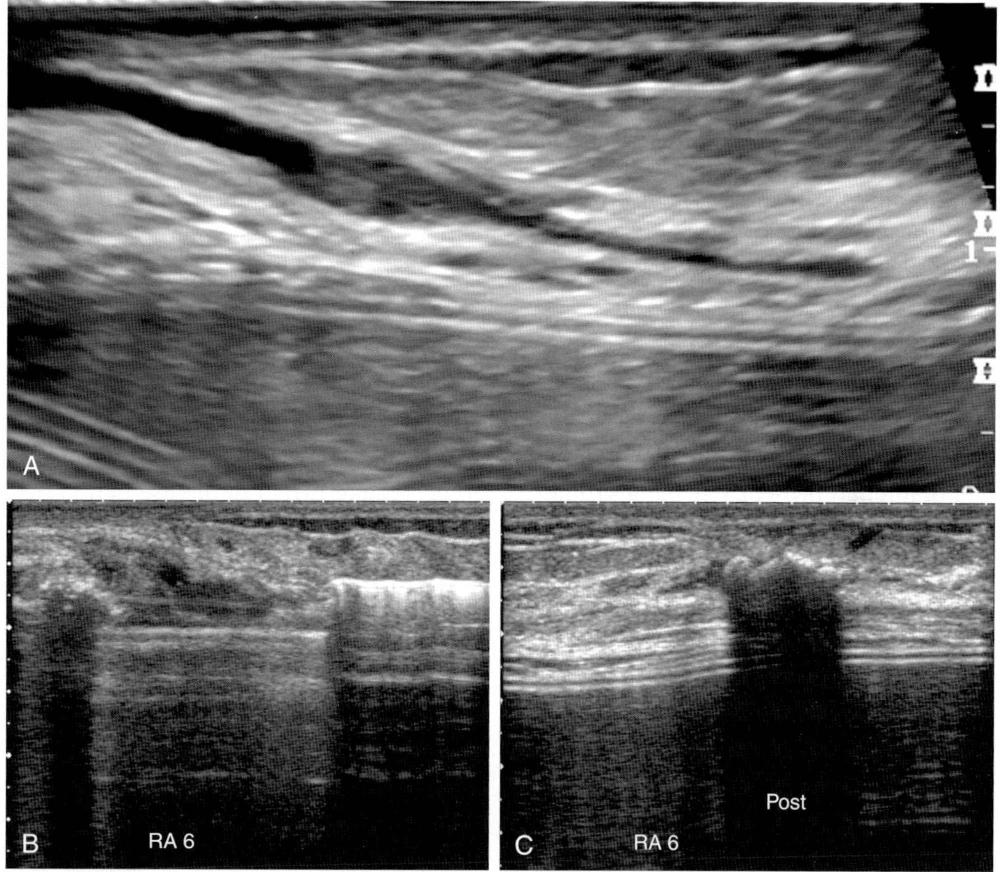

■ **FIGURE 10-6** A, Sonography shows a small and mildly expansile intraductal papillary lesion lying anterior to a mammary implant. **B,** The directional vacuum assisted probe has been placed between the lesion and the implant. Its aperture is directed anteriorly, toward the lesion and away from the implant and is open. **C,** A postbiopsy sonogram shows a marker that was placed through the directional vacuum-assisted biopsy (DVAB) device at the completion of the biopsy. (Histology indicates a benign large duct papilloma).

the other hand, are quite comfortable assessing papillary lesions removed at DVAB. We get a definitive diagnosis in all cases. Furthermore, while DVAB is approved for diagnosis, not treatment, in the process of removing enough of the papillary lesion to make an accurate histologic diagnosis, the discharge is terminated permanently in 90% of the patients.

Short Interval Follow-Up of Lesions

Once we characterize lesions as BI-RADS 3-probably benign, the patient will have to return for follow-up scans at 6 months, 1 year, and 2 years. As more and more patients undergo follow-up, a larger percentage of future breast ultrasounds will be done for purposes of short interval follow-up.

Additionally, we perform 6 month or 1-year follow-up exams on patients in whom biopsy was performed on lesions that were BI-RADS 3 or 4, but the histology was benign and considered concordant.

We prefer to use mean diameter rather than maximum diameter on short interval follow-up examinations. It helps to minimize variation due to measurement errors. It is important to measure the same way on each exam. In ultrasound, we measure different structures in different ways—some inside-to-inside, some outside to outside, some leading edge-to-leading edge, and some middle to middle. Changing measurement method from exam to exam can create false changes in size or create a false sense of stability. We prefer outside-to-outside measurements on all exams because that method includes the capsule or pseudo-capsule the surrounds the lesion. The capsule is water density, will be indistinguishable from the lesion on mammography, and thus, will be included in the lesion measurements mammographically. We must measure sonographically the same way we measure a lesion mammographically in order to obtain the best size correlation between mammography and sonography.

Short interval follow-up exams are usually quick and accurate for single lesions, but can be long and tedious when there are multiple lesions in each breast. There is no consistent definition of what constitutes a significant change in the size of the lesion, but we generally consider our measurements to be plus or minus 10%. Thus, by gestalt, it seems appropriate to use 20% change in mean diameter as being significant. Lesions that enlarge 20% or more during follow-up create a dilemma. Approximately, 20% of fibroadenomas will grow over time, so enlargement does not prove that the lesion malignant (Fig. 10-7). A growing lesion might still merely be a benign fibroadenoma. However, growth raises concern that a lesion might be malignant or might represent a phyllodes tumor. Therefore, a lesion that on follow-up is seen to have grown should be recharacterized sonographically to see if it has developed any suspicious characteristics. Of course, if its category has changed to BI-RADS 4a or higher, biopsy should be recommended. On the other hand, if its characteristics remain BI-RADS 3, we inform the patient that we still think the lesion is most likely a fibroadenoma, but that it is growing and biopsy is indicated.

Determining Extent of the Suspicious or Malignant Lesions

Characterizing solid breast nodules requires using multiple suspicious findings within a rigorous algorithm. The suspicious findings can be classified as surface, shape, and internal characteristics. They can also be classified as the following: (1) hard findings, that are signs of invasion; (2) soft findings that are signs of carcinoma in situ (CIS); and (3) mixed findings that can be seen with either invasive or in situ components of the lesion.

Classifying findings as hard and soft can be very useful for several reasons. Firstly, most invasive breast malignancies are not purely invasive, but also contain in-situ components. In many cases the invasive components are centrally located, while the CIS components lie on the surface and extend for various distances into the surrounding tissues. Thus, in many cases, the CIS components rather than the invasive components of the lesion may create the surface and shape characteristics of the lesion. This is particularly true of circumscribed carcinomas, which are usually high-grade invasive ductal carcinomas. This can also be true of special type tumors such as medullary colloid, or invasive papillary carcinomas. Including soft components in our algorithm has several benefits. It will improve our sensitivity for lesions such as circumscribed invasive lesions that have CIS components, and pure CIS lesions that have only soft findings (Fig. 10-8); it can also allow us to determine extent of disease better. Determining extent of disease requires identifying both invasive (hard findings) and CIS components (soft findings) of the lesion.

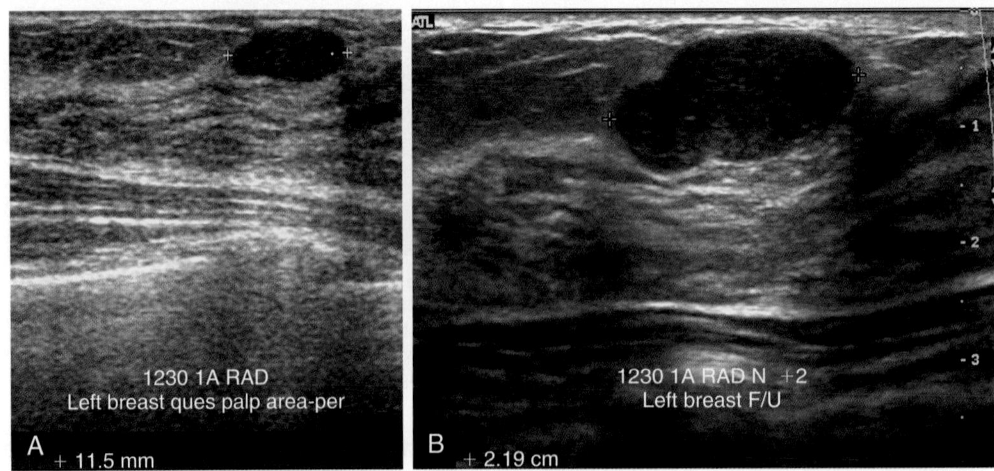

■ **FIGURE 10-7** **A,** This oval, circumscribed, hypoechoic solid mass (Breast Imaging Reporting and Data System (BI-RADS) 3) on baseline examination has a maximum diameter of 11.5 mm. **B,** On short interval follow-up examination 7 months later, the maximum diameter has almost doubled and the volume has increased nearly fourfold. However, the findings remain those of a probably benign (BI-RADS 3) lesion. Such rapid growth was considered highly suspicious for a phyllodes tumor, which can have a BI-RADS 3 appearance on mammography and ultrasound. Biopsy showed a benign fibroadenoma with cellular stroma. At least 20% of benign fibroadenomas do show growth on follow-up examination.

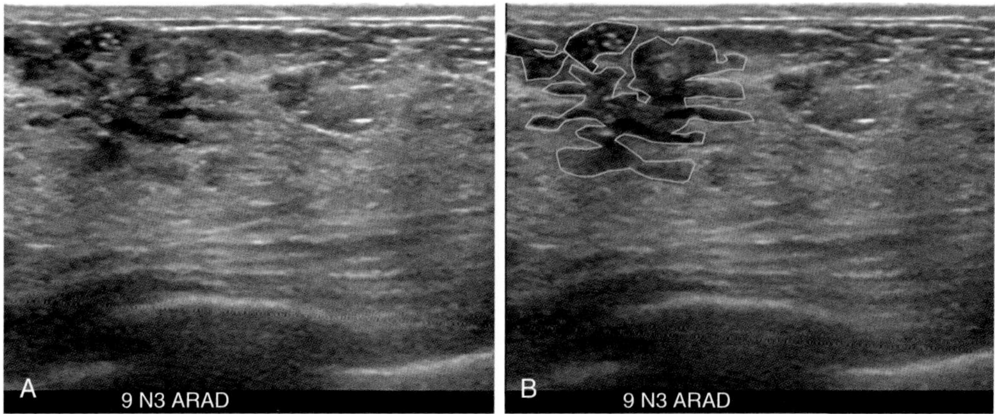

■ **FIGURE 10-8** **A,** This micropapillary carcinoma in situ (CIS) shows only multiple echogenic foci compatible with microcalcifications and enlarged irregular ducts. Micropapillary CIS secretes fluid, so the ducts are often fluid filled. **B,** As is often the case, the extent of calcifications (yellow outline) greatly underestimates the true extent of the disease (yellow plus aqua outlines).

In the tumor-lymph node-metastasis (TNM) classification system, the maximum diameter of an invasive breast malignancy is the maximum diameter of the index invasive lesion. However, the extent of disease is different from the maximum diameter. It includes the CIS components. Thus, a lesion that has a 2 cm invasive lesion with 2 cm of CIS extending toward the nipple from the invasive lesion and 2 cm of CIS growing peripherally away from the nipple would have a TNM maximum diameter of 2 cm, but would have an extent of 6 cm. The maximum TNM diameter and the extent of malignant disease represent radically different assessments of the size of the lesion. Medical oncologists may use the TNM diameter (or prognostic diameter) of the lesion to determine into which chemotherapeutic trial to enter their patients, but surgeons must consider the extent of the disease in deciding the type and extent of surgery if they hope to obtain clean margins, minimize re-excisions, and minimize local recurrences.

The hard findings can help identify the invasive part of the lesion and maximum TNM diameter, while the soft findings help determine the extent of the lesion, including its CIS components (Fig. 10-9). This is especially important in cases such as the earlier example, where there are great differences in the TNM diameter and extent of the disease. Recognizing the difference between the index invasive lesion and the surrounding CIS components of the lesion is especially important when the lesion is growing irregularly or asymmetrically within the breast or has extensive intraductal (CIS) components.

Assessment of Regional Lymph Nodes in Patients with Suspicious Breast Lesions Undergoing Biopsy

In any patient who has a suspicious or malignant nodule (BI-RADS 4 or 5) for which we will recommend image-guided biopsy, we extend the sonographic evaluation to include regional lymph nodes of the breast. We usually assess level 1 axillary and internal mammary lymph nodes. However, in some cases we will expand the search to higher level (levels 2 and 3) axillary lymph nodes, Rotter nodes, supraclavicular nodes, and internal jugular lymph nodes. We do this to help stage malignant disease. If a

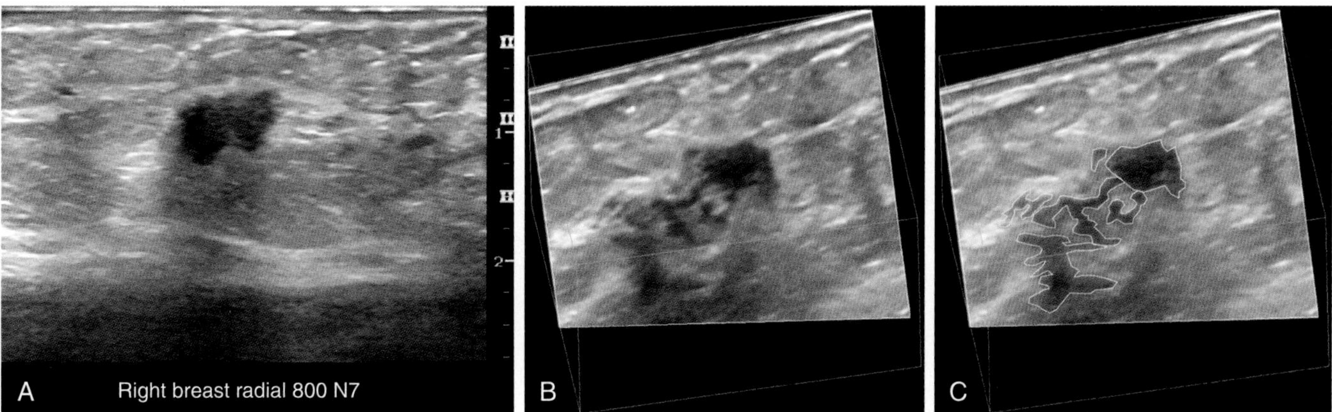

■ **FIGURE 10-9** **A,** Conventional sonographic view of this oval, microlobulated hypoechoic, shadowing solid mass shows numerous suspicious findings: microlobulation, hypoechoic echogenicity and mild acoustic shadowing. While the findings on this view accurately characterize the lesion as invasive, they do not show its true extent. **B,** A virtually reconstructed plane from a 3D volume acquisition shows numerous abnormally large and irregular ducts that represent carcinoma in situ extending into the surrounding tissues along the left posterior side of the invasive component of the lesion. **C,** Same image as in **B** with the in situ components outlined.

lymph node is suspicious for metastasis, we perform ultrasound-guided biopsy. A positive biopsy obviates a sentinel lymph node procedure and enables the surgeon to proceed straight to axillary dissection. Obviously, ultrasound cannot detect microscopic metastatic disease. Therefore, a normal ultrasound does not exclude metastatic disease. A negative ultrasound or an ultrasound that is abnormal with a biopsy revealing only a benign reactive lymph node does not prevent a planned sentinel lymph node procedure. Thus, a positive ultrasound and ultrasound guided biopsy is far more useful than a negative ultrasound or negative biopsy.

In evaluating lymph nodes we have the following two goals: (1) to distinguish normal from abnormal lymph nodes; and (2) to determine whether abnormal lymph nodes are more likely to be reactive or metastatic based upon their morphology and the morphology of surrounding lymph nodes.

There are many different criteria used to determine whether a lymph node is normal or not. These include a minimum diameter of 1 cm or greater, an abnormally round shape, abnormally hypoechoic cortex, and cortical thickening (particularly eccentric cortical thickening), obliteration of the hilum or mediastinum of the node, increased blood flow, particularly non-hilar vessels, and abnormally high resistance flow. While all of these findings are valid, eccentric cortical thickening has the best combination of sensitivity and positive predictive values of all of the findings and is the finding we rely upon the most. Size is unquestionably the least reliable of the findings, and the finding we choose to ignore in most cases. We commonly see normal fatty replaced lymph nodes that have minimum diameters of 3 or even 4 cm that have very thin cortices and are morphologically normal. On the other hand, we often see small metastatic nodes with maximum diameters well under 1 cm, but that are abnormally morphologically because of gross cortical thickening. Abnormally round shape has a good positive predictive value, but low sensitivity compared to cortical thickening, because all nodes with abnormally round shape have cortical thickening, but not all nodes with cortical thickening are abnormally round in shape. Some metastatic lymph nodes have an abnormally hypoechoic cortex, but this is generally a late finding, and all such nodes already have an abnormally thick cortex. Additionally, the use of digitally encoded harmonics makes the cortex of all lymph nodes hypoechoic. We routinely use harmonics because it makes the lymph nodes more conspicuous and easier to distinguish from surrounding axillary fat. We can find more lymph nodes more quickly with harmonics than without harmonics. Because we routinely use harmonics, we do not use hypoechogenicity as a finding. Color or power Doppler and pulse Doppler spectral analysis are less sensitive than the gray scale imaging findings, but can be helpful in a small number of cases as a tie-breaker to distinguish metastatic from benign reactive lymph nodes.

Cortical thickening is the key finding that enables us to accomplish goal number one: distinguishing normal from abnormal lymph nodes. Eccentric cortical thickening is the key finding that enables us to accomplish goal number two: distinguishing benign reactive lymph nodes from metastatic lymph nodes.

Understanding the anatomy and physiology of lymph nodes and how metastases affect the lymph node is paramount to understanding why cortical thickening is the key to the sonographic diagnosis of lymph node metastases. Afferent lymphatic vessels enter the lymph node not through the hilum, but from the periphery of the node. Lymph fluid flows from the afferent lymphatic vessels into the subcapsular sinusoids of the lymph node, then to the cortical sinusoids, the medullary sinusoids, and finally, exits the lymph node hilum through the efferent lymphatic vessels. Metastases tend to implant within the subcapsular and cortical sinusoids. (Foreign bodies, such as extravasated silicone gel, on the other hand, tend to be trapped within the medullary sinusoids initially.) Sonographically visible metastases manifest as cortical thickening because they implant within the subcapsular and cortical sinusoids.

The appearance of the cortical thickening varies, depending upon whether the initial implantation site is subcapsular, the center of the cortical sinusoids, or the inner part of the cortical sinusoids (Fig. 10-10). Metastases that implant within the subcortical sinusoids tend to present with an outward bulge of the cortex, often presenting as a "Mickey Mouse" ear appearance. Metastases that implant within the

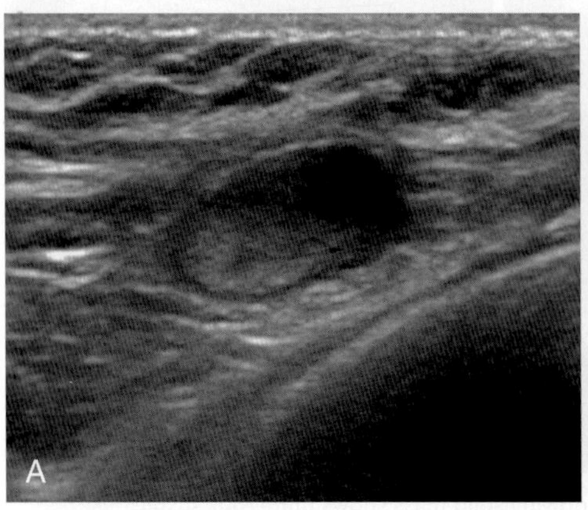

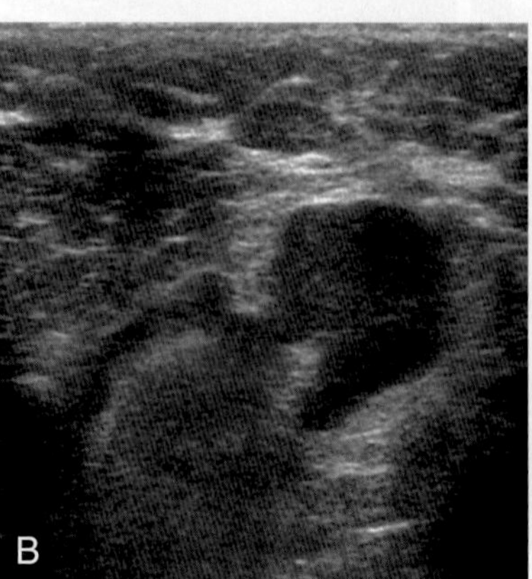

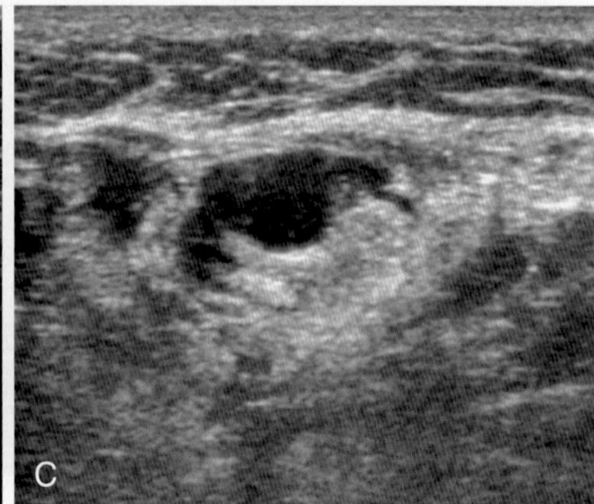

■ **FIGURE 10-10** **A,** When the metastasis implants in the mid cortical sinusoid, it causes approximately equal inward and outward thickening of the cortex. **B,** When the metastasis implants in the subcapsular sinusoids, the cortical thickening bulges outward from the lymph node in a "Mickey Mouse" ear configuration. **C,** When the metastasis implants along the inner side of the cortical sinusoid or in the medullary sinusoids, the metastasis bulges inwardly into the mediastinum of the lymph node in a "rat bite" configuration.

mid cortical sinusoids tend to thicken the cortex equally in inward and outward directions. Metastases that implant within the inner part of the cortical sinusoids tend to present with a focal bulge of the cortex into the mediastinum of the lymph node, creating a "rat bite" appearance.

When metastases extensively fill the cortical sinusoids of a lymph node they may cause uniform symmetrical thickening of the cortex, an appearance that is indistinguishable from that of most benign reactive lymph nodes (Fig. 10-11). In such cases we have several "tie-breakers" that we can use to help make the distinction. These include the following: (1) comparing the cortical thickness in adjacent lymph nodes; (2) comparing to contralateral axillary lymph nodes at the same level; (3) looking at vascular patterns with color or power Doppler; and (4) assessing the pulsed Doppler spectral waveform appearance. In most cases, comparing to adjacent lymph nodes is sufficient to make the distinction. It is almost always possible to rotate the ultrasound transducer in a manner that allows visualization of two adjacent axillary lymph nodes at the same time. If the lymph node adjacent to the one with symmetrical cortical thickening shows normal cortex, the node with thickened cortex is more likely to be metastatic than reactive (Fig. 10-12). If the lymph node next to the one with symmetrically thickened cortex shows eccentric cortical thickening or more severe cortical thickening, metastasis is more likely than reactive nodes. However, if the adjacent lymph node has a similar degree of cortical thickening, the lymph nodes might be either metastatic or reactive. In such cases, comparing to the mirror image level lymph nodes on the contralateral side might be helpful. An approximately equal degree of involvement of axillary lymph nodes on both sides favors a benign reactive process, while right to left asymmetry favors metastatic disease.

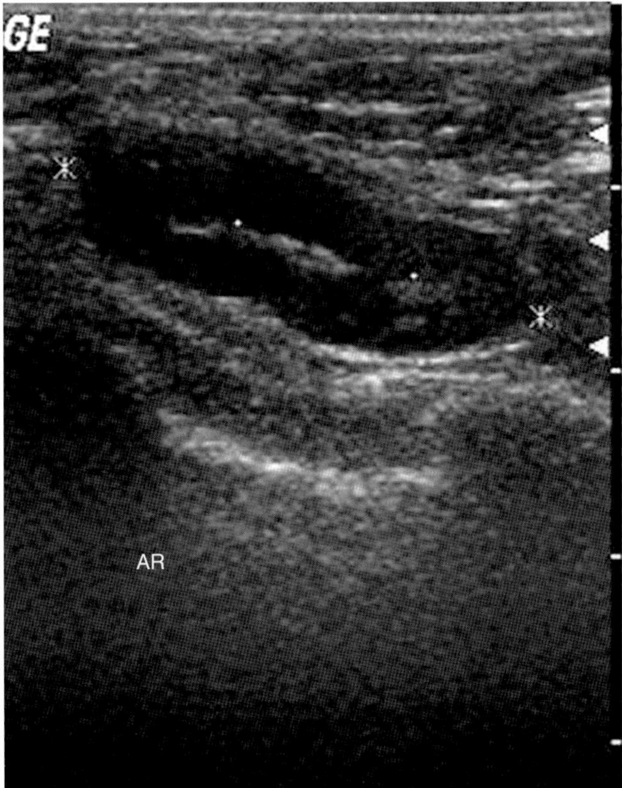

■ **FIGURE 10-11** Lymph nodes that show symmetrical and circumferential cortical thickening (> 3 mm) are abnormal, but can be either benign reactive or metastatic. Making the distinction between a reactive or metastatic etiology requires the use of other features that act as tiebreakers.

Doppler can be used to help distinguish between uniform cortical thickening caused by metastasis and the symmetrical thickening that occurs in a benign inflamed or reactive lymph node. Blood flow patterns differ between benign reactive and metastatic lymph nodes because of where metastases implant within the node. Because metastases tend to implant in the cortical and subcapsular sinusoids, any neovascularity that they incite tends to enter the node from the periphery rather than from the hilum. Thus, the presence of vessels that enter or exit through the capsule of the lymph node rather than the hilum (nonhilar vessels or transcapsular vessels) favors the node being metastatic or a high grade lymphoma rather than reactive. Reactive nodes may have increased blood flow, but all feeding arteries and draining veins are dilated, but otherwise normal, hilar vessels. (The same is true of low-grade lymphomas.)

Pulsed Doppler spectral waveforms can also help distinguish benign reactive from metastatic lymph nodes. The pulsed Doppler waveforms obtained from vessels within a metastatic lymph node tend to have a high sharp systolic peak and have high impedance. On the other hand, waveforms obtained from vessels within a reactive lymph node tend to have low and rounded systolic peaks and have low impedance.

Complete obliteration of the mediastinum of the lymph nodes requires special mention. While benign reactive nodes can occasionally present with complete obliteration of the mediastinum, 93% of such nodes are metastatic.

We are quite effective at distinguishing abnormal from normal nodes, but we are less effective at determining whether the cortical thickening represents metastasis or inflammation. However, every effort should be made to make this distinction. A biopsy of an abnormal, but benign reactive lymph node is just an extra procedure that does not change surgical management. If the surgeon had planned on performing a sentinel node procedure before the ultrasound-guided benign biopsy, he or she will still have to perform it. Only an abnormal ultrasound with an ultrasound guided biopsy revealing metastatic disease can prevent a planned sentinel lymph node procedure. We should not be overly aggressive about ultrasound-guided biopsy of lymph nodes. We should perform ultrasound-guided biopsy for lymph nodes whose sonographic appearance. blood flow, or both, is highly suspicious for metastatic disease.

Internal mammary lymph nodes lie in a parasternal location, adjacent to the internal mammary vessels. Sonographic demonstration of these nodes was used in the past to indicate that they were abnormal. However, with today's improved equipment and scan techniques this is no longer true. We now can demonstrate normal internal mammary lymph nodes in up to 90% of patients (Fig. 10-13). Like axillary nodes, they are oval shaped, but they are much smaller than axillary lymph nodes. The maximum diameter is

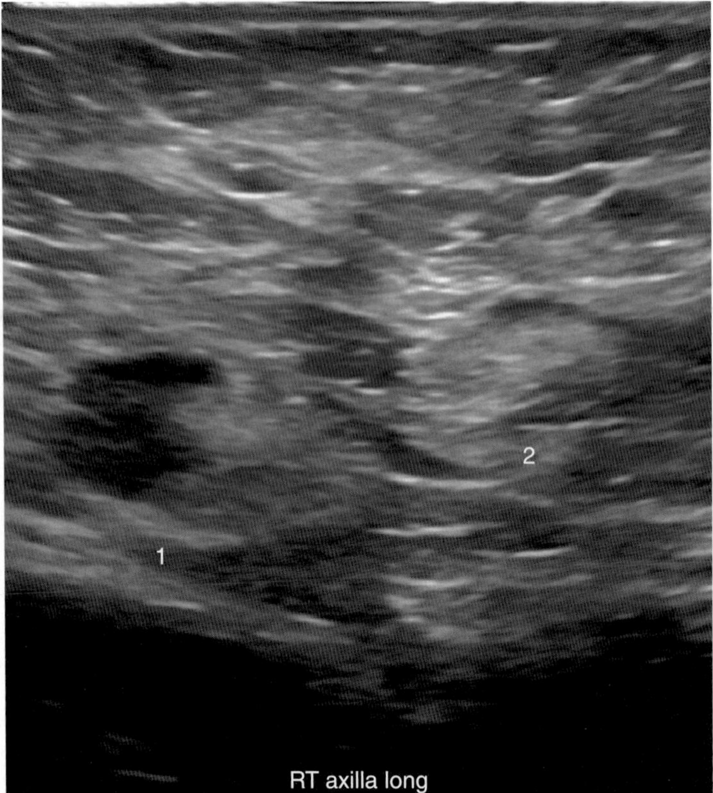

■ FIGURE 10-12 The relationship of adjacent lymph nodes is the "first tiebreaker" that we use to help distinguish a metastatic from a benign reactive lymph node. When two adjacent axillary nodes show differing degrees of cortical thickening, as in this case, the findings favor a metastasis in the node with the thicker cortex (#1).

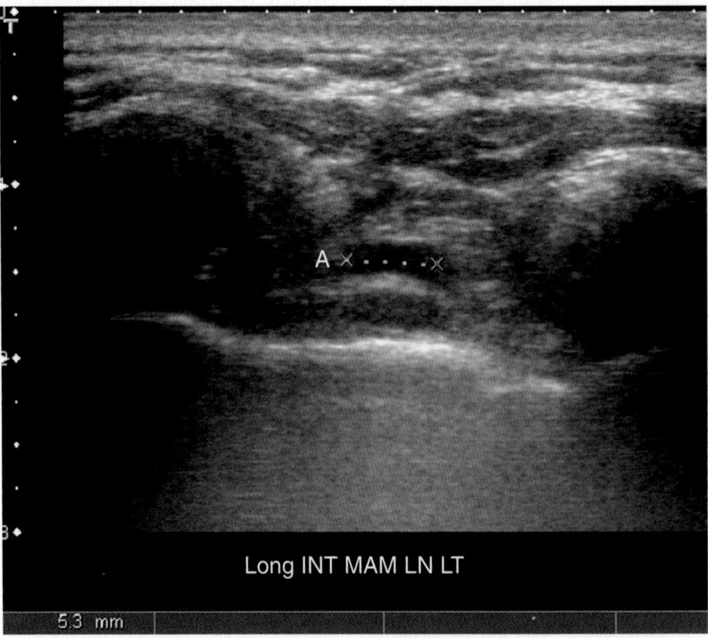

■ FIGURE 10-13 At least one normal internal mammary lymph node can be detected in most patients with current equipment. These lymph nodes are smaller than axillary nodes and generally do not have a demonstrable hyperechoic mediastinum. They are most easily demonstrated in the second and third intercostal spaces and are 5 to 7 mm in maximum diameter.

between 5 and 7 mm. An echogenic mediastinum is much less frequently demonstrable than it is in axillary lymph nodes. Internal mammary lymph nodes are best seen in the second and third intercostal spaces. Blood flow is almost never demonstrable within them. They can be difficult to distinguish on gray scale ultrasound from dilated tortuous internal mammary veins that occur in elderly patients who have congestive right heart failure. Color or power Doppler may be helpful in making this distinction. Metastases to internal mammary lymph nodes are much less common than are metastases to the axillary nodes because most of the breast drains to the periareolar lymphatic plexus (Sappey plexus) and then to the axilla. Generally, only the deep medial parts of the breast drain directly to the internal mammary lymph nodes. Metastases to internal mammary lymph nodes occur most commonly when gross metastatic disease to the axillary nodes causes "tumor damming" and collateral flow to the internal mammary nodes, or with large deep medial lesions. However, there are enough variations in drainage that isolated internal mammary lymph nodes metastases can occur. Therefore, the internal mammary lymph nodes should routinely be evaluated in patients who have suspicious breast lesions that will require image-guided biopsy. The presence of internal mammary lymph node metastasis can be confirmed by ultrasound-guided fine-needle aspiration (FNA) or positron emission tomography-computed tomography (PET CT). Metastases to internal mammary lymph nodes are most important to the radiation oncologist, who no longer routinely treats these nodes with radiation due to delayed pericardial, myocardial, and coronary complications that occurred when they were routinely radiated in the past. Today, however, in a patient with known or suspected internal mammary lymph node metastases, most radiation oncologists believe the risk is warranted and will employ an internal mammary field. Most radiation oncologists accept either a positive FNA or a positive PET CT as adequate evidence for treatment of the internal mammary nodes, but some also accept MRI or ultrasound evidence as adequate.

The level of axillary lymph nodes is determined by the margins of the pectoralis minor muscle (not the pectoralis major). Axillary nodes that lie inferior and lateral to the lateral edge of the pectoralis muscle are level 1 nodes. Nodes that lie posterior to the pectoralis minor are level 2 nodes, and nodes that lie superior and medial to the medial margin of the muscle are level 3 nodes (also called infraclavicular nodes). The spread of metastases tends to occur step by step from level 1 to level 2, from level 2 to level 3, and from level 3 to internal jugular and or supraclavicular nodes. Only rarely would metastases go to level 2 or 3 nodes directly. We generally examine only level 1 nodes. If level 1 nodes are sonographically normal, we do not evaluate level 2 or 3 nodes. However, we always try to examine one level higher than we see abnormal lymph nodes. Thus, if level 1 nodes are abnormal, we assess level 2. If level 2 nodes are abnormal we examine level 3 (Fig. 10-14). If level 3 nodes are abnormal, we are obligated to evaluate the supraclavicular and internal jugular nodes. We do not need to biopsy all levels. We will generally biopsy a level 1 node and a node from the highest level where we see abnormal nodes.

Either core biopsy or FNA of lymph nodes can be effective. We prefer core biopsy for level 1 axillary lymph nodes and FNA for higher level axillary, internal mammary, and all lymph nodes above the clavicle. However, FNA would be sufficient for most level 1 axillary lymph nodes, with the following two exceptions: (1) suspected perinodal invasion; and (2) suspected Hodgkin disease.

Suspected perinodal invasion matters to the surgeon and radiation oncologist. Surgeons normally perform axillary dissection as part of the staging of breast cancer, but when they know perinodal invasion is present, axillary dissection may be performed more aggressively as a treatment procedure. Likewise, radiation oncologists may be more aggressive in radiating the axilla to minimize recurrence. When sonographic findings are suspicious for perinodal invasion, a core biopsy rather than FNA should be performed. Fine-needle aspiration (FNA) can only document the presence

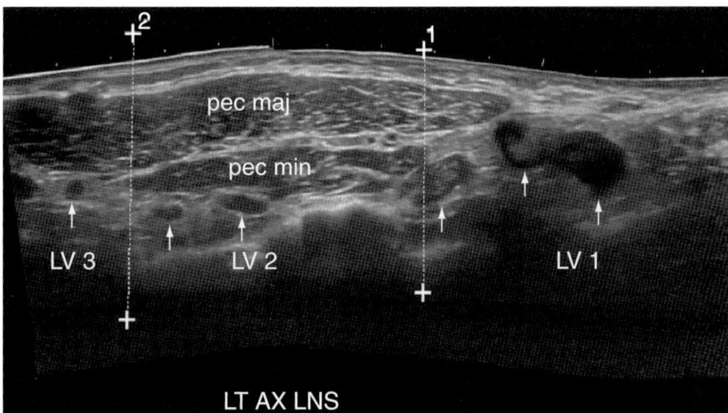

■ **FIGURE 10-14** The edges of the pectoralis minor muscle determine the levels of axillary lymph nodes. Nodes that lie inferior and lateral to the edge of the pectoralis minor are level 1 nodes. Nodes that lie posterior to the pectoralis minor muscle are level 2 nodes, and nodes that lie superior and medial to the superomedial edge of the pectoralis minor muscle are level 3 nodes. The pectoralis muscle position varies with arm position, so assessment of lymph node level is best performed with the arm 90 degrees abducted, as it is during breast surgery. We reserve evaluation of level 2 and 3 nodes for cases where level 1 nodes are grossly abnormal.

or absence of metastasis, while a properly targeted core biopsy can confirm suspected perinodal invasion. The following are sonographic findings that are suspicious for perinodal invasion: (1) loss of the thin-echogenic lymph node capsule; (2) irregular, angulated or spiculated cortical margins; and (3) the presence of perinodal edema. When we suspect perinodal invasion and want to confirm it on core biopsy, we must specifically place our sample volume so that it is half within the lymph node cortex and half within the surrounding perinodal fat. This is easiest to do with devices that allow placement of the inner stylet and fire only the outer sheath (Achieve or Temno core biopsy devices[CareFusion, San Diego, Calif.]).

Ultrasound Correlation with Magnetic Resonance Imaging ("Second-Look Ultrasound" after MRI)

The use of ultrasound to correlate with suspicious findings on MRI (second look ultrasound) has become the fastest growing area of ultrasound in recent years. Contrast enhanced MRI is the most sensitive modality we have for detecting breast cancer and is our best modality for locoregional staging of breast cancer. However, like mammography and ultrasound, MRI has false positives, enough that definitive treatment should not be based upon MRI findings alone. Instead, treatment should be based upon histologic mapping biopsies obtained from either second look ultrasound and subsequent ultrasound guided biopsy, MRI guided biopsy, or a combination of both. Correlative ultrasound is usually tried prior to proceeding to MRI guided biopsy for the following reasons: (1) If the lesion can be found on ultrasound, ultrasound-guided biopsies are generally quicker and cheaper than are biopsies guided by MRI; (2) MRI-guided biopsies tie up a machine (often a limited resource) that is essential for performing other imaging studies; (3) ultrasound guidance for biopsy is truly real-time, while MRI guidance is not; (4) the compression used during MRI-guided biopsy, despite being less than that used during mammography, can decrease the amount of contrast enhancement and make it more difficult to demonstrate the lesion for MRI guidance; (5) the contrast enhancement during MRI lasts for only a short time, and any delay in performing the MRI- guided biopsy can mean that the contrast is gone by the time the biopsy is completed; and (6) unlike specimen radiography or specimen sonography, there is no practical way to perform specimen MRI. The potential for MRI-guided biopsy misses is greater than for ultrasound guided biopsy. However, while ultrasound can be used to minimize false positives on MRI, ultrasound has more false negatives than does MRI, particularly for CIS. Therefore, a negative ultrasound should not dissuade us from MRI-guided biopsy if the MRI findings are suspicious for malignancy. The false negative rate for second look ultrasound varies greatly, but is probably between 10% to 20% even in the best hands. This is so important that facilities that are not capable of performing MRI-guided biopsies should not be performing contrast-enhanced breast MRI. Facilities that cannot perform high-quality second look ultrasound will likely have less optimal breast MRI efficacy than will facilities that are adept at it.

Second look ultrasound requires meticulous correlation between mammographic, sonographic, MRI, clinical, and pathologic findings. The process of correlating so much data is often tedious and time consuming. In many cases there are multiple foci of enhancement unilaterally or even bilaterally that essentially require sonographic evaluation of the whole breast on both sides. Identifying additional foci of invasive carcinoma shown by MRI is much less of a problem for second look ultrasound than is identifying CIS components of a lesion or additional foci of CIS. Sonographic hard findings that are signs of invasion and that have high positive predictive value, but lower sensitivity for cancer, can be used to detect these additional invasive lesions. The sonographic hard findings associated with invasive malignancy look very similar on ultrasound and MRI and are the findings we are most used to looking for in both diagnostic and screening ultrasound situations (Fig. 10-15). Hard findings are more evident than soft findings because they

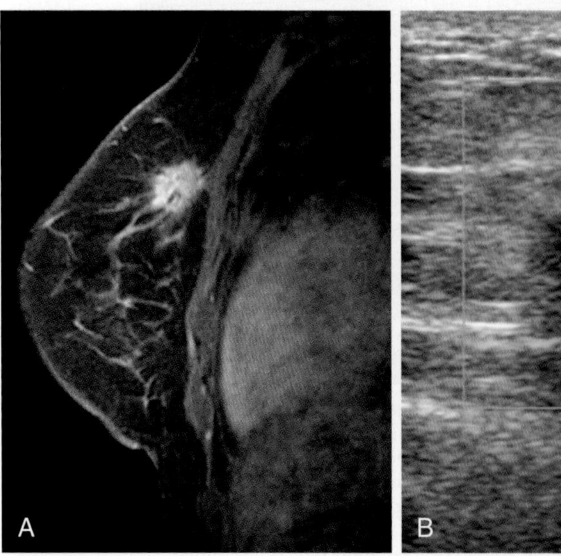

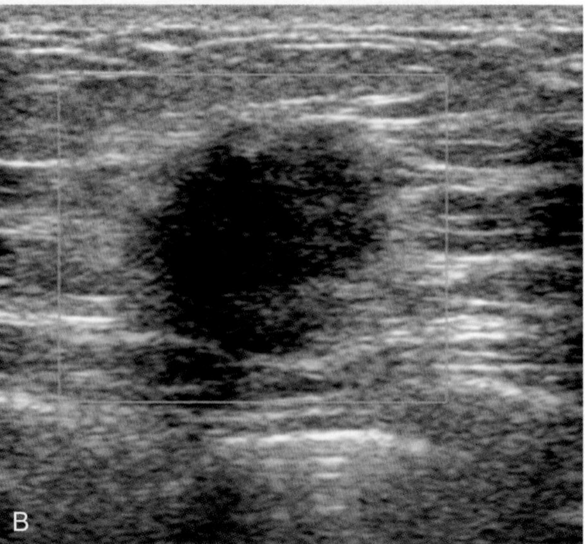

■ FIGURE 10-15 The sonographic findings look similar on ultrasound–B, and magnetic resonance imaging (MRI)–A. Both show an oval spiculated mass.

usually represent some degree of destruction of normal anatomic planes. Identifying CIS components of lesions on second look ultrasound can be very difficult, indeed, and often represent a paradigm shift for the breast radiologist. In most cases, patients with CIS do not present with a mass on either ultrasound or MRI. On MRI it is seen as non–mass-like enhancement, "clumped" enhancement, or ductal enhancement. On ultrasound, it is present as enlargement and distortion of ducts and lobules or increased numbers of ducts or lobules, with or without sonographically visible microcalcifications. The classic finding is microcalcifications within the center of microlobulations or ducts (Fig. 10-16). These are soft findings of CIS. The sensitivity is higher, but the positive predictive value is much lower than for hard findings. Soft findings distort the anatomy, but do not necessarily destroy it. They overlap much more with the ductal and lobular changes that occur in benign fibrocystic change or benign proliferative disorders than do hard findings. Such findings, if not associated with hard findings, might be considered normal if encountered during a screening ultrasound where the risk of cancer is only 4 per 1000 or even during a diagnostic ultrasound where the risk is 40 per 1000. However, when encountered in a patient with known cancer and suspicious contrast enhancement on MRI, where the risk of cancer is 40%, such findings must be considered positive, and biopsied. The 100-fold difference in the pre-test probabilities of cancer between screening and second look ultrasound populations demands that different rules of interpretation be used in each of these groups. In the screening group we are mainly looking for invasive carcinomas, and rely primarily on hard findings. In the second look ultrasound group, where additional lesions or additional components of the index lesion are quite often CIS, soft findings are important. Subtle soft findings that would have to be ignored on a screening examination must be considered positive in the setting of second-look ultrasound. In the diagnostic study, we use primarily hard findings, but do assess soft findings that are associated with a suspicious nodule.

Our approach to findings discovered during second look ultrasound varies depending upon our certainty about their correlation with the MRI findings. In cases where we are confident that our sonographic findings definitely explain the suspicious MRI findings (ultrasound and MRI findings are concordant) we proceed to ultrasound-guided biopsy. In cases where we cannot find a sonographic correlate to the suspicious MRI findings, we biopsy the lesion with MRI guidance. In cases where we think the findings explain the MRI findings, but are uncertain, (probably concordant, but not certain) we perform MRI-guided biopsy rather than ultrasound-guided biopsy. When performing ultrasound-guided biopsy of suspicious lesions found on second look ultrasound, the type of biopsy and best biopsy device depends on the findings present. Lesions that appear to be mass-like and have irregular shapes and peripheral enhancement on MRI can undergo ultrasound-guided core biopsy. On the other hand, lesions that show non–mass-like enhancement with clumped, linear, or branching morphology on MRI or soft finding of focally enlarged ducts or terminal duct lobular units (TDLUs) or too many ducts on ultrasound, should be biopsied with large vacuum-assisted biopsy devices, preferably 7- or 8-gauge rather than 10- or 11-gauge. As is the case for all other ultrasound-guided biopsies, we always deploy a marker into the biopsy site after biopsy and before removing the biopsy probe.

The difference between the prone position used for contrast-enhanced breast MRI and the supine position use for ultrasound creates difficulties when correlating second-look ultrasound with breast MRI. It has also created problems in trying to perform breast ultrasound-MRI fusion imaging, but "GPS" systems have been developed to facilitate fusion imaging and correlation of ultrasound with MRI. There is hope that newer diffusion weighted scans that can be performed in the supine position will make co-registered fusion imaging between breast MRI and second look ultrasound easier.

Ultrasound-Guided Interventional Procedures

Ultrasound-guided interventional procedures are limited only by our imagination. Any lesion that can be seen on ultrasound can be aspirated, biopsied, or localized under ultrasound guidance. Ultrasound-guided procedures include FNA, core biopsy, directional vacuum-assisted biopsy, cyst aspiration, abscess aspiration, hematoma, seroma, or lymphocele drainage, needle localization, foreign body removal and thrombosis of pseudoaneurysm within the breast. Ultrasound-guided core needle biopsy or FNA of axillary lymph nodes can also be performed.

Interventional procedures can be particularly difficult in certain lesions because of their locations, but performing hydrodissection with local anesthetic can usually create adequate space for needle procedures. Sites that can make

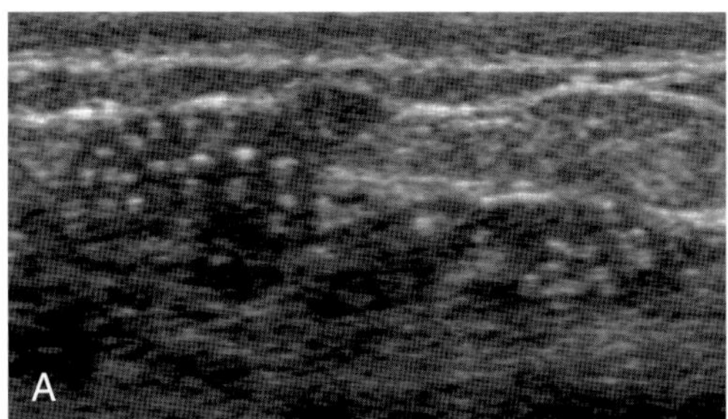

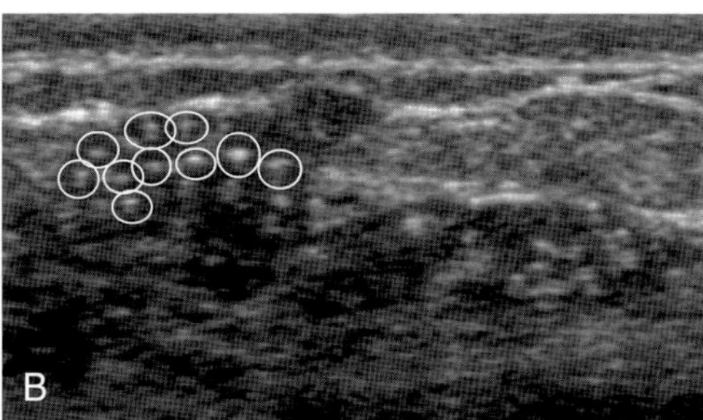

■ **FIGURE 10-16** **A,** Non–mass-like enhancement on magnetic resonance imaging (MRI) is more difficult to assess with ultrasound. It correlates with nonspecific findings of enlarged and irregular ducts and lobules with or without calcifications. The most specific sonographic finding of carcinoma in situ is microcalcifications. **B,** Same image as in A with calcium outlined in white.

biopsies technically difficult include locations that are subareolar, immediately deep to the skin, immediately superficial to implants and adjacent to the chest wall. We deploy clips in all lesions and structures that we biopsy. This is necessary not only to help localize the lesion for subsequent image-guided needle localization should the lesion prove to be atypical or malignant, but also aids in interpreting follow-up screening and diagnostic mammography.

Core biopsies of the breast are usually performed with a 14-gauge needle. Early studies by Parker and colleagues showed fewer inadequate specimens in fatty and fibrous tissues with a 14-gauge than with an 18-gauge needle. However, 18-gauge core needles are quite adequate for lymph node biopsies, particularly the variety in which the aperture first can be pre-positioned precisely, with only the outer cannula being fired in order to obtain the specimen.

We use two basic sizes of direction vacuum-assisted needles 10 to 11 gauge or 7 to 9 gauge. The smaller needles are used for smaller nodules while the larger bore needles are used to biopsy more widely spread calcifications, for lesions that correlate with non-mass-like enhancement on MRI, and to remove larger probably benign lesions.

While there are no hard and fast rules for when to use core biopsy and when to use directional vacuum-assisted biopsy, we do have some general guidelines. In general, we use a 9 to 11 gauge DVAB device for all lesions 10 mm or less in maximum diameter, because studies by Parker and colleagues showed fewer insufficient and false negative results (compared with surgical excisional biopsy) for DVAB devices than for core needle biopsy in such cases. In general, a 14-gauge core device is adequate to diagnose lesions 1.5 cm or larger. However, we will use a 7, 8, or 9 gauge DVAB device to attempt to completely remove all imaging evidence of probably benign lesions if that is the patient's choice (Fig. 10-17). It should be remembered that removing imaging evidence of a breast lesion is not the same as removing all histologic evidence of the lesion. Large bore vacuum devices are approved for diagnosis, not treatment. Thus, a marker must always be deployed, even when a lesion appears to have been completely removed. For lesions that are 11 to 14 mm, we usually perform DVAB. In cases of non-mass-like enhancement, clumped or ductal enhancement on MRI that correspond only to prominent ducts or lobules on second look ultrasound, we usually deploy 7- to 9-gauge DVAB devices.

Even when a lesion appears to have been completely removed, microscopic bits and even parts of the lesion may remain. Shadowing caused by large bore vacuum needles and bleeding that occurs during biopsy can both obscure residual areas of a biopsied lesion. For malignant or atypical lesions, even when DVAB appears to have removed all imaging evidence of the lesions, an ultrasound-guided needle localization excisional biopsy will still be necessary. Thus, a marker should be deployed on all biopsies to help localize the lesion for later excision.

The markers deployed at ultrasound-guided biopsies usually contain a substance that is hyperechoic enough to be visible on ultrasound and a metal clip that can be visualized on mammography and MRI. When multiple biopsies are being performed in a breast, metal clips of different shapes can be used to distinguish biopsy sites from each other on postmammography. Postbiopsy mammograms are obtained in all cases. Most of the time postbiopsy mammograms are obtained immediately after the biopsy. However, if there has been bleeding or development of a hematoma during biopsy, we wait 2 or 3 days before obtaining the postbiopsy mammograms. The ultrasound visible portion of the marker usually is visible for only a period of time. This varies from a few weeks to a few months between marker types. The stainless steel or titanium clip contained within gel or Gelfoam, however, remains permanently visible on mammography. Titanium markers, however, can be difficult to see on MRI.

When ultrasound guidance is used to biopsy microcalcifications, specimen radiographs and postbiopsy mammograms should be obtained. The specimen radiograph confirms that there are microcalcifications within the specimen, and the postbiopsy marker mammograms confirm that some or all of the calcifications have been removed and that the clip is in the immediate vicinity of the suspicious calcifications (Fig. 10-18).

When ultrasound guidance is used for needle localization, specimen ultrasound can be helpful to confirm that the suspicious lesion is contained within the surgical specimen.

Screening

A detailed discussion of how to interpret breast ultrasound is beyond the scope of this chapter, but a general overview of the principles guiding interpretation is not. We must consider general and specific goals, the range of normal anatomy, and how pathology alters or destroys the normal anatomy. We must also be aware of the great heterogeneity of both invasive and non-invasive cancer and how this affects our interpretation.

Goals

It is essential to have realistic goals for diagnostic breast ultrasound. It is unreasonable to expect that sonography will enable us to distinguish between benign and malignant lesions in all situations. We have never been able to do this in the past, cannot accomplish it now, and likely never will be able to achieve this. However, it is realistic to think that we can correctly assign a suspicious or malignant category (BI-RADS 4 or 5) to 98% or more of all malignant lesions. Furthermore, it is realistic to think that we can identify some subset of all benign nodules that can be characterized as benign with 98% or greater certainty (BI-RADS 3). It is also quite reasonable to expect that we can identify normal structures or definitively benign lesions as the cause of palpable or mammographic abnormalities in a large majority of cases.

Identifying Structures

It is important to identify normal anatomic structures such as ducts, lobules (TDLUs), dense interlobular stromal fibrous tissue, loose periductal and intralobular stromal fibrous tissues, Cooper ligaments and other septae, anterior and posterior mammary fascia, and the superficial fascia. While it is generally appropriate to classify water density

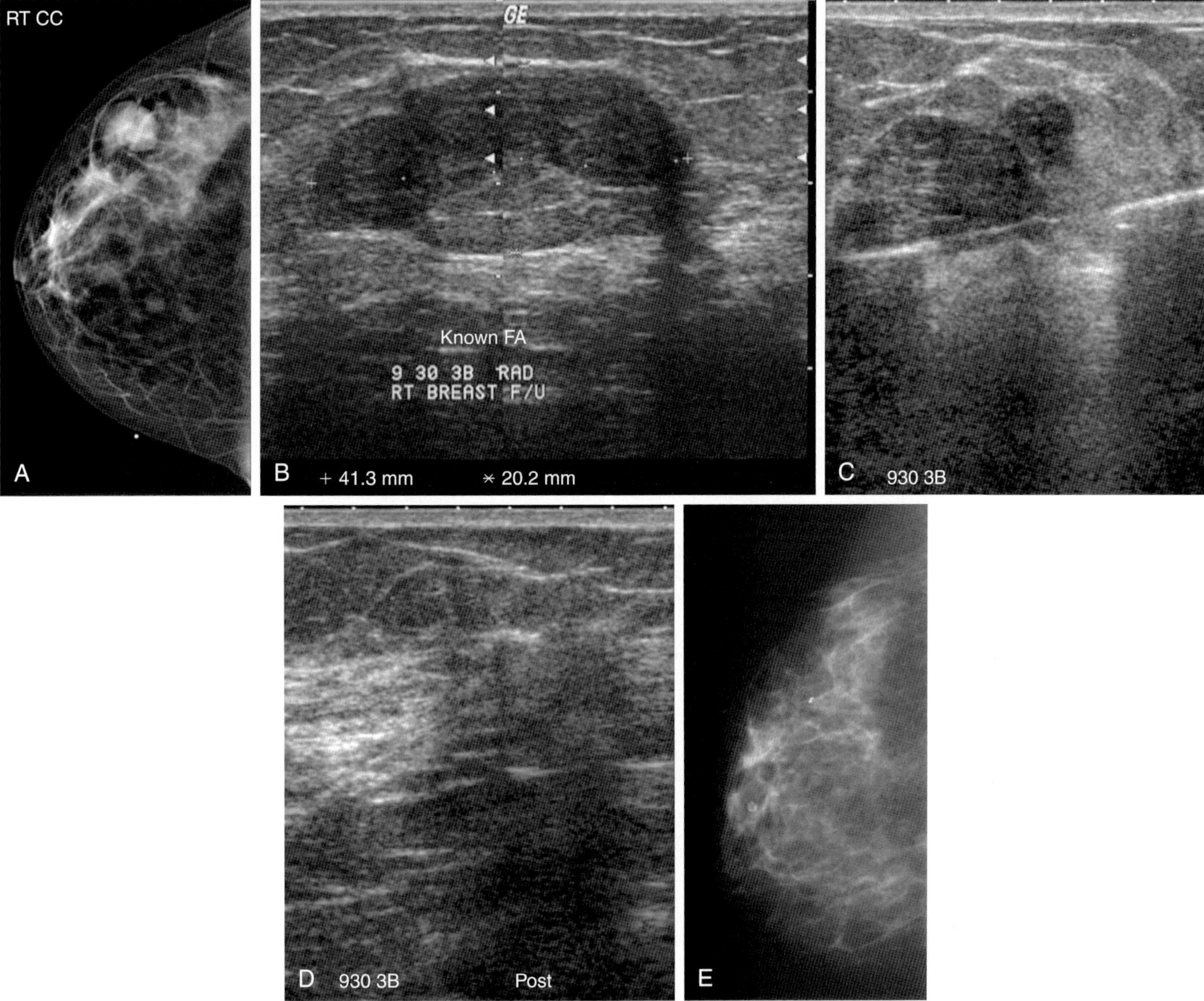

■ **FIGURE 10-17** **A,** Mammogram shows a large lobular, circumscribed mass. **B,** Diagnostic ultrasound shows a 4.1 cm oval, circumscribed hypoechoic solid mass with a thin echogenic border (Breast Imaging Reporting and Data System (BI-RADS) 3) compatible with a large fibroadenoma. **C,** Image obtained at the start of ultrasound guided directional vacuum-assisted biopsy (DVAB) shows the probe deep to the lesion. **D,** Postbiopsy sonogram shows no imaging evidence of a residual lesion. **E,** Postbiopsy mammogram confirms that there is no imaging evidence of a residual lesion and also, that despite the large size of the lesion prebiopsy, there is no postbiopsy hematoma.

tissue seen on mammography as *fibroglandular*, to do so is insufficient for sonography. Sonography can show four different echogenicities for water density and thus, it can more specifically identify the individual elements of the breast than can mammography in most cases. The identification of TDLUs is important because approximately 90% of all benign and malignant breast pathology arises within the lobule. The identification of ducts is important because about 10% of benign and malignant breast processes arise within the ducts and because breast cancer can use the ductal framework as one method of growing and spreading. The anterior and posterior mammary fascia are important because between them lies the mammary zone, where all of the ducts and virtually all of the TDLUs lie. Thus, almost all true breast pathology arises within the mammary zone (Fig. 10-19). Understanding this enables us to place our focal zones where they will do the most good. Cooper ligaments are important, because their bases are points of low resistance to invasion and a frequent site for development of angular margins that we find so useful in characterizing solid breast nodules. The superficial mammary fascia is important because Cooper ligaments insert into it and because there is a rich network of lymphatics just superficial to it (Fig. 10-20). Cancers that arise superficially near the superficial fascia and those that arise more deeply in the breast but invade up Cooper's ligaments to the superficial fascia are especially likely to invade the rich lymphatics there and to be associated with positive lymph nodes in a high percentage of cases. Almost all benign aberrations of normal development and involution (ANDIs) arise from and alter the shape, size, echogenicity, and/or sound transmission through the ducts and lobules. Most, but not all, in situ malignant lesions alter the ducts and lobules to a greater extent than do benign ANDIs.

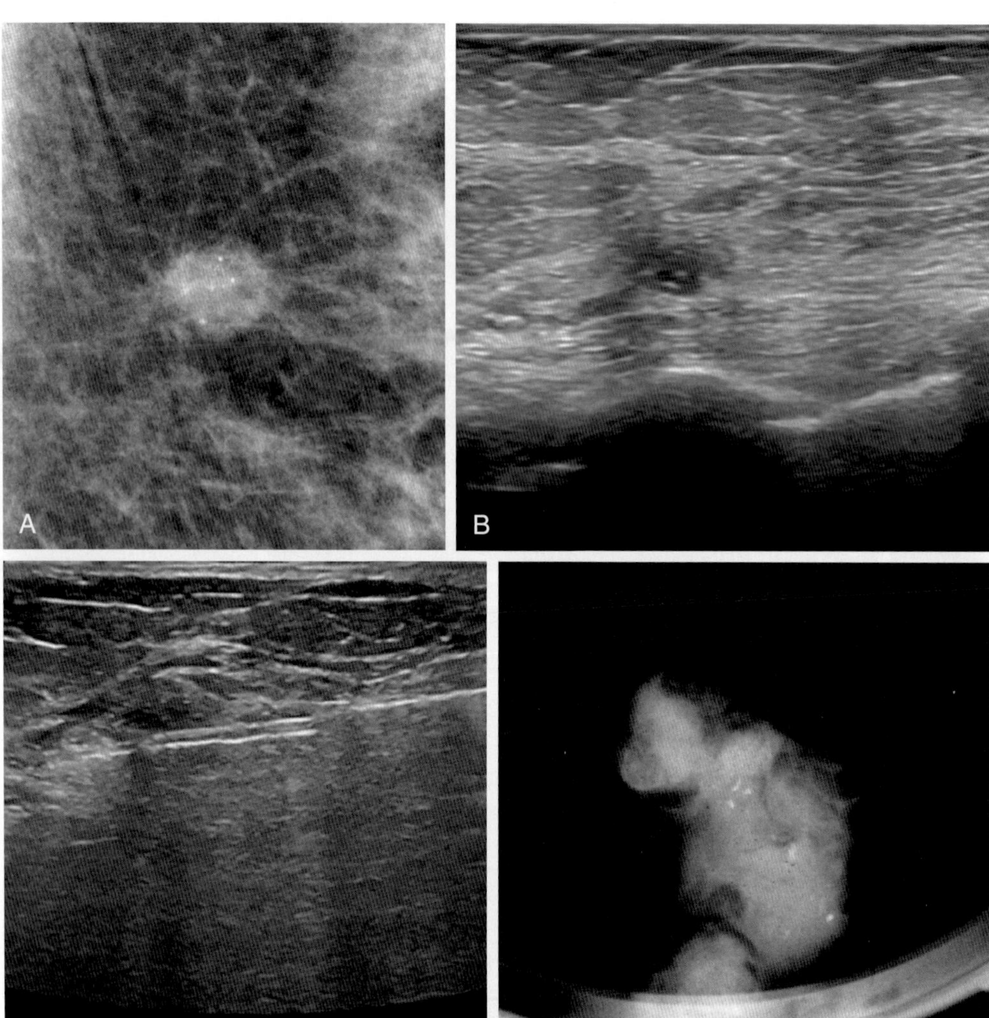

■ **FIGURE 10-18** **A,** Mammography shows a small round indistinct mass with microcalcifications. **B,** Ultrasound shows a small oval indistinct mass containing microcalcifications. **C,** Imaging obtained during ultrasound guided directional vacuum-assisted biopsy (DVAB) shows the mass within the aperture immediately prior to beginning. **D,** Specimen radiography confirms that the calcifications are within the specimen.

Invasive malignant lesions usually have associated in situ components that alter ducts and lobules, but the invasive components tend to destroy normal fascia and tissue planes as well. Recognizing the range of normal anatomy and when anatomy is altered beyond normal or even destroyed, is the key to diagnosing small killing cancers. Recognizing the range of normal is important in avoiding unnecessary further work-up or biopsy.

Solid Breast Nodules

When a lesion is large enough that it can no longer be recognized as being within normal ducts or lobules, we classify it as a mass or nodule and characterize it to assess its risk for being malignant and to determine the need for biopsy. The rules that we use for characterizing solid breast nodules are not unique to ultrasound. In fact, the use of multiple findings, six of the nine major findings we use, and the algorithm in which we use the findings were all developed first for mammography and merely borrowed by and applied to ultrasound. The general principle is that because of the heterogeneity of breast cancer, single findings can only identify a fraction of malignant breast nodules. To correctly classify 98% or more of all malignant nodules as BI-RADS 4 or 5 requires the use of multiple different findings that together achieve a sensitivity of 98% or greater even though none of the individual findings can do so. Some findings must be good for spiculated lesions, while others must be good for circumscribed invasive or in situ lesions. The suspicious findings can be characterized as shapes, surface characteristics, or internal characteristics. They can also be characterized as hard, soft, or indeterminate. Hard findings involve the destruction of normal anatomy and correlate with the presence of invasive carcinoma. Hard findings include spiculation, thick, echogenic halo, angular margins, and acoustic shadowing (Fig. 10-21). Soft findings represent distortion of normal anatomy without its destruction. Soft findings include effects on ducts within the tissues that surround the lesion (duct extension and branch pattern), microcalcifications, and most microlobulations (Fig. 10-22). The positive

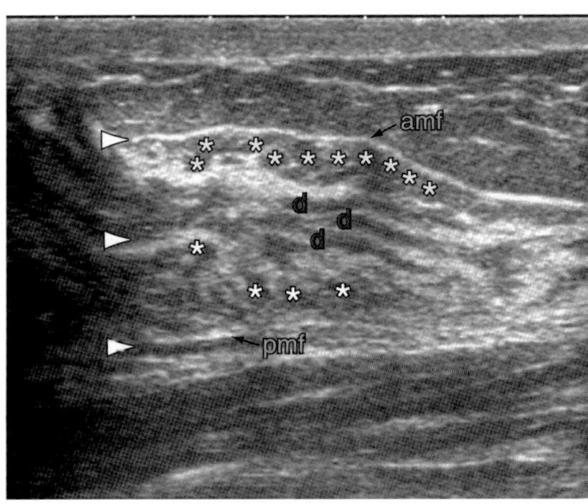

■ **FIGURE 10-19** The mammary zone lies between the anterior mammary fascia (amf) and the posterior mammary fascia (pmf). The mammary zone has a hilar-like structure similar to that of lung or kidney. The lobules (*asterisks*) are located around the periphery of the zone and the ducts (d) lie primarily within the center of the mammary zone. In most patients lobules are more numerous anteriorly than posteriorly. In this patient the anterior lobules are so numerous that some of them touch each other, obscuring the hyperechoic fibrous tissue between them and forming a continuous sheet of isoechoic tissue. Virtually all true breast pathology arises within the mammary zone from either lobules (90%) or ducts (10%). Thus, the transmit focusing that the sonographer or sonologist can control should be optimized within the entire mammary zone when in survey mode. Optimally focusing the entire mammary zone usually requires 3 transmit zones, one at the amf one at the pmf and one near the middle of the mammary zone (*white triangles*). The depth and spacing of the focal zones will vary from one patient to another and will also vary with the distance from the nipple.

predictive values of soft findings are better if soft findings are combined, especially if microcalcifications occur within ducts or microlobulations (Fig. 10-23). Soft findings can be seen with circumscribed invasive carcinoma and/or pure in situ carcinoma. There are nonspecific findings that can occur with either invasive carcinoma or CIS: non-parallel (taller-than-wide) orientation; and markedly hypoechoic texture, in comparison to fat (Fig. 10-24).

The algorithm first requires a search for each suspicious finding. If even a single suspicious finding is present, the nodule should be characterized as at least suspicious (BI-RADS 4), and the lesion should be recommended for biopsy. If no suspicious finding is present, specific benign findings should be sought. The classical probably benign findings of fibroadenomas are an oval or gently lobulated shape, an orientation that is wider than tall or parallel to the skin, and a circumscribed margin with a thin, echogenic pseudocapsule of compressed fibrous tissue (Fig. 10-25). Lesions that have no suspicious features and have the above reassuring findings have been benign 97.3% of the time in my experience.

Cysts

Cysts that are simple are benign in all cases. Cysts that are not simple generate much anxiety in patients, referring physicians, sonographers, and radiologists. In general cysts give rise to more concern than is merited in most cases. Good general rules are that: (1) Almost all cysts, simple or non-simple are benign; (2) malignant breast cysts are relatively rare; (3) most malignant cystic lesions really appear to be solid nodules that have undergone cystic or hemorrhagic infarction; and (4) a malignant breast cyst that could be mistakenly characterized as benign is truly exceedingly rare. However, as reassuring as these general rules may be in a population of patients, they may be far less reassuring in individual patients, many of whom are convinced that they are the exception to the rule. Thus, we must have a systematic way of assessing breast cysts that are not simple. First, we use features of ultrasound equipment and sonographic techniques that minimize artifact within cysts

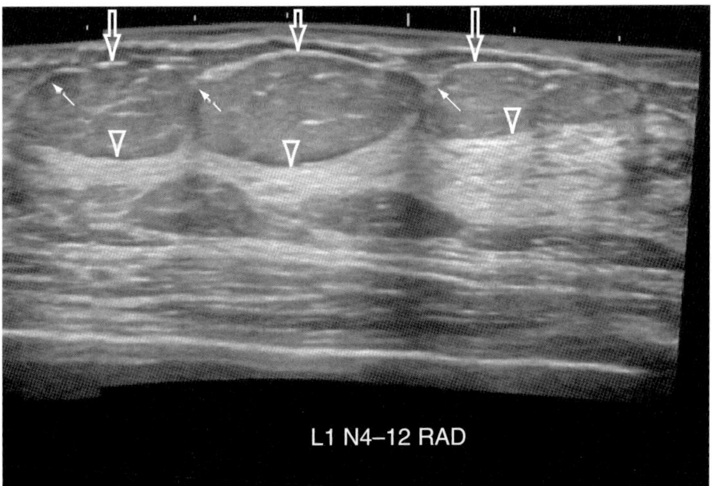

■ **FIGURE 10-20** The Cooper ligaments, which are formed by two layers of anterior mammary fascia, (*hollow arrowheads*) attach (*white arrows*) to the superficial fascia (*hollow arrows*) anteriorly. The superficial fascia is important because a rich network of lymphatics surrounds it. Malignant lesions that arise superficially near the superficial fascia and lesions that arise within the mammary zone, but invade superficially up Cooper ligaments to the superficial fascia, are particularly likely to have invaded lymphatic channels and metastasized to axillary lymph nodes.

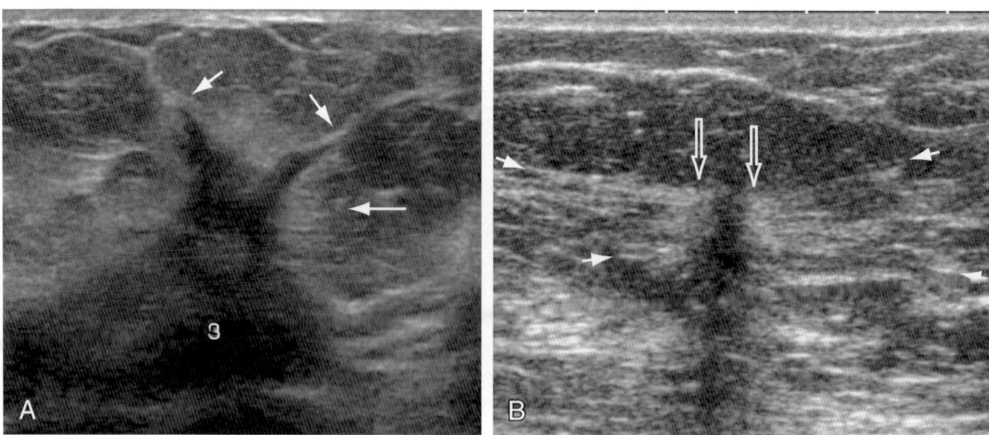

■ **FIGURE 10-21** **A,** The lesion on the left shows multiple highly suspicious (hard) findings that include: angular margins within the bases of Cooper ligaments (*short white arrows*), hyperechoic spiculation (*long white arrows*), and partial acoustic shadowing (*s*). Most malignant masses have more than one suspicious feature. **B,** The mass on the right is an irregular, hypoechoic mass with posterior acoustic shadowing and has a thick echogenic halo adjacent to the mass (*large hollow arrows*). Farther from the mass the individual spicules (*small arrows*) can be identified.

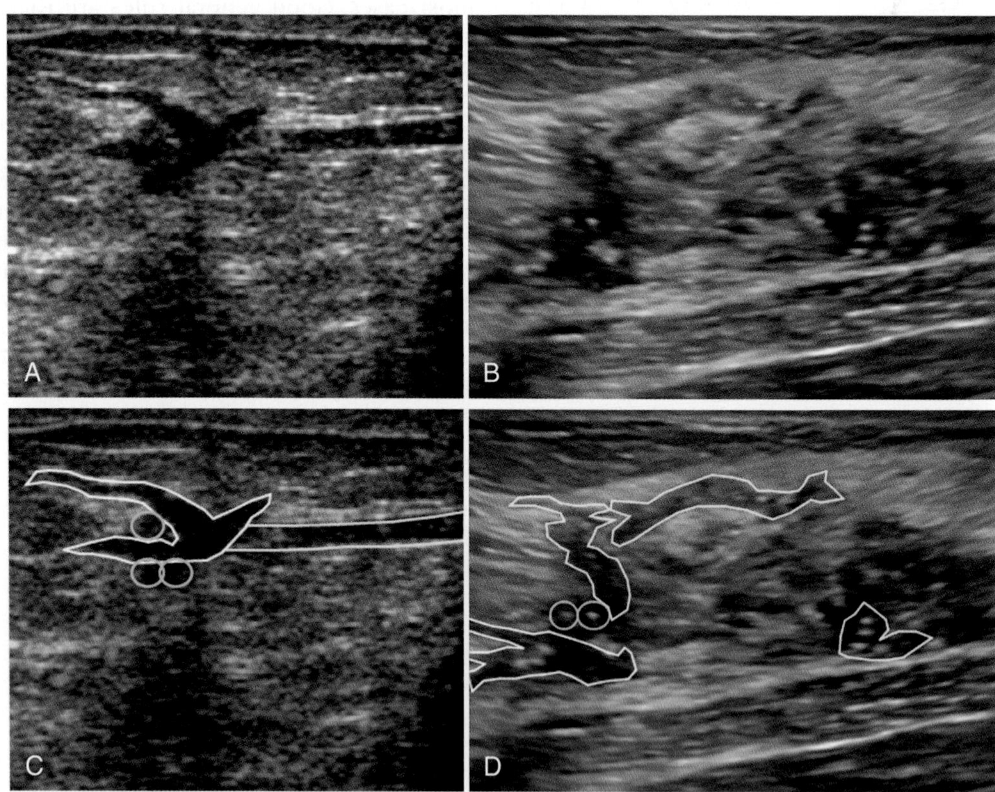

■ **FIGURE 10-22** Less suspicious (soft findings) are usually associated with carcinoma in situ. Soft findings include duct extension, branch pattern, microlobulations, and microcalcifications. The most predictive microcalcifications occur within other soft findings. **A** and **B,** Two lesions. **C** and **D,** the same two lesions with the pertinent findings outlined in color. **C,** duct extension (*yellow outline*), branch pattern (*white outline*), and microlobulation (*aqua outline*). **D,** multiple microcalcifications, some within the mass, but many within affected ducts that lie at the edge of the mass or within the surrounding tissues. Also shown are duct extensions (*yellow outline*), branching ducts (*white outline*), and microlobulations (*aqua outline*).

to exclude *pseudo-non-simple* cysts. Features that minimize artifact include digitally encoded tissue harmonics, spatial compounding, and speckle reduction algorithms. Once we have minimized artifact, we divide the true non-simple cysts into complicated and complex categories. Complicated cysts have echogenic fluid, floating or dependent debris (Fig. 10-26). Cysts with low level internal echoes caused by fatty or proteinaceous material within the fluid are complicated and almost always benign. In a small percentage of cases it may be difficult

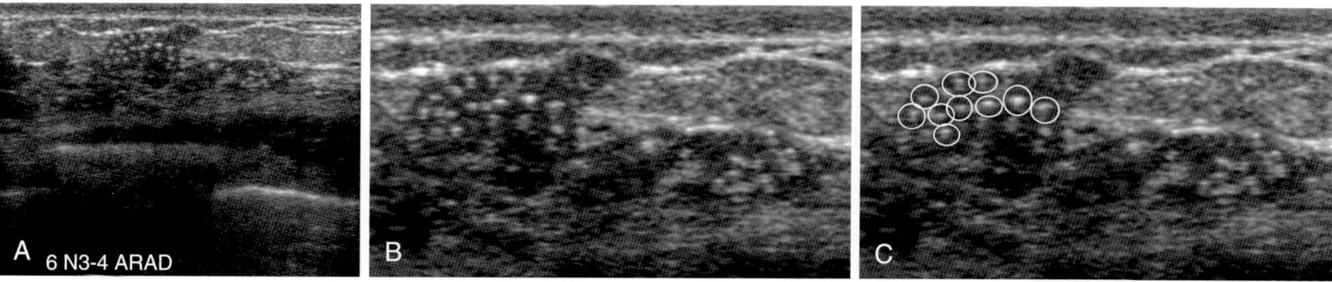

■ **FIGURE 10-23** **A,** Soft findings have better positive predictive value when combined, particularly when calcifications occur within microlobulations. **B,** That the calcifications lie within microlobulations is more evident when the image is magnified. Each microlobulation represents a carcinoma in situ (CIS)-distended duct that has necrosis within its lumen and calcifications within the necrosis. **C,** Several microlobulations have been outlined on the magnified views.

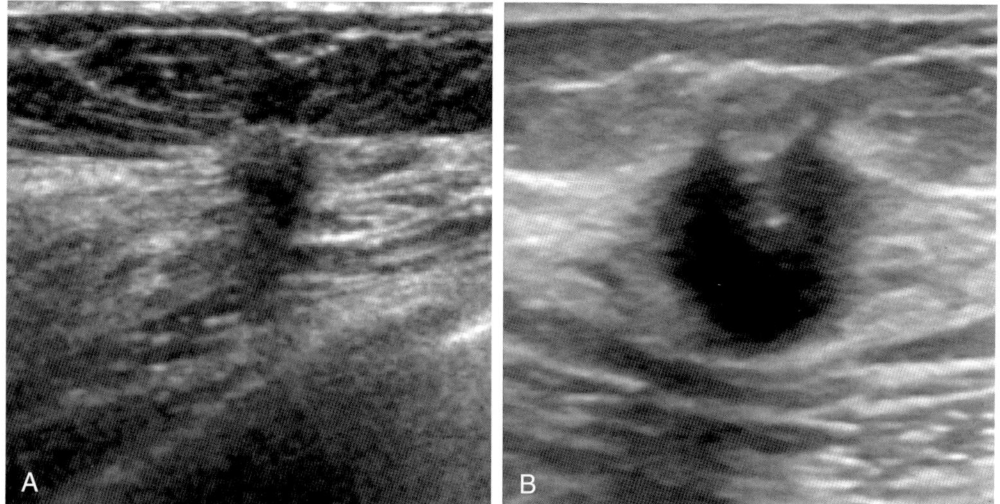

■ **FIGURE 10-24** **A,** This small grade 1 invasive ductal carcinoma is seen as an irregular, spiculated mass oriented perpendicular to the skin, and therefore, can be classified as not parallel to the skin or taller-than-wide. This is a very typical orientation of small breast carcinomas at a stage when they affect a single terminal duct lobular unit (TDLU). Note that the shape is that of an enlarged and distorted anterior TDLU. **B,** This round, indistinct mass with an echogenic collar is a grade 2 invasive ductal carcinoma but is markedly hypoechoic compared with the surrounding fat.

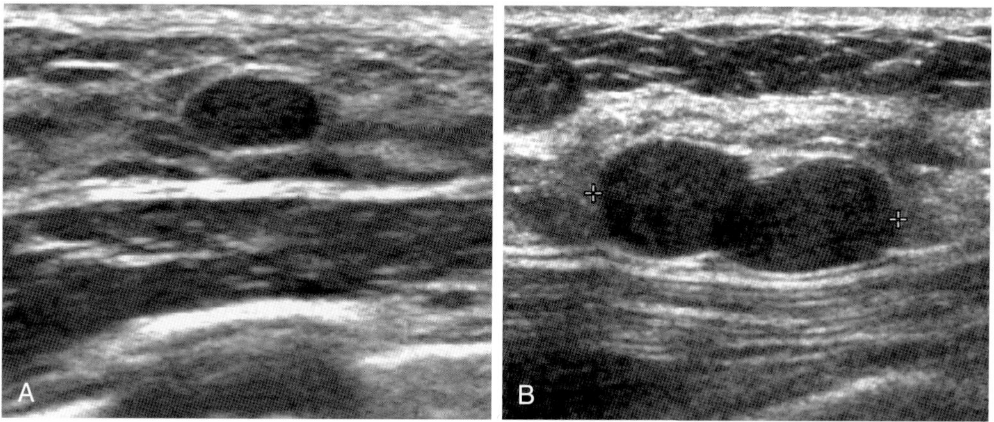

■ **FIGURE 10-25** **A,** The findings of mildly hypoechoic to isoechoic solid nodule that is oval in shape, parallel in orientation, well-circumscribed, with a delimiting thin hyperechoic pseudocapsule of compressed tissue comprise one classical appearance of fibroadenoma. **B,** The findings of a gently lobulated solid nodule that is oriented parallel to the skin, well-circumscribed, and encompassed by a thin hyperechoic pseudocapsule comprise the other classical appearance of fibroadenoma.

to distinguish a complicated cyst with low-level internal echoes from a solid nodule such as a fibroadenoma with either gray scale or Doppler techniques and attempted aspiration has been necessary to make this distinction. Preliminary data suggest that shear wave elastography should be able to make this distinction and should make attempted aspiration unnecessary. Cysts with fat-fluidlevels and fluid-debris levels are almost always benign as well (as long as the wall is thin and there are no mural nodules or thick septi). Cysts that have small bright

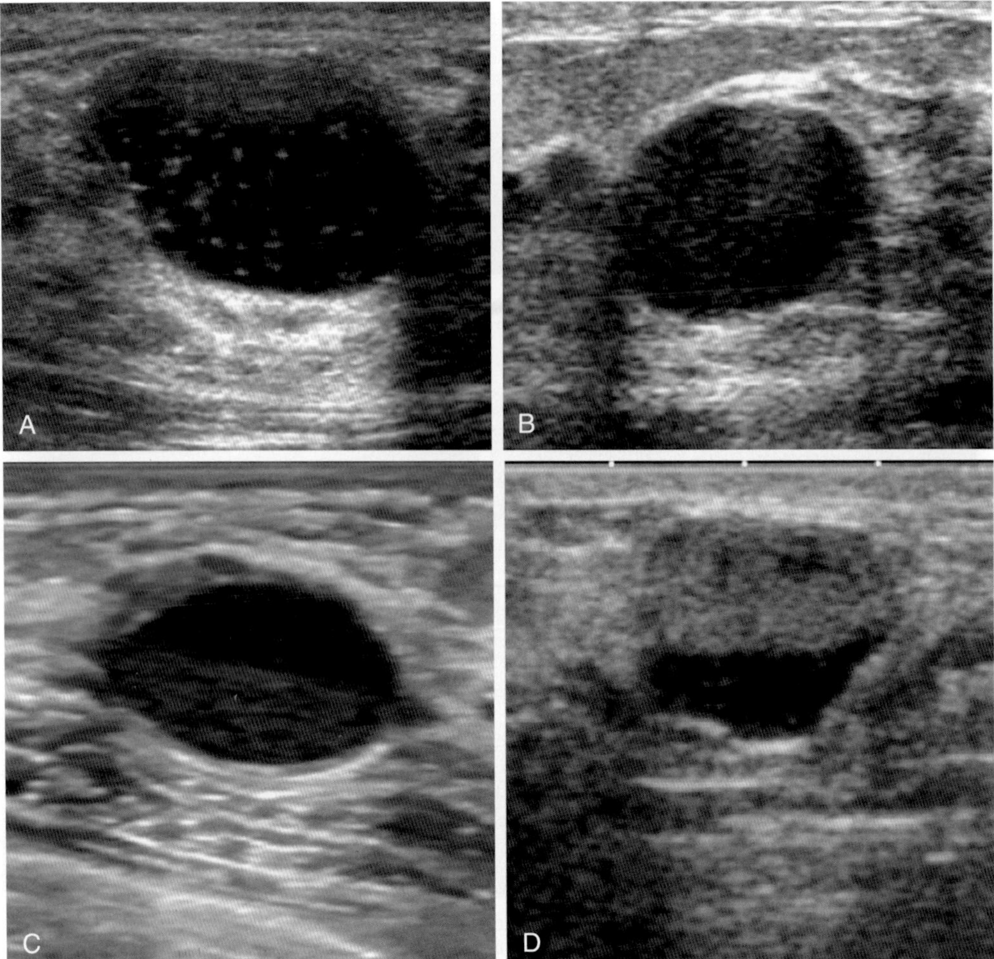

■ **FIGURE 10-26** Four examples of complicated cysts which are common entities within the benign fibrocystic change spectrum. **A,** Cyst with scintillating echoes. These bright echoes are subcellular in size and are pushed posteriorly by the energy of the ultrasound beam, particular when viewed with color or power Doppler. **B,** Cyst with diffuse low-level internal echoes that are caused by either proteinaceous or lipid material within the cyst fluid. Occasionally, it can be difficult to determine whether a lesion is a cyst with low-level internal echoes or a solid nodule. Tumefactive debris can simulate a mural nodule. **C,** Cyst with a fluid-debris level. The debris is proteinaceous in most cases, but can represent blood or pus in others. **D,** Cyst with a fat-fluid level. Such cysts are commonly lined by apocrine cells that release fat into the cyst fluid. The echogenic lipid layer, like a debris layer, can simulate a mural nodule.

echoes that move with the energy of the ultrasound or Doppler beam (acoustic radiation force), called *scintillating echoes*, also are complicated cysts. The particles that create these mobile echoes are subcellular in size and almost invariably associated with benign fibrocystic change or ANDIs. Complex masses manifest irregular wall thickening, mural nodules, or thick septations (Fig. 10-27). When malignant, they may be associated with enlarged or too numerous ducts, or both, within the tissues surrounding the cysts (Fig. 10-28). Complex masses have a higher risk of being papillomatous or malignant than do complicated cysts. Certain clustered microcysts, those with suspended microcalcifications and internal blood flow, are at increased risk for malignancy, specifically micropapillary CIS. While complex masses and some microcysts are at higher risk for malignancy than are complicated cysts, most complex masses and most clusters of microcysts are merely manifestations of benign fibrocystic change with associated florid apocrine metaplasia. In some cases a nonsimple cyst may demonstrate both complicated and complex features. In such cases, we must err on the side of caution and characterize the cyst as complex. Most simple and benign complicated cysts require no further imaging and do not require aspiration, except for relief of pain. Complicated cysts that are incidental, multiple, and/or bilateral are almost always benign, can be classified as BI-RADS 2, and do not require follow-up. Dominant complicated cysts that present as palpable lumps or mammographic abnormalities may be classified as BI-RADS 3 and followed. Tender complicated cysts may be aspirated for symptomatic relief. Complex masses that are suspicious for intracystic papilloma or intracystic carcinoma should not be assessed with aspiration and fluid

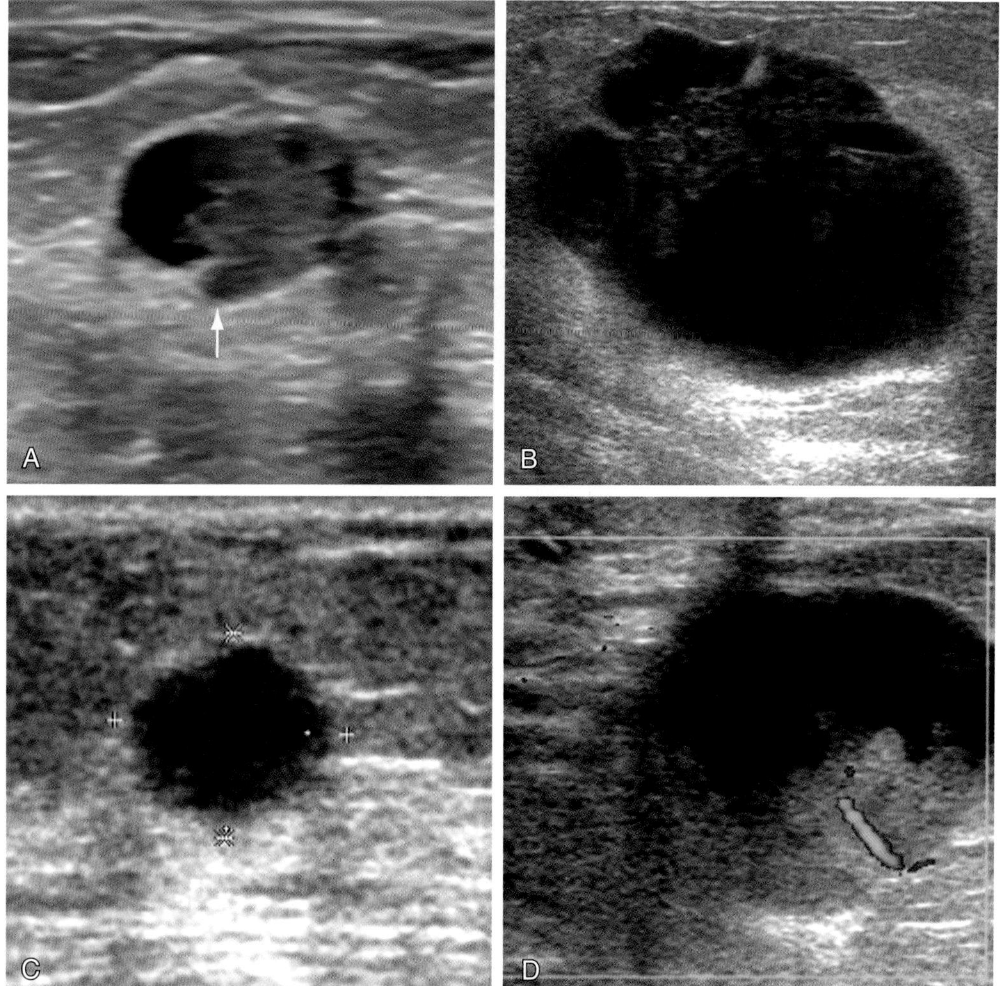

■ **FIGURE 10-27** Four examples of complex masses. These are more likely to contain papillomas or malignancy, although papillary apocrine metaplasia can also give rise to such lesions. **A,** An intracystic papilloma presents as a complex mass with a mural nodule that is growing out of the cyst into a duct (*arrow*). **B,** An intracystic carcinoma in situ (CIS) presents as a complex mass with a thick isoechoic septation containing microcalcifications (echogenic foci). **C,** An intracystic invasive ductal carcinoma presents with diffuse irregularity of the cyst wall. **D,** An intracystic papilloma has a prominent vascular stalk. Both intracystic papillomas and intracystic carcinomas tend to be very vascular unless they have undergone infarction. Apocrine metaplasia, the other cause of mural nodules, thick septations, and irregular walls, does not have demonstrable vascularity.

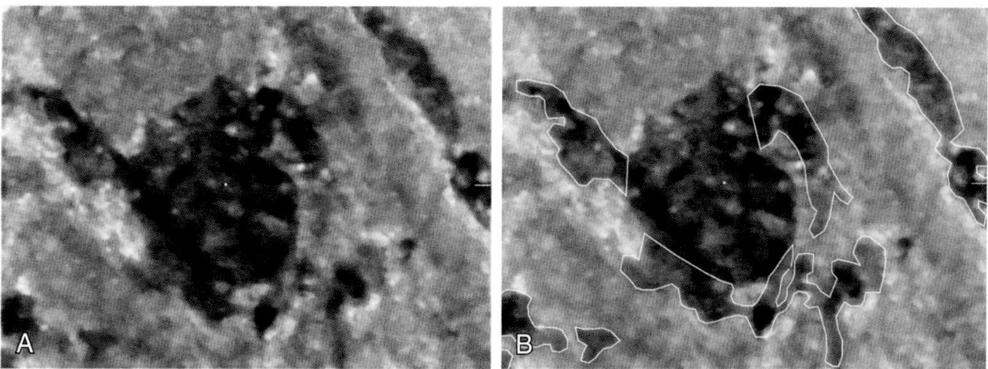

■ **FIGURE 10-28** **A,** Coronal reconstructed view of this micropapillary carcinoma in situ (CIS) shows extensive involvement of ducts surrounding the index lesion by micropapillary CIS. **B,** The affected ducts have been outlined.

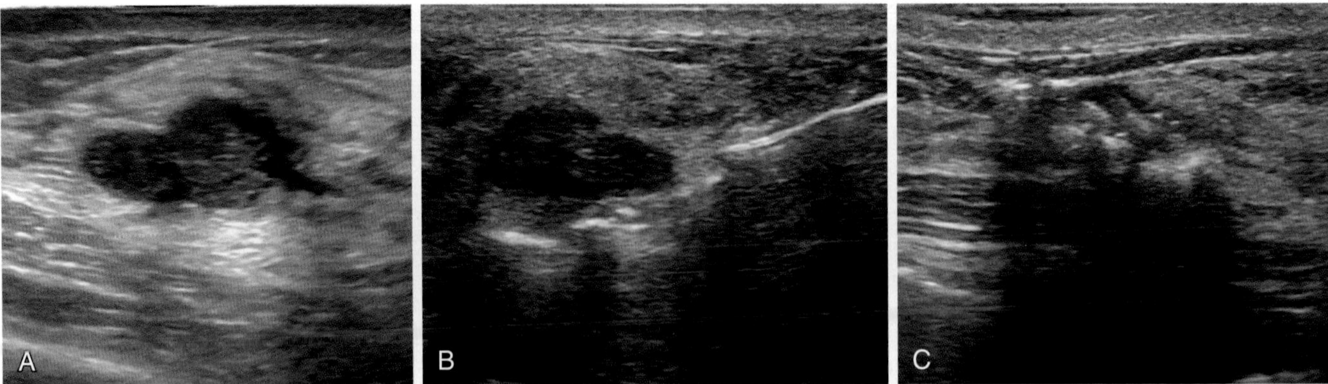

■ **FIGURE 10-29** Histology is preferable to cytology for complex masses. Directional vacuum-assisted biopsy (DVAB) is preferable to core biopsy for histologic evaluation of complex masses. A marker should always be deployed in case histology is malignant or atypical and requires excision. **A,** Bilobed intracystic papillary lesion. **B,** DVAB device has been placed deep to the lesion with the aperture directed anteriorly. **C,** Postbiopsy image shows lesion is gone. A Gelfoam marker has been placed.

cytology, as there are too many false positive and false negative results with fluid cytology. Suspicious complex masses require histologic evaluation. We prefer ultrasound-guided directional vacuum-assisted biopsy with deployment of a marker (Fig. 10-29), in case atypical or malignant histology requires later surgical resection. At sites where pathologists are reticent to diagnose papillary lesions from minimally invasive biopsy, ultrasound-guided needle localized excisional biopsy may be necessary for histologic diagnosis.

KEY POINTS

- Ultrasound of the breast is the main diagnostic test performed after mammography.
- Ultrasound is useful in assessing the cause of palpable and mammographic abnormalities and can be expected to show normal or definitively benign findings in more than 90% of cases that can make further work-up or biopsy unnecessary.

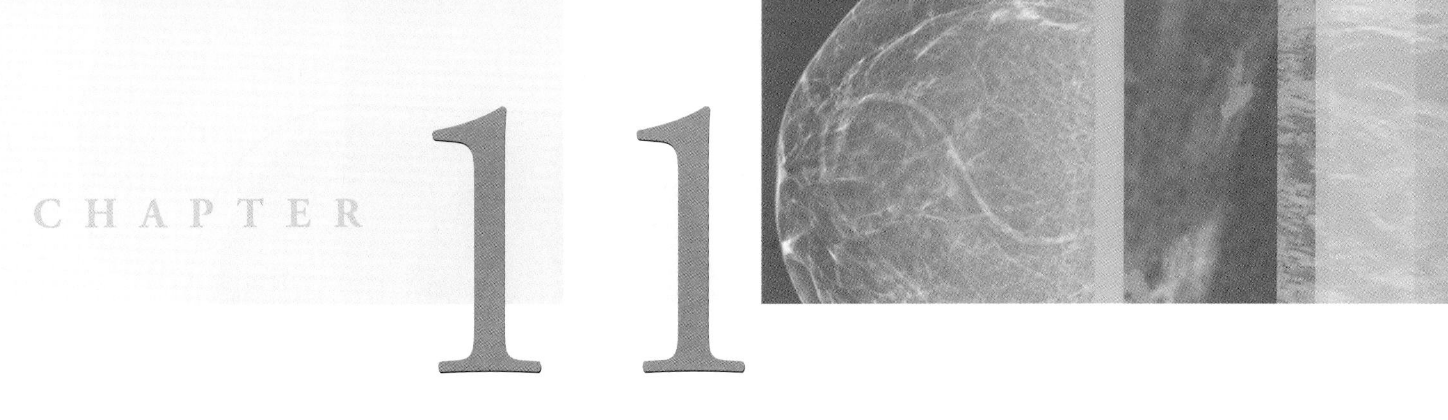

CHAPTER 11

Magnetic Resonance Equipment and Techniques

Thomas Oshiro, Helmuth Schultze-Haakh, and Jennifer Little

The foundations of magnetic resonance imaging (MRI) originate from a chemical analysis technique that incorporates the transmission and reception of radiofrequency (RF) signals within a high magnetic field. While Felix Bloch and Edward Purcell developed the analysis technique in the 1940s known as MR spectroscopy, in the 1970s, Paul Lauterbur and Peter Mansfield developed an imaging system based on Bloch and Purcell's theories.

With its ability to display soft tissue contrast, MRI has been shown to be useful in several areas of breast imaging including determining implant ruptures, performing needle guided biopsy procedures and breast cancer detection.

This chapter will focus on the technology behind the acquisition and will discuss the pulse sequences typically performed during an evaluation for breast cancer. As we will show, there are many factors involved when establishing breast MR protocols, evaluating the images and selecting equipment. Finally, some general guidelines for patient encountering and positioning will be reviewed. But before covering the specifics of breast MRI, we'll briefly cover the basic science of MR physics.

THE BASICS OF MAGNETIC RESONANCE THEORY

Magnetic Signal

The main component of an MRI system is the high strength magnet field created by a superconducting electromagnet (Fig. 11-1). Most clinical MR systems have magnet strengths ranging from 0.5 to 3 Tesla (5000-30,000 gauss). Higher field whole body systems are in use as research tools,[1] but are not yet approved by the U.S. Food and Drug Administration (FDA).

The signal acquired from MRI systems predominately comes from the hydrogen protons within the body, specifically, those from water and fat. All protons inherently have a nuclear "spin" and a resulting intrinsic magnetic field (Fig. 11-2A). Figure 11-2B shows the vector diagram with respect to the main magnetic field (B_0) of the magnet. The green arrow symbolizes the magnetization perpendicular to the B_0 field.

As protons (^1H nuclei) in the body are placed inside the strong external magnetic field (B_0), two phenomena occur. Firstly, the protons will orient either with (parallel) or against (anti-parallel) the B_0 field as shown in Figure 11-3. The excess amount of nuclei oriented parallel with the external magnetic field is known as the *net magnetization* (M_0) and is the basis for the MR signal. The green perpendicular magnetization vectors will cancel out due to their random orientation. The resulting M_0 is parallel to the main magnetic field. Stronger field strengths will produce a larger percentage of nuclei in alignment with the B_0 field and M_0 will be larger. Secondly, the proton "spins" will naturally precess around the external magnetic field at a frequency dependent on the external magnetic field strength. (Fig. 11-2C) Table 11-1 shows precessional frequencies (ω_0) for different field strengths.

The challenge for signal detection arises from how to distinguish this small magnetization created by the nuclei (M_0) from the larger main magnetic field (B_0) as shown in Figure 11-3.

Magnetic Resonance

When RF energy is applied at the precessional frequency of the proton within the main magnetic field, individual spins will absorb energy and rotate to the anti-parallel

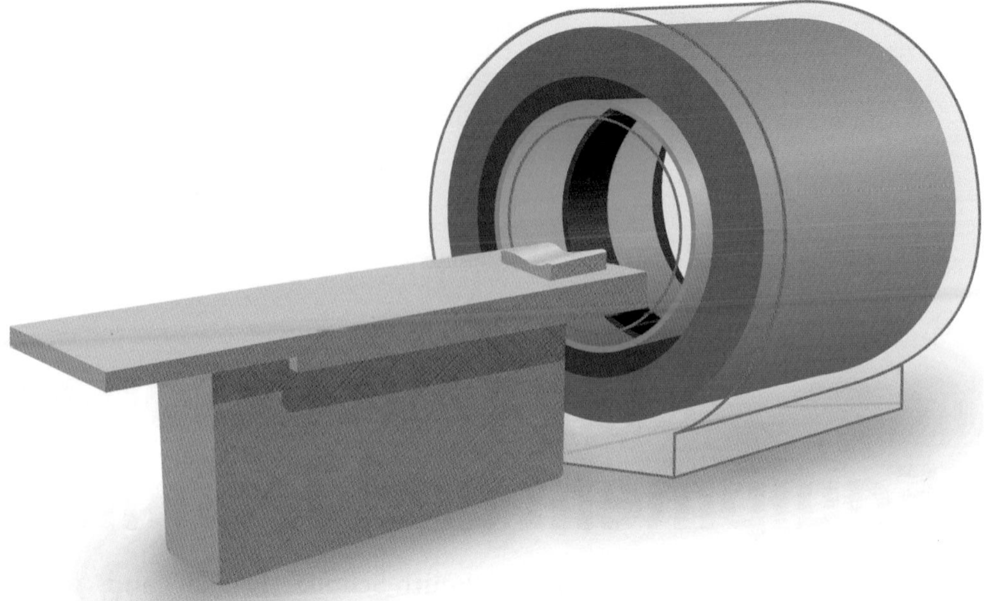

■ **FIGURE 11-1** Magnetic resonance scanner configuration. The magnetic field (B_0) is in the direction of the bore.

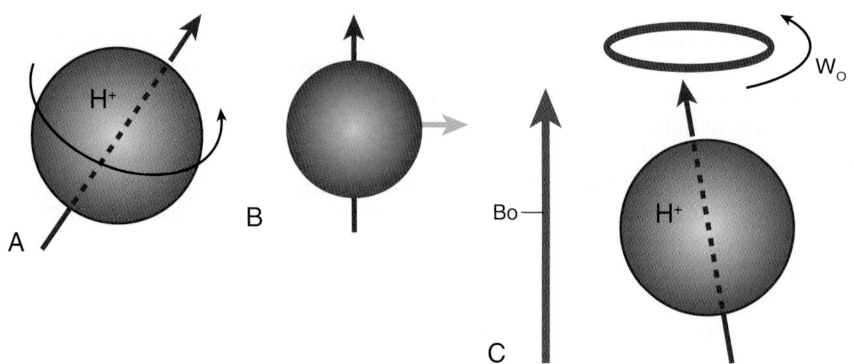

■ **FIGURE 11-2** A, The magnetic field (red) produced by spinning charge of a proton. **B**, Vector diagram of magnetization. **C**, Precession of proton due to the influence of external magnetic field (B_0)

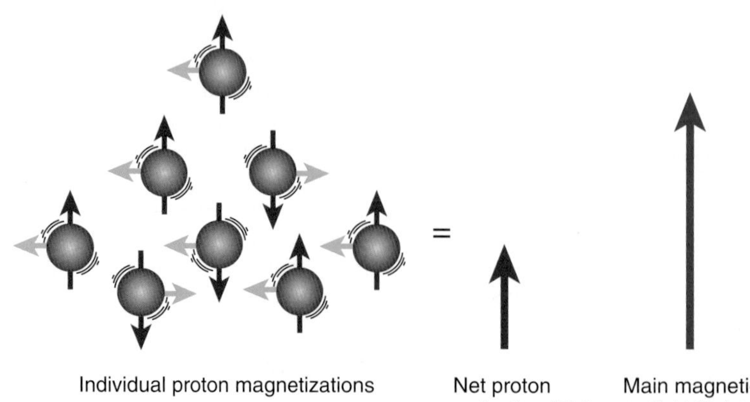

■ **FIGURE 11-3** Parallel and anti-parallel spins under the influence of the main magnetic field.

TABLE 11-1. Magnetic Field Strength and Precessional Frequency

Magnetic Field Strength	Precessional Frequency
0.5T	21.29 MHz
1.0T	42.57 MHz
1.5T	63.86 MHz
3.0T	127.71 MHz

position (transverse plane). As a result, the net magnetization also pulls away from the main magnetic field towards the anti-parallel position (Fig. 11-4). The angle between the main magnetic field (B_0) and the net magnetization (M_0) created by the RF pulse is called the *flip angle* (θ).

To apply the RF energy, RF coils located inside the MR system are tuned to the precessional frequency of the nuclei. A body coil is located in the surrounding structure of the MR system (see Fig. 11-1). However, close proximity of the coil to the anatomy will increase the signal-to-noise ratio (SNR) of the acquired image. Hence, anatomy specific coils are most often used for MR scanning. Figure 11-5 shows extremity, shoulder and head coils and Figure 11-6 shows a dedicated breast coil used for bilateral imaging.

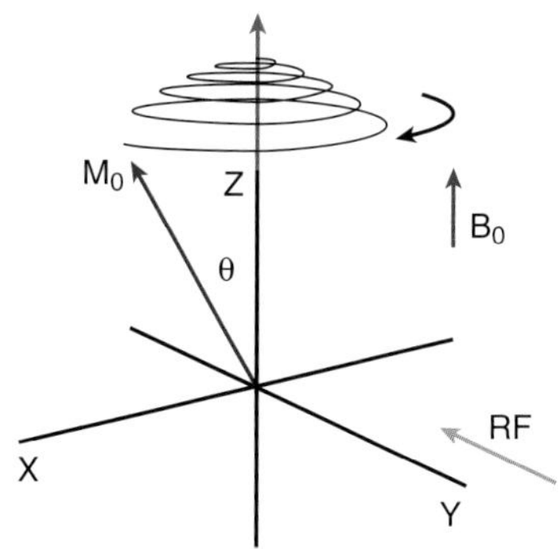

■ **FIGURE 11-4** Application of radiofrequency (RF) pulses causes the net magnification (M_0) to tip away from the magnetic field (B_0) by a flip angle (theta).

Relaxation

When the RF energy has stopped, the spins will "relax" back to their steady state position aligned with the external magnetic field (Fig. 11-7). There are two parameters of this relaxation process: T1 and T2. T1 relaxation (spin-lattice) is an indicator of how quickly protons will re-align with the main magnetic field as indicated by the blue arrow in Figure 11-7B. T2 (spin-spin) relaxation indicates how quickly the spins will be out of coherence due to

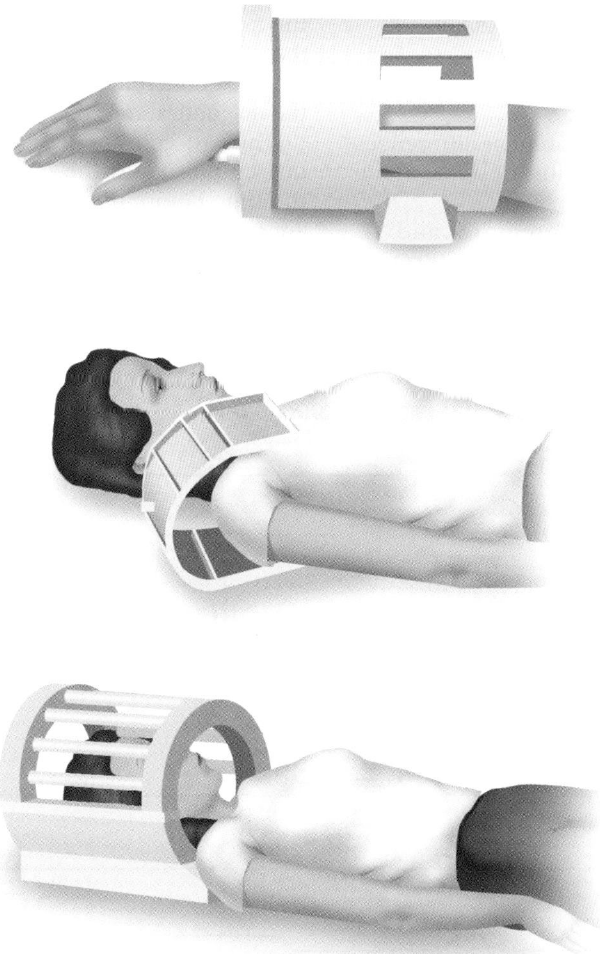

■ **FIGURE 11-5** Anatomy specific magnetic resonance (MR) coils.

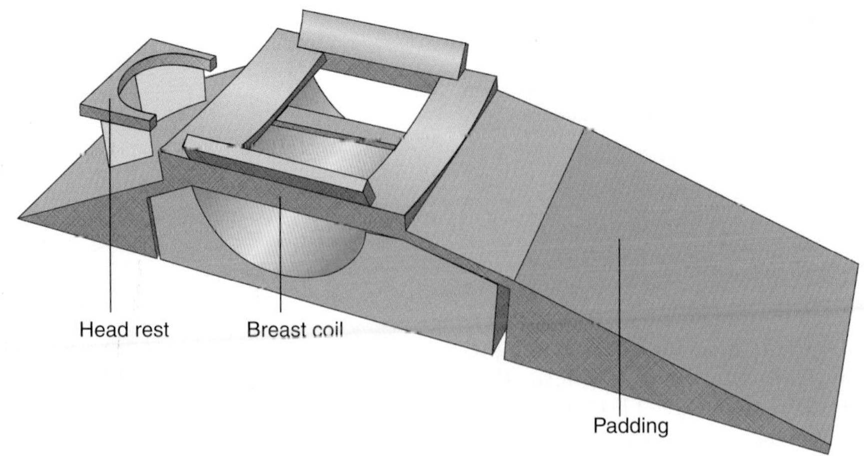

■ **FIGURE 11-6** Dedicated bilateral breast coil.

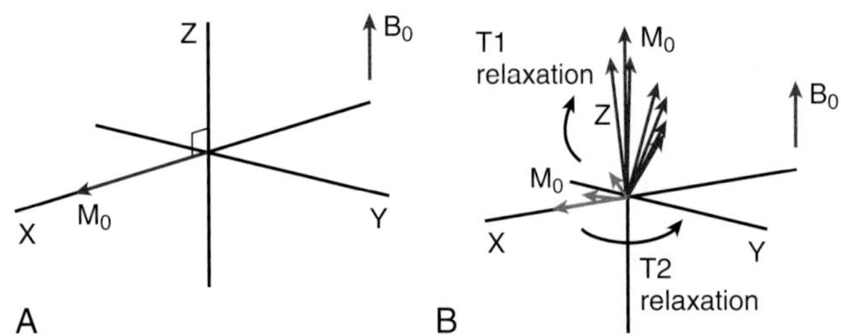

■ **FIGURE 11-7** **A**, Net magnetization position after application of a 90 degree flip angle. **B**, Net magnification (M_0) returns to magnetic field (B_0) alignment after radiofrequency (RF) energy terminates.

local magnetic field and chemical environment differences between the spins. This is shown as the loss of signal in the x-y direction (green arrow).

Different tissues will exhibit different T1 and T2 relaxation parameters and will be used to determine the contrast in the final image. Usually, T1 is much larger than T2.

Spin Echo Sequence

While used infrequently in breast MRI, the basic spin echo pulse sequence shown in Figure 11-8 demonstrates how the net magnetization is detected. The large body RF coil that is integrated into the bore of the magnet (see Fig. 11-1) is used to apply a 90 degree RF pulse. This is followed by a short time delay (TE/2) and then a 180 degree RF pulse is applied. The 180 degree pulse causes the net magnetization to refocus in the x-y direction and the T2 spin-spin decay reverses. Once the TE/2 delay time has again passed, the magnetization has regained coherence to a point where the RF coil can detect the magnetization. This re-coherent signal is called an *echo*.

Time to echo (TE) is the time between the initial 90 degree pulse and the echo time. Repetition time (TR) is the time before this sequence repeats. Typically, TE values are much shorter than TR. These variables along with the flip angle of the RF pulses (90 degrees for the spin echo sequences) are under the user's control and are used to modify the contrast of different tissues.

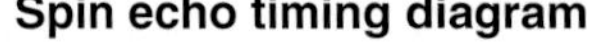

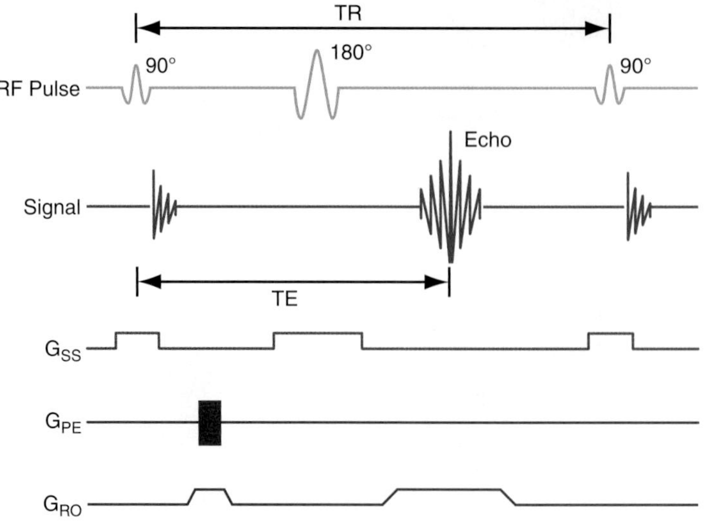

■ **FIGURE 11-8** Spin echo timing diagram.

The following equation determines the intensity of the received signal and tissue weighting for a spin echo sequence:

$$SI = \rho(1 - e^{\frac{-TR}{T1}})e^{\frac{-TE}{T2}}$$

Contrast between tissues with T1 differences (T1 weighting) can be accomplished by reducing the TE and TR values. T2 weighted imaging can be achieved by using a long TE and long TR value to reduce the T1 influence. Finally, a proton weighted sequence that minimizes both T1 and T2 relaxation effects can be achieved by using a short TE with a long TR.

While traditional spin echo sequences are not commonly used clinically, the general methodology for applying RF pulses and receiving the echo is applied in all pulse sequences. Faster sequences such as fast (turbo) spin echo and gradient echo sequences are more commonly used because of the increase in acquisition speed.

Image Formation

During the MR acquisition, three distinct magnetic gradient coils are activated at specific time points. These gradients spatially vary the external magnetic field based. The *slice select* gradient (G_{SS}) is switched on during the RF pulses (see Fig. 11-8). As a result, only protons in an anatomical "slice" are stimulated. A second set of gradient coils are activated during readout of the echo (G_{RO}) and a third set of coils will change the phase of the spins based on spatial positioning(G_{PE}). These gradients are known as the readout and phase encode gradients and are spatially applied orthogonally to each other.

Figure 11-9 shows the effect on the resonant frequency with respect to the readout gradient. As the gradient is applied, the spins experiencing a higher magnetic field will precess faster and those experiencing a lower magnetic field will precess slower. The echo is obtained while the readout gradient is active and therefore the location of spins can be discriminated via the resonant frequency of the echo.

Figure 11-10 shows the phase encode gradient applied in an orthogonal direction to the readout gradient. From Figure 11-8, the gradient (G_{PE}) is applied between the initial 90 degree RF pulse and the 180 degree refocusing pulse. Each time the spin echo sequence is repeated, the phase encode gradient is changed slightly in amplitude.

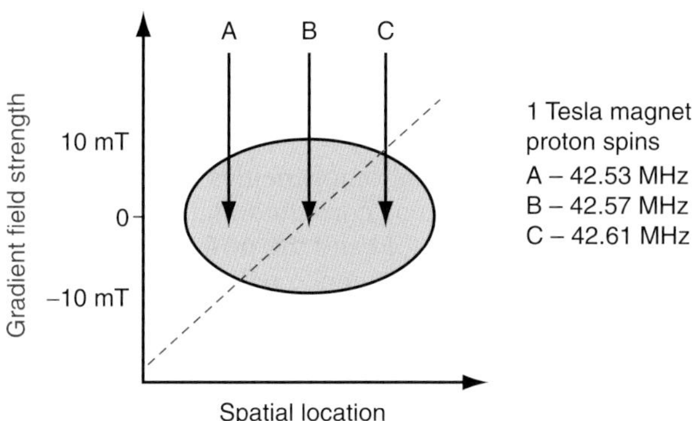

■ **FIGURE 11-9** Readout gradient effect on the resonant frequency.

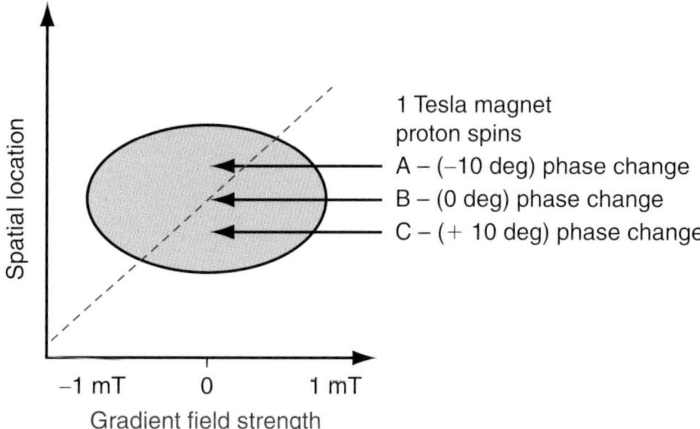

■ **FIGURE 11-10** Phase changes from the gradient applied in the phase encoding direction.

Every echo that is acquired will fill one line of data that is used to reconstruct the final image.

The spatial information received in an echo is based on the resonant frequency shift based on the readout gradient. This raw frequency domain image information is known as *k-space* and is shown in Figure 11-11. Once all k-space lines are filled, an inverse two-dimensional (2D) Fourier transform is applied to convert the frequency data back to spatial data for presentation (Fig. 11-12).

Three dimensional (3D) acquisitions are acquired by the application of an additional phase encode gradient in the slice-thickness direction. A 3D k-space data set is obtained and reconstructed into an image data set by the application of a 3D Fourier transform.

BREAST MAGNETIC RESONANCE PROTOCOLS

While there are several variations in breast MR protocols for the evaluation of breast cancer, a sample protocol is listed here.

1. Scout (localizer)
2. T1 weighted series without fat saturation and without contrast
3. T2 weighted images, with fat saturation and without contrast
4. Dynamic T1 weighted 3D images with fat saturation and with contrast injection

Each sequence will be discussed. However, it is important to note that there are differing opinions on the clinical benefits of viewing the morphology of a lesion with higher resolution scanning versus high temporal resolution (low scan time) contrast enhancement analysis. Large-scale clinical studies have yet to determine the optimal imaging sequence to improve specificity and sensitivity. In this context, Table 11-2 shows some generally agreed upon equipment standards for breast imaging and Table 11-3 shows image acquisition standards for the protocols mentioned above.

The scout (localizer) acquisition verifies correct positioning and field of view. An axial, coronal and sagittal set are acquired in the scout scan. Based on these scans, the MR technologist will determine the appropriate field of view and anatomical coverage. Hyperintense areas due

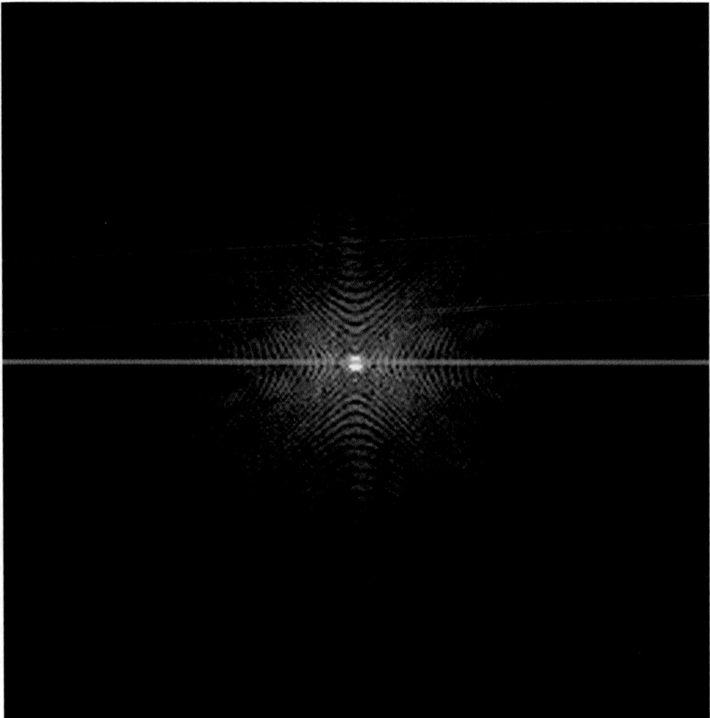

■ **FIGURE 11-11** K-space. Each acquired echo represents one line of information (highlighted).

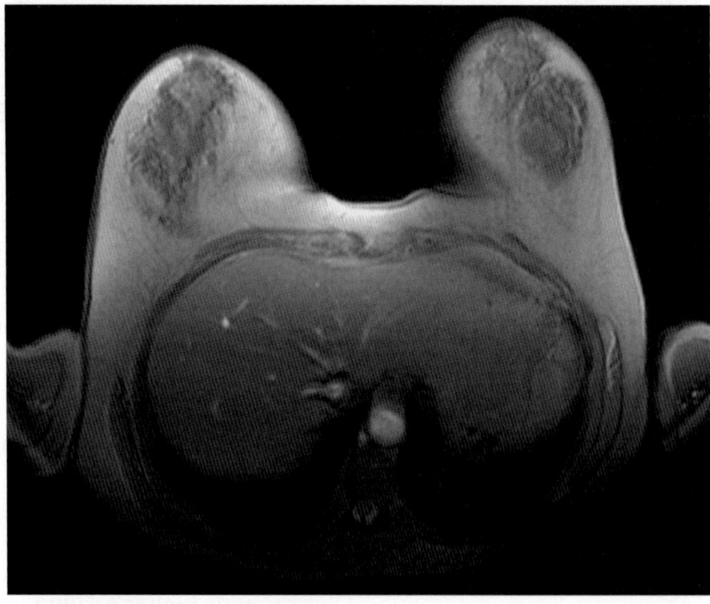

■ **FIGURE 11-12** An MR image that is reconstructed from k-space.

TABLE 11-2. Breast Magnetic Resonance Equipment Factors

Minimum field strength	1.5 Tesla
Minimum gradient strength	15 mT/m
Patient coil	Dedicated bilateral coil (multichannel)
Contrast injector	MR compatible power injector

to RF or magnetic field inhomogeneities can also be identified and positioning can be corrected. Figure 11-13 shows a breast with a large skin fold and the post-correction image.

The 3D T1 weighted sequence without fat suppression and without contrast shown in Figure 11-14 establishes a baseline T1 image for comparison of the contrast enhanced and fat suppressed sequences. Because of the lack of fat suppression, the hypointense areas of glandular content are easily identified within the breast.

TABLE 11-3. Typical Resolution and Imaging Requirements for Breast Magnetic Resonance Imaging

Parameter	T1 Weighted w/o fat saturation no contrast	T2 Weighted with fat saturation no contrast	T1 weighted with fat saturation with contrast
Sequence Type	3D gradient echo	3D turbo spin echo	3D gradient echo
In plane resolution	< 1 mm	< 1 mm	<1 mm
Slice Thickness	< 1.5 mm	< 5 mm	< 3 mm
Field of View	300 mm	300 mm	320 mm
Resolution Matrix	512 × 512	512 × 512	512 × 512
Typical Imaging Time	2 minutes	5 minutes	<2 minutes per scan, 6 minutes total

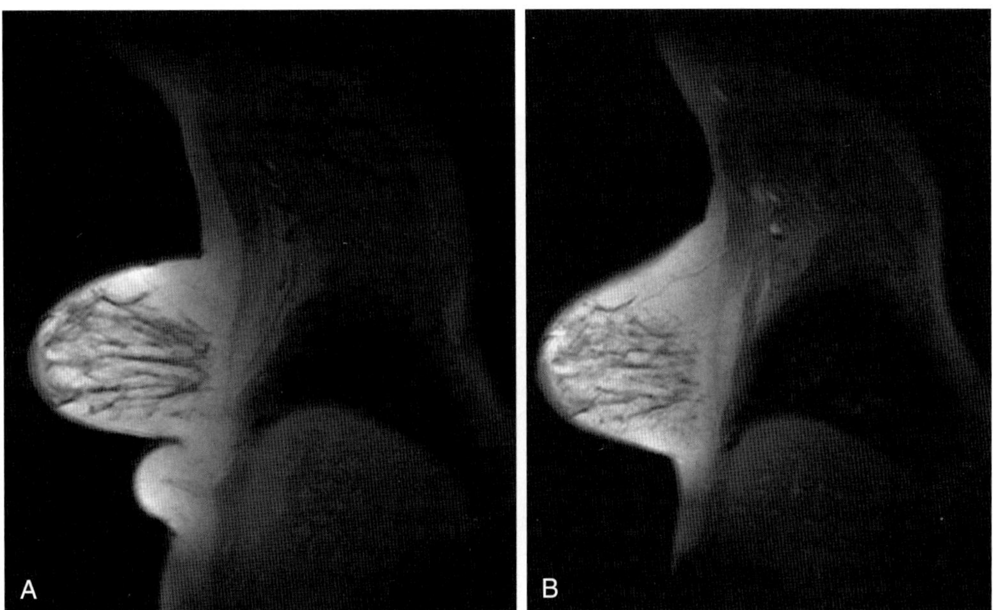

■ **FIGURE 11-13** **A**, A scout image showing an incorrectly positioned patient with a skin fold. **B**, Removal of the skin fold after repositioning.

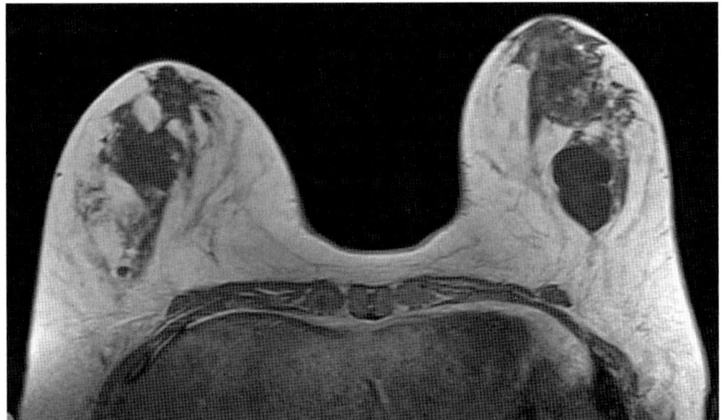

■ **FIGURE 11-14** A T1 weighted magnetic resonance (MR) image. Adipose tissue will be bright on T1 images due to the short T1 relaxation time compared with glandular tissue.

T2 weighted images, with fat saturation and without contrast will aid in diagnosing cysts, edema or hematomas. Figure 11-15 shows the cyst on a T2 image that is brighter than the glandular tissue due to the longer T2 value of fluid (water). The cyst is easily identified compared with the T1 image series (see Fig. 11-14) where the cyst appears only slightly darker compared with the glandular tissue.

Fat Suppression

As seen in Figure 11-14, fat appears hyperintense compared with glandular tissue on T1 weighted MR images. In T2 and contrast enhanced T1 images, visualization of small lesions in the glandular tissue can be difficult when in proximity to a strong fat signal. Therefore, suppression of the signal from fat is necessary in breast imaging.

There are several methods for suppressing the fat signal.[2] Chemical saturation using off resonance RF pulses, subtraction techniques, and the inversion recovery sequence are commonly used in breast imaging.

Chemical Saturation

Water and fat resonate at different frequencies in the same magnetic field due to different chemical environments in the molecular structure. The resonant frequency of fat is located 3.5 ppm from water. This difference is graphically shown in Figure 11-16. For a 1.5 Tesla magnet, there will be a 220 Hz resonant frequency difference and at 3T, the difference will be 440 Hz.

Figure 11-17 shows the additional RF pulse used to suppress the fat signal in the spin echo pulse sequence. To suppress the fat signal, a 90 degree RF pulse is applied exactly at the fat resonance frequency prior to the start of a standard spin echo sequence. This selectively flips the protons in fat to 90 degrees while leaving the water protons unaffected. The spin echo 90 degree pulse will

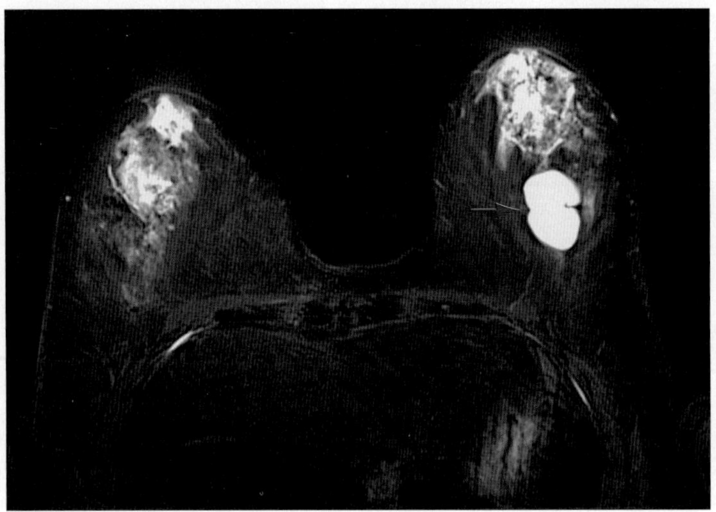

■ **FIGURE 11-15** A T2 weighted image. Fluid-filled cysts (*arrow*) will have longer T2 values and will be appear bright compared with the surrounding tissue.

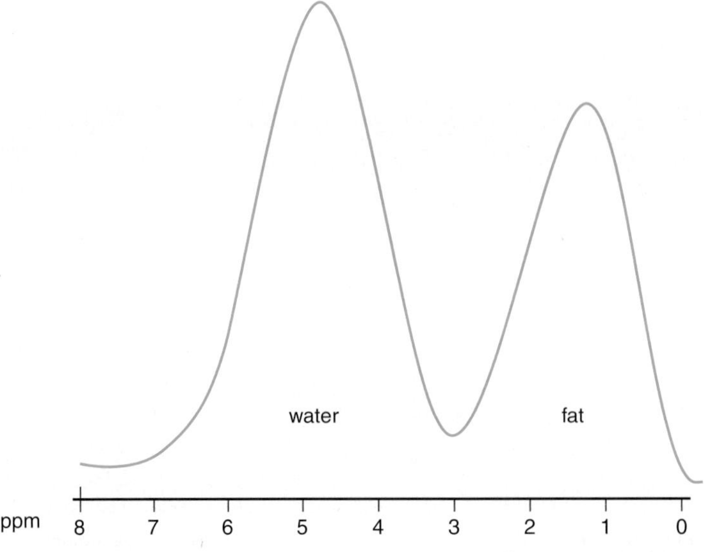

■ **FIGURE 11-16** A fat-water resonance spectra. Fat and water have slightly different resonant frequencies.

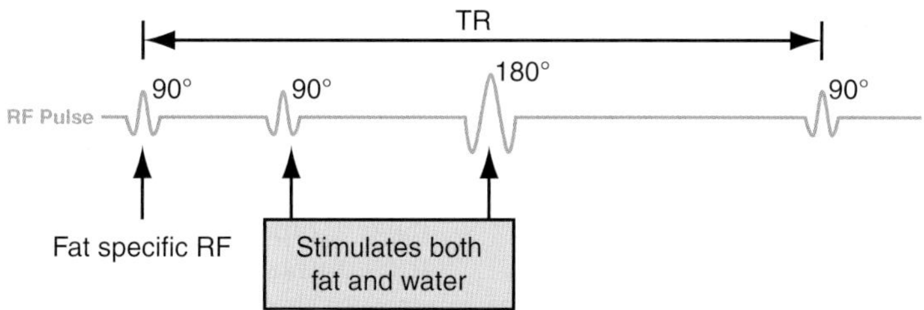

■ **FIGURE 11-17** A pulse sequence diagram showing a fat saturation pulse prior to the start of a standard spin echo sequence.

rotate both water and fat protons. Water protons rotate to 90 degrees but fat protons will rotate to 180. This process shifts the fat protons to an undetectable region by the RF receive coils during the echo and the signal from fat is minimized.

When using chemical saturation, prior to the acquisition, it is recommended that the MR technologist review a sample spectrum to confirm the frequency adjustment between the water and fat. Coils may inadvertently tune to the incorrect center frequency if the breast has a high fat content. Figure 11-18 shows the resonant peaks when there is a larger fat signal. In this case, a manual adjustment may be needed to center the frequency on water rather than fat.

Inversion Recovery

As with the chemical saturation pulse, the method used with inversion recovery attempts to isolate the proton spins from fat away from the glandular spins. Inversion recovery sequences rely on the differences between the T1 relaxation times between tissues to create this separation.

The sequence starts by initially applying a global 180 degree flip angle, so fat and glandular spins are flipped. As the spins experience T1 relaxation, fat protons will relax faster than the glandular tissue. At a certain time point, the fat signal passes by the 90 degree point. When this occurs, the fat spins are oriented at 90 degrees, which is similar to the chemical saturation sequence. The traditional spin echo sequence begins and the fat is removed from the received echo.

This method of removing the fat signal is not always perfect and residual fat signal can remain from the T1 relaxation of fat signal or inhomogeneities of the RF coil or magnet. Further reduction of the signal from fat can be obtained with image subtraction when processing contrast enhanced images.

Dynamic Contrast-Enhanced Scans

A malignant lesion can create new blood vessels when more than a few millimeters in size. This is known as *neoangiogenesis*. Vessels that form in these conditions are often abnormal and more porous than normal vasculature. Therefore, a higher perfusion rate exists in carcinomas compared with normal parenchyma. To visualize this perfusion on MR scans, a gadolinium based contrast agent is administered intravenously.

Gadolinium is a paramagnetic compound that will distort the local magnetic field. This local field disturbance causes the nearby protons to relax faster in both T1 (spin-lattice) and T2 (spin-spin) components. Therefore the T1 and T2 relaxation values are lower. These shortened T1 tissue values will appear brighter on a T1 weighted scan.

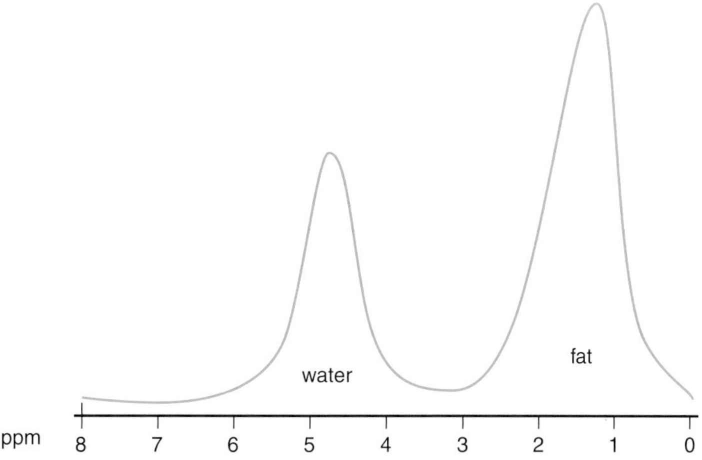

■ **FIGURE 11-18** Magnetic resonance (MR) spectra of breast tissue with a higher adipose content. Magnetic resonance (MR) systems may inadvertently tune to the stronger fat signal.

TABLE 11-4. Gadolinium Compounds

Chelate acronym	Generic Name
Gd-DTPA	Gadobenic acid
Gd-BOPTA	Gadopentetic acid
Gd-DOTA	Gadoteric acid

Gadolinium, a rare earth element, is normally is toxic in the body.[3] In order to reduce its toxicity and improve water solubility, gadolinium is chelated (Gd-ch) with another compound that reduces the reactivity within the body. Table 11-4 shows some common chelates used in MR imaging.

As the gadolinium compound is injected into the vessels, it will perfuse into the tumor at a higher rate compared with the normal parenchyma. Figure 11-19 shows the higher intensity of the signal from the enhancing regions compared with the image prior to contrast injection. By subtracting the contrast and non-contrast image, these areas can be easily visualized.

It has been shown that almost all malignancies will enhance after injection. Sensitivities of MR to contrast uptake in many clinical studies have been shown to be 94% or greater.[4,5] However, relying on a single post-uptake scan may give a high amount of false positives that can result in a lower specificity (37%).[6]

Specificity has been improved by analyzing the uptake and washout of contrast within the tissue at several time points after injection. Figure 11-20 shows the generalized characteristics of uptake curves. Carcinomas typically have a rapid uptake of contrast and exhibit washout of the contrast agent characterized by a sharp rise and then drop in signal intensity. Benign lesions will uptake contrast at a slower rate and form a signal that increases with time (persistent curve). When designing the pulse sequences, the practitioner should ensure that the kinetic sequences are acquired quickly enough to capture the initial wash-in phase of the enhancement curve. It is generally accepted that sequences of 2 minutes or less per scan be used.

For the dynamic T1 weighted scans with contrast injection, some clinical practitioners advocate higher spatial resolution dynamic scans while others prefer a higher temporal resolution.[7,8] Each imaging parameter comes with a sacrifice. Higher spatial resolution images require an increase in acquired k-space lines and longer sequences result. (Acquisition time = TR × number of k-space lines). Longer scans will reduce the amount of data points taken during uptake, and this potentially could cause a mischaracterization

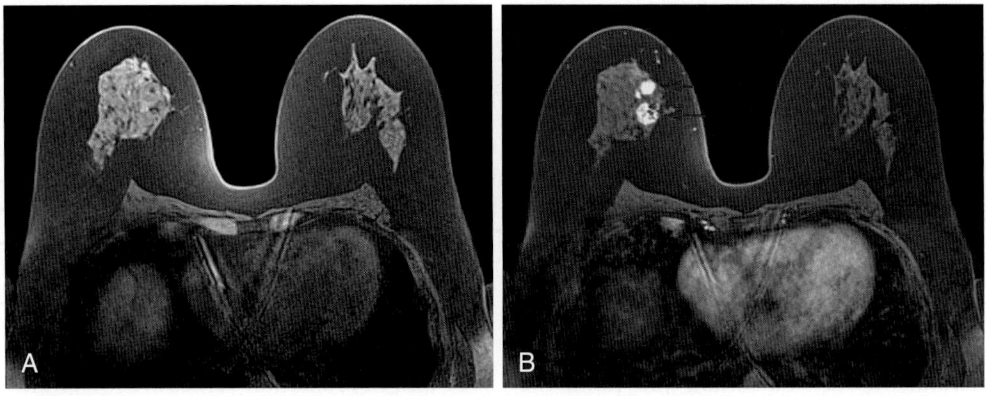

■ **FIGURE 11-19** **A,** A T1 weighted image prior to contrast injection. Note that this is a fat suppressed sequence. **B,** A T1 weighted image after contrast injection. Focal enhancement is seen in two regions (*arrows*).

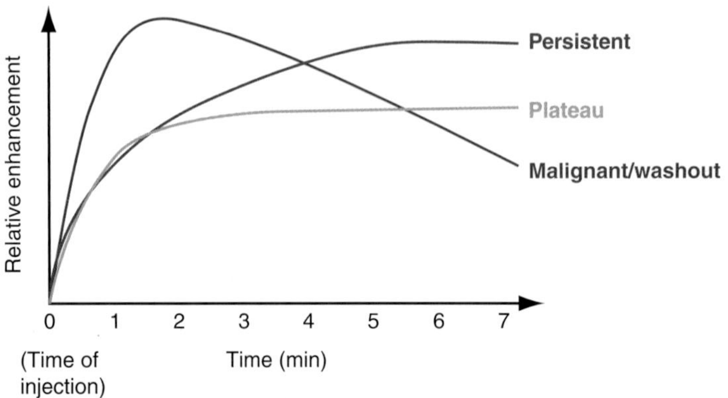

■ **FIGURE 11-20** Uptake curve characteristics. Malignant lesions are characterized by a high uptake followed by a wash-out phase.

of the lesion. In addition, because of the lower amount of signal per pixel with higher resolution images there will also be a decrease in the SNR.

Contrast injections of 0.1 mmol per kilogram of body weight are pushed at a rate of 2 to 3 cc/sec and are typically followed by a saline flush (20 cc). Power injectors (Fig. 11-21) are used to standardize injection rates and timing with pulse sequences.

The type of contrast chelation may make a difference in diagnostic efficacy of these scans.[9,10] Gadobenate dimeglumine (DTPA) is currently the standard contrast agent for breast MRI over gadopentetate dimeglumine (BOPTA).

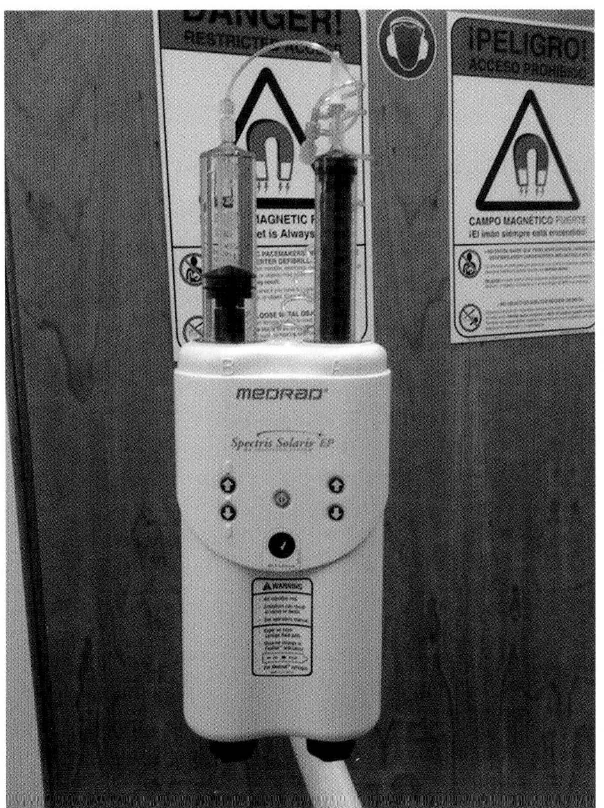

■ **FIGURE 11-21** Magnetic resonance (MR) compatible power injector

It is important to follow the recommended concentrations per patient weight and to properly screen the patient for contrast contraindications.

Processing and Uptake Analysis

Dedicated workstations are used for the analysis of the 3D dynamic T1 weighted scans with contrast injection. While many of the algorithms used in the software packages are proprietary, the overall goal is to analyze the uptake and washout curves and to characterize them into potential malignant and benign categories.

Once images are transferred from the MRI system, subtraction images are created from the difference between the contrast-enhanced and non–contrast-enhanced T1 images. Automated motion correction algorithms also are applied. This will reduce the amount of errors produced by misregistration of images. Areas of significant uptake are color coded and overlaid on a non-subtracted MR image. Figure 11-22 shows the T1 enhanced image and the color coded image on a CADstream reconstruction workstation. Red areas identify the areas of concern. In addition, the physician can mark a region of interest (ROI) in the color coded section and the curve of contrast enhancement is shown (similar to Fig. 11-20).

Some software packages allow for variability in the ROI size. While there is no standard for the optimum ROI size to create, it is important to note that it can affect the sensitivity and specificity of the results. Sardanelli and colleagues[11] noted that reducing the size and placing it on the most vascularized area will increase sensitivity and decrease specificity. If the ROI includes low vascularized areas, this will decrease sensitivity while increasing specificity.

RECENT HARDWARE ADVANCEMENTS AND TECHNIQUES

Higher Field Strengths

Most clinical MR scanners are 1.5 Tesla in strength. Using field strengths lower than 1.5T for breast MRI uptake scans may reduce the image quality and increase

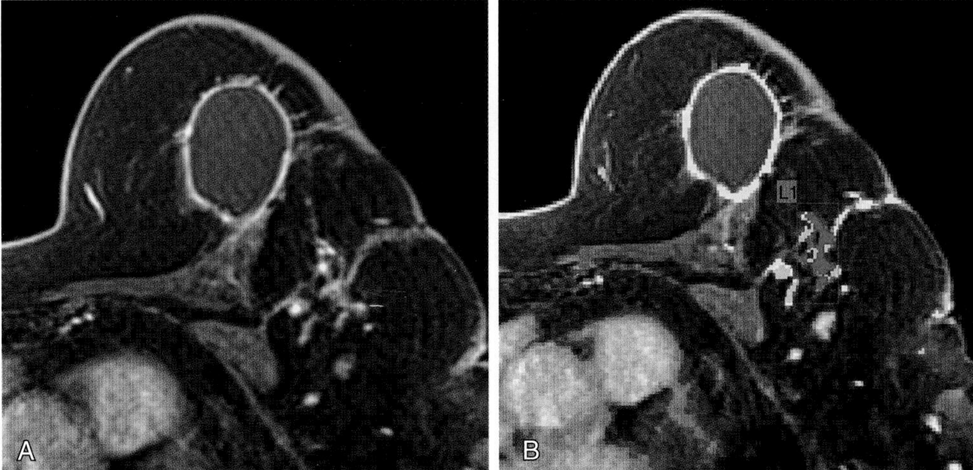

■ **FIGURE 11-22** A, T1 subtracted images showing enhancement. **B,** Post processing color coding showing areas of potential malignancy.

the requisite time needed for each dynamic set. As a result, a lower number of time points may be taken during dynamic imaging, to achieve the requisite image quality. Therefore, imaging lower than 1.5T is often not recommended.[7,12]

While the majority of breast MR studies have been performed on 1.5 Tesla scanners, higher field strength 3 Tesla systems are becoming integrated into clinical practices. It is important to note some of the major issues that arise when transitioning to higher field strengths.

The main improvement in using a higher field strength magnet is the increase in SNR.[13] As field strengths increase, additional protons become aligned with the main magnetic field and therefore the amount of signal from tissue increases. This potentially allows for faster acquisitions or improvements in the spatial resolution of the individual acquisitions.

There are issues to consider if a facility is transitioning into a higher field strength system. Scanning protocols will need to be modified (TE, TR, flip angles) from existing ones because of the differences in T1 and T2 tissue relaxation times in the 3T environment. Rakow-Penner and coworkers have shown that the SNR increases by a factor of 2 and the T1 times will increase for fatty and glandular breast tissue when using the 3T scanner.[14] As a consequence of these T1 changes, a longer TR time is typically necessary to visualize the same contrast changes compared with the 1.5T system. This in turn will increase the acquisition time.

Because of the higher field strength, there are additional safety concerns for all objects within the MR environment. Care must be taken even with MR compatible instruments. There have been concerns with equipment that has been deemed MR safe or compatible for the 1.5T environment. In the 3T environment, there is significant pull or torque on the instruments or implants.[15] The facility should ensure that all equipment used in the magnet room is safe for use at the higher field strength.

The specific absorption ratio (SAR) is a measure of RF energy deposition in tissue. At higher resonant frequencies, there is a higher absorption rate of RF energy in tissue. As a result, higher power is needed to transmit into areas of the body. While most breast MR protocols do not use high RF deposition sequences (turbo spin echo), the SAR should be reviewed when the protocols are established.

The chemical shift between water and fat will be larger at higher field strengths and therefore will increase the amount of pixel mismapping for a given gradient strength. Susceptibility artifacts will also be increased in size on a 3T scanner.

Initial studies show promise with 3T.[16,17] Kuhl and colleagues have found the image quality improvement to be statistically significant. This preliminary study noted that the enhancement ratio was not superior, but rather on par with 1.5T images due to the changes in flip angles and TR needed for proper T1 weighting in the image. Large-scale studies and optimization of parameters still need to validate whether images at 3T will improve diagnostic ability.

Multi-Channel Bilateral Breast Coils

The amount of noise in an image is proportional to the volume covered inside the coil. Body coils are not used as receive coils in breast imaging because they will receive the noise from the other parts of the body. By reducing the size of the coil and increased proximity of the coil to the tissue, the signal is increased and the amount of noise detected is reduced.[18]

Multi channel arrays are comprised of several coils placed in proximity to the anatomical region. These coils are oriented such that there is overlapping anatomical coverage. The system reconstructs the different regions of the image using preferential weighting from coils with strongest signal. Figure 11-23 highlights these coils within the support apparatus.

Figure 11-24 shows an example of multi-channel imaging of a series of brain images from an 8-channel coil. Each coil contributes to the final image. A higher SNR is achieved due to the proximity of the coils to the anatomical region.

Current breast coils are manufactured using 4 to 16 channels. As additional channels are added, the signal-to-noise values should increase. In turn, the amount of scan time reduction possible using parallel imaging improves as well.

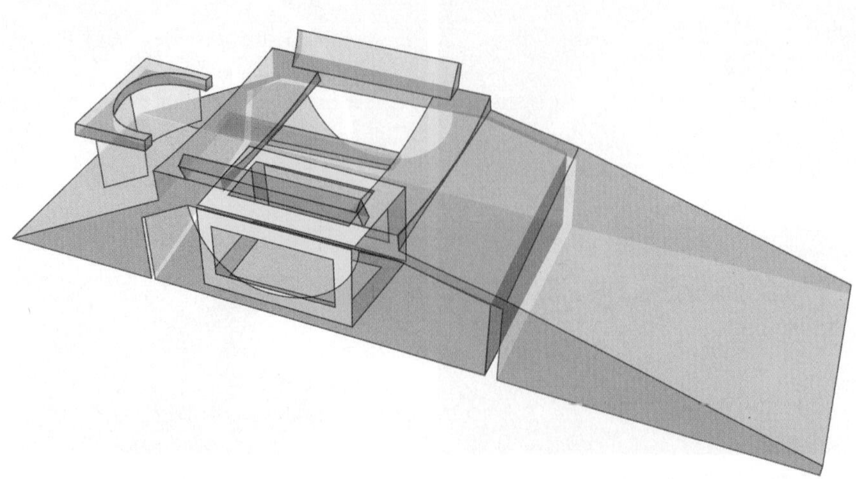

■ FIGURE 11-23 Breast multi channel coils highlighted in yellow.

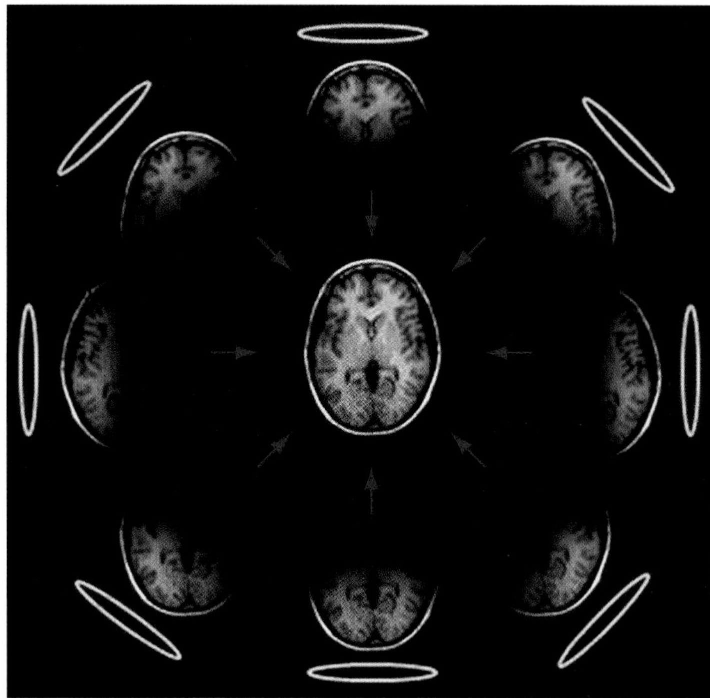

■ **FIGURE 11-24** Multichannel reconstruction example.

Parallel Imaging

Parallel imaging is a method for improving the temporal resolution (reducing scan time) by reducing the amount of k-space data required per image. A reduced k-space data set is obtained, and by using signal profile information from each independent RF coil in a phased array (multi-channel) setup, algorithms are used to calculate the remaining data.

The two most common methods apply algorithms on either the spatial information (sensitivity encoding [SENSE]) or frequency information (generalized autocalibrating partially parallel acquisition [GRAPPA]) in order to estimate the missing data from the reduced k-space acquisition. Both methodologies require the use of a reference scan using the body coil to determine each coil's sensitivity profile and tissue signal intensity from the patient.

An acceleration factor (R) represents the time savings achieved with parallel imaging; R is based on the reduction of k-space lines acquired. For example, if 128 out of 256 lines were acquired, the acceleration factor would be two. An acceleration factor can be achieved up to the amount of RF coils in the phased array (an 8 channel RF coil is able to achieve an acceleration factor of 8).

While parallel imaging techniques are able to improve the acquisition time, there are SNR losses associated with these scans. Depending on the coil and anatomy location, there is also a potential for wraparound artifacts.

Parallel imaging is showing promise compared with traditional acquisitions.[19,20] Because of the ability to decrease the scan time with minor reductions in SNR, the ability to acquire high resolution images in conjunction with high temporal resolution scans becomes possible.

ARTIFACT AVOIDANCE

There are several imaging pitfalls that arise when imaging the breast. In this section, some common breast MR artifacts will be discussed.

Motion and Misregistration

Unlike x-ray mammography, diagnostic breast MR procedures are performed without significant compression to aid in immobilization. This is in part due to the reduction in perfusion while under compression. Unfortunately, patient motion may take place between the dynamic scans, and can cause misregistration of images during subtraction. Figure 11-25 shows the effect of misregistration. A poorly subtracted image will cause problems on the uptake evaluation. Many reconstruction software packages can correct for motion artifacts (see Fig. 11-25). However, if motion is excessive, the study will need to be repeated.

In addition, motion in the phase encode direction can cause ghosting artifacts along the same direction. Heart motion can cause ghosting and can obscure the breast tissue if the phase direction is along the anteroposterior (AP) direction. By modifying the phase encode direction to the left-right direction, the heart motion artifacts can avoid the breast tissue.

Fat Saturation Errors

Some fat saturation techniques involve a chemically selective RF pulse prior to the start of each pulse sequence. However, if the RF coil has been inappropriately tuned to the fat peak instead of water because of the large amount of adipose tissue in the breast, the saturation pulse will be located at the incorrect frequency and fat will not be saturated.

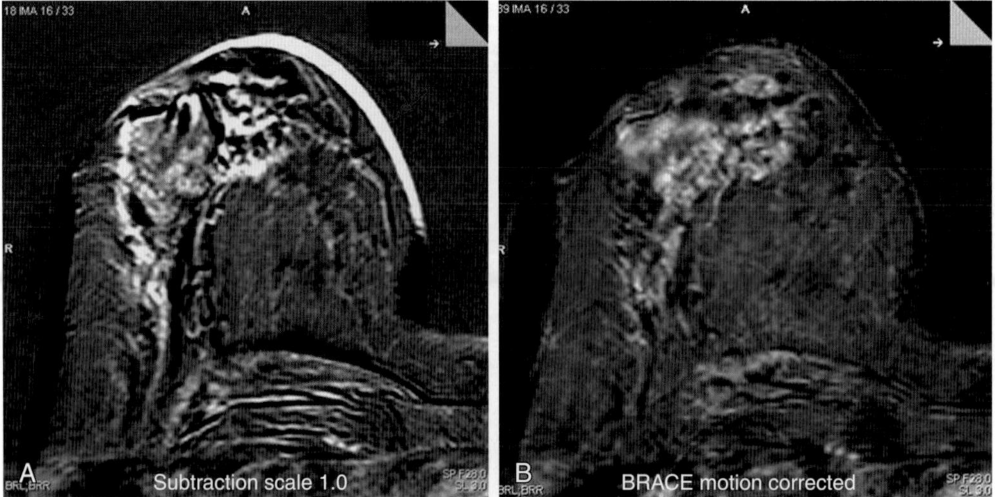

■ **FIGURE 11-25** A, Hyper and hypo intense areas on subtracted images due to patient motion (*arrows*). B, Subtracted images after application of motion correction algorithms

To avoid this situation, technologists often review the fat/water peak spectra (see Fig. 11-18) and if the coil has inadvertently tuned to fat, they can manually shift the tuning back to the water peak.

In addition, if there are coil inhomogeneities, there may be areas of inadequate fat suppression. Figure 11-26 shows an example of this. In some cases, the process of subtracting images can reduce the severity of this artifact.

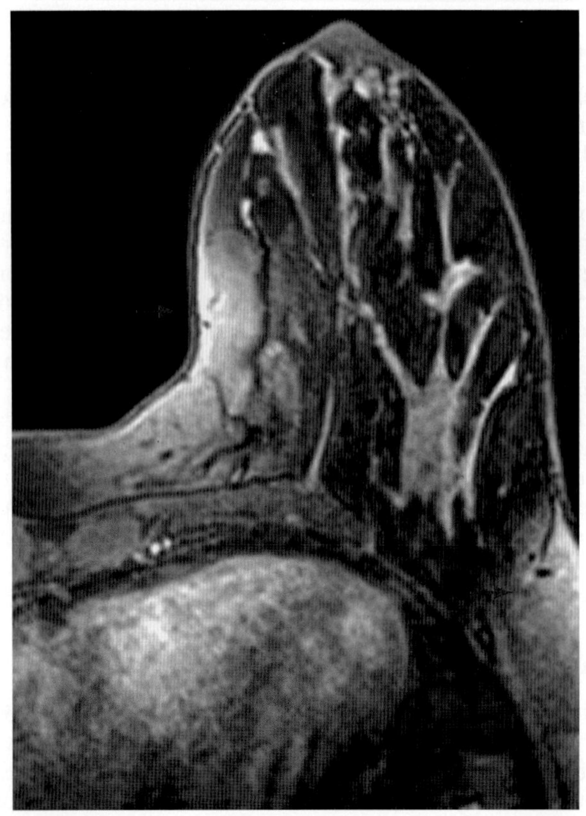

■ **FIGURE 11-26** T1 weighted images showing poor fat suppression in two areas (*arrows*).

Magnet and Coil Inhomogeneities

Within the bore of the magnet, inhomogeneities of the field can cause the resonant frequency to be off in certain areas. This may result in an image distortion or incorrect signal intensity in the final image. Coil inhomogeneities can cause hyper or hypo intense areas on the image.

Figure 11-27 shows a hyperintense area on a fat saturated T1 weighted image. Hot spots near the coil surface can arise when larger patients fill the entirety of the breast coil. The adverse effect on the dynamic uptake scans may be reduced due to the subtraction. However these spots may still be seen after subtraction and have the potential to be misdiagnosed as contrast uptake as shown in Figure 11-27.

To reduce the errors associated with these hot spots, care must be taken when positioning the patient, and when these artifacts are seen, the patient should be repositioned within the breast coil if possible. If there are magnetic field homogeneity issues, additional shimming of the magnet may be necessary in order to improve the field consistency.

Gadolinium Contrast—Missed Uptake

The dynamic uptake scans must be timed correctly with contrast injection to capture the uptake and washout phase of the enhancement curve. Problems that arise during contrast injection such as extravasation, accidental cannula removal or power injector malfunction may cause insufficient enhancement or no enhancement to be seen on the uptake scans. Also, if the incorrect injection rate is applied, then the uptake curve may not exhibit the correct characteristics.

Chemical Shift Artifacts

A chemical shift artifact manifests itself as a mismapping of fat signal on the reconstructed MR image in the readout direction. As mentioned previously, fat and water have frequency differences of 3.5 ppm and at 1.5 Tesla, this frequency shift will be 225 Hz.

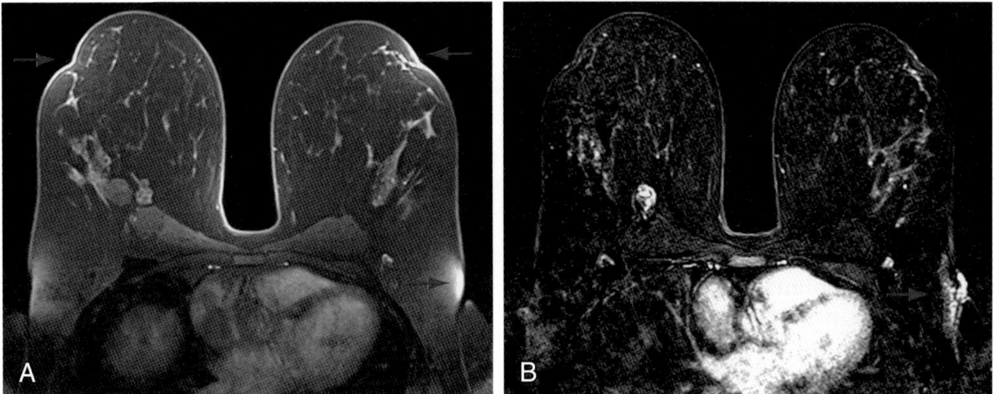

■ **FIGURE 11-27** A, Poor fat suppression from radiofrequency (RF) coil inhomogeneities. **B**, After subtraction, some RF inhomogeneities are removed, while the bottom hot spot remains. This can be mistaken as contrast update during analysis.

During acquisition of the echo, a readout gradient is applied. The system relates the frequency change to a spatial change along the readout direction. Because of the inherent frequency difference compared with water, the fat signal is received at 225 Hz lower than water. If the readout gradient is low in strength, the bandwidth (Hz/pixel) associated with each pixel will be low. When this occurs, and the frequency shift of fat exceeds the bandwidth per pixel, the fat signal will be mapped incorrectly on the final image and will be displaced in the readout direction.

By increasing the bandwidth, the resonant frequency difference can be reduced to a value less than a single pixel value. However it should be noted that higher bandwidths, especially with higher field strength systems, might not be achievable due to the higher gradient strength requirements. In addition, increasing the bandwidth will also reduce the SNR ratio of the images.

Metallic Clips

Diamagnetic or paramagnetic items within the body such as surgical clips can cause a change in the magnetic field and T1 and T2 in the area surrounding the object. This most commonly manifests itself as a signal void in the breast (Fig. 11-28). However, as shown in Figure 28, the local field change results in a reduction of T1 and shows signal enhancement.

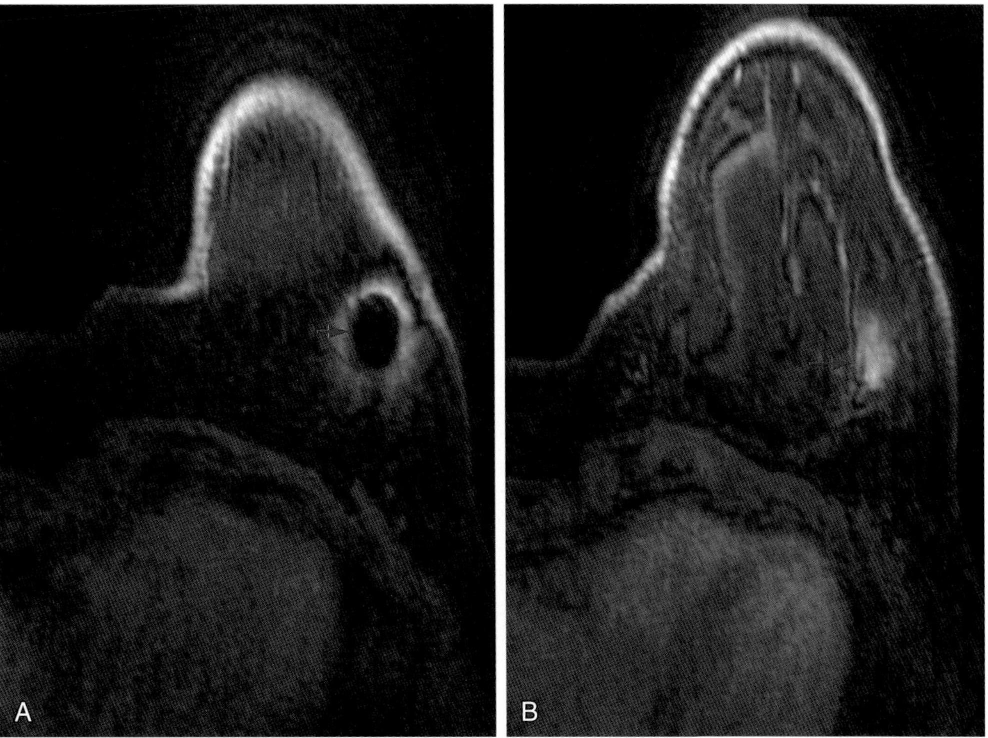

■ **FIGURE 11-28** **A,** Signal void seen from a metallic biopsy marker (*arrow*). **B**, Signal enhancement seen on a nearby slice caused by a reduction of T1 relaxation (*arrow*).

Previous surgeries or biopsies in the area should be noted. It is possible to reduce the strength and size of the signal void by modifying the pulse sequences to include a spin echo series. However, oftentimes it is not practical due to the fast imaging necessary for the dynamic scans.

PATIENT PREPARATION

As important as it is to have optimal MR equipment and sequences for breast imaging, patient cooperation is often essential to produce a high quality diagnostic exam. Lying face down on a table can be challenging for many patients, and therefore choosing a coil that is designed for comfort will help improve patient tolerance for the duration of the exam and reduce motion artifacts during the dynamic scans. Coils should provide adequate cushioning and allow the patient's back to be parallel to the table. Additionally, the design should allow enough room for larger breasts; provide adequate head support and even good arm support to allow the patient to relax.

MR scanners can have some limitations due to the bore size. A traditional bore diameter is approximately 60 cm with a weight limit of 300 to 450 lbs. In some cases, newer machines have diameters of 70 cm with weight limits of 550 lbs. It's important to note that while some patients may fit in the scanner in the supine position, they may have difficulties with breast procedures because of the prone positioning on the breast apparatus that elevates them above the table by 6 to 8 inches.

While patient comfort is essential for tolerance of the exam, proper patient positioning is essential to obtain a diagnostic scan. Most breast coils are designed such that the patient is in a prone position, which allows the breast to hang from the chest wall. Because of the difficulties in prone positioning on a table, some assistance in adjusting the breast may be needed. For MR technologists who are new to breast imaging, it is often helpful to gain assistance from mammography technologists in both patient encountering and positioning.

Eliminating the excess adipose tissue from the ribs and abdomen can be achieved by having the patient raise one side of their body and pulling down on the tissue to reduce any skin folds. Elevating the feet slightly can often relieve any strain on the patient's lower back. A head support with a mirror allows the patient to see out of the magnet bore, which decreases the claustrophobia sensation. Additionally, music can be played through most MR systems, which can reduce the anxiety levels.

Some positioning protocols specify that arms be raised above the head during the exam. With the limited bore size of 60 cm this may initially feel very comfortable for the patient and can allow more room in the magnet. In this position, adequate pillows should be placed under the arms in order to reduce the strain on the shoulders. However, this arm position may become uncomfortable over an extended period of time. It is not uncommon for patients to experience pain near the end of the exam during the dynamic uptake series where minimal motion is necessary for proper image registration. The technologist should communicate often with patients to ensure they are comfortable enough to tolerate the remainder of the exam.

Having the patient's arms down by her side can be better tolerated for the entire duration of the exam. However in this position, pulse sequence phase oversampling may be needed to eliminate phase wrap artifacts from the arms. This will result in an increase in the scan time. Additionally, some practitioners believe this produces inadequate coverage of breast tissue within the coil, especially on larger breasted women. While this may be a more comfortable position for the majority of patients and potentially reduces motion artifacts, the decision on whether to use "arms up" or "arms down" should be made in conjunction with the technologist and interpreting physician.

IV Placement and Training

Breast MRI requires the insertion of an IV. A minimum of a 20 gauge angiocatheter is suggested to withstand the pressure of the contrast injector and reduce the chance of the IV being dislodged while the patient is positioned. If the IV is in the antecubital vein, the patient should try to keep her arm straight as she lowers herself into position to keep the catheter in place. This will decrease the chance of extravasation.

In many cases, a trained technologist can perform the venipunctures. States such as California certify technologists for upper extremity venipuncture procedures for the sole purpose of contrast administration. These certificates vary from state to state and therefore it is best to check with local health agencies for regulatory guidance.

Contraindications

All patients are screened prior to the examination for contraindications related to the MR scan and contrast injection. Table 11-5 shows three categories of patient related items: safe, conditional, and unsafe. All "conditional" implanted devices should be confirmed for their safety before the patient enters the magnetic field. Although jewelry and removable dental work may not be ferrous, it should still be removed due to the risk of image susceptibility artifacts or RF burns.[21] If a family member is allowed to stay with the patient during the exam, he or she must also be screened in a similar fashion.

TABLE 11-5. Screening Items for Magnetic Resonance Safety

Safe	Conditional	Unsafe
Artificial joint replacements	Aneurysm clips	All loose ferrous objects
Cotton hospital gowns	Breast tissue expander	Pacemaker
Post surgical hardware	Copper and stainless steel IUDs	Pacing wires
Sutures	Implanted drug pump	Swanz-Gantz IV access catheters
Titanium surgical clips/staples	Stents/coils/filters	Vagal nerve stimulator

In addition, MR compatible instrumentation such as power injectors, IV equipment, tray tables and carts and wheelchairs must be made of non-magnetic materials to avoid the magnetic field from pulling equipment and potentially injuring patients, staff, and MR equipment.

Creatinine and Glomerular Filtration Rate

A new contraindication that needs to be addressed is the association between Gd-chelates and the risk of nephrogenic systemic fibrosis (NSF).[22] NSF is a non-curable disorder that causes fibrosis of the skin and other organ systems and has been linked to the gadolinium contrast injection in patients with severe kidney failure.

In order to screen for potential risk of developing NSF, patients should be initially screened for a history of diabetes, hypertension, or kidney disease. If a patient has any risk factors associated with NSF, the patient's glomerular filtration rate is estimated (eGFR) by obtaining their blood serum creatinine level along with their age, sex and ethnicity.[23] Creatinine levels can be affected by kidney disease, diabetes, high blood pressure, congestive heart failure, liver disease, and nonsteroidal anti-inflammatory drugs taken on a regular basis. Once calculated, if the eGFR is found to be less than 60 mL/min/1.72 m^2, then a review of the case is necessary by the radiologist in order to proceed with the examination.

Claustrophobia

Lastly, the biggest issue concerning breast imaging with MRI is claustrophobia. Claustrophobia has a wide range of severity. MRI can usually be tolerated with either open communication between the technologist and the patient, moral support from a family member or a sedative taken prior to the MRI.

SUMMARY

When establishing a breast MR program, there are numerous factors to consider including specific MR equipment, pulse sequences and image processing factors. It is important to understand how these technical factors can affect the overall diagnosis of the patient.

In addition to the technology factors, proper management of the patient experience can also help obtain high quality diagnostic images. Patient and staff safety issues must also be considered because of the strong magnetic field and contrast reactions.

Breast MRI has matured as an essential modality for the comprehensive diagnosis of the breast. As developments are made on the basic science level, we will continue to see further improvements in breast MR imaging.

KEY POINTS

- Equipment and technique selection is essential for diagnostic quality images.
- Pulse sequences should balance spatial resolution and acquisition time.
- Image artifacts in breast MR can cause errors in categorization of lesions.
- Patient positioning is a critical step in producing a high quality diagnostic image.
- Safety issues must be addressed when working in the MR environment.
- Patient contraindications must be considered prior to the exam.

REFERENCES

1. Robitaille PM, Warner R, Jagadeesh J, Abduljalil AM, Kangarlu A, Burgess RE, et al. Design and assembly of an 8 tesla whole-body MR scanner. *J Comput Assist Tomogr* 1999;**23**:808–20.
2. De Kerviler E, Leroy-Willig A, Clément O, Frija J. Fat suppression techniques in MRI: an update. *Biomed Pharmacother* 1998;**52**:69–75.
3. Cacheris WP, Quay SC, Rocklage SM. The relationship between thermodynamics and the toxicity of gadolinium complexes. *Magn Reson Imaging* 1990;**8**:467–81.
4. Liberman L, Morris EA, Lee MJ, Kaplan JB, LaTrenta LR, Menell JH, et al. Breast lesions detected on MR Imaging: features and positive predictive value. *AJR Am J Roentgenol* 2002;**179**:171–8.
5. Orel SG, Schnall MD. MR imaging of the breast for the detection, diagnosis, and staging of breast cancer. *Radiology* 2001;**220**:13–30.
6. Harms SE, Flamig DP, Hensley KL, Meiches MD, Jensen RA, Evans WP, et al. MR imaging of the breast with rotating delivery of excitation off resonance: clinical experience with pathologic correlation. *Radiology* 1993;**187**:493–501.
7. Kuhl C. The current status of breast MR imaging. Part I. Choice of technique, image interpretation, diagnostic accuracy, and transfer to clinical practice. *Radiology* 2007;**244**:356–78.
8. Goto M, Ito H, Akazawa K, Kubota T, Kizu O, Yamada K, et al. Diagnosis of breast tumors by contrast-enhanced MR imaging: comparison between the diagnostic performance of dynamic enhancement patterns and morphologic features. *J Magn Reson Imaging* 2007;**25**:104–12.
9. Pediconi F, Catalano C, Padula S, Roselli A, Dominelli V, Cagioli S, et al. Contrast-enhanced MR mammography: improved lesion detection and differentiation with gadobenate dimeglumine. *AJR Am J Roentgenol* 2008;**191**:1339–46.
10. Knopp MV, Bourne MW, Sardanelli F, Wasser MN, Bonomo L, Boetes C, et al. Gadobenate dimeglumine-enhanced MRI of the breast: analysis of dose response and comparison with gadopentetate dimeglumine. *Am J Roentgenol* 2003;**181**:663–76.
11. Sardanelli F, Fausto A, Iozzelli A, Rescinito G, Galabrese M. Dynamic breast magnetic resonance imaging. Effect of changing the region of interest on early enhancement using 2D and 3D techniques. *J Comput Assist Tomogr* 2004;**28**:642–6.
12. Rausch DR, Hendrick RE. How to optimize clinical breast MR imaging practices and techniques on your 1.5-T system. *Radiographics* 2006;**26**:1469–84.
13. Machann J, Schlemmer HP, Schick F. Technical challenges and opportunities of whole-body magnetic resonance imaging at 3T. *Phys Med* 2008;**24**:63–70.
14. Rakow-Penner R, Daniel B, Yu H. Relaxation times of breast tissue at 1.5T and 3T measured using IDEAL. *J Magn Reson Imaging* 2006;**23**:87–91.
15. Shellock FG. Biomedical implants and devices: assessment of magnetic field interactions with a 3.0-Tesla MR system. *J Magn Reson Imaging* 2002;**16**:721–32.
16. Pinker K, Grabner G, Bogner W, Gruber S, Szomolanyi P, Trattnig S, et al. A combined high temporal and high spatial resolution 3 Tesla MR imaging protocol for the assessment of breast lesions: initial results. *Invest Radiol* 2009;**44**:553–8.

17. Kuhl CK, Jost P, Morakkabati N, Zivanovic O, Schild HH, Gieseke J. Contrast-enhanced MR imaging of the breast at 3.0 and 1.5 T in the same patients: initial experience. *Radiology* 2006;**239**:666–76.
18. Wolfman NT, Moran R, Moran PR, Karstaedt N. Simultaneous MR imaging of both breasts using a dedicated receiver coil. *Radiology* 1985;**155**:241–3.
19. Orlacchio A, Bolacchi F, Rotili A, Cossu E, Tanga I, Cozzolino V, et al. MR breast imaging: a comparative analysis of conventional and parallel imaging acquisition. *Radiol Med* 2008;**113**:465–76.
20. Dougherty L, Isaac G, Rosen MA, Nunes LW, Moate PJ, Boston RC, et al. High frame-rate simultaneous bilateral breast DCE-MRI. *Magn Reson Med* 2007;**57**:220–5.
21. Shellock FG, Crues JV. MR procedures: biologic effects, safety, and patient care. *Radiology* 2004;**232**:635–52.
22. Grobner T, Prischl FC. Gadolinium and nephrogenic systemic fibrosis. *Kidney Int* 2007;**72**:260–4.
23. Shellock FG, Spinazzi A. MRI safety update 2008: part 1, MRI contrast agents and nephrogenic systemic fibrosis. *AJR Am J Roentgenol* 2008;**191**:1129–39.

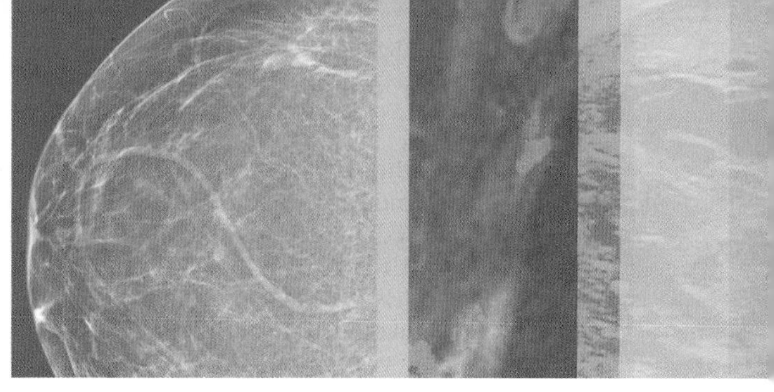

CHAPTER 12

Magnetic Resonance Imaging: Indications and Interpretation

Colin J. Wells and Nanette D. DeBruhl

HISTORY

In 1986, Heywang and colleagues[1] first reported the use of gadolinium dimeglumine intravenous contrast agents with magnetic resonance imaging (MRI) of the breasts. Before this time MRI of the breasts was almost exclusively performed for implant evaluation because the differences in signal intensity between malignancies and normal breast tissue without contrast were usually insufficient for adequate tumor analysis. Heywang and colleagues found that malignant tumors enhanced after injection of gadolinium contrast agents, thus increasing their conspicuity, whereas normal breast tissue either did not enhance or only mildly enhanced. Subsequent research confirmed these findings.

Work by Kaiser and coworkers[2] extended the use of contrast-enhanced (dynamic) scanning by optimizing temporal resolution using fast repeat scanning and graphing changes in signal intensity within a lesion over an extended period of time, thus creating time-signal intensity curves.

Because early technology was limited in its ability to yield high spatial resolution and high temporal resolution images simultaneously (both of which are needed for modern breast MRI) Harms and associates[3] approached improving contrast-enhanced breast MRI by optimizing spatial imaging, using a novel pulse sequence to produce higher-resolution fat-suppressed images. Because it is well known that malignant lesions often demonstrate specific morphologic features different from benign lesions, using Harms and associates' approach or similar approaches that optimize spatial imaging could improve specificity and sensitivity of breast MRI.

By the early to mid 1990s, sequential dynamic and high resolution morphologic scanning was being done, and by the mid to late 1990s, MRI technology and pulse sequences had developed to the point that simultaneous scanning was possible, achieving both high spatial resolution and high temporal resolution at the same time. This led to a combined interpretation model melding evaluation of both morphology and contrast enhancement characteristics from the same scan sequences. This approach uses shape and margin analysis as well as contrast enhancement kinetics to locate and differentiate benign from malignant lesions. This combined model improved sensitivity and specificity of breast MRI, and subsequent studies confirmed that this approach was highly predictive for determining outcome. In our practice, we use this combined approach to evaluate lesions using both morphology and kinetics for diagnosis. We have also found that the combined approach yields higher sensitivity and specificity than using either alone. Averaging across various reports shows the sensitivity for breast MRI is 85% to 90%, with average sensitivity of 65% to 80%.

PATHOPHYSIOLOGY OF ENHANCEMENT

The interpretation of breast MRI examinations can be challenging because benign lesions and malignant lesions can share both morphologic and contrast enhancement characteristics. The largest overlap seems to be with contrast enhancement characteristics.

The vascular pathophysiology that causes benign and malignant enhancement has been examined but has not yet been fully clarified. Research has shown that malignant lesions possess and release angiogenic factors. The most frequently reported is vascular endothelial growth factor (VEGF), which stimulates the growth of preexisting capillaries and induces new vessel formation. This new vasculature is abnormal, exhibiting anomalous vessel wall architecture with leaky endothelial linings and arteriovenous shunt formation. The increased number of abnormal vessels leads to increased vascular density and permeability, which, in turn, can lead to rapid increased influx and efflux of contrast material. Unfortunately, although extensive research has been done examining the correlation between vessel density, signal intensity, and patterns of enhancement in postcontrast images, results have been conflicting. For example, invasive ductal carcinoma (IDC) as well as high-grade ductal carcinoma in situ (DCIS) are associated with high VEGF expression whereas infiltrating lobular carcinoma (ILC) has low VEGF expression. There is no significant difference in the vascular density between these two types of invasive cancers, however, suggesting other factors are stimulating vessel density in ILC. In addition, vessel density is not specific for malignancy. Some benign lesions display unexpectedly high vessel density with locally increased permeability and therefore can mimic malignant-type contrast enhancement. This prominent vascularity appears to be related to their growth. Conversely, up to 10% of cancers, usually of the true lobular, scirrhous, and desmoplastic types, can show less enhancement than expected. This is most likely related to low vessel density. Although it is clear that there is a correlation between high vessel density in known cancers and the percentage of maximal signal increase after contrast agent injection, it is also clear that there are other causes of differences in signal intensity. Those differences include variations in biologic presentation, tumor composition, tissue relaxation times, interstitial pressure gradients, and probably other as yet undetermined factors that are also important in determining contrast enhancement, in addition to abnormal vessel architecture and abnormal vessel permeability. This contrast enhancement variability can be a source of frustration for interpreting radiologists and supports the premise that interpretation based on contrast enhancement alone for determining malignancy is not sufficient. Nevertheless, dynamic contrast enhancement patterns have proven useful in contrast-enhanced breast MRI interpretation.

ADVANTAGES AND DISADVANTAGES

Contrast-enhanced MRI has several important benefits in evaluating the breasts. Ionizing radiation is not used, thus eliminating the potential for radiation-induced cancers. To date, MRI has not been linked to breast cancer induction. In reality this benefit is not convincing because the incidence of mammographically induced breast cancer is unknown, if indeed it exists at all. Current mammography technology and the federal regulation of mammography has ensured safe x-ray doses. In addition, if radiation risk exists it probably affects only a small high-risk population. Furthermore, mammography is still necessary for correlation with MRI examinations.

An additional benefit of MRI is the ability to use various pulse sequences, including tissue-suppression techniques, to optimize lesion visualization. Computer-aided postprocessing algorithms allow further image manipulation, which can aid in the detection and characterization of breast lesions. Both of these techniques can be useful in differentiating benign from malignant lesions. MRI provides a more complete three-dimensional (3D) evaluation of the breasts and therefore can aid in determining the extent of disease, thus affecting staging and treatment options.

MRI may be used in women with a history of previous excisional breast biopsies or lumpectomies to differentiate recurrent/residual malignancy from postsurgical and/or postradiation changes when mammography or ultrasonography are inconclusive. Contrast-enhanced breast MRI can occasionally be helpful when mammograms and/or ultrasound images are problematic or inconclusive. Contrast-enhanced breast MRI is more sensitive than mammography or ultrasonography. For example, Berg and coworkers[4] reported a 94% sensitivity for breast MRI but sensitivities of 67.8% and 83%, respectively, for mammography and ultrasonography. Other authors have reported similar results, with sensitivities ranging from 75% to 95%.

MRI has disadvantages as well. The most important disadvantage is lower specificity, generally reported to be between 65% and 80%. In addition there is cost; length of time to complete the scan; continued limited availability in some areas of the country; nondepiction of most calcifications due to poorer resolution than mammography; lack of standardized scanning techniques, which can make second opinion interpretation or comparison review at another institution very difficult or impossible; contrast injection requirements; and medical constraints. Dynamic contrast-enhanced breast MRI examinations are expensive, usually ranging from $2500 to more than $5000. Moreover, in our experience, some third-party payers may still not reimburse for breast MRI examinations. For these reasons, the information derived from MRI must be clinically useful and not obtainable by less expensive means. In addition to financial cost, MRI imposes a time cost of between 30 to 45 minutes per patient even with a modern scanner.

Contraindications to MRI include all of the general contraindications to any MRI examination. These include, but are not limited to, implantable devices that are not MRI compatible (e.g., cardiac pacemakers and automatic defibrillators), non-MRI-compatible metallic aneurysm clips, neurocutaneous stimulators, cochlear implants, insulin delivery pumps, and so on. If there is any question about the MRI compatibility of a specific device or implant, the manufacturer's literature should be consulted before scanning. Current and comprehensive Internet-based resources also are available for reference and can be located through Internet search engines. We consider the presence of a postmastectomy reconstruction tissue expander a contraindication to breast MRI. Older tissue expanders can become quite hot during an MRI evaluation, to the point of causing severe burns. Although heat generation is less of a problem with newer tissue expanders, the susceptibility artifact caused by these prostheses is so extensive that it precludes adequate evaluation of the ipsilateral and contralateral breasts. Figure 12-1 demonstrates marked susceptibility artifact from a reconstruction tissue expander.

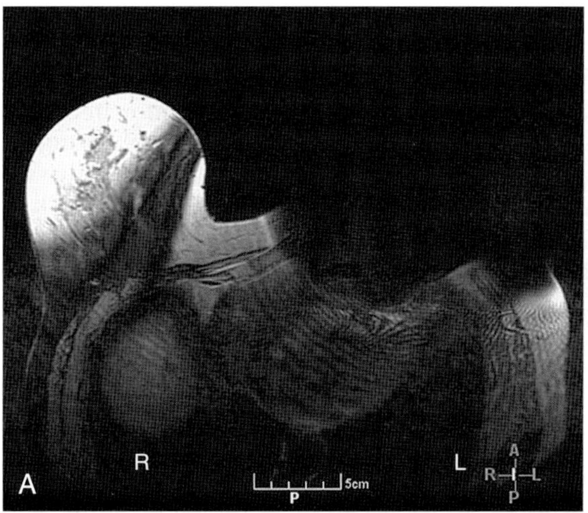

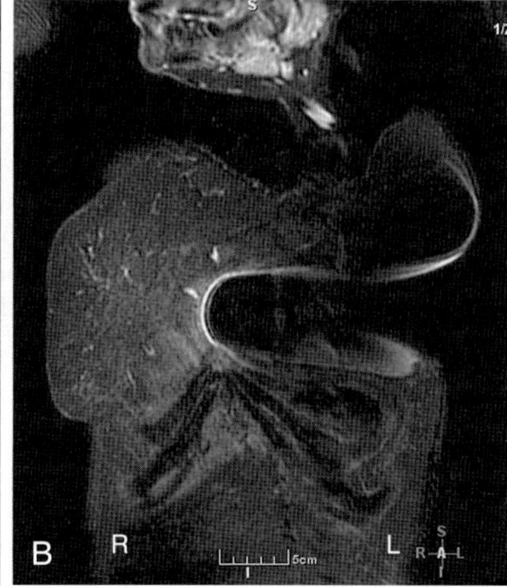

■ **FIGURE 12-1** **A,** Axial, high-resolution, T1-weighted, fat-suppressed MR image of a patient with a left reconstruction tissue expander showing marked susceptibility artifact obscuring the reconstructed left breast and causing marked inhomogeneity of fat saturation in the right breast. **B,** Coronal, short tau inversion recovery (STIR) coronal chest image of a patient with a left reconstruction tissue expander showing marked susceptibility artifact and image distortion obscuring the reconstructed left breast and sternum.

The left reconstructed breast is completely obscured, and marked distortion of the contralateral breast makes visualization and interpretation of any breast pathologic process very difficult, if not impossible.

As with any MRI examination the possibility of contrast reaction must be considered. Gadolinium-containing contrast agents have been approved by the U.S. Food and Drug Administration (FDA) since 1988. These agents have been proven safe and are well tolerated. However, they are not completely free from adverse reactions. Reviewing the literature, Weinreb[5] reported a 0.03% to 0.2% incidence of allergic-like reactions compared with an incidence of 0.23% to 0.7% for iodinated contrast materials. Li and associates[6] reported a total adverse reaction rate of 0.48%, 45 reactions in 9528 examinations over a 6-year period. Most reactions in their study were mild or moderate, requiring only supportive care or oral diphenhydramine. They did experience one severe anaphylactoid reaction (0.01% incidence) and had no deaths.

Because of the rare possibility of nephrogenic systemic fibrosis, chronic renal failure may preclude contrast-enhanced breast MRI. In our practice, any patient with an elevated creatinine concentration or with a glomerular filtration rate less than 30 mL/min/1.73 m^2 is not scanned unless cleared for gadolinium contrast agents by a nephrologist and the patient's primary care physician. Every attempt is made to find a noncontrast solution to the diagnostic imaging problem before performing a contrast-enhanced breast MRI in these patients. The benefits of the scan must clearly outweigh any risks involved.

Medical constraints, such as claustrophobia, make it difficult for some patients to complete any MRI procedure. Another limitation of contrast-enhanced breast MRI is nondepiction of most calcifications, including those that are associated with DCIS. Calcifications are best demonstrated mammographically, but the tissues involved with DCIS will frequently enhance. MRI of the breast may provide a more complete picture of the extent of DCIS involvement than can be determined mammographically, but occasionally mammograms show calcifications in a larger area than is seen by MRI. For this reason it is important to compare the breast MRI findings with the mammographic findings.

Breast MRI scanning protocols have become more standardized than in the past, but variations still persist. Imaging results cannot always be clearly reproduced from one facility to another because of differences in imaging technique. This can make it difficult or impossible to adequately interpret examinations not done at one's own facility. For this reason our policy is to not reinterpret contrast-enhanced breast MRI examinations done at outside facilities. If our clinicians are not willing to accept the outside interpretation we repeat the examination using our protocols.

MR units can vary from 0.3 T (Tesla) to 3.0 T. Currently, most breast imaging is performed with 1.5 T scanners; breast scanning should not be done on magnets of less than 1.0 T and preferably not on scanners less than 1.5 T. Three-Tesla scanners are increasingly replacing 1.5-T units for breast imaging. Because of the complexity of breast MRI examinations these studies should be interpreted at a workstation capable of displaying high-quality images for morphologic evaluation and also capable of providing dynamic data. We prefer to interpret breast MR images at a workstation with software that provides both 3D reconstructions for improved morphologic evaluation and color-coded dynamic data for kinetic evaluation of breast lesions.

Except in rare instances, at this time, breast MRI is not a stand-alone modality for breast cancer detection. Contrast-enhanced breast MRI does have an important auxiliary role in breast cancer diagnosis and surveillance.

INDICATIONS

The current clinical indications for MRI of the breast include the following:

- Evaluation of known breast malignancy
- Screening of high-risk patients

- Evaluation of tumor response to neoadjuvant chemotherapy
- Evaluation of difficult or equivocal mammographic, ultrasound, or other breast imaging modalities
- Imaging of the augmented breast

It must be emphasized that at this time the contrast-enhanced breast MRI examination is an adjunct method of breast evaluation. High-quality mammography, ultrasonography, and clinical breast examination should be done before MRI is performed.

EVALUATION OF KNOWN BREAST MALIGNANCY

Dynamic contrast-enhanced breast MRI is more reliable than mammography, ultrasonography, or clinical breast examination in determining the extent of newly diagnosed breast cancer.[4,7] In general, both mammography and ultrasonography underestimate the true size of breast malignancies. Numerous studies have found that multifocal and multicentric disease are better demonstrated by MRI than by other breast imaging modalities.[8] Mammography and clinical breast examinations also are limited when evaluating lesions located posteriorly in the breast and in evaluation of the chest wall. Contrast-enhanced breast MRI is much better at demonstrating the posterior breast and chest wall and at demonstrating invasion of the chest wall by tumor. Figure 12-2 shows a posteriorly located IDF with chest wall involvement. There is enhancement in both the cancer and in the intercostal muscles that extend to the pleura. Because breast cancer treatment is dependent on the extent and stage of disease, better evaluation of the extent of disease can affect presurgical planning but the long-term benefits (or liabilities) of these changes (e.g., converting lumpectomy to mastectomy or vice versa) have not yet been determined.

Historically, immediate postoperative imaging evaluation for residual disease has been performed using spot compression magnification mammography to evaluate for residual malignant microcalcifications. Breast MRI can also be used after lumpectomy to assess the postoperative bed for residual tumor because it is not limited either by benign postsurgical changes such as patient discomfort or increased postoperative tissue density or overlap, by imaging plane, or by lack of microcalcifications. In the past there was debate as to the optimal time interval between breast conservation surgery and follow-up MRI. The answer to this question is moot. Because margin involvement is rarely present, if ever, the clinical question to be answered (pathology reports include presence or absence of margin involvement), when margins are positive the question is, "Is there other disease in the breast that must be addressed when re-excision surgery is necessary?" MRI should be performed as soon as is practical after the initial surgery to localize any other residual disease in the breast that should be addressed at the time of re-excision. This is no longer a problem we frequently encounter in our practice since we prefer to scan our patients *before* surgery, preoperatively ascertaining the extent of disease and aiding surgical planning, reducing the incidence of positive margins and the need to look for additional disease after surgery. We prioritize our scanning schedule to facilitate this. It can take six or more months for postoperative changes to resolve, so it is best to wait at least this long before follow-up scanning when looking for recurrent disease.

One of the disadvantages of early breast MRI technology was the inability to simultaneously scan both breasts. This problem has been overcome with modern scanner and coil technology, and there is no longer any indication to do a unilateral scan for breast malignancy unless the patient is absent one breast. The incidence of contralateral breast cancer found mammographically and by physical examination is 4% to 5%. Evaluation of the contralateral breast in patients with known unilateral breast cancer is a subset of scanning for extent

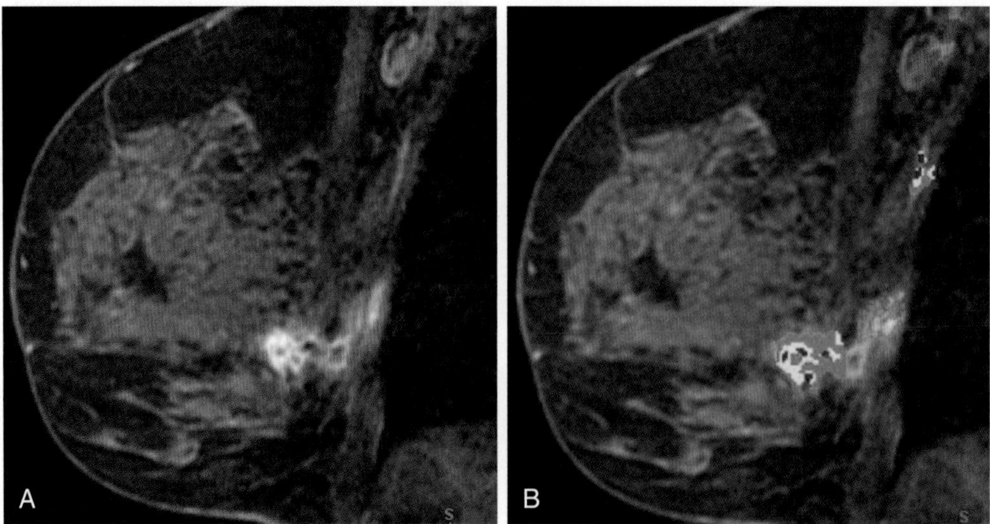

■ FIGURE 12-2 **A,** High-resolution, fat-suppressed, T1-weighted sagittal MR image showing a posteriorly located oval, irregular rim enhancing mass returned from biopsy as infiltrating ductal carcinoma (IDC) with chest wall invasion. **B,** Same image as A demonstrating color coding of dynamic data, which makes it easier to evaluate posterior invasion of the tumor into the chest wall.

of disease. Lehman and colleagues[9] reported finding 30 (3.1%) contralateral breast cancers in 969 patients with negative mammograms and clinical breast examinations that were scanned because of a recent diagnosis of breast cancer. Lee and coworkers[10] reported that finding contralateral breast cancer changed the original treatment plan in approximately 30% of cases.

Occult primary breast cancer is unusual, comprising less than 1% of all breast malignancies. Unfortunately, the ability of mammography and ultrasonography to find these lesions is disappointing, ranging from 0% to 50%. A recent review of six studies by Van Goethem and associates[7] has shown an overall sensitivity of 94% for contrast-enhanced breast MRI in detecting ipsilateral breast cancer presenting as malignant axillary lymph adenopathy. Figure 12-3 shows the digital right craniocaudal (CC) and mediolateral oblique (MLO) mammograms of a 59-year-old woman with a suspicious palpable right axillary lymph node and no palpable abnormalities in the breast. The MLO image demonstrates the palpable lymph node, but no masses or calcifications are identified in the breast. Figure 12-3 shows the same slice images of a fat-suppressed axial T1 image and an initial subtraction image with color display of the right breast showing this patient's occult cancer.

Breast MRI demonstrates both intramammary and low axillary lymph nodes. If a coronal water-sensitive sequence is added to the scan protocol, lymph nodes in the entire axilla as well as the internal mammary chain lymph nodes and supraclavicular and infraclavicular and low cervical lymph nodes can be evaluated for lymphadenopathy. Level 2 and 3 axillary lymph nodes cannot be palpated, and breast MRI can be especially helpful in evaluating these areas. Figure 12-4 is a coronal short tau inversion recovery (STIR) chest image showing marked right axillary metastatic adenopathy from levels I to III. Figure 12-5 is a STIR image from a different patient with metastatic cervical lymph adenopathy.

SCREENING MAGNETIC RESONANCE IMAGING

Initially, screening contrast-enhanced breast MRI was discouraged because there had not been any randomized clinical trials examining the effect of breast MRI on survival and because of its cost. Numerous subsequent studies have shown better sensitivity (with moderate specificity) for breast MRI when compared with mammography and ultrasonography. Because of these newer data, the American Cancer Society (ACS) has published

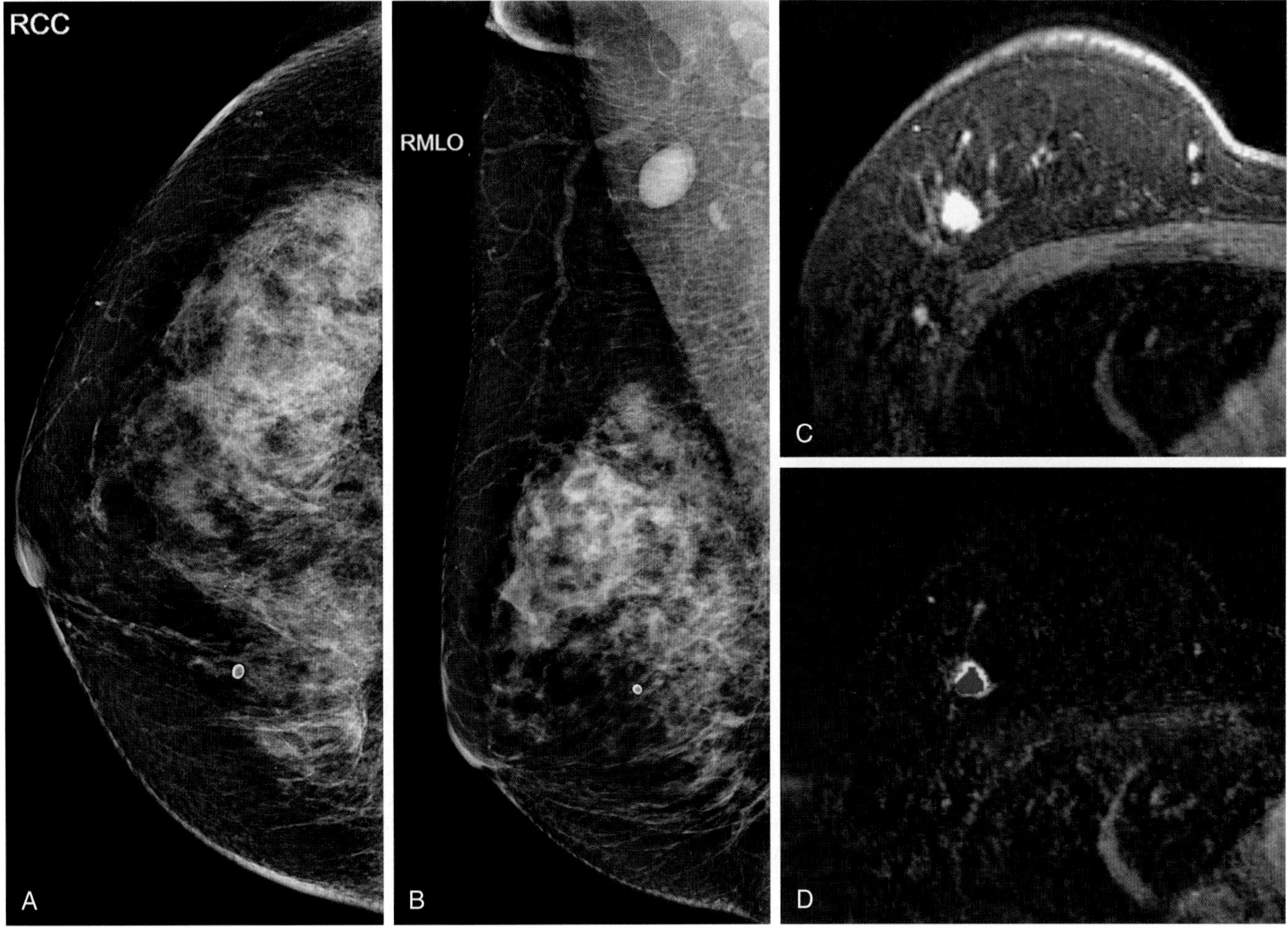

■ **FIGURE 12-3** Occult cancer. **A,** Right craniocaudal (CC) digital mammogram showing no evidence of mass or calcification. **B,** Right mediolateral oblique (MLO) digital mammogram showing a palpable abnormal right axillary lymph node. **C,** Axial fat-suppressed T1-weighted MR image of the right breast showing a round mass with spiculated margins and homogeneous enhancement not identified on mammography. **D,** Axial initial subtraction T1-weighted MR image in the same plane.

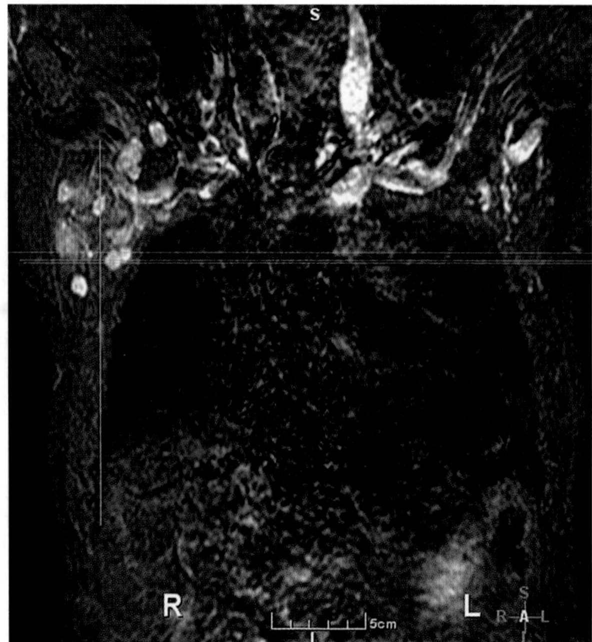

■ **FIGURE 12-4** Coronal short tau inversion recovery (STIR) chest image showing marked right axillary metastatic lymph adenopathy.

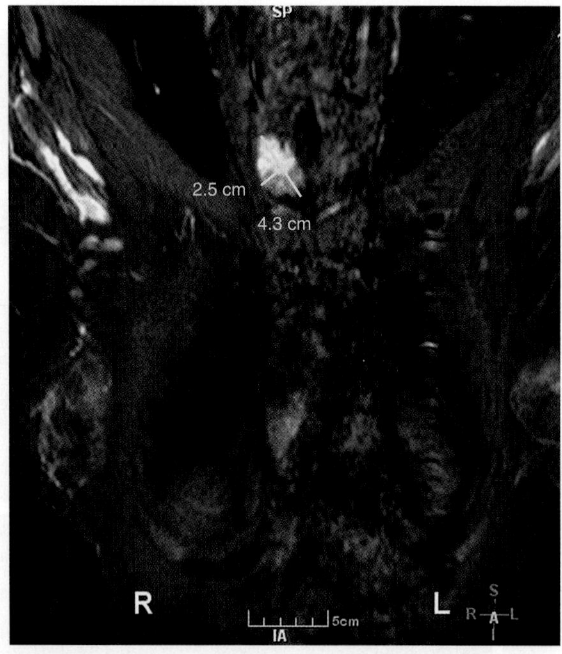

■ **FIGURE 12-5** Coronal short tau inversion recovery (STIR) chest image showing cervical metastatic lymph adenopathy.

consensus guidelines for high-risk breast MRI screening (Box 12-1).[11] Based on current available data, the ACS panel divided their recommendations into the following four categories: (1) recommended annual MRI screening based on evidence; (2) recommended annual MRI screening based on consensus opinion; (3) cases with insufficient evidence to recommend for or against annual MRI screening; and (4) recommendation against screening MRI based on consensus opinion.

Based on current research, the ACS panel recommended annual contrast MRI screening for any woman with a 20% to 25% lifetime risk or more of breast cancer. In addition to the evidence-based recommendation for annual screening breast MRI, the panel, by consensus opinion, also recommended annual breast MRI to patients who received chest radiation between the ages of 10 and 30 years, usually for Hodgkin disease, and to those patients with Li-Fraumeni, Cowden, and Bannayan-Riley-Ruvalcaba syndromes and first-degree relatives of those patients. The committee recommended against adding contrast-enhanced breast MRI to the screening regimen for women with less than a 15% lifetime risk of breast cancer. Because there did not yet appear to be sufficient evidence to recommend either for or against screening breast MRI for patients with a risk between 15% and 20% to 25% the committee recommended that those patients should discuss the potential benefits, limitations and risks, including the risk of false-positive findings, of adding breast MRI to their surveillance regimen with their health care providers with decisions made on a case-by-case basis. Finally, breast MRI is an adjunct to, not a substitute

BOX 12-1 American Cancer Society Breast Magnetic Resonance Image Screening Guidelines

RECOMMENDED ANNUAL MRI SCREENING (BASED ON EVIDENCE*)

BRCA gene mutation

First-degree relative of *BRCA* carrier, but untested

Lifetime risk about 20% to 25% or greater, as defined by BRCAPRO (statistical model for assessing probability of deleterious mutation of the *BRCA1* and *BRCA2* genes) or other models that are largely dependent on family history

RECOMMENDED ANNUAL MRI SCREENING (BASED ON EXPERT CONSENSUS OPINION†)

Radiation to chest between age 10 and 30 years

Li-Fraumeni syndrome and first-degree relatives

Cowden and Bannayan-Riley-Ruvalcaba syndromes and first-degree relatives

INSUFFICIENT EVIDENCE TO RECOMMEND FOR OR AGAINST MRI SCREENING‡

Life-time risk 15% to 20%, as defined by BRCAPRO or other models that are largely dependent on family history

Lobular carcinoma in situ (LCIS) or atypical lobular hyperplasia (ALH)

Atypical ductal hyperplasia (ADH)

Heterogeneously or extremely dense breast on mammography

Women with a personal history of breast cancer, including ductal carcinoma in situ (DCIS)

RECOMMEND AGAINST MRI SCREENING (BASED ON EXPERT CONSENSUS OPINION)

Women at less than 15% lifetime risk.

**Evidence from nonrandomized screening trials and observational studies.*
†Based on evidence of lifetime risk for breast cancer.
‡Payment should not be a barrier. Screening decisions should be made on a case-by-case basis, because there may be particular factors to support MRI. More data on these groups are expected to be published soon.
From Saslow D, Boetes C, Burke W, Harms S, Leach MO, Lehman CD, et al: American Cancer Society guidelines for breast screening with MRI as an adjunct to mammography. CA Cancer J Clin 2007;57:75-89.

for, screening mammography. For women in the high risk category (20% - 25% lifetime risk) both breast MRI and mammography should be done annually, beginning at age 30, at a facility capable of providing acceptable quality studies and able to provide MRI-guided biopsy of any suspicious lesions that cannot be identified by other imaging modalities. In women at intermediate risk for breast cancer in whom screening MRI has been chosen, no recommendations for what age to begin MRI screening or the frequency of these examinations were made by the committee. In lieu of adequate data it seems reasonable to follow the recommendations for screening mammography and begin these studies at age 40 and then screen annually.

In Britain, the National Institute for Health and Clinical Excellence (NICE) has published similar recommendations.[12] NICE adds the following to the ACS recommendations. Women with known *TP53* mutation should begin both mammography and contrast-enhanced breast MRI at age 20. Annual MRI surveillance is recommended for women aged 30 to 39 years with a 10-year risk of more than 8%, for women ages 40 to 49 years with a 10-year risk greater than 20%, and for women aged 40 to 49 with a 10-year risk greater than 12% and mammographically dense breasts.

EVALUATION OF TUMOR RESPONSE TO NEOADJUVANT CHEMOTHERAPY

Neoadjuvant chemotherapy is chemotherapy given to breast cancer patients before surgery with the goal of reducing tumor size and improving overall survival by treating undetected micrometastasis as well as improving postsurgical cosmetic results. There are two applications for dynamic contrast-enhanced breast MRI with neoadjuvant chemotherapy. The first is monitoring early response to treatment, potentially allowing for quick change in therapy in patients not responding to a given protocol. The second application is in determining the extent of residual disease after completion of therapy.

Response to neoadjuvant chemotherapy can be difficult to evaluate mammographically, by ultrasonography, or by physical examination because differentiating residual tumor from fibrotic changes or identifying small nonpalpable disease may be difficult or impossible. A number of studies have shown that MRI is more accurate in estimating overall tumor volume both before and after neoadjuvant chemotherapy; and because contrast-enhanced breast MRI provides some functional information, such as qualitative tumor angiogenesis,[13] it can be used to evaluate response to neoadjuvant chemotherapy more accurately than mammography, ultrasonography, or physical examination.

Our current practice protocol includes a pretherapy scan to evaluate and document tumor size, location, number of lesions, and contrast enhancement characteristics. The first follow-up scan is obtained after the second cycle of chemotherapy to re-evaluate the tumor for these parameters. Findings consistent with response to chemotherapy include a decrease in overall contrast enhancement, improvement in the enhancement curves, and reduction of tumor size. Nonresponders show either no change or increasing tumor size and no change or worsening contrast enhancement curves.[14,15] We will typically order another scan after chemotherapy has concluded to document residual disease before surgery. Because neoadjuvant chemotherapy can suppress contrast enhancement of primary, residual, and recurrent malignancy without completely eliminating the tumor we advocate waiting at least 6 months after completion of chemotherapy before follow-up scanning to evaluate for residual disease. A negative scan sooner may be due to tumor suppression, not tumor elimination.

EVALUATION OF A DIFFICULT OR EQUIVOCAL MAMMOGRAM, ULTRASOUND IMAGE, OR CLINICAL FINDINGS

Using dynamic contrast-enhanced breast MRI as a problem-solving tool is controversial. In our practice it is rare that we recommend MRI of the breasts because mammography, ultrasonography, or other methods of breast evaluation are inconclusive. Generally, we treat inconclusive or questionable findings as suspicious and recommend appropriate follow-up, usually tissue sampling.

Because occasionally mammography and ultrasonography can be limited in the evaluation of the postsurgical breast, MRI examination can be helpful in patients with a remote history of surgery and equivocally changing postoperative scarring. We have also found breast MRI occasionally helpful in the postirradiated breast for similar reasons. Very uncommonly we have used MR to further evaluate possible asymmetry or focal asymmetry, possible architectural distortion and for further evaluation of mammographic/ultrasound images and sometimes clinical breast examination discordance. Before resorting to breast MRI, it is imperative that a complete, high-quality evaluation of the breasts is completed using the more standard modalities of mammography and ultrasonography. Dynamic contrast-enhanced breast MRI should never be used to avoid biopsy of any suspicious lesion seen mammographically or by ultrasonography or of any clinically suspicious palpable lesion.

IMAGING THE AUGMENTED BREAST

There is a twofold purpose for evaluating the augmented breast. Evaluating silicone implant integrity was one of the earliest uses of breast MRI. Although to some extent ultrasonography can be used to evaluate silicone implants and to a lesser extent mammography can also be used, MRI is the most effective method for the detection of both intracapsular or extracapsular implant rupture. The integrity of saline implants is readily determined by physical examination, mammography, and ultrasonography. MRI should not be used to evaluate saline implants for rupture. Figure 12-6 shows axial and sagittal inversion recovery water saturation images of a ruptured silicone implant. Please see Chapter 35 for additional information about implant imaging.

Evaluation of the breasts for malignancy is the second reason for evaluating the breasts with MRI. The standard CC and MLO mammographic views are limited in their evaluation of the breast tissue due to the implants themselves, and this limits breast cancer detection. Although

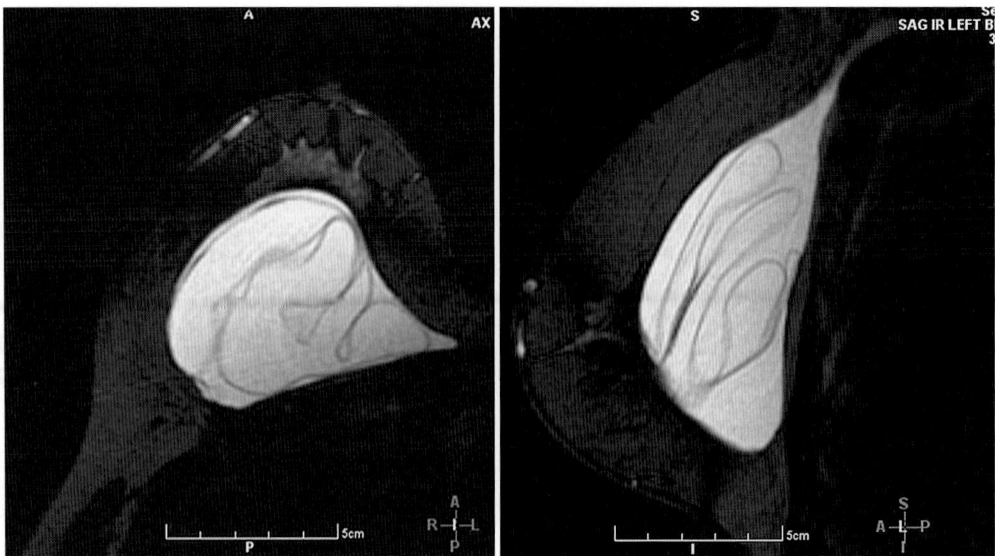

■ **FIGURE 12-6** Axial and sagittal inversion recovery water saturation images of a ruptured silicone implant demonstratting the "linguine" sign.

implant-displaced views improve the mammographic evaluation of the augmented breast, sensitivity is still lower with implants because cancers may still be hidden from view. Physical examination of the breasts and ultrasonography of palpable areas in conjunction with mammography offer additional benefits in breast cancer detection, but both ultrasonography and physical examination can be problematic. When results of physical examination, mammography, and ultrasonography are inconclusive, MRI has proven useful in tumor detection because the implant does not obscure breast tissue. Protocols for imaging the augmented breast and the nonaugmented breast for malignancy are essentially the same. At our facility, all patients coming for MRI implant evaluation are scanned for malignancy, too. We add inversion recovery sequences of the breasts with water suppression, in both the axial and sagittal planes, for assessment of implant integrity, in addition to our standard tumor protocols.

In addition to the screening indications discussed, MRI can play an important role in patients with ruptured implants or silicone injections. The standard methods of breast assessment, clinical breast examination, mammography, and ultrasonography are limited in patients with silicone injections or large volumes of free silicone in the breast from implant rupture. Silicone granulomas are poorly penetrated on mammography, and the mammogram can be extremely dense and show marked architectural distortion with limited visualization of breast tissue (Fig. 12-7). Ultrasound is scattered by free silicone and silicone granulomas, making it difficult if not impossible to adequately visualize underlying breast tissue. Although breast MRI will also demonstrate silicone masses and architectural distortion, dynamic scanning can reveal areas of enhancement suggestive of malignancy. In our practice this is one of the rare instances when we rely on contrast enhancement almost exclusively for clues to pathology because morphology can be difficult or impossible to evaluate because of architectural distortion and masses caused by silicone masses and granulomas, just as in mammography and ultrasonography.

TECHNIQUES

The key to high-quality breast MRI interpretation is simultaneous high quality temporal and spatial imaging with high signal-to-noise ratios to achieve the best morphologic and dynamic evaluation of any pathologic process that may be present. It is beyond the scope of this text to provide specific protocols for dynamic contrast-enhanced breast MRI. For specific techniques it is best to consult either an MRI physicist or the scanner manufacturer's applications support group.

Most breast MR images are currently obtained using high field strength 1.5-T scanners but 3.0-T imaging is increasingly being used. Dynamic contrast-enhanced breast MRI should not be performed on scanners of less than 1.0 T. Because of differences in imaging philosophy and differences in MRI scanner capabilities, breast MRI techniques vary from center to center across the world. As a general rule, however, most MR imagers now follow the same fundamentals. A dedicated surface breast coil capable of scanning both breasts at the same time is a necessity. Closed coils generally give slightly better signal-to-noise ratios but open coils facilitate MRI-guided biopsy. At this time, using modern scanners and protocols when evaluating for malignancy, there is no indication for unilateral breast scanning unless the patient is postmastectomy. As with mammography, comparison to the contralateral breast can improve sensitivity and specificity. In our practice we scan bilaterally when evaluating implant integrity as well, unless requested not to by the patient or her primary care provider.

The patient is scanned in the prone position with the breasts pendulous. Care must be taken by the MRI technologist to ensure that the breasts are properly positioned in the coil. The entire breast should be in the wells of the coil with the nipples pointed straight down. Improper positioning can obscure portions of the breast, simulate pathologic processes, or alter contrast enhancement characteristics. Some investigators use mild compression to support the breasts and minimize involuntary

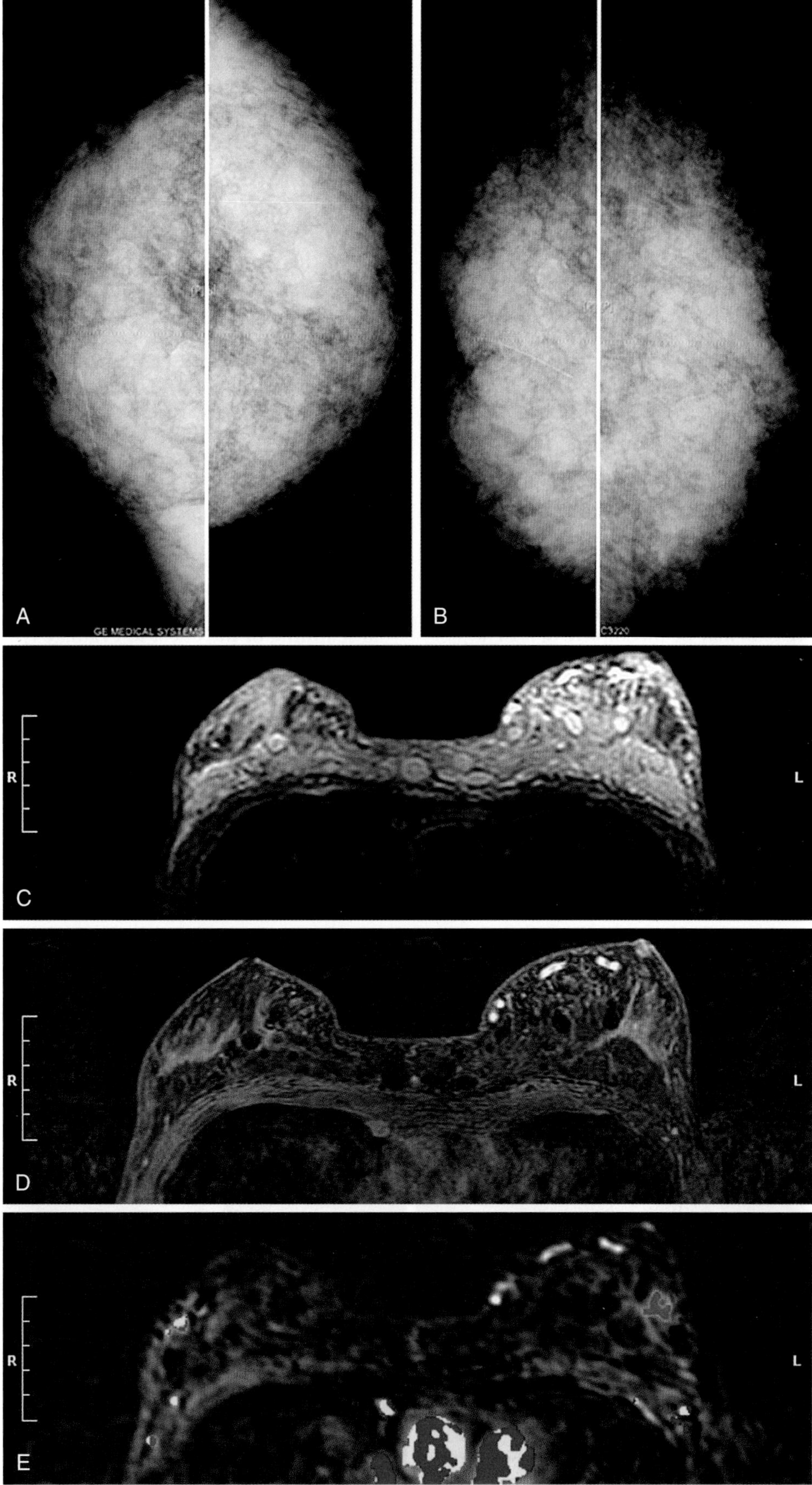

■ **FIGURE 12-7** Bilateral craniocaudal (**A**) and mediolateral oblique (**B**) mammography views in a patient who had silicone injections in both breasts in the 1960s. There is marked increased density of the breasts. Parts **C** to **E** are at the same slice location from the dynamic contrast-enhanced breast MRI of the same patient as in A and B. Both the axial short tau inversion recovery (STIR) (**C**) and fat-suppressed T1-weighted image (**D**) demonstrate marked parenchymal distortion. The dynamic image (**E**) shows focal, clumped enhancement bilaterally. Both areas were sampled. The enhancement in the right breast was caused by infiltrating ductal carcinoma (IDF) and the contrast enhancement in the left breast was inflammatory.

patient movement. Others believe this is not necessary and if improperly done could alter contrast enhancement characteristics.

Using a modern high-speed scanner, two basic sequence acquisitions are obtained. A water-sensitive two-dimensional (2D) sequence of the breasts is performed before administration of a contrast agent (either fast spin-echo T2-weighted or STIR) to evaluate for cysts and the water content of breast tissue and tumors, and a T1-weighted, fat-suppressed, 3D volume combined dynamic and high-resolution acquisition. A 3D volume acquisition minimizes partial volume averaging by allowing thinner slices and eliminating the interslice gap, which improves spatial resolution. Voxel size should be no greater than 1 × 1 mm in plane, and slice thickness should be no greater than 3 mm. Most modern scanners can achieve nearly isotropic voxel size. Volume acquisition also facilitates reconstruction of images in any of the standard orthogonal planes. Fat suppression enhances the conspicuity of enhancing lesions; it is easier to see and evaluate a white or light gray abnormality against a dark or black ground than it is to see it against a background of light gray or white. The MRI technologist should manually confirm the correct peak has been chosen; otherwise, fat suppression may be incomplete or absent.

Patient motion is most noticeable in the phase-encoding direction of the scan. For this reason it is important to ensure that for axial scanning phase, encoding is left to right and for sagittal or coronal scanning phase, encoding should be craniocaudal. This will generally place cardiac pulsation artifact posterior to the breasts.

Most laboratories use 0.1 mmol/kg of one of the gadolinium-based contrast agents. Patients should be weighed before scanning and the dose adjusted accordingly. The contrast agent is injected manually or by using a power injector at a rate of 2.0 mL/sec to 3.0 mL/sec, followed by a 20-mL saline flush. A precontrast sequence is obtained, followed by timed sequential sequences at 60, 90, or 120 seconds, depending on the scanner used and radiologist preference, for 5 to 6 minutes. This basic scanning protocol provides both high-resolution morphologic data and dynamic data simultaneously. On older scanners the dynamic and morphologic imaging was performed separately. High-resolution morphologic sequences were obtained either after or in some cases during the dynamic scan. Although the method of separate scanning is not optimal, at this time it is still considered acceptable. Because there is still some loss of information with reconstruction, each interpreting radiologist must choose the initial scan plane he or she is most comfortable with for initial evaluation. In our practice, initial imaging is usually in the axial projection for both of these basic sequences; in some laboratories initial scans are done in the sagittal plane. Because of the complexity of breast MRI interpretation and the number of images both obtained and reconstructed, these studies should be interpreted at a computer-aided detection (CAD) workstation. This allows the reader to view and manipulate images in the sagittal, coronal, and axial planes, which facilitates lesion evaluation and allows correlation of size, location, and enhancement characteristics. Use of other scan sequences, such as water-sensitive coronal scanning of the chest to evaluate lymph nodes and fat-suppressed or non-fat-suppressed precontrast sequences, are at the discretion of the interpreting radiologist.

For patients who are claustrophobic, conscious sedation can be achieved with oral or sublingual short-acting hypnotics or antianxiety medications to diminish symptoms. In more severe cases, intravenous sedation can be used, although we rarely use any of these in our practice.

Because the breasts are metabolically active in premenopausal women, these patients should be scanned between days 7 and 12 of the menstrual cycle (some laboratories use a day 5 to 15 schedule or scan during the second week of the menstrual cycle) when possible (Fig. 12-8). The breasts are also metabolically active in postmenopausal women

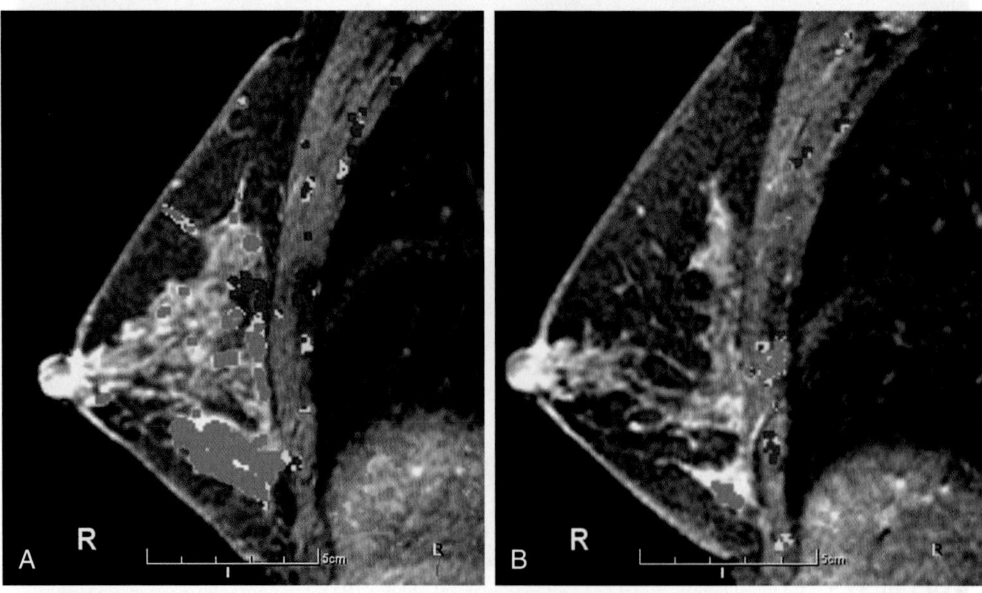

■ **FIGURE 12-8** A 46-year-old premenopausal high-risk patient scanned on day 20 (**A**) of her menstrual cycle and again on day 9 (**B**). The color overlay shows considerable contrast enhancement in the breast on day 20 and considerably less on day 9, demonstrating the marked differences in physiologic enhancement seen at different times in the menstrual cycle.

using hormone replacement therapy (HRT). It can take up to 8 weeks for the effects of HRT to resolve, so, if possible, HRT should be discontinued for approximately 2 months before scanning. We try to follow these guidelines in our practice and are reasonably dogmatic for our screening examinations. However, any woman with biopsy-proven cancer is scanned as quickly as possible, usually within 1 or 2 days of the request, regardless of her menstrual or HRT status. Immediately postoperatively, it is best to wait at least 4 weeks before scanning for residual disease and at least 6 months after chemotherapy or surgery when scanning for residual malignancy (Table 12-1).

TABLE 12-1. Ideal Dynamic Contrast Enhanced Breast Scanning Times

Best Breast Magnetic Resonance Imaging Scanning Times	
Premenopausal	Days 7-12 (5-15)
Postmenopausal using HRT	8 weeks or more after HRT stopped
Postoperative	≥ 4 weeks
Post chemotherapy	≥ 6 months
Post radiation therapy	1 year

HRT, hormone replacement therapy.

IMAGE ASSESSMENT AND REPORTING

In an effort to standardize breast MRI analysis and reporting, the American College of Radiology (ACR) has published guidelines for lesion analysis and for reporting breast MRI findings (Table 12-2).[16] The report requirements include clinical history, comparison with old studies, MRI techniques, terminology for describing lesion morphology, enhancement characteristics and kinetic characteristics, breast composition, the final impression, recommendations including treatment recommendations, and overall

TABLE 12-2. Lesion Classification Form for Magnetic Resonance Imaging*

	Lesion Type (select one)	
A. Focus/Foci (tiny spot of enhancement, <5 mm); if only finding, *GO TO SECTION E*		
B. Mass (three-dimensional space-occupying lesion that is one process, usually round, oval, or irregular in shape)		
	Shape *(select one)*	**Description**
☐	Round	Spherical or ball-shaped
☐	Oval	Elliptical or egg-shaped
☐	Lobular	Undulating contour
☐	Irregular	Uneven shape (not round, oval, or lobulated)
	Margin *(select one)*	**Description**
☐	Smooth	Well-circumscribed and well-defined margin
☐	Irregular	Uneven margin can be round or jagged (not smooth or spiculated)
☐	Spiculated	Characterized by radiating lines
	Mass Enhancement *(select one)*	**Description**
☐	Homogeneous	Confluent uniform enhancement
☐	Heterogeneous	Nonspecific mixed enhancement
☐	Rim enhancement	Enhancement more pronounced at the periphery of mass
☐	Dark internal septation	Dark nonenhancing lines within a mass
☐	Enhancing internal septation	Enhancing lines within a mass
☐	Central enhancement	Enhancement more pronounced at center of mass
C. Non-Mass-like Enhancement (in an area that is not a mass)		
	Distribution Modifiers *(select one)*	**Description**
☐	Focal area	Enhancement in a confined area, less than 25% of quadrant
☐	Linear	Enhancement in a line that may not conform to a duct
☐	Ductal	Enhancement in a line that may have branching, conforming to a duct
☐	Segmental	Triangular region of enhancement, apex pointing to nipple, suggesting a duct or its branches
☐	Regional	Enhancement in a large volume of tissue not conforming to a ductal distribution, geographic
☐	Multiple regions	Enhancement in at least two large volumes of tissue not conforming to a ductal distribution, multiple geographic areas, patchy areas of enhancement
☐	Diffuse	Enhancement distributed uniformly throughout the breast
	Internal Enhancement *(select one)*	**Description**
☐	Homogeneous	Confluent uniform enhancement
☐	Heterogeneous	Nonuniform enhancement in a random pattern
☐	Stippled, punctate	Punctate, similar-appearing enhancing foci, sand-like or dot-like
☐	Clumped	Cobblestone-like enhancement, with occasional confluent areas
☐	Reticular, dendritic	Enhancement with finger-like projections extending toward nipple, especially seen on axial or sagittal images, in women with partly fatty-involuted breasts

Continued

TABLE 12-2. Lesion Classification Form for Magnetic Resonance Imaging—Cont'd

D. Symmetrical or Asymmetrical (bilateral scans only)

	Symmetrical or Asymmetrical (*select one*)	Description
☐	Symmetrical	Mirror-image enhancement
☐	Asymmetrical	More in one breast than in the other

E. Other Findings (select all that apply)

☐	None apply	Edema
☐	Nipple retraction	Lymphadenopathy
☐	Nipple invasion	Pectoralis muscle invasion
☐	Pre-contrast high ductal signal	Chest wall invasion
☐	Skin thickening (focal)	Hematoma/blood
☐	Skin thickening (diffuse)	Abnormal signal void
☐	Skin invasion	Cysts

F. Kinetic Curve Assessment

	Kinetic Curve Assessment (*select one*)	Description
☐	Initial rise	Slow, medium, rapid
☐	Delayed phase	Persistent, plateau, washout

G. Assessment Category

	Assessment Category (*select one*)	Description
☐	**Category 0**– Incomplete: Need additional imaging evaluation	Finding for which additional evaluation is needed
	Final Assessment	
☐	**Category 1**–Negative	No abnormal enhancement, no lesion found (routine follow-up)
☐	**Category 2**–Benign finding	Benign, no malignant features; i.e., cyst (routine follow-up)
☐	**Category 3**–Probably benign finding	Probably benign finding (short interval follow-up)
☐	**Category 4**–Suspicious abnormality	Low to moderate suspicion for malignancy (biopsy should be considered)
☐	**Category 5**–Highly suggestive of malignancy	High probability of malignancy (appropriate action should be taken)
☐	**Category 6**–Known cancer	Biopsy-proven malignancy diagnosis on the imaged finding prior to definitive therapy (appropriate action should be taken)

*American College of Radiology Breast Imaging Reporting and Data System (BI-RADS). Instructions to user: For each of the following categories, select the term that best describes the dominant lesion feature. Wherever possible, definitions and descriptions used in BI-RADS for mammography will be applied to MRI of the breast. This form is for data collection and does not constitute a written MRI report.

From American College of Radiology: ACR BI-RADS-Magnetic Resonance Imaging. In ACR Breast Imaging Reporting and Data System, Breast Imaging Atlas. Reston Va., American College of Radiology, 2003, p. 111-113.

assessment using the ACR Breast Imaging Reporting and Data System (BI-RADS) assessment codes. To these recommendations, in our reports, we add information about background enhancement of the breasts because this may affect the sensitivity of an examination.

Before beginning the interpretation of a dynamic contrast-enhanced breast MRI study it is imperative to have available a recent accurate breast history and physical examination as well as have available for viewing all current mammograms and ultrasound images and other breast imaging studies (e.g., prior breast MR images) with their written reports. The breast history should include a current menstrual history. From this information the time the breast MRI was performed within the menstrual cycle can be calculated. This should be reported and, if relevant, a discussion of how timing of the examination within the menstrual cycle might affect the sensitivity and specificity of the interpretation should be included. If the patient is postmenopausal and using HRT, this should be reported as well, again with a discussion of its pertinence to interpretation. The history should also include other medications that might influence interpretation (e.g., tamoxifen, raloxifene, herbal supplements, vitamins).

The presence and location of any palpable masses should be noted in the history, as should any relevant mammographic or ultrasound findings. Nipple discharge or other nipple abnormalities are also important to report because MRI evaluation of the nipple and periareolar region can be difficult.

Dates and locations of prior breast surgeries and any history of needle biopsies, including pathology results, should be identified. If markers were left in the breast from prior biopsies, their locations should be noted for later correlation with susceptibility artifact findings on the breast MRI.

Any personal history of breast cancer, including DCIS as well as nonmalignant pathologic abnormalities such as ADH, ALH, and lobular carcinoma in situ (LCIS) should be reported. *BRCA* gene status, if known, should be included as well. This information may be obtained from the patient's primary care provider, other referring provider, or from the patient herself via questionnaire.

The first step in image analysis is a technical review of all the sequences performed to confirm appropriate patient positioning in the scanner and that correct scan protocols were followed, including sequences obtained and sequence timing, as well as contrast dose, speed of injection, and timing in the scan cycle. Contrast or injection problems are usually readily apparent by looking at the cardiac enhancement and venous enhancement in the breasts. Lack of cardiac enhancement and late-phase venous enhancement are clues to injection or contrast problems. Any technical problems such as marked patient motion, failure of fat suppression, or inhomogeneous fat suppression should be noted because these can complicate or contravene adequate interpretation.

Use of a CAD workstation, especially one that can color code dynamic data can significantly improve productivity by shortening interpretation time. Color coding of contrast enhancement generally makes it easier to find lesions quickly and provides all relevant kinetic data in an easy-to-interpret format without having to take time to draw multiple kinetic curves. When first beginning interpretation of contrast-enhanced breast MRI studies, color coding of physiologic changes and/or artifact (primarily motion artifact) can cause confusion, but with experience most of these findings are recognized for what they are, either artifact or benign physiologic enhancement. There are preliminary reports that interpretation using a CAD workstation can increase the positive predictive value (PPV) of contrast-enhanced breast MRI.

After ensuring that all scan parameters are correct, the 3D Maximum Intensity Projection (MIP) reformatted images are reviewed first to get a general overview of the breasts, background enhancement, and any possible pathologic process. The water-sensitive (T2-weighted or STIR) images (axial and, if obtained, coronal chest) are then examined looking for cysts and other fluid collections in the breasts, including recent postoperative changes if present. These scans are also useful for evaluating lymph nodes.

Depending on the technique used (STIR or fast spin-echo T2), benign and malignant masses can have varying levels of T2 intensity. Some investigators prefer fast spin-echo T2-weighted imaging because malignancies tend to show less signal intensity than they do on STIR imaging, thus providing an additional parameter to help in diagnosis. For other investigators this is of less concern.

The high-resolution dynamic sequences are then reviewed for lesion characteristics. In our practice we use the ACR BI-RADS reporting system (see Table 12-1).[16] The first determination is whether the finding is caused by a mass or is due to non-mass-like enhancement. Each mass is evaluated first for morphology, including shape, margins, and location, including distance from the nipple, and then for internal enhancement characteristics. As in mammography, shape and margin characteristics are most important.[17-20] Any shape can be seen in malignancy, but an irregular shape is more often seen in breast cancers.[18-20] Margin characteristics are the most predictive of malignancy, and of the three BI-RADS descriptors, spiculated margins have a PPV of 91%.[18,19] Of the six internal enhancement characteristics described in the BI-RADS lexicon, rim enhancement is most predictive of malignancy.[18-20] Figure 12-9 shows an infiltrating ductal carcinoma demonstrating all of the most predictive findings of malignancy: irregular shape, spiculated margins, rim enhancement, and fast wash-out enhancement.

After evaluating any masses that may be present, non-mass-like enhancement is assessed. The BI-RADS lexicon defines a number of different types of non-mass-like enhancements that are cataloged in Table 12-1.[16] Of these different types of enhancements the most suspicious for malignancy are ductal (Fig. 12-10), segmental (Fig. 12-11), and clumped (Fig. 12-12).[18-21] These non-mass-like contrast enhancement patterns are more likely to indicate DCIS. Ductal enhancement is linear enhancement that may or may not branch and that points toward the nipple. It may be smooth or irregular.

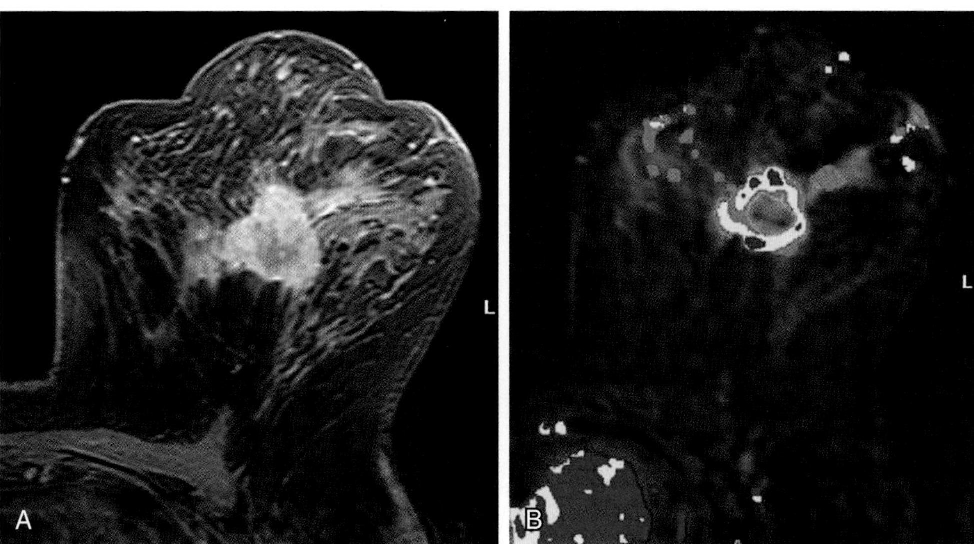

■ **FIGURE 12-9** **A,** Infiltrating ductal carcinoma showing an irregular shape with spiculated margins and rim enhancement. **B,** Same slice location, subtraction image with color overlay showing heterogeneous enhancement with three small foci of fast wash-out enhancement (*red*).

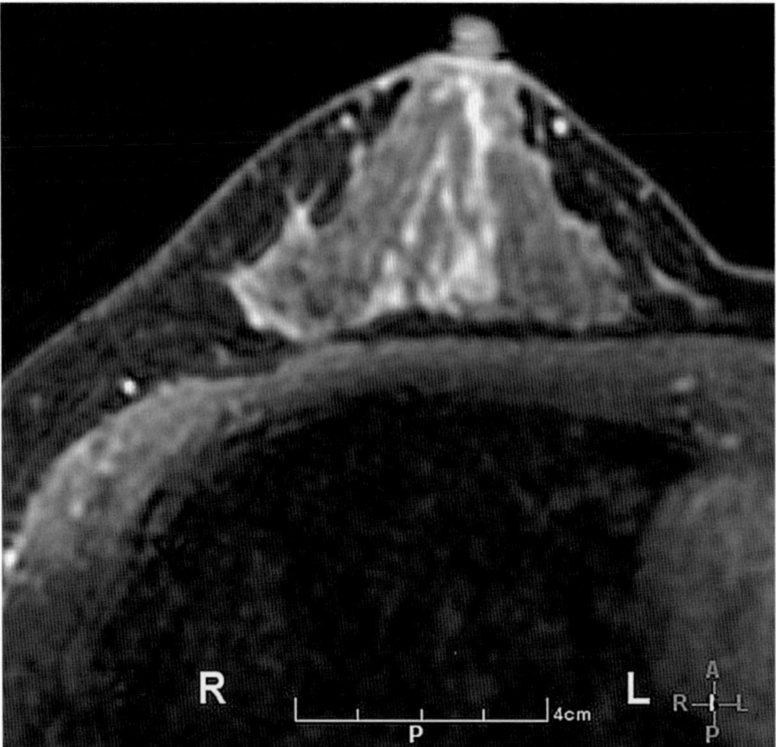

■ **FIGURE 12-10** Axial high-resolution, T1-weighted, fat-suppressed MR image showing ductal enhancement (DCIS).

The appearance of segmental enhancement is triangular or cone shaped owing to enhancement in a single ductal distribution. The apex of the cone or triangle points toward the nipple. Clumped enhancement is difficult to define. It has been described as "cobblestone" in appearance and sometimes confluent or like a bunch of grapes; if it is more linear, it may appear like beads or a string of pearls.

After morphology, internal contrast enhancement characteristics and non-mass-like enhancement have been completely evaluated, lesion kinetics are reviewed. For reporting purposes the signal intensity time graph is divided into two parts: an initial portion and a delayed portion. The initial portion of the graph is defined as the initial slope within the first 2 minutes (or when the curve starts to change) after contrast injection, and the delayed portion of the graph is defined as the slope of the curve after 2 minutes (or when the curve starts to change) until scanning is completed, usually 5 to 6 minutes.[16] This is more of a semi-quantitative analysis than has been published by some authors. The three descriptors

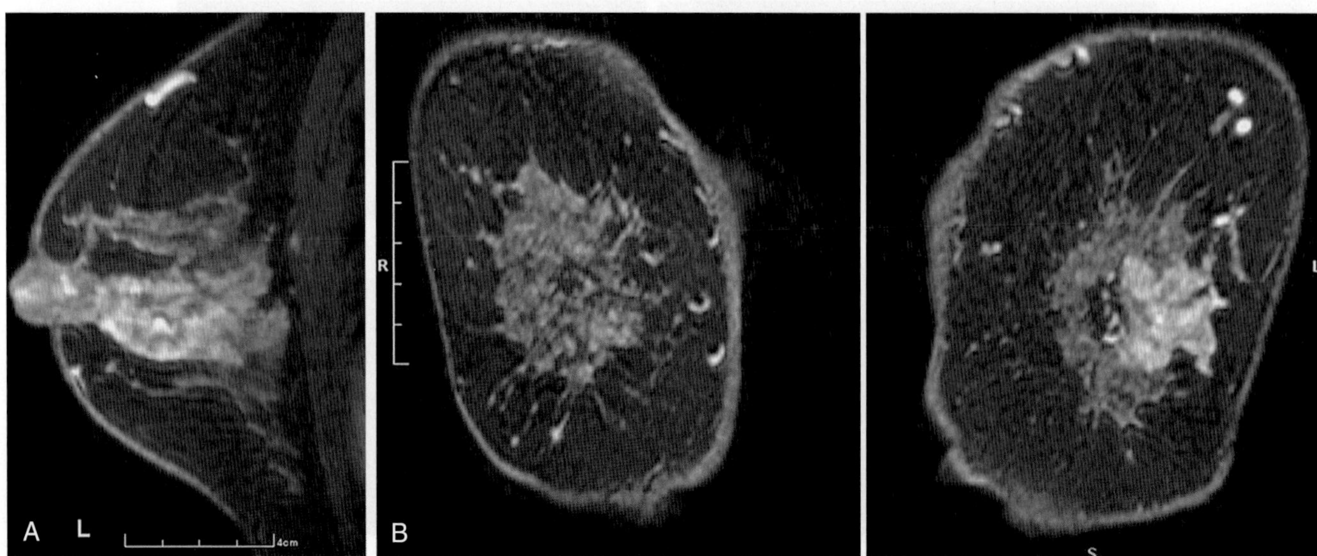

■ **FIGURE 12-11** Sagittal reformatted (**A**) and coronal reformatted (**B**) T1-weighted, fat-suppressed MR images in the same patient as in Figure 12-10 showing segmental enhancement (DCIS). Note on the coronal image that the enhancement is asymmetric.

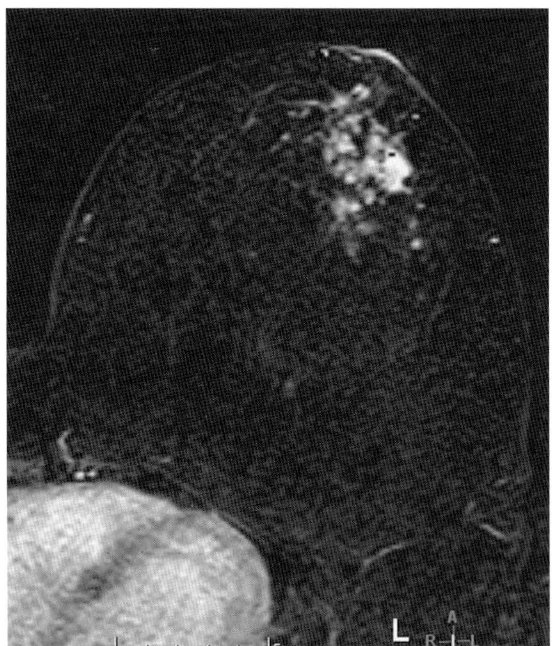

■ **FIGURE 12-12** Ductal carcinoma in situ (DCIS): segmental clumped enhancement.

for initial enhancement are as follows: (1) fast (or rapid); (2) medium; and (3) slow. The lexicon does not define the amount of change that must occur for any of these terms. Percent change in signal intensity is defined as $(SI_{post} - SI_{pre} / SI_{pre}) \times 100$, where SI_{post} is signal intensity at a given time point after contrast injection and SI_{pre} is signal intensity before contrast injection. In our practice we define fast (or rapid) initial enhancement as any signal change of 100% or greater, medium initial enhancement as a 50% to 100% change in signal intensity during the initial portion of the curve, and slow initial enhancement as less than 50% change in signal intensity. Lehman and associates[22] have reported that using a 100% change threshold decreases false-positive findings by 50%. The BI-RADS lexicon provides three descriptors for the delayed portion of the contrast enhancement curve as follows: (1) wash out; (2) plateau; and (3) persistent. *Wash out* describes the rapid decrease in signal intensity during the delayed portion of the contrast enhancement curve. *Plateau* means that signal intensity does not change during the delayed portion of the contrast enhancement curve, and *persistent* enhancement is defined as continued rise in signal intensity during the delayed portion of the contrast enhancement curve. Generally this continued increase in signal intensity is at a lesser rate than that seen during the initial portion of the curve. The worst curve for any significant lesion should be reported.

A number of authors have demonstrated that a wash-out enhancement pattern is the most suspicious enhancement curve for malignancy.[20,23] Whereas both IDC and ILC frequently demonstrate this enhancement pattern, any malignancy, including DCIS, can show any enhancement pattern, and most tumors demonstrate heterogeneous contrast enhancement; that is, several different curve patterns will be seen in different portions of the lesion. There also is evidence of different contrast enhancement characteristics between high-grade and non–high-grade DCIS.[24,25]

Findings suggesting a lesion is benign include the lack of any visible lesion (PPV ≤ 96%), no enhancement at all (PPV ≤ 95%), mass with smooth margins (PPV ≤ 95%), dark internal septations (PPV = 95%), and minimal enhancement (PPV < 89%).[8,17-19] The classic appearance of benign breast tumors on contrast-enhanced MR imaging, if such can be said to exist, is a nonenhancing or slowly enhancing smoothly margined round or oval lesion that may have dark internal septations. For example, fibroadenomas in postmenopausal women typically show either slow enhancement or no enhancement, have circumscribed margins, and frequently have dark internal septations. Benign lesions usually, but not always, show slow or medium persistent enhancement. Unfortunately, breast cancers can demonstrate benign findings and occasionally benign lesions will have a malignant or suspicious appearance just as they do on mammography.[18] Figures 12-13 and 12-14 show two fibroadenomas. The fibroadenoma in Figure 12-13 is oval with dark internal septations. Kinetic curve analysis (not shown) demonstrated medium persistent enhancement. Biopsy, at patient request, showed a fibroadenoma. Figure 12-14 also shows dark internal septations, but this lesion is irregular with heterogeneous contrast enhancement. Kinetic curve analysis (not shown) demonstrated heterogeneous medium persistent and plateau enhancement. This lesion was classified 4B and sampled because of the irregular margins and heterogeneous enhancement.

Contrast enhancement is an unreliable indicator of metastatic lymph adenopathy. Lymph nodes should be evaluated by their morphology alone. Normal lymph nodes have an appearance similar to that seen on other

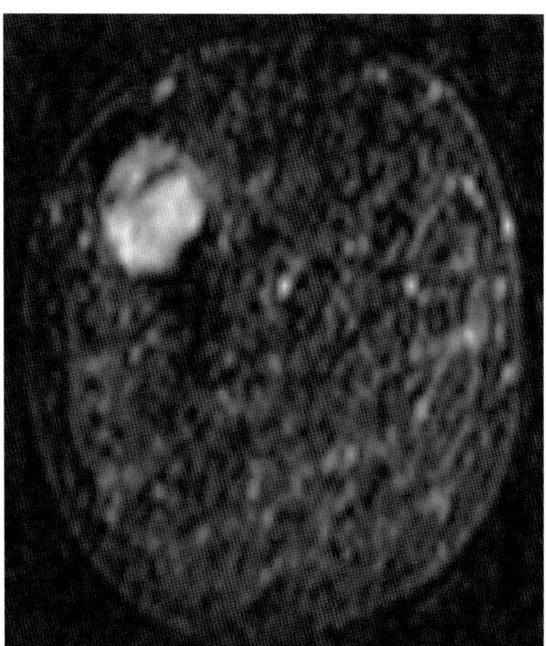

■ **FIGURE 12-13** Fibroadenoma: coronal reformatted image showing dark internal septations.

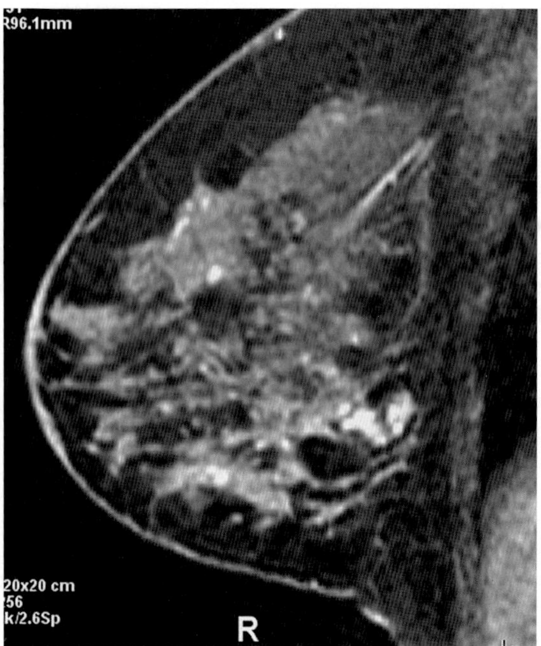

■ **FIGURE 12-14** Fibroadenoma: sagittal reformatted image showing irregular margins and dark internal septations.

imaging modalities, that is, they are oval or reniform with smooth, usually thin, cortical margins and well-defined, normal-appearing hilar fat. Abnormal lymph nodes become more spherical; the cortex thickens and becomes irregular, "lumpy," or "bumpy;" and there is marked loss or absence of hilar fat. As with mammography, size is not a criterion for diagnosing metastatic disease when evaluating axillary, supraclavicular or infraclavicular, or neck nodes. In the axilla, metastatic lymph nodes can be quite small whereas very large lymph nodes that have smooth cortical margins, a reniform shape, and well-defined fatty hilum can be benign. Evaluating the internal mammary lymph nodes is more difficult. Because it is unusual to visualize internal mammary chain lymph nodes on MRI, any time they are seen metastatic disease should be considered. Although the literature is sparse, Kinoshita and coworkers[26] reported a 90.7% accuracy in differentiating benign internal mammary lymph nodes from metastatic disease using size criteria of greater than or less than 5 mm.

Often the most problematic enhancement seen on dynamic contrast-enhanced breast MRI is the small spot or dot of enhancement, now called a focus. This is defined as "a tiny punctate enhancement that is nonspecific, is too small to be characterized morphologically, and has no corresponding finding on the pre-contrast scan … a focus is usually smaller than 5 mm."[16] A focal area is a larger nonspecific area of contrast enhancement usually measuring less than 25% of a breast quadrant volume.[16] In our practice the significance of these foci is often determined by the context of the scan and the size of the focus or focal area. Liberman and colleagues[27] have reported that the frequency of malignancy increases with increasing size of these lesions and that lesions measuring less than 5 mm have a 3% frequency of malignancy. A decision to dismiss, follow, or biopsy a focus or foci is determined by the indications for the scan, the patient's breast history, other findings on the scan, and the pretest probability of malignancy.

After reporting all of the relevant mass and non-mass-like enhancement findings, ancillary abnormalities such as skin thickening, nipple retraction, duct dilation, cysts, postsurgical architectural distortion, and so on, should be documented. As with mammography, our experience has shown that skin thickening and the nipple-areolar complex are frequently overlooked.

MAGNETIC RESONANCE IMAGING-GUIDED BIOPSY AND WIRE LOCALIZATION

MRI of the breast is very sensitive in detecting both breast cancers and benign breast lesions. Whenever a lesion is identified that has not already been documented by another imaging modality we recommend targeted second-look ultrasonography for further evaluation. It is rare that an abnormality detected on MRI cannot be found this way. For those few lesions seen only by MRI, a method must be available to localize the finding for either presurgical wire localization or image-guided percutaneous core needle biopsy. It is for this reason that we believe any laboratory performing contrast-enhanced breast MRI must have the ability to do MRI-guided biopsies.

Breast MRI-guided interventional procedures have been modified from the standard methods utilized in mammography and stereotactic biopsy. Many of the methods are similar and include image localization of the lesion, immobilization of the breast, appropriate access to the lesion using a grid or coordinate system, needle placement and image confirmation of needle placement, and a method of marking the biopsy site for future reference. Today MR-guided interventions are done with the patient in the prone position using a dedicated breast biopsy coil and vacuum-assisted devices. Initially, commercially available breast coils allowed access only from the lateral approach, but modern breast coils allow both a lateral and medial approach, which facilitates biopsy of more medial lesions without having to traverse most of the breast.

Review of the MRI-guided breast biopsy literature by Eby and Lehman[28] showed an overall success rate of between 91% and 100%, an average of 97% with overall cancer yields ranging from 0% to 80%, and an average of 37% positive biopsy rate across the studies, which is comparable with the yields reported for mammography and ultrasonography for similar procedures. These large-bore core needle biopsy systems for MRI have the same risks and complications as in mammography or ultrasonography, but they do eliminate the complications of open surgical biopsy.

There are limitations to MRI-guided breast biopsy. One of these is the inability to document the removal of these lesions with specimen radiography. The only method currently available to verify that the breast lesion was removed after needle biopsy is to document a signal void in the region of the lesion on a postprocedural scan. In our practice we routinely leave a tissue marker at the biopsy site so the biopsy location can be demonstrated mammographically. Additional limitations include limited access to areas of interest that are located posteriorly or near the chest wall and lesions located near the breast skin surface, but these limitations are similar to stereotactic biopsy and ultrasonography. Limited magnet time, cost, and patient limitations such as claustrophobia as well as small breasts can make MRI-guided breast biopsy difficult or impossible. As mentioned earlier, at our institution if a lesion is found on MRI, targeted ultrasonography is recommended. We frequently identify the abnormality on ultrasound imaging, and if the lesion is suspicious, a biopsy is performed under ultrasound guidance. When there is a question of concordance between what is seen at ultrasonography and MRI, we will place a stainless steel tissue marker within the lesion under ultrasound guidance and confirm the location of the susceptibility artifact with contrast-enhanced MRI. We prefer stainless steel markers to titanium markers because we often have not been able to find titanium markers on MRI after placement. Modern stainless steel markers usually show some susceptibility artifact allowing us to confidently identify the biopsy site while the artifact is not so large as to obscure pathology. Percutaneous MRI-guided interventional procedures are thus limited to the few cases when other imaging modalities are unable to visualize the suspicious lesion. Reports in the literature support this approach.[29]

The MRI-guided localization/core biopsy procedure requires 45 to 60 minutes (including setup, intravenous access, breast positioning, lesion localization, biopsy, confirmation of postprocedural signal void, and postprocedural mammography for marker placement).

A preliminary scan is performed to confirm all technical parameters such as patient comfort, positioning, and appropriate fat suppression. Gadolinium is then injected, and the breast is scanned. After lesion visualization, localization is confirmed and plotted. This can be done either manually using a worksheet or using software built into currently available CAD systems. These coordinates are transferred to the patient, local anesthesia is achieved, and vacuum-assisted biopsy is performed. Lesion conspicuity usually remains high throughout the procedure without the need for a second injection; however, occasionally a lesion may require additional injections of gadolinium to ensure adequate visualization of the lesion during the entire procedure. A final postprocedural scan is then done to document appropriate signal void in the location of the lesion, and a radiopaque marker is left in place. We have found that the key to successful MRI-guided breast biopsy is thorough knowledge of the breast's and lesion's anatomic appearance on sagittal MRI.

SUMMARY

Breast MRI began in the early 1980s but was not successful for tumor evaluation until the development of more modern scanners and contrast-enhancement techniques. Today it is an important adjunct breast imaging procedure for patients with known malignancy and is increasingly being used for screening patients at high risk for the development of breast cancer. Advances in both spatial and temporal resolution, imaging sequences, pharmacokinetics of contrast uptake, use of dedicated breast coils, and gadolinium-based contrast agents have played significant roles in the evolution of contrast-enhanced breast MRI.

Current clinical indications include presurgical evaluation of the breast, screening of high risk patients, and postsurgical, postchemotherapy, and postirradiation evaluation and surveillance, and imaging of the augmented breast. Evaluation of inconclusive findings from other breast imaging modalities is more controversial. Standardized guidelines for reporting breast MRI have been published by the ACR. The ACR BI-RADS lexicon has improved reporting, communication, and collection of data.

KEY POINTS

- High sensitivity and moderate specificity make dynamic contrast-enhanced breast MRI an important adjunct technique in breast imaging.
- Meticulous attention to technique is necessary to obtain quality images.
- Indications for contrast-enhanced breast MRI include the following: (1) evaluation of known breast malignancy; (2) screening of high-risk patients; (3) evaluation of tumor response to neoadjuvant chemotherapy; (4) evaluation of difficult or equivocal mammographic, ultrasound, or other breast imaging modalities; and (5) imaging of the augmented breast.
- Laboratories providing contrast-enhanced breast MRI should also be capable of MRI-guided biopsy.

SUGGESTED READINGS

Bazzocchi M, Zuiani C, Panizza P, et al. Contrast-enhanced breast MRI in patients with suspicious microcalcifications on mammography: results of a multicenter trial. *AJR Am J Roentgenol* 2006;**186**:1723-32.

DeMartini W, Lehman C. A review of current evidenced-based clinical applications for breast magnetic resonance imaging. *Top Magn Reson Imaging* 2008;**19**:143-50.

Eby PR, Lehman CD. Magnetic resonance imaging-guided breast interventions. *Top Magn Reson Imaging* 2008;**19**:143-50.

Kuhl CK. Current status of breast MR imaging. Part 2. Clinical applications. *Radiology* 2007;**244**:672-91.

Kuhl C. The current status of breast MR imaging: I. Choice of technique, image interpretation, diagnostic accuracy, and transfer to clinical practice. *Radiology* 2007;**244**:356-78.

Macura KJ, Ouwerkerk R, Jacobs MA, Bluemke DA. Patterns of enhancement on breast MR images: interpretation and imaging pitfalls. *Radiographics* 2006;**17**:19-34.

Orel S. Who should have breast magnetic resonance imaging evaluation? *J Clin Oncol* 2008;**26**:703-11.

Turnbull LW. Dynamic contrast-enhanced MRI in the diagnosis and management of breast cancer. *NMR Biomed* 2009;**22**:28-39. Available at *www3.interscience.wiley.com/journal/120841456/abstract*.

Van Goethem M, Tjalma W, Schelfout K, Verslegers I, Biltjes I, Parizel P. Magnetic resonance imaging in breast cancer. *Eur J Surg Oncol* 2006;**32**:901-10.

REFERENCES

1. Heywang SH, Hahn D, Schmidt H, Krischke I, Eiermann W, Bassermann R, et al. MR imaging of the breast using gadolinium-DTPA. *J Comput Assist Tomogr* 1986;**10**:199-204.
2. Kaiser WA, Zeitler E. MR imaging of the breast: fast imaging sequences with and without Gd-DTPA: Preliminary observations. *Radiology* 1989;**170**:681-6.
3. Harms SE, Flamig DP, Hesley KL, Meiches MD, Jensen RA, Evans WP, et al. MR imaging of the breast with rotating delivery of excitation off resonance: clinical experience with pathologic correlation. *Radiology* 1993;**187**:493-501.
4. Berg WA, Gutierrez L, NessAiver MS, Carter WB, Bhargavan M, Lewis RS, et al. Diagnostic accuracy of mammography, clinical examination, US, and MR imaging in preoperative assessment of breast cancer. *Radiology* 2004;**233**:830-49.
5. Weinreb JC. Which study when? Is gadolinium-enhanced MR imaging safer than iodine-enhanced CT? *Radiology* 2008;**249**:3-8.
6. Li A, Wong CS, Wong MK, Au Yeung MC. Acute adverse reactions to magnetic resonance contrast media-gadolinium chelates. *Br J Radiol* 2006;**79**:368-671.
7. Van Goethem M, Tjalma W, Schelfout K, Verslegers I, Biltjes I, Parizel P. Magnetic resonance imaging in breast cancer. *Eur J Surg Oncol* 2006;**32**:901-10.
8. Schnall MD, Blume J, Bluemke DA, Deangelis GA, Debruhl N, Harms S, et al. MRI detection of distinct incidental cancer in women with primary breast cancer studied in IBMC 6883. *J Surg Oncol* 2005;**92**:32-8.
9. Lehman CD, Gatsonis C, Kuhl CK, Hendrick RE, Pisano ED, Hanna L, et al. MRI evaluation of the contralateral breast in women with recently diagnosed breast cancer. *N Engl J Med* 2007;**356**:1295-303.
10. Lee JM, Orel SG, Czerniecki BJ, Solin LJ, Schnall MD. MRI before reexcision surgery in patients with breast cancer. *AJR Am J Roentgenol* 2004;**182**:473-80.
11. Saslow D, Boetes C, Burke W, Harms S, Leach MO, Lehman CD, et al. American Cancer Society guidelines for breast screening with MRI as an adjunct to mammography. *CA Cancer J Clin* 2007;**57**:75-89.
12. National Institute for Health and Clinical Excellence. *Quick reference guide familial breast cancer*. 2006. Available at *www.nice.org.uk/nicemedia/pdf/CG41quickrefguide1.pdf*.
13. Delille JP, Slanetz PJ, Yeh ED, Halpern EF, Kopans DB, Garrido L. Invasive ductal breast carcinoma response to neoadjuvant chemotherapy: noninvasive monitoring with functional MR imaging pilot study. *Radiology* 2003;**228**:63-9.
14. Loo CE, Teertstra HJ, Rodenhuis S, van de Vijver MJ, Hannemann J, Muller SH, et al. Dynamic contrast-enhanced MRI for prediction of breast cancer response to neoadjuvant chemotherapy: initial results. *AJR Am J Roentgenol* 2008;**191**:1331-8.
15. Padhani AR, Hayes C, Assersohn L, Powles T, Makris A, Suckling J, et al. Prediction of clinicopathologic response of breast cancer to primary chemotherapy at contrast-enhanced MR imaging: initial clinical results. *Radiology* 2006;**239**:361-74.
16. ACR BI-RADS Committee (ed). *ACR BI-RADS-ACR Breast Imaging Reporting and Data System, Breast Imaging Atlas*. 4th ed. Reston, Va: American College of Radiology; 2003.
17. Liberman L, Morris EA, Lee MJ, Kaplan JB, LaTrenta LR, Menell JH, et al. Breast lesions detected on MR imaging: features and positive predictive value. *AJR Am J Roentgenol* 2002;**179**:171-8.
18. Nunes LW, Schnall MD, Orel SG. Update of breast MR imaging architectural interpretation model. *Radiology* 2001;**219**:484-94.
19. Nunes LW, Schnall MD, Orel SG, Hochman MG, Langlotz CP, Reynolds CA, et al. Breast MR imaging: interpretation model. *Radiology* 1997;**202**:833-41.
20. Schnall MD, Blume J, Bluemke DA, DeAngelis GA, DeBruhl N, Harms S, et al. Diagnostic architectural and dynamic features at breast MR imaging: multicenter study. *Radiology* 2006;**238**:42-53.
21. Jansen SA, Newstead GM, Abe H, Shimauchi A, Schmidt RA, Karczmar GS. Pure ductal carcinoma in situ: kinetic and morphologic MR characteristics compared with mammographic appearance and nuclear grade. *Radiology* 2007;**245**:684-91.
22. Lehman CD, Peacock S, DeMartini WB, Chen X. A new automated software system to evaluate breast MR examinations: improved specificity without decreased sensitivity. *AJR Am J Roentgenol* 2006;**187**:51-6.
23. Yabuuchi H, Matsuo Y, Okafuji T, Kamitani T, Soeda H, Setoguchi T, et al. Enhanced mass on contrast-enhanced breast MR imaging: lesion characterization using combination of dynamic contrast-enhanced and diffusion-weighted MR images. *J Magn Reson Imaging* 2008;**28**:1157-65.
24. Facius M, Renz DM, Neubauer H, Böttcher J, Gajda M, Camara O, et al. Characteristics of ductal carcinoma in situ in magnetic resonance imaging. *Clin Imaging* 2007;**31**:394-400.
25. Neubauer H, Li M, Kuehne-Heid R, Schneider A, Kaiser WA. High grade and non-high grade ductal carcinoma in situ on dynamic MR mammography: characteristic findings for signal increase and morphological pattern of enhancement. *Br J Radiol* 2003;**76**:3-12.
26. Kinoshita T, Odagiri K, Andoh K, Doiuchi T, Sugimura K, Shiotani S, et al. Evaluation of small internal mammary lymph node metastases in breast cancer by MRI. *Radiat Med* 1999;**17**:189-93.
27. Liberman L, Mason G, Morris EA, Dershaw DD. Does size matter? Positive predictive value of MRI-detected breast lesions as a function of lesion size. *AJR Am J Roentgenol* 2006;**186**:426-30.
28. Eby PR, Lehman CD. Magnetic resonance imaging-guided breast interventions. *Top Magn Reson Imaging* 2008;**19**:151-62.
29. LaTrenta LR, Menell JH, Morris EA, Abramson AF, Dershaw DD, Liberman L, et al. Breast lesions detected with MR imaging: utility and histopathologic importance of identification with US. *Radiology* 2003;**227**:856-61.

CHAPTER 13

BI-RADS, Reporting, and Communication

Carl J. D'Orsi, Edward A. Sickles, Ellen B. Mendelson, and Elizabeth A. Morris

The American College of Radiology Breast Imaging Reporting and Data System (ACR BI-RADS) was initiated in 1988 at the request of our clinical colleagues who were troubled by the lack of uniformity of the mammography reports they received. The vague management recommendations placed them at increased risk of poor quality of care for their patients and also exposed them to increased medical-legal consequences. In response, the ACR established a committee to address these concerns and develop a lexicon of terminology to standardize reporting and management recommendations. A recently published history of BI-RADS is available for those who are interested.[1]

The fourth edition of BI-RADS underwent many changes from the initial earlier editions, including the addition of terminology and management options for breast ultrasound and breast magnetic resonance imaging (MRI). Although not as mature as the mammography portion of BI-RADS, these additions have helped expand and develop breast ultrasound and MRI, just as it did for mammography years ago. As much as is feasible, BI-RADS is data driven. When data is not available, consensus between general radiologists and those dedicating all of their time to breast imaging, either community based or in academics, is used. BI-RADS has been instrumental in developing an area of medicine that is arguably one of the most standardized and data driven specialties, with dramatic health benefits for the female population. Additionally it has allowed research in breast imaging to accelerate by providing standard terminology and defining benchmarks that provide clear and understandable definitions for sensitivity and specificity, which are basic to all areas of medical research. The ACR has an ongoing BI-RADS committee that accepts questions and issues related to BI-RADS. There is an overall chair of the committee and co-chairs for each of the subdivisions of BI-RADS. Since BI-RADS was meant to evolve as new data becomes available and practice patterns change, this committee welcomes any comments on issues related to BI-RADS.

The purpose of this chapter is not to reiterate what is in the current fourth edition but to review substantive changes in the fifth edition. This chapter begins with a short section on communication to underscore the need for clear concise reporting with standardized language to the health care provider. This is followed by a review of the changes in BI-RADS from the fourth edition to the fifth edition.

THE IMPORTANCE OF THE COMMUNICATION PROCESS

Communication among health professionals and the people for whom they care plays a critical role in the delivery of health care, influencing the quality of care and its outcomes. Effective communication is an essential part of quality assurance and risk management, promoting satisfaction among the women served, ensuring compliance with follow-up and long term screening recommendations, and minimizing physician-patient conflict and the potential for malpractice claims.

The very nature of the delivery of breast imaging services, especially screening mammography, is unique. Screening mammography is performed on a healthy woman as part of her regular regimen of health maintenance. The delivery of breast imaging care can involve a host of health care professionals and support staff, including the referring health care provider, interpreting physician (usually the radiologist), pathologist, surgeon, radiologic technologist, radiologic physicist, nurse, and receptionist. Effective communication lies at the core. A woman may not recognize the importance of combining mammography with a clinical breast examination, the need to convey her previous medical history and clinical signs and symptoms to the imaging personnel, or even the need to follow the recommendations of the interpreting physician. To combat potential misunderstanding by the patient, specific communication efforts must be made at every stage of the process. Good communication at one stage increases the probability of improved communication at the next, with an enhanced opportunity to achieve early detection and effective treatment of breast cancer.

Reporting the results of the mammography examination occurs at two levels: the technical or medical report to the woman's health care provider and the communication of results and recommendations in lay language to the woman. The interpreting physician, the referring health care provider, and the woman are all responsible for ensuring that the mammography results are communicated in an effective and timely manner and that the accompanying recommendations are carried out.

The Final Regulations of the Mammography Quality Standards Act (MQSA) mandate that facilities send each woman a summary of the mammogram report in lay language within 30 days of the mammographic examination. If the final assessment is for *suspicious* or *highly suggestive of malignancy* findings, the facility must make reasonable attempts to ensure that the results are communicated to the patient as soon as possible. Similar attempts should be made to communicate suspicious findings to the woman's health care provider as soon as possible (usually within 48 hours), in addition to the technical report.

Direct communication of mammography results to the woman by the imaging facility affects compliance with follow-up recommendations in a positive manner. Communication of the results of screening mammography only through the referring health care provider often leads to inadequate follow-up of abnormal results.[2] The impression that "no news is good news" can have adverse consequences for women with abnormal mammography results. Problems in communicating abnormal results can produce confusion about the next steps to be taken and cause delays in diagnosis and treatment, with consequences that may limit treatment options. Providing the results directly to the woman is a sound risk-management procedure and is a key component in facilitating communication between physicians and the women to whom they provide medical care. Many women, especially those who have little interaction with health care delivery systems, may be unaware of the need for follow-up with their regular health care providers or may make incorrect or unrealistic assumptions about the involvement of the imaging facility in this process. The fine points of physician interrelationships among the different specialties and their relative levels of responsibility for patient management are not as clear to the general public as they are to the provider community. The more explicit the instructions about follow-up, the greater the likelihood that they will be heeded. Improved physician-patient communication can also reduce the number of legal actions against the interpreting physician and the referring health care provider.

Results should be communicated clearly, promptly, and in simple lay language. The written communication should document the name of the interpreting physician and, in the case of abnormal results, should detail the next steps the woman should take. Priyanath and colleagues[3] evaluated patient satisfaction, timely report delivery, anxiety, and follow-up on recommendations before and after the passage of the Mammography Quality Standards Act of 1998 (MQSA) using a telephone survey. Although the MQSA improved patient satisfaction and report delivery, it had no effect on reducing anxiety about or fully understanding follow-up recommendations. This finding underscores the need for both patient and physician education about the expectations of mammography and its impact on breast cancer mortality.

The written report to the referring health care provider should be concise and understandable. A well-written report increases the use of both screening and diagnostic mammography. BI-RADS is intended to standardize terminology in the mammography report as well as to outline the organization of the report. This technical report should begin with a brief statement concerning the reason for the examination, followed by a brief description of the composition of the breast; significant findings, if any, using standard terminology; results of comparison with prior examinations, if applicable; and, finally, an impression that encompasses an overall assessment and recommendations. In the mammography report, any clinical concern should be specifically dealt with, and all verbal communications with the woman, her health care provider, or both should be documented.

The use of standardized terminology and a system such as BI-RADS facilitates the medical audit and outcome monitoring, which provides important peer review and quality assurance data to improve the quality of patient care. Because this information is used in peer review, it is considered confidential and must be collected and reported in a manner that complies with applicable statutory and regulatory peer review procedures.

MAMMOGRAPHY

Breast Density

The fourth edition of BI-RADS, unlike previous editions, indicated quartile ranges of percentage dense tissue (increments of 25%) for each of the four density categories, with the expectation that the assignment of breast density would be distributed more evenly across categories than the historical distribution of 10% fatty, 40% scattered, 40% heterogeneously and 10% extremely dense. However, it has since been demonstrated in clinical practice that there has been essentially no change in this historical distribution across density categories. This absence of change in clinical practice may reflect the reality that a few coalescent areas of dense tissue may be present in breasts with as little as 10% dense tissue, whereas primarily fatty areas may be present in breasts with as much as 90% dense tissue. The fifth edition of BI-RADS no longer indicates ranges of percentage dense tissue for the four density categories.

The BI-RADS committee is aware of recent and continuing investigations of percentage breast density as an indicator for breast cancer risk, and by eliminating percentage ranges we do not intend to compromise or impede any such research. We simply recognize the reality that interpreting physicians will continue to use density categories in mammography reports as they have done over the past many years, independent of BI-RADS guidance. We further recognize that both subjective estimates and planimetry measurements of breast density based on area as depicted on (two-dimensional) mammograms are imprecise indicators of the volume of dense tissue, which may be precisely measured using (three-dimensional) cross-sectional breast imaging modalities.[4] We await publication of robust volume-based breast density data, using percentage cut points that are readily and reproducibly determined at imaging, before again indicating percentage ranges for BI-RADS density categories.

Some breasts may appear more or less dense when imaged using full-field digital mammography compared with screen-film mammography. The superior depiction of the skin line by digital mammography provides the observer with a more accurate (and usually larger) estimate of the extent of the subcutaneous fat, thereby resulting in generally lower estimates of percentage dense tissue, especially for breasts with abundant dense tissue anteriorly. As the use of digital mammography continues to increase relative to screen-film mammography, we may observe a clinical-practice shift in the historical distribution across density categories to the less frequent use of higher-density categories.

Masses and Asymmetries

A mass is a space-occupying lesion seen on two different projections. If a potential mass is seen only on a single projection it should be called an asymmetry until its three-dimensionality is confirmed. Asymmetries have different border contours than true masses and also lack the conspicuity of masses. Indeed, asymmetries appear similar to other discrete areas of benign fibroglandular tissue except that they are unilateral, with no mirror-image correlate in the opposite breast. An asymmetry demonstrates concave-outward borders and usually is interspersed with fat, whereas a mass demonstrates completely or partially convex-outward borders and (when radiodense) appears denser in the center than at the periphery. As a descriptor of specific mammographic findings, use of the term *asymmetry* rather than *density* avoids potential confusion, insofar as *density* also is used to describe the attenuation characteristics of masses.

The new fifth edition includes clarification of asymmetry including a solitary dilated duct. The BI-RADS atlas describes four types of asymmetry: asymmetry, global asymmetry, focal asymmetry and developing asymmetry.[5] The term *asymmetry* is used to define a discrete but asymmetric area of fibroglandular tissue that is visible on only one mammographic projection. This finding is usually identified at screening mammography, when only one mediolateral oblique (MLO) and one craniocaudal (CC) view is obtained of each breast. When such a finding reaches the interpreting radiologist's threshold for recall, additional mammographic views should be obtained to establish or exclude the diagnosis of summation artifact (superimposition of normal breast structures). This is because research has demonstrated that up to 80% of screening-detected asymmetries represent summation artifact.[6] Twenty-nine percent of these were characterized as superimposition artifact after recall and diagnostic workup. Global asymmetry is a real finding (visible on two different mammographic projections), involving a large portion of the breast, defined as at least one quadrant. In the absence of a palpable correlate, global asymmetry usually is a normal variant or due to contralateral excision of a large volume of dense fibroglandular tissue, and is assessed as benign (BI-RADS category 2) with a recommendation for routine screening. A focal asymmetry differs from global asymmetry only in the size of the volume of the breast involved, occupying less than one quadrant. Despite its smaller size, focal asymmetry is of more concern than global asymmetry, because a small (especially < 1 cm) focal asymmetry may be nonpalpable yet malignant. Robust clinical research indicates that there is a 0.5% to 1.0% likelihood of malignancy for a solitary focal asymmetry identified at screening, with no associated architectural distortion, microcalcifications or underlying mass identified at subsequent diagnostic mammography and ultrasound examination.[7-11] Therefore, it is reasonable to assess such a finding as probably benign (BI-RADS category 3) with a recommendation for short-interval follow-up imaging and surveillance imaging.

Comparison with previous examinations is critical in evaluating asymmetries. Research indicates a near-zero likelihood of malignancy for focal asymmetries that are stable at imaging over at least a 2-year to 3-year interval.[7-11] However, more recent research has demonstrated that when a focal asymmetry is new or appears larger or more conspicuous than on a previous examination, the likelihood of malignancy is substantial.[12] Based on this evidence, the term *developing asymmetry* has been added to the lexicon. A developing asymmetry requires additional imaging evaluation in the absence of a history of surgery, trauma or infection at the site of the finding. Unless shown to be characteristically benign (for example, representing a simple cyst at ultrasound), it is reasonable to assess an unexplained developing asymmetry as suspicious (BI-RADS category 4) with a recommendation for tissue diagnosis.

Solitary dilated duct is another discrete mammographic finding for which recent research suggests a change in assessment and management from what was recommended previously.[13] Although rarely encountered, the frequency of malignancy is approximately 10% when a solitary dilated duct is identified (without associated mass, architectural distortion or microcalcifications). Therefore, although previous editions of the BI-RADS atlas indicated that this finding is usually of minor clinical significance, we now recommend additional imaging evaluation leading to tissue diagnosis unless a benign etiology is demonstrated.

Calcifications

With the fifth edition of BI-RADS, the *intermediate* category for calcifications will be eliminated. The two categories will be *typically benign* and *suspicious*. The former will retain the same list of calcifications as described in the fourth edition. The latter will now list *amorphous* and *coarse heterogeneous* in the suspicious category.

Amorphous calcifications appear sufficiently small or hazy, or both, that a more specific morphologic classification cannot be determined. Amorphous calcifications in a clustered, linear or segmental distribution are suspicious and generally warrant biopsy. Bilateral, diffuse (scattered) amorphous calcifications usually may be dismissed as benign, although baseline magnification views may be helpful.

In two recent studies,[14,15] the positive predictive value (PPV) of amorphous calcifications is reported to be approximately 20%. Therefore, calcifications of this morphology appropriately would be placed into BI-RADS assessment category 4B (PPV range, >10% to ≤50%). Coarse heterogeneous calcifications are between 0.5 mm and 1.0 mm in size and variable in size and shape, but are smaller than the similarly-shaped less than 1 mm *dystrophic* calcifications that occur in response to injury. When present as multiple bilateral groupings, coarse heterogeneous calcifications are almost always due to fibrosis or fibroadenomas, and benign assessment may be appropriate. Over time, these tend to coalesce into typically benign calcifications. However, when present as a solitary isolated group (cluster), coarse heterogeneous calcifications have a small but significant likelihood of malignancy in 20% of cases, especially when occurring together with even smaller, fine pleomorphic calcifications.[15] Among the several types of grouped calcifications that vary in size and shape, there is a continuum from *fine pleomorphic* to *coarse heterogeneous* to *coarse or popcorn-like* and *dystrophic*, based on increasing size of the largest, most coalescent calcific particles in the group. Assessment may be challenging at or close to the cut points for particle size (0.5 mm, 1.0 mm) among these different types of calcifications.

Distribution modifiers are used to describe the arrangement of calcifications in the breast. Multiple similar groups may be indicated in the report when there are more that are similar in morphology and distribution. In evaluating the likelihood of malignancy for calcifications, distribution is at least as important as morphology. A recent study involving 146 consecutive imaging-guided biopsies for calcifications, demonstrated that none of the calcifications in diffuse (scattered) or regional distribution represented malignancy, whereas 22% of calcifications in clustered, 50% of calcifications in linear and 56% of calcifications in segmental distributions represented malignancy.[15] The fifth edition more clearly defines the difference between *grouped (clustered)* and *regional*. The regional distribution will now include calcifications in a 2 cm or greater area and grouped within 2 cm. There was confusion with the prior definition in clearly separating grouped, formerly described within a 1 cm distribution, and regional, 2 cm and greater, leaving a gap of 1 cm. It is hoped this will clarify that distinction, which can be an extremely important one when deciding whether to sample or not sample calcifications.

Assessment and Management

In previous editions of the BI-RADS atlas, management recommendations were included with the text used to describe several of the assessment categories. In the fifth edition, we have removed the management recommendations from the text in order to provide more flexibility for several specific clinical scenarios for which a seemingly discordant management recommendation might still be appropriate for a given assessment. However, except for a few scenarios described below, the management recommendation should be fully concordant with the assessment. Assessment-management concordance is a hallmark of appropriate interpretation. To do otherwise invites confusing the referring clinician, the patient, or both, with the potential for producing incorrect treatment.

The most common clinical scenario in which the appropriate management recommendation may appear to be discordant with the proper BI-RADS assessment category occurs when there are no imaging findings in a patient who has a palpable breast abnormality. In this situation, it would seem that the breast imaging report should indicate a negative assessment (BI-RADS category 1), because there are indeed no imaging findings to describe. However, to cover the possibility that a palpable cancer might not be visible at breast imaging, the interpreting radiologist may want to suggest surgical consultation or tissue diagnosis, management recommendations that are discordant with a negative assessment. The correct approach to reporting in this scenario is to provide a negative (BI-RADS category 1) assessment with a concordant management recommendation for routine mammography screening, but to follow this with a sentence recommending surgical consultation or tissue diagnosis if clinically indicated. The presence of certain other mammographically occult clinical findings also may require a recommendation for prompt action by the referring clinician, such as suspected Paget's disease of the nipple without a suspicious finding at imaging. Another seemingly discordant clinical scenario involves the simple (characteristically benign) cyst that is either tender or painful, for which therapeutic aspiration is recommended for symptomatic relief, given that the recommendation for an interventional procedure is discordant with a benign assessment. The correct approach to reporting in this scenario is to provide an assessment of benign (BI-RADS category 2) with a concordant management recommendation for routine mammography screening, but to follow this with a sentence recommending aspiration to relieve the discomfort produced by the cyst. Still another scenario that involves an assessment-management discordance occurs in the woman who has a ruptured implant but no imaging findings suggestive of malignancy. The seemingly appropriate benign assessment would be discordant with a recommendation for surgical consultation leading to implant removal and possible replacement with a new implant. The correct approach to reporting in this scenario is to provide an assessment of benign (BI-RADS category 2) with a concordant management recommendation for routine mammography screening, but to follow this with a sentence recommending surgical consultation that addresses proper treatment for the ruptured implant. The presence of certain other benign imaging findings also may require a recommendation for prompt action by the referring clinician, such as breast abscess, edema of the breast (when not suspicious for malignancy), new hematoma, new clinically relevant foreign body, and gynecomastia in a male patient.

It should be clear from the previous examples that the correct approach to reporting for all seemingly discordant interpretive scenarios is that the assessment category reflect the imaging findings of the case, that a concordant management recommendation be provided for this assessment, and that an additional sentence be added to clarify the apparently discordant assessment and management options for the appropriate scenarios. This approach provides the flexibility in reporting to allow for both concordant and discordant components of management to be associated with the imaging-appropriate assessment.

Audit

While there are no major changes planned for most of the audit section there are three that deserve mention. The first relates to the positive predictive value of an exam recommended for biopsy (PPV_2) which is meant as a follow-up to a diagnostic exam that is placed into BI-RADS category 4 or 5 to determine how often that management will result in a breast cancer diagnosis. The second refers to benchmarks for the various metrics that can be calculated in an audit of a breast imaging practice. The third relates to use of BI-RADS category 3 in the audit.

PPV_2 is the percentage of all diagnostic examinations recommended for tissue diagnosis or surgical consultation (BI-RADS categories 4 and 5) that result in a tissue diagnosis of cancer within 1 year. A true positive (TP) is a recommendation for biopsy and a cancer is discovered within the year, and the false positive (FP_2) is a recommendation for biopsy that does not lead to a diagnosis for cancer within the year ($PPV_2 = TP / TP + FP_2$). Note that although PPV_2 is a metric designed to evaluate diagnostic imaging examinations, some published studies of screening outcomes also report PPV_2 data. In the screening context, PPV_2 is based on a variant of the definition of FP_2, in which positive examinations include the screening examination at which tissue diagnosis is recommended (BI-RADS categories 4 and 5), as well as the screening examination at which recall examination is recommended (BI-RADS category 0) followed by a diagnostic examination at which tissue diagnosis is recommended for the same lesion (BI-RADS categories 4 and 5). Therefore, PPV_2 at screening is meant to indicate the downstream outcomes of tissue diagnoses that result from positive screening examinations, even if the recommendation for tissue diagnosis is made at diagnostic imaging examination by a different interpreting physician than the screening interpreter who recommended only recall imaging. As such, PPV_2 at screening is more pertinent as a measure of screening practice in general than as a direct measure of the performance of the interpreting physician who interpreted the screening examination.

BI-RADS category 3 counts as a negative reading on the diagnostic mammogram. However there are a substantial number of BI-RADS categories 3, 4 and 5 given on screening examinations. In order to assess this unintended use of categories 3, 4 and 5, a positive screening mammogram will now include any screening exam assessed as category 0, 3, 4 or 5. Basically it is any action recommended from a screen that occurs within the normal year interval to the next screening exam. Thus, if a reader feels that there is enough information to issue a BI-RADS 3 recommendation without a diagnostic workup and no malignancy is discovered within the year, it will be counted as a false positive for screening audit purposes. Thus, the substantive change is counting a category 3 as a positive exam from a screen. This does not affect its status as a negative exam when issued after a diagnostic exam.

ULTRASOUND

The ultrasound (US) and MRI sections were new additions to the fourth edition of BI-RADS in recognition of the important role they play in breast imaging. The first US and MRI editions emphasized the similarity of their terminology to that of mammography whenever possible as well as introducing new feature categories and descriptors unique to each of these imaging modalities. Although not as mature as the mammography section of BI-RADS, data are rapidly accumulating regarding the feature characteristics that contribute to assessments of US and MRI imaging. The fifth edition for mammography and second editions of US and MRI will incorporate recent advances in feature analysis and refine the lexicon terminology with an overall goal of harmonizing the entire document.

The second edition of US BI-RADS has additional sections related to technical factors with examples illustrating optimal as well as poor technique. To obtain US images of diagnostic quality, minimizing its vaunted operator dependence, some guidelines for adjusting imaging parameters such as field of view, gray scale and contrast settings, compound scanning will be included.

Technical Considerations

The *ACR Practice Guideline for the Performance of the Breast Ultrasound Examination* suggests use of a linear array transducer with a center frequency of at least 10 MHz.[16] Higher frequency transducers provide higher resolution images in the near field but with decreased penetration of deeper tissues, compensated for by the lower end frequencies of ranges such as 17 to 5 MHz. Transducers with overall lower frequency ranges such as 10 to 5 MHz may produce images with insufficient clarity to allow accurate interpretation or, in some cases, may result in failure to detect lesions altogether. The field of view refers to setting the depth of tissue that will display on the monitor. When searching for lesions, the depth should generally be set deep enough so that all of the breast tissue can be seen back to the pectoralis muscle but shallow enough to minimize the unhelpful amount of lung that is displayed. When a lesion is identified, the field of view should be set small enough to maximize the potential resolution of the display screen. When the field of view is set too deep, detail in small lesions may not be perceived. For larger lesions, extended field of view (EFOV) imaging can be helpful to visualize the entire lesion. EFOV can also be useful to demonstrate the geographic relationship between multiple lesions or between a lesion and a structure such as the nipple. Automated ultrasound systems in development also depict the entire breast, and distance between lesions can be estimated, as well as relationship of a lesion to an anatomic reference point. The focal zone defines the depth of tissue where the ultrasound beam is most focused and where resolution is optimized. One or more focal zones can be electronically set at the depth of the area being investigated. Artifacts and blur caused by suboptimal placement of the focal zone can cause misinterpretation of breast lesions. For deeper lesions, the active frequency of a broad bandwidth linear transducer will be reduced to allow penetration when the focal zone is adjusted to the lesion's depth (the greatest depth). The gray scale gain and dynamic range set the overall brightness of the image by controlling the extent of echo amplification. Gray scale gain should be set so normal breast parenchyma varies in echogenicity using much of the gray-scale range. If fat is gray, not black, the gray scale is set appropriately. The gain may be set too high if the tissue appears as varying shades of white or too low if the fat and hypoechoic lesions appear black, creating a situation where hypoechoic masses can be mistaken for simple cysts. Real-time spatial compound imaging creates a single ultrasound frame by averaging three to nine overlapping ultrasound images obtained at slightly different angles of insonation. The different angles are obtained by electronically steering the transducer array. The process is repeated rapidly to create a real-time technique. Compound imaging provides improved depiction of important features of a mass centered in the image-shape and margins, while ultrasound artifacts such as speckle and clutter are suppressed. Posterior shadowing and enhancement will be less apparent with spatial compounding, although they remain perceptible once the eye is trained, and the speckle reduction and improved marginal definition in lesion analysis far outweigh the importance of intense enhancement and shadowing. In some instances, the posterior features may look conical rather than columnar, representing the crossing points of the angulated beams in a compound scan.

The new edition will continue to focus on the first edition triumvirate of three important feature categories for US: shape, margin, and orientation. In addition to the section on technique, the second edition will expand some of the feature categories and change others to make the lexicon more user-friendly in lesion assessment. There will be expanded coverage of anatomy, lymph nodes, and cystic lesions, for example. A new section, substituting for the current, *Surrounding Tissue*, will be called *Associated Findings*. This section will include many of the features such as duct changes, Cooper ligament changes, edema, architectural distortion, and skin thickening, retraction, and irregularity. The descriptors for the current feature categories of *Vascularity* and *Border zone* (e.g., echogenic halo) will be relocated in *Associated Findings* along with an entry on elastography. Much recent work has been done on using ultrasound to assess stiffness of a mass compared with the normal tissue around it. The theory of elastography is that malignant masses are harder and stiffer than benign masses and will deform less either when manually compressed with the transducer or when supersonic wavelengths are utilized, although some cancers are soft. Elastography may also have value in confirming identity of some masses as cysts. Sensitivities and specificities of the different methods used to evaluate *hardness* or *softness* are areas of current research.

In summary, the expanded and revised fifth BI-RADS edition (the second edition of BI-RADS for US) will re-emphasize through many examples the power of combined analysis of three feature categories in determining an assessment category for a breast lesion: shape (oval, round, irregular), orientation (parallel, not parallel), and margin (circumscribed, not circumscribed), the current descriptors provided within parentheses.

MAGNETIC RESONANCE IMAGING

The fourth edition of the ACR BI-RADS-MRI is the product of development and testing by the international group of MRI experts. This edition includes a section on definitions and illustrations of each morphologic feature described in the ACR BI-RADS-MRI nomenclature, technical aspects of acquiring breast MRI examinations, and illustrations of dynamic curve data. The objective of the ACR BI-RADS-MRI lexicon is to standardize the language used in breast MRI reporting, to aid clinicians in understanding the results of the breast MRI tests for subsequent patient management, and to aid scientific research by enabling investigators to compare studies based on similar breast MRI terminology.

Background enhancement

The amount of breast tissue present and the degree of background parenchymal enhancement should be reported. The enhancement of glandular tissue plays a very similar role to breast density in mammography. As background enhancement increases, the ability for detection of cancers decreases. The enhancement patterns should be indicated as follows:

Breast parenchymal enhancement

1. None/Minimal
2. Mild
3. Moderate
4. Marked

Further clarification of the definitions of each of these categories will be included in the fifth edition.

Focus or Foci

A *focus* is a tiny punctate enhancement that is nonspecific, is too small to be characterized morphologically, and has no corresponding finding on the precontrast scan. These can be seen frequently, but should be evaluated in the clinical context of the exam. *Multiple foci* are tiny but widely separated small dots of enhancement. A focus is usually smaller than 5 mm and could be benign or malignant. *Stippled* refers to multiple, often innumerable, punctate foci that are approximately 1 to 2 mm in size and appear scattered throughout an area of the breast that does not conform to a duct system. Stippled enhancement is more characteristic of benign normal variant parenchymal enhancement or fibrocystic changes.

Dynamic Contrast Enhancement

Kinetic techniques analyze the lesion enhancement rate by analyzing the signal intensity on a pixel-by-pixel basis over time. More acquisitions obtained after intravenous contrast administration results in more points on the enhancement curve. Additionally, the faster the acquisition, the more potential information is obtained about the curve. The most suspicious aspect of the lesion should be used to generate this information. The kinetic information needed for a time intensity curve can be obtained by placing an region of interest (ROI) of at least three pixels on a computer-aided software program. Signal intensity (SI) increase is measured relative to the baseline signal-intensity value $[(SI_{post} - SI_{pre})/SI_{pre}] \times 100\%$. SI_{pre} = baseline signal intensity, and SI_{post} = signal intensity after contrast injection.

Kinetic techniques generate time/signal-intensity curves (TIC). The information derived from these curves can be interpreted by defining a threshold level for determination of malignancy. In general the immediate phase of the curve represents the enhancement that occurs in the first 2 minutes post contrast enhancement or when the initial portion of the curve begins to change. This initial change may be termed *rapid* if the increase is equal to or greater than 100% enhancement from baseline, *medium* if it is 50% to 100% of baseline, or *slow* if it is less than 50% of baseline. In addition to the degree of enhancement in the initial phase of the curve, the shape of the curve over more delayed time points is also important to help separate benign from malignant findings. There are three general types of curves. The delayed-phase enhancement pattern occurs after 2 minutes, or after the curve starts to change, and in general will be used to describe the overall curve shape.

A *persistent* curve shows continuous enhancement increasing with time in its delayed phase. A *plateau curve* shows maximum signal intensity approximately 2 to 3 minutes after injection, and the signal intensity then remains constant at this level. A *washout* curve shows decreasing signal intensity after peak enhancement has been reached within 2 to 3 minutes. In general, for the delayed phase, persistent is 10% or more of the initial enhancement; plateau is equal to the initial enhancement; and washout is 10% or less of the initial enhancement. There is overlap between malignant and benign lesions, however. As a general rule, most benign lesions follow persistent curves, and most malignant lesions follow washout curves. A plateau curve can be seen with both benign and malignant lesions. These kinetic definitions of enhancements are evolving, and what is presented are representative guidelines. Morphologically benign-appearing lesions may benefit most from enhancement kinetics, since enhancement kinetic data may influence the decision to biopsy a benign-appearing mass. On the other hand, suspicious morphologic features should prompt biopsy in appropriate clinical settings regardless of kinetic analysis. It should be emphasized that kinetic analysis is one aspect of interpretation and management should not be based solely on kinetic features.

CONCLUSION

This chapter reflects the maturity and updates related to BI-RADS for each of the subdivisions of mammography, breast US and breast MRI. The mammography subdivision, as the oldest, reflects more data related to BI-RADS validation, as well as changes related to issues that arise in clinical practice of breast imaging. As use of the US and MRI lexicons becomes more frequent, research in these divisions, as it relates to BI-RADS validation, will be forthcoming and future editions of BI-RADS are anticipated to demonstrate these positive evolving changes.

KEY POINTS

- Breast density measurement definitions will not be by quartiles as currently described.
- When a focal asymmetry is new or appears larger likelihood of malignancy is substantial.
- When a solitary dilated duct is encountered, frequency of malignancy is about 10%.
- Calcifications will be placed in either a *benign* or *suspicious* category with elimination of the *intermediate* category.
- Coarse heterogeneous calcifications have a 20% chance of malignancy when grouped.
- Final assessment and management recommendations will be separated for certain defined scenarios to accommodate clinically important issues with negative or benign imaging.

SUGGESTED READINGS

Burnside E, Sickles EA, Bassett LW, Rubin DL, Lee CH, Ikeda DM, et al. The ACR BI-RADS experience: learning from history. *J Am Coll Radiol* 2009;**6**:851-60.

D'Orsi CJ, Newell MS. BI-RADS decoded: detailed guidance on potentially confusing issues. *Radiol Clin North Am* 2007;**45**:751-63.

REFERENCES

1. Burnside E, Sickles EA, Bassett LW, Rubin DL, Lee CH, Ikeda DM, et al. The ACR BI-RADS experience: learning from history. *J Am Coll Radiol* 2009;**6**:851-60.
2. Cardenosa G, Eklund GW. Rate of compliance with recommendations for additional mammographic views and biopsies. *Radiology* 1991;**181**:359-61.
3. Priyanath A, Feinglass J, Dolan NC, Haviley C, Venta LA. Patient satisfaction with the communication of mammographic results before and after Mammography Quality Standards Reauthorization Act of 1998. *AJR Am J Roentgenol* 2002;**178**:451-6.
4. Kopans DB. Basic physics and doubts about relationship between mammographically determined tissue density and breast cancer risk. *Radiology* 2008;**246**:348-53.
5. Mendelson EB, Berg WA, Merritt CR. Toward a standardized breast ultrasound lexicon, BI-RADS: ultrasound. *Semin Roentgenol* 2001;**36**:217-25.
6. Sickles EA. Findings at mammographic screening on only one standard projection: outcomes analysis. *Radiology* 1998;**208**:471-5.
7. Sickles EA. Periodic mammographic follow-up of probably benign lesions: results in 3,184 consecutive cases. *Radiology* 1991;**179**:463-8.
8. Varas X, Leborgne F, Leborgne JH. Nonpalpable, probably being lesions: role of follow-up mammography. *Radiology* 1992;**184**:409-14.
9. Helvie MA, Pennes DR, Rebner M, Adler DD. Mammographic follow-up of low-suspicion lesions: compliance rate and diagnostic yield. *Radiology* 1991;**178**:155-8.
10. Vizcaíno I, Gadea L, Andreo L, Salas D, Ruiz-Perales F, Cuevas D, et al. Short-term follow-up results in 795 nonpalpable probably benign lesions detected at screening mammography. *Radiology* 2001;**219**:475-83.
11. Varas X, Leborgne JH, Leborgne F, Mezzera J, Jaumandreu S, Leborgne F. Revisiting the mammographic follow-up of BI-RADS category 3 lesions. *Am J Roentgenol* 2002;**179**:691-5.

12. Leung JW, Sickles EA. Developing asymmetry identified on mammography: correlation with imaging outcome and pathologic findings. *AJR Am J Roentgenol* 2007;**188**:667-75.
13. Chang CB, Lvoff NM, Leung JW, Brenner RJ, Joe BN, Tso HH, et al. Solitary dilated duct identified at mammography: outcomes analysis. *AJR Am J Roentgenol* 2010;**194**:378-82.
14. Berg WA, Arnoldus CL, Teferra E, Bhargavan M. Biopsy of amorphous breast calcifications: pathologic outcome and yield at stereotactic biopsy. *Radiology* 2001;**221**:495-503.
15. Bent C, Bassett LW, D'Orsi CD, Sayre JW. The positive predictive value of BI-RADS microcalcifications descriptors and final assessment categories. *AJR Am J Roentgenol* 2010;**194**:1378-83.
16. American College of Radiology. *Practice guideline for the performance of a breast ultrasound examination*. Reston, Va: American College of Radiology; 2007.

SECTION

THREE

Imaging of the Normal Breast

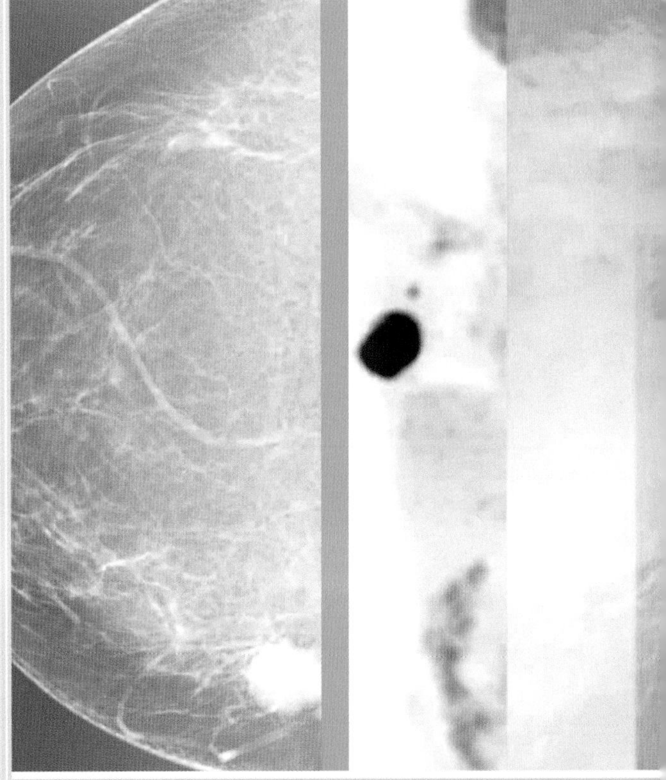

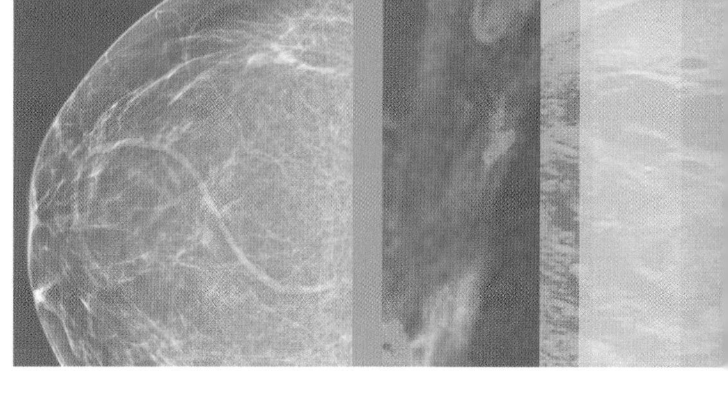

CHAPTER 14

The Normal Breast

Neda A. Moatamed, Lawrence W. Bassett, and Sophia Kim Apple

Traditionally, physiology, and morphology of the normal organs have been described before pathologic changes. At the present, understanding of the molecular biology of the cells has become increasingly crucial in diagnosis, treatment, and prognosis of breast disorders. Therefore, in this chapter, attempts have been made to explore some constitutional molecular aspects of the breast tissue cells pertinent to the current and emerging gene-targeted therapies.

EMBRYOLOGY AND DEVELOPMENT

Breast development starts at the fifth week of fetal life when a series of highly ordered events involving interactions among a number of distinct cell types are encountered. An array of systemic and local factors such as growth factors and hormones regulate these complex interactions. Development of the organ is initially identical among males and females of the same species.

During the fifth week of gestation, the remnant of the mammary ridge ectoderm begins to proliferate. This *primary mammary bud* subsequently begins growth downward as a solid diverticulum into the underlying dermis during the seventh week. Initially, a pair of *milk streaks* or *milk lines*, a primitive thickening of the ectoderm, appears on the ventral surface of the fetus, extending from the axillae to the groins.

In normal human development, the milk lines disappear except at the level of the fourth intercostal space on the anterior thorax, where the mammary gland subsequently develops. Failure of the regression of the milk lines in areas other than the thoracic region can result in ectopic breast tissues, including supernumerary nipples anywhere along the mammary milk line.[1,2] The primary mammary bud subsequently begins growth downward as a solid diverticulum into the underlying dermis during the seventh week. By the 10th week, the primary bud begins to branch, yielding secondary buds by the 12th week, which eventually develop into the mammary lobules of the adult breast.

This initial downgrowth and subsequent branching has been shown to occur as the result of an inductive influence of the extracellular matrix of the mesoderm on the primary mammary bud. This epithelial-mesenchymal signaling is probably through paracrine and juxtacrine mechanisms where the underlying mesoderm produces growth factors and hormones that interact with receptors on the overlying ectodermal cells of the primary mammary bud. The adipose tissue in the underlying mesoderm represents a significant store of lipids for the production of hormones and growth factors, which are then available to promote and regulate growth of the developing mammary gland.

During the remainder of gestation these buds continue lengthening and branching. During the 20th week, small lumina develop within the buds that coalesce and elongate to form the lactiferous ducts. The canalization of the mammary buds with formation of the lactiferous ducts is induced by placental hormones entering the fetal circulation. These hormones include progesterone, growth hormone, insulin-like growth factor, estrogen, prolactin, adrenal corticoids, and triiodothyronine. At term, 15 to 20 lobes of glandular tissue have formed, each containing a lactiferous duct. The supporting fibrous connective tissue, Cooper ligaments, and fat of the mammary gland develop from the surrounding mesoderm.[3]

Until the age of puberty, the breast consists of lactiferous ducts without evidence of alveolar differentiation, although some developed rudimentary lobular structures may persist.[4]

In the female, the onset of menstrual cycles and the secretion of sex hormones at puberty stimulate the ducts to proliferate and the lobules to form. The stroma accumulates fatty tissue.[5]

Adipose tissue and lactiferous ducts grow in response to estrogen. Progestrone stimulation results in lobular growth and alveolar budding. Thelarche, or the onset of pubertal breast development, occurs between the ages of 11 and 11.5 years. The anomaly of breast development includes amastia (absence of breast), supernumerary breast/polythelia (accessory nipples) and polymastia (accessory breast), hypomastia (excessively small breast), and macromastia (excessively large breast).[6]

ANATOMY, HISTOLOGY, AND ULTRASONOGRAPHY OF NORMAL BREAST TISSUE

The breast lies on the anterior chest wall over the pectoralis major muscle and extends from the second to the sixth rib in the midclavicular line (Fig. 14-1). The breast tissue spreads from the lateral edge of the sternum to the anterior axillary line and often extends into the axilla as the tail of Spence.[4] The presence of axillary breast tissue is important because it signifies the possibility of benign and malignant lesions in the axilla. Fibrous strands that extend from the deep dermis into the underlying breast tissue, called the suspensory ligaments of Cooper, provide support to the breast and attach the breast to the underlying fascia and pectoral muscles.[5]

The breast consists of 15 to 20 lobes, each emptying into a separate major duct terminating in the nipple. Each lobe is surrounded by connective tissue and is divided into many lobules[4] (Fig. 14-2). A lobe comprises all of the lobules and excretory ducts that drain via one lactiferous duct at the nipple. The branching system ends at the terminal duct lobular unit (TDLU), which consists of an interlobular duct and an associated

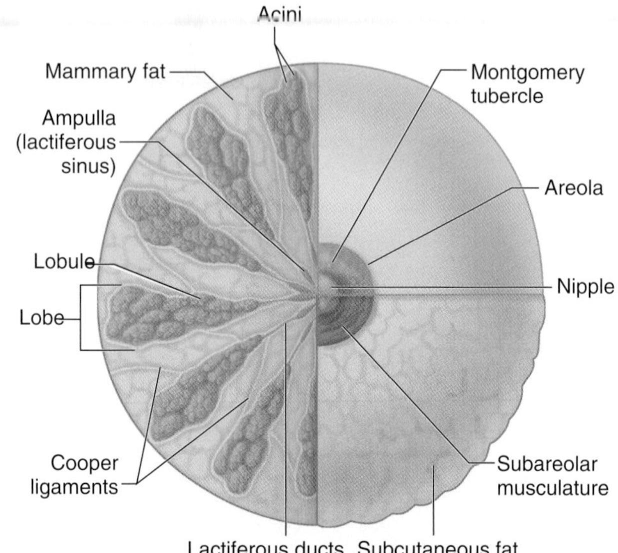

■ **FIGURE 14-2** Frontal section of the breast. A lobe includes all of the ducts that terminate at a single orifice at the nipple. In reality, the lobes are poorly defined subdivisions that may overlap and have no real anatomic delineation. The tubercles of Montgomery are small, rounded elevations on the surface of the areola.

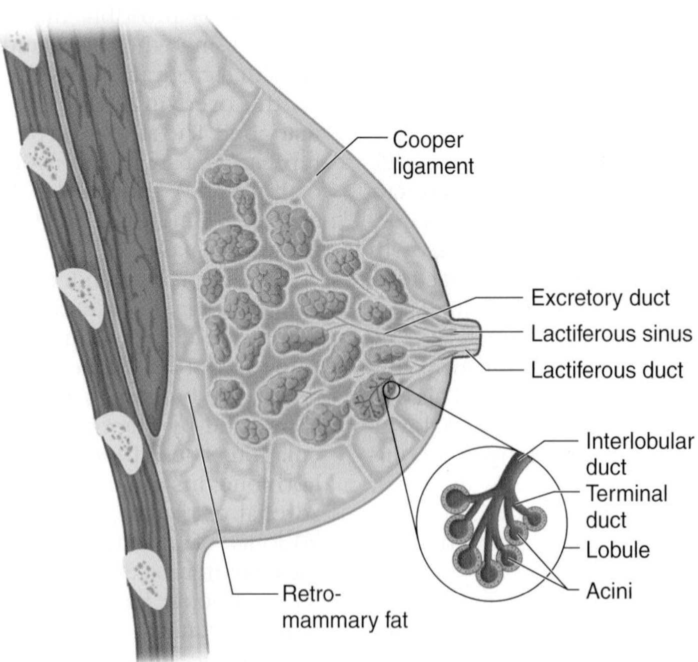

■ **FIGURE 14-1** Sagittal section of the breast. The breast lies primarily on the pectoralis muscle and extends from approximately the second to the sixth rib. Retroglandular fat lies behind the fibroglandular tissue. The pyramid of fibroglandular tissue contains the ducts, which extend from the nipple posteriorly as lactiferous ducts, lactiferous sinuses, and excretory ducts, dividing and subdividing to end in the lobule. The functional unit of the breast, the lobule, is composed of terminal ducts and acini. Cooper ligaments are supporting ligaments that extend from the deep fascia to the skin of the breast.

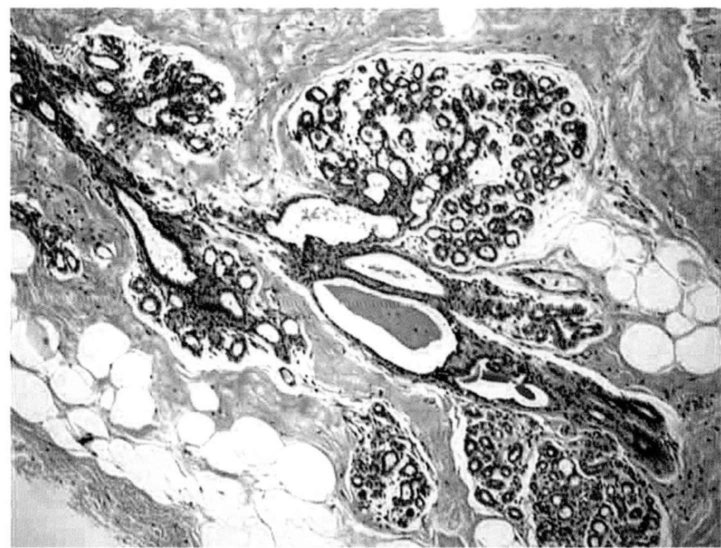

■ FIGURE 14-3 A low-power view of an interlobular duct. Note the two cell layers in the terminal duct lobular units (TDLUs).

lobule (Fig. 14-3). The lobule itself is composed of terminal ducts and acini (sometimes called ductules and terminal ductules, respectively). The secretory product drains from the acini to the terminal ducts, interlobular ducts, excretory ducts, lactiferous sinus, lactiferous duct, and nipple.[5]

Histologically, the breast tissue in women consists of ducts, ductules, and lobuloacinar structures surrounded by basement membrane and collagenous stroma with fibroblasts, vessels, and fat. The immature mammary ductular and alveolar lining consists of a two-cell-layered basal cuboidal and low cylindrical surface epithelium.[7] All normal glandular tissue, including the ducts, terminal ducts, and acini, have a two-cell epithelial layer, an inner layer of secretory cells, and an outer layer of myoepithelial cells (Fig. 14-4). The myofilaments in the myoepithelial layer provide contractility to squeeze the secretory product toward the nipple.

The lobule is the functional unit of the breast. Histologically, it is composed of terminal ducts and acini (Fig. 14-5A). During the resting phase, acini may become inconspicuous and the lobules may be composed largely of terminal ductules. During the secretory phase of the menstrual cycle the lobule undergoes hyperplasia. After childbirth, the hyperplastic lobules begin to produce milk. Myoepithelial cells in the outer layer of ducts and acini can be identified by immunohistochemical stains for smooth muscle actin and p63 protein (Fig. 14-5B). After menopause, atrophy results in a decrease in the size and number of lobules and a relative increase in stromal hyalinization and fibrosis (Fig. 14-6A) in comparison to the perimenopausal lobule (see Fig. 14-6B).

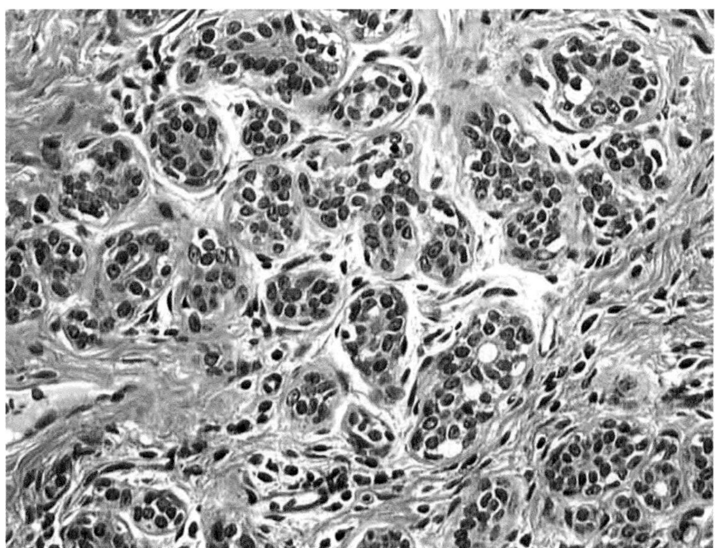

■ FIGURE 14-4 High-power view (400x, H&E stain) of a duct showing two cell layers of epithelial lining. All normal glandular tissues, including ducts and acini, are characterized by an inner layer of either cuboidal or columnar cells and an outer layer of myoepithelial cells.

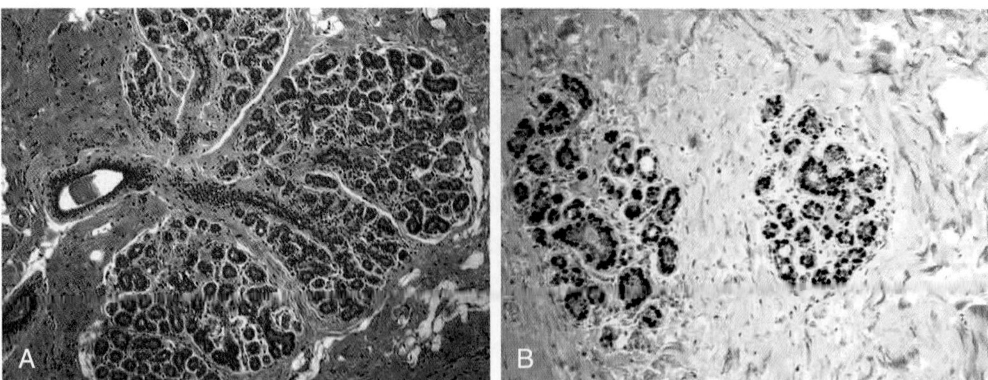

■ **FIGURE 14-5** A, The terminal duct lobular unit consists of a terminal duct and acini (40x, H&E stain). **B**, Immunohistochemical stains for p63 identify myoepithelial cells in the outer layer of the duct and acini.

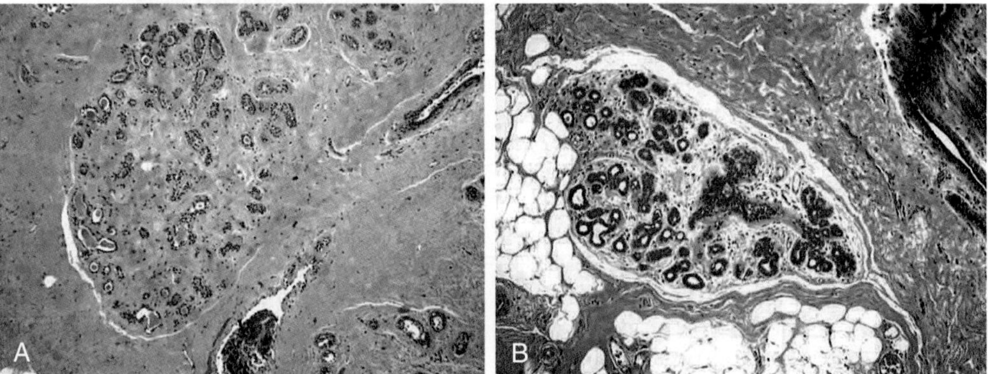

■ **FIGURE 14-6** A, Lobule in postmenopausal woman. The lobule is involuted with a smaller number of acini and more sclerosis of surrounding stroma compared with the perimenopausal lobule (40x, H&E stain). **B**, Lobule in a perimenopausal woman (40x, H&E stain).

The sensitivity of mammography is inversely related to the tissue composition or ratio of dense tissue to fatty tissue. The fatty breast tissue serves as a lucent background against which radiodense abnormalities can be identified, whereas normal fibroglandular tissue can obscure a mass (Fig. 14-7). Therefore, the tissue composition is important for the referring physician to know because it correlates with the ability of mammography to detect lesions in the breast. The four categories of tissue composition are as follows: (1) almost entirely fat; (2) scattered fibroglandular densities; (3) heterogeneously dense tissue (in which the sensitivity of mammography may be lower); and (4) extremely dense tissue (which could obscure a lesion on a mammogram). As tissue density increases, sensitivity of mammography decreases.[5]

Normal anatomic variations in the breast can be seen on mammography and are important to recognize (Fig. 14-8). Accessory breast tissue can be seen anywhere along the milk line but is most often observed in the axilla. It can be either in continuity with or separate from the breast (Fig. 14-9). The sternalis muscle runs parallel to the sternum and can be seen on the craniocaudal (CC) view but not the mediolateral oblique (MLO) projection (see Fig. 14-9). A variant, visualization of the sternalis muscle on the MLO projection, is present in less than 10% of people.[5]

NORMAL ULTRASONOGRAPHIC ANATOMY

We described the normal anatomy of the breast here to provide a foundation for the understanding of breast ultrasonography (Fig. 14-10). The normal skin measures 3 mm or less and consists of parallel white lines beneath the lines produced by the transducer. Below the skin is a layer of subcutaneous fat, followed by intervening layers of fibroglandular tissue and fat. The fibroglandular tissue is hyperechoic (white) compared with the fatty tissue (gray to black). Beneath the fibroglandular tissue is the retromammary fat, which is superficial to the chest wall. The chest wall contains the pectoralis muscle, the ribs, and the parietal pleura that encases the thoracic cavity. These structures can be readily identified with ultrasonography.[5]

PATHOLOGY OF THE BREAST

Only basic pathology of the breast is discussed here; more detailed pathologic descriptions of common entities appear elsewhere in this text. A wide variety of benign lesions in ducts and lobules are observed in the breast. Most of these lesions are identified mammographically, or less commonly they present as a palpable mass. These changes have been divided into the

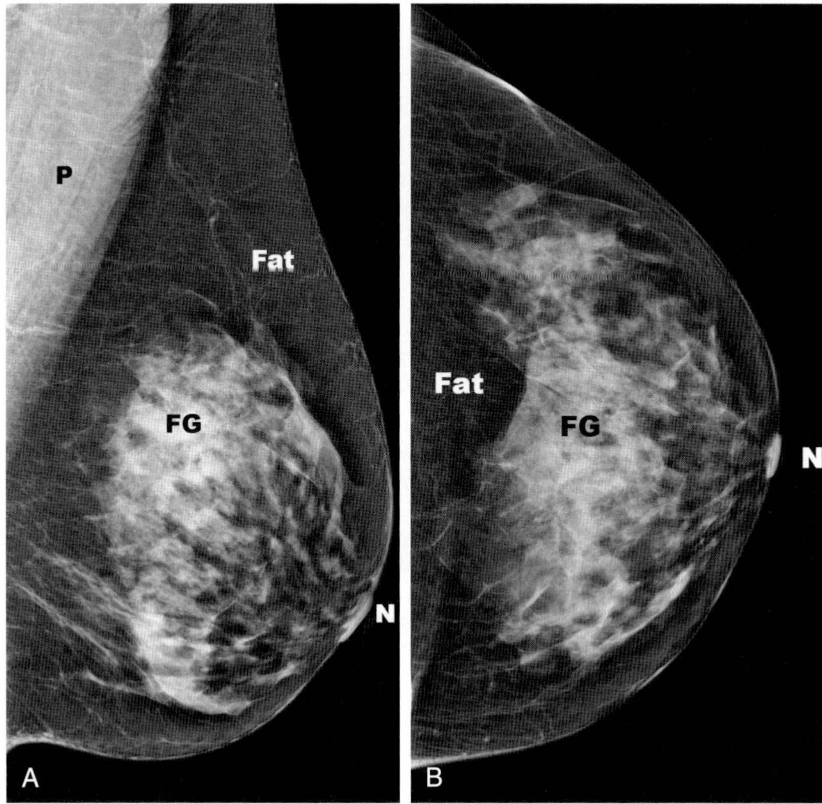

■ **FIGURE 14-7** A, Normal mammogram, mediolateral oblique projection. Fibroglandular tissue (FG) is radiodense (*white*) and may obscure an underlying lesion. In this case there are prominent ducts arising at the nipple (**N**). Fat is radiolucent. P, pectoral muscle. **B,** Normal mammogram, craniocaudal projection. FG, fibroglandular tissue; N, nipple.

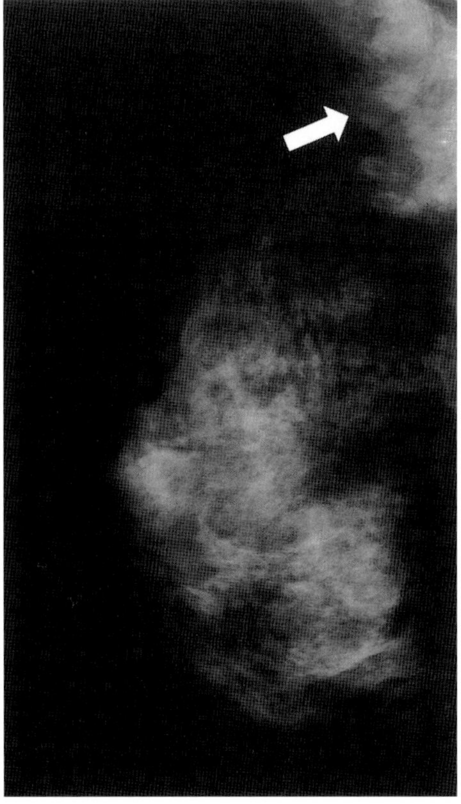

■ **FIGURE 14-8** Accessory breast tissue in the axilla (*arrow*) seen in mediolateral oblique mammogram.

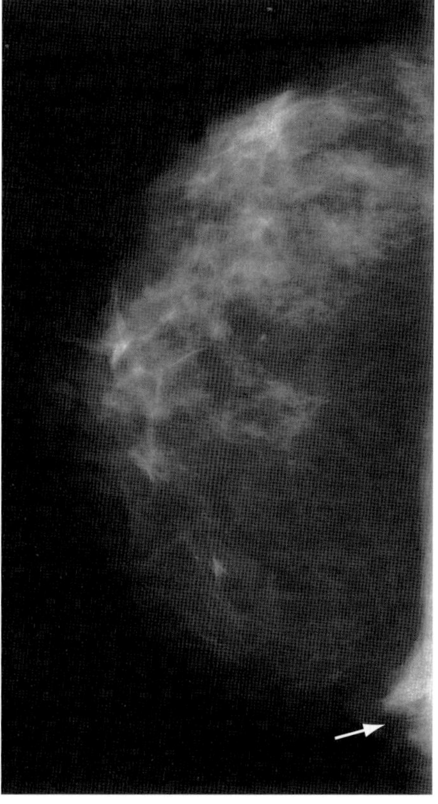

■ **FIGURE 14-9** Sternalis muscle (*arrow*) seen on craniocaudal mammogram.

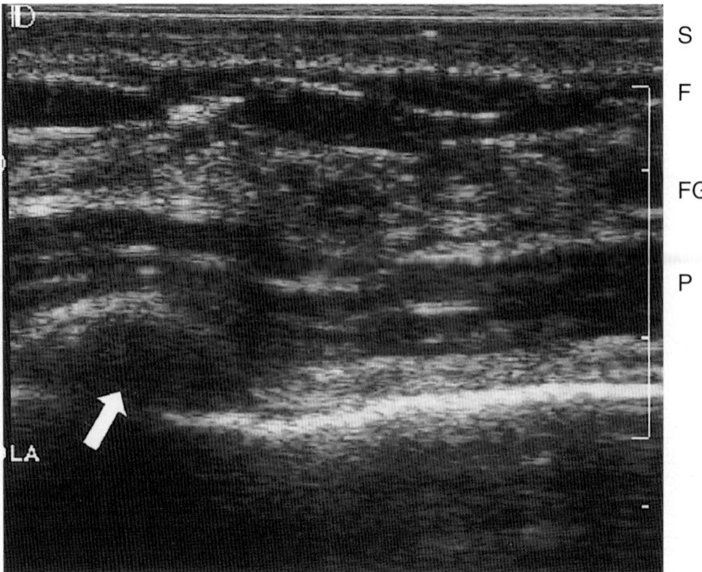

■ **FIGURE 14-10** Normal ultrasound image. Structures with different echogenicities are shown from superficial to deep. Subcutaneous fat (F), fibroglandular tissue (FG), pectoralis muscle (P), rib (*arrow*), skin (S),.

following three groups, according to the subsequent risk of developing breast cancer: (1) nonproliferative breast changes; (2) proliferative breast disease; and (3) atypical hyperplasia. Nonproliferative breast changes or fibrocystic changes include cysts, fibrosis, and adenosis.[8] In a study of normal breasts in unselected forensic postmortem cases, grossly evident cysts and fibrosis were found in 20% and histologic changes were present in 59% of women.[9] Therefore, nonproliferative changes are most likely part of the spectrum of histologic features that can be observed in the normal breast.[8] Proliferative breast diseases without atypia include hyperplasia, adenosis, papilloma, and fibroadenomas. These changes rarely form palpable masses. They are more commonly detected as mammographic densities or calcifications (e.g., sclerosing adenosis) or incidental findings (e.g., hyperplasia). Large duct papillomas present as nipple discharge. Proliferative breast disease with atypia includes atypical ductal hyperplasia (ADH) and atypical lobular hyperplasia (ALH). Occasionally, ADH is associated with calcifications; more commonly it is adjacent to another calcifying lesion. ALH is an incidental finding.[8] The relative risk for women with atypical hyperplasia is four to five times that of women with no proliferative disease. When this finding is combined with other known risk factors, about 20% of women who have atypical hyperplasia and a family history of breast cancer will experience breast cancer over a 15-year follow-up period, compared with 8% of women with atypical hyperplasia but no family history. The comparable rates are 4% for women with proliferative changes without atypia and 2% for women without any evidence of proliferative changes.[5] In subsequent studies, Dupont and Page reported that the highest risk for the development of invasive breast carcinoma in these women occurs during the first 10 years after biopsy and the risk decreases thereafter.[10,11]

Carcinoma of the breast is the most common solid epithelial malignant tumor in women. It can occur at any age but is rare in patients younger than 25 years and older than 80 years; the peak incidence is 45 to 60 years. The incidence and mortality are high in most developed countries, especially the United Kingdom and United States. The frequency is increasing in younger age groups. Breast carcinoma is more than 200 times more common in women than in men.[12] Affected males tend to be somewhat older.[13] It is conventional to subdivide carcinoma of the breast into two main pathologic categories: in situ carcinoma and invasive carcinoma.[12] Almost all breast carcinomas are adenocarcinomas, with all other types (i.e., squamous cell carcinoma, metaplastic carcinomas, phyllodes tumors, sarcomas, and lymphomas) making up fewer than 5% the total. Carcinoma in situ refers to a neoplastic population of cells limited to ducts and lobules by the basement membrane. Invasive carcinomas have invaded beyond the basement membrane into stroma. Carcinoma in situ was originally classified as ductal or lobular on the basis of the resemblance of the involved spaces to ducts and lobules.[8] Ductal carcinoma in situ (DCIS) may be of low, intermediate, or high grade.[5] Historically, DCIS has been divided into five architectural subtypes: comedocarcinoma, solid, cribriform, papillary, and micropapillary. Some cases of DCIS have a single growth pattern, but the majority have a mixture of patterns.[8] Rare variants of DCIS are small cell solid, apocrine, neuroendocrine, signet ring, hypersecretory DCIS.[12] DCIS usually presents as calcifications on mammography and less commonly as a density or mass. Lobular carcinoma in situ (LCIS) is characterized by solid filling of the lobules with relatively small, uniform cells.[5] LCIS is usually an incidental finding in a biopsy for another reason, because LCIS is usually not associated with calcifications or a stromal reaction that would form a density.[8]

In the absence of mammographic breast screening, the great majority of invasive carcinomas are detected because of a palpable mass. The mass can be found anywhere in the breast, but the outer upper quadrant is the most frequent site. Many cases are now detected by mammography screening before they are palpable.[5]

The histologic appearance of the tumors cannot fully reveal the underlying complex genetic alterations and the biologic events involved in their development and progression. Malignant tumors are caused by a multiplicity of genetic disturbances in normal cells. The analysis of somatic mutations is greatly facilitated by advances in molecular biology and technology. Development of a new classification based on key molecular events involved in the process of carcinogenesis has provided a molecular explanation for the different morphologic phenotypes and behavior. Recent genomic studies have offered the opportunity to challenge the molecular complexity of breast cancer and have provided evidence for an alternative method for classifying breast cancer into biologically and clinically distinct groups based on gene expression patterns.[14,15] No karyotypic hallmarks (the number and visual appearance of the chromosomes in the cell nuclei) of breast cancer have been identified. There is not yet even a cytogenetic marker for any of the histologic subtypes of breast cancer. Nonetheless, several hundred primary tumors have been karyotyped to date, allowing some general patterns to be discerned.[16] An increased modal chromosome number is the most conspicuous characteristic in many tumors, in keeping with the finding that approximately two thirds of all breast cancers have a hyperploid DNA content in flow-cytometric analysis. Unbalanced translocations are most often seen as recurrent changes, with the i(1)(q10) and the del(1;16)(q10;p10) the most prominent. For the latter, it is not clear whether loss of 16q or gain of 1q is the selective change or whether both are. Other conspicuous changes are I(8)(q10) and subchromosomal deletions on chromosomes 1 (bands p13, p22, q12, q42), 3(p12-p14), and 6(q21). No specific genes have been associated with any of these changes. Classic cytogenetic analysis had already indicated that double minute chromosomes and homogeneously staining regions are a frequent occurrence in breast cancer. These regions were later shown to contain amplified oncogenes. Comparative genomic hybridization (CGH) has identified more than 20 chromosomal subregions with increased DNA-sequence copy number, including 1q31-q32, 8q24, 11q13, 16p13, 17q12, 17q22-q24, and 20q13. For many of these regions with increased copy number there is often a span of tens of megabases, suggesting the involvement of more than one gene. Loss of chromosomal material is also detected by CGH, and this pattern is largely in agreement with loss of heterozygosity data. A number of genes have been identified as critical targets for DNA amplifications by a combination of CGH and gene expression analysis.[17]

Loss of Heterozygosity (LOH)

Loss of heterozygosity (LOH) has been found to affect all chromosome arms in breast cancer to varying degrees. LOH is interpreted in the light of Knudson's two-hit model for the inactivation of a tumor suppressor gene. Numerous studies have attempted to map common regions of LOH on chromosome arms with frequent LOH. Such a region could flag the position of a tumor suppressor gene more accurately, aiding its identification.[18]

Tumor Suppressor Genes

There have been few tumor suppressor genes identified in breast cancer. Listed by chromosomal site, they are:

6q26: ***IGF2R*** gene, encoding the insulin-like growth factor II (IGF-II)/mannose 6-phosphate receptor, is frequently inactivated during carcinogenesis.[17]

7q31: ***ST7*** (for suppression of tumorigenicity 7) is a gene with unknown cellular function. A role of *ST7* in primary breast cancer has been questioned.[19]

8q11: ***RB1CC1.*** The RB1CC1 protein is a key regulator of the tumor suppressor gene *RB1.*

16q22: ***CDH1.*** The cell-cell adhesion molecule E-cadherin acts as a strong invasion suppressor in experimental tumor cell systems. Frequent inactivating mutations have been identified in *CDH1* in more than 60% of infiltrating lobular cancers but not in ductal carcinomas.[20]

17p13: ***TP53*** encodes a nuclear protein of 53 kD, which binds to DNA as a tetramer and is involved in the regulation of transcription and DNA replication. Normal p53 may induce cell cycle arrest or apoptosis, depending on the cellular environment.[17] Mutations, which inactivate or alter either one of these functions, are found in approximately 20% of breast carcinomas.[21] Most of these are missense changes in the DNA-binding domain of the protein; a small proportion (~20%) are frame shifting. The large majority of these mutations are accompanied by loss of the wild type allele (LOH).[17]

Microsatellite Instability (MSI)

Microsatellite instability (MSI) is a genetic defect caused by mutations in mismatch repair genes (*MLH1, MSH2, MSH6, PMS1, and PMS2*), reflected by the presence of multiple alleles at loci consisting of small tandem repeats or mononucleotide runs. MSI in breast cancer is negligible, with possible exception of breast cancer arising in the context of the inherited colon cancer syndrome. Somatic mutations in the mismatch repair genes have not yet been detected in breast cancer.[17]

Gene Expression Patterns

Although the field of gene expression patterns is in its infancy, five distinct patterns were discerned among 115 tumors—one basal-like, one *erbB2* overexpression, two luminal-like, and one normal breast tissue-like subgroup.[14]

Breast cancer in general is believed to arise most often from luminal epithelial cells of the TDLU of the breast. Recent microarray studies have identified a small but significant subpopulation of breast cancers with a basal epithelial-like cell-like gene expression profile. Although a clear working definition for basal carcinoma is lacking, there are a number of features reported to be associated with this type of tumor. Morphologically, they are

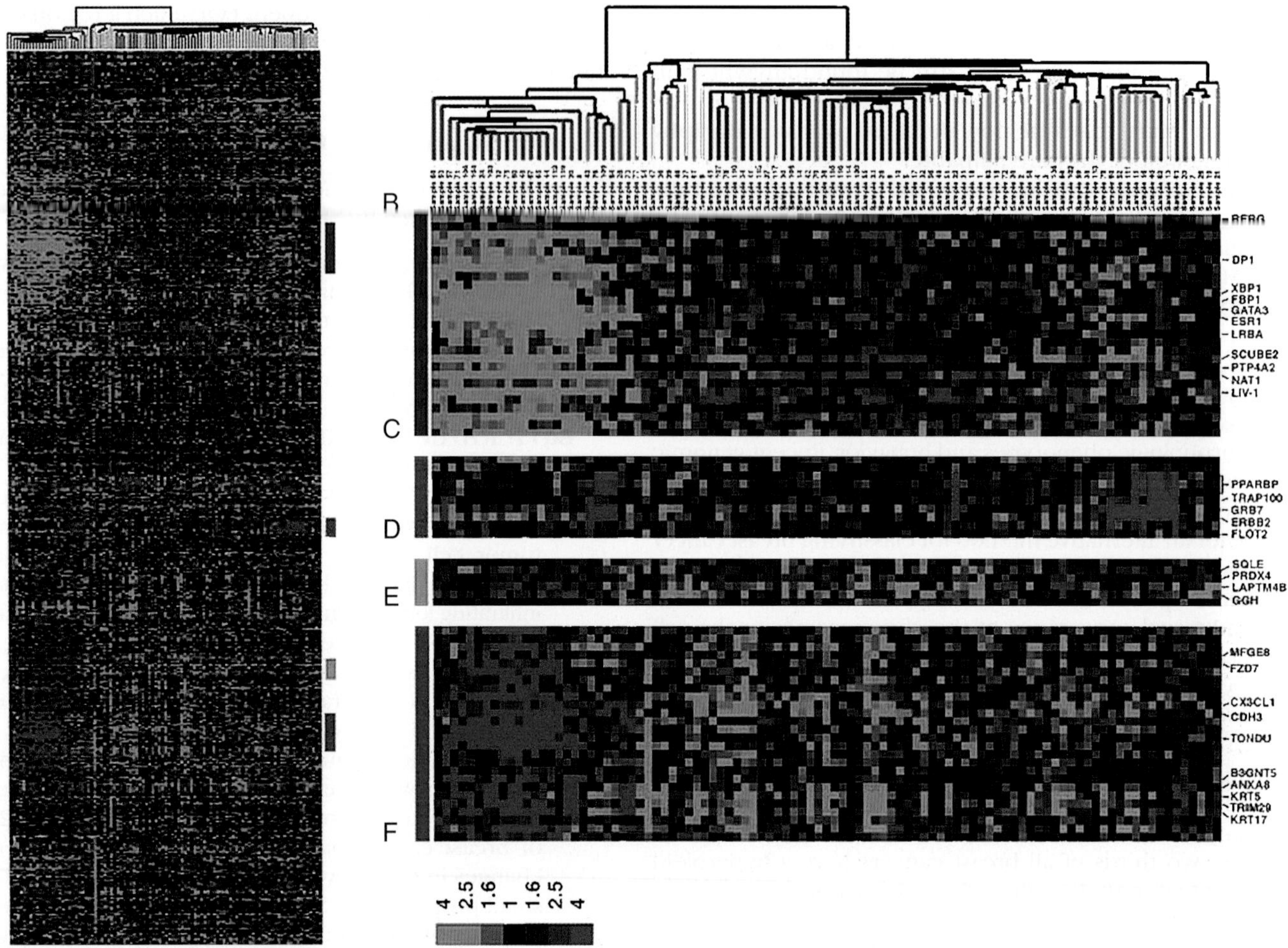

■ **FIGURE 14-11** Hierarchical clustering of 115 tumor tissues and 7 nonmalignant tissues using the intrinsic gene set. **A**, A scaled-down representation of the entire cluster of 534 genes and 122 tissue samples based on similarities in gene expression. **B**, Experimental dendrogram showing the clustering of the tumors into five subgroups. Branches corresponding to tumors with low correlation to any subtype are shown in gray. **C**, Gene cluster showing the *erbB2* oncogene and other coexpressed genes. **D**, Gene cluster associated with luminal subtype B. **E**, Gene cluster associated with the basal subtype. **F**, A gene cluster relevant for the normal breast-like group. Scale bar represents fold change for any given gene relative to the median level of expression across all samples. *(Courtesy of David Botstein.[22])*

usually high grade, and some of them have been reported to contain large central acellular zones comprising necrosis, tissue infarction, collagen, and hyaline material. These tumors show positivity for intermediate filament such as cytokeratin (CK) 5/6 or CK14. Immunohistochemically, as well as expressing a number of myoepithelial markers, these tumors are often estrogen receptor (ER), progesterone receptor (PR), and HER-2 negative, an immunophenotype resembling *BRCA1* tumors.[12] The erb2 group also expresses several other genes in the erb2 amplification, such as *GRB7*. The normal breast-like group shows a high expression of genes characteristic of adipose tissue and other nonepithelial cell types. Cluster analyses of two published, independent data sets representing different patient cohorts from different laboratories uncovered the same breast cancer subtypes (Fig. 14-11).[22]

GENETIC SUSCEPTIBILITY: FAMILIAL RISK OF BREAST CANCER

Virtually every study has found significantly elevated relative risk of breast cancer for female relatives of breast cancer patients. However, the magnitude has varied according to the number and type of affected relatives of breast cancer, age at diagnosis of the proband(s), laterality, and overall study design.

A number of studies have found increased risk for other cancers among relatives of breast cancer probands. The most commonly reported are ovarian, uterine, prostate, and colon cancers. Undoubtedly, the majority of the associations detected in these population studies are due to the *BRCA1* gene, known to be involved in a large proportion of extended kindreds with clearly inherited susceptibility to breast and ovarian cancer. It is likely that some of the discrepancies in results are linked to the frequency of *BRCA1* deleterious alleles in the respective data sets.[17]

Five percent to 10% of breast cancers are of hereditary origin, and two major breast cancer susceptibility genes have been identified: *BRCA1* and *BRCA2*.

BRCA1 and *BRCA2* explain only a minority of the overall familial risk of breast cancer, although they may contribute much more substantially to the fourfold increased risk at younger ages. *BRCA1*-derived breast cancers display certain histopathologic characteristics, such as well-circumscribed tumor, high nuclear grade, and predominant lymphoplasmacytic infiltrates, "triple negative" tumors (ER,

PR, and HER-2/neu negative) that may aid in the diagnosis of *BRCA1* tumors; however, these tumors do not constitute an entirely uniform group. *BRCA2* breast cancers make up a considerably more heterogeneous group also. One can assume an overall twofold increased risk among first-degree female relatives of breast cancer cases and that, as is likely, these genes act in an additive manner with the other loci involved, resulting in a familial risk of 1.8 to be explained by other genes and/or correlated family environment. There could be several genes similar to *BRCA1* and *BRCA2*, with lower breast cancer risks or a set of more common polymorphisms in biologically relevant genes, each associated with only a small increased risk, or something in between. Genes are not the only factors that could cause the observed familial correlation. Shared lifestyle or environmental risk factors would also cause some degree of familial clustering; however, it can be demonstrated that the known environmental risk factors for breast cancer are unlikely to contribute significantly to the overall familial risk.[23]

Based on a model of the contribution of the overall familial risk, it can be estimated that variation in as few as 70 of the 30,000 genes in the human genome may contribute to breast cancer susceptibility. Of course, this model is based on a number of unverifiable assumptions and does not include potential gene-gene and gene-environment interactions and so should be interpreted cautiously.[17]

Prognosis and Predictive Factors

Age

The prognostic significance of age and menopausal status in patients with breast carcinoma is controversial. Younger patients have been found to have a poor prognosis.[24] A favorable outcome or no correlation has been found with age by other studies.[25,26] These discrepancies may be due to differences in patient selection, age grouping, and other factors, including high grade, vascular invasion, extensive in-situ component, steroid receptor negativity, high proliferation, and *TP53* abnormalities.[17]

Pregnancy

Breast cancer developing during pregnancy is generally considered to have an unfavorable prognosis. There are, however, conflicting data as to whether this is an independent factor.[17]

Lymph Node Status

The status of axillary lymph nodes is the single most important prognostic factor for patients with breast cancer. Numerous studies have shown that disease-free and overall survival rates decrease as the number of positive nodes increase.[17]

Tumor Size

Tumor size is an important prognostic factor. Even among patients with breast cancers 1 cm and smaller (T1a and T1b), size is an important prognostic factor for axillary lymph node involvement and outcome.[17]

Histologic Type

Some special histologic types of breast cancer are associated with a particularly favorable clinical outcome. These include tubular, invasive cribriform, mucinous, and adenoid cystic carcinomas.[17]

Histologic Grade

Grading is recommended for all invasive carcinomas of the breast, regardless of morphologic type. Higher rates of distant metastasis and poorer survival are seen in patients with higher grade (poorly differentiated) tumors, independent of lymph node status and tumor size.[17]

Tumor Cell Proliferation

Markers of proliferation have been extensively investigated to evaluate prognosis. Mitotic count is part of histologic grading. Other methods include DNA flow cytometry measurement of S-phase fraction (SPF). Many studies indicate that high SPF is associated with inferior outcome. Ki67/MIB-1 is a labile, non-histone nuclear protein detected in the G1 through M phases of the cell cycle but not in resting cells and is therefore a direct indicator of the growth fraction. The percentage of Ki67 positivity can be used to stratify patients into good and poor survivors. Quantitative reverse transcription polymerase chain reaction (RT-PCR) in detecting the mRNA level has also been introduced, as well as array-based quantification of proliferation.[17]

Lymphatic and Blood Vessel Invasion

Lymphatic vessel invasion has been shown to be an important and independent prognostic factor, particularly in patients with T1, node-negative breast cancers. Its major value is in identifying patients at increased risk of axillary lymph node involvement and adverse outcome.[17]

Perineural Invasion

Perineural invasion is sometimes observed in invasive breast cancers, but it has not been shown to be an independent prognostic factor.[17]

Tumor Necrosis

In most studies the presence of necrosis has been associated with an adverse effect on clinical outcome.[17]

Inflammatory Cell Infiltrates

The presence of a prominent mononuclear cell infiltrate has been correlated in some studies. The significance of this finding is controversial, with some studies noting an adverse effect on clinical outcome and others observing either no significant effect or a beneficial effect.[17]

Extent of Ductal Carcinoma in Situ

The presence of an extensive intraductal component is a prognostic factor for increased local recurrence in patients with conservative surgery and radiation therapy, when status of the excision margins is unknown.[17]

Steroid Hormone Receptors (Estrogen Receptor And Progesterone Receptor)

Approximately 60% of breast carcinomas express the ER protein. Initially, ER-positive tumors were associated with an improved prognosis, but studies with long-term follow-up have suggested that ER-positive tumors, despite having a slower growth rate, do not have a lower metastatic potential. Nonetheless, ER status remains very useful in predicting the response to adjuvant tamoxifen. ER/PR-positive tumors have a 60% to 70% response rate compared with less than 10% for ER/PR-negative tumors.[17]

HER-2 *Oncogene*

The prognostic value of *erbB2* overexpression was first reported in 1987.[27] *ErbB2* overexpression is a weak to moderately independent predictor of survival, at least for node-positive patients. Gene amplification or overexpression is a weak to moderately independent predictor of survival, at least for node-positive patients.[17]

TP53 *Mutations*

Approximately 25% of breast cancers have mutations in the tumor suppressor gene tumor protein 53 (*TP53*), most of which are missense mutations (a point mutation in which a single nucleotide is changed), leading to the accumulation of a stable, but inactive protein in the tumor cells. Studies using DNA sequencing all showed a strong association with survival, whereas those using only immunohistochemistry did not, or did only so weakly. Loss of heterozygosity (LOH) at the *TP53* has been shown to be a marker for prognosis and predictor of response to certain therapies.[17]

DNA Amplification

Amplification of the fibroblast growth factor receptor 1 (*FGFR1*) gene on 8p12 has been correlated with reduced disease-free survival, especially if the gene is amplified together with the cyclin D1 gene.[17] The *MYC* gene on 8q12 is amplified in approximately 20% of breast cancers, which is associated with ER negativity, locally advanced disease, and poor prognosis.[28]

Expression Profiling

Much recent work has been focused on the potential of gene expression profiles to predict the clinical outcome of breast cancer. These studies, although heterogeneous in patient selection and numbers of tumors analyzed, have indicated that gene expression patterns can be identified that associate with lymph node or distant metastasis and that are capable of predicting disease course in individual patients with high accuracies. A remarkable feature of the expression signatures identified in these studies is that they usually involve fewer than 100 genes (Fig. 14-12). Further comparative studies are required to elucidate the critical components of poor prognosis signature.[29]

A large number of genetic and phenotypic alterations have been suggested in breast cancer. However, only a handful have been fully identified and brought to clinical study (Fig. 14-13). In the next decade, the research emphasis in breast cancer will probably focus on the molecular basis of treatment, invasion, angiogenesis, metastases, and resistance to chemotherapy. The development of new targeted therapy rests on the identification of well-defined molecular targets in breast cancer growth and metastases. Understanding genetic and phenotypic alterations from normal cells to malignant cells in breast cancer is critical in terms of designing drugs to target specific molecular pathways. New targeted drugs that are currently available are listed in Table 14-1.[30]

SUMMARY

In this chapter we have described the anatomy, histology, imaging, and molecular aspects of the normal breast. In addition, we have introduced some of the basics of the abnormal breast, which are elaborated on in future chapters.

KEY POINTS

- Histologically, the breast tissue in women consists of ducts, ductules, and lobuloacinar structures surrounded by basement membrane and collagenous stroma with fibroblasts, vessels, and fat.
- The imaging features of the normal breast are represented on mammography based on the density of the structures.
- The imaging features of the normal breast are represented on ultrasound based on the echogenicity of the tissue interfaces.
- A large number of genetic and phenotypic alterations are believed to be associated with breast cancer.
- Understanding genetic and phenotypic alterations from normal cells to malignant cells in breast cancer is critical in terms of designing drugs to target specific molecular pathways.

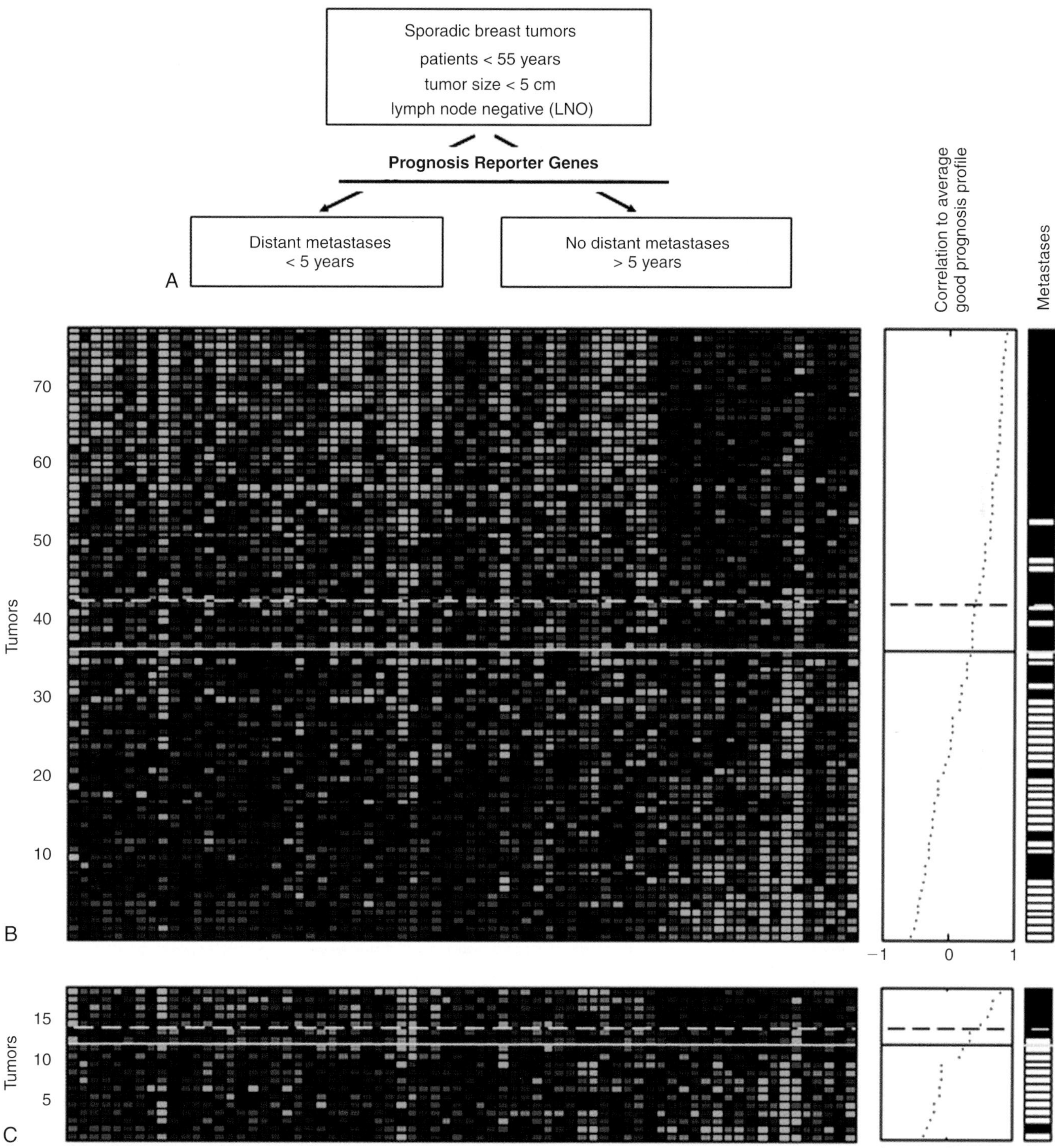

■ **FIGURE 14-12** Supervised classification of prognosis signature. **A**, use of prognostic reporter genes to identify optimally two types of disease outcome from 78 sporadic breast tumors into a poor and a good prognosis group. **B**, Expression data matrix of 70 prognostic marker genes from tumors of 78 breast cancer patients (*left panel*). Each row represents a tumor and each column a gene. Genes are ordered according to their correlation coefficient with the two prognostic groups. Tumors are ordered by the correlation to the average profile of the good prognosis group (*middle panel*). *Solid line,* prognostic classifier with optimal accuracy; *dashed line,* with optimized sensitivity. Above the dashed line patients have a good prognosis signature; below the dashed line the prognosis signature is poor. The metastasis status for each patient is shown in the *right panel: white* indicates patients who developed distant metastasis within 5 years after the primary diagnosis; *black* indicates patients who continued to be disease free for at least 5 years. **C**, Same as for **B**, but the expression data matrix is for tumors of 19 additional breast cancer patients using 70 optimal prognostic marker genes. Thresholds in the classifier (*solid and dashed lines*) are as **B**. *(Courtesy of Stephen H. Friend.*[29]*)*

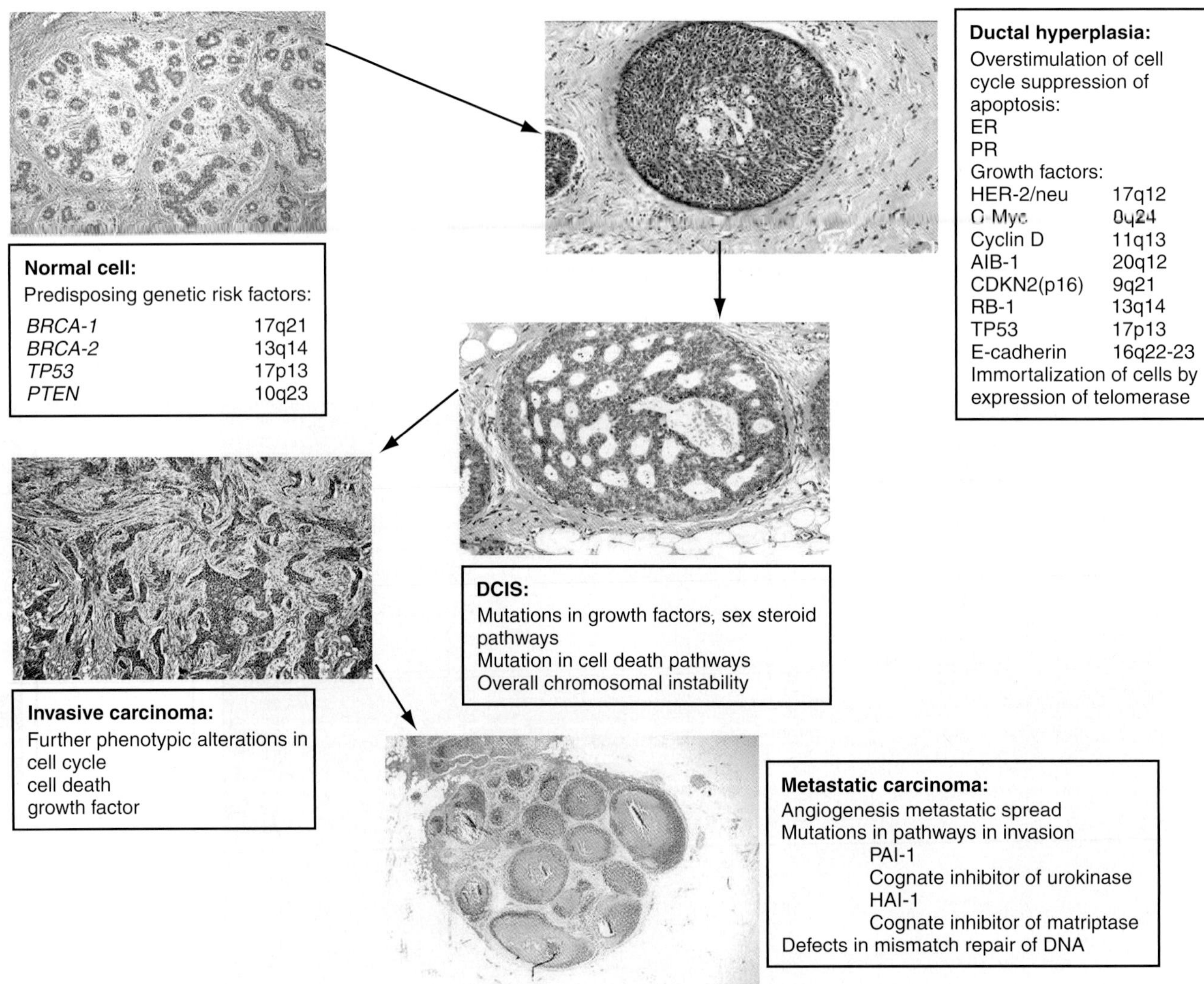

Ductal hyperplasia:
Overstimulation of cell cycle suppression of apoptosis:
ER
PR
Growth factors:
HER-2/neu 17q12
C Myc 8q24
Cyclin D 11q13
AIB-1 20q12
CDKN2(p16) 9q21
RB-1 13q14
TP53 17p13
E-cadherin 16q22-23
Immortalization of cells by expression of telomerase
Normal cell:
Predisposing genetic risk factors:
BRCA-1 17q21
BRCA-2 13q14
TP53 17p13
PTEN 10q23
DCIS:
Mutations in growth factors, sex steroid pathways
Mutation in cell death pathways
Overall chromosomal instability
Invasive carcinoma:
Further phenotypic alterations in
cell cycle
cell death
growth factor
Metastatic carcinoma:
Angiogenesis metastatic spread
Mutations in pathways in invasion
PAI-1
Cognate inhibitor of urokinase
HAI-1
Cognate inhibitor of matriptase
Defects in mismatch repair of DNA

■ **FIGURE 14-13** Summary of the currently known genetic and phenotypic alterations in breast cancers.

TABLE 14-1. Modified Pathways Related to Cell Growth and Metastases and Targeted Agents

Pathways	Target	Agent
Epidermal growth factor receptor	EGFR	Cetuximab, ABX-EFG
	Selective erbB-1 (HER-1) tyrosine kinase inhibitors	Erlotinib, gefitinib
	ErbB-2 (HER-2) inhibitors	Trastuzumab (Herceptin)
	Pan-erbB inhibitors	CI-1033, GW572016, EKB-569
Ras/RAF/mitogen-activated protein kinase	Farnesyl transferase inhibitors	Tipifarnib (Zarnestra, R115777)
PI3K/AKT and MTOR	Rapamycin analogs	CCI-779, RAD001, AP23573
Apoptosis	Bcl-2	Oblimersen (G3139, Genasense)
	Tumor necrosis factor-related apoptosis ligand (TRAIL)	TRM-1
Histone deacetylase inhibitors		LAQ824, suberoylanilide, depsipeptide, MS-275, CI-994 hydroxamic acid
Angiogenesis inhibitors	Anti-vascular endothelial growth factor (VEGF) antibody	Bevacizumab (Avastin), CP-547, 632, PTK787/ZK222584
	VEGF tyrosine kinase inhibitors	ZD6474, SU11248

From Rowinsky S. The new generation of targeted therapies of breast cancer. *Oncology*. 2003;17:1339-1351.

SUGGESTED READINGS

Sorlie T, Tibshirani R, Parker J, Hastie T, Marron JS, Nobel A, et al. Repeated observation of breast tumor subtypes in independent gene expression data sets. *Proc Natl Acad Sci U S A* 2003;**100**:8418-23.

Van't Veer LJ, Dai H, van de Vijver MJ, He YD, Hart AA, Mao M, et al. Gene expression profiling predicts clinical outcome of breast cancer. *Nature* 2002;**415**:530-6.

REFERENCES

1. Tavassoli FA. Normal Development and Anomalies. In: Tavassoli FA, editor. *Pathology of the Breast*. 2nd ed. Stamford: Appleton & Lange; 1999. p. 1-25.
2. Rosen PP. Anatomy and physiologic morphology. In: Rosen PP, editor. *Rosen's breast pathology*. 2nd ed. Philadelphia: Lippincott Williams & Wilkins; 2001. p. 1-21.
3. Robinson GW. Cooperation of signalling pathways in embryonic mammary gland development. *Nat Rev Genet* 2007;**8**:963-72.
4. Collins LC, Schnitt SJ. Breast. In: Mills SE, editor. *Histology for pathologists*. 3rd ed. Philadelphia: Lippincott Williams & Wilkins; 2007. p. 57-71.
5. Fu KL, Fu YS, Lopez JK, Cardall SY, Bassett LW. The normal breast. In: Bassett LW, Jackson VP, Fu KL, Fu YS, editors. *Diagnosis of diseases of the breast*. 2nd ed. Philadelphia: Elsevier; 2005. p. 391-7.
6. De Silva NK, Brandt ML. Disorders of the breast in children and adolescents, Part 1: Disorders of growth and infections of the breast. *J Pediatr Adolesc Gynecol* 2006;**19**:345-9.
7. McCarty KS, Nath M. Breast. In: Sternberg SS, editor. *Histology for pathologists*. 2nd ed. Philadelphia: Lippincott & Raven; 1997. p. 71-84.
8. The breast. In: Kumar V, Abbas AK, Fausto N, editors. *Robbins & Cotran pathologic basis of disease*. 7th ed. Philadelphia: Elsevier Saunders; 2004. p. 1119-54.
9. Bartow SA, Black WC, Waeckerlin RW, Mettler FA. Fibrocystic disease: a continuing enigma. *Pathol Annu* 1982;**17**(Pt 2):93-111.
10. Dupont WD, Page DL. Relative risk of breast cancer varies with time since diagnosis of atypical hyperplasia. *Hum Pathol* 1989;**20**:723-5.
11. Page DL, Dupont WD. Premalignant conditions and markers of elevated risk in the breast and their management. *Surg Clin North Am* 1990;**70**:831-51.
12. Ellis IO, Pinder SE, Lee AHS. Tumors of the breast. In: Fletcher CDM, editor. *Diagnostic histopathology of tumors*. 3rd ed. Philadelphia: Churchill Livingstone Elsevier; 2007. p. 903-69.
13. Donegan WL, Redlich PN. Breast cancer in men. *Surg Clin North Am* 1996;**76**:343-63.
14. Perou CM, Sorlie T, Eisen MB, van de Rijn M, Jeffrey SS, Rees CA, et al. Molecular portraits of human breast tumours. *Nature* 2000;**406**:747-52.
15. Wang Y, Klijn JG, Zhang Y, Sieuwerts AM, Look MP, Yang F, et al. Gene-expression profiles to predict distant metastasis of lymph-node-negative primary breast cancer. *Lancet* 2005;**365**:671-9.
16. Mitelman database of chromosome aberrations in cancer. 2008, May 23; Available at *http://cgap.nci.nih.gov/Chromosomes/Mitelman*.
17. Ellis IO, Schnitt SJ, Sastre-Garau X, et al. Invasive breast carcinoma. In: Tavassoli FA, Devilee P, editors. *Tumors of the breast and female genital organs*. 1st ed. Lyon: IARC Press; 2003. p. 13-59.
18. Devilee P, Cleton-Jansen AM, Cornelisse CJ. Ever since Knudson. *Trends Genet* 2001;**17**:569-73.
19. Brown VL, Proby CM, Barnes DM, Kelsell DP. Lack of mutations within ST7 gene in tumour-derived cell lines and primary epithelial tumours. *Br J Cancer* 2002;**87**:208-11.
20. Berx G, Cleton-Jansen AM, Nollet F, de Leeuw WJ, van de Vijver M, Cornelisse C, et al. E-cadherin is a tumour/invasion suppressor gene mutated in human lobular breast cancers. *EMBO J* 1995;**14**:6107-15.
21. Pharoah PD, Day NE, Caldas C. Somatic mutations in the p53 gene and prognosis in breast cancer: a meta-analysis. *Br J Cancer* 1999;**80**:1968-73.
22. Sorlie T, Tibshirani R, Parker J, Hastie T, Marron JS, Nobel A, et al. Repeated observation of breast tumor subtypes in independent gene expression data sets. *Proc Natl Acad Sci U S A* 2003;**100**:8418-23.
23. Hopper JL, Carlin JB. Familial aggregation of a disease consequent upon correlation between relatives in a risk factor measured on a continuous scale. *Am J Epidemiol* 1992;**136**:1138-47.
24. Albain KS, Allred DC, Clark GM. Breast cancer outcome and predictors of outcome: are there age differentials? *J Natl Cancer Inst Monogr* 1994;35-42.
25. Rutqvist LE, Wallgren A. Influence of age on outcome in breast carcinoma. *Acta Radiol Oncol* 1983;**22**:289-94.
26. Hibberd AD, Horwood LJ, Wells JE. Long term prognosis of women with breast cancer in New Zealand: study of survival to 30 years. *Br Med J (Clin Res Ed)* 1983;**286**:1777-9.
27. Slamon DJ, Clark GM, Wong SG, Levin WJ, Ullrich A, McGuire WL. Human breast cancer: correlation of relapse and survival with amplification of the HER-2/neu oncogene. *Science* 1987;**235**:177-82.
28. Berns EM, Klijn JG, van Putten WL, van Staveren IL, Portengen H, Foekens JA. c-myc amplification is a better prognostic factor than HER2/neu amplification in primary breast cancer. *Cancer Res* 1992;**52**:1107-13.
29. Van't Veer LJ, Dai H, van de Vijver MJ, He YD, Hart AA, Mao M, et al. Gene expression profiling predicts clinical outcome of breast cancer. *Nature* 2002;**415**:530-6.
30. Syed SR. The new generation of targeted therapies of breast cancer. *Oncology* 2003;**17**:1339.

SECTION

FOUR

Imaging of the Benign Breast Disease

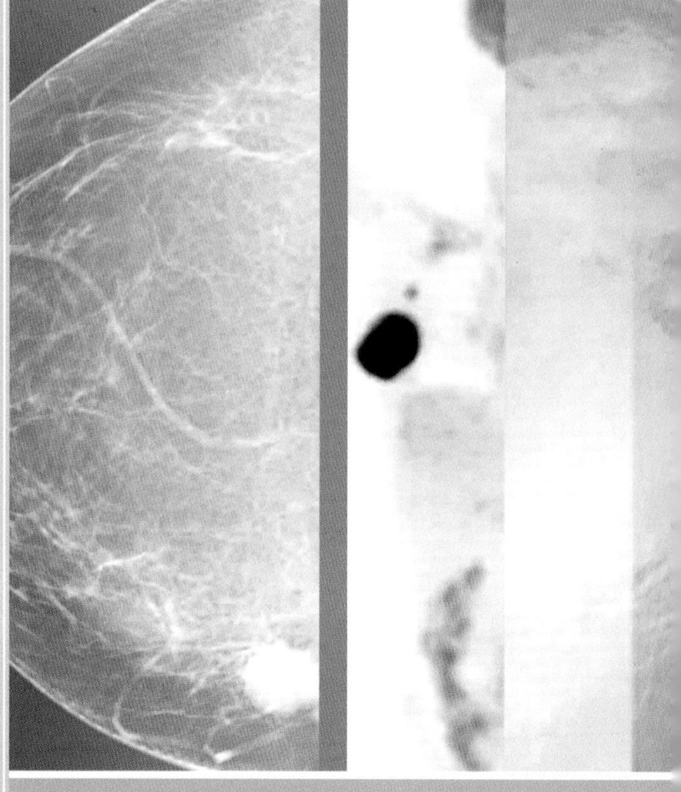

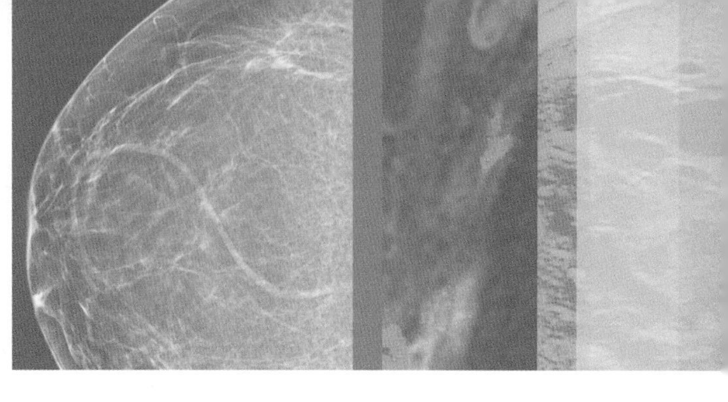

CHAPTER 15

Benign Cystic Lesions of the Breast

Sophia Kim Apple, Laura Doepke, and Lawrence W. Bassett

The vast majority of cystic lesions in the breast are benign. In this chapter, we discuss epidermal inclusion cyst, sebaceous cyst, galactocele, duct ectasia, and fibrocystic changes of the breast. Although abscess can present as a cystic lesion of the breast, it is discussed in the chapter on infection.

EPIDERMAL INCLUSION CYSTS AND SEBACEOUS CYSTS

Definition

In the American College of Radiology (ACR) Breast Imaging Reporting and Data System (BI-RADS) cystic lesions are divided into three types: simple cyst (Fig. 15-1), complicated cyst (Fig. 15-2), and complex mass. Simple cysts are benign lesions; complicated cysts have a very low potential for malignancy involving the wall. Complex masses may be benign or malignant and have both a cystic and solid component, thus core needle biopsy or excisional biopsy is recommended. Pathologically, cystic lesions are divided into two types according to the lining of the cysts: simple cyst or pseudocyst. A simple or so-called true cyst is a cyst lined by epithelial cells, and a pseudocyst is a cyst devoid of an epithelial cell lining, but which forms cystic spaces with or without luminal contents.

Prevalence and Epidemiology

Epidermal inclusion cysts are not common in the breast but may occur especially after reduction mammoplasty or after other iatrogenic procedures. Sebaceous cysts are rare within the breast parenchyma.

Etiology and Pathophysiology

Epidermal inclusion cysts usually arise from obstruction of the infundibular portion of the hair follicle, hence the term *infundibular cyst.* Epidermal inclusion cysts can also arise by traumatic implantation or squamous metaplasia of a sweat duct.[1] They are predominantly found on the face, neck, torso, and, rarely, breast. Sebaceous cysts are retention cysts and are believed to arise from the acral surface of the skin by implantation of the epidermis into the dermis. At times, these cysts can rupture and cause significant discomfort. Sebaceous cysts are also called *pilar* or *richilemmal* cysts and occur predominantly on the scalp.

Manifestations of Disease

Clinical Presentation

Sebaceous cysts and epidermal inclusion cysts are benign breast lesions that can arise from the skin of the breast. Clinical presentations of both entities are similar and present as an asymptomatic, palpable mass on the superficial or subcutaneous skin. When the cyst is ruptured, pain may be associated with the lesion.

Imaging Indications and Algorithm

Because patients with sebaceous cysts and epidermal inclusion cysts often present with palpable masses, diagnostic mammography and ultrasonography should be performed. During positioning of the breast for mammography, the palpable abnormality should be marked with a metallic BB before imaging. The lesions are also usually apparent on physical examination.

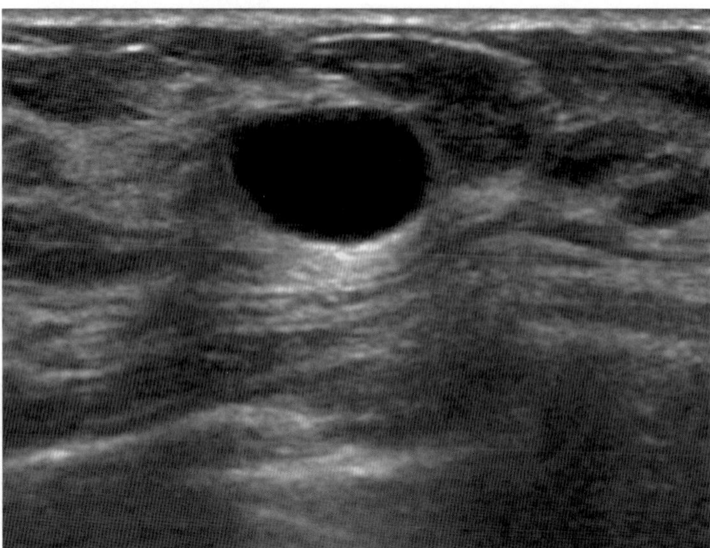

■ **FIGURE 15-1** Simple cyst. Ultrasound features include an anechoic circumscribed mass with imperceptible walls, enhanced through-transmission, and no septations or solid components.

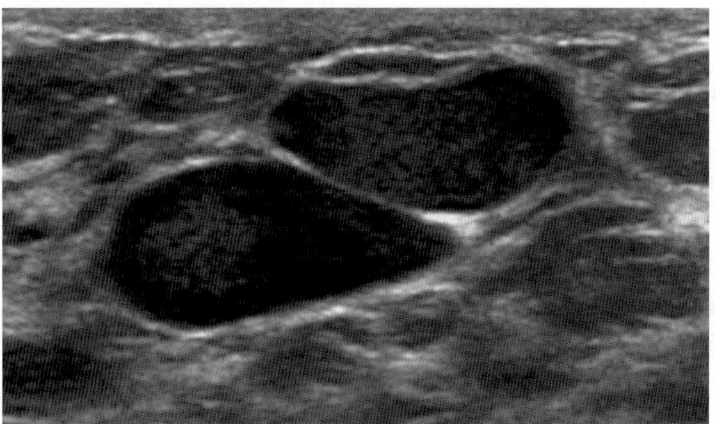

■ **FIGURE 15-2** Ultrasound of two complicated cysts. These cysts contain echogenic internal debris without evidence of solid components to suggest a complex mass.

Imaging Findings by Modality

Mammography

On mammography, epidermal inclusion cysts and sebaceous cysts are circumscribed, round masses that may be projected over the breast parenchyma on any view. Often, a portion of the border is ill defined (Fig. 15-3).

Ultrasonography

On ultrasonography, epidermal inclusion cysts and sebaceous cysts arise from the skin or immediate subcutaneous tissue of the breast. At times the appearance of the skin surrounding the mass is described as the *claw sign*. Most epidermal inclusion and sebaceous cysts are circumscribed and contain low-level internal echoes, produced by the thick material within these lesions (Figs 15-4 and 15-5).

Magnetic Resonance Imaging

The magnetic resonance imaging (MRI) findings are nonspecific.

Differential Diagnosis

From Clinical Presentation

Epidermal inclusion cysts and sebaceous cysts can vary significantly in size, some measuring up to several centimeters. They can also be fixed to the skin and clinically resemble carcinoma. If ruptured, there may be pain associated with the lesion.

From Imaging Findings

Epidermal inclusion cysts and sebaceous cysts usually present as circumscribed masses with mammography and

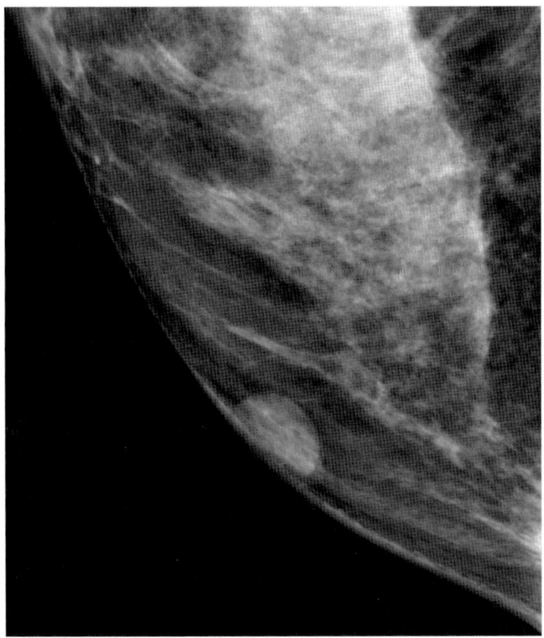

■ **FIGURE 15-3** Sebaceous cyst. Mammogram demonstrates a dermal-based, circumscribed oval mass.

with ultrasonography and can be mistaken for carcinoma or fibroadenoma.

From Pathology Findings

Epidermal inclusion cysts are usually circumscribed dermal masses immediately underlying the epidermis. Fine-needle aspiration (FNA) is useful for diagnosis because the cytologic features are diagnostic with abundant anucleated squames and keratin debris. When infected, numerous inflammatory cells and multinucleated giant cells are seen adjacent to the cystic structure. On excisional biopsy, a typical cut section of the gross specimen expresses "cheese-like" material, which is keratinizing debris. Microscopically, an epidermal inclusion cyst is a circumscribed subcutaneous lesion lined by keratinizing squamous epithelium with luminal contents of anucleated squamous debris. When these cysts rupture, the inflammatory reaction causes multinucleated giant cells along with acute and chronic inflammation (Figs 15-6 and 15-7). Sebaceous cysts are usually located in the mid to deep reticular dermis of the skin. The epithelial lining is composed of three to four layers of keratinocytes with peripheral palisading nuclei without the intercellular bridges seen in the epidermal inclusion cyst. The cyst consists mostly of anucleated squamous debris, similar to an epidermal inclusion cyst. Sebaceous cysts are extremely rare within the breast.

Synopsis of Treatment Options

Various treatment options are available for epidermal inclusion cysts and sebaceous cysts. Conservative observation is one option. Surgical treatment techniques include lasers, incision and drainage, traditional or mini-excision, and trephination. Excisional biopsy is the most definitive treatment to prevent recurrence, and is the most preferred method to treat infected or fibrosed cysts. Other techniques may result in an increased recurrence rate.

GALACTOCELE

Definition

A galactocele is a benign milk-filled cyst.

Prevalence and Epidemiology

Galactoceles almost always occur in women during or just after cessation of lactation [3] and rarely occur in men.[2-4]

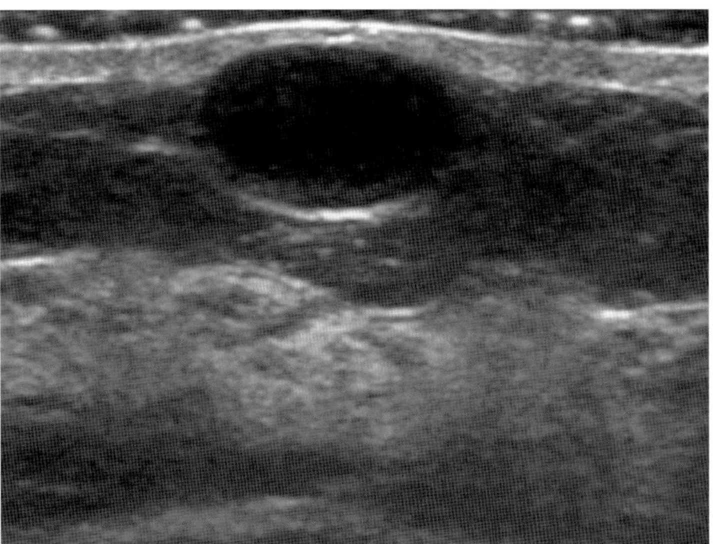

■ **FIGURE 15-4** Ultrasound of a sebaceous cyst. Note the intradermal nature of the mass. A standoff pad made of gel was used to better evaluate the dermal based mass.

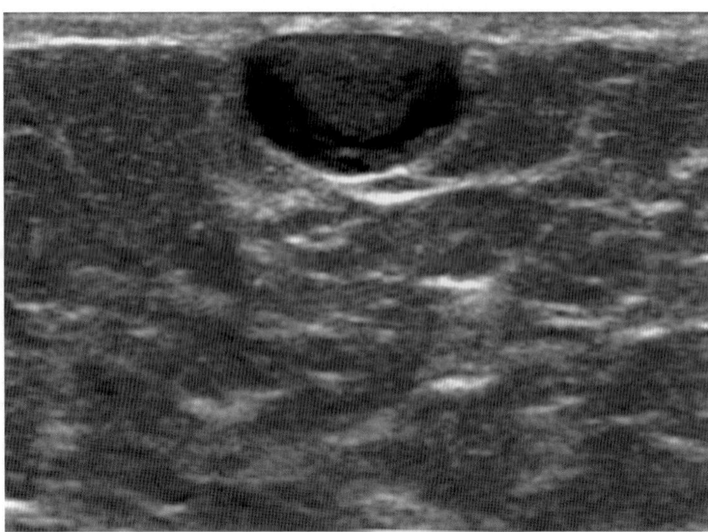

■ **FIGURE 15-5** Ultrasound of a sebaceous cyst in a different patient from Fig. 15-4. Again note the intradermal nature of the mass.

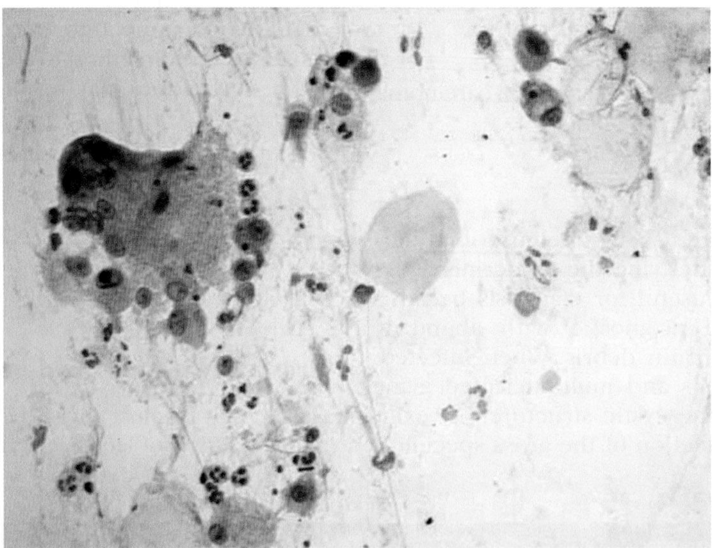

■ **FIGURE 15-6** Fine-needle aspiration (FNA) of epidermal inclusion cyst aspirated from the nipple area showing multinucleated giant cells and anucleated squames with inflammatory cells in the background (Papanicolaou [PAP] stain, × 400).

Etiology and Pathophysiology

A galactocele is presumably caused by ductal obstruction. It is not a common lesion but can be seen in pregnancy or in the setting of chronic galactorrhea caused by a pituitary adenoma.

Manifestations of Disease

Clinical Presentation

Galactoceles often present as a nontender, firm, freely mobile palpable mass.They may be solitary or multiple circumscribed masses, unilateral or bilateral, and often lack evidence of an acute inflammatory process.

Imaging Indications and Algorithm

Diagnostic mammography and ultrasonography may be performed in women age 30 years or older.

Imaging Technique and Findings

Mammography

The need for breast imaging in pregnant or lactating women depends on patient's age and clinical findings. Although galactoceles may be one of the most common conditions encountered in pregnant or lactating women, carcinoma arising in association with pregnancy has first to be ruled out. Because galactoceles mimic fibroadenoma or carcinoma on physical

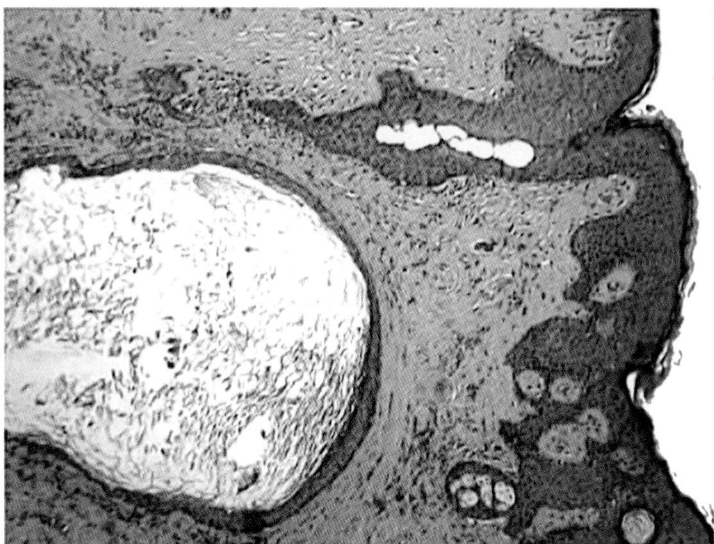

■ **FIGURE 15-7** Epidermal inclusion cyst in the nipple. The cyst is located in the dermis lined by squamous epithelium and the contents are laminated anucleated keratin debris (H&E, ×100).

examination, imaging is often performed. The mammographic appearance depends on the amount of fat and proteinaceous material within the milk. If the fat content is very high, the mass may be completely radiolucent, mimicking a lipoma.[5,6] The mammographic finding of a circumscribed mass with a fat-fluid level on upright horizontal (mediolateral or lateromedial) beam film is diagnostic (Fig. 15-8). This finding will not be as apparent on a mediolateral oblique view (MLO) because it is not a horizontal beam film.

Ultrasonography

Galactoceles have a variable appearance on ultrasound. Some are circumscribed with low-level internal echoes and posterior acoustic enhancement, similar to circumscribed solid breast tumors.[6] Others contain a fluid-debris level, with the proteinaceous debris appearing highly echogenic and the liquid fat appearing anechoic.[7] The ultrasound appearance is not specific or diagnostic (Fig. 15-9).

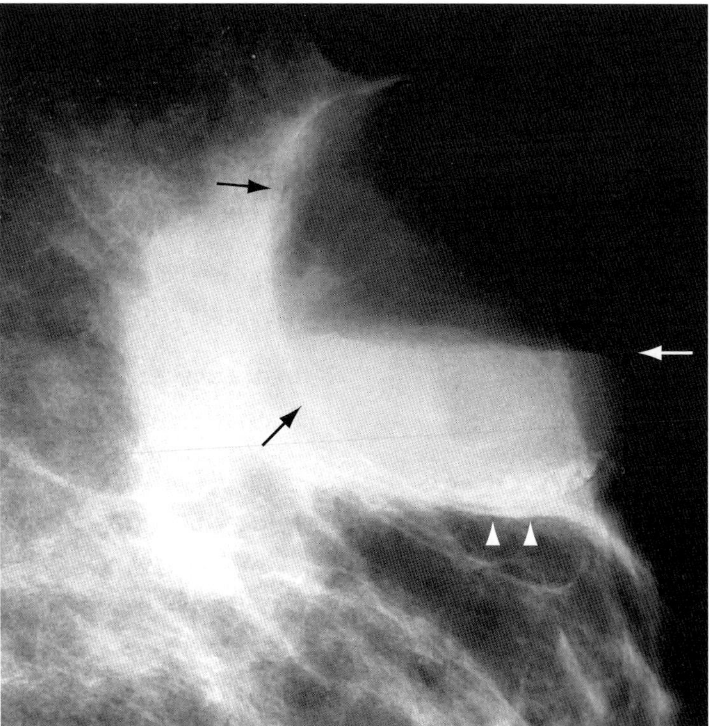

■ **FIGURE 15-8** Galactocele. Mediolateral mammogram of a 4 cm palpable mass (*black arrows*) in the left breast of a lactating woman. A fat/fluid level (*white arrow*) and layering calcifications (*white arrowheads*) are present.

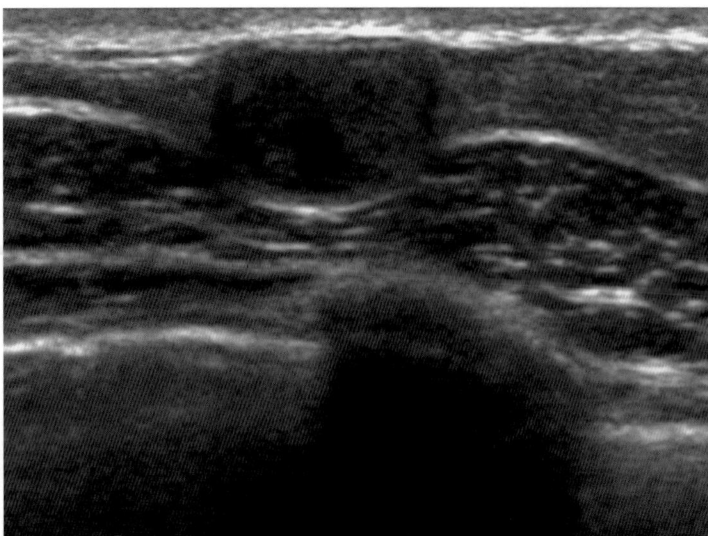

■ **FIGURE 15-9** Galactocele in a 28-year-old breastfeeding woman who presented with a palpable abnormality. Ultrasound demonstrates an isoechoic oval mass with a circumscribed margin. Fine-needle aspiration (FNA) demonstrated a galactocele.

Magnetic Resonance Imaging

The specific MRI appearance of galactoceles is not well described, as MRI is often unnecessary in these patients. The diagnosis can be established by mammography, ultrasound or aspiration.[8]

Classic Signs

A circumscribed mammographic mass with a fat-fluid level on a mediolateral or lateromedial projection is diagnostic.

Differential Diagnosis

From Clinical Presentation

Because galactoceles often present as palpable masses, the differential diagnosis would include malignancy or solid benign masses.

From Imaging Findings

The differential diagnosis would include hamartoma or lipoma.

From Pathology Findings

Galactoceles are composed of either single or, more commonly, multiple small cysts with fluid contents resembling milk. Microscopically, galactoceles are either solitary or multiple cystic dilatations of large ducts lined by low to tall cuboidal inner epithelial cells and outer myoepithelial cells. Within the cystic lumen, necrotic debris and inflammatory cells including degenerative macrophages can be seen. On FNA smears of galactoceles may demonstrate single or loose clusters of foamy degenerative macrophages with multivacuolated droplets in a background of proteinaceous material consistent with milk contents (Fig. 15-10).

Synopsis of Treatment Options

Once malignancy has been ruled out, most patients with galactoceles are treated with aspiration of the cyst contents if clinically indicated. No therapy is necessary with the classic presentation of galactoceles. A fistula formation with milk is a rare complication of incomplete surgical excision.

Excisional biopsy is diagnostic and provides adequate therapy if clinically indicated for symptomatic cases.

DUCT ECTASIA

Definition

Duct ectasia is a nonspecific dilation of the major subareolar ducts, with occasional involvement of smaller ducts. The various anatomic features of this disease have led to many different descriptive diagnostic terms, including *plasma cell mastitis, obliterate mastitis,* and *comedomastitis.*

Prevalence and Epidemiology

Duct ectasia has been found in women of all ages and is rarely seen in men.

Etiology and Pathophysiology

The cause of duct ectasia is unknown. It has been suggested that the initiating event is the inflammatory process, which leads to destruction of the elastic network of the duct and, hence, duct ectasia and periductal fibrosis. Others have suggested that the dilation is primary, perhaps caused by obstruction of the duct, and that the inflammation is a secondary phenomenon related to leakage of duct contents. Parity and lactation are not factors predisposing to the development of duct ectasia.

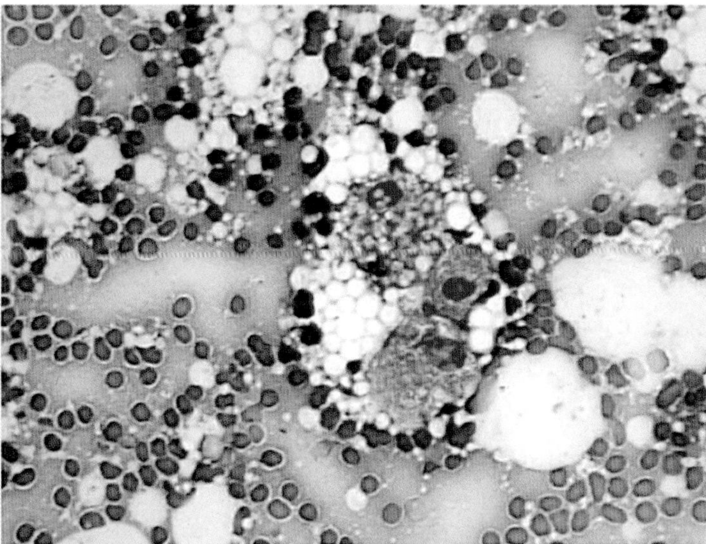

■ **FIGURE 15-10** Fine-needle aspiration (FNA) of galactoceles showing scattered single foamy macrophages with multivacuolated cytoplasm and proteinaceous background of milk contents (May-Grunewald Giemsa [MGG] stain, ×400).

Manifestations of Disease

Clinical Presentation

The majority of patients are asymptomatic but the distended ducts may be palpable on examination. If clinical manifestations do occur, however, the earliest sign is spontaneous and intermittent nipple discharge. Most nipple discharge is a clear to yellow fluid. If the patient presents with spontaneous clear or bloody nipple discharge, papilloma or malignancy must be excluded. Nipple inversion or retraction can occur in the later stage of duct ectasia; however, other causes of nipple inversion such as malignancy should be excluded.

Imaging Indications and Algorithm

Because most patients with duct ectasia are asymptomatic, this disorder is often diagnosed on annual screening mammography. However, if the patient presents with a palpable abnormality or spontaneous nipple discharge, then diagnostic mammography, ultrasonography, and possibly ductography should be performed, because patients with high-risk lesions such as intraductal papillomas or malignancies may present in a similar fashion.

Imaging Technique and Findings

Mammography

When ectatic ducts are filled with thick secretions and cellular debris, the material often calcifies. The typical secretory calcifications seen on mammography are dense, solid, and rod-like; they are usually bilateral and diffuse (Fig. 15-11). The calcifications may also contain internal lucencies when the duct secretions surround the duct itself. Such calcifications are of no clinical consequence to the patient and do not elevate the woman's risk of breast cancer. Occasionally, early focal secretory calcifications may mimic malignant microcalcifications, leading to biopsy. If asymmetrically dilated ducts represent an interval change or contain pleomorphic calcifications, biopsy should be considered.

Ultrasonography

Ultrasonography often demonstrates dilated ducts that may be filled with anechoic fluid, echogenic debris, or both (Fig. 15-12).

Magnetic Resonance Imaging

The specific MRI appearance of duct ectasia is not well described because MRI is often unnecessary in these patients. The diagnosis can often be made by mammography and ultrasonography.

Classic Signs

Rod-like calcifications are evident and usually are bilateral and diffuse on mammography.

Differential Diagnosis

From Clinical Presentation

The differential diagnosis from the clinical presentation would include malignancy or intraductal papilloma, if the patient presents with nipple discharge.

From Imaging Findings

The differential diagnosis based on the imaging findings is limited. Occasionally, early focal secretory calcifications can mimic malignancy and would lead to biopsy for accurate diagnosis.

From Pathology Findings

Duct ectasia is a benign condition with unknown etiology and patients present with spontaneous and intermittent

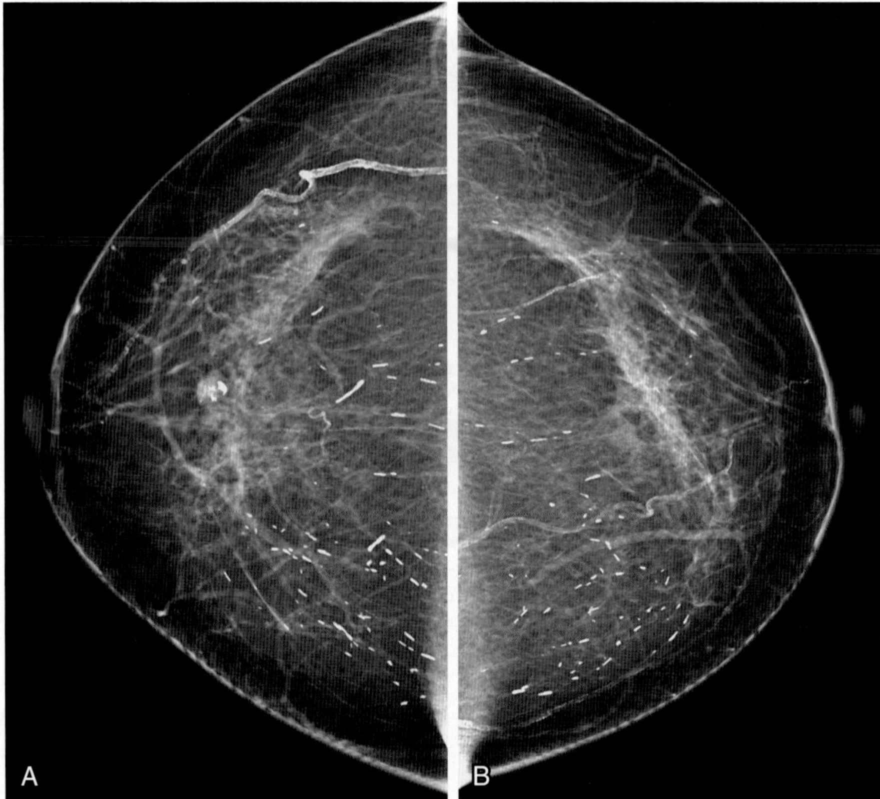

■ **FIGURE 15-11** A and B, Screening mammogram in an asymptomatic woman demonstrates bilaterally symmetric, large rod-like calcifications consistent with secretory calcifications. Incidental note is made of an involuting fibroadenoma in central right breast on the craniocaudal view.

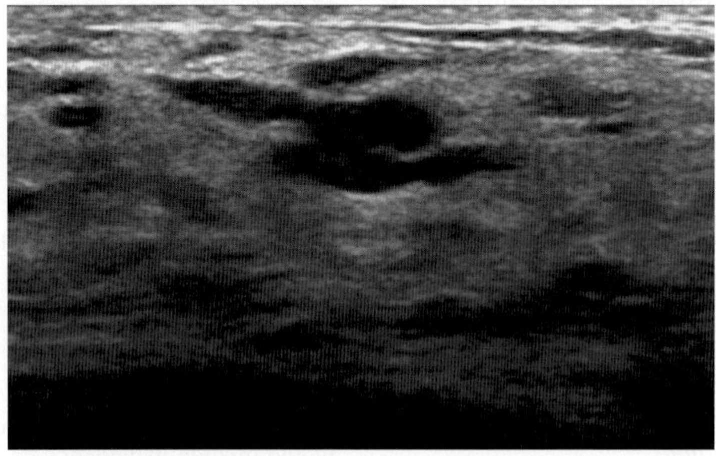

■ **FIGURE 15-12** Screening ultrasound in an asymptomatic patient demonstrates dilated, prominent ducts in both breasts.

nipple discharge that can be clear to brown. It is a nonspecific dilatation of the major subareolar or smaller ducts, which contain proteinaceous material in the lumen. The epithelial cells are attenuated and flattened, and myoepithelial cells are seen at the periphery. Epithelial proliferation or hyperplasia is not a feature of duct ectasia. Luminal contents also commonly show foam cells, desquamated duct epithelial cells, and cholesterol clefts. Periductal stromal fibrosis with mixed inflammatory cells can be seen, especially with ruptured ectatic ducts (Figs 15-13 and 15-14).

Synopsis of Treatment Options

Mammary duct ectasia often improves without treatment or with antibiotic treatment if clinically indicated. Clinical presentation and imaging studies may not be sufficient to provide a specific diagnosis of duct ectasia

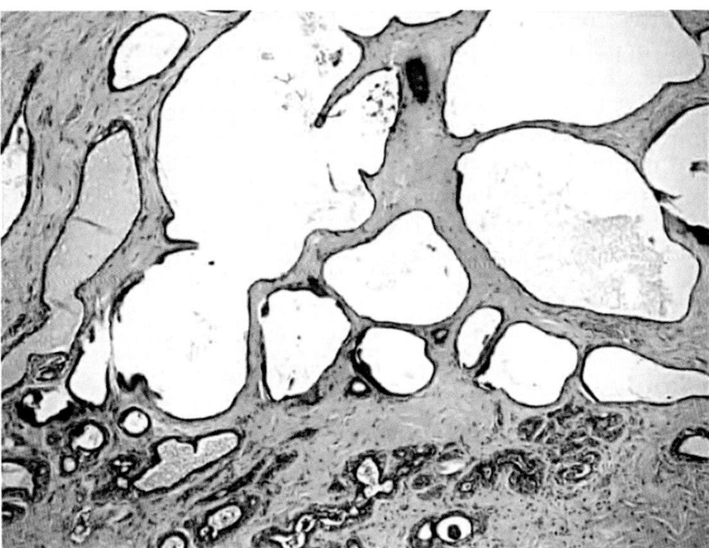

■ **FIGURE 15-13** Duct ectasia with several dilated ducts forming microcysts (H&E, ×100).

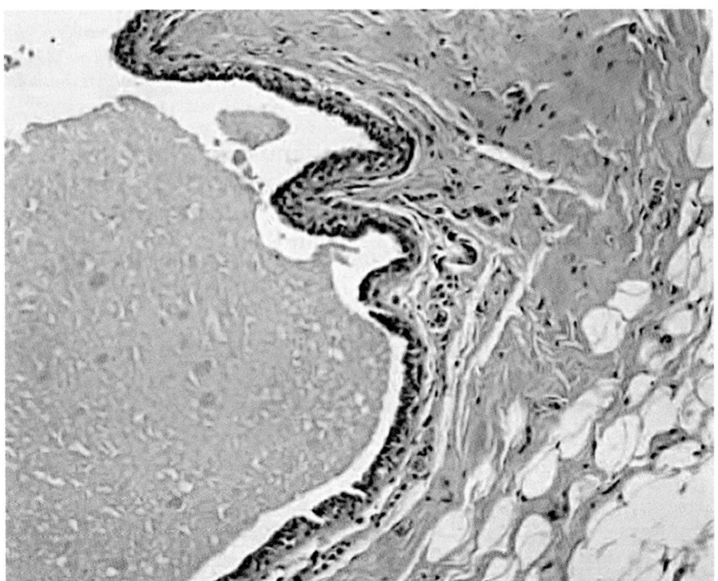

■ **FIGURE 15-14** Luminal proteinaceous material lined by attenuated ductal cells. Stromal fibrosis and periductal inflammatory cells are seen (H&E, ×200).

and confidently rule out carcinoma. The diagnosis of duct ectasia can be established by excisional biopsy through a tiny incision at the edge of the nipple areolar complex with removal of a conical segment of the involved dilated ducts.

FIBROCYSTIC CHANGE

Definition

Fibrocystic change is not a disease but refers to a constellation of benign histologic findings. It was previously referred to as *fibrocystic disease*, a name that should no longer be used because the symptoms are within the normal spectrum of hormone-related changes in the breast. However, despite attempts to rename this condition, the term *fibrocystic disease* appears to be ingrained in clinical usage, even though there is no "disease" component in the condition.

Prevalence and Epidemiology

Fibrocystic change is a common finding in younger and premenopausal women. There is no increased risk for the subsequent development of breast cancer in women with nonproliferative fibrocystic breast changes. When there is ductal hyperplasia, a proliferative process within fibrocystic changes, the relative risk of developing breast cancer is increased to 1.5 to 2 times that of women without proliferative changes. If there is atypia found within the fibrocystic changes, the relative risk of development into breast cancer is increased 5 times (Box 15-1). For these reasons, the term *fibrocystic changes* should not be used as a catch-all phrase; the lesions in this category should be considered separately.

BOX 15-1 Relative Risk for Invasive Breast Carcinoma Based on Pathologic Examination of Benign Breast Tissue

NO INCREASED RISK

- Adenosis
- Apocrine metaplasia
- Cysts (macrocysts, microcysts, or both)
- Duct ectasia
- Hyperplasia, mild
- Mastitis
- Periductal mastitis
- Squamous metaplasia

SLIGHTLY INCREASED RISK (1.5 TO 2 TIMES)

- Hyperplasia, moderate or florid, solid or papillary
- Papilloma with fibrovascular core

MODERATELY INCREASED RISK (5 TIMES)

- Atypical ductal hyperplasia
- Atypical lobular hyperplasia

Modified from Hutter RVP. Cancer Committee of the College of American Pathologists: consensus meeting: is "fibrocystic disease" of the breast precancerous? Arch Pathol Lab Med 1986; 110:171-173. Copyright 1986, American Medical Association.

Etiology and Pathophysiology

Fibrocystic changes are known to be associated with hormonal shifts in estrogen and progesterone, which affect the breast tissue. During the progesterone phase of the menstrual cycle, the breasts enlarge as the milk glands and ducts increase in size and the breasts retain water, causing tenderness. After menstruation the breast swelling abates and the breasts return to normal.

Manifestations of Change

Clinical Presentation

Most common symptoms are palpable irregular nodules in the breasts, cyclic pain and tenderness, swelling, and fullness. The breast tissue may feel dense with areas of thicker tissue having an irregular or ridge-like surface. Women may experience sensitivity to touch with a burning sensation, and for some the pain is so severe that it limits exercise or the ability to lie prone. Fibrocystic changes usually occur in both breasts, most often in the upper outer quadrant where most of the milk-producing glands are located.

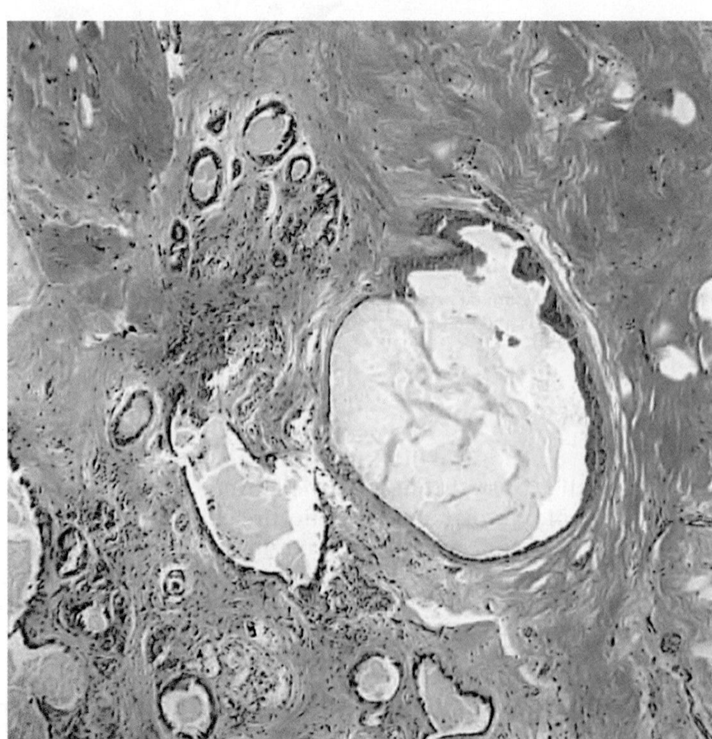

■ **FIGURE 15-15** Fibrocystic changes of the breast showing cysts, apocrine metaplasia, nonproliferating ducts, and stromal fibrosis (H&E, ×40).

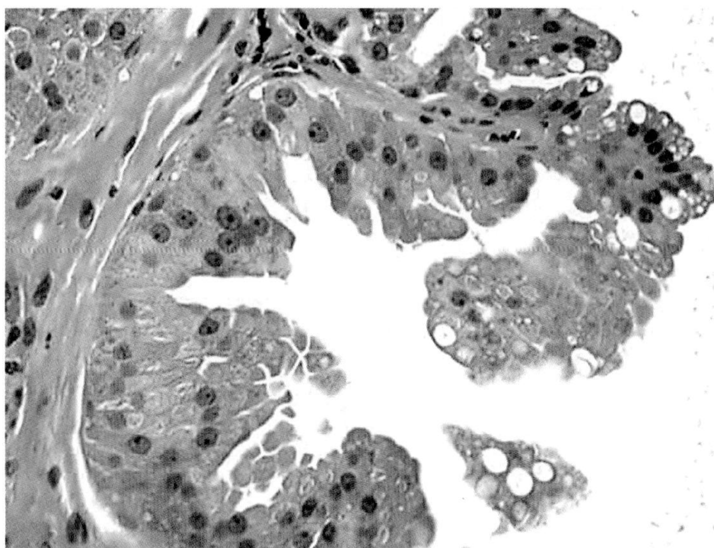

■ **FIGURE 15-16** Within fibrocystic changes, apocrine metaplasia is seen. The cells have round nuclei with central prominent nucleoli with abundant pink granular cytoplasm. Apical snouts of cytoplasmic products are protruding into the lumen (H&E, ×400).

Imaging Indications and Algorithm

If a woman presents with a palpable abnormality, it should be evaluated with diagnostic mammography and ultrasonography. In the case of focal and unrelenting pain, mammography with or without ultrasonography may be performed.

Imaging Technique and Findings

No specific mammographic, ultrasound, or MRI appearance has been documented, because these are normal breast tissue responses to hormonal changes.

Differential Diagnosis

From Clinical Presentation

Most breast carcinomas do not present as pain, nor do they typically change with the menstrual cycle. Although rare cases of breast carcinoma have been reported with pain, it is reassuring that if a woman presents with cyclic tenderness and fullness of the breast bilaterally, the condition is most likely a benign process.

From Imaging Findings

There are no specific imaging findings associated with fibrocystic changes.

From Pathology Findings

Histologically, fibrocystic changes of the breast include a variety of benign mammary alterations and patients may present with microscopic cysts, apocrine metaplasia, nonproliferative ducts and/or ductal hyperplasia without atypia, stromal fibrosis, and, occasionally, a mild degree of adenosis. Fibrocystic changes are commonly seen and are incidental findings in breast biopsy specimens (Figs 15-15 and 15-16).

Synopsis of Treatment Options

Most women with fibrocystic change do not need surgical treatment. Conservative medical treatment is recommended. Although there is no definitive, medically proven treatment for breast pain caused by fibrocystic changes, there are various remedies that patients can try. Reducing fat in the diet may be helpful while the use of supportive brassieres may supply immediate relief.

KEY POINTS

- Sebaceous cysts and epidermal inclusion cysts are benign breast lesions that arise from the skin of the breast.
- Galactoceles are single or more commonly multiple benign cysts with fluid contents resembling milk.
- Mammary duct ectasia is a nonspecific dilatation of the major subareolar or smaller ducts and represents a collection of dilated ducts with proteinaceous material within the lumen.
- Fibrocystic changes refer to a constellation of benign histologic findings, including microscopic cysts, apocrine metaplasia, nonproliferative ducts and/or ductal hyperplasia without atypia, stromal fibrosis, and, occasionally, a mild degree of adenosis.

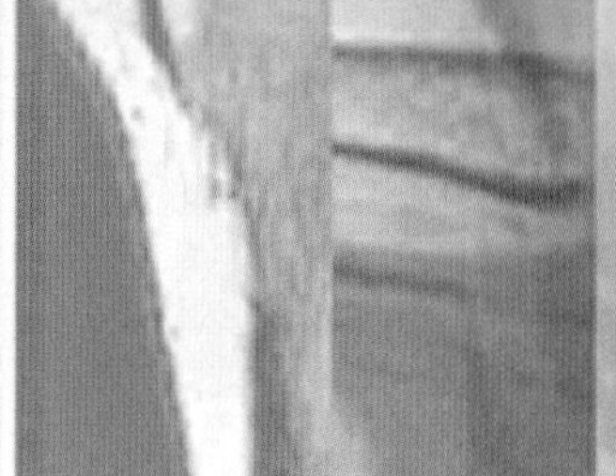

CASE STUDY

Chapter 15 Benign Cystic Lesions of the Breast

PATIENT HISTORY

A 40-year-old woman presented with a painful palpable abnormality in the right breast.

FINDINGS

A partially obscured oval mass near the inframammary fold is seen on the cleavage and craniocaudal (CC) views (Fig. 15-17). Ultrasonography (Fig. 15-18) demonstrates a superficial complex mass, possibly of dermal origin.

DIFFERENTIAL DIAGNOSIS

A dermal-based mass such as epidermal inclusion cyst or sebaceous cyst is possible. Malignancy is much less likely.

DIAGNOSIS

Fine-needle aspiration demonstrated cellular material with anucleated keratin debris in aggregates with numerous neutrophils and multinucleated giant cells (Figs. 15-19 and 15-20). The diagnosis was a ruptured epidermal inclusion cyst.

Core needle biopsy showed a benign epidermal inclusion cyst with evidence of rupture into adjacent soft tissue. Benign keratinized squamous epithelium with hyperkeratosis was noted within the dermis of the breast skin. The cystic contents were anucleated keratinized debris. The ruptured areas showed predominant mixed acute and chronic inflammatory cells and multinucleated giant cells engulfing the keratin debris (Figs 15-21 and 15-22).

IMPRESSION

The clinical presentation of pain is not uncommon in patients with epidermal inclusion or sebaceous cysts that have ruptured. Ultrasound-guided core needle biopsy was performed that demonstrated a ruptured epidermal inclusion cyst.

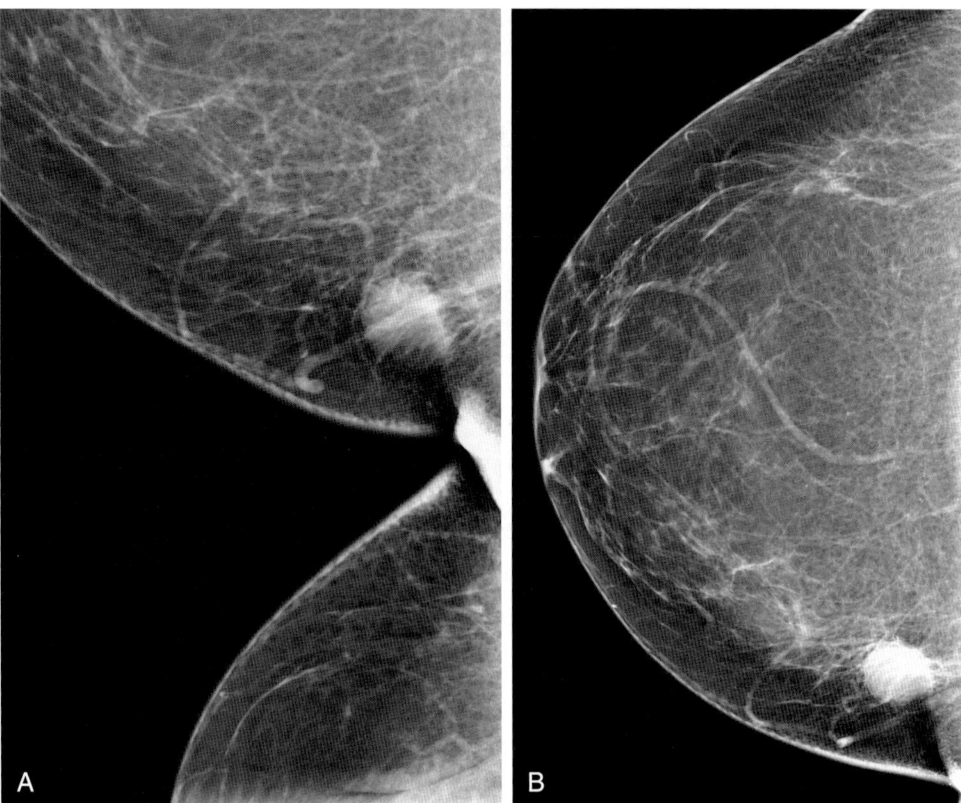

■ **FIGURE 15-17** Example of epidermal inclusion cyst mammogram. A partially obscured oval mass near the inframammary fold is seen on the cleavage (**A**) and craniocaudal (**B**) views.

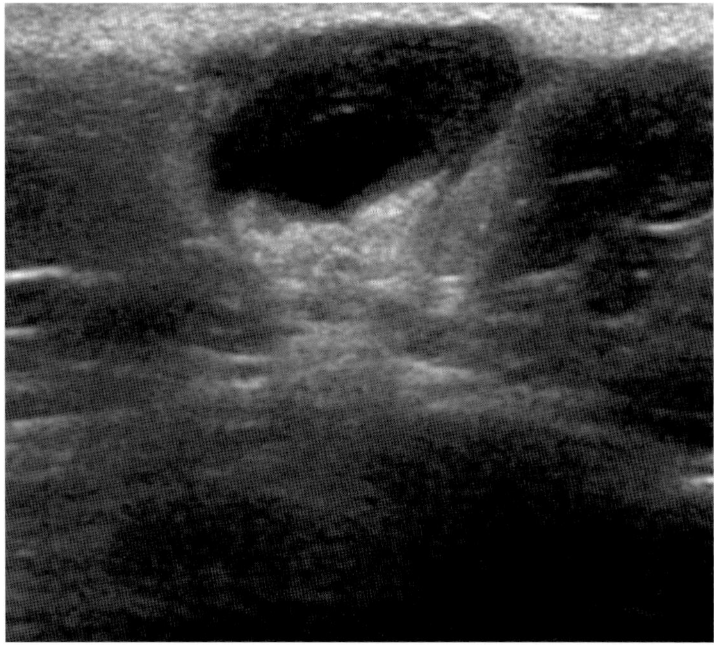

■ **FIGURE 15-18** Ultrasound image of the same patient as in Fig. 15-17 demonstrates a superficial complex intradermal mass.

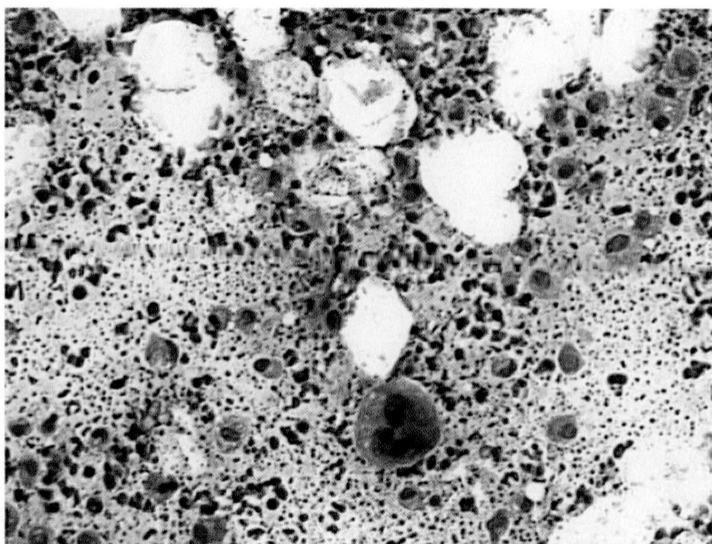

■ **FIGURE 15-19** Fine-needle aspiration (FNA) smear showing cellular materials with anucleated keratin debris with numerous neutrophils and multinucleated giant cells (May-Grunewald Giemsa [MGG] stain, ×100).

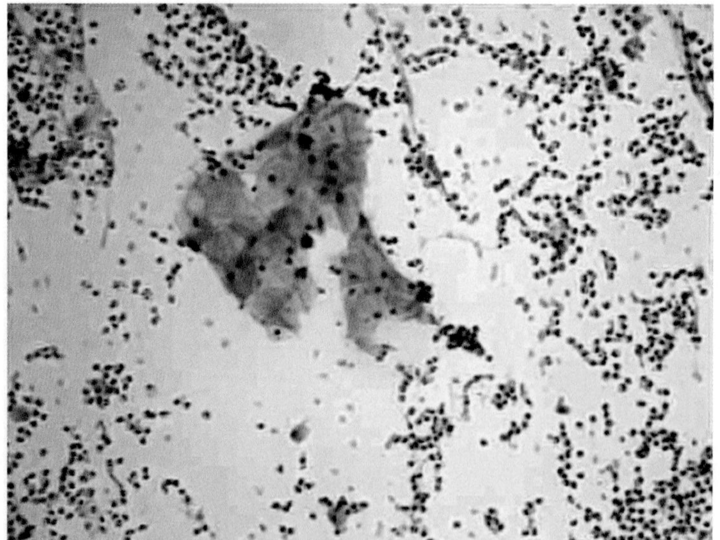

■ **FIGURE 15-20** Fine-needle aspiration (FNA) smear showing cellular materials with anucleated keratin debris in aggregates with numerous neutrophils and multinucleated giant cells (Papanicolaou [PAP] stain, ×100).

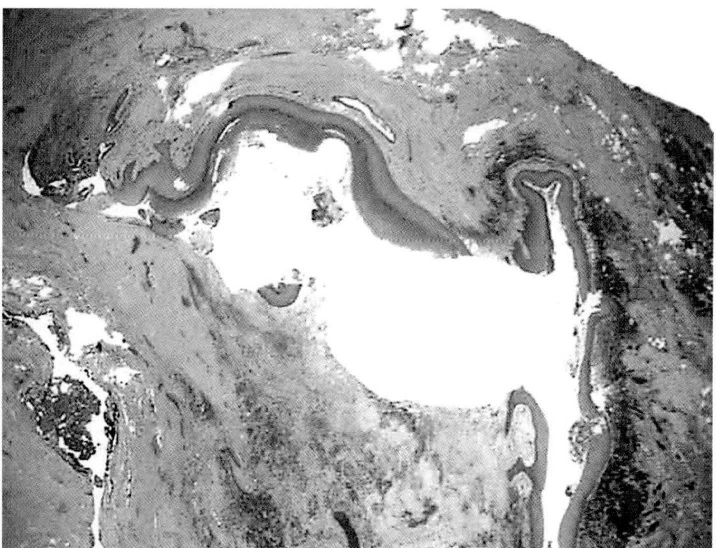

■ **FIGURE 15-21** Benign epidermal inclusion cyst with evidence of rupture of its contents into the adjacent soft tissue. Benign keratinized squamous epithelium with hyperkeratosis with luminal keratin debris is noted within the dermis of the breast skin (H&E, ×100).

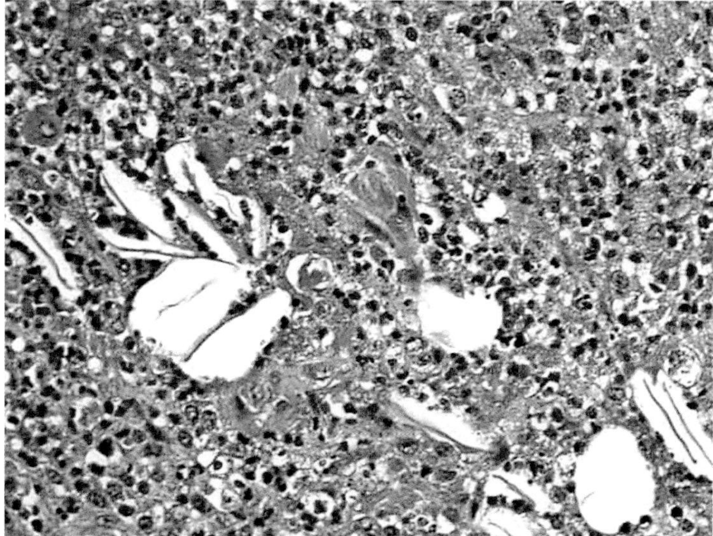

■ **FIGURE 15-22** The ruptured areas showed predominant mixed acute and chronic inflammatory cells, and multinucleated giant cells engulfing the keratin debris (H&E, ×400).

SUGGESTED READINGS

Houssami N, Irwig L, Ung O. Review of complex breast cysts: implications for cancer detection and clinical practice. *ANZ J Surg* 2005;**75**:1080-5.

Norwood SL. Fibrocystic breast disease. An update and review. *J Obstet Gynecol Neonatal Nurs* 1990;**19**:116-21.

Sabate JM, Clotet M, Torrubia S, Gomez A, Guerrero R, de las Heras P, et al. Radiologic evaluation of breast disorders related to pregnancy and lactation. *RadioGraphics* 2007;**27**(Suppl. 1):S101-24.

Sehgal CM, Weinstein SP, Arger PH, Conant EF. A Review of breast ultrasound. *J Mammary Gland Biol Neoplasia* 2006;**11**:113-23.

REFERENCES

1. Chantra PK, Tang JTC, Stanley TM, Bassett LW. Circumscribed fibrocystic mastopathy with formation of an epidermal cyst. *AJR Am J Roentgenol* 1994;**163**:831-2.
2. Golden GT, Wangensteen SL. Galactocele of the breast. *Am J Surg* 1972;**123**:271-3.
3. Winkler JM. Galactocele of the breast. *Am J Surg* 1964;**108**:357-60.
4. Bessman SP, Lucas JC. Galactocele in a male infant. *Pediatrics* 1953;**11**:109-12.
5. Feig SA. Breast masses. Mammographic and sonographic evaluation. *Radiol Clin North Am* 1992;**30**:67-92.
6. Kopans DB. Pathologic, mammographic, and ultrasonographic correlation. In: Kopans DB, editor. *Breast Imaging*. 2nd ed. Philadelphia: Lippincott-Raven; 1997. p. 511-615.
7. Salvador R, Salvador M, Jimenez JA, Martinez M, Casas L. Galactocele of the breast: radiologic and ultrasonographic findings. *Br J Radiol* 1990;**63**:140-2.
8. Kopans DB. Histologic, pathologic and imaging correlation. In: Kopans DB, editor. *Breast imaging*. 3rd ed. Philadelphia: Lippincott Williams & Wilkins; 2006. p. 824-6.

CHAPTER 16

Solid Benign Lesions of the Breast

Sophia Kim Apple, Jane M. Dascalos, and Lawrence W. Bassett

The majority of solid lesions of the breast are benign. Benign processes may be asymptomatic or have clinical manifestations, which include nodularity, thickening, a palpable mass, pain, inflammation, or nipple discharge. However, many of the signs and symptoms of breast disease are nonspecific and must be evaluated further with imaging and sometimes biopsy to determine whether the lesion is benign or malignant.

In this chapter, we will discuss benign solid lesions of the breast including fibroadenoma, intramammary lymph node, hamartoma, lipoma, fibromatosis, fibrosis, adenosis, diabetic mastopathy, granular cell tumor, fat necrosis, silicone breast prostheses, hemangioma, pseudoangiomatous stromal hyperplasia, myofibroblastoma, adenomyoepithelioma, and nipple adenoma.

FIBROADENOMA

Definition

A fibroadenoma is a benign fibroepithelial proliferative tumor with the hallmark of a concurrent proliferation of glandular and stromal elements.

Prevalence and Epidemiology

Fibroadenomas are the most common breast masses encountered in women younger than 35 years of age and the most common solid masses found in women of all ages.

Etiology and Pathophysiology

The exact etiology of fibroadenomas is unknown. They seem to be influenced by estrogen levels. They are most often seen in premenopausal or pregnant women, or in women who are postmenopausal and taking hormone replacement therapy.

Manifestations of Disease

Clinical Presentation

Clinically apparent fibroadenomas are round, oval, freely mobile masses that may change with the menstrual cycle or pregnancy. Fibroadenomas can be multiple. Most fibroadenomas are less than 3 cm, but giant fibroadenomas are large and can exceed 6 cm in diameter. The tumor is not fixed to the adjacent skin, pectoralis muscle, or axillary lymph nodes, so they are mobile within the breast on palpation. Many fibroadenomas undergo hyalinization, degeneration, and calcification after menopause and may become smaller.

Imaging Indications and Algorithm

Because fibroadenomas often present as palpable findings in young patients, the workup is dependent on the patient's age. In patients younger than 30 years of age, ultrasonography is the initial study of choice. In patients older than 30, mammography and ultrasonography are performed. If the classic appearance is not present, tissue diagnosis is often performed. Surgical excision may be performed if the lesion is large or if it is desired by the patient. An enlarging solid mass should be worked up to rule out malignancy and should not be assumed to be a fibroadenoma.

Imaging Technique and Findings

Mammography

On mammography, fibroadenomas are usually circumscribed, round to oval masses (Fig. 16-1) or lobular (Fig. 16-2), low to equal density radiopaque masses. Involuting fibroadenomas have typical coarse calcifications, which usually begin at the periphery of the mass and coalesce and increase, often completely replacing the soft tissue mass itself. When calcifications are present within the mass, ultrasonography is not necessary.

Ultrasonography

The typical ultrasound finding is an oval, circumscribed (Fig. 16-3), homogeneous solid mass with internal echoes, often isoechoic or slightly hypoechoic to fat. Posterior acoustic enhancement is sometimes seen (see Fig. 16-3). Atypical findings seen in some fibroadenomas include microlobulated (Fig. 16-4) or indistinct (Fig. 16-5) margins. In the case of an involuting fibroadenoma, acoustic shadowing is seen because of calcification. In some cases it is difficult to differentiate a fibroadenoma from a fat lobule.

Magnetic Resonance Imaging

The MRI appearance of a fibroadenoma varies depending on the percentage of myxoid and fibrous components. With increasing age the fibrous components increase. The classic MR appearance is of an oval mass with smooth margins and low signal septations on enhanced T1- or T2-weighted images. They usually grow parallel in orientation to Cooper ligaments. Homogeneous enhancement is usually present, with more heterogeneous enhancement seen with increasing fibrosis and sclerosis. The enhancement kinetics are most commonly that of rapid persistent enhancement. Sclerotic fibroadenomas are of low signal intensity on T2-weighted images, and the septations are often not visible.

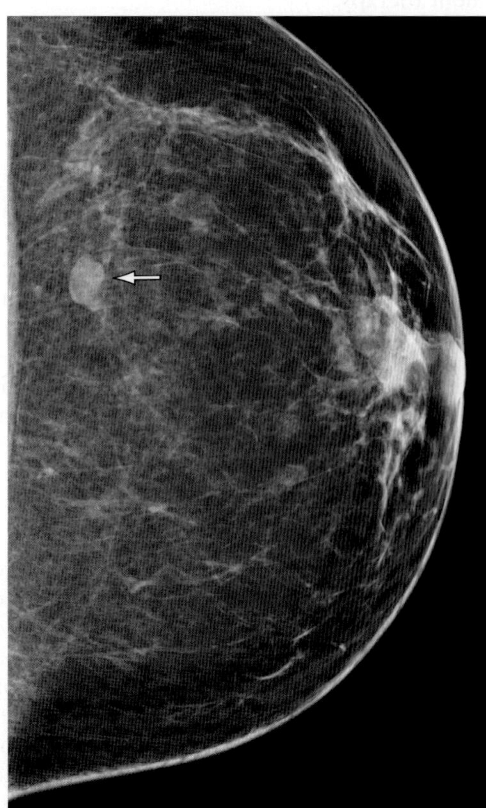

■ **FIGURE 16-1** Fibroadenoma. Screening mammography shows an oval circumscribed mass in the left breast (*arrow*).

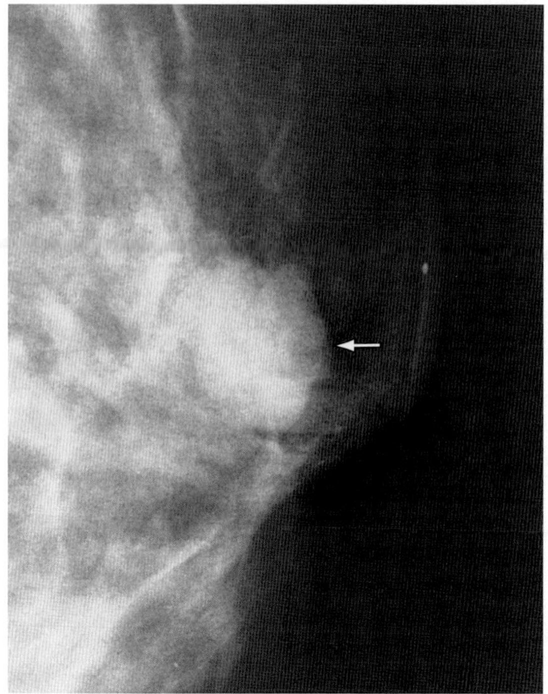

■ **FIGURE 16-2** Fibroadenoma. A 1.2-cm subareolar lobular mass with circumscribed margins (*arrow*).

Classic Signs

The classic sign is an ultrasonographically visible oval isoechoic to hypoechoic mass with circumscribed margins.

Pathology Findings

A fibroadenoma is a benign fibroepithelial proliferative lesion that usually is noted to be a localized palpable tumor. Patients occasionally present with a nonpalpable radiographically detected tumor. The origin of the tumor is from the epithelium of the terminal ductal lobular unit and interlobular stroma. Thus, the hallmark of a fibroadenoma is concurrent proliferation of glandular and stromal elements. There are mainly two growth patterns: intracanalicular and pericanalicular (Figs 16-6 and 16-7). Fibroadenomas seen in younger women tend to be more cellular in stroma and myxoid in appearance. Aged fibroadenomas can have appearance of fibrotic and less cellular stroma and calcifications, and at times ossifications can be seen within the lesions (Figs 16-8 and 16-9). Mitotic figures are extremely rare. The epithelial component can have florid ductal hyperplasia, squamous metaplasia, and papillary apocrine metaplasia. When adenosis and or sclerosing adenosis are seen within the fibroadenoma, it has been designated as

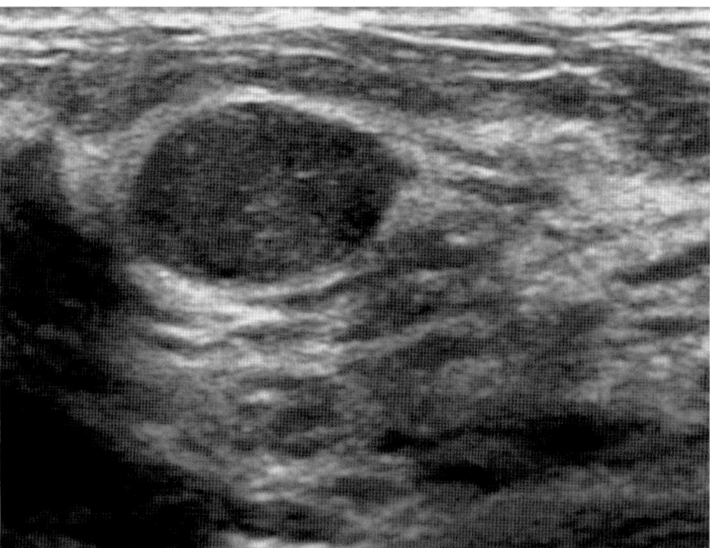

■ **FIGURE 16-3** Fibroadenoma. Ultrasonogram of a classic-appearing fibroadenoma that is oval, with circumscribed margins and isoechoic to slightly hypoechoic with low-level internal echoes. In this case, posterior acoustic enhancement is seen.

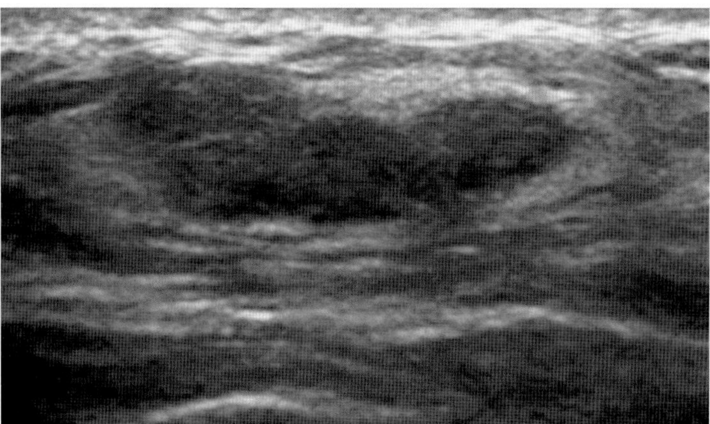

■ **FIGURE 16-4** Fibroadenoma. Margins of the mass are microlobulated on ultrasonogram.

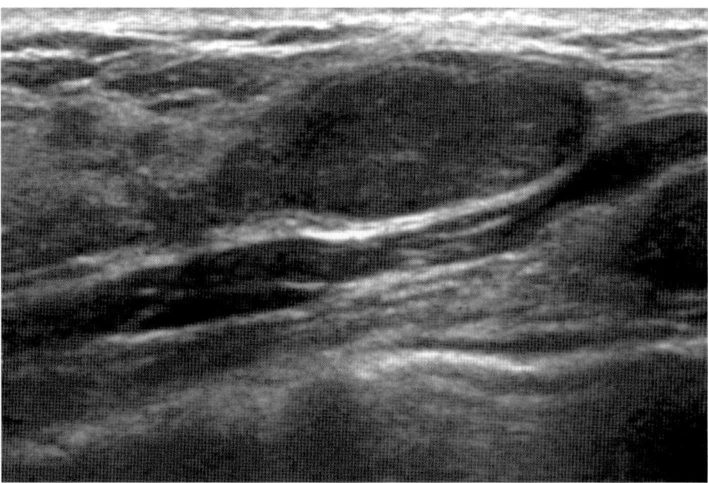

■ **FIGURE 16-5** Fibroadenomas. Margins of the mass on ultrasonogram are somewhat indistinct compared with that of Fig. 16-3.

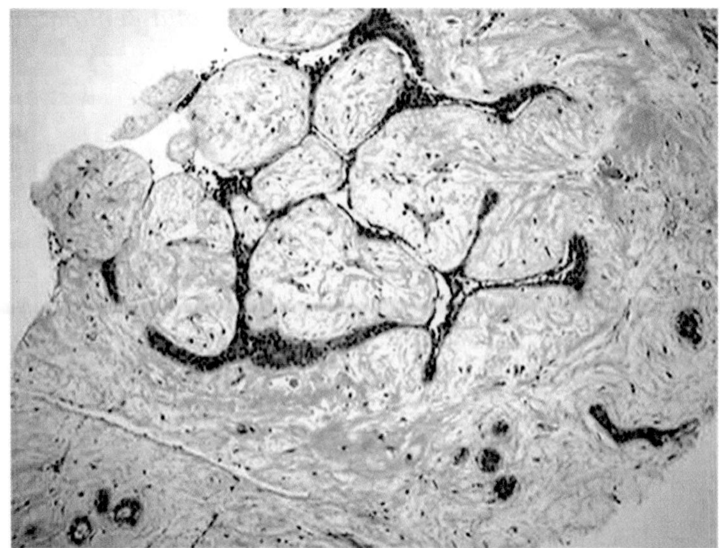

■ **FIGURE 16-6** The intracanalicular growth pattern is formed by myxoid stroma compressing epithelial slit-like spaces (H&E, ×100).

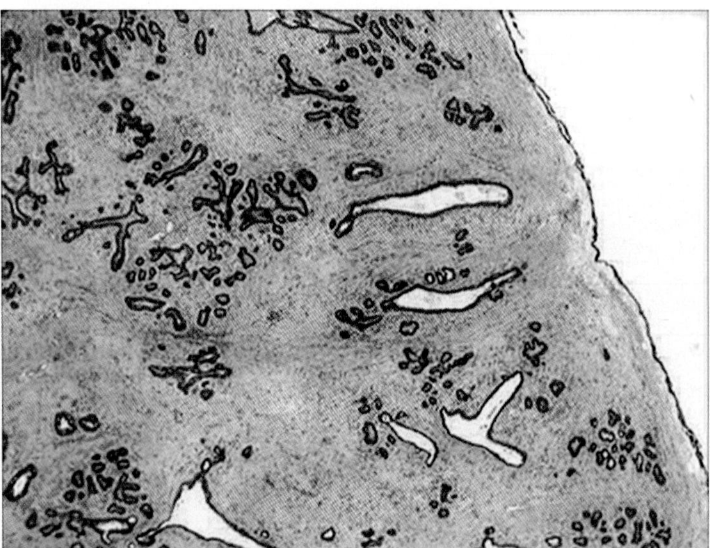

■ **FIGURE 16-7** A pericanalicular growth pattern is formed by fibrous stroma arranged in a circumferential area of glands without significant degree of compressed ducts (H&E, ×40).

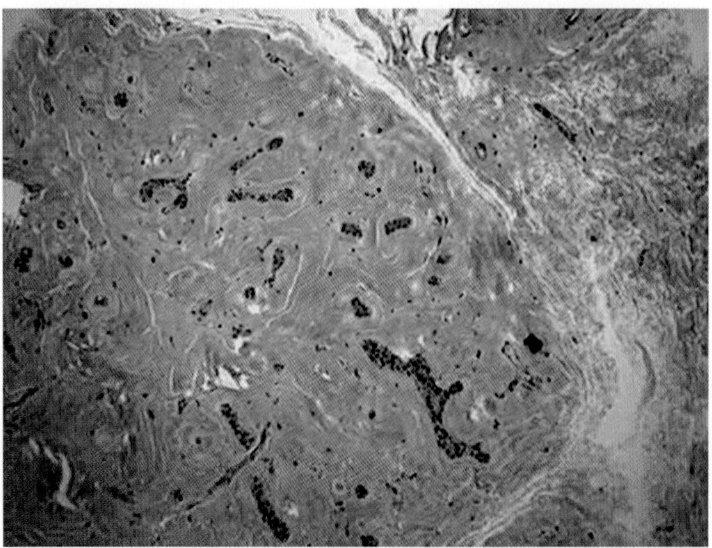

■ **FIGURE 16-8** Fibrosed (old) fibroadenoma with intracanalicular pattern in hyalinized fibrotic stroma. No myxoid stroma is seen (H&E, ×40).

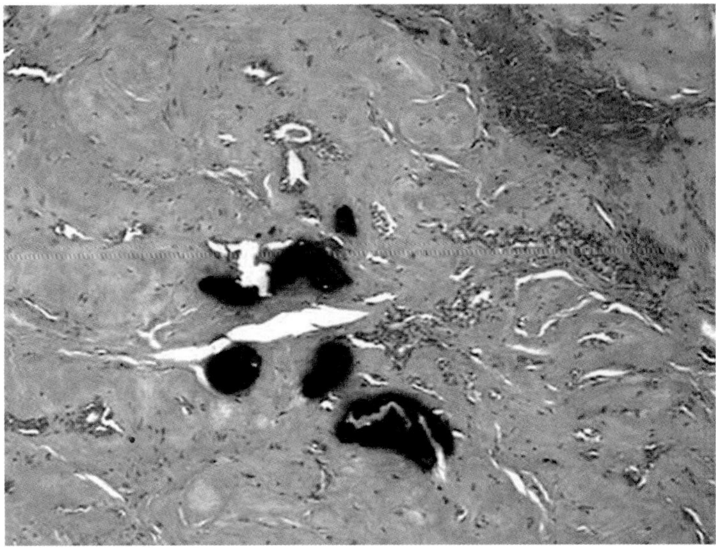

■ **FIGURE 16-9** Fibrosed (old) fibroadenoma with calcifications (H&E, ×200).

"complex fibroadenoma." Rarely, fibroadenomas can be seen with epithelial atypia such as atypical ductal hyperplasia (ADH), ductal carcinoma in situ (DCIS) (Fig. 16-10), and lobular carcinoma in situ (LCIS). There are no helpful clinical features suggesting which fibroadenomas may have high-risk epithelial atypia. However, there may be changes in calcification pattern via mammographic analysis especially when comedo-type DCIS is seen within the fibroadenoma. Many fibroadenomas do not require excisional biopsy unless there is concern about the nature of the lesion. Some patients' desire to remove palpable lesions may lead to excisional biopsies of fibroadenomas. The lesion is most typically "shelled out" without adjacent surrounding breast tissue during the excision. Some fibroadenomas will recur. Most fibroadenomas can be diagnosed readily in breast core needle biopsy and fine-needle aspiration (FNA) biopsy. Fibroadenomas on FNA show the following three classic features: (1) abundant epithelial fragments composed of tight clusters of uniform bland-appearing cells, some showing antler-horn like appearance; (2) numerous naked nuclei in the background that are known to be myoepithelial cells; and (3) fragments of stromal cells (Figs 16-11 and 16-12). However, cellular fibroepithelial lesions seen in FNA or even core needle biopsies can make it difficult to distinguish between cellular fibroadenomas and phyllodes tumors. Excisional biopsy should be recommended in these cases.

Juvenile fibroadenomas usually occur in women younger than 20 years of age but have been reported in adults as old as 72 years. They usually present as a rapidly growing, well-circumscribed mass that can be large (up to 20 cm). Juvenile fibroadenomas have higher stromal cellularity and epithelial hyperplasia with a more commonly pericanalicular and gynecomastia-like growth pattern (Fig. 16-13). The differential diagnosis of juvenile fibroadenoma is phyllodes tumor. However, unlike the phyllodes tumor,

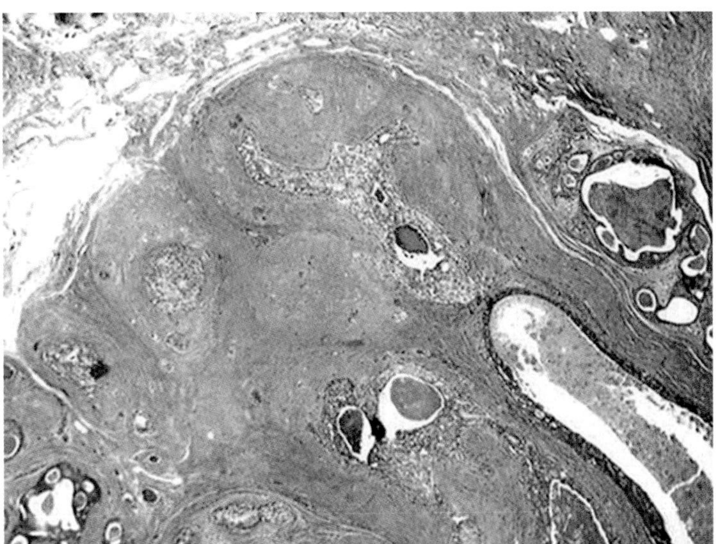

■ **FIGURE 16-10** Ductal carcinoma in situ (DCIS), comedo type, with central necrosis within fibroadenoma (H&E, ×100).

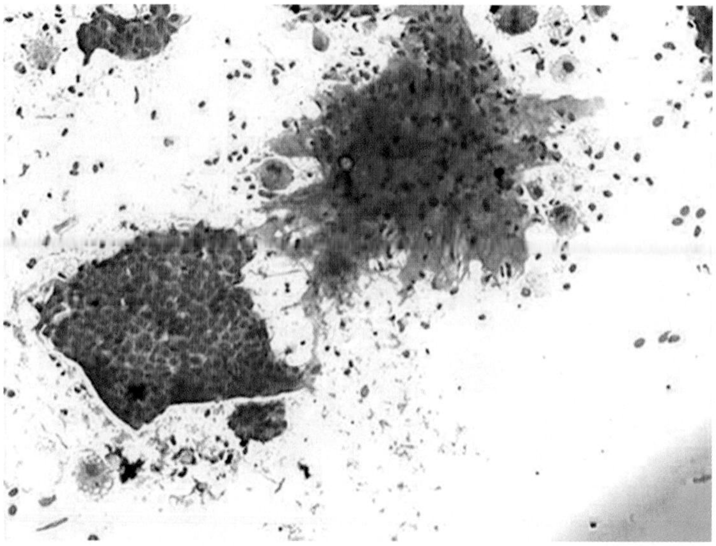

■ **FIGURE 16-11** Fibroadenoma showing honeycomb pattern of bland-appearing epithelial cells, stromal fragments and numerous bare nuclei in the background (fine-needle aspiration, May-Grunwald Giemsa [MGG] stain, ×200).

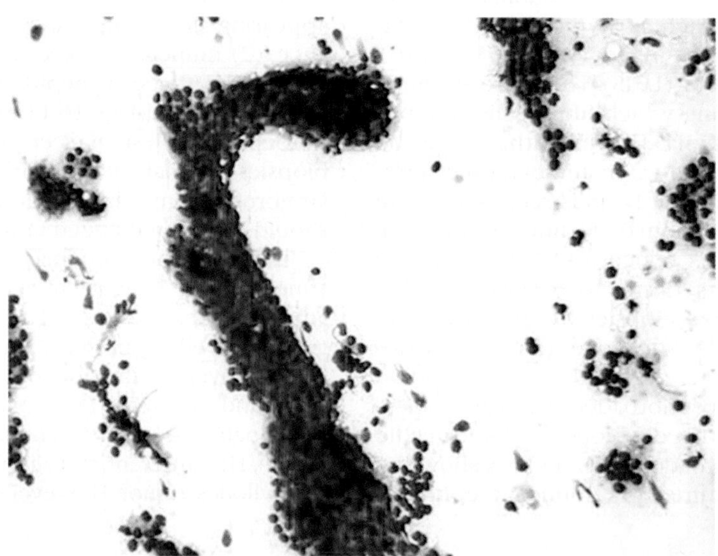

■ **FIGURE 16-12** Some of the epithelial cells in fibroadenoma are elongated with blunt-ended structure resembling antler-horn pattern (Fine-needle aspiration, May-Grunwald Giemsa [MGG], ×200).

juvenile fibroadenomas lack marked stromal nuclear pleomorphism and cleft-like spaces with broad fronds. Mitotic figures are rare to absent, and myxoid stroma is absent in juvenile fibroadenomas. Most patients with juvenile fibroadenoma are managed by excisional biopsy.

The risk of development of carcinoma within fibroadenomas is no higher than the risk of breast carcinoma in the general population. Many of the reported cases of fibroadenomas associated with cancer have had DCIS or LCIS adjacent to the fibroadenoma, but several cases of carcinoma truly within fibroadenomas have been reported.

Synopsis of Treatment Options

Some fibroadenomas will recur. Most fibroadenomas can be diagnosed readily by breast core needle biopsy and FNA. If imaging studies correlate well with either procedure, there is no need to excise the mass unless the lesion is large or the patient desires its removal. However, cellular fibroepithelial lesions seen in FNA or even core needle biopsy can be difficult to distinguish versus phyllodes tumor. Conservative excisional biopsy should be recommended in these cases. Most patients with juvenile fibroadenomas are managed by excisional biopsy.

INTRAMAMMARY LYMPH NODE

Definition

An intramammary lymph node is a lymph node found within the breast parenchyma at any quadrant, excluding axillary lymph nodes.

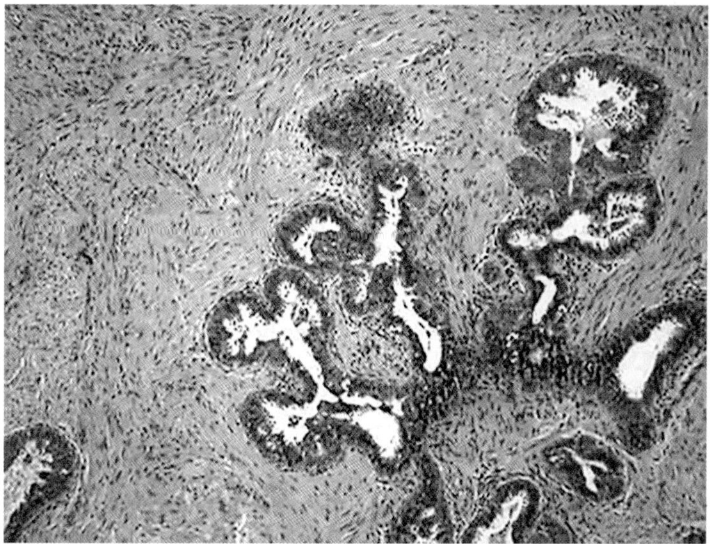

■ **FIGURE 16-13** Juvenile fibroadenoma showing a higher stromal cellularity and epithelial hyperplasia (H&E, ×200).

Prevalence and Epidemiology

Lymph nodes are commonly encountered on mammograms. The vast majority seen on mammography are in the upper outer quadrant of the breast, the axillary tail, and the axilla, but lymph nodes can be found within any quadrant of the breast.

Etiology and Pathophysiology

Intramammary lymph nodes are usually a normal, incidental finding. Occasionally, they may be involved with inflammation, granulomatous processes, or metastatic carcinoma. Coarse calcifications are sometimes seen in lymph nodes involved with granulomatous disease such as histoplasmosis (Fig. 16-14), tuberculosis, or sarcoidosis. Rarely, primary lymphoma can involve an intramammary lymph node. Faint metallic deposits simulating microcalcifications can be seen in patients with rheumatoid arthritis secondary to gold therapy (Fig. 16-15). The focus here is on normal intramammary lymph nodes and benign involved lymph nodes.

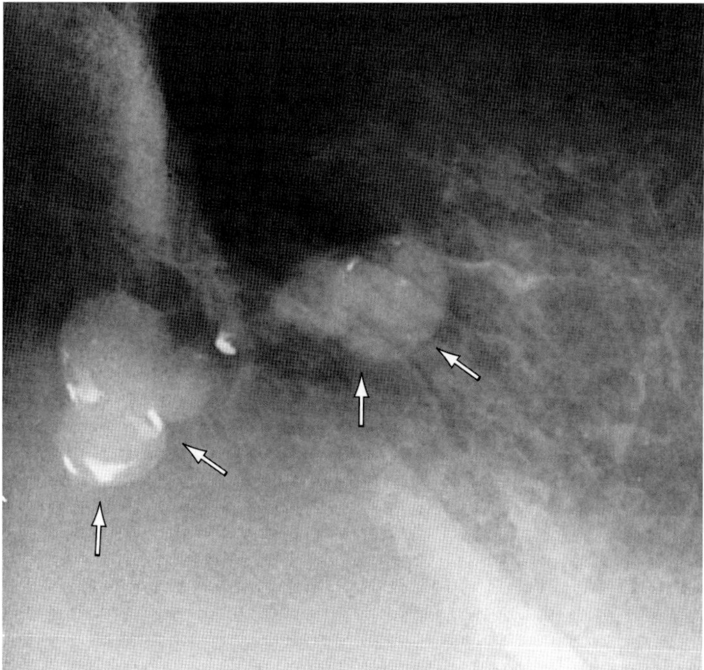

■ **FIGURE 16-14** Histoplasmosis. Enlarged axillary lymph nodes with dystrophic peripheral calcifications (*arrows*) in a woman with a history of disseminated histoplasmosis. Other granulomatous diseases may produce identical calcifications.

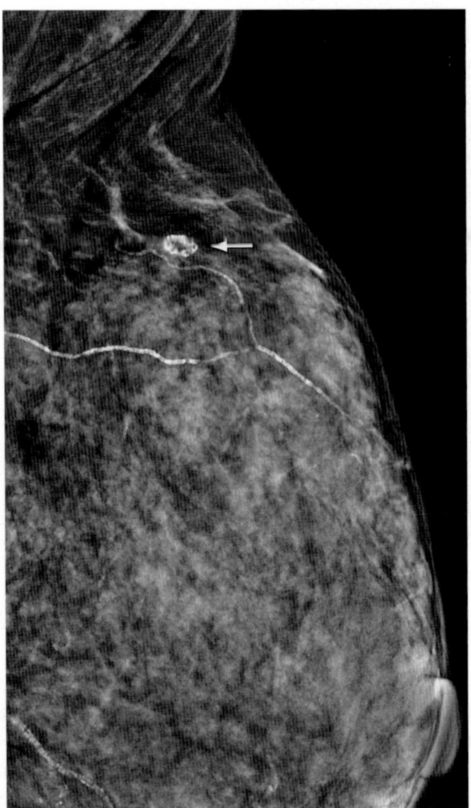

■ **FIGURE 16-15** Gold deposits. This woman had gold injections for rheumatoid arthritis. The metallic particles simulate microcalcifications in a lymph node (*arrow*).

Manifestations of Disease

Clinical Presentation

Normal intramammary lymph nodes are usually not apparent clinically and are seen incidentally on imaging studies. Involved lymph nodes can present as a palpable finding.

Imaging Indications and Algorithm

Most intramammary lymph nodes are less than 1 cm in greatest dimension, whereas normal axillary lymph nodes may be 2 cm or more. Regardless of the size, when the typical mammographic appearance is seen, the lymph node can be regarded as being benign and no further workup is needed. In some cases, the diagnosis is not obvious on the standard views, and additional mammographic workup is necessary to demonstrate fat within the structure. An involved lymph node might appear abnormal on mammography and require additional evaluation with ultrasonography and possibly biopsy. In some normal lymph nodes, the classic radiologic appearance is not demonstrated and follow-up mammography or biopsy may be indicated.

Imaging Findings by Modality

Mammography

Normal intramammary lymph nodes usually appear on mammography as oval or reniform, circumscribed noncalcified masses. The fat within the hilum of the lymph node is often seen as a lucency at the periphery when viewed in tangent or in the central portion of the mass when viewed en face (Fig. 16-16).

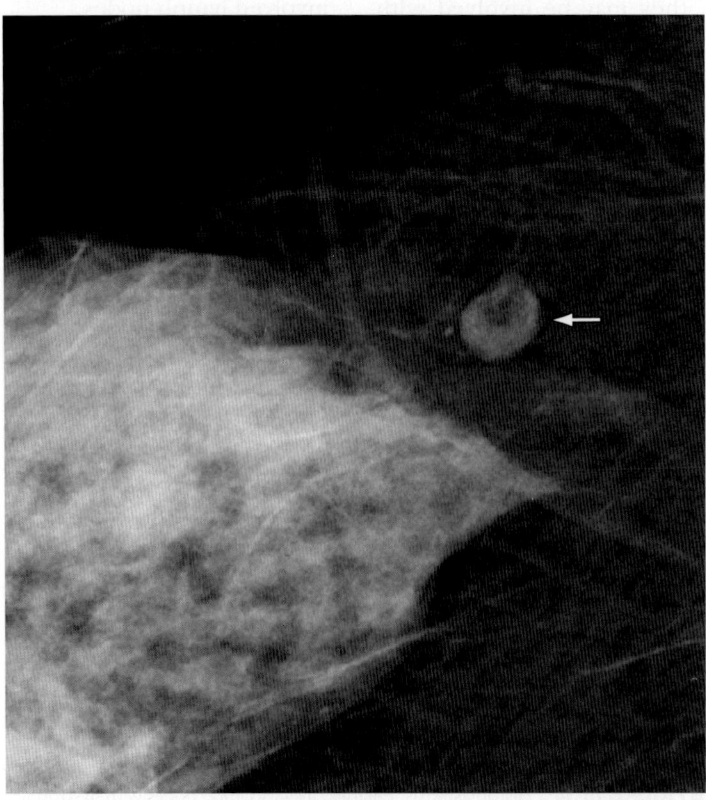

■ **FIGURE 16-16** Intramammary lymph node (*arrow*). In this case, the fatty hilum is seen en face.

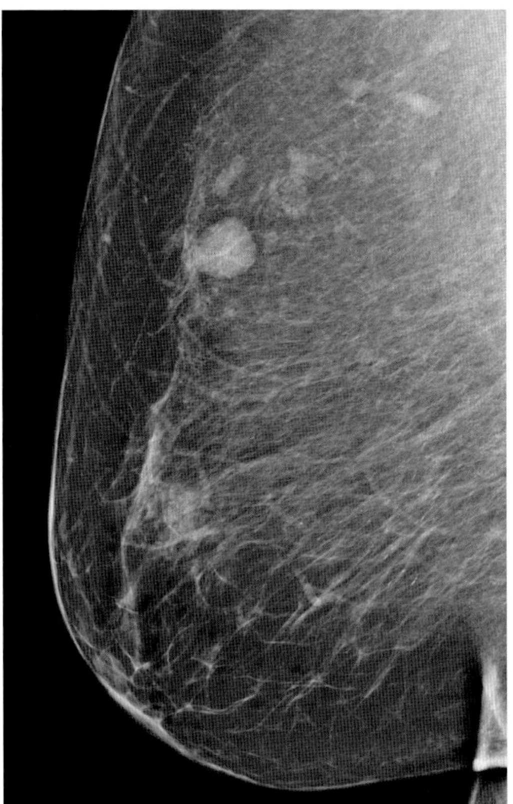

■ **FIGURE 16-17** Reactive lymph node. This 69-year-old female had an incidentally enlarged lymph node seen in the right breast on screening mammography and a history of left breast carcinoma. Core biopsy was performed.

On mammography, most involved lymph nodes are round, enlarged, and abnormally dense and lack a visible fatty hilum. They may be seen to originate at the site of a previously identified, mammographically normal-appearing lymph node. Reactive inflammatory lymph nodes usually maintain circumscribed margins (Fig. 16-17). This is in contrast to metastatic lymph nodes, which may develop indistinct or spiculated margins and occasionally microcalcifications.

Ultrasonography

On ultrasonography, the periphery of a normal intramammary lymph node is hypoechoic relative to fat and fibroglandular tissue. The fatty hilum is highly echogenic (Fig. 16-18). In reactive processes, the normal architecture tends to be preserved within the enlarged node and the echogenic hilum often remains visible. (Fig. 16-19).

Magnetic Resonance Imaging

The MRI appearance of a normal intramammary lymph node is of a kidney-shaped structure. The enhancement pattern is variable but most commonly demonstrates rapid washout kinetics. For this reason it is important to look for the high signal intensity of fatty hilum on the non-fat suppressed T1-weighted images. Lymph nodes are of high signal on T2 weighted sequences, which can be a very helpful diagnostic feature, given their enhancement pattern. The combination of an oval mass with smooth margins, and the fat signal intensity of the fatty hilum, with high signal on T2 weighted images is virtually diagnostic of an intramammary lymph node. Replacement of the fatty hilum, especially in the setting of breast carcinoma, is suspicious, as is thickening of the cortex.

Classic Signs

The fatty hilum of a normal intramammary lymph node is classically described as notched on mammography with a kidney-shaped architecture and is often located in association with a vessel.

Differential Diagnosis

From Clinical Presentation

When an intramammary lymph node is palpable, the clinical differential diagnosis includes both breast carcinoma and solid benign tumors.

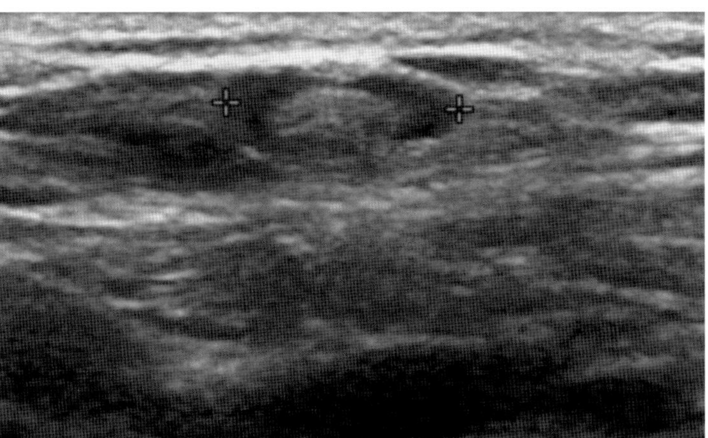

■ **FIGURE 16-18** Intramammary lymph node. Ultrasonogram of a normal lymph node. The peripheral lymphoid tissue is hypoechoic relative to fat. The fatty hilum is echogenic.

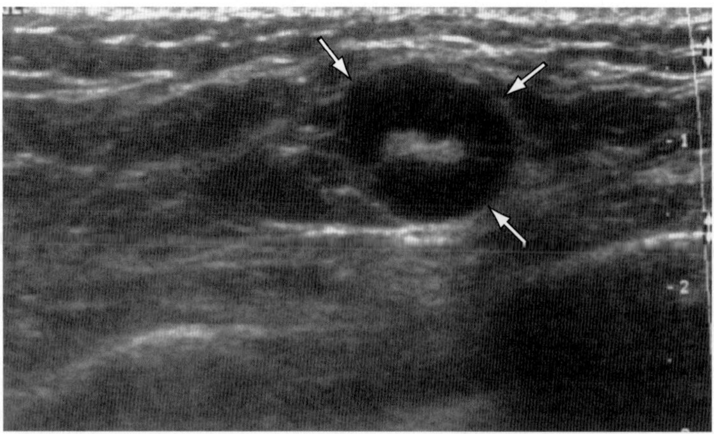

■ **FIGURE 16-19** Reactive intramammary lymph node in a patient with psoriasis. On ultrasonography, the echogenic fatty hilum is visible and the peripheral lymphoid tissue is diffusely thickened (*arrows*) but the normal architecture is preserved.

From Imaging Findings

When classic in radiologic appearance, a normal intramammary lymph node has no differential diagnosis. When atypical or frankly abnormal, other solid lesions of the breast with circumscribed margins are also in the differential diagnosis, including fibroadenoma, lipoma, and breast carcinoma as well as pathologic intramammary lymph nodes.

Pathology Findings

Intramammary lymph nodes are usually found in the lateral aspect of the breast and axillary tail. Lymph nodes found within the breast parenchyma are usually located deep in the outer quadrants of the breast. Intramammary lymph nodes may become involved with inflammation, granulomatous processes, lymphoma, or metastatic tumors. Reactive lymph nodes can present as lymphadenopathy. Histologically, the reactive lymph nodes appear round and enlarged and maintain the normal architecture of a typical lymph node (Fig. 16-20). Sometimes, the entire lymph node can be replaced by fatty metamorphism where most of the lymph node is replaced by adipocytes with only a rim of lymphoid tissue and subcapsular sinus (Fig. 16-21). Granulomatous adenopathy can be seen due to tuberculosis, histoplasmosis, rheumatoid arthritis, sarcoidosis, or an unknown cause.

Synopsis of Treatment Options

When typical mammographic features are present, one can confidently make the diagnosis of an intramammary lymph node and no further intervention is required. In the unusual situation in which the lesion is palpable and the patient is bothered by the mass, excision can be considered. In such cases, local excision is sufficient. A short-term interval follow-up may be indicated for cases with unusual mammographic and ultrasonographic features.

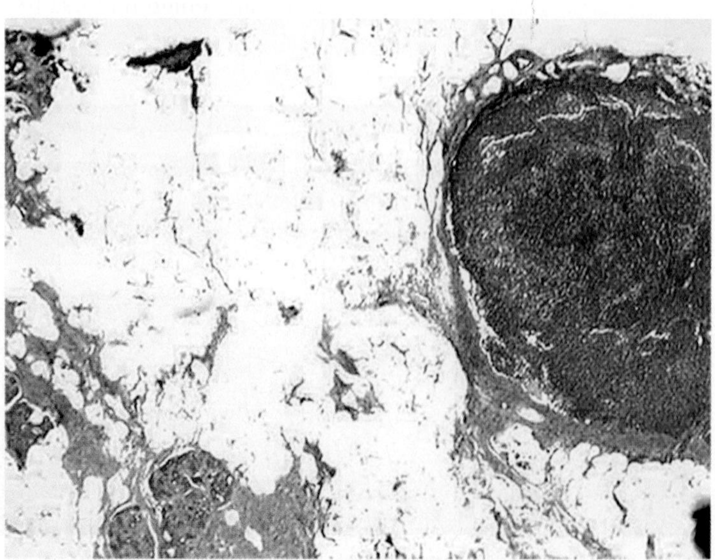

■ **FIGURE 16-20** Intramammary lymph node is found within the adjacent normal breast lobules, ducts and fatty tissue (H&E, ×40).

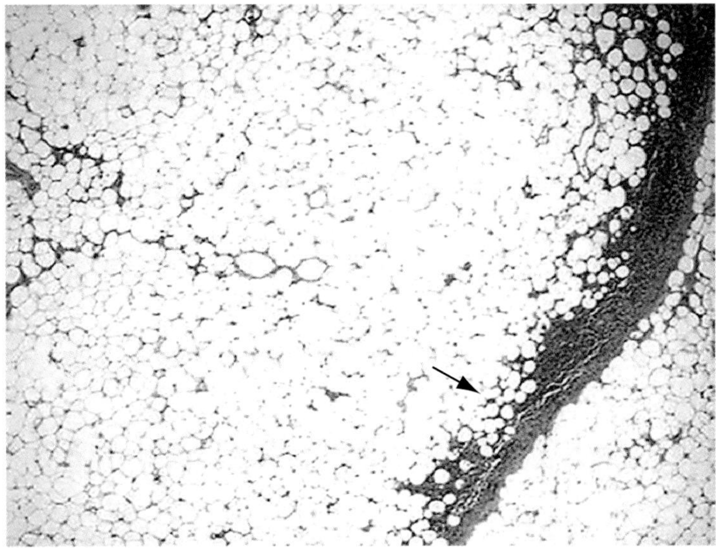

■ **FIGURE 16-21** Fatty metamorphism of lymph node. Most of the lymph node is replaced by mature adipose tissue with only a narrow rim of lymphoid tissue and underlying subcapsular tissue (*arrow*) (H&E, ×100).

HAMARTOMA

Definition

Hamartomas are benign well-circumscribed breast lesions composed of variable normal constituents of breast tissue, including fat, glandular tissue, and fibrous connective tissue. Other names such as fibroadenolipoma and lipofibroadenoma have been used to reflect the dominant component of tissue type within the mass.

Prevalence and Epidemiology

The majority of the hamartomas are detected in women older than 35 years of age.

Etiology and Pathophysiology

The pathogenesis is unclear. The lesion may be a result of dysgenesis rather than a true tumor.[1]

Manifestations of Disease

Clinical Presentation

Hamartomas are often asymptomatic, but some are palpable and are usually painless. Large predominantly fatty hamartomas are often nonpalpable, whereas lesions with a large fibrous component often mimic fibroadenomas or well-circumscribed carcinomas clinically.

Imaging Indications and Algorithm

The patient may present with a palpable finding where diagnostic mammography would be the initial step. If the classic mammographic appearance is demonstrated, no further workup is indicated. If it is atypical in appearance, it would require close interval follow-up mammographically, additional imaging with ultrasound, or even biopsy depending on the lesion's size, imaging features, and clinical findings.

Imaging Technique and Findings

Mammography

The classic mammographic appearance of a breast hamartoma is virtually diagnostic. The lesion is circumscribed and contains both fat and soft tissue density surrounded by a thin radiopaque capsule, which is visible when fat is identified on both sides (Fig. 16-22). The appearance is similar to a "cut sausage" on radiography or a "breast within a breast." Although many of these lesions do not have a true fibrous capsule, a thin radiopaque pseudocapsule is usually seen around at least a portion of the mass. Hamartomas containing predominantly fibrous tissue density are more difficult to diagnose. Some have only a small amount of fat beneath the capsule and others have so little fat that they mimic a fibroadenoma or carcinoma.

Ultrasonography

When the typical mammographic appearance is present, there is no indication for ultrasonography. For lesions that present atypically as a circumscribed mass, however, ultrasonography is usually performed to distinguish between a cyst and a solid mass. The ultrasonographic appearance is variable. The lesion may contain areas of low-level internal echogenicity interspersed with irregular areas of hyperechogenicity (Fig. 16-23). In some cases, the fatty tissue within the lesion may be highly echogenic. The appearance may also mimic a fibroadenoma.

Magnetic Resonance Imaging

The MRI appearance is that of an encapsulated mass with a heterogeneous appearance (Figs 16-24 and 16-25). If there are prominent glandular elements, some contrast enhancement can be seen on T1-weighted contrast-enhanced imaging (Fig. 16-26).

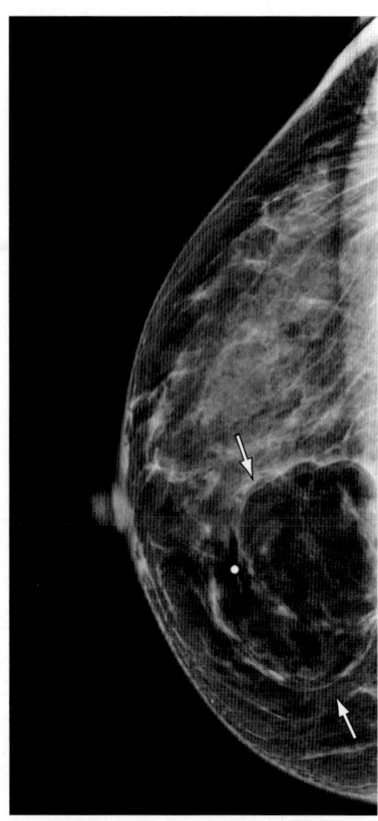

■ **FIGURE 16-22** Hamartoma. Craniocaudal mammogram demonstrates a round, circumscribed mass (*arrows*) containing both fat and soft tissue density with a palpable marker overlying.

Classic Signs

Hamartomas seen on mammography are classically described as "cut sausage" or a "breast within a breast" due to the presence of both fat and soft tissue density.

Pathology Findings

Hamartomas of the breast are benign, well-circumscribed masses that consist of mammary glandular structures with prominent lobular architecture, fibrous stroma, smooth muscle tissue, and fat in variable proportions. The size of the tumor varies from less than 1 cm to 17 cm with breast distortion. Clinical and imaging findings may be similar to fibroadenomas; however, histologically, hamartomas are not fibroepithelial tumors, unlike fibroadenomas. Hamartomas are at least partially or completely encapsulated masses composed of normal constituents of breast tissue. Lobules and ductules present within the lesion are structurally normal without proliferation (Fig. 16-27) The other variants of hamartoma are myoid hamartoma with smooth muscle differentiation, adenolipoma, and chondrolipoma. Of note, a small sample of a hamartoma seen on a core biopsy can be diagnosed as benign breast tissue, particularly when the knowledge of the clinical and imaging studies is not included during the pathologic examination.

Synopsis of Treatment Options

When typical mammographic features are present, one can confidently make the diagnosis of a hamartoma, and

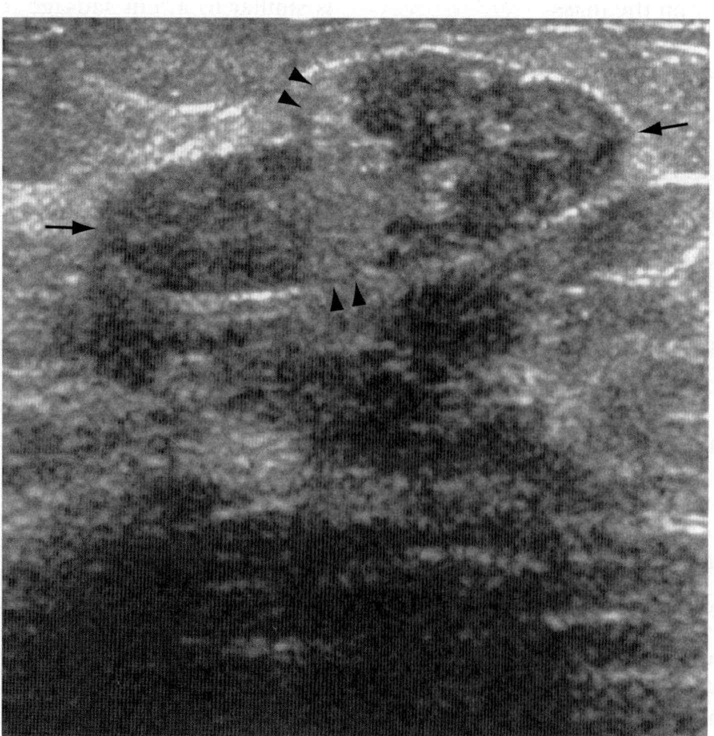

■ **FIGURE 16-23** Hamartoma. Ultrasonogram demonstrates a 3-cm oval circumscribed mass with mixed iso and hypoechoic echogenicity (*arrows*). Some of the fatty tissue within the lesion is isoechoic (*arrowheads*), although this is not seen in all hamartomas. *(Courtesy of James Youker, Milwaukee, Wis.)*

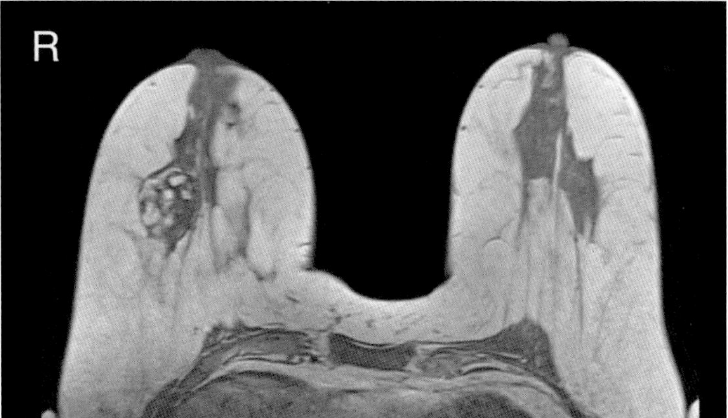

■ **FIGURE 16-24** Hamartoma. T1-weighted non-fat suppressed breast MR image demonstrates an oval mass with smooth margins in the right breast with both fat and soft tissue signal intensity.

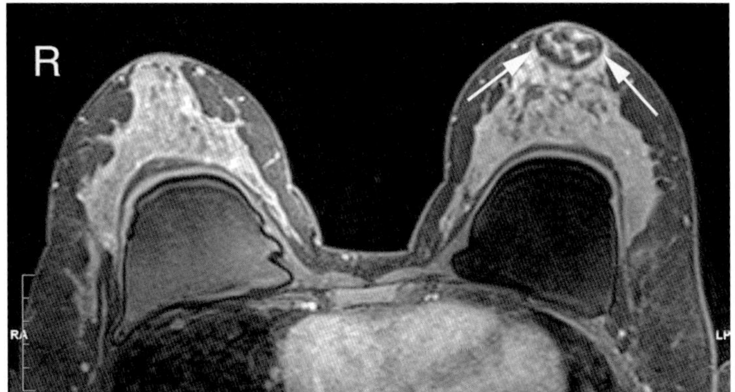

■ **FIGURE 16-25** Hamartoma. T1-weighted fat-suppressed breast MR image demonstrates an oval mass with smooth margins in the left breast (*arrows*) with both fat and soft tissue signal intensity. Bilateral breast prostheses also are present.

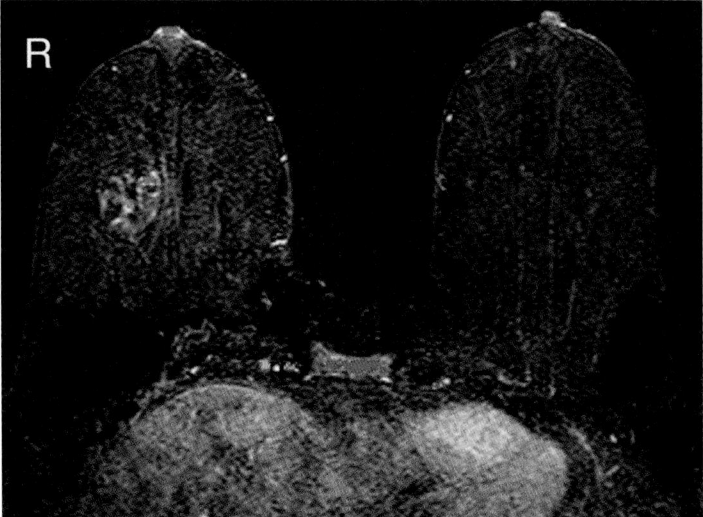

■ **FIGURE 16-26** Hamartoma T1-weighted subtraction right breast MR image shows prominent glandular elements with some contrast enhancement.

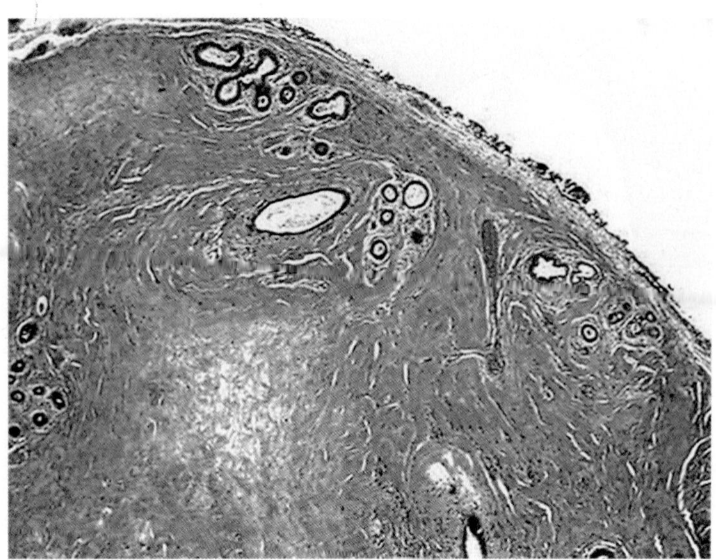

■ **FIGURE 16-27** Hamartoma. A well-circumscribed mass with pseudoencapsulated fibrous tissue and normal breast lobules and ducts with fibrous stroma (H&E, ×40).

no further follow-up or intervention is required. In the unusual situation in which the lesion is palpable and the patient is bothered by the mass, excision may be considered. In such cases, local excision is sufficient because there is no risk of recurrence or malignant transformation. Malignancy within a hamartoma is so rare that an aggressive approach to the management of these lesions is not indicated.

LIPOMA

Definition

Lipomas are benign fatty tumors that may occur anywhere within the breast.

Prevalence and Epidemiology

Lipomas occur in 1% of the population and may develop in virtually all organs throughout the body. Lipomas occur frequently in the breast but not as frequently as expected, considering the extent of fat that is present.

Etiology and Pathophysiology

The etiology of lipomas is unknown.

Manifestations of Disease

Clinical Presentation

Lipomas can be solitary or multiple. Most lipomas are located in the subcutaneous fat. When palpable, they are usually soft and freely movable. A lipoma is one of the more common causes of a palpable finding in a male patient.

Imaging Indications and Algorithm

If the patient presents with a palpable finding, the workup should begin with mammography in patients older than age 30. With the classic mammographic appearance, no further workup is indicated. When the patient presents with a palpable abnormality with a normal mammogram, ultrasonography is performed as the next step.

Imaging Technique and Findings

Mammography

On mammographic examination, a lipoma is a fat-containing, completely radiolucent lesion surrounded by a thin radiopaque capsule. This appearance is diagnostic for a benign lesion, and further workup or intervention is not necessary (Fig. 16-28).

Ultrasonography

If the mammographic appearance is classic, ultrasonography is not necessary. However, sometimes the radiopaque capsule is subtle and difficult to visualize mammographically, especially in a heterogeneous breast. In these cases, ultrasonography is performed. The ultrasonographic appearance varies and can be completely isoechoic (to adjacent fat lobules) (Fig. 16-29), mildly hyperechoic (Fig. 16-30), or isoechoic with numerous thin, internal echogenic septa that course parallel to the skin (Fig. 16-31). Softness of the lipoma can be demonstrated by physical examination or compression with the ultrasound transducer.

Magnetic Resonance Imaging

A lipoma presents as an oval mass with smooth margins and has high signal intensity on T1-weighted imaging.

Classic signs

The radiolucent mammographic appearance with a thin radiopaque capsule is classic.

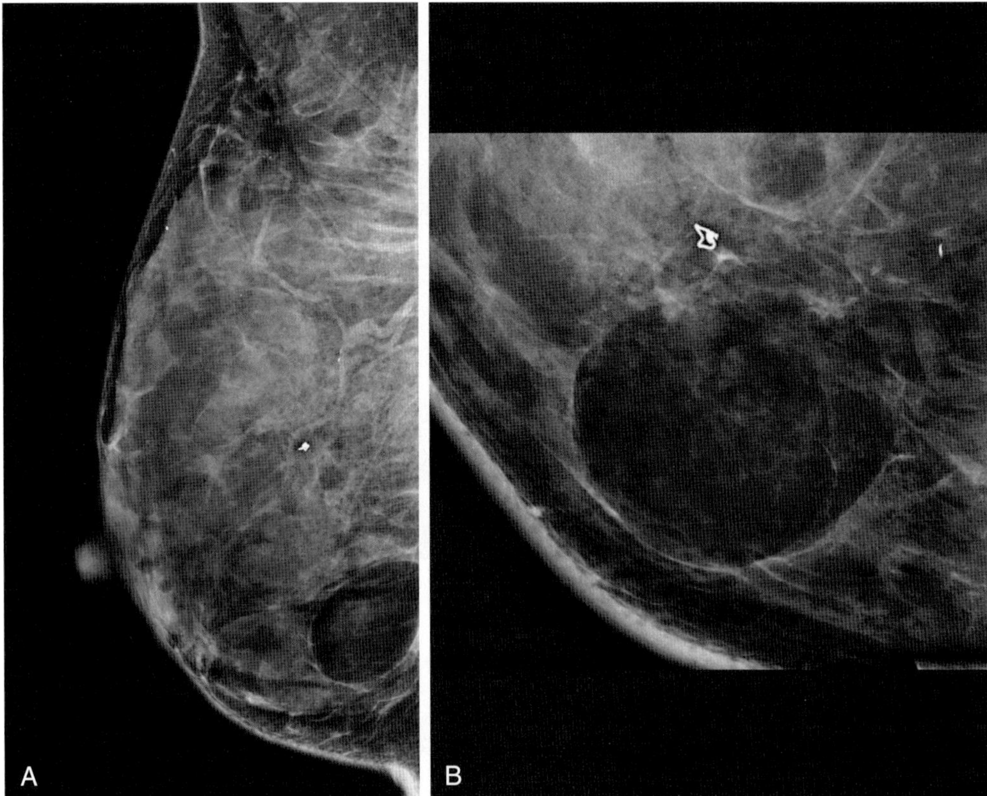

■ **FIGURE 16-28** Lipoma. **A**, Oval circumscribed mass with thin radiopaque capsule in the lower inner quadrant of the right breast on the mediolateral mammogram. **B**, Spot craniocaudal image shows the lateral portion of radiopaque capsule obscured by fibroglandular tissue (*arrow*).

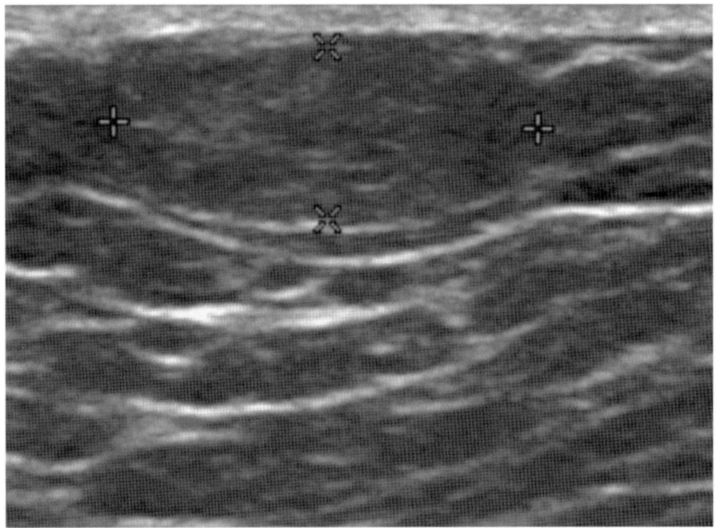

■ **FIGURE 16-29** Lipoma. Oval circumscribed isoechoic mass on ultrasonography. Note the lack of conspicuity of the mass since it is isoechoic with fat.

Pathology Findings

Lipoma of the breast is usually a solitary tumor located predominately in the subcutaneous fat. Lipomas are circumscribed masses composed of mainly mature adipocytes. Because fat tissue is a normal part of breast tissue, a clinically palpable mass proven to be composed of entirely mature fat would be a lipoma. There are many variants of lipoma, such as hibernomas composed of brown fat, fibrolipomas composed of fat and collagenous stroma, spindle cell lipomas composed of mixed spindly myofibroblasts and variable collagenous stroma and fat tissue, and angiolipomas composed of capillary-sized vascular proliferation often with fibrin clot and fat tissue (Fig. 16-32).

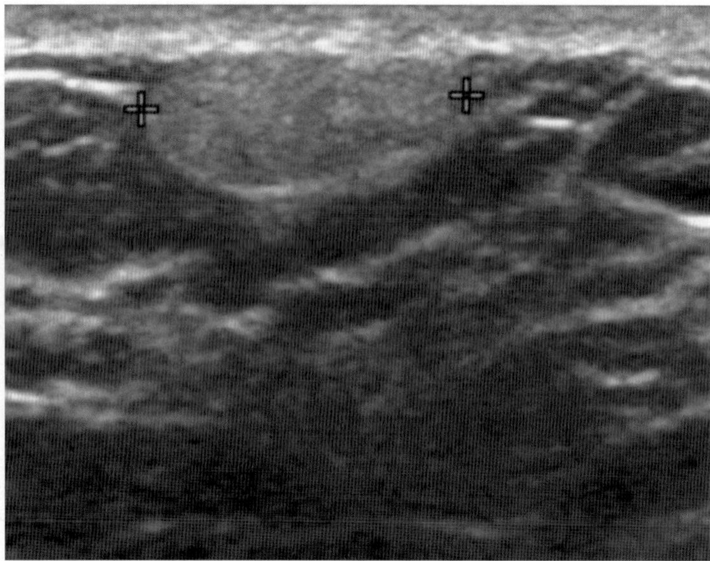

■ **FIGURE 16-30** Lipoma. Oval circumscribed hyperechoic mass on ultrasonography.

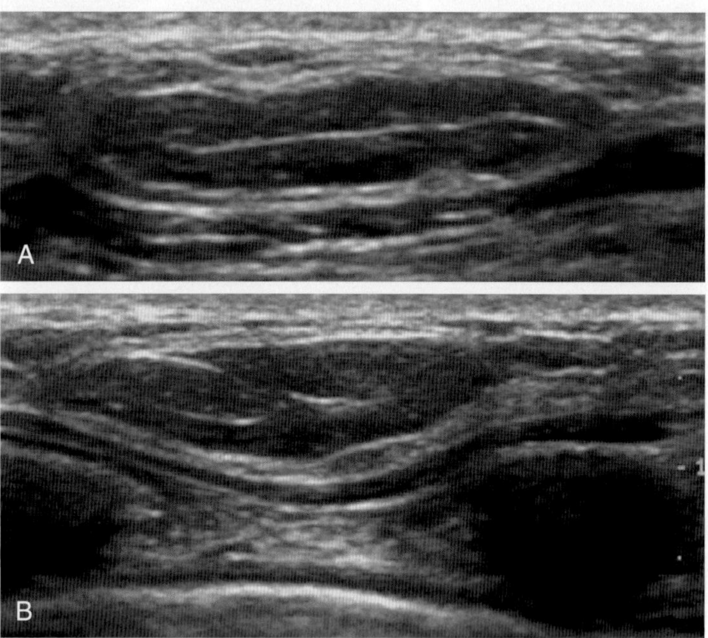

■ **FIGURE 16-31** Lipoma. Longitudinal image (**A**) shows an oval circumscribed mass (*arrows*) with a central echogenic septa. Transverse image (**B**) of the same lipoma (*arrowheads*) shows internal echogenic septa (*arrows*) that course parallel to the skin line. Also shown are the ribs (R).

Synopsis of Treatment Options

Lipomas are usually slow-growing tumors. Excision may be required if the mass is large and continuously growing. Surgical margins of lipomas can be difficult to assess because the normal breast parenchyma also has fatty tissue. Conservative excision is recommended.

FIBROMATOSIS

Definition

Fibromatosis of the breast (extra-abdominal desmoid tumor) is a benign localized proliferation of fibroblasts that is nonmalignant but does have a tendency to recur after excision.

Prevalence and Epidemiology

Fibromatosis usually occurs in the abdominal wall and superficial muscular-aponeurotic tissues of the extremities. Pathologic diagnosis of fibromatosis of the breast is extremely rare, with an incidence as low as 0.2% of breast tumors. It may arise from the pectoralis muscle/fascia or mammary tissue as a primary tumor.[2] All cases reported in the literature have been in women after the onset of puberty, with an average reported age of 30 to 40 years.[3]

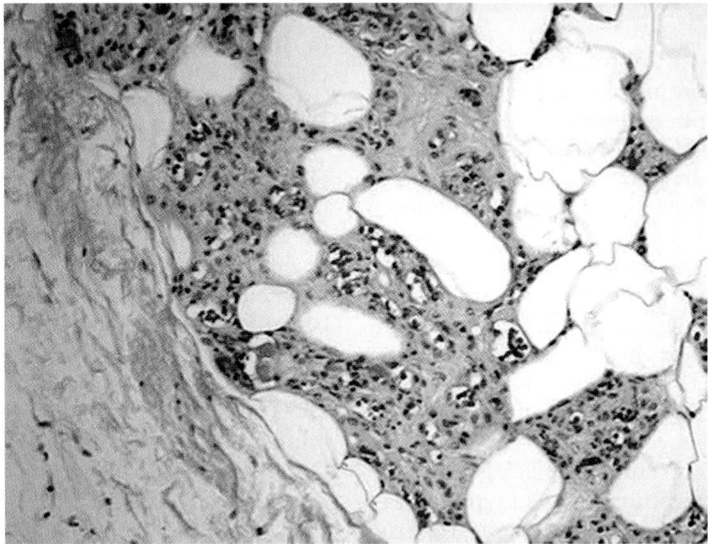

■ **FIGURE 16-32** Angiolipoma presented as a well-circumscribed mass lesion. Small capillary size vessels are seen with fibrin thrombi admixed with fatty tissue (H&E, ×100).

Etiology and Pathophysiology

The etiology of breast fibromatosis is unknown. A few reported cases suggest that trauma, sex steroid hormones, and Gardner syndrome may play a role.[4] The majorities of cases are spontaneous with no history of trauma or Gardner syndrome and are hormone-receptor negative.[4]

Manifestations of Disease

Clinical Presentation

Clinical presentation is that of a firm, freely mobile, nontender, palpable mass with occasional skin retraction or fixation to the pectoralis muscle.

The most common presenting complaint is skin tethering. This is caused by fibrous tissue contraction versus desmoplastic reaction, which is attributable to tethering associated with malignancy.[5]

Imaging Indications and Algorithm

Because fibromatosis presents as a palpable mass, the workup is that of mammography, followed by ultrasonography, and core biopsy.

Imaging Technique and Findings

Mammography

Mammographic findings include a circumscribed or a spiculated mass without microcalcifications that can be indistinguishable in appearance from carcinoma.

Ultrasonography

On ultrasound evaluation, fibromatosis usually presents as an irregular hypoechoic mass with indistinct margins similar to that seen with malignancy (Fig. 16-33).

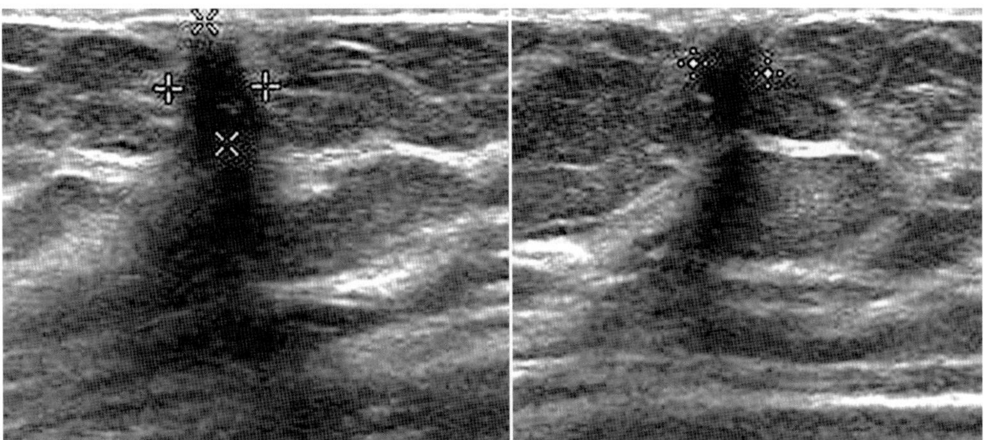

■ **FIGURE 16-33** Fibromatosis. Ultrasonogram demonstrates a irregular hypoechoic mass with indistinct margins, an echogenic collar and posterior acoustic shadowing. *(From Povoski SP, Jimenez RE. Fibromatosis (desmoid tumor) of the breast mimicking a case of ipsilateral metachronous breast cancer. World J Surg Oncol 2006;4:57.)*

Magnetic Resonance Imaging

There are a few case reports of fibromatosis findings on MRI. In one case report of fibromatosis on breast MRI, the mass showed isointensity on unenhanced T1-weighted images. On T2-weighted images, the mass was variable in signal intensity. High-signal areas on T2-weighted images were correlated with prominent myxoid change, and low-signal areas were correlated with dense collagenous tissue in the tumor. On contrast-enhanced fat-suppressed T1-weighted images, the mass had irregular margins and heterogeneous enhancement. Dynamic MRI demonstrated a type I (persistent) curve thought to reflect the significant amount of collagenous tissue in and myxoid change of the tumor. MRI findings in this case were not typical of a breast carcinoma.[6]

An additional case of recurrent fibromatosis showed that on dynamic MRI, kinetic features showed type II (plateau) and type III (washout) curves.[7] Previous reports on musculoskeletal fibromatosis have described a more aggressive behavior of fibromatosis recurrences, which might explain the enhancement pattern observed in this case.[7]

A third published case mimicked breast carcinoma in its morphologic and pharmacokinetic features of enhancement.[8]

Pathology Findings

Fibromatosis is a rare neoplastic tumor composed of fibroblastic and myofibroblastic cells. Gross examination of the tumor shows an infiltrative firm gray-white lesion that resembles scar formation. Microscopically, the lesion is characterized by bland-appearing spindle cells arranged in broad fascicles intermixed with thick fibrous collagenous bands. The tumor borders are not sharply delineated but highly infiltrative to the adjacent breast parenchyma (Fig. 16-34). Presence of an abundant amount of collagen may mimic scars from areas of healed prior surgery (Fig. 16-35). Other differential diagnoses include nodular fascitis, myofibroblastoma, and metaplastic carcinoma.

Nodular fascitis is characterized by regionally variable cellularity; centrally the lesion is more acellular with myxoid changes, and peripherally it appears more cellular with spindle to round plump cells and frequent mitotic figures. Abnormal mitosis is rare.

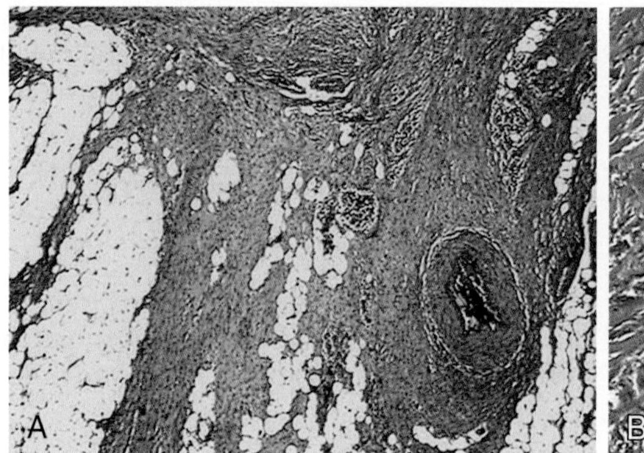

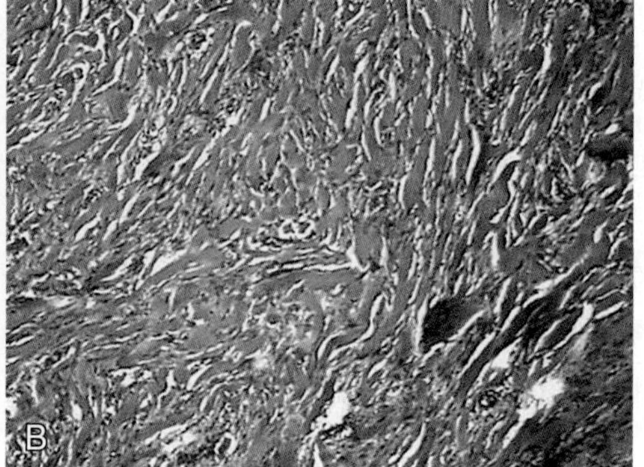

■ FIGURE 16-34 **A,** Fibromatosis showing infiltrative margin to the adjacent breast parenchyma and fat (H&E, ×40). **B,** Fibromatosis showing spindle cells in a mixed thick collagenous stroma mimicking keloidal scar (H&E, ×200).

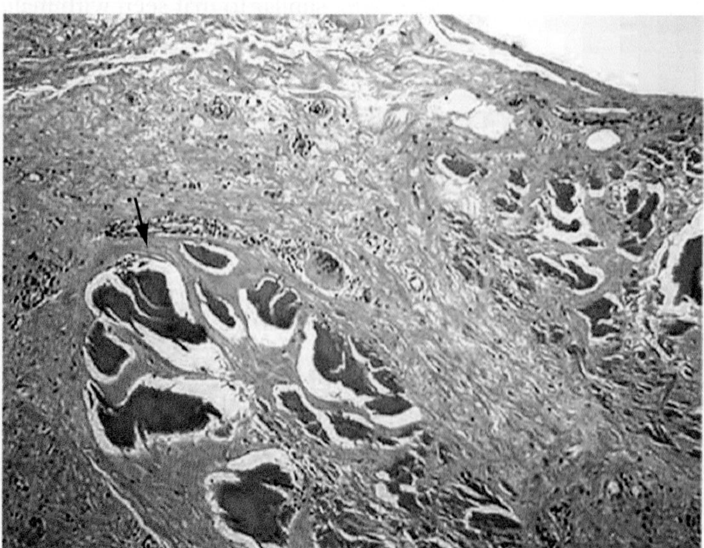

■ FIGURE 16-35 Keloid scar formation with multinucleated giant cells and chronic inflammatory infiltrates from the previous surgical site (H&E, ×100).

Synopsis of Treatment Options

Fibromatosis is important to distinguish from other benign stromal tumors because it tends to recur in about 27% of cases.[9] Wide local excision is a treatment of choice to prevent local recurrence.[9]

FIBROSIS

Definition

Fibrosis is a benign proliferation of fibrous connective tissue of the breast. Stromal fibrosis has been described by a variety of terms including *focal fibrous disease of the breast*, *fibrosis of the breast*, *fibrous mastopathy*, *fibrous tumor of the breast*, and *focal fibrosis of the breast*.

Prevalence and Epidemiology

The diagnosis has become increasingly common with increased screening mammography and may represent as much as 2.1% to 9% of lesions found in patients who undergo image-guided core biopsy.[10]

Etiology and Pathophysiology

The etiology of fibrosis includes a history of trauma with scar tissue, a surgical history, and a history of insulin-dependent diabetes mellitus. It has been suggested that the fibrous tumor is the end result of an inflammatory process that leads to atrophy and obliteration of the glandular tissue, with fibrosis accompanying and following the inflammation.

Manifestations of Disease

Clinical Presentation

Patients with focal fibrosis may present with a palpable mass or may be asymptomatic.

Imaging Indications and Algorithm

Fibrosis may present as a palpable mass or as a screening mammographic abnormality seen in asymptomatic patients. If the patient presents with a palpable mass, workup with mammography and ultrasonography is performed. Because of the non-specific imaging findings, biopsy is often necessary. If a mammographic finding is seen in an asymptomatic patient on screening mammography, recall for diagnostic mammography and ultrasound evaluation would be performed, with possible biopsy.

The low incidence (2.7%) of missed cancers in a case series suggests that patients diagnosed after core biopsy as having stromal fibrosis can be treated conservatively with a short-term follow-up protocol.[10] However, it would be prudent to continue to recommend either a second core biopsy or an excisional biopsy for imaging features that cannot be reliably differentiated from malignancy.[10]

Imaging Technique and Findings

Mammography

The mammographic findings are nonspecific and include an irregular mass with spiculated margins (Fig. 16-36), architectural distortion, or a benign-appearing circumscribed mass (Fig. 16-37).

Ultrasonography

On ultrasonography, fibrosis can be highly echogenic or identical in appearance to normal fibroglandular tissue. However, it is not unusual for ultrasonography to demonstrate an oval hypoechoic mass. Because the imaging findings often mimic malignancy, biopsy should be

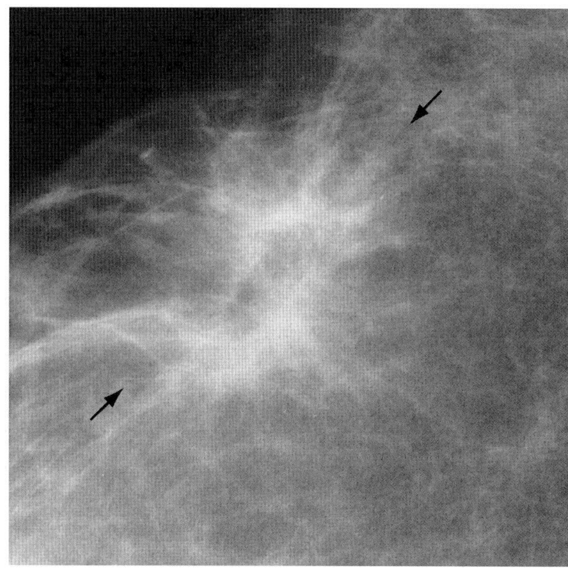

■ **FIGURE 16-36** Fibrosis. A 2 cm irregular speculated mass (*arrows*), simulating carcinoma. Suggestion of fat within.

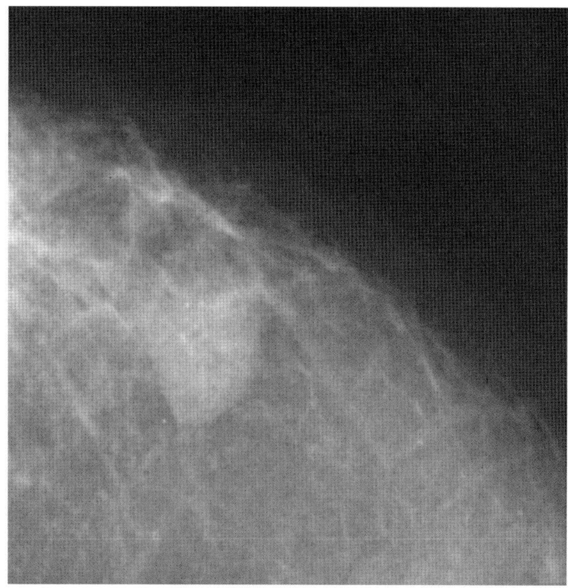

■ **FIGURE 16-37** Focal fibrosis. A 1.3-cm oval mass with partially circumscribed and partially obscured margins.

considered unless one has a reliable history of previous biopsy or trauma to that area, in which case close follow-up would be warranted.

Magnetic Resonance Imaging

On MRI, most cases of fibrosis present as small enhancing masses or areas of non-mass-like enhancement that are most often focal or regional in distribution.

Classic Signs

The imaging of fibrosis does not have a classic appearance and is usually diagnosed pathologically after biopsy.

Pathology Findings

Nodular fibrosis, otherwise known as fibrous tumor of the breast, is a benign condition that presents as a discrete mass composed of collagenized mammary stroma with the presence of often atrophic lobules. Core biopsy specimen of this lesion will be reported with the nonspecific description of *focal fibrosis*. Fibrous tumor has the appearance of a discrete nodule without encapsulation. Histologically, fibrous tumor consists of hypocellular hyalinized and collagenous stroma with scattered fibroblasts and absent to scant amounts of atrophic lobules.

Synopsis of Treatment Options

Treatment options are excision or close follow-up depending on the individual circumstances.

ADENOSIS

Definition

Adenosis is a spectrum of histologic lesions ranging from hyperplasia of the lobule to sclerosing adenosis with fibrosis and calcifications. In this section, tubular adenomas and lactating adenomas are described. Tubular adenomas and lactating adenomas are most likely variants of the pericanalicular fibroadenoma with an exceptionally prominent or florid adenosis-like epithelial proliferation. Some authors describe these lesions as florid adenosis.

Prevalence and Epidemiology

The age distribution in women with these lesions is similar to that of fibroadenomas, occurring during the reproductive years.

Etiology and Pathophysiology

Lactating adenomas may represent the same lesion as tubular adenomas but under different physiologic conditions. Lactating adenomas are often associated with pregnancy and puerperium. Lactating adenomas are the most prevalent pregnancy-associated breast lesions, typically arising during the third trimester of gestation; although most lactating adenomas spontaneously involute after delivery, the diagnosis is not always straightforward and surgical resection may be required for definitive diagnosis.

Manifestations of Disease

Clinical Presentation

In most cases, the presenting symptom is a painless, firm, circumscribed, solitary tumor found by the patient. When palpable, tubular adenomas tend to be softer than the average fibroadenoma. Nonpalpable lesions are often found as an incidental mammographic finding.

Imaging Indications and Algorithm

The imaging workup includes initial ultrasonography in patients younger than age 30 and pregnant patients. Ultrasonography is the primary tool in the diagnostic workup of a breast lump during pregnancy because of its accuracy in discriminating between solid and cystic lesions, such as galactoceles, and its safety due to the lack of ionizing radiation. Mammography and ultrasonography should be performed in nonpregnant patients older than age 30.

Imaging Technique and Findings

Mammography

Mammographic findings are similar to those of fibroadenomas of the breast. The most common finding is an oval circumscribed mass.

Ultrasonography

The ultrasound appearance of both lactating and tubular adenomas is similar to that of fibroadenomas, presenting as an oval isoechoic to slightly hypoechoic mass (Fig. 16-38) with circumscribed margins. Posterior acoustic enhancement can be present.

Magnetic Resonance Imaging

A published case of a pathologically proven lactating adenoma seen on MRI has been described.[11] The lesion appeared as an oval mass, with smooth margins, and significant contrast enhancement, displacing the normal breast parenchyma and the nipple/areolar complex inferiorly and compressing the galactiferous ducts almost completely.[11]

Pathology Findings

A tubular adenoma is a well-circumscribed mass often occurring in the reproductive age and clinically resembling fibroadenoma. Tubular adenoma may be a variant of fibroadenoma and is a benign lesion composed of compact epithelial cells in small round tubules with luminal secretions and lined by myoepithelial cells. The intervening stroma is usually scant. The longitudinal glandular proliferation has a pattern that resembles tubular adenosis. The smaller glandular tubular proliferation has a pattern that resembles florid adenosis (Figs. 16-39 and 16-40).

A lactating adenoma is seen more commonly during pregnancy and lactation and, rarely, in postmenopausal women on hormone replacement therapy and nonhormonal drugs such as digitalis, phenytoin (Dilantin), and reserpine. Lactational changes are commonly seen and involve and expand the terminal ductal lobular unit,

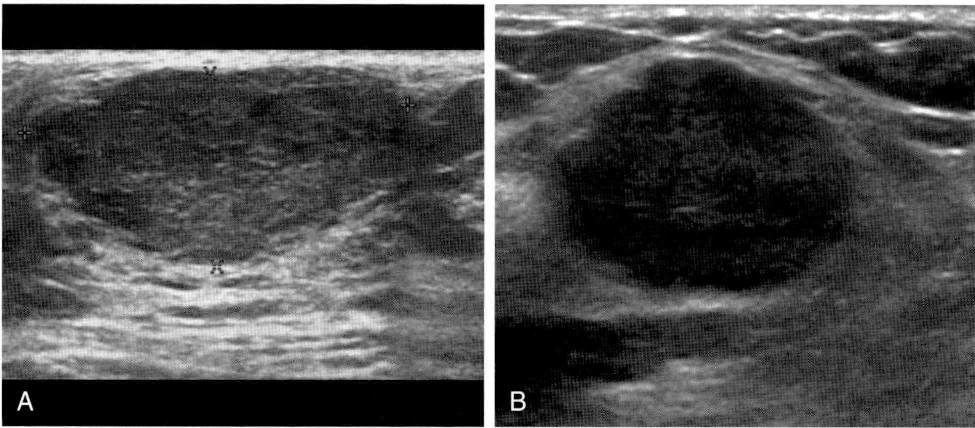

■ **FIGURE 16-38** Ultrasound of lactating adenoma (**A**) and tubular adenoma (**B**). Oval/round slightly hypoechoic circumscribed masses. Note the posterior acoustic enhancement in **A**.

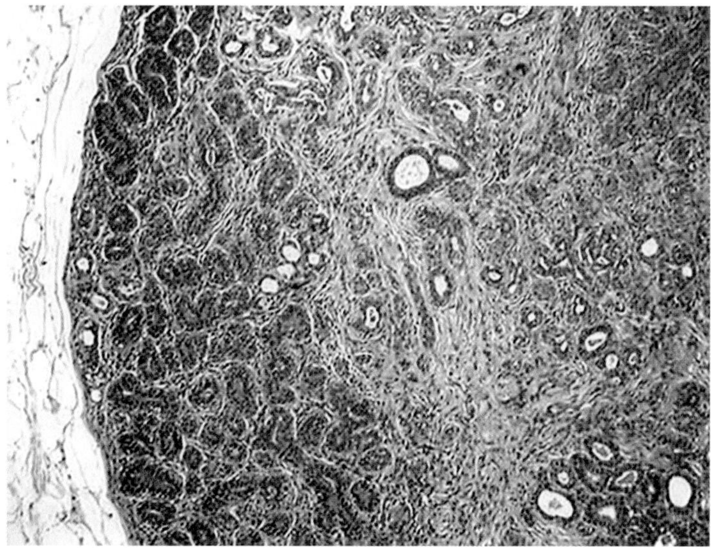

■ **FIGURE 16-39** Tubular adenoma showing a well-circumscribed nonencapsulated mass composed of compact proliferations of small tubules and intervening sparse collagenous stroma (H&E, ×40).

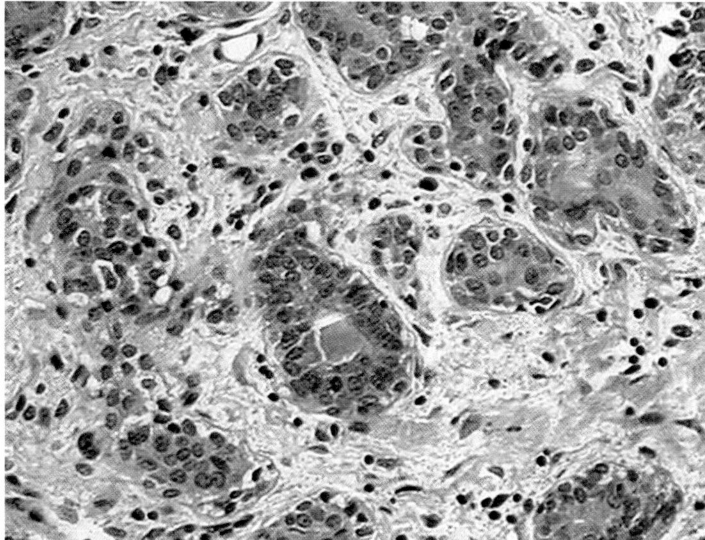

■ **FIGURE 16-40** Higher-power view of tubular adenoma showing luminal non-distended eosinophilic secretion with epithelial and myoepithelial cells. Some of the epithelia cells show prominent nucleoli (H&E, ×400).

resembling the Arias-Stella reaction in the endometrium. (Arias-Stella reaction is a focal decidual change in endometrial epithelium that consists of intraluminal budding, nuclear enlargement, and hyperchromatism with cytoplasmic swelling and vacuolation and is associated with pregnancy.) Similar changes can be seen in the breast tissue with dilated acini with luminal secretions and are lined by plump epithelial cells with prominent nucleoli and vacuolated cytoplasm. These changes are recognizable in both FNA smears and excisional biopsy (Figs. 16-41 and 16-42). Many cells show a hobnail appearance, and distended acini contain detached cells sometimes with multinucleated and pyknotic nuclei (Fig. 16-43).

When predominant populations of cells are apocrine, this lesion is referred to as an apocrine adenoma. It is a localized nodular focus of apocrine cells with papillary and cystic structures.

Synopsis of Treatment Options

Treatment options include excision versus close follow-up depending on the individual circumstances.

DIABETIC MASTOPATHY

Definition

Diabetic mastopathy is a condition in which stromal proliferation forms fibrous tumors predominately in patients with insulin-dependent diabetes mellitus.

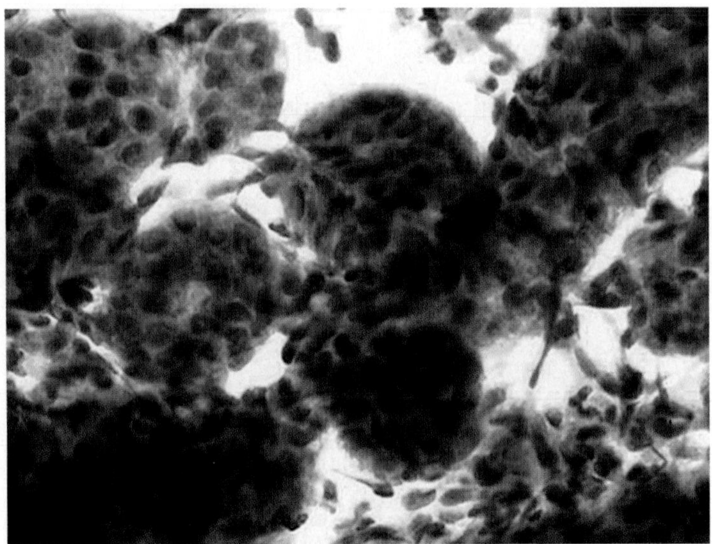

■ **FIGURE 16-41** Lactating adenoma seen from a pregnant woman. Round acini structures are seen with nuclear overlapping (fine-needle aspiration, Papanicolaou stain).

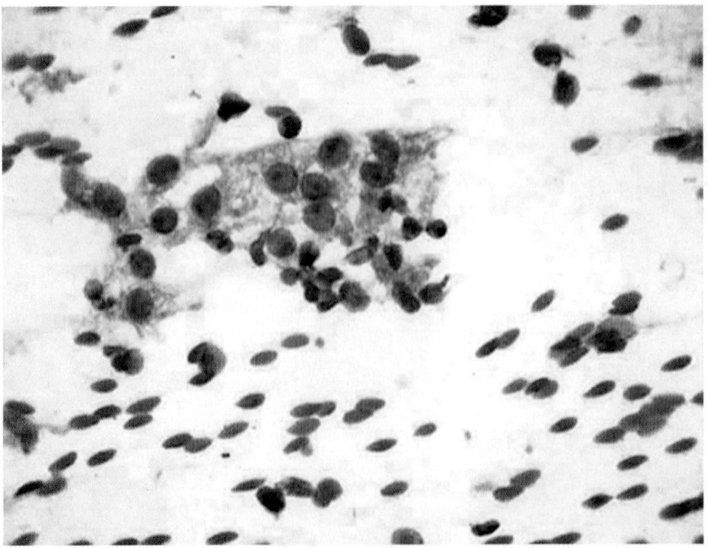

■ **FIGURE 16-42** Lactating adenoma showing finely vacuolated wispy cytoplasm with round nuclei and prominent nucleoli (fine-needle aspiration, Papanicolaou stain).

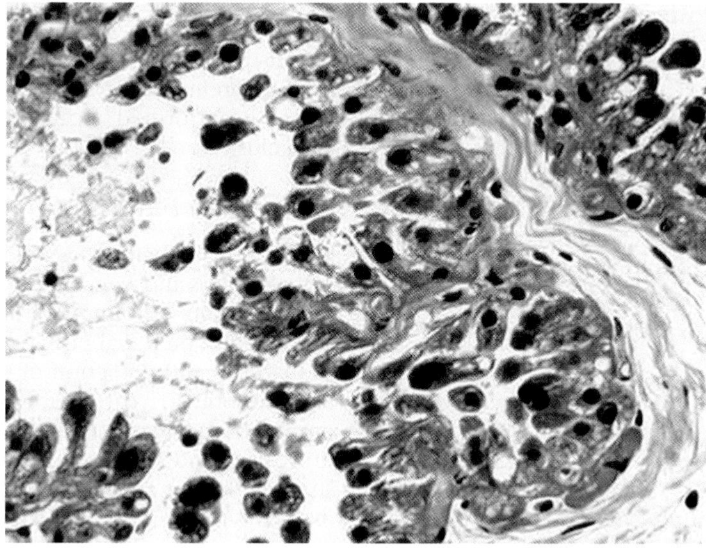

■ **FIGURE 16-43** Core biopsy sample of lactating adenoma. The glandular cells have vacuolated cytoplasm and a hobnail appearance (H&E, ×400).

Prevalence and Epidemiology

Diabetic mastopathy is most commonly seen in women with insulin-dependent diabetes mellitus. However, it also has been reported rarely in males as well as in non-insulin-dependent diabetic patients and in non-diabetic patients with histocompatibility locus antigen (HLA)-associated autoimmune diseases.

Etiology and Pathophysiology

The disease probably represents an immune reaction to the abnormal accumulation of altered extracellular matrix in the breast, which is a manifestation of the effects of hyperglycemia on connective tissue.[12,13] This is likely due to the inability to degrade glycosylation as well as an increase in the intermolecular cross-linkages, which leads to accumulation of fibrous tissue in insulin-dependent diabetes mellitus.

Manifestations of Disease

Clinical Presentation

The most common clinical symptom is a nontender palpable, firm to hard mass detected in one or both breasts. It mimics breast cancer owing to the extent of fibrosis.

Imaging Indications and Algorithm

Because the patient often presents with a palpable finding, diagnostic mammography and ultrasonography are performed in patients older than age 30. Diabetic mastopathy is also seen in patients younger than age 30, in whom ultrasonography should be the initial examination. Because of its nonspecific appearance, diabetic mastopathy should be sampled, because breast carcinoma is a diagnosis of exclusion.

Imaging Technique and Findings

Mammography

Mammography often reveals a focal asymmetry or a heterogeneous parenchymal pattern (Fig. 16-44). In some cases, the mammographic appearance is that of a mass

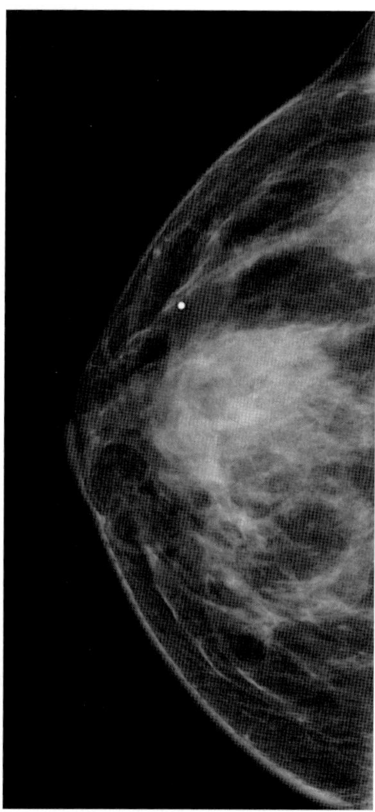

■ **FIGURE 16-44** Diabetic mastopathy. Craniocaudal mammogram with radiopaque marker (BB) in a insulin-dependent diabetic patient presenting with a palpable lump. A focal asymmetry was present.

that resembles carcinoma with indistinct or spiculated margins or rarely, an oval or irregular mass with obscured margins.

Ultrasonography

In a series of eight cases of diabetic mastopathy, a heterogeneous hypoechoic mass with indistinct margins (Fig. 16-45) was identified on high-frequency gray-scale ultrasound evaluation in all lesions.[14] Marked posterior acoustic shadowing was present in seven of eight (88%) lesions.[14] Six lesions interrogated with color flow ultrasonography showed absence of Doppler signal.[14]

Magnetic Resonance Imaging

Diabetic mastopathy is isointense to glandular tissue on breast MRI, but a mass can be visualized on the non-fat-suppressed T1-weighted imaging (Fig. 16-46). MRI shows minimal nonspecific stromal enhancement (Fig. 16-47).

Classic Signs

Because of its nonspecific appearance and similarity to breast carcinoma on clinical examination and imaging, biopsy is performed because breast cancer is the diagnosis of exclusion.

Pathology Findings

Diabetic mastopathy is also known as sclerosing lymphocytic lobulitis and seen in type I insulin-dependent diabetes mellitus, other autoimmune disorders related to HLA-DR4, and, rarely, type II diabetes. The interval between the onset of diabetes and detection of the breast lesion is reported to be about 20 years. Hard firm masses are detected in one or both breasts. Grossly, the lesion is somewhat distinct, firm, and homogeneous. Microscopically, the lesions show abundant collagenous stroma with keloidal features, mature lymphocytic infiltrates around small-sized vessels and/or around atrophic lobules (Figs. 16-48 and 16-49).

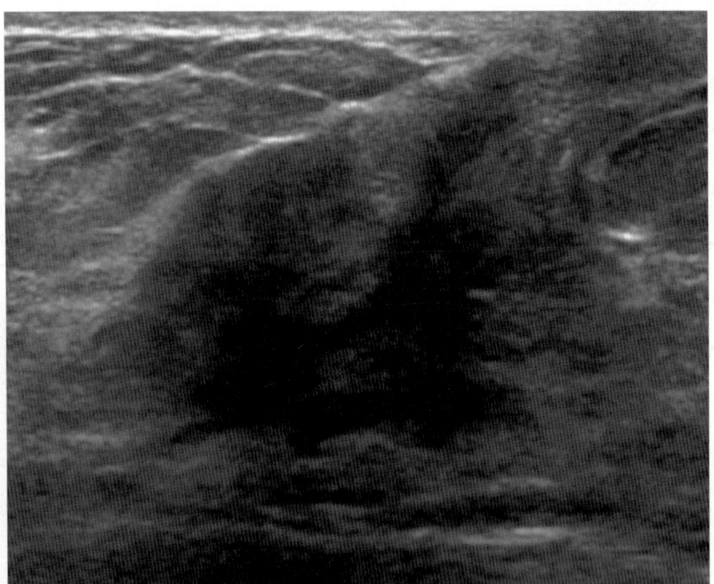

■ FIGURE 16-45 Diabetic mastopathy. Ultrasonogram of same patient as Figure 16-31 shows an irregular iso- and hypoechoic mass with indistinct margins.

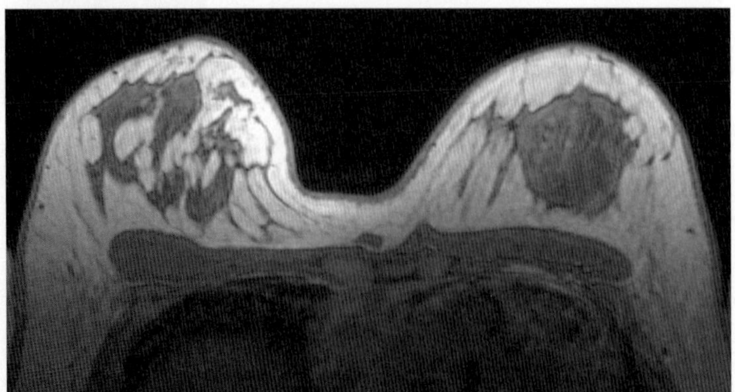

■ FIGURE 16-46 Diabetic mastopathy. T1-weighted non-fat-suppressed MR image shows an isointense round mass with slightly irregular margins in the left breast.

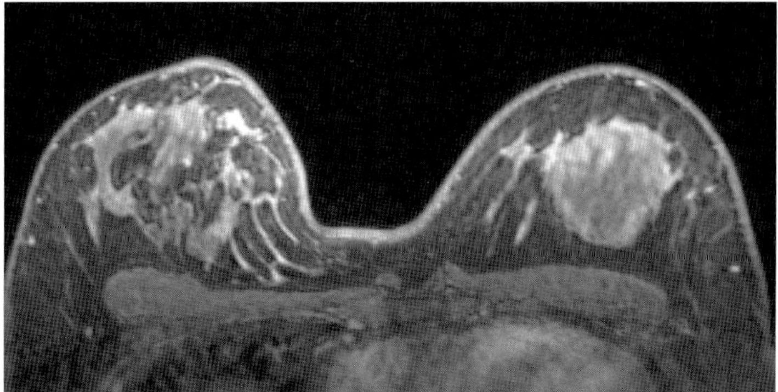

■ **FIGURE 16-47** Diabetic mastopathy. T1-weighted contrast-enhanced MR image shows minimal contrast enhancement of the left fibrous mass.

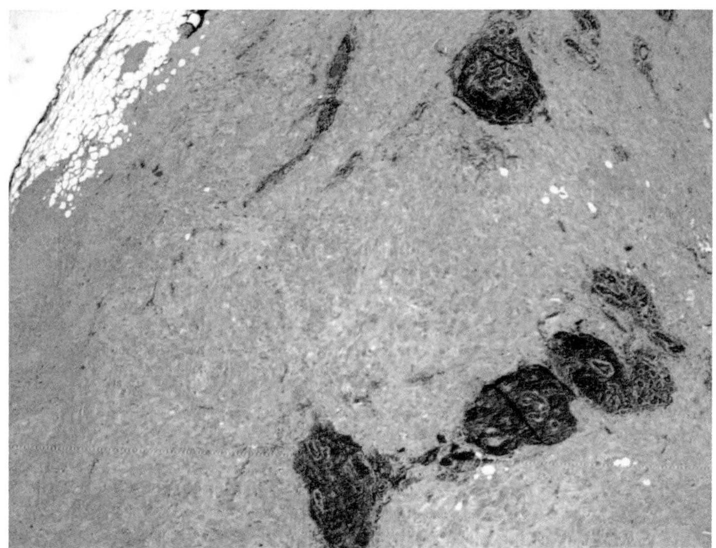

■ **FIGURE 16-48** Diabetic mastopathy. Nodular mass-like lesion with prominent fibrosis resembling a keloid-like stroma and myofibroblasts proliferation (H&E, ×40)

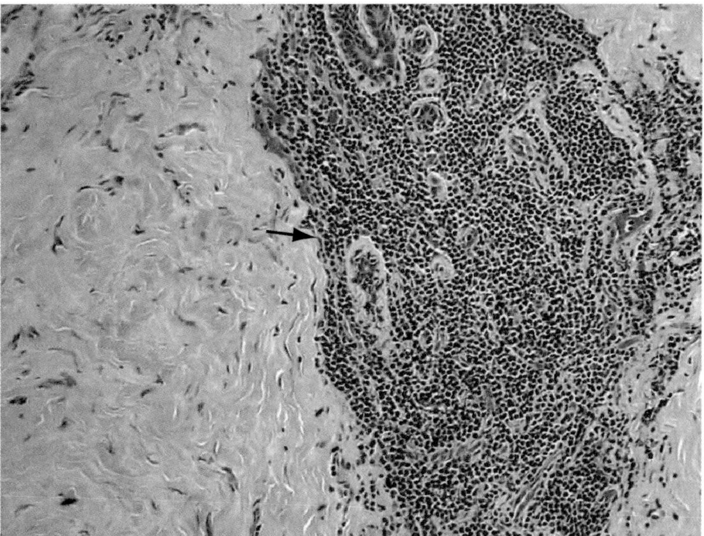

■ **FIGURE 16-49** Diabetic mastopathy. Perivascular and perilobular infiltrate of mature lymphocytes and myofibroblasts in surrounding fibrotic stroma (*arrow*) (H&E, ×200).

Synopsis of Treatment Options

Treatment options include excision versus close follow-up, depending on the individual circumstances. There is no evidence to suggest that patients with diabetic mastopathy have higher incidences of mammary carcinoma or stromal neoplasm.

GRANULAR CELL TUMOR

Definition

Granular cell tumor is an uncommon, usually benign tumor originating from Schwann cells. Granular cell tumor was initially thought by Abrikossoff in 1926 to be of myogenic origin and originally was labeled granular cell myoblastoma.[15]

Prevalence and Epidemiology

Five percent to 6% of granular cell tumors occur in the breast.[16] The most common site of this tumor is in the head and neck region, particularly the tongue. In a published report of 10 cases, 9 tumors occurred in female patients and 1 occurred in a male patient. The mean patient age was 51.8 years, and the mean lesion size was 1.57 cm.[17] Other sources list a younger presenting age, with granular cell tumor occurring in middle-aged premenopausal women.[18-19]

Etiology and Pathophysiology

The etiology of granular cell tumor is unknown.

Manifestations of Disease

Clinical Presentation

On clinical examination, granular cell tumor simulates carcinoma due to fixation to the skin and a hard mass-like lesion on palpation. Skin ulceration can be seen.

It appears most commonly in the upper inner quadrant of the breast, in contrast to breast carcinoma, which is found more commonly in the upper outer quadrant.[18]

Imaging Indications and Algorithm

Mammography, ultrasonography, and biopsy are all indicated.

Imaging Technique and Findings

Mammography

On mammography, the mass is usually irregular with spiculated margins (Fig. 16-50). However, it can less commonly present as a mass with circumscribed margins. Microcalcifications have not been reported in these lesions.

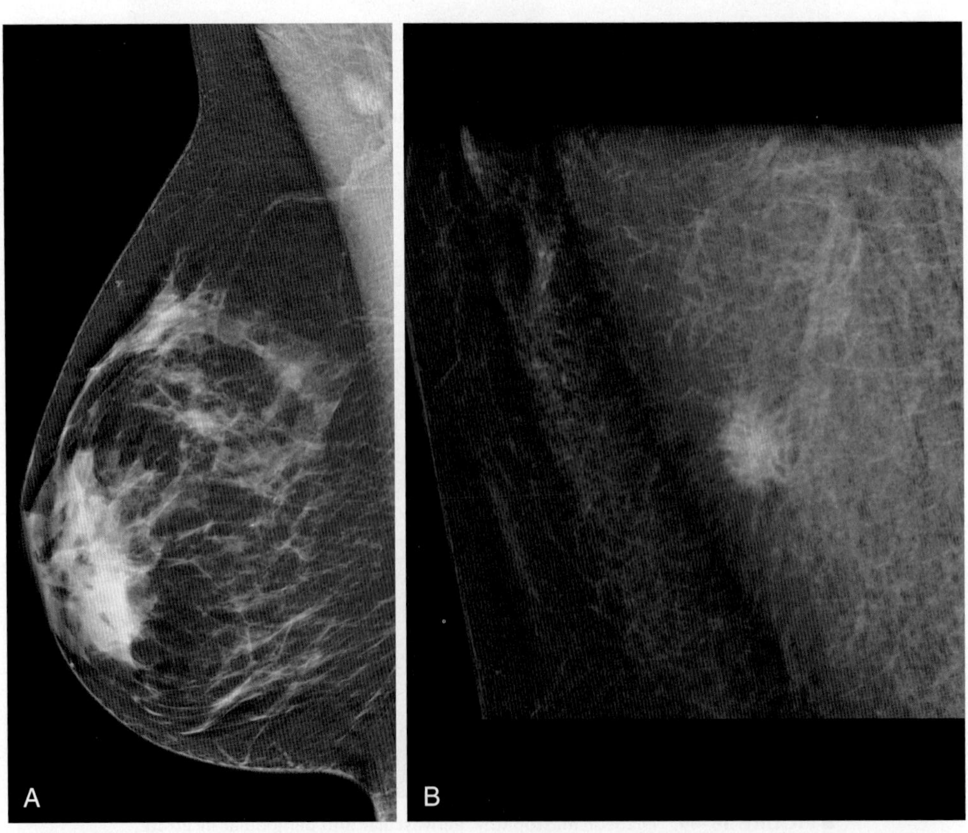

■ **FIGURE 16-50** Granular cell tumor. Mammogram mediolateral oblique (**A**) and spot (**B**) images of the right breast demonstrate an oval, spiculated mass.

Ultrasonography

In the report of 10 cases of granular cell tumors, 7 tumors visualized on ultrasonography were hypoechoic masses.[17] Posterior acoustic enhancement was noted in three tumors, and posterior shadowing was noted in two tumors (Fig. 16-51). Two of the seven tumors did not show any posterior enhancement or shadowing, and two were taller than wide.[17]

Another report of seven granular cell tumors showed that the ultrasonographic features mimicked those of carcinoma, including heterogeneous echotexture, indistinct margins, and hypervascularity.[20] Hyperechogenicity was noted in five of the seven tumors (71%) in this series.[20]

Magnetic Resonance Imaging

There are few anecdotal reports on the MRI findings of granular cell tumor of the breast. Kohashi and colleagues[21] described the features as homogeneously enhancing masses on T1-weighted imaging showing a high signal intensity rim on the T2-weighted sequences. Scaranelo and associates[22] demonstrated granular cell tumor of the breast as a round mass with irregular margins that was slightly hypointense compared with the breast parenchyma on T1-weighted imaging and that was not seen on T2-weighted imaging. After gadolinium injection, the enhancement was more pronounced in the periphery of the lesion. The visual analysis of the time course of enhancement was categorized as persistent.[22]

Classic Signs

The classic clinical presentation is a firm, fixed mass with overlying skin changes.

The appearance is indistinguishable mammographically and clinically from that of breast carcinoma.

Pathology Findings

Granular cell tumor is an uncommon, usually benign tumor that occasionally involves the breast. Grossly this tumor has ill-defined borders and is firm in consistency. Microscopically, the tumor is ill defined with infiltrative borders. The most distinct histologic feature is the abundant granular eosinophilic cytoplasm with small round nuclei and inconspicuous to small prominent nucleoli. Tumor cells are arranged in bundles, cords, and nests in a dense fibrous stroma. Mitotic figures are rare. The differential diagnosis includes metastatic renal cell carcinoma and apocrine carcinoma of breast. Granular cell tumor is usually positive for S-100 protein, NSE, and CEA and negative for cytokeratin by immunohistochemical stains (Figs 16-52 to 16-54). Renal cell carcinoma and apocrine carcinoma are usually positive for cytokeratin stain.

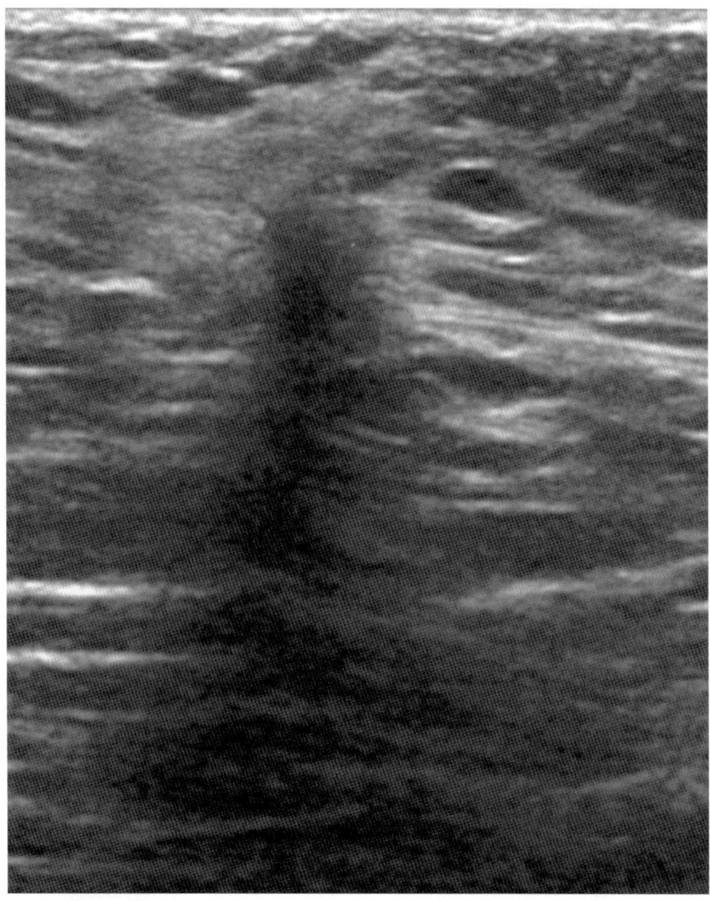

■ **FIGURE 16-51** Granular cell tumor. Ultrasonogram demonstrates an irregular, indistinct hypoechoic mass with posterior acoustic shadowing.

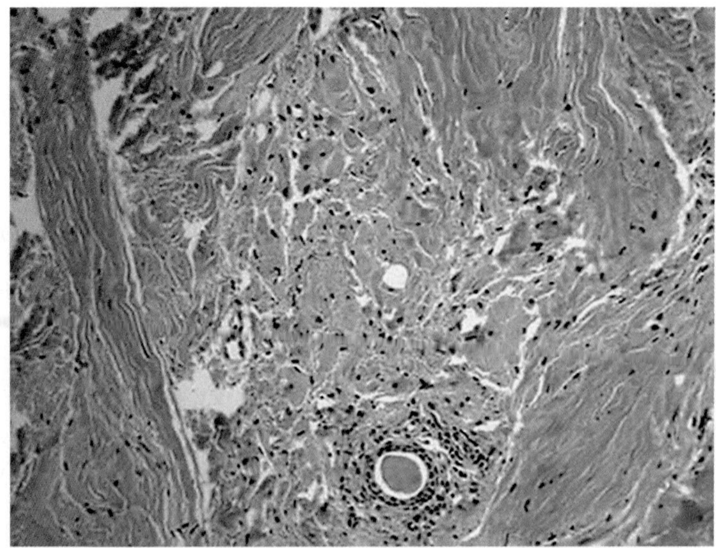

■ **FIGURE 16-52** Granular cell tumor of the breast. Tumor cells are arranged in cords and nests separated by prominent fibrous septa giving the appearance of infiltration (H&E, ×200).

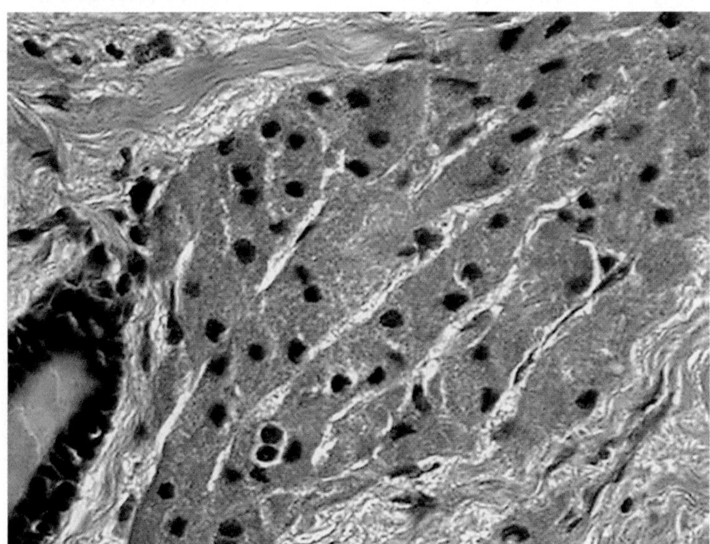

■ **FIGURE 16-53** Granular cell tumor of the breast. Tumor cells show small round nuclei with abundant granular eosinophilic cytoplasm (H&E, ×400).

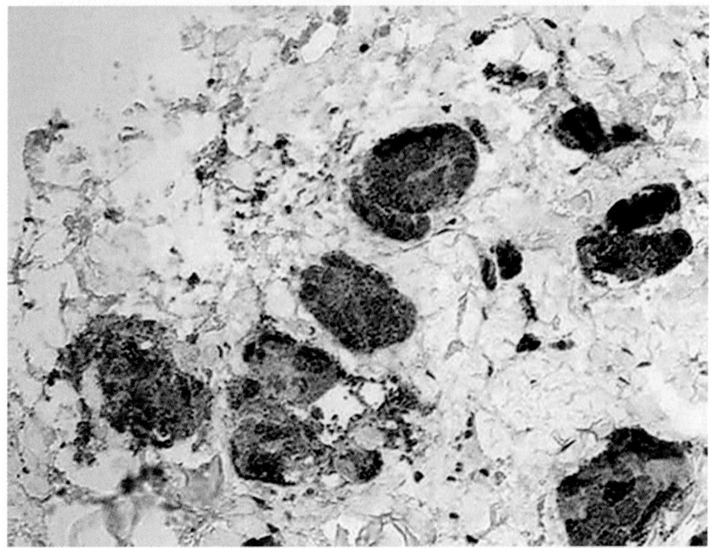

■ **FIGURE 16-54** Granular cell tumor (S-100 immunohistochemical stain, ×400).

Synopsis of Treatment Options

Wide local excision is the treatment of choice for both benign and malignant granular cell tumors. Less than 1% of granular cell tumors are reported to be malignant. A complete local excision results in cure, although it can be challenging to get a clear margin because of the infiltrative nature of this tumor. Complete removal may require inclusion of muscle and other adjacent structures, and histologically it is recommended that the margins be completely free of tumor. Incomplete excision may result in local recurrences. Adjuvant therapy is not given unless the tumor is malignant.[19]

FAT NECROSIS

Definition

Fat necrosis involves necrosis of adipose tissue and is characterized by the formation of small quantities of calcium soaps when fat is hydrolyzed into glycerol and fatty acids.

Prevalence and Epidemiology

Fat necrosis is a common benign condition.

Etiology and Pathophysiology

Fat necrosis occurs after trauma (including surgery) to the breast.

Manifestations of Disease

Clinical Presentation

Fat necrosis may present as a palpable mass, pain, skin thickening, or nipple retraction that may mimic carcinoma. Some patients may not recall trauma to the area. Fat necrosis is commonly seen after lumpectomy and radiation therapy for breast carcinoma and after extensive surgery such as reduction mammoplasty.

Some patients may be asymptomatic, with fat necrosis detected incidentally during screening mammography.

Imaging Indications and Algorithm

Fat necrosis is often seen incidentally on screening mammography, and if it has the characteristic appearance, no further workup is indicated. If the patient presents with a palpable finding, diagnostic mammography is performed and infrequently ultrasonography and biopsy, depending on the imaging characteristics.

Imaging Technique and Findings

Mammography

Fat necrosis may have a variety of mammographic appearances. In most cases, these findings are diagnostic of a benign lesion. The lesion can present as an oval mass containing fat density (Fig. 16-55). One common and characteristic finding is a radiolucent or mixed fat and soft tissue density circumscribed mass with a calcified or noncalcified rim, known as a lipid or oil cyst[23] (Fig. 16-56). In most cases, the location of the calcifications at the periphery of a fat-density circumscribed mass is sufficient to establish the benign diagnosis.

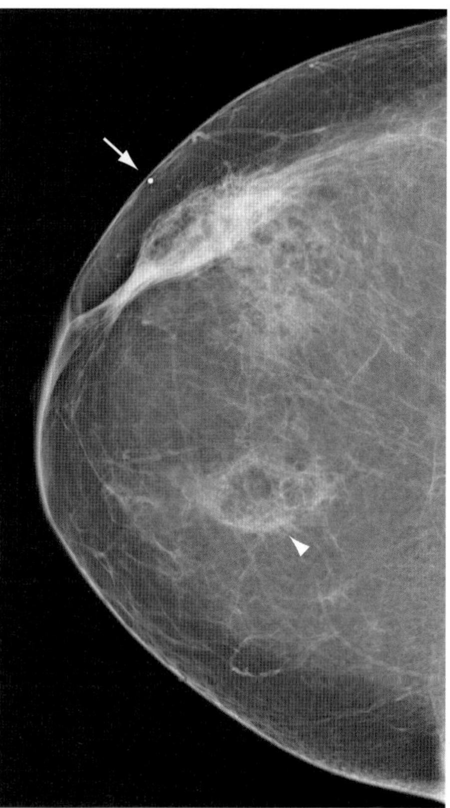

■ **FIGURE 16-55** Fat necrosis. A 46-year-old woman presented with a history of reduction mammoplasty 1 year prior and a palpable lump (site of radiopaque marker indicated by *arrow*). The craniocaudal mammogram demonstrated an oval, indistinct fat-containing mass corresponding to the palpable finding (see Figure 16-47 for ultrasound image). A second site of fat necrosis (*arrowhead*) was also noted.

However, sometimes the findings mimic carcinoma including spiculated masses, sometimes with microcalcifications and architectural distortion (Fig. 16-57).[24] Early peripheral calcifications may mimic microcalcifications of malignancy (Fig. 16-58).

Ultrasonography

Ultrasonography is not performed when the mammographic features are typical for fat necrosis, but it is often performed for cases for which the mammogram shows a soft-tissue mass. Early fat necrosis is usually manifested as an indistinct uniform hyperechoic area, usually in the superficial tissue of the breast (Fig. 16-59). As fat necrosis progresses, it can have a heterogeneous appearance (Fig. 16-60). Calcified fat necrosis demonstrates ultrasonographic shadowing (see Chapter).

Magnetic Resonance Imaging

The most common MRI appearance is that of a lipid cyst. A round or oval mass with hypointense T1-weighted signal on fat-saturated images is typical.[25]

The rim of the mass commonly enhances, although to varying degrees. The extent and avidity of enhancement may vary with the proportion of acute and chronic

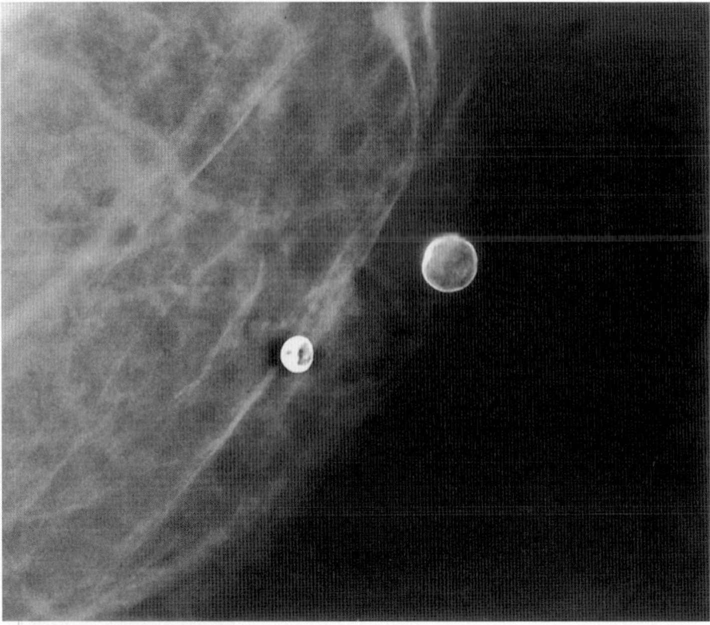

■ **FIGURE 16-56** Mammogram of small eggshell/lucent centered calcifications from fat necrosis. This patient had no known trauma.

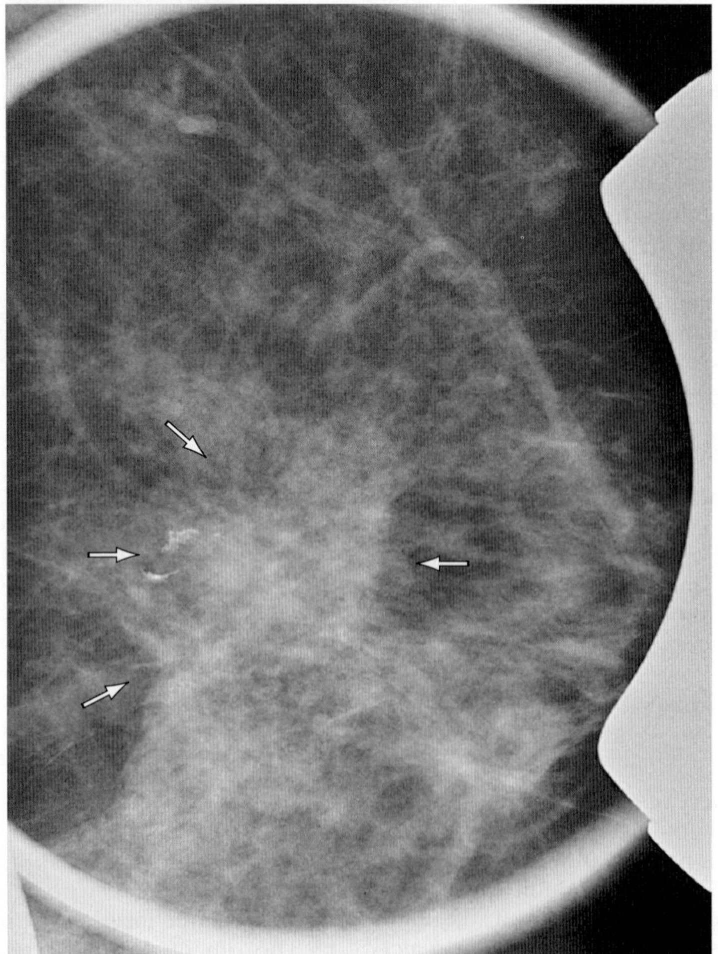

■ **FIGURE 16-57** Mammogram shows fat necrosis with architectural distortion (*white arrows*) and a few rim calcifications.

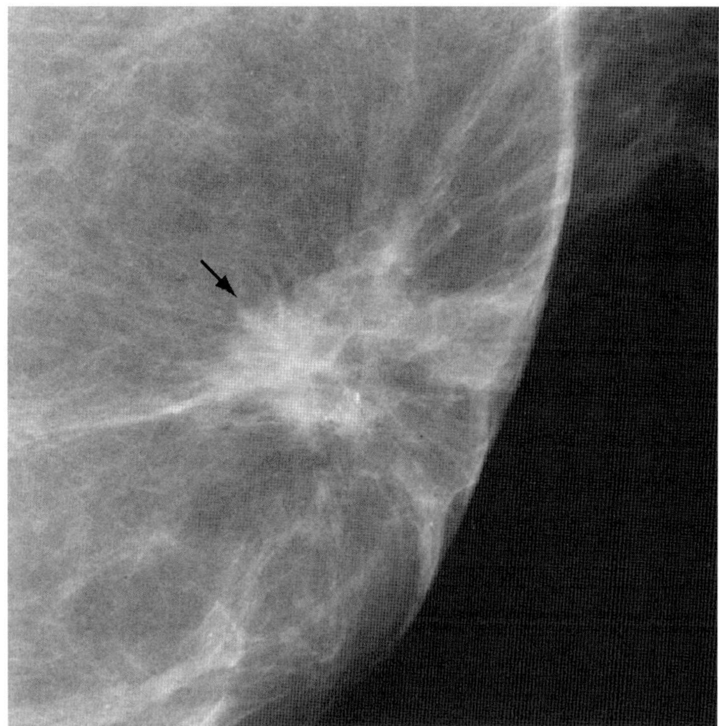

■ **FIGURE 16-58** Mammogram of fat necrosis. The irregular, spiculated mass (*arrow*) has a few peripheral microcalcifications.

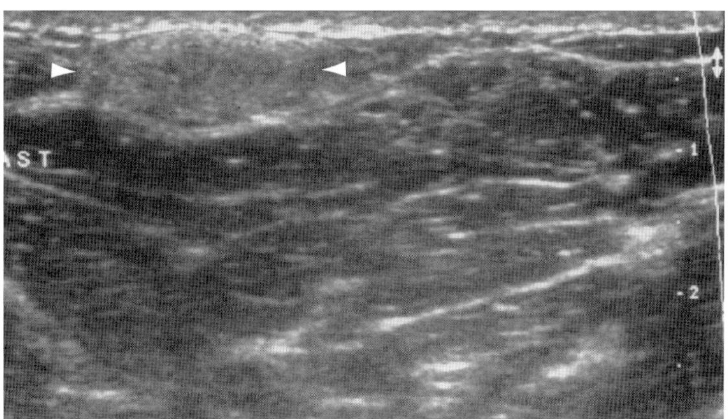

■ **FIGURE 16-59** Ultrasound image of fat necrosis. The superficial hyperechoic mass (*arrowheads*) developed after blunt trauma to the breast and resolved on follow-up examination.

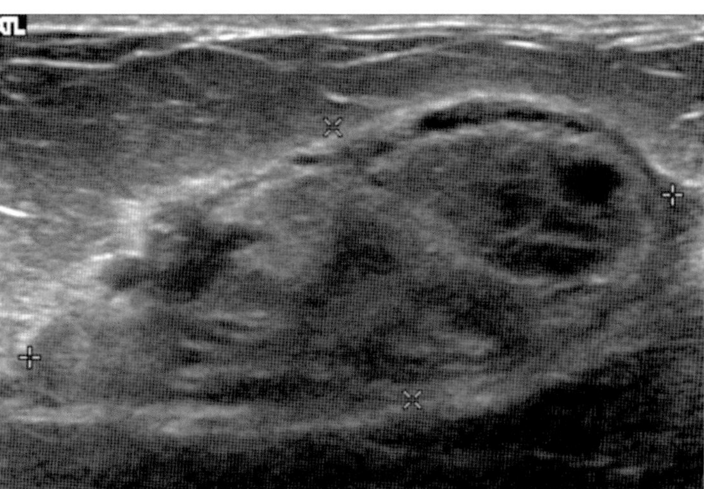

■ **FIGURE 16-60** Fat necrosis. Ultrasound image shows an oval, circumscribed mass with heterogeneous echotexture (same patient as in Fig. 16-42) corresponding to the patient's mammographic and palpable abnormality.

inflammatory changes and granulation tissue. A thin rim of enhancement is common. However, the rim may also be thick, irregular, or spiculated, which are features that may be seen with recurrent or residual cancer. Thin enhancing internal septations are also possible.[25]

The key to diagnosis is assessing internal signal characteristics and enhancement of the mass: fat necrosis is usually nearly isointense to fat elsewhere in the breast. Occasionally, the T1-weighted signal may be lower than that of fat elsewhere in the breast, perhaps because of hemosiderin deposition and inflammatory changes.[26] Non-fat-suppressed T1-weighted images are particularly helpful in diagnosing fat necrosis where fat necrosis is seen as an area of high signal.

Classic Signs

The most classic appearance of fat necrosis is that of an oil cyst.

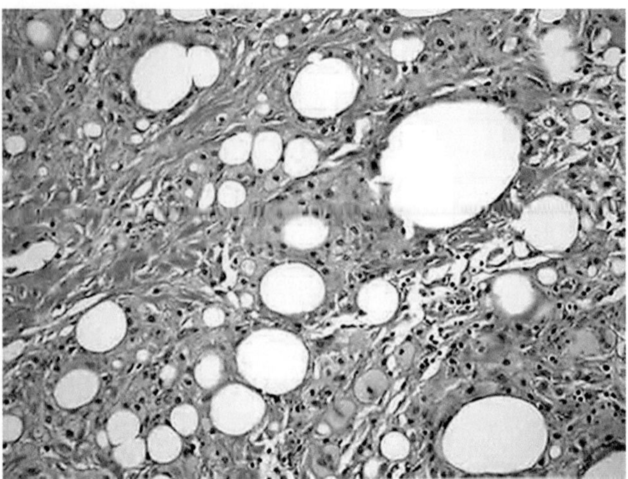

■ **FIGURE 16-61** Fat necrosis. Histiocytes, multinucleated giant cells, and variable lymphocytes and plasma cells are noted around degenerated lobulated fat (H&E, ×200).

Pathology Findings

Fat necrosis may mimic carcinoma clinically, by imaging studies, and by gross pathologic examination. It is associated with trauma to the breast, surgical intervention, and radiotherapy. The excised lesion has ill-defined borders, a firm consistency in the periphery, and yellow to golden brown, soft, and sometimes liquefied material in the center resembling necrotic invasive breast carcinoma. Microscopically, fat necrosis is characterized by the loss of nuclei and fusion of adipocytes, resulting in irregular variable sized empty spaces that are lined by foamy histiocytes, lymphoplasmacytic infiltrates, multinucleated giant cells, cholesterol clefts, and fibrosis. The fatty acid released by necrotic cells is removed by alcohol during tissue processing, resulting in empty spaces (Fig. 16-61). Microcalcifications eventually deposit in fibrous tissue over a period of several months (Fig. 16-62). Calcifications sometimes occur within the necrotic fat.

Synopsis of Treatment Options

When the diagnosis of fat necrosis is made via imaging studies no tissue diagnosis is necessary. If the diagnosis is made via FNA or core biopsy, there is no need for subsequent excisional biopsy.

SILICONE BREAST PROSTHESES

Definition

Silicone breast prostheses (implants) are frequently used in breast augmentation. Complications of silicone implants include rupture, leakage, fibrous or calcified contracture of the tissue capsule that forms around the implants, localized pain, and paresthesia. When both the implant shell's integrity and the surrounding fibrous tissue capsule are breached (extracapsular rupture), silicone content leaks into the breast and can

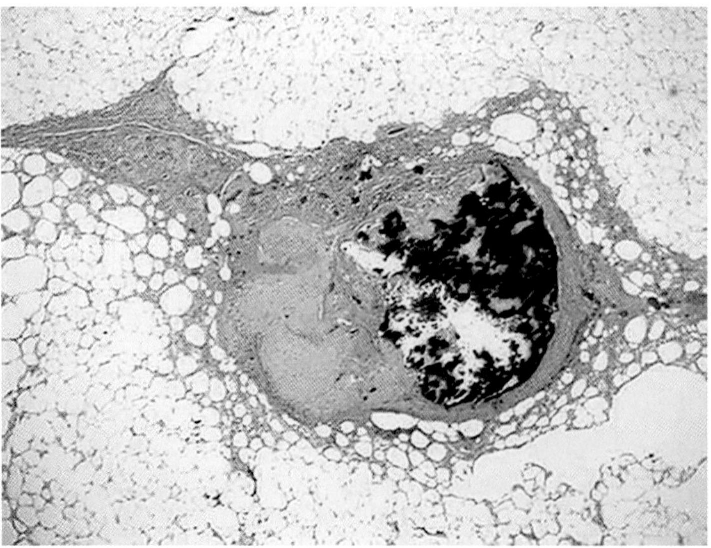

■ **FIGURE 16-62** Later changes in fat necrosis showing fibrosis and calcification (H&E, ×200).

cause silicone mastitis and silicone granulomas and can drain into the axillary lymph nodes, causing silicone lymphadenitis.

Prevalence and Epidemiology

The incidence of silicone breast implant rupture is variable depending on the age and brand of breast implant. Silicone mastitis, granuloma, and lymphadenitis are only seen with extracapsular silicone implant rupture.

Etiology and Pathophysiology

Extracapsular silicone implant leakage causes a foreign-body giant cell reaction.

Manifestations of Disease

Clinical Presentation

When a silicone implant ruptures, it does not deflate like a saline implant would and is usually not clinically apparent.

Imaging Indications and Algorithm

Extracapsular silicone can be seen on screening mammography as high-density material distant from the implant. It can be indistinguishable from a high density breast mass, in which case ultrasonography and sometimes biopsy are necessary.

Imaging Technique and Findings

Mammography

Extracapsular silicone can be seen on screening mammography as an irregular high-density mass with circumscribed or indistinct margins distant from the implant (Fig. 16-63).

Ultrasonography

Silicone granulomas are seen as hyperechoic or hypoechoic nodules with loss of distal ultrasonographic information (Fig. 16-64) and shadowing often described as the snowstorm effect.

Magnetic Resonance Imaging

Extracapsular silicone can be detected on silicone selective sequences with breast MRI. The optimal sequence suppresses the signal from fat and water while maintaining high signal from silicone (see Chapter).

Classic Signs

The classic appearance of a silicone granuloma on ultrasonography demonstrates loss of distal ultrasonographic information.

Pathology Findings

Silicone mastitis and lymphadenitis may present as solid mass lesions in the breast and lymph node, respectively.

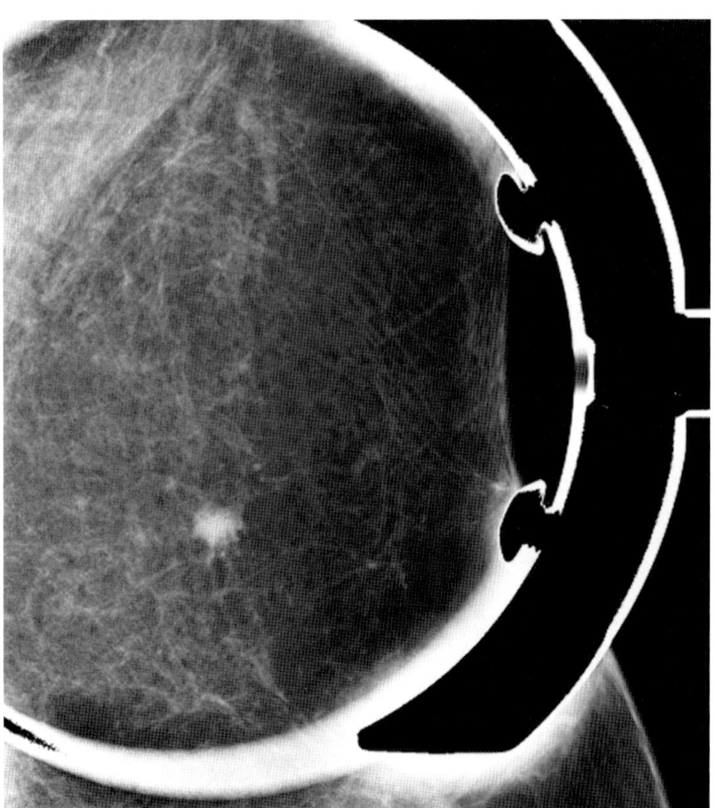

■ **FIGURE 16-63** Silicone granuloma. Spot view mammography in a patient with silicone breast implants demonstrates an oval, microlobulated high density mass.

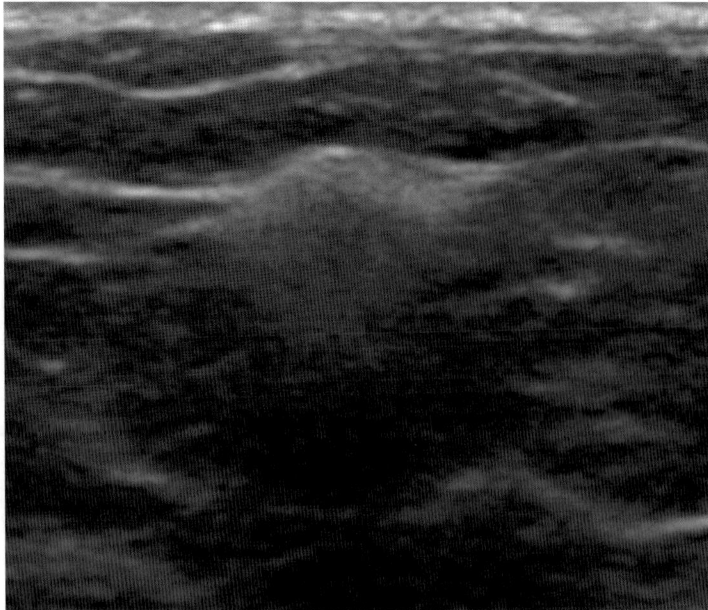

■ **FIGURE 16-64** Silicone granuloma. Ultrasonogram of the lesion in Fig. 16-50 demonstrates a hyperechoic mass with distal loss of ultrasonographic information.

Silicone implant leakage or injection of silicone causes a foreign-body giant cell reaction. Silicone mastitis typically shows clear spaces of variable vacuole size with macrophages, chronic inflammatory cells, plasma cells, and multinucleated giant cells. The clear spaces are often refractile and birefringent but not polarizable under a polarizing lens. Silicone mastitis resembles fat necrosis by microscopic appearance in a low-power view. The main differences between the two conditions are that the size of vacuoles are quite variable and birefringent crystalline material is seen in multinucleated giant histiocytes in silicone granuloma but not in fat necrosis due to trauma. Silicone lymphadenitis is caused by silicone material draining into the axillary lymph nodes (Figs. 16-65 and 16-66).

HEMANGIOMA

Definition

Hemangiomas are benign vascular tumors.

Prevalence and Epidemiology

Hemangiomas are commonly seen in women aged 19 to 82 (mean, 60 years).[27] Breast hemangiomas are found in

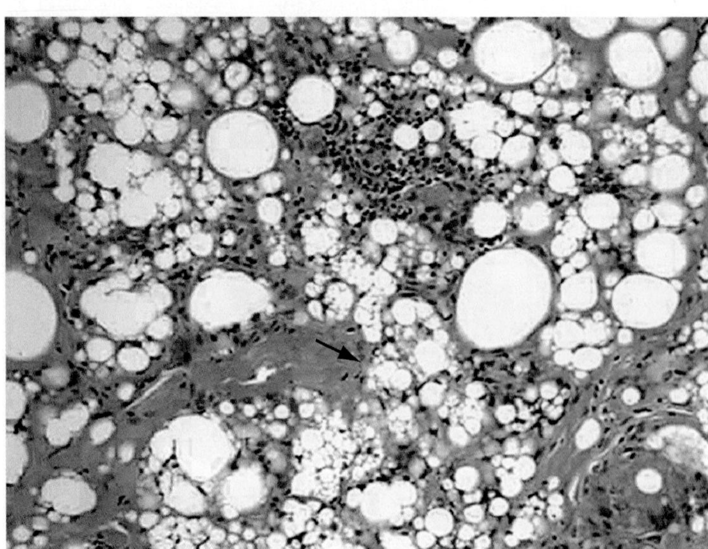

■ **FIGURE 16-65** Breast silicone mastitis. Clear spaces with variable vacuole size and inflammation is the reaction to silicone (*arrow*) (H&E, ×200).

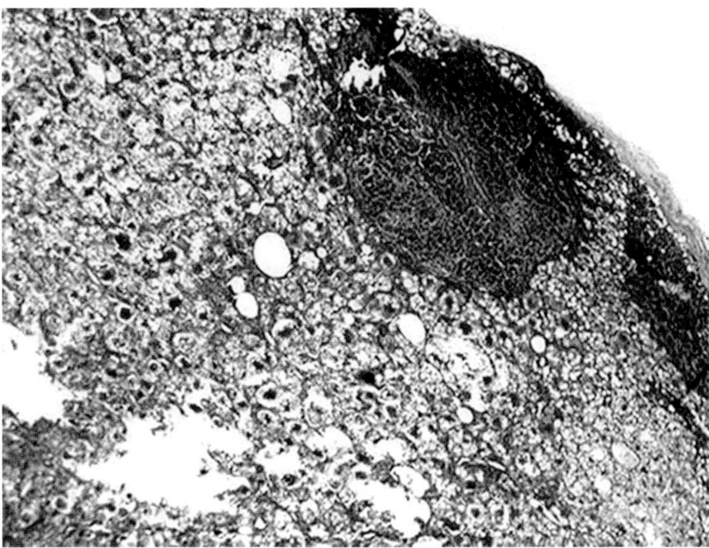

■ **FIGURE 16-66** Silicone lymphadenitis in the axillary lymph node (H&E, ×100).

1.2% of mastectomy specimens and 11% of postmortem specimens of the female breast.[27]

Etiology and Pathophysiology

The etiology of hemangiomas is unclear. Angiogenesis likely plays a role in the vascular excess present. Cytokines, such as basic fibroblast growth factor (bFGF) and vascular endothelial growth factor (VEGF), are known to stimulate angiogenesis. Excesses of these angiogenic factors or decreases of angiogenesis inhibitors (e.g., gamma-interferon, tumor necrosis factor-beta, transforming growth factor-beta) have been implicated in the development of hemangiomas.[28]

Manifestations of Disease

Clinical Presentation

Most hemangiomas are small and asymptomatic and nonpalpable clinically, and the vast majority of such lesions are detected incidentally by mammography. Females occasionally present with large hemangiomas. Males present with palpable and, on average, larger-sized hemangiomas. A small incidental hemangioma may not be visible mammographically.

Imaging Indications and Algorithm

Because hemangiomas are usually found incidentally on mammography, the next step is diagnostic mammography and ultrasonography. Many lesions will meet the criteria for American College of Radiology (ACR) Breast Imaging Reporting and Data System (BI-RADS) 3. However, if they do not meet the criteria for BI-RADS 3, core biopsy may be necessary.

Imaging Technique and Findings

Mammography

A published series of 16 pathologically proven hemangiomas described the mammographic characteristics of breast hemangiomas.[29] Most were oval or lobular isodense masses with circumscribed margins. Superficial location is another characteristic of these lesions. Microcalcifications in the mass are rarely seen, but likely represent phleboliths.[29]

Ultrasonography

Ultrasonography usually shows an oval solid mass with circumscribed or microlobulated margins, parallel orientation, and variable echotexture but is usually hypoechoic, isoechoic, or heterogeneous.

Magnetic Resonance Imaging

MRI demonstrates a variable appearance, depending on the size and subtype of the hemangioma. Large cavernous hemangiomas are quite heterogeneous in appearance owing to different stages of thrombosis.[30]

Small incidental hemangiomas demonstrate focal areas of intense enhancement simulating malignancy, which when seen on histology represent areas of capillary hemangioma (Figs. 16-67 and 16-68).

Pathology Findings

Benign hemangiomas in the form of capillary, cavernous, and venous types can occur in the breast parenchyma and are usually small and incidentally found on excisional biopsy for other lesions. These are benign, localized growths without infiltration. The lining endothelial cells are flat to low cuboidal cells and may show reactive changes, but nuclear atypia or mitotic figures are absent. Thrombus formation for luminal congestion is common. Perilobular hemangioma is partially or completely within the lobular stroma adjacent to, but not invading the terminal ductal lobular unit. They can be identified at low-power view because they usually contain many red blood cells (Fig. 16-69). The vessel size may vary from capillary size to miniature cavernous channels. Cavernous

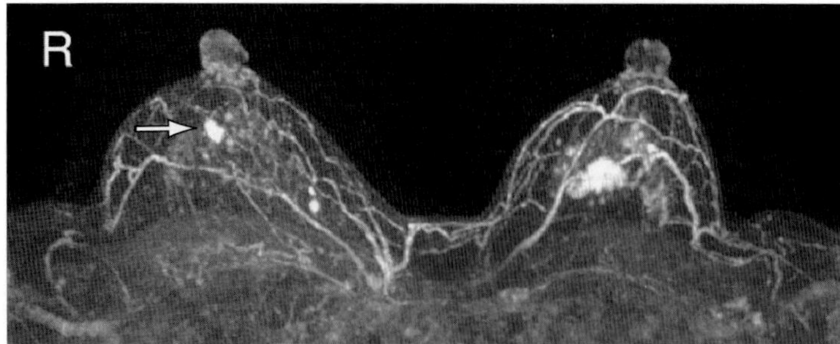

■ **FIGURE 16-67** Hemangioma. A 50-year-old female patient presented with biopsy-proven left breast invasive ductal carcinoma for breast MRI to evaluate extent of disease. Three-dimensional maximum intensity projection image shows an incidental 8 × 4 mm homogeneously enhancing oval irregularly marginated mass present in the anterior right breast at the 6 o'clock position (*arrow*). An MRI-guided biopsy was recommended. (See Fig. 16-55.)

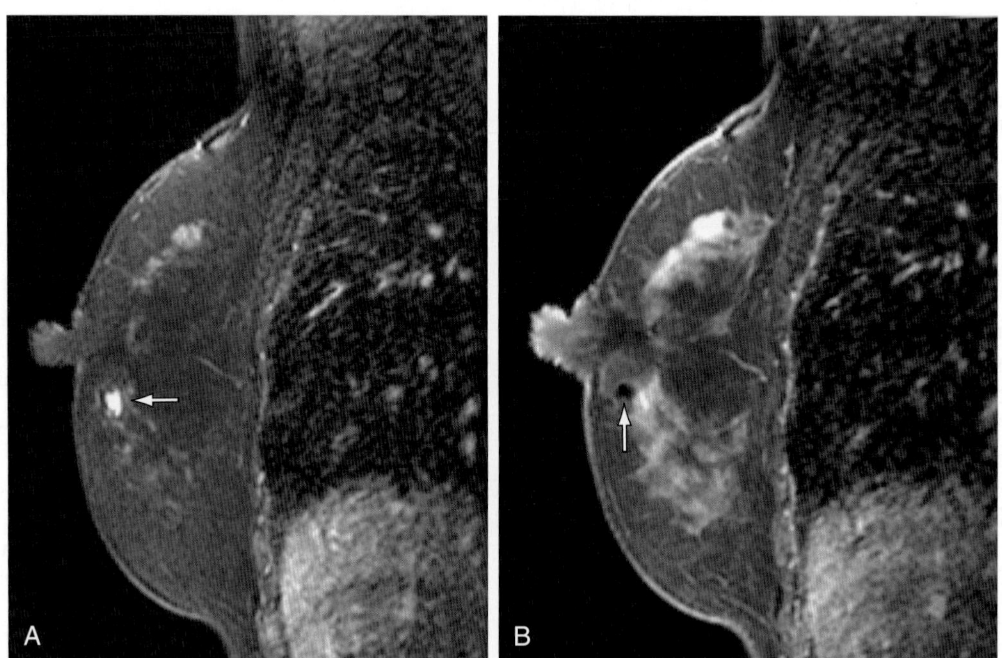

■ **FIGURE 16-68** Hemangioma (*arrow,* **A**). MRI-guided biopsy. Sagittal T1-weighted gadolinium enhanced MR images before (**A**) and after (**B**) biopsy. Note the postbiopsy susceptibility artifact (*arrow,* **B**) that can be secondary to the microclip or air.

hemangiomas are the most common type of mammary hemangioma. Grossly, the lesion is typically well circumscribed, dark-red or brown, and spongy. Microscopically, a compact mass lesion separated by distended and congested vascular channels is seen. Endothelial cells are attenuated and are inconspicuous. Lumens are dilated with red blood cells, and sometimes organizing blood clot is seen (Fig. 16-70) The differential diagnosis of any type of hemangioma within the breast is well-differentiated angiosarcoma. The vast majority of vascular tumors arising in the breast are malignant. An infiltrative pattern, terminal ductular lobular unit involvement, nuclear atypia, and the presence of mitotic figures are key features of angiosarcoma.

Synopsis of Treatment Options

Because the vast majority of vascular tumors arising in the breast are malignant, any questionable vascular lesions of the breast should be completely excised for complete evaluation.

PSEUDOANGIOMATOUS STROMAL HYPERPLASIA

Definition

Pseudoangiomatous stromal hyperplasia (PASH) is a proliferative, benign disorder of breast stromal tissue. Its appearance histologically mimics a vascular lesion, hence

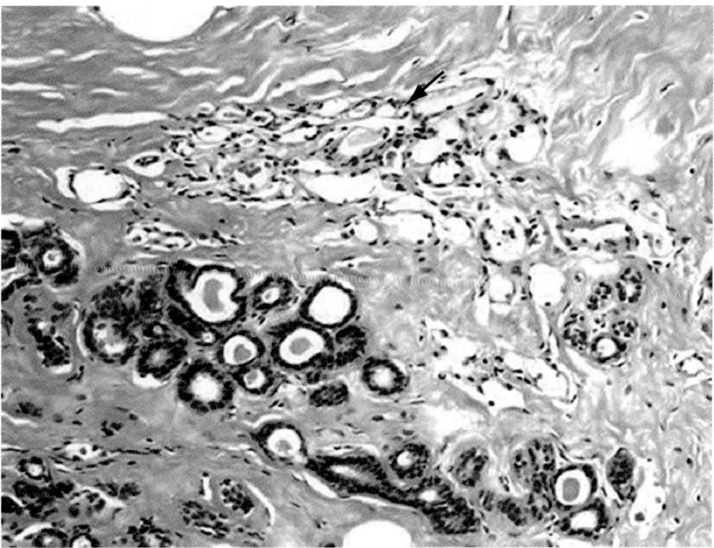

■ **FIGURE 16-69** Perilobular hemangioma. Capillary-size vessels are adjacent to lobules and composed of congested red blood cells and lined by flattened endothelial cells (H&E, ×40).

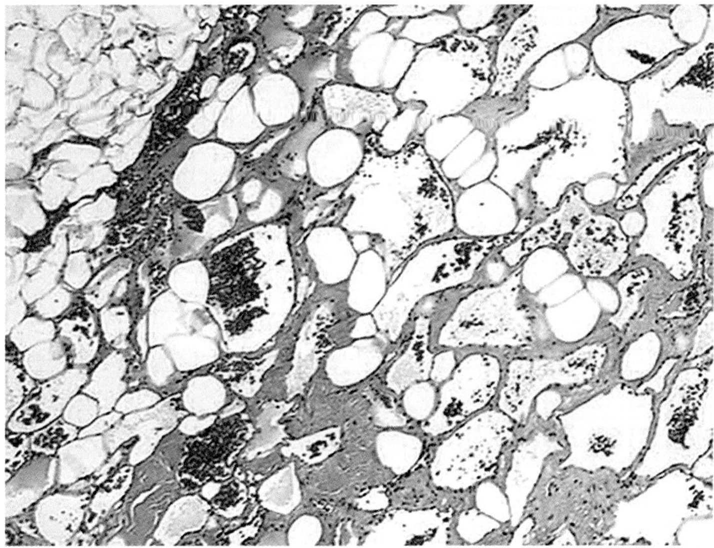

■ **FIGURE 16-70** Cavernous hemangioma of breast. Dilated and congested vascular spaces line attenuated and flattened endothelial cells (H&E, ×200).

the term *pseudoangiomatous*, and it can be mistaken for angiosarcoma histologically.

Prevalence and Epidemiology

A study of 1661 breast biopsies identified PASH in 0.4% of subjects.[31]

Usually, PASH is found in native breast tissue (breast or axillary) of premenopausal females or, less commonly, in postmenopausal females on hormone replacement therapy. PASH can also be an incidental component of gynecomastia in males.

Etiology and Pathophysiology

The etiology of PASH remains uncertain, but aberrant reactivity of myofibroblasts to endogenous or exogenous hormones is likely to be an important factor. It is theorized that it is hormonally related because of its occurrence in premenopausal women and postmenopausal women taking estrogen replacement as well as men with gynecomastia. Also, its appearance is similar to the normal changes in mammary stroma during the luteal phase.

PASH is considered a neoplastic process due to its ability to recur. However, it is not known to be premalignant. In-situ or invasive carcinoma within a PASH mass has not been reported.

Manifestations of Disease

Clinical Presentation

PASH is frequently a microscopic incidental finding in breast biopsies performed for benign or malignant disease.

However, when it presents clinically, it does so as a mass lesion (nodular PASH). These women usually present with a palpable, nontender, unilateral mass that is firm and rubbery, clinically similar to a fibroadenoma. Any area of the breast may be affected. PASH has frequently been misdiagnosed at clinical examination as a fibroadenoma.

Imaging Indications and Algorithm

Mammography and directed ultrasonography are indicated if the patient presents with a palpable abnormality. Both the mammographic and ultrasonographic features in PASH are nonspecific, so core biopsy of these lesions is necessary to exclude a malignancy. Simple excision is adequate treatment initially and for infrequent recurrences. Diffuse PASH occasionally presents a difficult management problem that may necessitate mastectomy.

Imaging Technique and Findings

Mammography

Because PASH most commonly presents pathologically as an incidental finding there is often no mammographic correlate. The mammographic appearance of nodular PASH is of a round or oval circumscribed mass (Fig. 16-71). Indistinct or obscured margins have also been reported as well-spiculated margins.

Ultrasonography

Nodular PASH presents as a hypoechoic solid mass (Fig. 16-72). The echotexture may be slightly heterogeneous. Posterior sound quality varies from moderate acoustic enhancement to mild shadowing.

Magnetic Resonance Imaging

PASH has a variable MRI appearance. Most cases present as areas of non–mass-like enhancement, which are most often focal or regional in distribution. This enhancement can be homogeneous, heterogeneous, or stippled. Enhancing masses can also be seen corresponding to nodular PASH.

Classic Signs

Although it can be a dominant mass, PASH more frequently presents as an incidental pathologic finding with other lesions.

Pathology Findings

PASH is a lesion of myofibroblasts and not vasoformative proliferation; hence the term *pseudoangiomatous* is used. Grossly, PASH can be an ill-defined to well-circumscribed mass with a homogeneous, tan, firm cut surface. Microscopically, PASH has an increased amount of stromal components intermixed by lobules and ducts. The most striking histologic finding is anastomosing spaces in the dense fibrous stroma resembling vascular spaces. These spaces have slit-like openings, are devoid of red blood cells, and involve both interlobular and extralobular stroma (Fig. 16-73). The most critical differentiation is from a low grade angiosarcoma. The lining cells are immunoreactive for CD34, vimentin, and smooth muscle actin (SMA) but not other vascular markers, such as factor VIII-related antigen, and they are negative for cytokeratin. PASH-like change can be seen within hamartomas, and the lesion can grow over time.

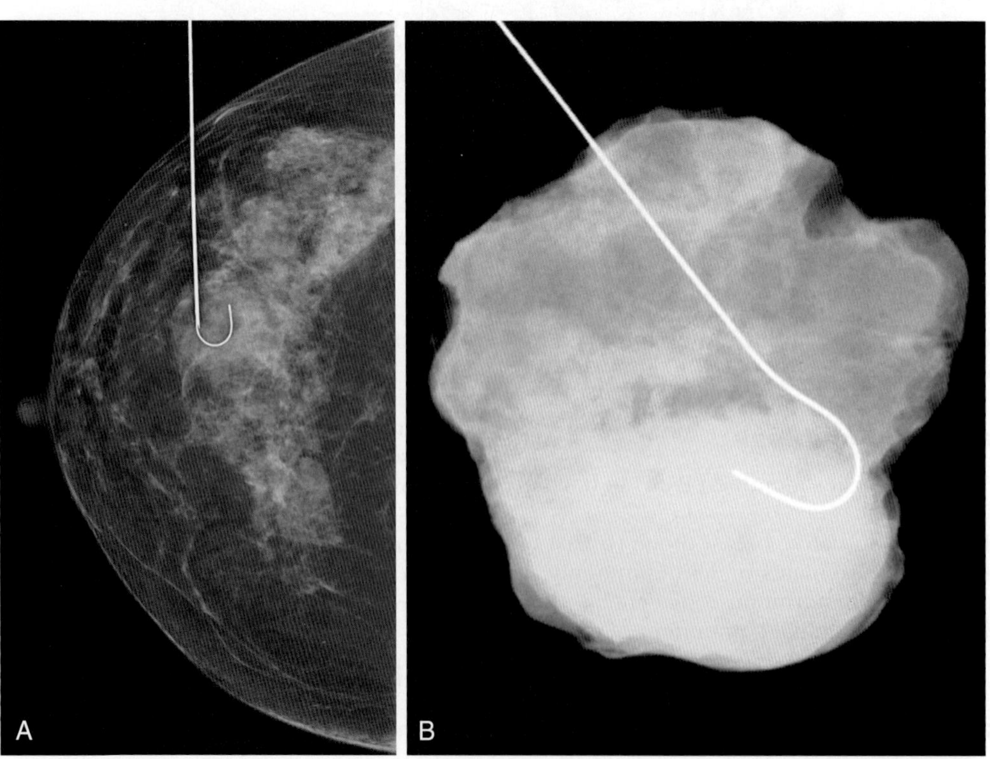

■ **FIGURE 16-71** Pseudoangiomatous stromal hyperplasia (PASH). Mammographic wire localization (**A**) and specimen radiograph (**B**) demonstrate nodular PASH presenting as an oval solid mass with obscured margins.

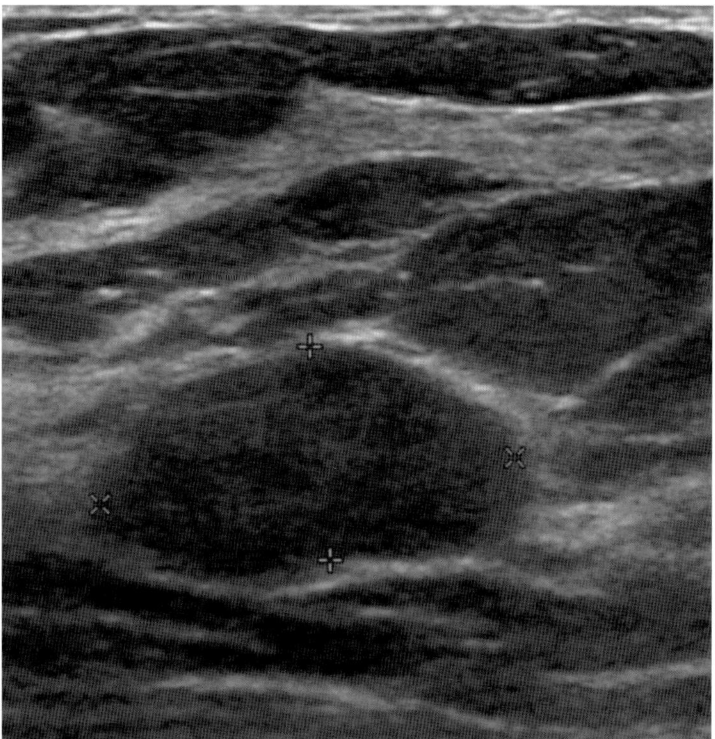

■ **FIGURE 16-72** Pseudoangiomatous stromal hyperplasia (PASH). Ultrasonogram of nodular PASH presenting as an oval isoechoic solid mass.

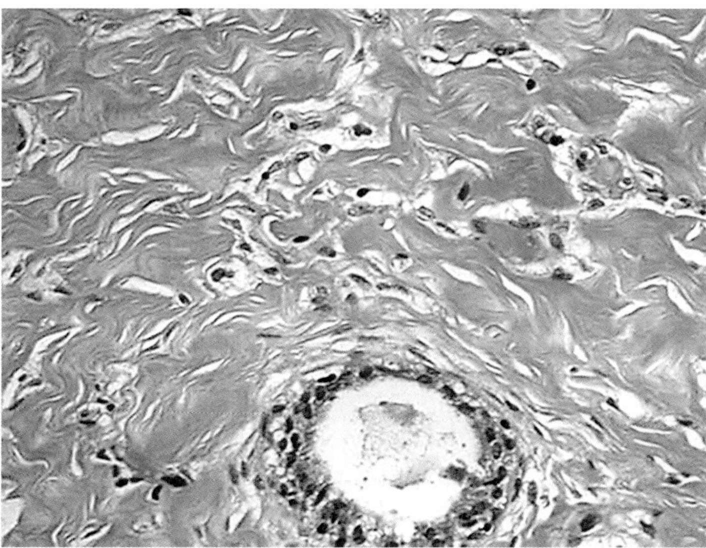

■ **FIGURE 16-73** Pseudoangiomatous stromal hyperplasia (PASH) involving interlobular area showing a diffuse complex network of vascular-like spaces lined by myofibroblastic cells (H&E ×200).

Synopsis of Treatment Options

The recommended treatment is wide local excisional biopsy. PASH can recur multiple times and occasionally presents as a large mass requiring mastectomy.

In the largest reported case series, 5 of 40 (12.5%) patients developed ipsilateral recurrent PASH after excision, with a mean follow-up of 4½ years.[32] In a second study, two of nine (22%) patients developed recurrent PASH after excisional biopsy with a follow-up extending to 30 months.[33]

MYOFIBROBLASTOMA

Definition

Myofibroblastoma is a benign mesenchymal tumor characterized by proliferation of myofibroblasts. Myofibroblastoma of the breast typically occurs as a unilateral, solitary lesion. These lesions are circumscribed, unencapsulated tumors characterized by spindle cells in fascicles that exhibit varying degrees of myogenic and fibroblastic differentiation without intervening epithelial components.

Prevalence and Epidemiology

Myofibroblastoma of the breast is an uncommon mass, more commonly encountered in men in their fifth to seventh decades. It is also seen in postmenopausal women.

Etiology and Pathophysiology

The pathogenesis of myofibroblastoma is unknown. Given the demographics of this lesion, the established trophic effect of steroid hormones, and the potential diagnostic utility of hormone receptor analysis in differentiating spindle cell tumors, immunohistochemical research has been done in testing for estrogen and androgen receptors.[34] The results showed strong nuclear antibody staining for the androgen receptor. It is postulated that the androgen receptor or its ligands may be pathologically related to the development of myofibroblastoma of the breast and diagnostically useful in differentiating it from other spindle cell lesions.[34]

Manifestations of Disease

Clinical Presentation

Physical examination discloses a solitary, unilateral, painless, freely movable, nontender nodule that is usually firm in consistency and has been growing slowly during the course of several months to years.[34]

Imaging Indications and Algorithm

Because of the higher prevalence in men, myofibroblastoma usually presents as a palpable finding, and therefore diagnostic mammography and ultrasonography are performed, followed by biopsy. Occasionally, myofibroblastoma is seen as an incidental mass on screening mammography in females and additional workup is advised.

Imaging Technique and Findings

Mammography

Mammographic findings usually consist of a circumscribed, round to oval, dense mass that is variable in size but frequently 1 to 4 cm in its greatest diameter. It is usually devoid of calcifications but, rarely, may show coarse calcifications within tumor.

Ultrasonography

Ultrasonography confirms the solid nature of the tumor, showing a well-circumscribed, homogeneous, slightly hypoechoic mass suggestive of fibroadenoma.[35] Also seen and more specific are mixed echogenicity and hyperechoic bands of collagen traversing the echolucent cellular foci, which may help narrow the differential possibilities.[35]

Magnetic Resonance Imaging

In the few cases where it was performed, MRI revealed a well-circumscribed nodular mass with homogeneous enhancement and internal septations.[36]

Pathology Findings

Myofibroblastoma is a rare benign mesenchymal tumor in the breast predominantly seen in males, composed of well-circumscribed spindle-shaped or fusiform cells probably originating from fibroblasts. Gross examination of myofibroblastoma shows a well-demarcated tumor with homogeneous cut surface, ranging from 1.0 to 5.0 cm without cystic and hemorrhagic changes. Myxoid changes can be seen. Microscopically, the classic myofibroblastoma is a well-defined lesion composed entirely of spindle cells devoid of ducts and lobules. The tumor is moderately cellular and composed of uniform ovoid to spindle-shaped cells interspersed by thick collagen. Mitotic figures are rare (Figs 16-74 and 16-75). Adipose tissue from the

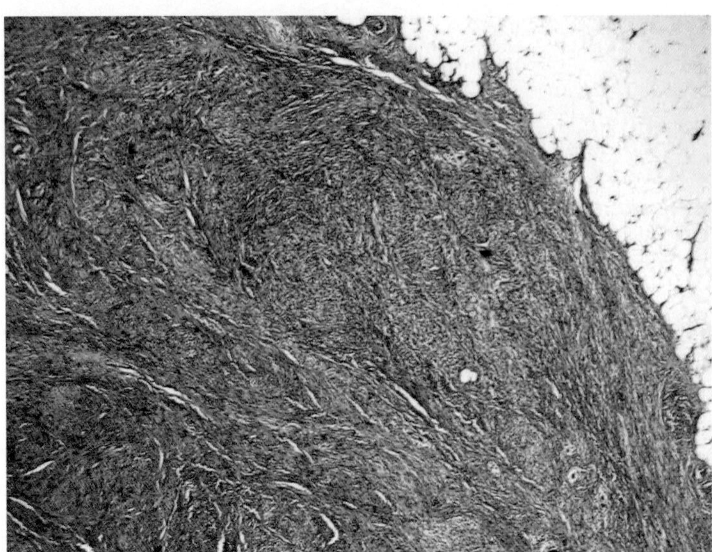

■ **FIGURE 16-74** Well-circumscribed lesion with spindle-shaped cells without ducts or acini of breast (H&E, ×40).

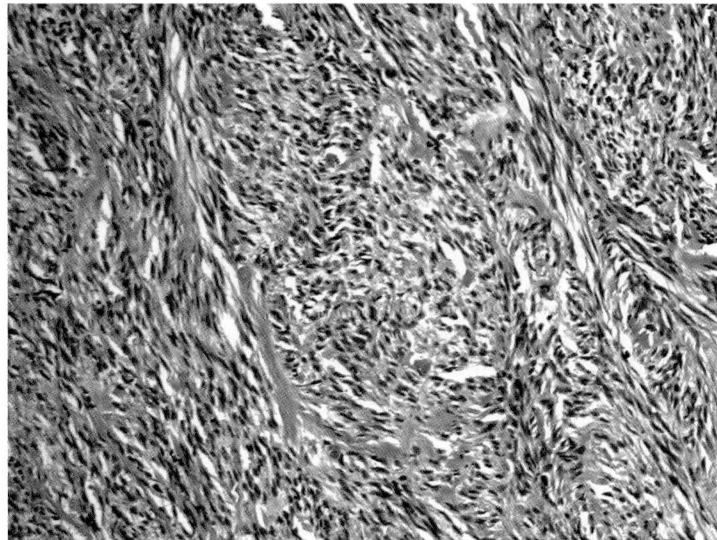

■ **FIGURE 16-75** Myofibroblastoma showing spindle cells arranged in clusters and fascicles separated by intervening bands of hyalinized collagen (×200).

breast can be incorporated into the lesions. There are many variants of myofibroblastomas. Epithelioid smooth muscle cell, cartilaginous, and osseous differentiation can be seen within the tumor. These features do not alter the clinical behavior. Immunohistochemical stains are variable depending on the constituent's smooth muscle cell differentiation; however, the majority of myofibroblastomas are immunoreactive for desmin, vimentin, actin and CD34.[34,35]

Synopsis of Treatment Options

Local excision is adequate treatment, and recurrences have not been reported.

ADENOMYOEPITHELIOMA

Definition

Adenomyoepithelioma is a benign biphasic tumor composed of both epithelial and myoepithelial proliferation.

Prevalence and Epidemiology

Adenomyoepithelioma of the breast is a rare tumor.

Etiology and Pathophysiology

The exact etiology of breast adenomyoepithelioma is unknown.

Manifestations of Disease

Clinical Presentation

Patients with breast adenomyoepithelioma present with a unilateral painless mass.

Imaging Indications and Algorithm

The lesion may be asymptomatic and seen on screening. When palpable, diagnostic mammography, ultrasonography, and biopsy are performed. Rapid enlargement of a mass is highly suggestive of malignant change.

Imaging Technique and Findings

Mammography

The imaging features of breast adenomyoepithelioma are not well described. Benign adenomyoepithelioma shows benign features, with the lesion appearing circumscribed and having no associated parenchymal distortion. In malignant adenomyoepitheliomas, mammography shows an indistinct lesion and marked distortion of the surrounding breast parenchyma.

Ultrasonography

Ultrasonography demonstrates a round hypoechoic mass with circumscribed margins. In malignant adenomyoepitheliomas, acoustic shadowing may be seen.

Magnetic Resonance Imaging

Contrast-enhanced MRI shows a round mass of low signal intensity on T1-weighted images with spiculated margins and rapid plateau enhancement.[37]

Classic Signs

The findings are not classic. The diagnosis of exclusion is breast carcinoma.

Pathology Findings

Adenomyoepithelioma is a benign biphasic tumor composed of both epithelial and myoepithelial proliferations.

Patients usually present with a solitary mass or multiple masses that are lobulated with pushing borders to adjacent breast parenchyma. There are many variants of adenomyoepithelioma: spindle cell, tubular, and lobulated types.[38] Occasionally, central necrosis due to infarct and dystrophic calcification with basophilic background stroma can be seen. The epithelial components often have apocrine metaplasia. Myoepithelial proliferation is commonly seen with clear, eosinophilic, or hyaline (plasmacytoid) cells compressing epithelial components. Mitotic figures are rarely seen and usually do not exceed 1 to 2 per 10 high-power fields (Figs 16-76 and 16-77). The myoepithelial cells frequently have clear cytoplasm and are shown immunohistochemically via positive staining for smooth muscle α-actin, smooth muscle myosin, and S-100 protein.

Synopsis of Treatment Options

Malignant transformation can occur in adenomyoepithelioma. Both benign and malignant adenomyoepitheliomas are known to have local recurrence after excision and may recur several years after the initial surgery.[37] The best predictor for local recurrence of a benign adenomyoepithelioma is an initial incomplete margin. The multinodular and peripheral extension of the lesion may contribute to local recurrence. If the excisional margin is narrow or incomplete, re-excision is recommended. Metastases may occur in malignant adenomyoepithelioma and can consist of one or both cellular components. Malignant adenomyoepithelioma has been reported to metastasize to lung, brain, and, in rare cases, thyroid.[39-41] Metastases from malignant

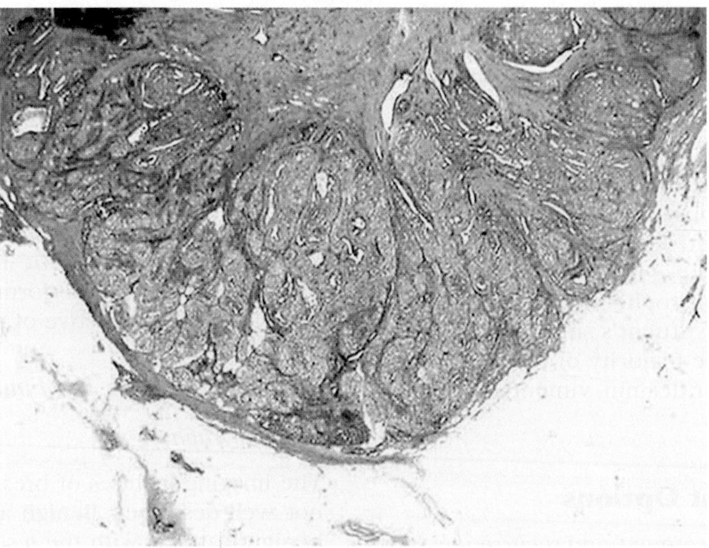

■ **FIGURE 16-76** Adenomyoepithelioma showing a well-circumscribed border composed of aggregated nodules (H&E, ×40).

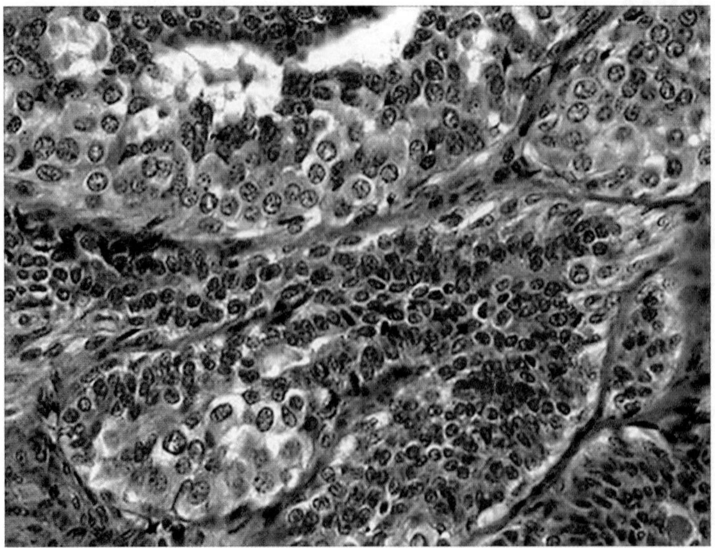

■ **FIGURE 16-77** Adenomyoepithelioma composed of small glandular lumen compressed by polygonal and clear myoepithelial cell proliferations. The contrast between the darkly stained luminal cells and the pale stained myoepithelial cells is striking (H&E, ×400).

adenomyoepithelioma appear to be hematogenous rather than lymphatic to the axillary lymph nodes.

NIPPLE ADENOMA

Definition

Nipple adenoma is a rare, benign neoplasm of breast lactiferous ducts that develops in the superficial portion of the nipple.

Prevalence and Epidemiology

Nipple adenomas are rare. Most lesions present during the patient's fifth decade of life.[42]

Etiology and Pathophysiology

The etiology of nipple adenoma is unclear.

Manifestations of Disease

Clinical Presentation

Patients with nipple adenoma present with a palpable tumor of the papilla of the nipple with clear or serosanguineous nipple discharge, skin ulceration, erythema, and nipple enlargement. The symptoms resemble those of Paget's disease. The lesion is usually unilateral and usually 0.5 to 1.5 cm in diameter.

Imaging Indications and Algorithm

In a patient with a new mass arising in conjunction with nipple discharge and abnormal findings at physical examination, the workup begins with mammography and ultrasonography and would also warrant biopsy. The differential diagnosis based on imaging findings includes a periareolar fibroadenoma, intraductal papilloma, or a subareolar abscess.

Imaging Technique and Findings

Mammography

Because of its small size and location, a nipple adenoma is usually not visualized on mammography but can appear as an indistinct oval density that is contiguous with the nipple. Because of its indistinct margins, the lesion can be indistinguishable from breast carcinoma and other solid masses.

Ultrasonography

The ultrasonographic appearance is not well described.

Magnetic Resonance Imaging

MRI demonstrates a mass in the nipple with intense and persistent enhancement kinetics.[42] Nipple abnormalities may be overlooked on breast MRI because of the prominent enhancement of the normal nipple. However, on bilateral breast MRI, the enhancement will be greater in the affected nipple.[42]

Classic Signs

Nipple adenoma appears clinically similar to Paget's disease.

Pathology Findings

Nipple adenoma is a benign lesion with many different names, including nipple duct adenoma, florid papillomatosis, papillomatosis of the nipple, subareolar duct papillomatosis, and erosive adenomatosis. Clinical presentation includes erosion of the nipple and nipple discharge with or without a mass lesion underlying the nipple. Gross examination of the nipple adenoma demonstrates a scaly lesion with ulceration. Cut surface shows a firm white-to-tan nodule with irregular edges. Microscopically, the nipple adenoma shows adenomatous glandular proliferation beneath the epidermis without atypia in a pseudoinfiltrative border. The overlying squamous epidermis may show ulceration or hyperplasia (Figs 16-78 and 16-79).

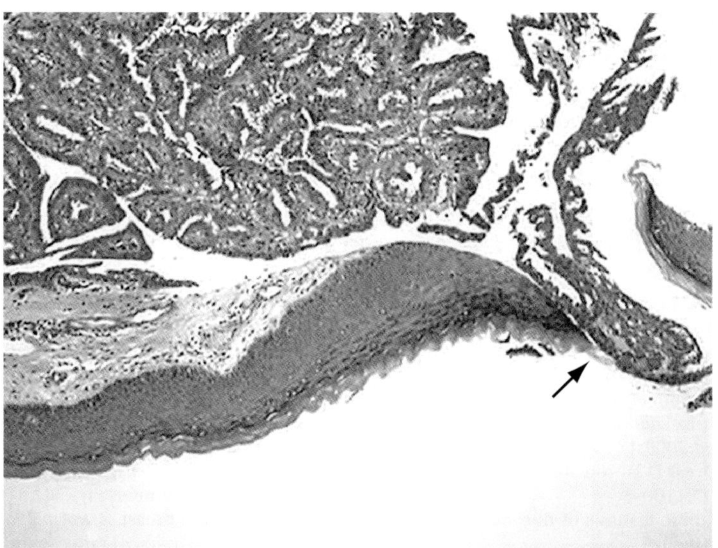

■ **FIGURE 16-78** Nipple adenoma showing erosion of overlying epidermis and an adenomatous proliferation of glandular structures (*arrow*) (H&E, ×40).

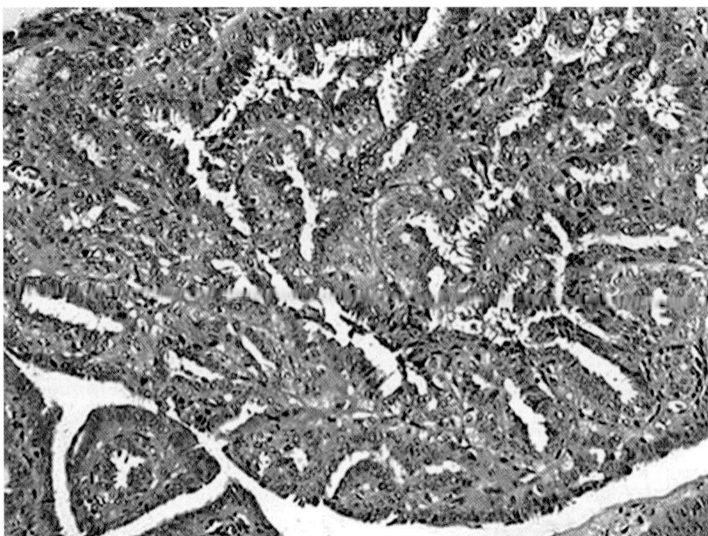

■ **FIGURE 16-79** Nipple adenoma showing ductal hyperplasia without atypia with intervening dense fibrous stroma (H&E, ×200).

The four variants of nipple adenoma, which depend on the epithelial hyperplasia forms, are as follows: (1) sclerosing papillomatosis pattern; (2) papilloma pattern; (3) adenosis pattern; and (4) mixed proliferative patterns. Squamous metaplasia and apocrine metaplasia are commonly seen with nipple adenomas. The differential diagnosis clinically is Paget's disease, but microscopically these two lesions are quite different. The microscopic differential diagnosis of nipple adenoma includes intraductal papilloma and subareolar involvement of ductal carcinoma in situ or ADH involving large lactiferous ducts.

Synopsis of Treatment Options

Complete excisional biopsy is recommended, which may require removal of the nipple. Local recurrence of nipple adenoma may occur after incomplete excision. There has been concomitant breast carcinoma in association with nipple adenoma,[43-45] but the evidence indicating that nipple adenoma is a precancerous lesion is less substantial.

KEY POINTS

- There are multiple lesions that can present as a solid mass in the breast. Circumscribed lesions include fibroadenoma, intramammary lymph node, hamartoma, lipoma, tubular/lactating adenomas, pseudoangiomatous stromal hyperplasia (PASH), myofibroblastoma, adenomyoepithelioma, and nipple adenoma.
- Irregular lesions include fibromatosis, fat necrosis, and granular cell tumor. Some cases of diabetic mastopathy and PASH also can present as irregular masses.

SUGGESTED READINGS

McMenamin ME, DeSchryver K, Fletcher CD. Fibrous lesions of the breast and a review. *Int J Surg Pathol* 2000;**8**:99-108.

REFERENCES

1. Guray M, Sahin AA. Benign breast diseases: classification, diagnosis, and management. *Oncologist* 2006;**11**:435-49.
2. Yiangou C, Fadi H, Sinnett HD, Shousha S. Fibromatosis of the breast or carcinoma? *J R Soc Med* 1996;**89**:638-40.
3. Devouassoux-Shisheboran M, Schammel MD, Man YG, Tavassoli FA. Fibromatosis of the breast: age-correlated morphofunctional features of 33 cases. *Arch Pathol Lab Med* 2000;**124**:276-80.
4. Matherne T, Green A, Tucker JA, Dyess D. Fibromatosis: The breast cancer imitator. *South Med J* 2004;**97**:1100-3.
5. Leibman AJ, Kossoff MB. Sonographic features of fibromatosis of the breast. *J Ultrasound Med* 1991;**10**:43-5.
6. Nakazono T, Satoh T, Hamamoto T, Kudo S. Dynamic MRI of fibromatosis of the breast. *AJR Am J Roentgenol* 2003;**181**:1718-9.
7. Mesurolle B, Leconte I, Fellah L, Feger C. Dynamic breast MRI in recurrent fibromatosis. *AJR Am J Roentgenol* 2005;**184**:696-7.
8. Schwarz GM, Drotman R, Rosenblatt L, Milner J, Shamonki, Osborne, M. Case reports. Fibromatosis of the breast: case report and current concepts in the management of an uncommon lesion. *Breast J* 2006;**12**:66-71.
9. McMenamin ME, DeSchryver K, Fletcher CD. Fibrous lesions of the breast and a review. *Int J Surg Pathol* 2000;**8**:99-108.
10. Sklair-Levy M, Samuels TH, Catzavelos C, Hamilton P, Shumak R. Stromal fibrosis of the breast. *AJR Am J Roentgenol* 2001;**177**:573-7.
11. Magno S, Terribile D, Franceschini G, Fabbri C, D'Alba P, Chiesa F, et al. Breast MRI in a case of "early onset" lactating adenoma: signal characteristics are similar to fibroadenomas. *Breast J* 2009;**15**:105-6.

12. Haj M, Weiss M, Herskovits T. Diabetic sclerosing lymphocytic lobulitis of the breast. *J Diabetes Complications* 2004;**18**:187-91.
13. Baratelli GM, Riva C. Diabetic fibrous mastopathy: sonographic-pathologic correlation. *J Clin Ultrasound* 2005;**33**:34-7.
14. Wong KT, Tse GM, Yang WT. Ultrasound and MR imaging of diabetic mastopathy. *Clin Radiol* 2002;**57**:730-5.
15. Abrikossoff A. Ueber Myome, Augesehend von der quergestreiften willkurlichen Muskulatur. *Virchows Arch Pathol Anat* 1926;**260**:215-33.
16. Montagnese MD, Roshong-Denk S, Zaher A, Mohamed I, Staren ED. Granular cell tumor of the breast. *Am Surg* 2004;**70**:52-4.
17. Irshad A, Pope TL, Ackerman SJ, Panzegrau B. Characterization of sonographic and mammographic features of granular cell tumors of the breast and estimation of their incidence. *J Ultrasound Med* 2008;**27**:467-75.
18. Tobin CE, Hendrix TM, Geyer SJ, Mendelson EB, Resnikuff LB. Breast imaging case of the day. *RadioGraphics* 1996;**16**:983-5.
19. Balzan SMP, Farina PS, Maffazzioli L, Riedner CE, Guedes Neto EP, Fontes PR. Granular cell breast tumour: diagnosis and outcome. *Eur J Surg* 2001;**167**:860-2.
20. Yang WT, Edeiken-Monroe B, Sneige N, Fornage BD. Sonographic and mammographic appearances of granular cell tumors of the breast with pathological correlation. *J Clin Ultrasound* 2006;**34**:153-60.
21. Kohashi T, Kataoka T, Haruta R, Sugino K, Marubayashi S, Yahata H, et al. Granular cell tumor of the breast: report of a case. *Hiroshima J Med Sci* 1999;**48**:31-3.
22. Scaranelo AM, Bukhanov K, Crystal P, Mulligan AM, O'Malley FP. Granular cell tumour of the breast: MRI findings and review of the literature. *Br J Radiol* 2007;**80**:970-4.
23. Bassett LW, Gold RH, Mirra JM. Nonneoplastic breast calcifications in lipid cysts: development after excision and primary irradiation. *AJR Am J Roentgenol* 1982;**138**:335-8.
24. Bassett LW, Gold RH, Cove HC. Mammographic spectrum of traumatic fat necrosis: the fallibility of "pathognomonic" signs of carcinoma. *AJR Am J Roentgenol* 1978;**130**:119-22.
25. Daly CP, Jaeger B, Sill DS. Variable appearances of fat necrosis on breast MRI. *AJR Am J Roentgenol* 2008;**191**:1374-80.
26. Chala LF, de Barros N, de Camargo Moraes P, Endo E, Kim SJ, Pincerato KM, et al. Fat necrosis of the breast: mammographic, sonographic, computed tomography, and magnetic resonance imaging findings. *Curr Probl Diagn Radiol* 2004;**33**:106-26.
27. Lesueur GC, Brown RW, Bhathal PS. Incidence of perilobular hemangioma in the female breast. *Arch Pathol Lab Med* 1983;**107**:308-10.
28. Chang J, Most D, Bresnick S, Mehrara B, Steinbrech DS, Reinisch J, et al. Proliferative hemangiomas: analysis of cytokine gene expression and angiogenesis. *Plast Reconstr Surg* 1999;**103**:1-9; discussion, 10.
29. Mesurolle B, Sygal V, Lalonde L, Lisbona A, Dufresne MP, Gagnon JH, et al. Sonographic and mammographic appearances of breast hemangioma. *AJR Am J Roentgenol* 2008;**191**:W17-22.
30. Kim SM, Kim HH, Shin HJ, Gong G, Ahn SH. Cavernous haemangioma of the breast. *Br J Radiol* 2006;**79**:e177-80.
31. Polger MR, Denison CM, Lester S, Meyer JE. Pseudoangiomatous stromal hyperplasia: mammographic and sonographic appearances. *AJR Am J Roentgenol* 1996;**166**:349-52.
32. Powell CM, Cranor ML, Rosen PP. Pseudoangiomatous stromal hyperplasia (PASH): a mammary stromal tumor with myofibroblastic differentiation. *Am J Surg Pathol* 1995;**19**:270-7.
33. Vuitch MF, Rosen PP, Erlandson RA. Pseudoangiomatous hyperplasia of mammary stroma. *Hum Pathol* 1986;**17**:185-91.
34. Wargotz ES, Weiss SW, Norris HJ. Myofibroblastoma of the breast: sixteen cases of a distinctive benign mesenchymal tumor. *Am J Surg Pathol* 1987;**11**:493-502.
35. Magro G, Bisceglia M, Michal M, Eusebi V. Spindle cell lipoma-like tumor, solitary fibrous tumor and myofibroblastoma of the breast: a clinicopathological analysis of 13 cases in favor of a unifying histologic concept. *Virchows Arch* 2002;**440**:249-60.
36. Vourtsi A, Kehagias D, Antoniou A, Moulopoulos LA, Deligeorgi-Politi H, Vlahos L. Male breast myofibroblastoma and MR findings. *J Comput Assist Tomogr* 1999;**23**:414-6.
37. Ruiz-Delgado ML, López-Ruiz JA, Eizaguirre B, Saiz A, Astigarraga E, Fernández-Temprano Z. Benign adenomyoepithelioma of the breast: imaging findings mimicking malignancy and histopathological features. *Acta Radiol* 2007;**48**:27-9.
38. Brogi E. Benign and malignant spindle cell lesions of the breast. *Semin Diagn Pathol* 2004;**21**:57-64.
39. Tavassoli FA. Myoepithelial lesions of the breast. Myoepitheliosis, adenomyoepithelioma, and myoepithelial carcinoma. *Am J Surg Pathol* 1991;**15**:554-68.
40. Loose JH, Patchefsky AS, Hollander IJ, Lavin LS, Cooper HS, Katz SM. Adenomyoepithelioma of the breast: a spectrum of biologic behavior. *Am J Surg Pathol* 1992;**16**:868-76.
41. Ahmed AA, Heller DS. Malignant adenomyoepithelioma of the breast with malignant proliferation of epithelial and myoepithelial elements: a case report and review of the literature. *Arch Pathol Lab Med* 2000;**124**:632-6.
42. Perzin KH, Lattes R. Papillary adenoma of the nipple (florid papillomatosis, adenoma, adenomatosis): a clinicopathologic study. *Cancer* 1972;**29**:996-1009.
43. Fornage BD, Faroux MJ, Pluot M, Bogomoletz W. Nipple adenoma simulating carcinoma: misleading clinical, mammographic, sonographic, and cytologic findings. *J Ultrasound Med* 1991;**10**:55-7.
44. Adusumilli S, Siegelman ES, Schnall MD. MR findings of nipple adenoma. *AJR Am J Roentgenol* 2002;**179**:803-4.
45. Tavassoli FA. Coexistence of nipple duct adenoma and breast carcinoma: A clinicopathologic study of five cases and review of the literature. *Mod Pathol* 1995;**8**:637-42.

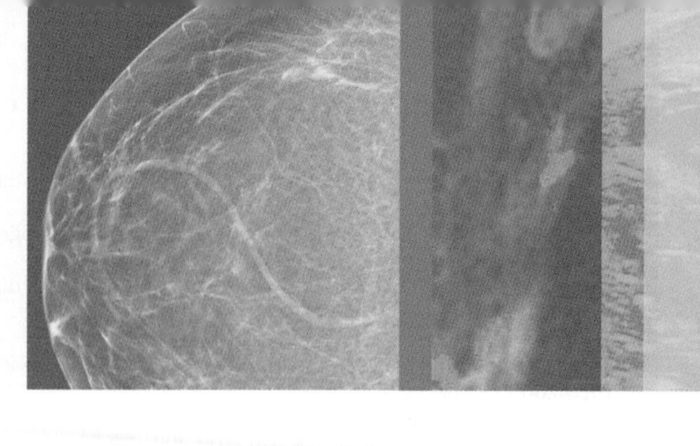

CHAPTER 17

Proliferative Lesions

Sophia Kim Apple, Jennifer M. J. Overstreet, and Lawrence W. Bassett

Benign breast lesions are generally classified into three categories: nonproliferative, proliferative without atypia, and proliferative with atypia. Nonproliferative lesions have no increased risk for the development of breast cancer and include benign cysts, apocrine metaplasia, and mild ductal hyperplasia. Proliferative lesions, in the absence of atypia, confer only a 1.5 to 2.0 relative risk (RR) for the development of breast cancer. Adenosis, radial scar, moderate to florid ductal hyperplasia of usual type, fibroadenoma, and gynecomastia are among proliferative lesions without atypia that are discussed in this chapter. Atypical proliferative lesions have four to five times increased risk for the development of breast cancer. Atypical ductal hyperplasia and lobular neoplasia, including atypical lobular hyperplasia and lobular carcinoma in situ, are described in detail in Chapter 19 on high-risk proliferative lesions.

ADENOSIS

Definition

Adenosis is a spectrum of histologic lesions ranging from hyperplasia of the lobule to sclerosing adenosis with fibrosis and calcification. Sclerosing adenosis is a benign breast lesion characterized by the lobulocentric proliferation of ducts and lobules with stromal fibrosis.

Prevalence and Epidemiology

Sclerosing adenosis has been seen in 3.1% of females at autopsy and in up to 12.5% in the noncancerous surgical specimen.[1,2]

Etiology and Pathophysiology

In the early stage of adenosis, under estrogenic stimulation, the lobules become hyperplastic and enlarged beyond the average range of 10 to 100 acini. This is essentially the change that occurs during pregnancy. Later, with the cessation of hormonal stimulation, the lobules regress. In addition, myoepithelial proliferation and stromal fibrosis occur, which can cause elongation and distortion of acini. In the final stage, the acini become few in number and the lobules become involuted with fibrosis, so-called *sclerosing adenosis*. The stromal fibrosis can cause increased density on the mammogram, which in combination with the calcifications may simulate malignancy.

Manifestations of Disease

Clinical Presentation

Sclerosing adenosis is most commonly clinically silent and asymptomatic. However, it may present as a palpable mass, most commonly in women between the ages of 45 and 55.

Imaging Indications and Algorithm

Screening mammography detects the majority of known cases of sclerosing adenosis. Less likely, when it presents as a palpable mass, a diagnostic workup ensues, including additional mammographic views and ultrasound evaluation.

Imaging Findings by Modality

Mammography

The mammographic findings of sclerosing adenosis are usually nonspecific and most commonly include clustered, round or punctuate calcifications. Other mammographic appearances include asymmetries, focal asymmetries, architectural distortion, and speculated masses with or without microcalcifications, mimicking breast carcinoma (Figs. 17-1 and 17-2) Similarly, the mammographic findings of adenosis are nonspecific, including ill-defined 3- to 5-mm nodular densities (Fig. 17-3).

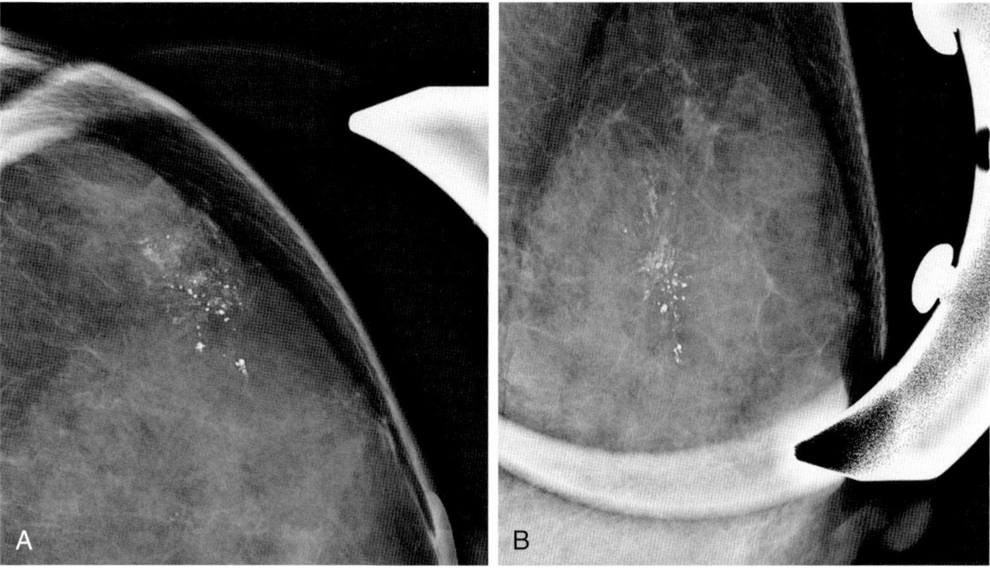

■ **FIGURE 17-1** Sclerosing adenosis. Craniocaudal (**A**) and mediolateral (**B**) digital magnification mammogram views of the left breast show punctuate and amorphous calcifications in a linear branching distribution in the upper outer quadrant.

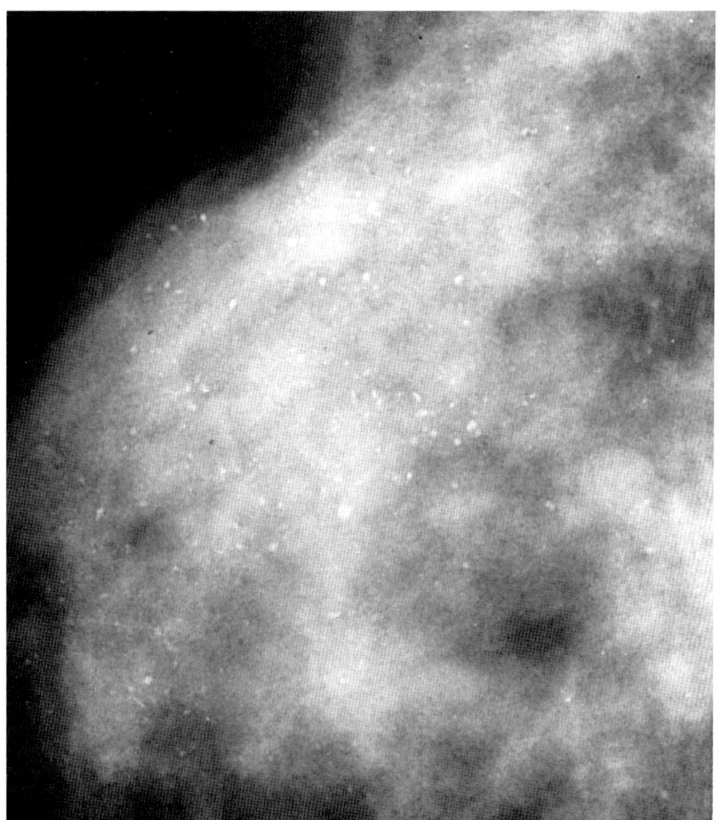

■ **FIGURE 17-2** Sclerosing adenosis. Mediolateral oblique mammogram of the right breast demonstrates multiple round and punctuate calcifications in a regional distribution associated with radiographically dense breast tissue.

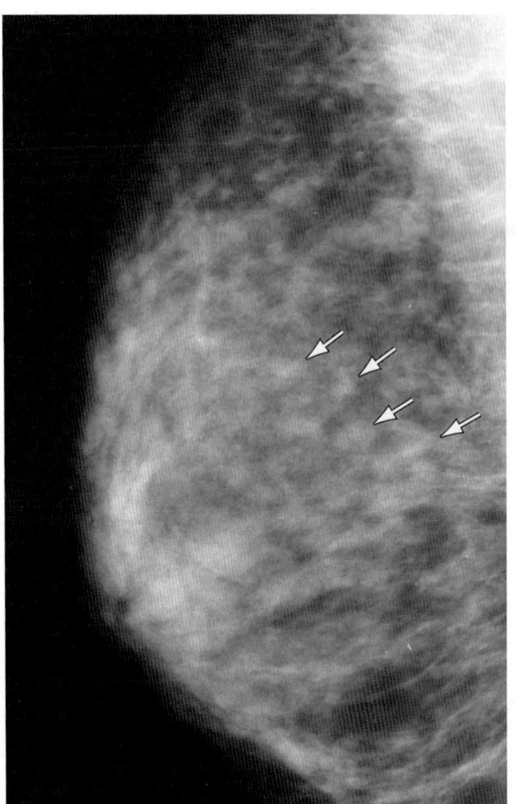

■ **FIGURE 17-3** Adenosis. Mediolateral oblique view mammogram of the right breast shows diffuse, scattered, indistinct 3- to 5-mm tiny masses (*arrows*) caused by hyperplasia of the lobules.

Ultrasonography

The ultrasonographic findings of sclerosing adenosis are usually nonspecific and include masses with circumscribed, microlobulated, or indistinct margins.

Magnetic Resonance Imaging

The MRI findings of sclerosing adenosis are usually nonspecific and include non-mass-like ductal enhancement.[3]

Classic Signs

Because of the lack of definitive imaging findings, sclerosing adenosis should be considered a histologic diagnosis, rather than an imaging diagnosis. When the imaging findings mimic carcinoma, biopsy is required.

Differential Diagnosis

From Clinical Presentation

Rarely, sclerosing adenosis presents as a palpable mass. As in all instances of a palpable breast mass, the differential diagnosis includes benign versus malignant etiologies.

From Imaging Findings

The differential diagnosis for the imaging features of sclerosing adenosis is broad, including both malignant and benign lesions. Specifically, the differential includes infiltrating carcinomas, ductal carcinoma in situ, postoperative scar, radial scar, and fat necrosis.

Pathology Findings

Sclerosing adenosis is a benign breast lesion characterized by lobulocentric proliferation of ductules/lobules and fibrous tissue. It is notable for its ability to mimic invasive carcinoma mammographically, grossly and microscopically, and has been seen in 3.1% of female breasts at autopsy. Within the surgical specimen, sclerosing adenosis has been reported in 12.5% of noncancerous and 5.3% to 7% of cancerous breasts.[4,5] Sclerosing adenosis can be focal or diffuse and florid within the breast. It is characterized by an organoid and lobulated pattern of proliferation of closely packed ductules and lobules with distortion by thick collagen compressing ductules and lobules (Fig. 17-4). The ductules and lobules are lined by myoepithelial cells. On high-power magnification, sclerosing adenosis has a two-cell layer: one inner layer of luminal epithelium and an outer layer of myoepithelial cells (Fig. 17-5). Sclerosing adenosis

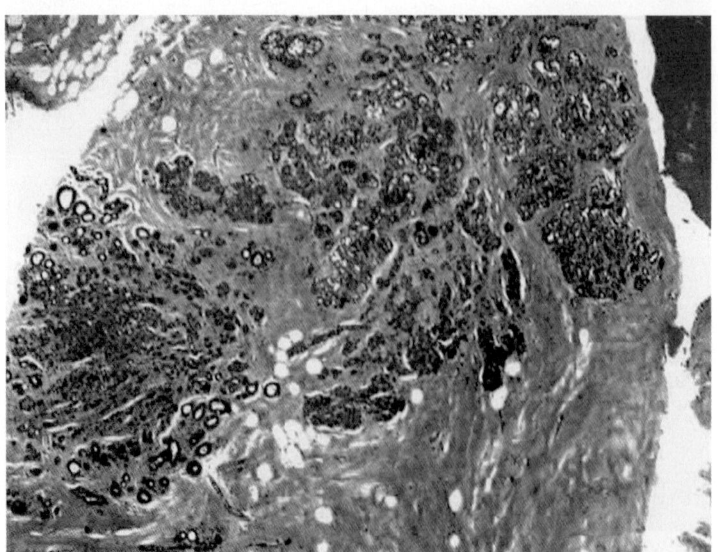

■ **FIGURE 17-4** Sclerosing adenosis has lobulated architecture with ductules and lobular proliferation with sclerotic dense fibrous tissue (H&E, ×40).

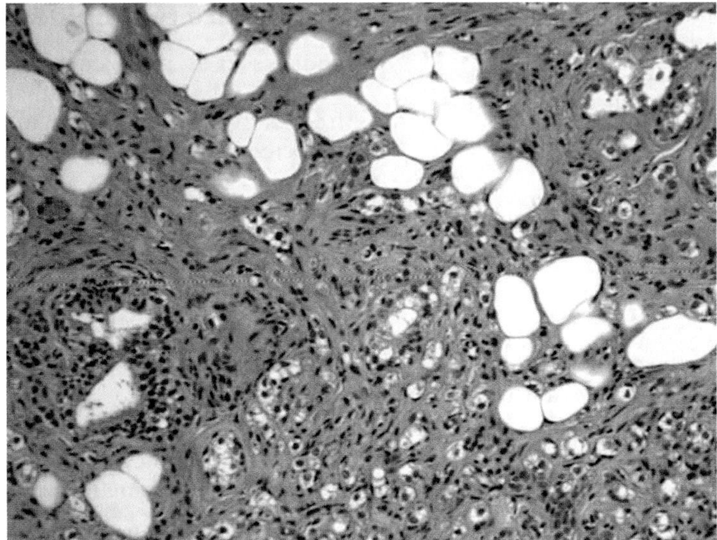

■ **FIGURE 17-5** In higher power view, sclerosing adenosis can appear as a haphazard pattern infiltrating in the fatty adipocytes (H&E, ×400).

can be associated with microcalcifications. In some cases, a massive proliferation of ductules and lobules occurs and presents as a palpable nodule. When a distinct nodule forms, the term *nodular sclerosing adenosis* or *adenosis tumor* can be used. When sclerosing adenosis extends beyond lobulocentric growth and into the fat tissue, the differential diagnosis of invasive carcinoma, especially tubular carcinoma, can be challenging. Other atypical neoplasia such as atypical ductal hyperplasia, ductal carcinoma in situ (DCIS), atypical lobular hyperplasia, or lobular carcinoma in situ (LCIS) can be seen in association with sclerosing adenosis, which can be even more difficult to distinguish from invasive carcinoma. Immunohistochemical stains to study presence or absence of myoepithelial cells can be extremely helpful. Most sensitive and specific myoepithelial cell markers are p63, smooth muscle myosin heavy chain (SMMHC), and calponin (Fig. 17-6). The presence of myoepithelial cells supports the diagnosis of benign sclerosing adenosis, and the absence of myoepithelial cells supports invasive carcinoma. Management for sclerosing adenosis diagnosed by core needle biopsy is controversial. Sclerosing adenosis is not known to be a precursor lesion of invasive carcinoma of the breast. An overall RR has been reported as 1.7 to 2.5.[4,5] When atypical proliferation is associated with sclerosing adenosis, the RR factor rises to as much as 6.7.[2] The presence of sclerosing adenosis without atypia in a core needle biopsy specimen does not require excisional biopsy.

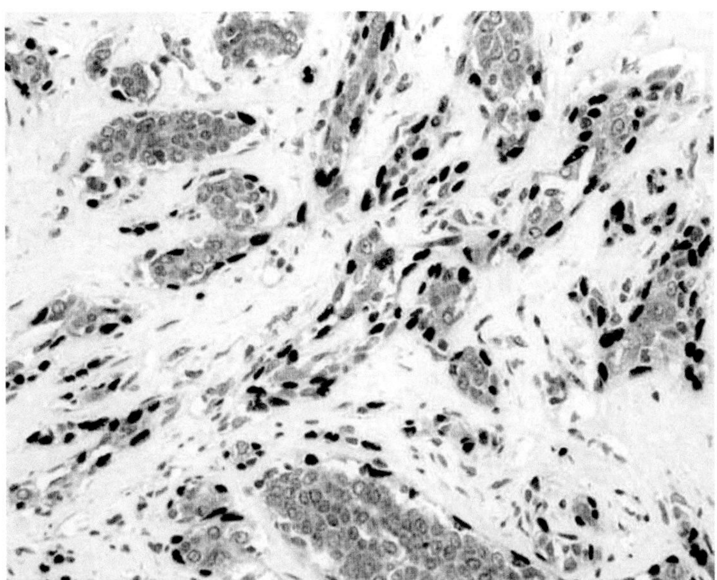

■ **FIGURE 17-6** Positive nuclear staining emphasizing the presence of myoepithelial cells surrounding ductules proliferation of sclerosing adenosis (P63 IHC stain, ×400).

There are differences in RR and absolute risk (AR). RR is calculated by dividing the number of cancers per number of subpopulation over the number of cancers per number of reference population. AR is number or percentage of cancers in number of years per individual patient.

$$RR = \frac{\text{No. cancers / No. in subpopulation}}{\text{No. cancers / No. in reference population}}$$

$$AR = \text{No. or \% cancers in No. years}$$

Since 1984, four large studies have been published using standardized criteria in pathology diagnosis with the subsequent risk of breast cancer: the Nashville study by Dupont and Page, the Nurse Health Study (NHS) by London and associates, the Breast Cancer Detection Demonstration Project (BCDDP) by Dupont and colleagues, and the Mayo Clinic study by Hartmann and associates. These studies contain more than 532,390 total population in the benign breast disease category. Other factors that may modify the risk of development of breast cancer include family history, postmenopausal hormone usage, and other coexisting benign lesions.

RADIAL SCAR

Definition

Radial scar is a benign lesion known by a variety of names in the literature, including infiltrating epitheliosis, nonencapsulated sclerosing lesion, indurative mastopathy, scleroelastic lesion, sclerosing papillary proliferation, benign sclerosing ductal hyperplasia, and radial sclerosing lesion. It is composed of a central sclerotic core and peripheral proliferative ducts.

Prevalence and Epidemiology

Radial scar is most commonly seen between the ages of 40 to 60 years and is uncommon before age 30. The frequency of radial scar in mastectomy specimens is reported between 4% and 26%.[7,8]

Etiology and Pathophysiology

The cause is unknown, but it is not related to previous surgery or trauma.

Manifestations of Disease

Clinical Presentation

Radial scar is clinically silent and, therefore, almost always detected at screening mammography.

Imaging Indications and Algorithm

Screening mammography detects the majority of known cases. A diagnostic study including magnification and spot compression views may follow.

Imaging Technique and Findings

Mammography

Most radial scars are spiculated masses or areas of architectural distortion, often with multiple long spicules and central areas of lucency.[9-11] These findings are nonspecific, however, and may be found in invasive ductal carcinoma, invasive lobular carcinoma, and many benign processes.[10,12] In addition, radial scars may have dense central regions and microcalcifications may be mammographically visible in up to 37% of cases (Figs. 17-7 to 17-9).[10,12]

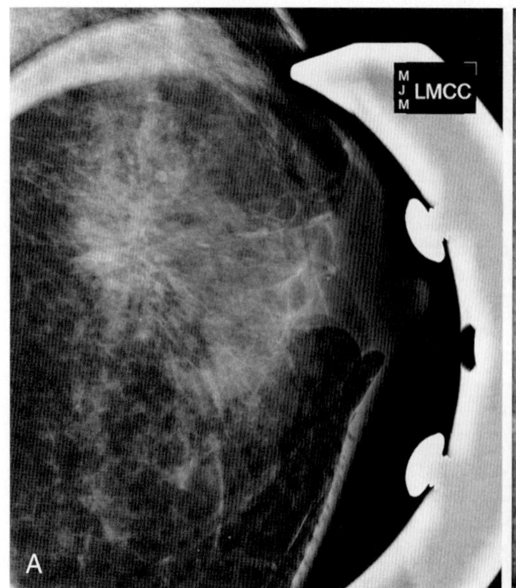

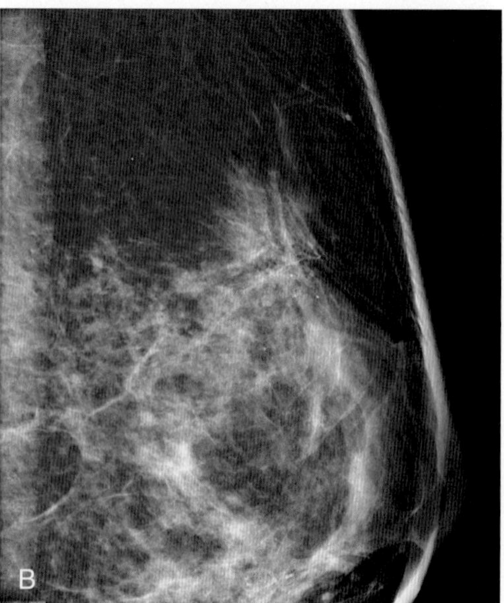

■ **FIGURE 17-7** Radial scar. Craniocaudal (**A**) and mediolateral (**B**) digital magnification mammogram views of the left breast show architectural distortion in the upper outer quadrant containing amorphous microcalcifications.

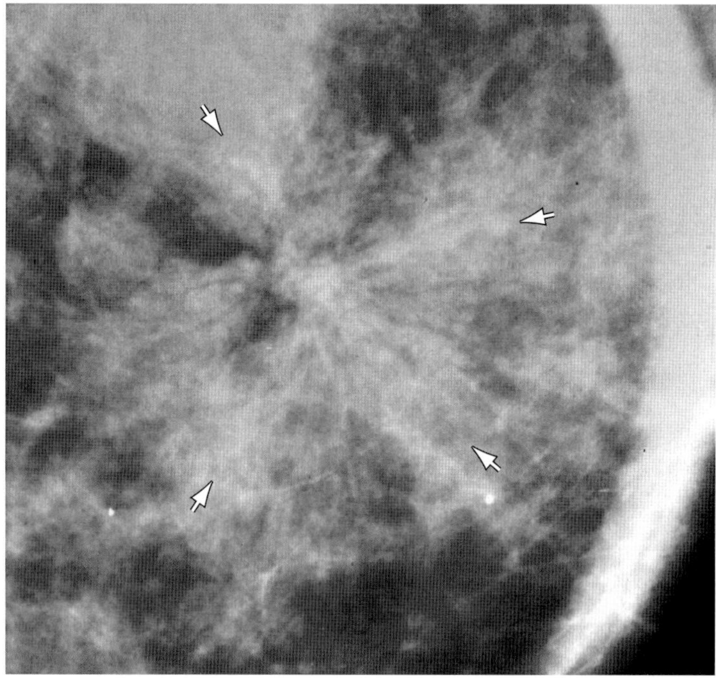

■ **FIGURE 17-8** Radial scar with area of central density (*arrows*) seen on mammogram.

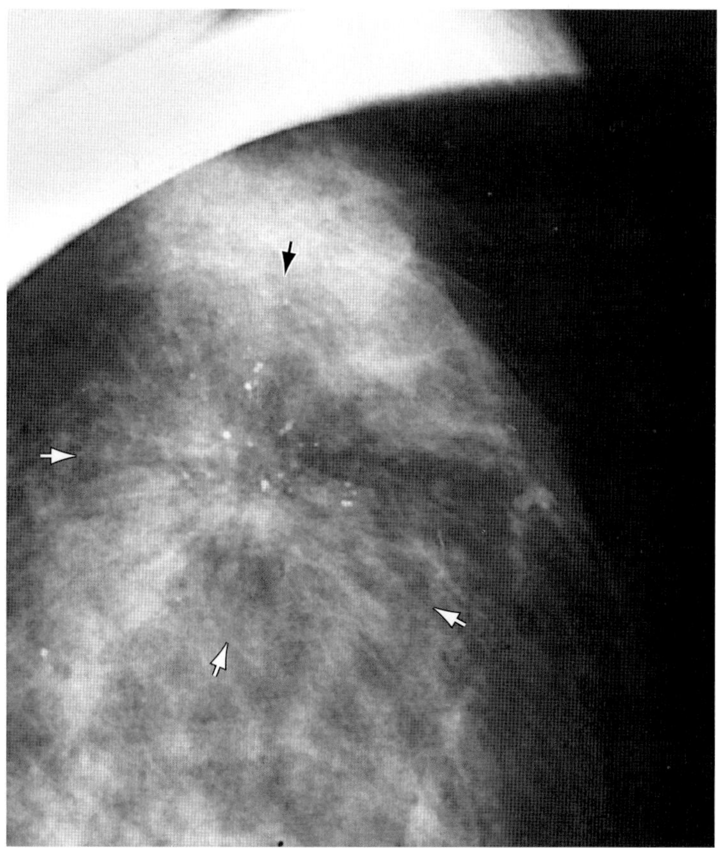

■ **FIGURE 17-9** Mammogram shows radial scar with pleomorphic microcalcifications.

Ultrasonography

The ultrasound appearance of radial scar is nonspecific, including an ill-defined mass with or without posterior acoustic shadowing (Fig. 17-10).[13]

Magnetic Resonance Imaging

The appearance of radial scar with MRI is not well documented. The literature suggests that the MRI appearance is variable, including non–mass-like ductal enhancement as well as enhancing masses with spiculated margins.[3,14]

Differential Diagnosis

From Clinical Presentation

Radial scar is clinically silent and asymptomatic.

From Imaging Findings

The differential diagnosis of radial scar includes benign versus malignant processes, including infiltrating carcinomas, ductal carcinoma in situ, postoperative scar, and sclerosing adenosis. It is not possible to differentiate between radial scar and breast carcinoma by imaging, and biopsy should be performed.

Pathology Findings

Radial scar is a benign breast lesion characterized by central distortion with area of scar and peripheral proliferative ducts (Fig. 17-11). These lesions have both gross and microscopic appearance as small invasive carcinomas of the breast. Grossly, most of radial scars lack a distinct mass-like lesion but present as a firm ill-defined area or rarely a mass. Microscopically, radial scar is characterized

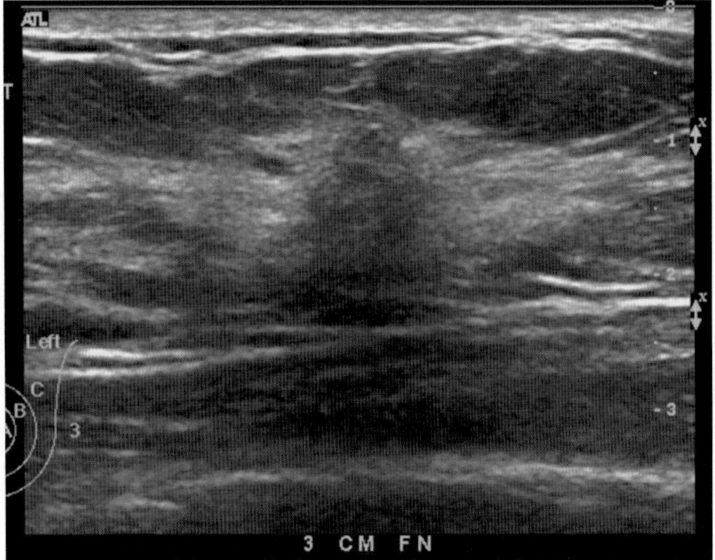

■ **FIGURE 17-10** Radial scar. Ultrasound image demonstrates an isoechoic, indistinct shadowing mass not parallel to the surface of the breast.

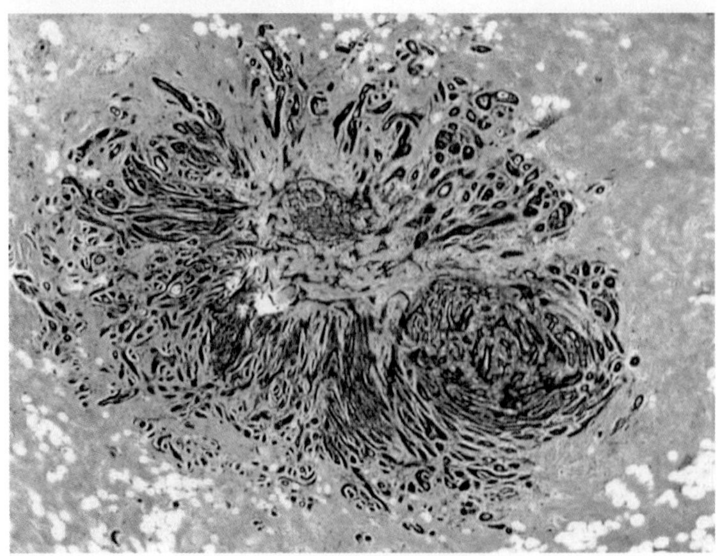

■ **FIGURE 17-11** Radial scar typically consists of a stellate central fibrotic core with radiating peripheral ductal and lobular proliferations (H&E, ×40).

by having a distinct sclerotic center containing entrapped ducts that resembles invasive ductal or tubular carcinoma (Figs. 17-12 and 17-13). The central area often contains elastosis and hyalinized fibrosis. Peripheral area of radial scar often shows florid ductal hyperplasia, microcysts, apocrine metaplasia, and adenosis radiating from a central nidus similar to spokes on a wheel, producing resultant distortion and retraction. Ductal hyperplasia seen at the periphery may have central luminal necrosis (Fig. 17-14).

Ductal hyperplasia of usual type with central luminal necrotic cellular debris is different from comedo necrosis in DCIS which shows ghost cells and contents that have a more granular appearance. The usual ductal hyperplasia rarely has central necrosis, but it is not uncommonly seen in ductal hyperplasia associated with radial scar. The peripheral zone of proliferative process may not be present or may be partially present especially in the core needle biopsy samples. Rarely, atypical proliferations of both ductal and lobular types including invasive carcinoma can be seen with radial scar. Tubular carcinoma is a main differential diagnosis to be considered, especially in the sclerotic areas with entrapped and sclerotic ducts and lobules. The entrapped central zone of radial scar will have myoepithelial cells, whereas tubular carcinoma will have absence of myoepithelial cells and "haphazard" glandular arrangement.

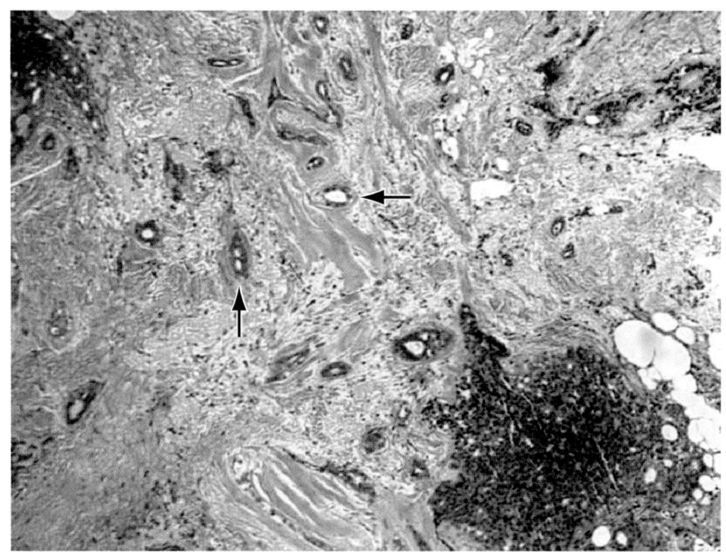

■ **FIGURE 17-12** Higher power view of radial scar with central fibrotic area with haphazard pattern of entrapped glands (*arrows*) mimicking invasive tubular carcinoma (H&E, ×400).

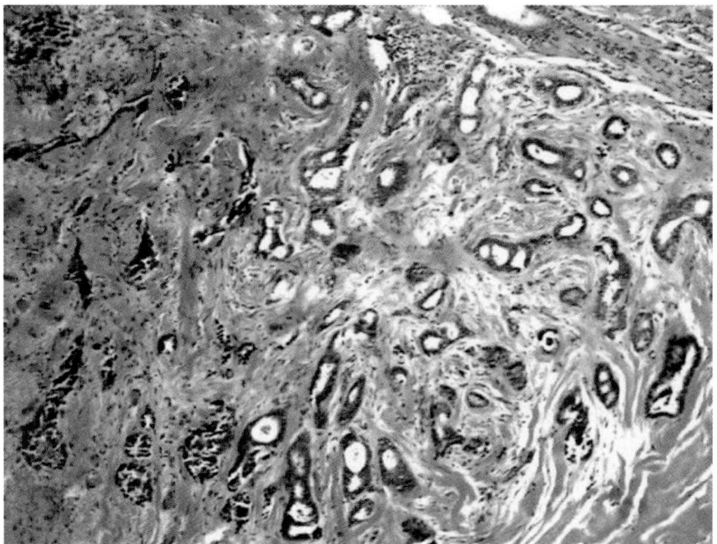

■ **FIGURE 17-13** Tubular carcinoma showing haphazard arrangement of glands (H&E, ×100).

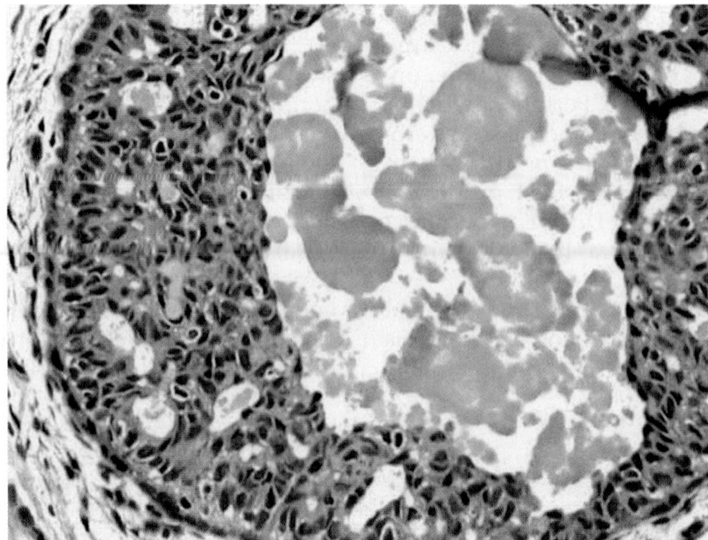

■ **FIGURE 17-14** Ductal hyperplasia of usual type seen at the periphery of radial scar can have luminal necrosis and concretions. The presence of luminal necrosis within ductal proliferation should not be mistaken for comedo necrosis of ductal carcinoma in situ (H&E, ×200).

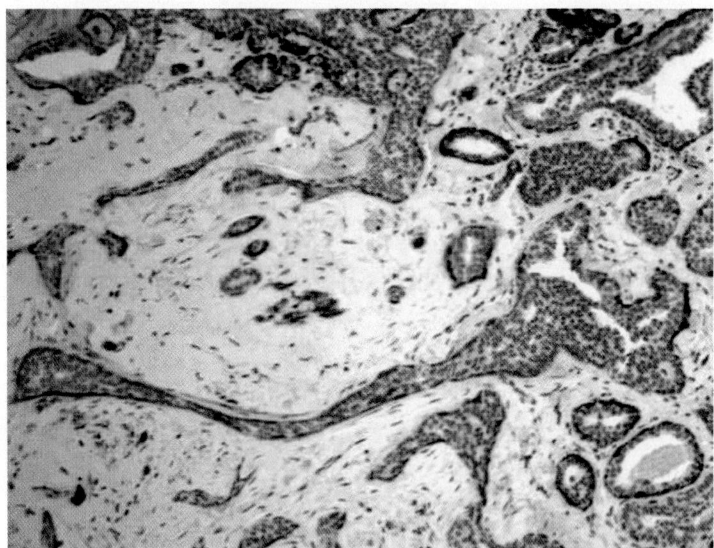

■ **FIGURE 17-15** Immunohistochemical stain for smooth muscle myosin heavy chain (SMMHC) shows the presence of myoepithelial cells with cytoplasmic positivity around the entrapped ducts, supportive of a noninvasive process.

Immunohistochemical stains may be helpful to delineate the presence or absence of myoepithelial cells (Figs. 17-15 and 17-16).

Carcinoma seen within the context of radial scar is well documented, especially when mammographic radial scar measures 2 cm or larger and patient age is older than 50 years.[15] A prospective cohort study of a large number of patients with a median follow-up of 12 years and a biopsy result of radial scars was found to have an independent risk factor for breast carcinoma.[16] The RR for carcinoma after radial scar in women was 1.8, and it increased to 5.8 when concurrent atypical hyperplasia was seen.[17]

Synopsis of Treatment Options

There has been controversy over the years regarding the appropriate biopsy method for lesions for which radial scar is high in the differential diagnosis. In the past, excisional biopsy, rather than needle biopsy, was usually recommended because of the sampling error associated with the use of 14-gauge automated Tru-Cut biopsy devices; problems with differentiating between radial scar and other lesions, such as tubular carcinoma, in the small histologic specimens; and the fact that radial scar has been shown to be associated with invasive ductal carcinoma (not otherwise specified), tubular

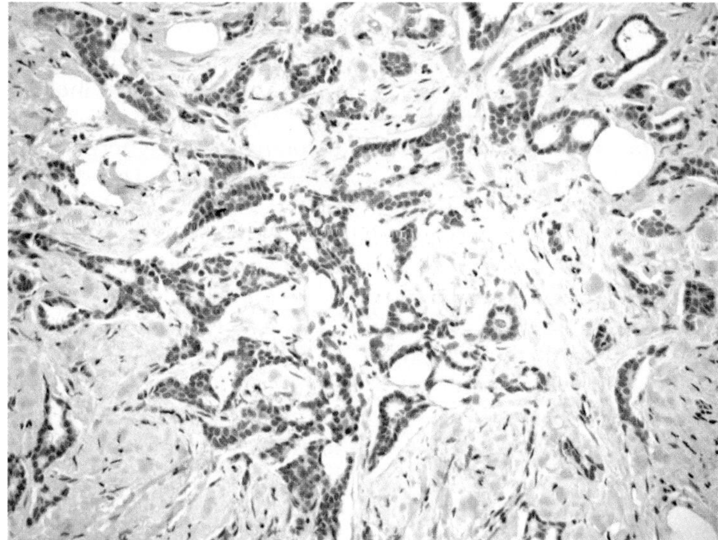

■ **FIGURE 17-16** Tubular carcinoma. Note absence of myoepithelial cell cytoplasmic staining around each gland (SMMHC IHC stain, ×200).

carcinoma, DCIS, LCIS, and atypical ductal hyperplasia.[18] Today, in many practices, needle biopsy with a stereotactic 11-gauge directional vacuum-assisted device is the preferred method. Many of these lesions are carcinoma, rather than radial scar, and subsequent definitive therapy can proceed in the usual manner. For those lesions for which the histologic diagnosis is radial scar on the needle biopsy, most mammographers and pathologists recommend excision of the lesion to exclude sampling error (missing of an associated malignancy). It is possible that radial scar may be definitively diagnosed by needle biopsy, particularly when large amounts of tissue are removed with the large-gauge vacuum-assisted devices.

When the radial scar is found on core needle biopsy, there is also controversy as to what is the appropriate follow-up management. This is because of divergent conclusions on the cancer risk when radial scars are found in the breast; the NHS study found that there is an increased risk, whereas the Nashville and Mayo Clinic studies found no increased risk.

An appropriate management of a patient who is found to have a diagnosis of radial scar after core needle biopsy should be individualized by correlating imaging findings to make sure that the targeted lesion was sampled. If there is any atypia associated with radial scar, excisional biopsy is recommended. If the targeted lesion was not sampled, excisional biopsy is recommended. If a large amount of tissue was removed by the large-gauge vacuum-assisted device and the diagnosis of radial scar was found, careful clinical follow-up may be necessary to rule out additional ipsilateral lesion in the future.

DUCTAL HYPERPLASIA OF USUAL TYPE

Definition

Ductal hyperplasia of usual type, or usual ductal hyperplasia, is a benign epithelial proliferation with an increase in the layers of epithelium lining the glands beyond the usual double cell layer. Epithelial hyperplasia has been categorized as either ductal or lobular. This can be misleading, because it tends to infer a site of origin for these lesions: lobular hyperplasia is thought to arise from the lobular units; ductal hyperplasias do not arise solely from the ducts. In fact, these ductal-pattern lesions usually occur within the terminal duct lobular unit. For this reason, some authors prefer the term *epithelial hyperplasia of usual type* or *of no special type* rather than ductal type.[19] Each type of epithelial hyperplasia has a spectrum of morphologic changes ranging from mild, with almost no increased risk of malignancy, to severe, with patterns approaching that of carcinoma in situ.

Prevalence and Epidemiology

Ductal hyperplasia of usual type is a frequently found lesion in the breast. It is often a common incidental finding seen from reduction mammoplasty to lumpectomy specimen for carcinoma of the breast.

Etiology and Pathophysiology

In response to hormonal stimulation and imbalances, the ductal epithelium can undergo hyperplasia or involution. In hyperplasia, the number of cells above the basement membrane in the glandular structures increases. The proliferating cells may form a variety of histologic patterns, including papillary projections, cribriform spaces, or solid sheets of cells with occlusion of the ductal lumen.

Manifestations of Disease

Clinical Presentation

Ductal hyperplasia of usual type is clinically silent and asymptomatic and, therefore, almost always detected at screening mammography when microcalcifications or masses are present.

Imaging Indications and Algorithm

Screening mammography may detect the presence of microcalcifications in association with ductal hyperplasia of usual type. A diagnostic study including magnification and spot compression views may then be obtained.

Imaging Technique and Findings

Mammography

Ductal hyperplasia of usual type is detected on mammography as tiny, punctate or amorphous clustered calcifications. With the use of digital screening mammography, the detection of such microcalcifications is increasing. Additionally, this lesion is incidentally detected on core needle biopsy of microcalcifications associated with other breast processes (Figs. 17-17 and 17-18).

Ultrasonography

There are no reported ultrasound findings associated with ductal hyperplasia of usual type.

Magnetic Resonance Imaging

There are no reported MRI findings associated with ductal hyperplasia of usual type.

Differential Diagnosis

From Clinical Presentation

Ductal hyperplasia of usual type is clinically silent and asymptomatic.

From Imaging Findings

The differential diagnosis for clustered punctuate or amorphous calcifications includes many benign processes, including apocrine metaplasia, columnar cell change, columnar cell hyperplasia, and calcification associated with microcysts. The differential diagnosis also includes high-risk lesions such as atypical ductal hyperplasia and flat epithelial atypia. Biopsy is often indicated to exclude these atypical lesions or DCIS.

Pathology Findings

Epithelial hyperplasia of ductal type is called usual ductal hyperplasia and occurs in response to hormonal stimulation. Normal breast ducts and lobules consist of one luminal cell layer and one peripheral myoepithelial cell layer (Figs. 17-19 and 17-20). The luminal epithelial layer becomes more than one layer thick in ductal hyperplasia, forming different patterns: gynecomastia-like pattern, papillary projections, cribriform spaces, and solid sheets of cells with occlusion of ductal lumen. Ductal hyperplasia of usual type can be mild, moderate, and florid depending on the degree of luminal epithelial cell proliferations. The characteristic features are epithelial proliferation with the typical streaming pattern and irregular size and shape of luminal fenestrations (Figs. 17-21 to 17-25). Ductal hyperplasia of usual type has a mixture of different size and shape of cells and contains both epithelial luminal and myoepithelial cells. Nuclei are crowded and overlapping without distinct cytoplasmic borders between each cell. Intranuclear inclusions are commonly observed.

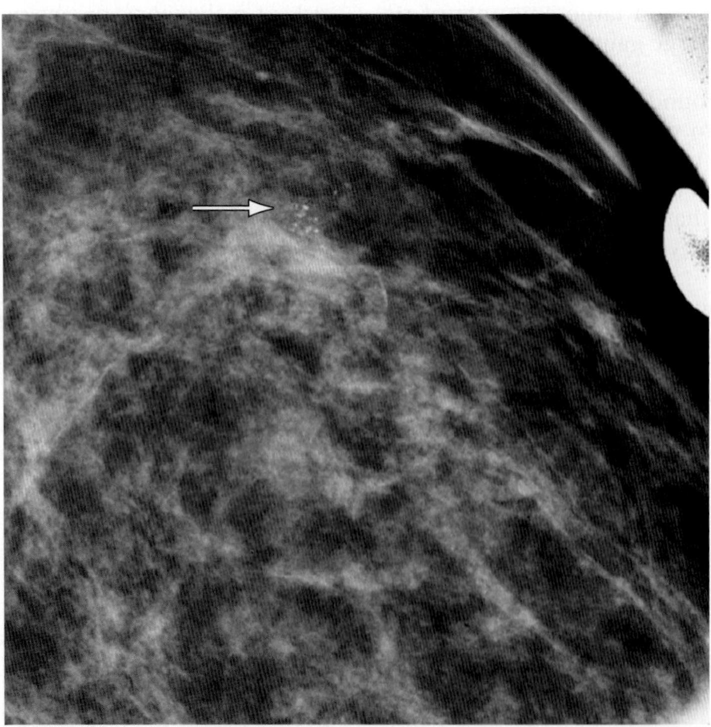

■ **FIGURE 17-17** Usual ductal hyperplasia. Craniocaudal digital magnification view mammogram of the left breast shows a 4-mm cluster of punctuate calcifications (*arrow*). Core needle biopsy demonstrated usual ductal hyperplasia and calcifications within benign ducts.

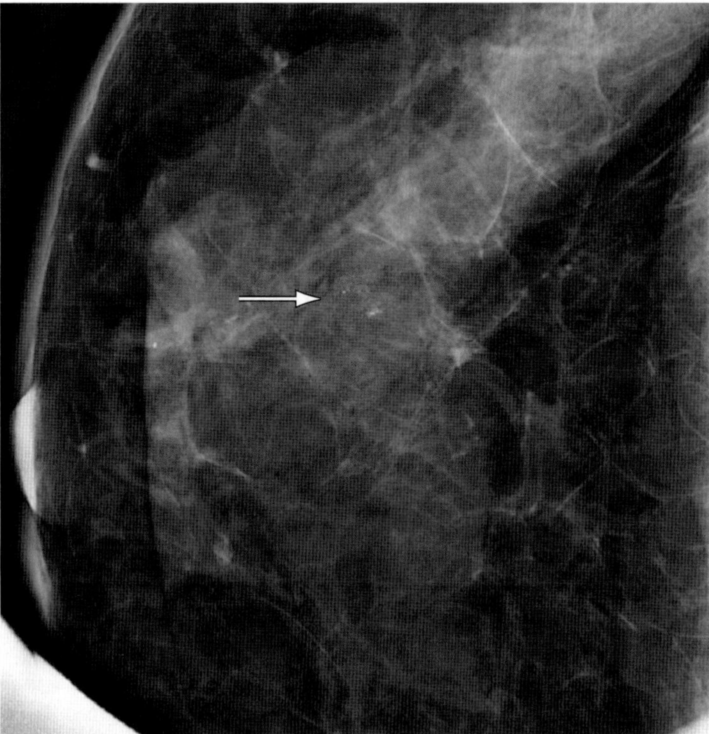

■ **FIGURE 17-18** Usual ductal hyperplasia. Craniocaudal digital magnification view mammogram of the right breast shows a 6-mm cluster of amorphous calcifications (*arrow*). Core needle biopsy demonstrated usual ductal hyperplasia and calcifications within benign ducts.

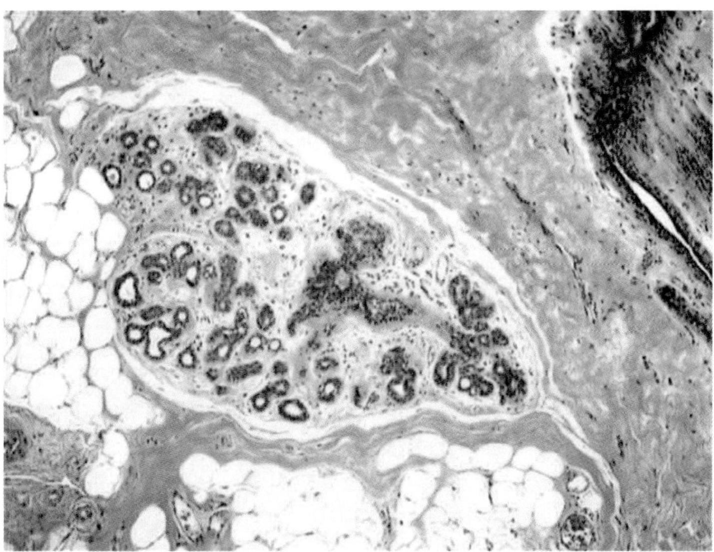

■ **FIGURE 17-19** Normal terminal ductal lobular unit (H&E, ×100).

Central necrosis is rare unless it is associated with radial scars. Mitotic figures are rare in ductal hyperplasia. Ductal hyperplasia is commonly seen with fibrocystic breast changes and is often an incidental finding in women of all ages. A mass lesion that incorporates ductal hyperplasia is seen in pseudoangiomatous stromal hyperplasia (PASH), radial scar, and papillary lesions. The differential diagnosis of usual ductal hyperplasia especially florid type is atypical ductal hyperplasia and low-grade DCIS. Distinction between atypical ductal hyperplasia and DCIS depends on the degree of architectural rigidity and monotonous cytologic atypia. Although architectural and cytomorphologic findings are distinguishable between ductal hyperplasia, atypical ductal hyperplasia and DCIS in most cases,

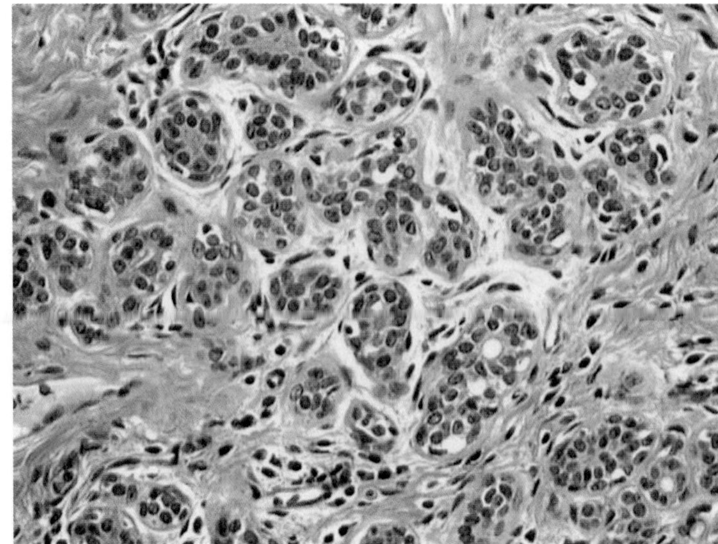

■ **FIGURE 17-20** Normal terminal ductal lobular unit with one layer of inner luminal epithelial cells and peripheral one layer of outer myoepithelial cells (H&E, ×400).

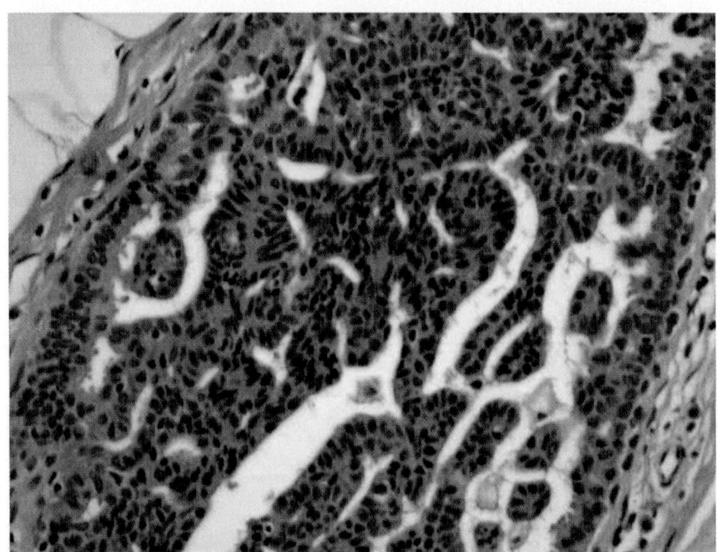

■ **FIGURE 17-21** Ductal hyperplasia of usual type showing florid proliferation of ductal cells filling the entire duct. Microlumens are unevenly distributed and vary in shapes and sizes (H&E, ×400).

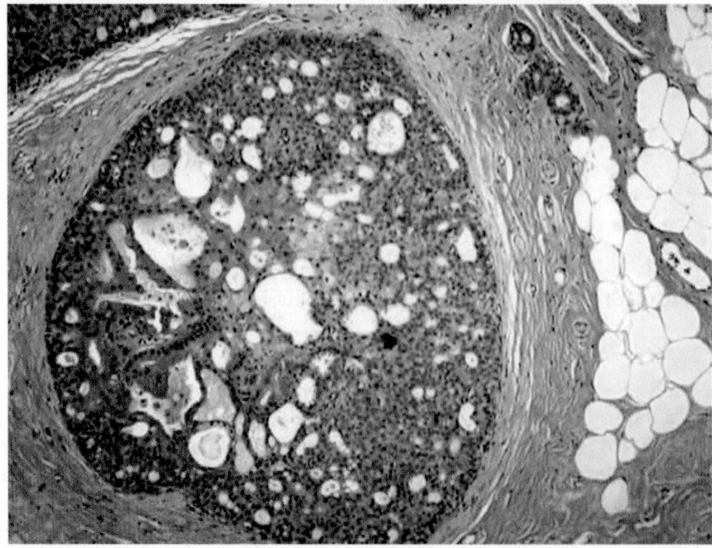

■ **FIGURE 17-22** Ductal hyperplasia of usual type with florid epithelial proliferation and central apocrine metaplasia (H&E, ×100).

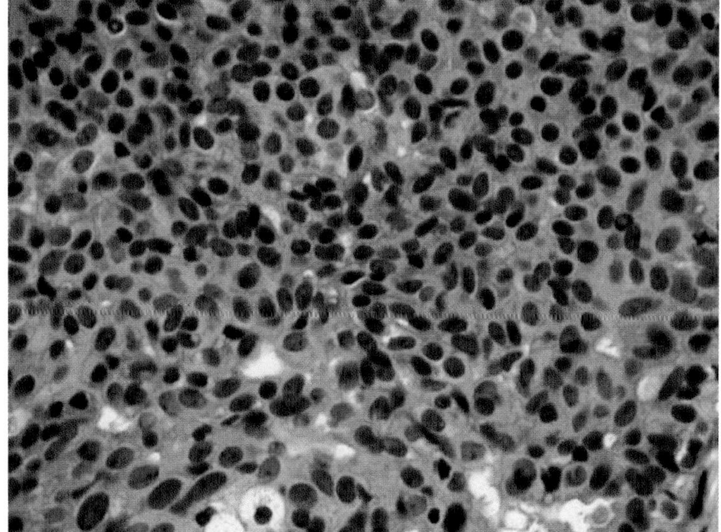

■ **FIGURE 17-23** Ductal hyperplasia of usual type in high-power view showing epithelial cells with overlapping nuclei, indistinct cytoplasmic borders, and polymorphic populations of cells with streaming pattern of growth (H&E, ×400).

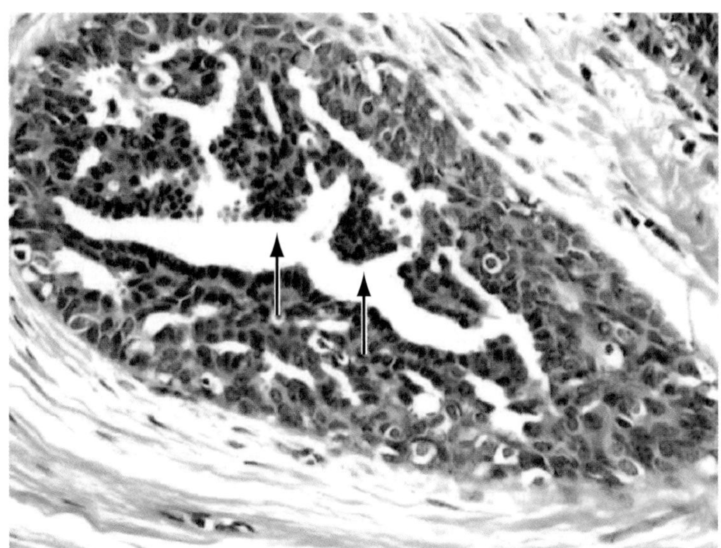

■ **FIGURE 17-24** Ductal hyperplasia of usual type with gynecomastia-like or micropapillary pattern (*arrows*). Epithelial cells traverse and tuft the duct lumen without central fibrovascular cores and secondary lumens are fenestrated (H&E, ×100).

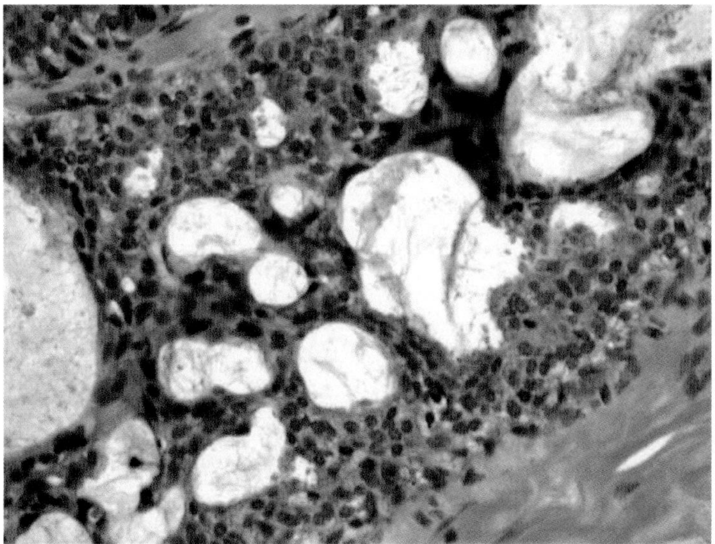

■ **FIGURE 17-25** Ductal hyperplasia of usual type with cribriform pattern showing irregular shapes and sizes of secondary lumens. Nuclei are not polarized (H&E, ×200).

immunohistochemical stains can be used to differentiate these entities. Ductal hyperplasia will have the presence of myoepithelial cells within the luminal proliferation and atypical ductal hyperplasia and DCIS will have none to small numbers of myoepithelial cells within the luminal contents. Immunohistochemical stains that may be helpful include CK34B12 (cytokeratin 903) and CK5/6; both are high-molecular-weight keratin markers. Strong and diffuse staining is helpful in the diagnosis of ductal hyperplasia of usual type. Epithelial hyperplasia is a polymorphic proliferation with a mixture of cell types (epithelial and myoepithelial), and the only important aspect of this lesion is to distinguish it from carcinoma in situ.

Pathologic diagnosis of ductal hyperplasia of usual type only on a core needle biopsy sample should raise a question as to whether the sampling was adequate because most ductal hyperplasia of usual type is an incidental finding. The clinical significance of this lesion is that it has a slight increased RR of 1.5 to 2 times for the subsequent development of breast cancer. The AR depends on the individual patient and includes family history, age, and other factors. Ductal hyperplasia of usual type with other proliferative lesions such as radial scar and sclerosing adenosis will further increase the RR of future development of breast cancer.

Synopsis of Treatment Options

No excisional biopsy is needed when ductal hyperplasia of usual type is diagnosed by core needle biopsy. The reason for the core needle biopsy, such as mass lesion or microcalcifications, has to correlate with the final pathologic diagnosis of ductal hyperplasia of usual type.

GYNECOMASTIA

Definition

Gynecomastia is enlargement of the male breast due to benign ductal and stromal proliferation so that the breast takes on a female form (Greek *gyne*, pertaining to women; *mastos*, breast).

Prevalence and Epidemiology

Approximately 85% of male breast masses are due to gynecomastia, which is the most common disorder in the male breast. It may be detected incidentally at the time of a routine physical examination as either a tender mass beneath the nipple or as a progressive painless enlargement of the breast.[20]

Etiology and Pathophysiology

The development of gynecomastia is believed to be due to hormone imbalance, with a relative excess of female hormones. Pathophysiologic mechanisms resulting in gynecomastia can be divided into the following four categories: (1) estrogen excess; (2) androgen deficiency; (3) androgen receptor defects; and (4) enhanced sensitivity of breast tissue to estrogenic hormones. Gynecomastia can be physiologic or due to underlying diseases, including medication effect. Hormonal manipulation, such as androgen and antiestrogen therapy for prostatic cancer, and drugs, such as digitalis, cimetidine, tricyclic antidepressants, and spironolactone can cause gynecomastia (Table 17-1). Braunstein reported that 25% of patients seeking consultation for gynecomastia are found to have idiopathic gynecomastia; another 25% have pubertal gynecomastia; 10% to 20% of cases are drug related; and 8% are associated with cirrhosis or malnutrition.[21]

TABLE 17-1. Conditions Associated with Gynecomastia

Predisposing Conditions
Estrogen excess
Gonadal origin
True hermaphroditism
Testicular estrogen-producing tumors
Nontesticular tumors
Adrenal cortical neoplasm
Lung carcinoma
Hepatocellular carcinoma
Liver disease
Nonalcoholic and alcoholic cirrhosis
Androgen deficiency
Aging
Hypoandrogen states
Primary testicular failure
Klinefelter syndrome (XXY)
Kallmann syndrome
Secondary testicular failure
Trauma
Orchitis
Cryptorchidism
Irradiation
Hydrocele
Varicocele
Spermatocele
Renal failure
Drug-Related Conditions
Drugs with estrogenic or estrogen-related activity
Anabolic steroids
Digitalis
Heroin
Drugs that inhibit the action and/or synthesis of testosterone
Antineoplastic agents (vincristine, nitrosoureas, methotrexate)
Cimetidine
D-Penicillamine
Diazepam
Flutamide
Ketoconazole
Phenytoin
Spironolactone
Drugs with unknown mechanisms for induction of gynecomastia
Amiodarone
Busulfan
Furosemide
Isoniazid
Methyldopa
Reserpine
Theophylline
Tricyclic antidepressants
Verapamil

Adapted from Bland KI, Page DL. Gynecomastia. In: Bland KI, Copeland EM III, editors. *The breast: comprehensive management of benign and malignant diseases.* Philadelphia, WB Saunders, 1991.

Manifestations of Disease

Clinical Presentation

Patients with gynecomastia are generally asymptomatic; however, breast tenderness is reported in 20% of cases. If present, nipple discharge should be viewed with suspicion because a much higher percentage of cases of male breast cancer demonstrate this feature compared with cases of gynecomastia. Physiologic gynecomastia has three distinct peaks in age distribution; they are neonatal, pubertal, and senescent.[22]

The physical appearance of the breasts of obese men may simulate gynecomastia through deposition of adipose tissue (pseudogynecomastia).

Imaging Indications and Algorithm

The gold standard for imaging gynecomastia is mammography. If a suspicious mass or calcifications are identified, further imaging may be obtained, including additional mammographic images (spot compression or magnification views) and ultrasonography. There is no role for ultrasound evaluation if the mammogram is diagnostic for gynecomastia in the absence of additional suspicious findings.

Imaging Technique and Findings

Mammography

Mammography of the normal breast shows a homogeneously radiolucent appearance with minimal strands of ductal or interlobar connective tissue. The mammographic hallmark of gynecomastia is the presence of a subareolar density concentrically distributed around the nipple.[22] Gynecomastia can be unilateral or bilateral and bilaterally symmetric or asymmetric. Three mammographic patterns of gynecomastia have been described. The first pattern is the *early nodular pattern* (florid phase on histopathology), which is seen in patients with gynecomastia of less than 1 year's duration.[22] In this type, a relatively well-demarcated mass under the nipple extends into the posterior fatty tissue of the breast in a fan-like configuration, evenly distributed above and below the midplane of the nipple. In more severe cases, the mass becomes triangular in appearance with the nipple at the vertex of the triangle or becomes a subareolar, disc-shaped mass. A later *dendritic pattern* (quiescent fibrous phase on histopathology) features a flame-shaped central subareolar opacity with prominent linear projections (dendrites) radiating into the deeper adipose tissue toward the upper outer quadrant of the breast. A *diffuse glandular* pattern features a diffuse, dense nodular parenchyma in an enlarged breast that mimics the density seen in a dense female breast. This pattern of gynecomastia is commonly seen in patients who receive exogenous estrogen, such as men who undergo a sex change operation and those who are treated for advanced prostatic carcinoma. In these situations, the relatively rapid breast enlargement usually has a conical or pyramidal contour, unlike the rather rounded or hemispheric shape found in women. Severe gynecomastia can also be distinguished from a dense female breast by the lack of Cooper ligaments (Figs. 17-26 and 17-27).

Pseudogynecomastia, an enlargement of the breast due to obesity, is readily differentiated from true gynecomastia by means of the preponderance of radiolucent fat and the absence of dense retroareolar tissue in pseudogynecomastia (Fig. 17-28).

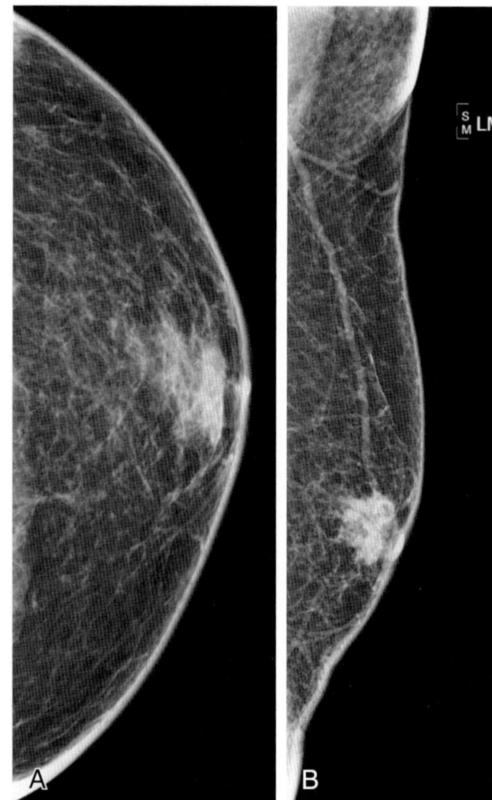

■ **FIGURE 17-26** Early gynecomastia. Craniocaudal (**A**) and mediolateral oblique (**B**) digital mammograms of the left breast in a male patient show glandular tissue in the retroareolar region.

Ultrasonography

The ultrasonographic appearance of gynecomastia demonstrates breast tissue in the subareolar palpable area and often mimics the ultrasonographic findings in developing female breasts.[23] The ultrasonographic appearance of gynecomastia can be directly correlated with the findings on mammographic and histologic examinations. Initially, there is small subareolar hypoechogenicity with a definable, slightly lobulated posterior border representing ductal hyperplasia of the nodular phase. In the dendritic phase, the posterior border of the subareolar hypoechoic change becomes angular with finger-like projections. Occasionally, it may be difficult to differentiate between early carcinoma and nodular gynecomastia because both conditions are hypoechoic. However, changes in gynecomastia are always subareolar in location and the hypoechogenicity is not associated with acoustic shadowing, a finding often seen in carcinoma. In the late stage, when more fibrosis develops, there is an increase in the echogenicity of the breast parenchyma, almost similar to the fibroglandular echogenicity in the female breast (Fig. 17-29).

Magnetic Resonance Imaging

Gynecomastia appears similar to female normal fibroglandular tissue characterized by homogeneous, non-mass-like enhancement and normal fibroglandular

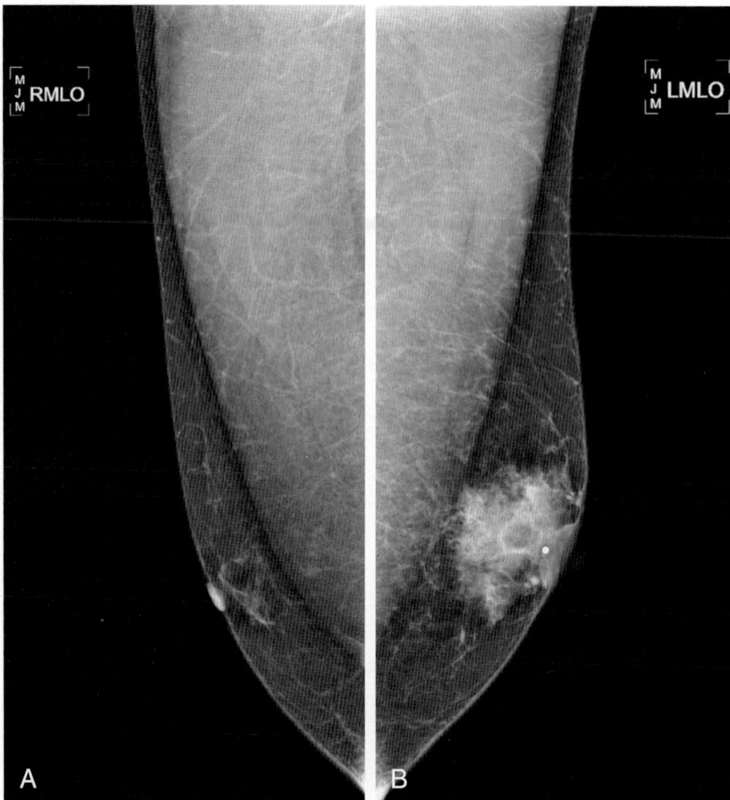

■ **FIGURE 17-27** Asymmetric gynecomastia. Bilateral mediolateral oblique (**A**) and (**B**) digital mammograms show moderate left gynecomastia and a normal right male breast. A BB denotes a palpable abnormality of the left breast.

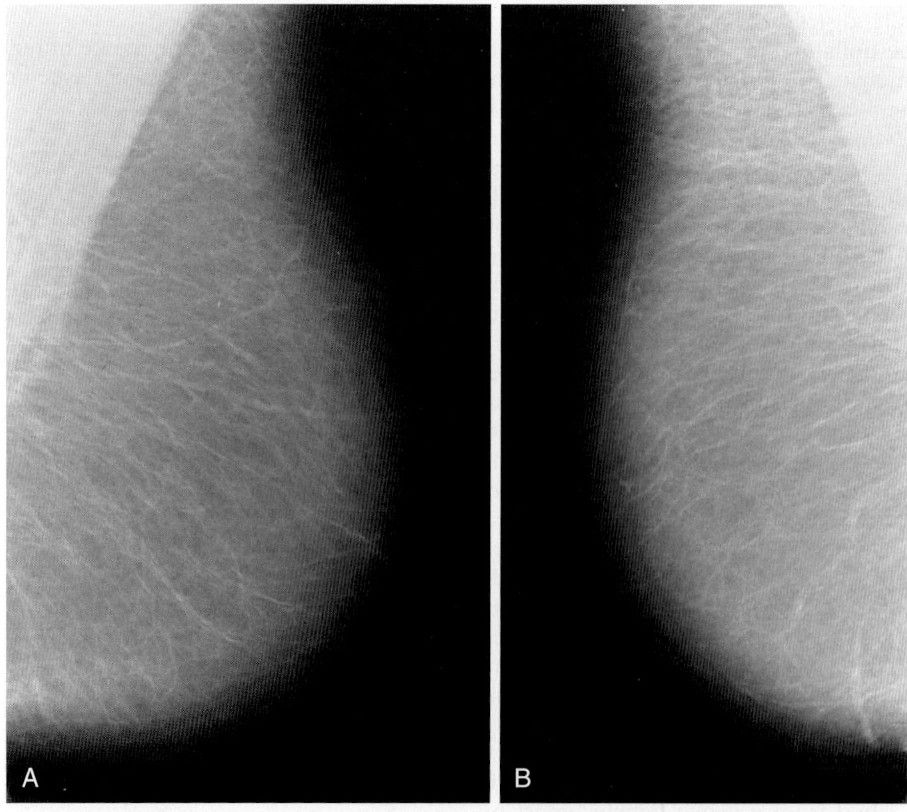

■ **FIGURE 17-28** Pseudogynecomastia in an obese man. Bilateral mediolateral oblique mammograms (**A and B**) show only fat, blood vessels, and supporting stroma. The absence of retroareolar densities ruled out true gynecomastia. *(From Chantra PK, So GJ, Wollman JS, Bassett LW. Mammography of the male breast. AJR Am J Roentgenol 1995;164:853-858.)*

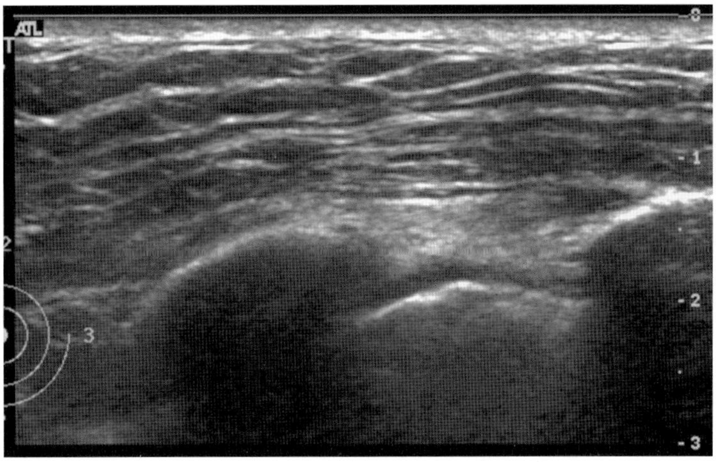

■ **FIGURE 17-29** Gynecomastia. Right breast ultrasound image shows fibroglandular tissue.

architecture. Kinetic analysis shows a slow initial phase and a persistent delayed phase.[24]

Classic Signs

Gynecomastia commonly appears as a flame-shaped central subareolar opacity on a mammogram.

Differential Diagnosis

From Clinical Presentation

The differential diagnosis for an enlarged breast or palpable mass in the male patient includes gynecomastia, pseudogynecomastia, and breast carcinoma. A complete physical examination should ensue. If clinical findings fail to differentiate among these, imaging is warranted.

From Imaging Findings

The purpose of mammography is to reliably differentiate between benign conditions and breast carcinoma. The differential diagnosis of benign breast conditions in a male breast includes gynecomastia, pseudogynecomastia, lipoma, duct ectasia, intraductal papilloma, fat necrosis, abscess, and epidermal inclusion cyst.

Pathology Findings

Gynecomastia is the most common breast lesion in the male. Gross examination of gynecomastia is soft to firm depending on the amount of fibrous tissue, gray to white without a mass lesion.

Microscopically, gynecomastia shows florid ductal hyperplasia of usual type with micropapillary tufting into the lumen, periductal stromal edema, and fibrosis. Changes similar to PASH are common (Figs. 17-30 and 17-31). There are two types of gynecomastia: active type with florid epithelial hyperplasia and fibrous type. Gynecomastia-like ductal hyperplasia seen in the female breast is indistinguishable microscopically from florid gynecomastia. Invasive carcinoma can be seen in conjunction with gynecomastia, but there is no evidence that gynecomastia is an

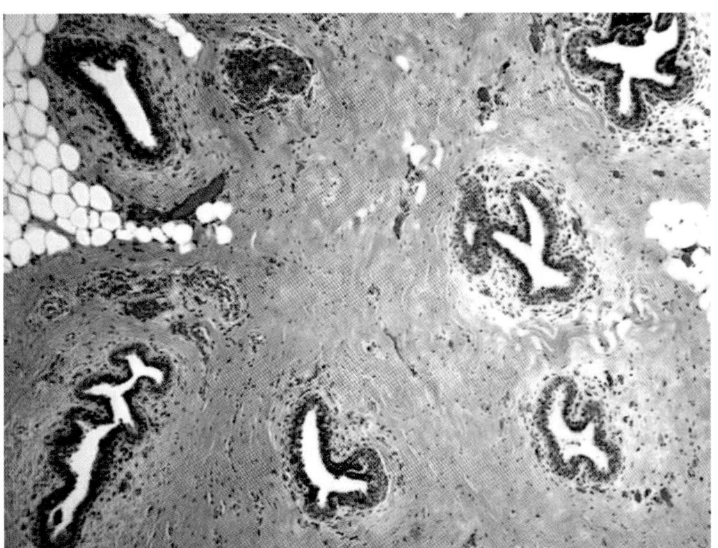

■ **FIGURE 17-30** Low power view of male gynecomastia. Mild degree of epithelial hyperplasia with periductal stroma edema and fibrotic stroma is seen (H&E, ×40).

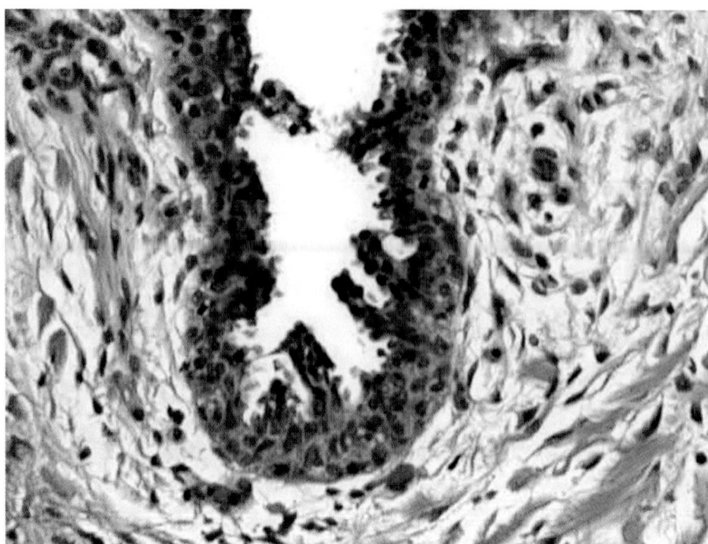

■ **FIGURE 17-31** Epithelial hyperplasia in gynecomastia shows luminal micropapillary tufting, which are finger-like projections (H&E, ×400).

obligatory precursor lesion to carcinoma. Gynecomastia is a self-limiting process. It often regresses when a specific etiology agent is withdrawn. In early gynecomastia, or in the florid histopathologic phase, proliferation of the ducts and formation of a loose, cellular, and richly vascular stroma with scattered mononuclear cells occur. The ductal system dilates and lengthens with an increase in the number of branches and typically shows epithelial hyperplasia. With time, the number of the ducts and the extent of epithelial hyperplasia become less prominent as fibrosis and hyalinization slowly replace the ductal system. The later fibrous quiescent phase takes place about a year after the onset of gynecomastia.

Synopsis of Treatment Options

When a patient is referred for evaluation of possible gynecomastia, a careful drug history should be taken. The breast and regional lymph nodes should be palpated, and physical signs of hyperthyroidism, liver failure, and testicular atrophy or tumor should be excluded.[25] Hormonal investigation (measurements of serum testosterone, estradiol, human chorionic gonadotropin, luteinizing hormone, prolactin, liver function, thyroid-stimulating hormone, and thyroxine) should be reserved for patients with recent breast enlargement and no identifiable cause. Depressed levels of luteinizing hormone or increased human chorionic gonadotropin and estradiol values are indications for testicular ultrasonography; if ultrasonographic findings are normal, chest radiography and abdominal computed tomography should be considered.

Most cases of gynecomastia are idiopathic and resolve spontaneously. In other cases, gynecomastia is reversible if the causative factors are removed in the early stages of development. The literature suggests that medical treatment with a trial of tamoxifen may be beneficial during the acute phase. However, once gynecomastia has evolved to the stage of extensive fibrosis, the process may be irreversible. Surgical management is often the treatment of choice.

MICROGLANDULAR ADENOSIS

Definition

Microglandular adenosis is a rare lesion of the breast and characterized by a proliferation of glandular epithelium that mimics invasive ductal carcinoma.

Prevalence and Epidemiology

Microglandular adenosis is a rare lesion of the breast. Carcinoma or DCIS is associated. Microglandular adenosis has been reported in women in all ages.

Etiology and Pathophysiology

The etiology of microglandular adenosis is unknown.

Manifestations of Disease

Clinical Presentation

Microglandular adenosis can present as a mass lesion or as an incidental finding.

Imaging Technique and Findings

There are no specific findings of microglandular adenosis evident in radiography.

Pathology Findings

Microglandular adenosis is a rare variant of adenosis of the breast and is characterized by a proliferation of glandular epithelium that mimics invasive ductal carcinoma. Grossly, microglandular adenosis is an ill-defined infiltrative tumor like invasive ductal carcinoma. Microscopically, it shows small glands in fibrous and fatty breast parenchyma without lobulocentric configurations and stromal desmoplasia. The most characteristic features are the presence of amorphous, eosinophilic globules in the lumen, which are usually periodic acid-Schiff (PAS) diastase-resistant-positive material, and round small glands lined by a single layer without myoepithelial cells (Figs. 17-32 to 17-35). Because microglandular adenosis lacks myoepithelial cells, immunohistochemical stains for myoepithelial cells also will be negative, which further complicates separation from well differentiated invasive ductal carcinoma or tubular carcinoma. Recognizing this entity is important. Microglandular adenosis is usually strongly positive with S-100, cytokeratin, E-cadherin, and cathepsin D. It is often negative for estrogen receptor (ER), progesterone receptor (PR), and human epidermal growth factor receptor 2 (HER2/neu). Well-differentiated ductal or tubular carcinomas are usually positive with ER and PR. Microglandular adenosis can be seen in association with sclerosing adenosis. Atypical microglandular adenosis is also seen with cytologically atypical epithelial proliferation. DCIS and invasive carcinoma have been described arising in microglandular adenosis (Figs. 17-36 and 17-37). Carcinomas arising from microglandular adenosis also tend not to express ER, PR and HER2/neu. Long-term follow-up studies are lacking in otherwise typical microglandular adenosis. Thus, in excisional biopsy it is recommended that a specimen with a clear margin be obtained, which may be difficult because of the infiltrative pattern of microglandular adenosis without stromal changes.

Synopsis of Treatment Options

A complete excision of microglandular adenosis is prudent, especially when there is associated atypia, because residual lesion can give rise to recurrent carcinoma in this setting.[26]

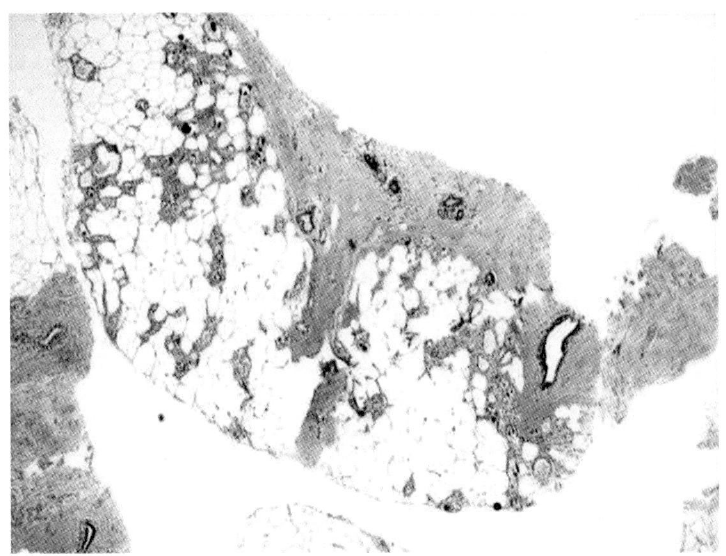

■ **FIGURE 17-32** Microglandular adenosis in core needle biopsy. Infiltrative pattern of round small glandular proliferations in fibrofatty stroma is shown (H&E, ×40).

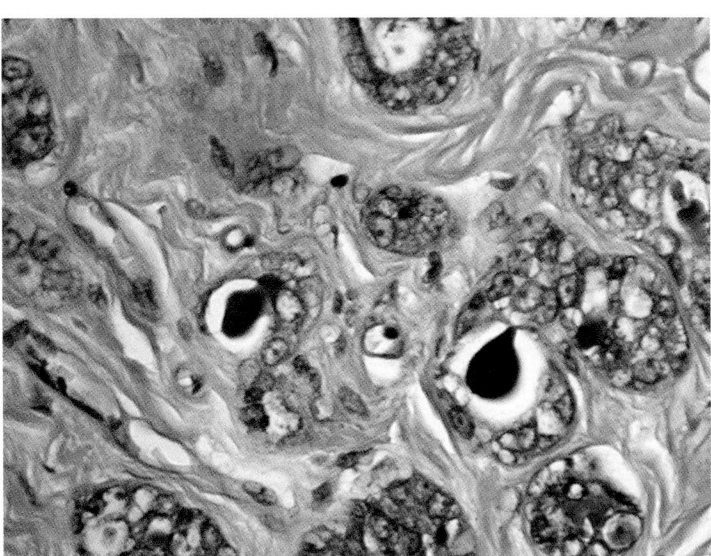

■ **FIGURE 17-33** Microglandular adenosis is positive with periodic acid-Schiff (PAS) stain in the luminal eosinophilic secretions (PAS, ×400).

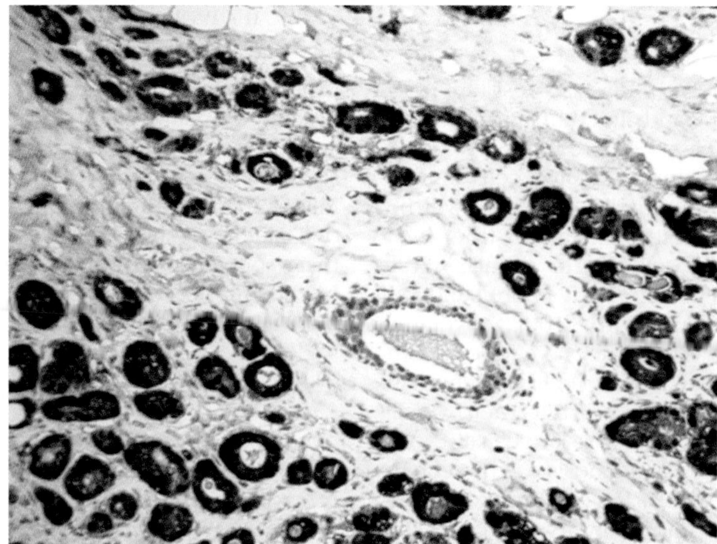

■ **FIGURE 17-34** Microglandular adenosis is strongly positive with S-100 protein stain (S-100 IHC, ×100).

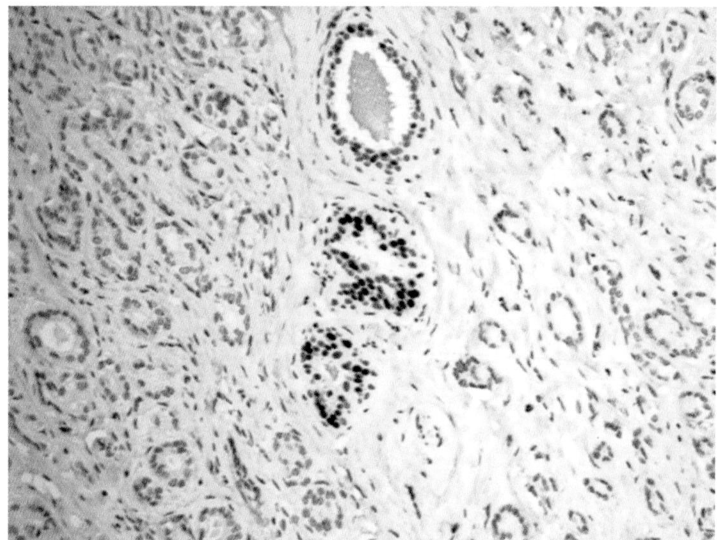

■ **FIGURE 17-35** Normal ducts are positive for estrogen receptor but microglandular adenosis is not positive with estrogen receptor (ER IHC stain, ×100).

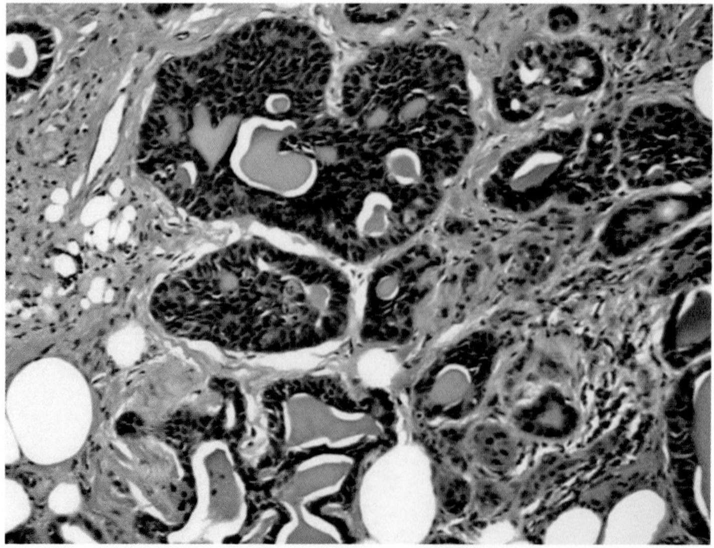

■ **FIGURE 17-36** Atypical microglandular adenosis showing cytologically atypical cell proliferation adjacent to the lesion (H&E, ×200).

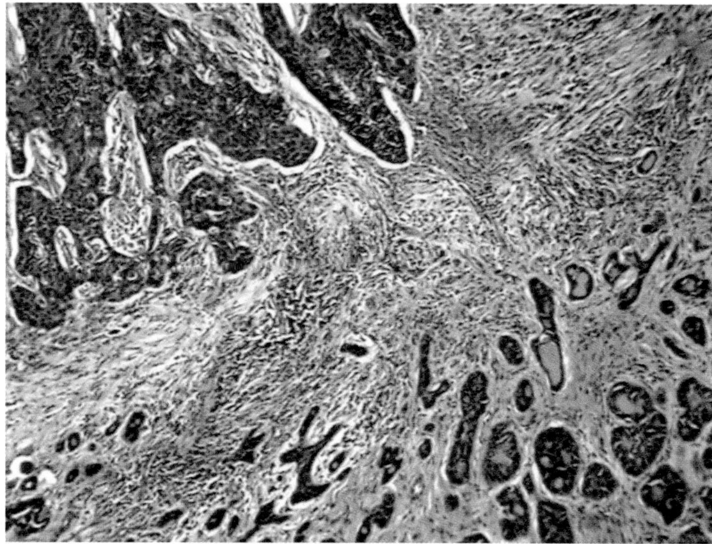

■ **FIGURE 17-37** Atypical microglandular adenosis and invasive ductal carcinoma are seen in the same slide (H&E, ×100).

KEY POINTS

- Radial scar and sclerosing adenosis are benign breast lesions characterized by sclerotic and hyalinized scar and proliferative ducts. Both lesions have imaging features and gross and microscopic appearances similar to invasive carcinoma of the breast.
- Ductal hyperplasia of usual type or epithelial hyperplasia is a benign epithelial proliferation with an increase in the layers of epithelium lining the glands beyond the usual double cell layer from the terminal ductal lobular units. Mammographically, this lesion may present as punctate or amorphous clustered calcifications; however, biopsy is often indicated to exclude high-risk pathology.
- Gynecomastia is enlargement of the male breast due to benign ductal and stromal proliferation so that the breast takes on a female form. It commonly appears as a flame-shaped central subareolar opacity on a mammogram.
- Microglandular adenosis is a rare lesion of the breast characterized by a proliferation of glandular epithelium that mimics invasive ductal carcinoma.

SUGGESTED READINGS

D'Orsi CJ, Feldhaus L, Sonnenfeld M. Unusual lesions of the breast. *Radiol Clin North Am* 1983;**21**:67-80.

Dupont WD, Page DL. Risk factors for breast cancer in women with proliferative breast disease. *N Engl J Med* 1985;**312**:146-51.

Dupont WD, Parl FF, Hartmann WH, Brinton LA, Winfield AC, Worrell JA, et al. Breast cancer risk associated with proliferative breast disease and atypical hyperplasia. *Cancer* 1993;**71**:1258-65.

Hartmann L, Sellers T, Frost MH, Lingle WL, Degnim AC, Ghosh K, et al. Benign breast disease and the risk of breast cancer. *N Engl J Med* 2005;**353**:229-37.

Jacobs TW, Byrne C, Colditz G, Connolly JL, Schnitt SJ. Radial scars in benign breast-biopsy specimens and the risk of breast cancer. *N Engl J Med* 1999;**340**:430-6.

Page D, Dupont W. Benign breast disease: indicators of increased breast cancer risk. *Cancer Detect Prev* 1992;**16**:93-7.

Page DL, Anderson TJ, Rogers LW. Epithelial hyperplasia. In: *The breast*. Edinburgh: Churchill Livingstone; 1987. p. 120-56.

REFERENCES

1. Foote FW, Stewart FW. Comparative studies of cancerous versus noncancerous breast. *Ann Surg* 1942;**121**:197-222.
2. Jensen RA, Page DL, Dupont WD, Rogers LW. Invasive breast cancer risk in women with sclerosing adenosis. *Cancer* 1898;**64**:1977-83.
3. Liberman L, Morris EA, Dershaw DD, Abramson AF, Tan LK. Ductal enhancement on MR imaging of the breast. *AJR Am J Roentgenol* 2003;**181**:519-25.
4. Dupont WD, Page DL. Risk factors for breast cancer in women with proliferative breast disease. *N Engl J Med* 1985;**312**:146-51.
5. Hrieger N, Hiatt RA. Risk of breast cancer after benign breast diseases: variation by histologic type, degree of atypia, age at biopsy, and length of follow-up. *Am J Epidemiol* 1992;**136**:619-31.
6. Jacobs TW, Connolly J, Schnitt S. Nonmalignant lesions in the breast needle core biopsies. To excise or not to excise? *Am J Surg Pathol* 2002;**26**:1095-110.

7. Fisher ER, Palekar AS, Kotwal N, Lipana N. A nonencapsulated sclerosing lesion of the breast. *Am J Clin Pathol* 1976;**71**:240–6.
8. Wellings SR, Alpers CE. An atlas of subgross pathology of the human breast with special reference to possible precancerous lesions. *J. Natl Cancer Inst* 1975;**55**:231–73.
9. Alder DD, Helvie MA, Oberman HA, Ikeda DM, Bhan AO. Radial sclerosing lesion of the breast: mammographic features. *Radiology* 1990;**176**:737–40.
10. Ciatto S, Morrone D, Catarzi S, Del Turco MR, Bianchi S, Ambrogetti D, et al. Radial scars of the breast: review of 38 consecutive mammographic diagnoses. *Radiology* 1993;**187**:757–756.
11. Tabar L, Dean PB. Stellate/speculated lesions. In: Tabar L, Dean PB, editors. *Teaching atlas of mammography*. 3rd ed. Stuttgart: Thieme; 2001. p. 93–147.
12. D'Orsi CJ, Feldhaus L, Sonnenfeld M. Unusual lesions of the breast. *Radiol Clin North Am* 1983;**21**:67–80.
13. Kopans DB. Pathologic, mammographic, and ultrasonographic correlation. In: Kopans DB, editor. *Breast imaging*. 2nd ed. Philadelphia: Lippincott-Raven; 1997. p. 511–615.
14. Nunes LW, Schnall MD, Orel SG, Hochman MG, Langlotz CP, Reynolds CA, et al. Correlation of lesion appearance and histologic findings for the nodes of a breast MR imaging interpretation model. *Radiographics* 1999;**19**:79–92.
15. Sloane JP, Mayers MM. Carcinoma and atypical hyperplasia in radial scars and complex sclerosing lesions: importance of lesion size and patient age. *Histopathology* 1993;**23**:225–31.
16. Jacobs TW, Byrne C, Colditz G, Connolly JL, Schnitt SJ. Radial scars in benign breast biopsy specimens and the risk of breast cancer. *N Engl J Med* 1999;**340**:430–6.
17. Jacobs TW, Connolly J, Schnitt S. Nonmalignant lesions in the breast needle core biopsies. To excise or not to excise. *Am J Surg Pathol* 2002;**26**:1095–110.
18. Brenner RJ, Jackman RJ, Parker SH, Evans WP 3rd, Philpotts L, Deutch BM, et al. Percutaneous core needle biopsy of radial scars of the breast: when is excision necessary? *AJR Am J Roentgenol* 2003;**179**:1179–84.
19. Page DL, Anderson TJ, Rogers LW. Epithelial hyperplasia. In: *The breast*. Edinburgh: Churchill Livingstone; 1987. p. 120–56.
20. Hill A, Yagmur Y, Tran KN, Bolton JS, Robson M, Borgen PI. Localized male breast carcinoma and family history. An analysis of 142 patients. *Cancer* 1999;**86**:821–5.
21. Braunstein G. Gynecomastia. *N Engl J Med* 1993;**328**:490–5.
22. Dershaw D. Male mammography. *AJR Am J Roentgenol* 1986;**146**:127–31.
23. Weinstein SP, Conant EF, Orel SG, Zuckerman JA, Bellah R. Spectrum of US findings in pediatric and adolescent patients with palpable breast masses. *Radiographics* 2000;**20**:1613–21.
24. Morakkabati-Spitz N, Schild HH, Leutner CC, von Falkenhausen M, Lutterbey G, Kuhl CK. Dynamic contrast-enhanced breast MR imaging in men: preliminary results. *Radiology* 2006;**238**:438–45.
25. Macmillan D, Dixon M. Gynaecomastia: When is action required? *Practitioner* 2000;**244**:785–7.
26. Resetkova E, Flanders DJ, Rosen PP. Ten-year follow-up of mammary carcinoma arising in microglandular adenosis treated with breast conservation. *Arch Pathol Lab Med* 2003;**127**:77–88.

CHAPTER 18

Typical Benign Calcifications

Sophia Kim Apple, Lawrence W. Bassett, and Erum W. Sethi

The vast majority of calcifications that occur within the breast are benign. The morphology and distribution of the calcifications help determine whether they are benign or suspicious. Typically, benign calcifications include vascular, dystrophic lucent-centered, or layered calcifications. A regional or diffuse distribution is more common with benign calcifications. Further evaluation is usually not necessary, but additional projections and magnification views can be performed for calcifications that appear indeterminate on the standard projections. Biopsy is usually not performed for these typical benign calcifications but may be done in cases for which the findings are not definitively determined.

MILK OF CALCIUM

Milk of calcium collects within the dependent portion of microcysts or macrocysts (Fig. 18-1) and has been observed in approximately 4% of patients.[1] On horizontal beam images (mediolateral or lateromedial), layering calcifications have a linear or crescent shape—the *teacup* sign (Fig. 18-2), whereas on vertical beam films (craniocaudal), the calcification is rounded or amorphous (Fig. 18-3).[1-4] It is critically important to obtain magnification views in the 90-degree lateral (mediolateral or lateromedial) and craniocaudal projections to best assess the configuration of the calcification. When all of the calcifications are typical for milk of calcium, the benign cystic nature of the lesion is confirmed and further evaluation (including ultrasonography) or intervention is not necessary.

DERMAL CALCIFICATIONS

Calcifications often occur within the sebaceous glands of the skin. They are not visible on inspection of the skin during physical examination and are of no clinical consequence. They may, however, cause confusion on mammography. Depending on their location, dermal calcifications may be projected peripherally on one or more mammographic views, or they may appear to be within the parenchyma. The most common appearance on mammography is faint spherical or polygonal lucent-centered calcifications, which are frequently clustered (Figs. 18-4 and 18-5).[5] They occur most often in the inferior and medial aspect of the breasts.

Some dermal calcifications do not have a characteristic appearance and appear only as nonspecific clustered microcalcifications.[5] Skin calcifications should be suspected when the calcifications appear to be quite superficial on at least one view. In these cases, further workup is necessary to determine whether they are dermal or parenchymal. This is most easily done with the use of a grid or fenestrated mammographic compression paddle.[6] The standard mediolateral oblique (MLO) and craniocaudal (CC) views are reviewed to determine the skin surface closest to the calcifications, and the breast from the woman is placed in the mammography unit with the grid or fenestrated paddle against that skin surface. A film in this projection is processed and reviewed while the breast remains in compression (Fig. 18-6A). The coordinates of the calcifications are used to guide placement of a metallic BB (Fig. 18-6B) on the skin before a tangential view is obtained (Fig. 18-6C).

It is important to distinguish between dermal and parenchymal calcifications if a recommendation for biopsy is contemplated, because dermal calcifications are always benign and breast biopsies do not usually include skin. Thus, specimen radiographs do not include the calcifications. Unnecessary biopsies can be avoided at the time of stereotactic needle biopsy by noting that the targeted calcifications are at the same depth as the skin or at the time of presurgical needle localization by placing a metallic BB at the skin entry site of the localizing needle. If the calcifications are located within the skin, their location will be

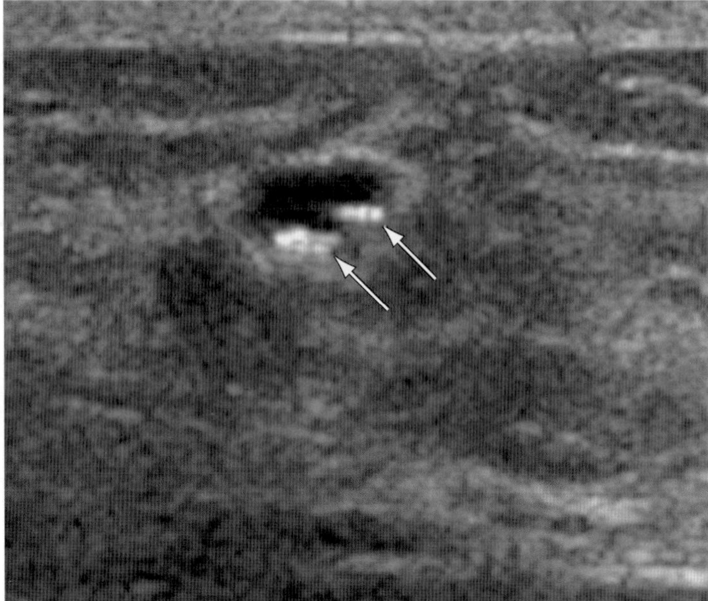

■ **FIGURE 18-1** Milk of calcium. Layering milk of calcium (*arrows*) within microcysts on ultrasonography.

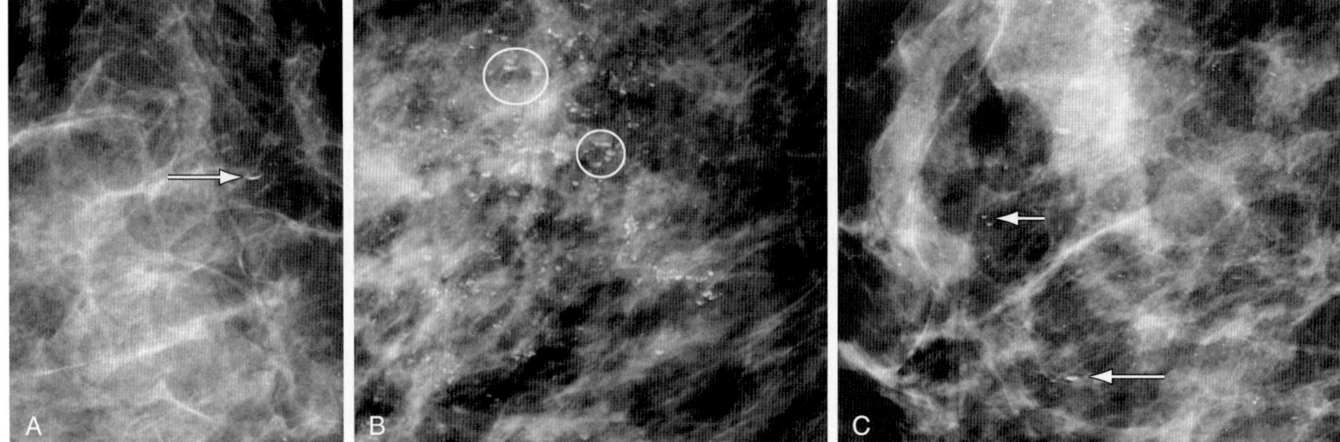

■ **FIGURE 18-2** Milk of calcium. Crescent-shaped milk of calcium (*arrow*) on the mediolateral projection: the *teacup* sign (**A**). Layering milk of calcium (**B**) (*circles*) and (**C**) (*arrows*) on the mediolateral projection.

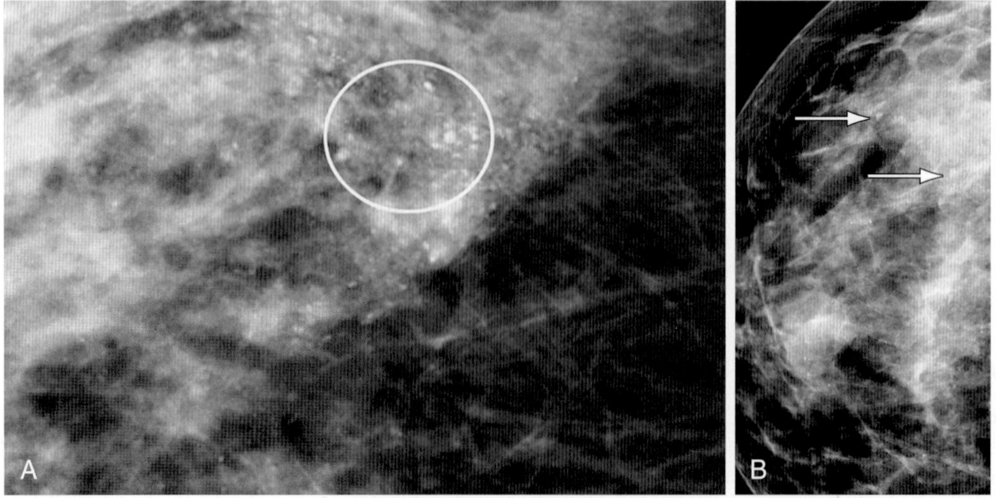

■ **FIGURE 18-3** Milk of calcium. **A,** Amorphous and round milk of calcium (*circle*) seen en face on the craniocaudal (CC) projection. **B,** Amorphous and round milk of calcium (*arrows*) seen en face is much more difficult to see on the CC projection.

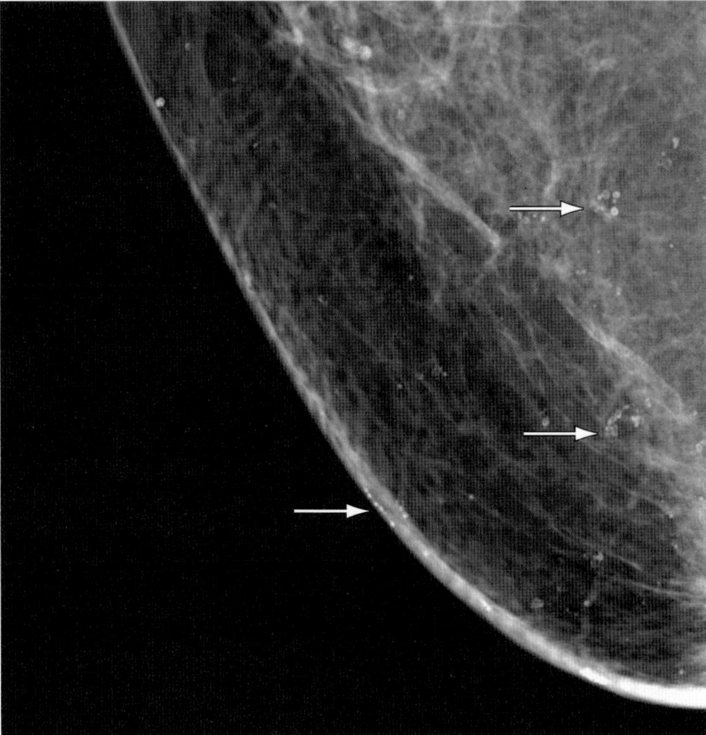

■ **FIGURE 18-4** Dermal calcifications. Lucent-centered, round dermal calcifications (*arrows*).

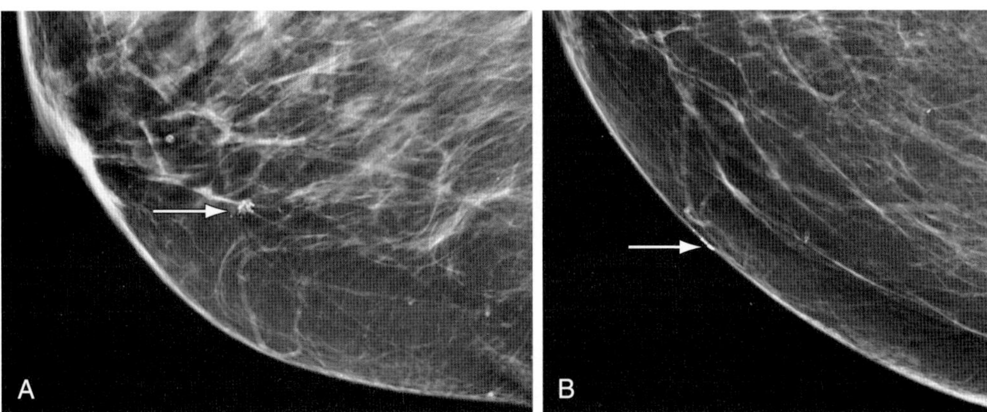

■ **FIGURE 18-5** Dermal calcifications. **A,** Cluster of punctate and round calcifications (*arrow*) on the craniocaudal (CC) projection. **B,** Cluster of calcifications (*arrow*) is clearly in the skin on the mediolateral oblique (MLO) projection.

obvious when the orthogonal view for needle placement is obtained with the BB in tangent. The needle then can be withdrawn and the biopsy canceled.[7] Unfortunately, some women have multiple unsuccessful surgical biopsies to remove clusters of dermal calcifications when the true location has not been recognized. Even today, some women are subjected to unnecessary anxiety if stereotactic biopsy is recommended for calcifications that are not recognized as dermal in location.

DERMATOMYOSITIS

Dermatomyositis is a condition of diffuse inflammation and degeneration involving the skeletal muscles and skin. It most frequently affects middle-aged women and may be manifested on mammography as subcutaneous calcifications. The calcifications are large, dense, clearly benign, and often bizarre (Figs. 18-7 and 18-8).[8] Fifteen percent to 25% of patients with dermatomyositis also have a malignancy. This situation most commonly occurs in men. In women, breast cancer has been reported to be one of the associated malignancies.[9,10]

SUBSTANCES ON THE SKIN

A number of materials that are applied to the skin are radiopaque. The best known is underarm antiperspirant, which contains aluminum chlorhydrate (Fig. 18-9). Plain deodorant does not contain metallic material and therefore is not visible on mammography. Although most facilities recommend that women not use antiperspirant before mammography, not all women follow this recommendation; it is also possible that some of the material may remain within skin crevices after

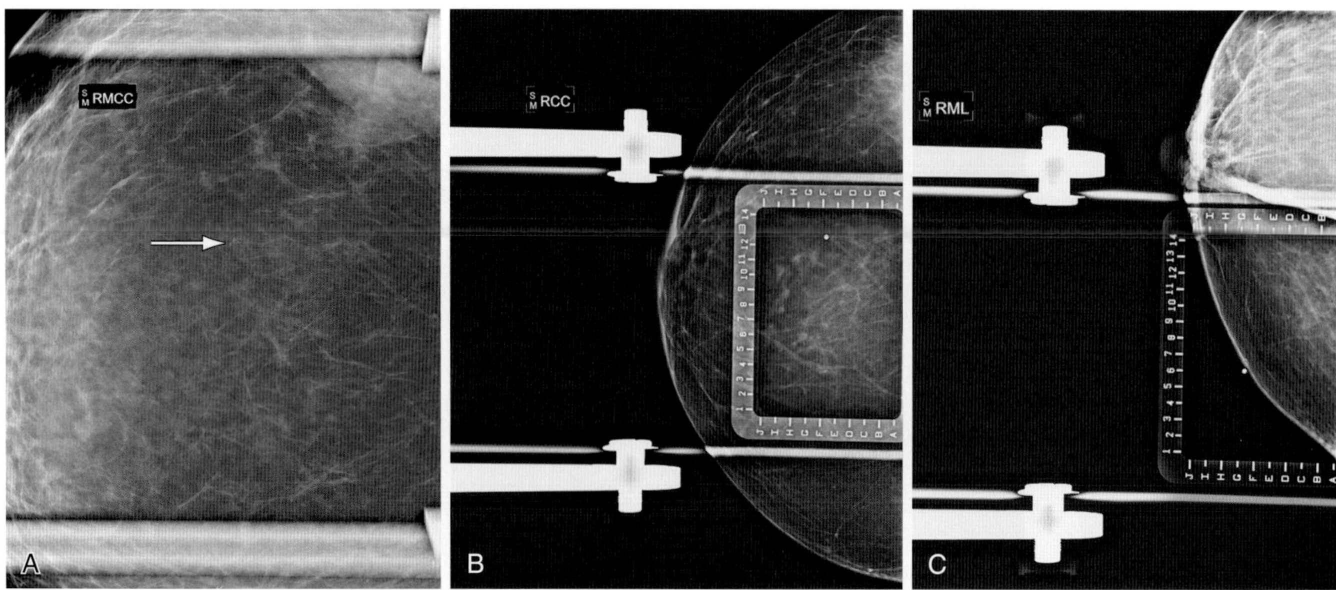

■ **FIGURE 18-6** Dermal calcifications. **A,** Amorphous cluster of microcalcifications (*arrow*) on this magnification craniocaudal (CC) projection. **B,** A grid compression paddle is used, and a metallic BB marker is placed at the coordinates of the targeted calcifications. **C,** A tangential view is performed that demonstrates that the cluster of calcifications is within the skin.

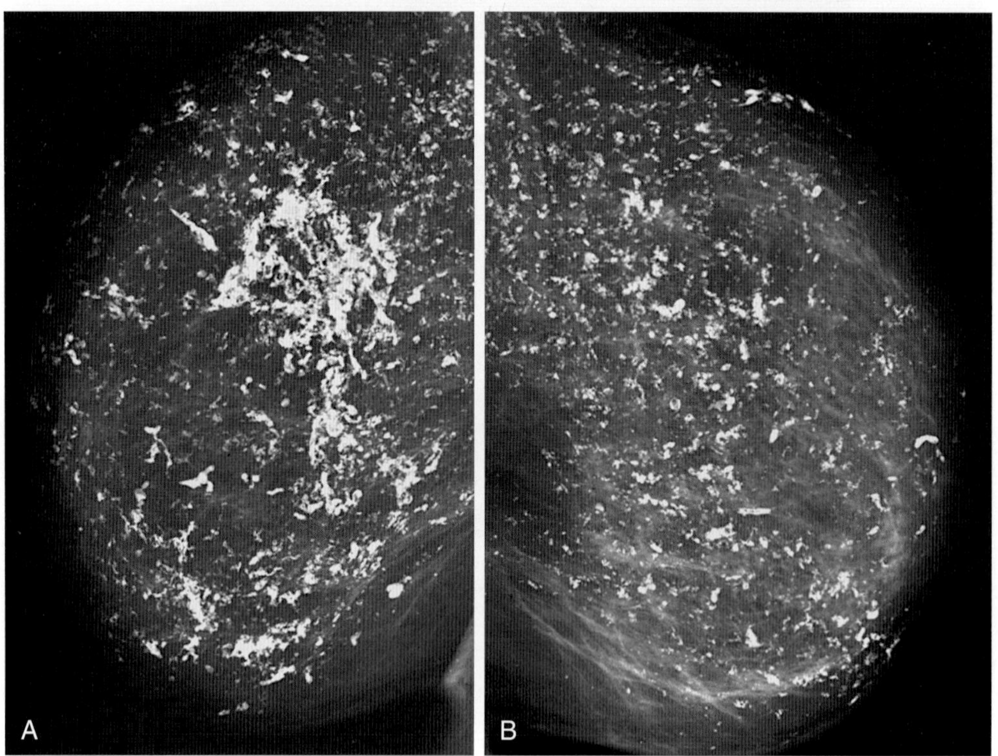

■ **FIGURE 18-7** Dermatomyositis. Right (**A**) and left (**B**) mediolateral oblique views demonstrate diffuse dystrophic superficial calcifications.

washing. It is not difficult to determine the cause of the densities when the material is in the axilla, but some women apply it in a wide area, including the area over the axillary tail of the breast, where it may simulate parenchymal calcifications. Some powders, creams, and ointments also contain radiopaque material, which can mimic suspicious microcalcifications on mammography (Fig. 18-10). Some pigments used in tattoos are radiopaque and can be mammographically visible (Fig. 18-11).[11] Substances in or on the skin should be suspected when the "calcification" is faint, has a bizarre configuration, is extremely peripheral in location, or extends into the axilla, or if the woman has skin lesions for which she might apply medication.

VASCULAR CALCIFICATIONS

The most common vascular lesion identified with mammography is found in the media and is known as Mönckeberg type of calcification (Fig 18-12). The classic

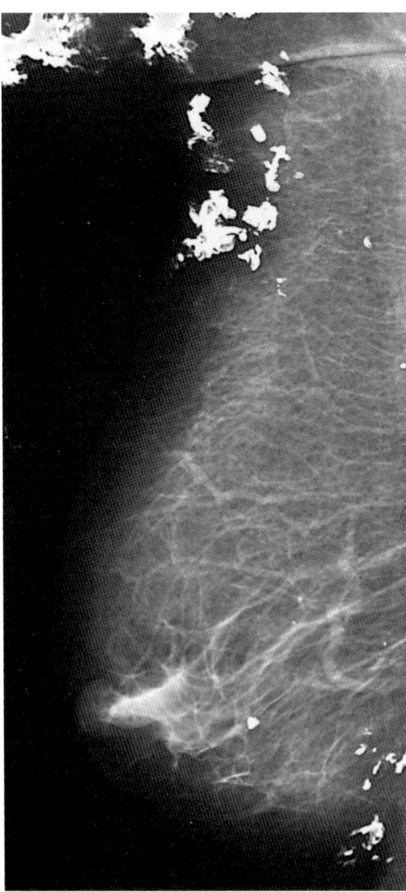

■ **FIGURE 18-8** Dermatomyositis. Right mediolateral oblique (MLO) view demonstrates coarse, dystrophic superficial calcifications in the axillary tail, upper arm, and inferior aspect of the breast.

tram-track appearance of two parallel calcific lines on mammography usually makes the diagnosis obvious (Fig. 18-13). In early atherosclerosis, however, the calcification may be seen on only one wall, and it can even mimic malignant ductal calcifications.

Arterial calcification is usually a finding of advancing age. Although it occurs more commonly in diabetic than nondiabetic women, the presence of arterial calcification is not an accurate predictor for this disease.[12] Mammographic demonstration of arterial calcification has been associated with systemic cardiovascular disease and increased risk for events such as myocardial infarction and stroke.[13] Extensive diffuse bilateral arterial calcifications are often seen in women with secondary hyperparathyroidism from chronic renal failure, particularly those on dialysis (Fig. 18-14).[14,15]

FAT NECROSIS

Clinical Aspects

Fat necrosis is a common benign condition that may be asymptomatic or may present as a palpable mass, pain, or associated findings, such as skin thickening or nipple retraction. The clinical findings may mimic carcinoma.

Imaging Features

Fat necrosis may have a variety of mammographic appearances. Many of the findings mimic carcinoma, including spiculated masses, microcalcifications, and architectural distortion.[16] One common and characteristic finding is a

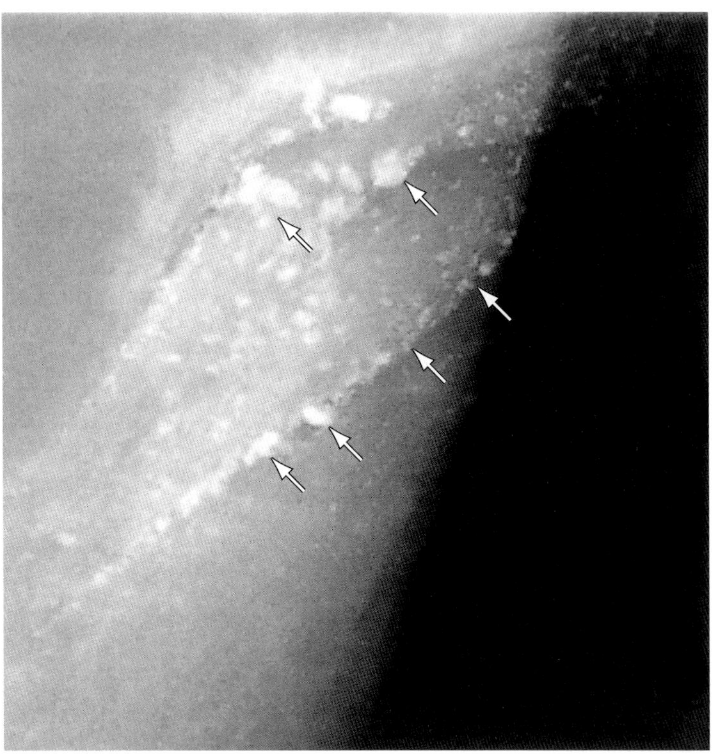

■ **FIGURE 18-9** Antiperspirant (*arrows*) in the axilla.

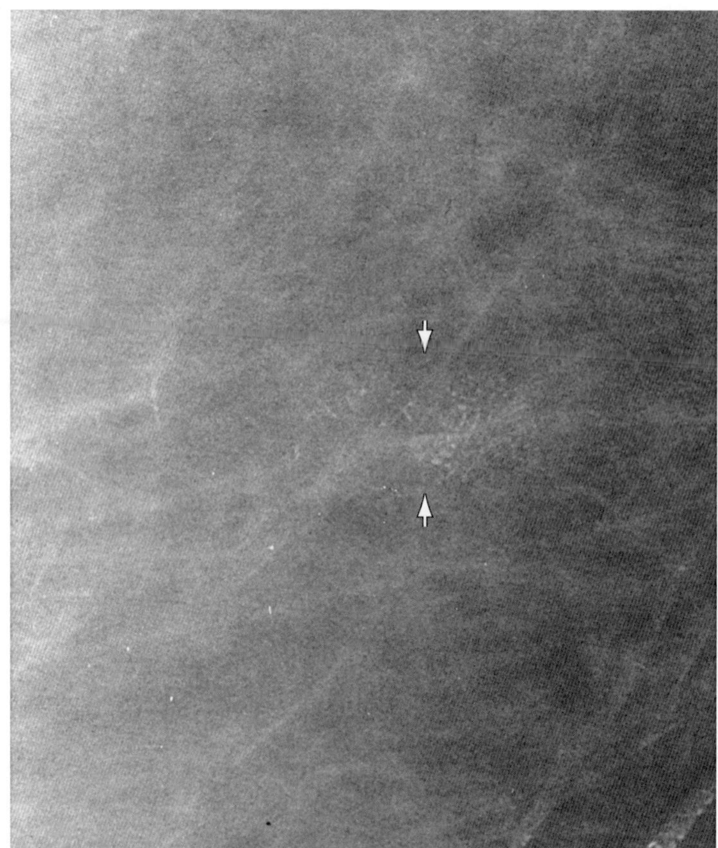

■ **FIGURE 18-10** Zinc oxide-containing ointment on the skin, producing faint amorphous radiopaque densities (*arrows*).

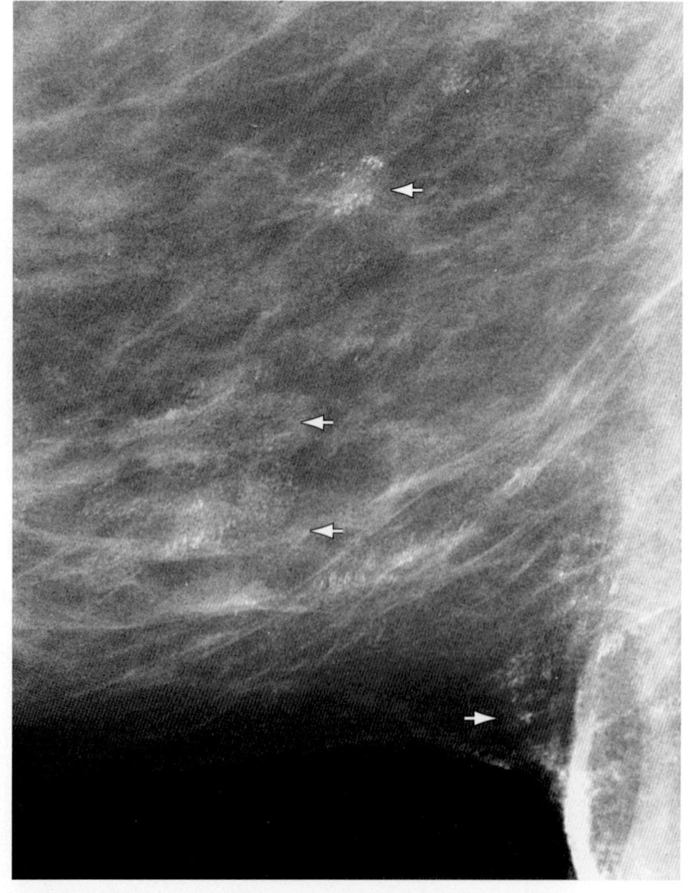

■ **FIGURE 18-11** Radiopaque pigments in skin tattoos (*arrows*).

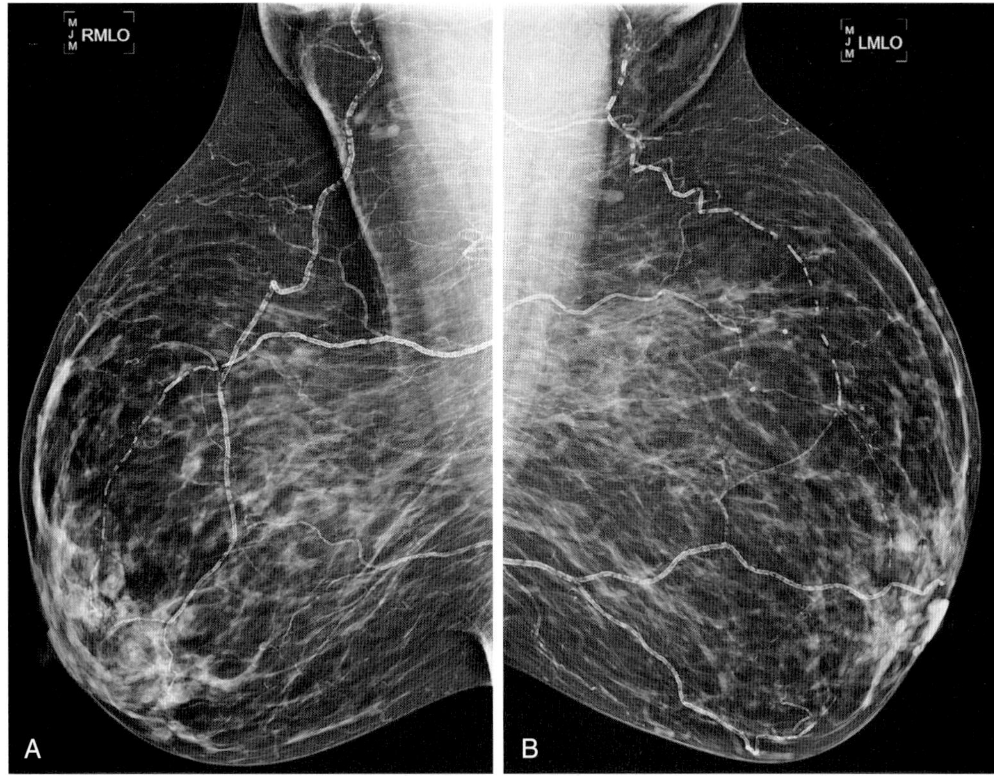

■ **FIGURE 18-12** Right (**A**) and left (**B**) mediolateral oblique (MLO) views demonstrate bilateral Mönckeberg type of calcifications.

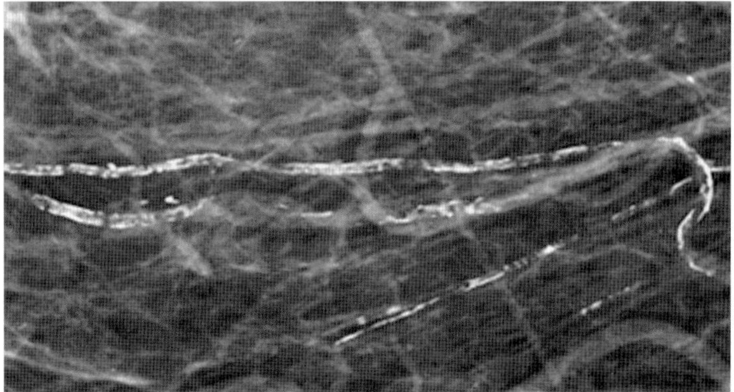

■ **FIGURE 18-13** Classic *tram-track* appearance of vascular calcifications.

radiolucent or mixed fat/soft tissue circumscribed mass with a calcified or noncalcified rim, known as a lipid or oil cyst (Fig. 18-15).[16-18] These can be seen after any trauma to the breast (Fig. 18-16), including surgery (Fig. 18-17). Fat necrosis is commonly seen after lumpectomy (Fig. 18-18) and radiation therapy for breast carcinoma and after extensive surgery such as reduction mammoplasty. In most cases, the mammographic findings are diagnostic of a benign lesion. Early peripheral calcification may mimic microcalcification of malignancy, however. Nonetheless, in most cases, the location of the calcifications at the periphery of a fat-density circumscribed mass is sufficient to establish the benign diagnosis.

Ultrasound (US) studies are not performed when the mammographic features are typical for fat necrosis, but US is often used when the mammogram shows a dense mass of soft tissue. In our experience, early fat necrosis is usually manifest as an ill-defined hyperechoic area, usually in the superficial tissue of the breast (Figs. 18-19 and 18-20 would better describe the US findings according to the American College of Radiology Breast Imaging Reporting and Data System [ACR BI-RADS]. Fig. 18-20B has architectural distortion on the US).

INVOLUTING FIBROADENOMAS

Clinical Aspects

Many fibroadenomas begin to involute in the postpartum period and after menopause, with hyaline degeneration and subsequent calcification.

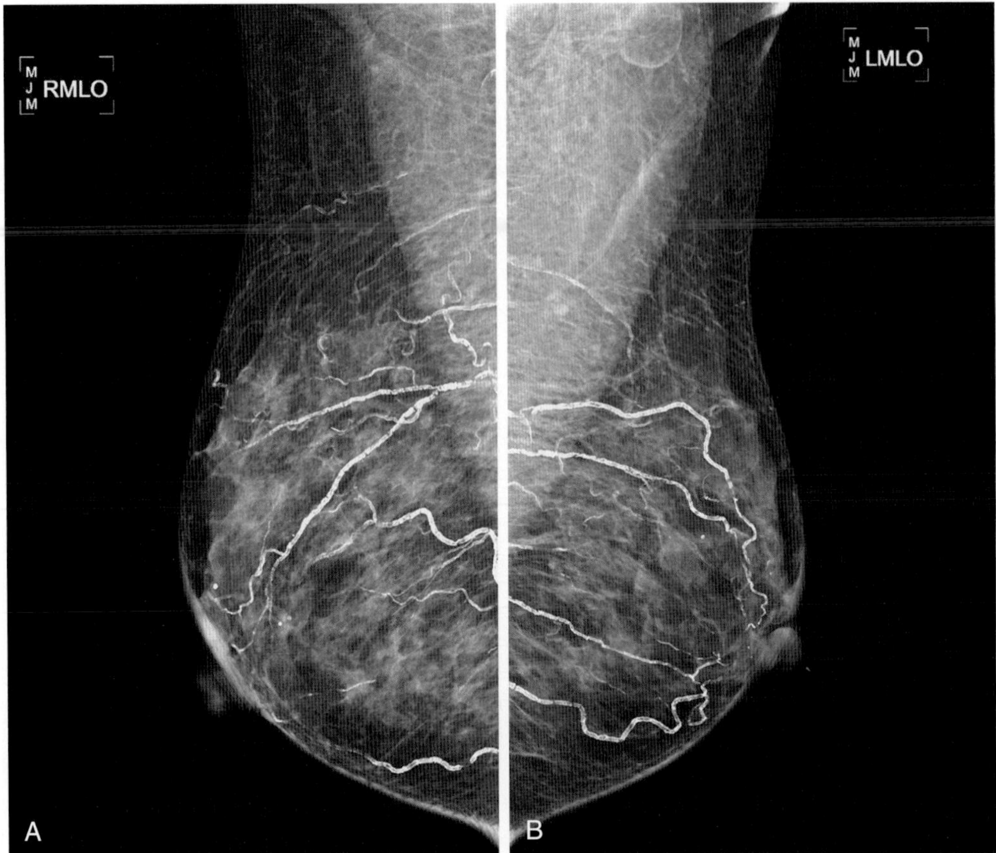

■ **FIGURE 18-14** Right (**A**) and left (**B**) mediolateral oblique (MLO) views demonstrate vascular calcifications in a 65-year-old women with chronic renal failure on hemodialysis.

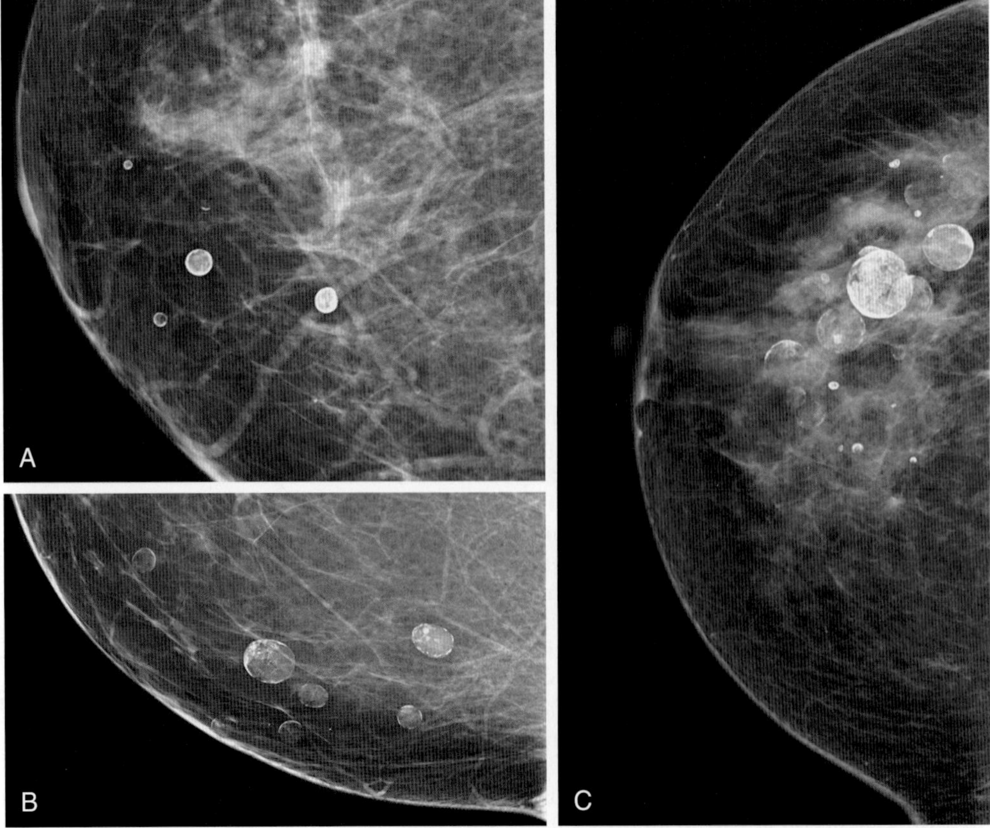

■ **FIGURE 18-15** Fat necrosis. **A** to **C**, Typical lucent oil cysts with calcified rim and lucent centers on mammogram.

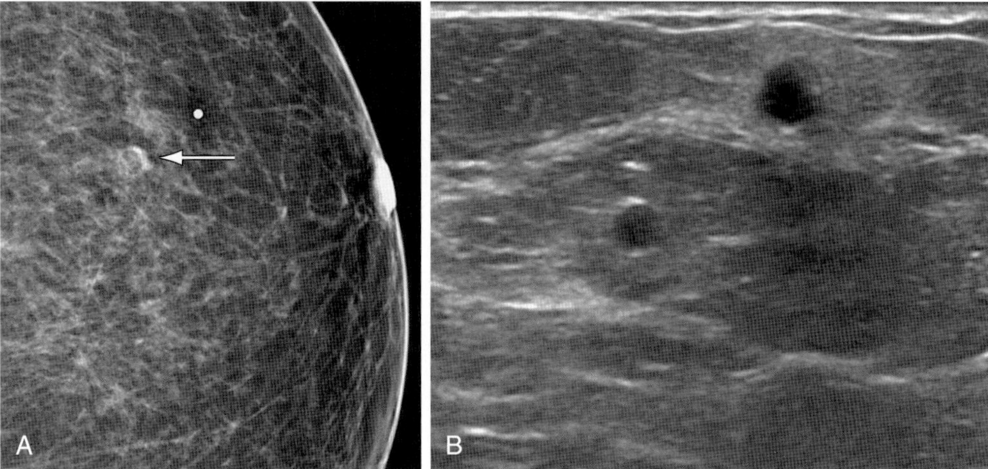

■ **FIGURE 18-16** Fat necrosis. Mammogram and ultrasound image of a patient who complained of a lump after a car accident with seatbelt injury. Mammogram (**A**) demonstrates a subtle round, circumscribed, fat containing mass (*arrow*) consistent with an oil cyst in patient's area of palpable abnormality. Directed ultrasound image (**B**) of this region demonstrates two hypo to anechoic round masses that correlate to the oil cysts.

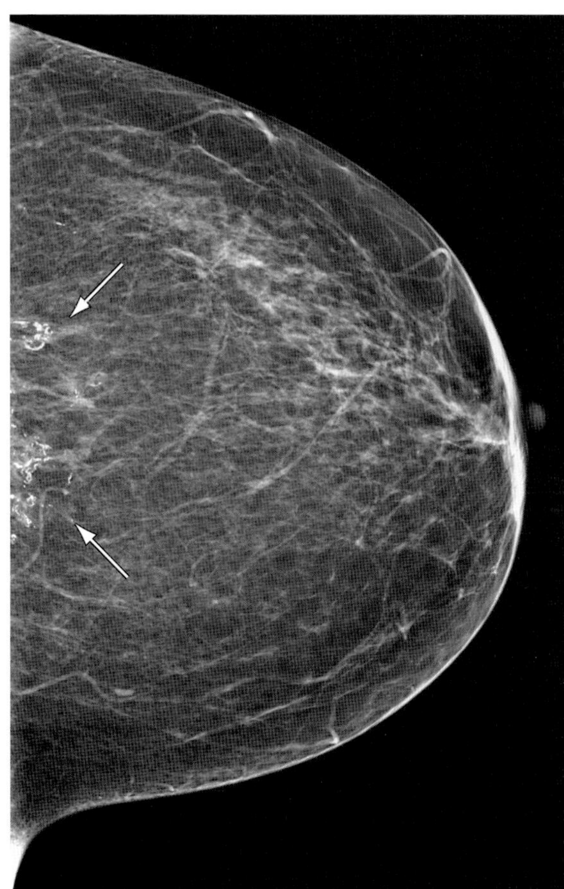

■ **FIGURE 18-17** Fat necrosis. Craniocaudal (CC) projection demonstrates partial eggshell calcifications compatible with fat necrosis (*arrows*) in the posterior breast seen in a patient who is status post lung transplant. The opposite breast showed similar findings.

Imaging Features

Involuting fibroadenomas have typical coarse calcification, which usually begins at the periphery of the mass and moves centrally, often completely replacing the soft tissue mass itself (Figs. 18-21 to 18-23). They often demonstrate the typical *popcorn* shape (Fig. 18-24). When calcifications are present within the mass, obviously US is not necessary (Fig. 18-25). Rarely, fibroadenomas have *atypical* mammographic appearances, mimicking carcinoma with irregular shapes, indistinct or spiculated margins, or pleomorphic microcalcifications.

DUCT ECTASIA WITH SECRETORY CALCIFICATIONS

Clinical Aspects

Duct ectasia is a nonspecific dilation of the major subareolar ducts, with occasional involvement of the smaller ducts. The various anatomic features of this disease have led to many different descriptive diagnostic terms, including *plasma cell mastitis*, *obliterative mastitis* and *comedomastitis*. The cause of duct ectasia is unknown. It has been suggested that the initiating event is the inflammatory process, which leads to destruction of the elastic network of the duct and, hence, duct ectasia and periductal fibrosis. Others have suggested that the dilation is primary, perhaps caused by obstruction of the duct, and that the inflammation is a secondary phenomenon related to leakage of duct contents.

Imaging Features

The distended ducts may be palpable or visible on mammography or US. They may be filled with fluid or with thick secretions and cellular debris.[19] The material within the ducts often calcifies, producing the typical secretory calcifications seen on mammography as dense, solid, rodlike calcifications, which are usually bilateral, symmetric, and diffuse (Figs. 18-26 and 18-27) but occasionally focal. The calcifications may also contain internal lucencies when the calcified material is outside, rather than within, the duct. Such calcifications are asymptomatic, are of no clinical consequence to the patient, and do not elevate

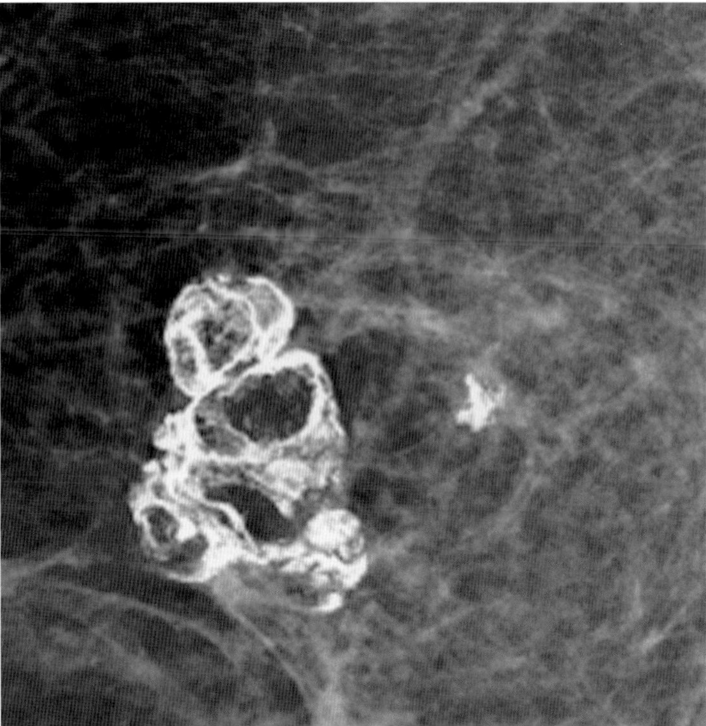

■ **FIGURE 18-18** Eggshell calcifications compatible with fat necrosis in a patient who is status post lumpectomy.

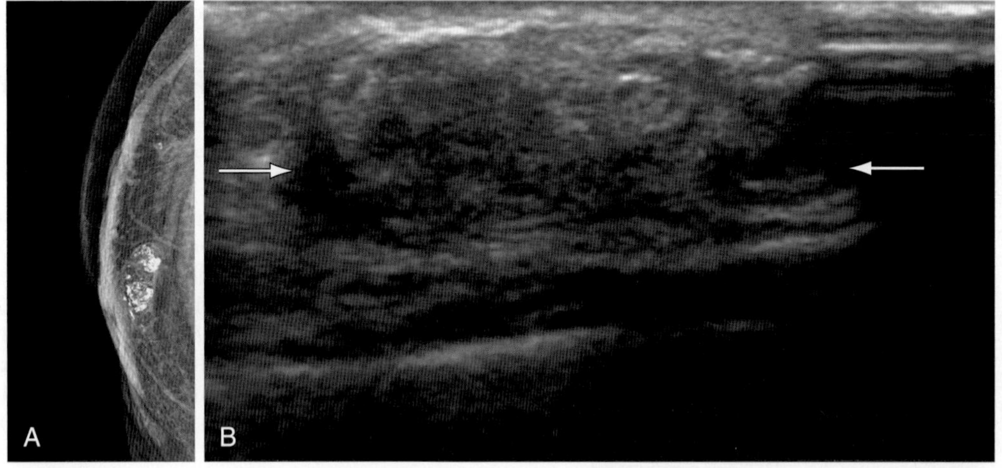

■ **FIGURE 18-19** Fat necrosis in a patient status post mastectomy on mammogram (**A**) and ultrasound image (**B**) (*arrows*).

the woman's risk of breast cancer. Occasionally, early focal secretory calcifications may mimic malignant microcalcifications, leading to biopsy. Additionally, if asymmetrically dilated ducts represent an interval change or contain pleomorphic microcalcifications, biopsy should be performed.[20]

FOREIGN BODY CALCIFICATIONS

The most common foreign bodies seen within the breast mammographically are metallic bullet fragments (Fig. 18-28). Occasionally, the particles are small enough to mimic microcalcifications, but careful attention to the very high radiographic density of the fragments should prevent confusion (Figs. 18-29 and 18-30). Other metal objects, such as sewing needles or fragments of localizing wires, are occasionally found (Fig. 18-31). One of the few nonmetallic foreign bodies that are mammographically visible is the retained Dacron cuff of a Hickman central venous catheter, which has a characteristic appearance (Fig. 18-32).[21] Foreign-body reaction or abscess formation around foreign bodies may produce an ill-defined or spiculated mass and mimic carcinoma.[22] The visualization of the foreign object within the mass should establish the benign diagnosis.

Calcified suture material results from delayed resorption of catgut sutures upon which calcium precipitates. It is most common in the radiated breast and appears as curvilinear or tubular calcifications in the region of previous surgery (Fig. 18-33).[23]

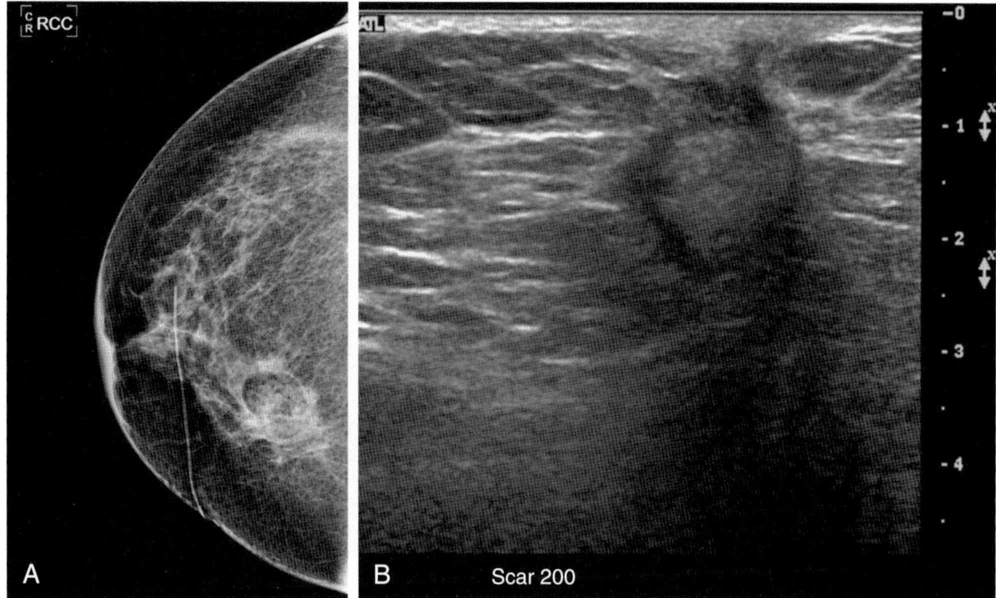

■ **FIGURE 18-20** Fat necrosis. Right craniocaudal (CC) projection demonstrates an oval partially circumscribed and partially obscured fat containing mass compatible with fat necrosis in a patient status post lumpectomy on mammogram (**A**) ultrasound image depicts an oval, angular mass with central hyperechogenicity and peripheral hypoechogenicity (**B**).

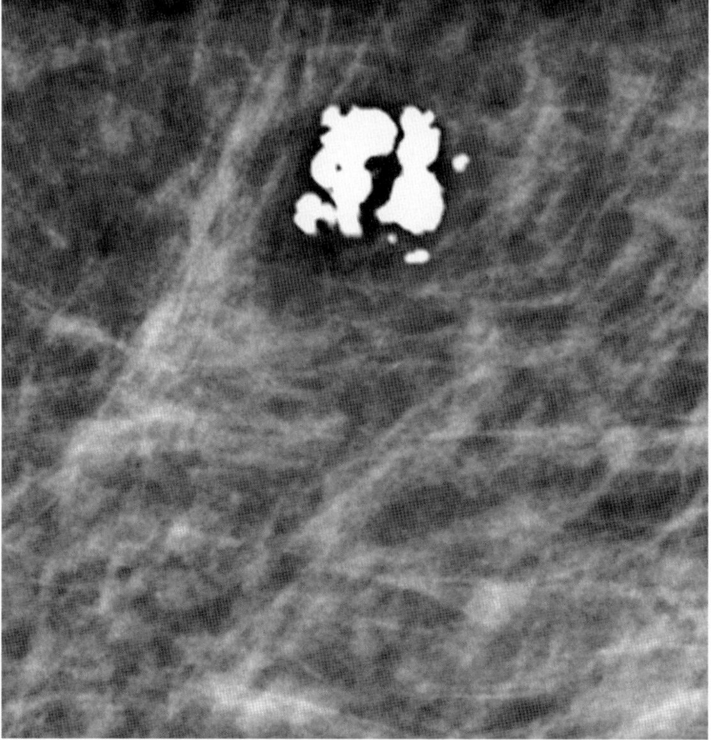

■ **FIGURE 18-21** *Popcorn*-shaped calcified fibroadenoma.

Gold deposits in axillary lymph nodes in patients with rheumatoid arthritis being treated with intramuscular gold therapy can simulate microcalcifications on mammograms. Gold deposits appear as multiple stippled densities in axillary lymph nodes (Fig. 18-34).[24]

Parasitic calcifications such as with echinococcosis,[25,26] schistosomiasis,[27] and loiasis,[28] are rare but can occur in the breast as tubular or curved calcifications (Fig. 18-35).

PATHOLOGY

Microcalcification is one of the most common causes for obtaining tissue diagnosis by core needle biopsy. There are two types of histologic calcifications. Most of the calcifications detected by mammograms are basophilic concretions of varying size composed of calcium phosphates. These calcifications appear as lamellar and concentric layers of a dark basophilic purple color on hematoxylin

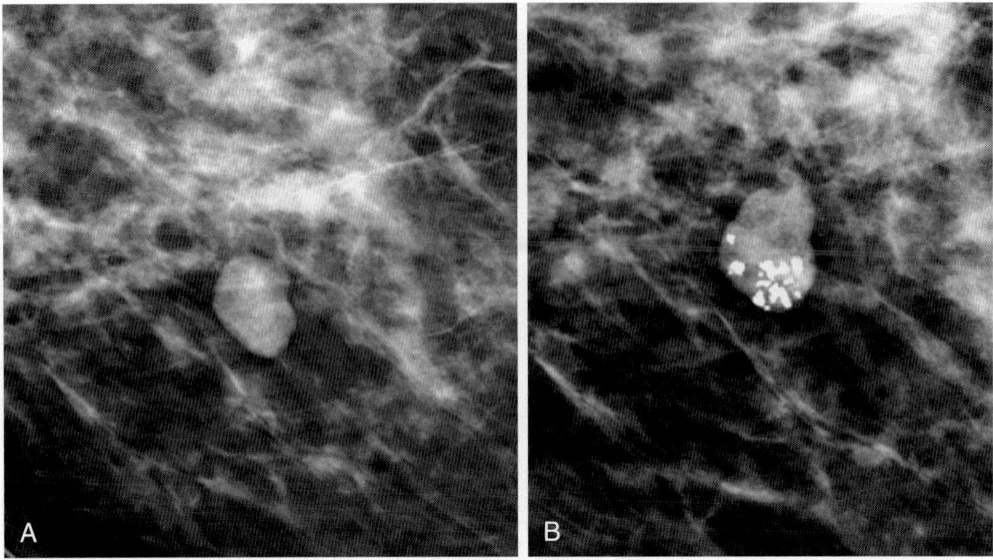

■ **FIGURE 18-22** Lobular, circumscribed mass on (**A**) mammogram that has developed typical dystrophic calcifications (**B**) 1 year later consistent with an involuting fibroadenoma.

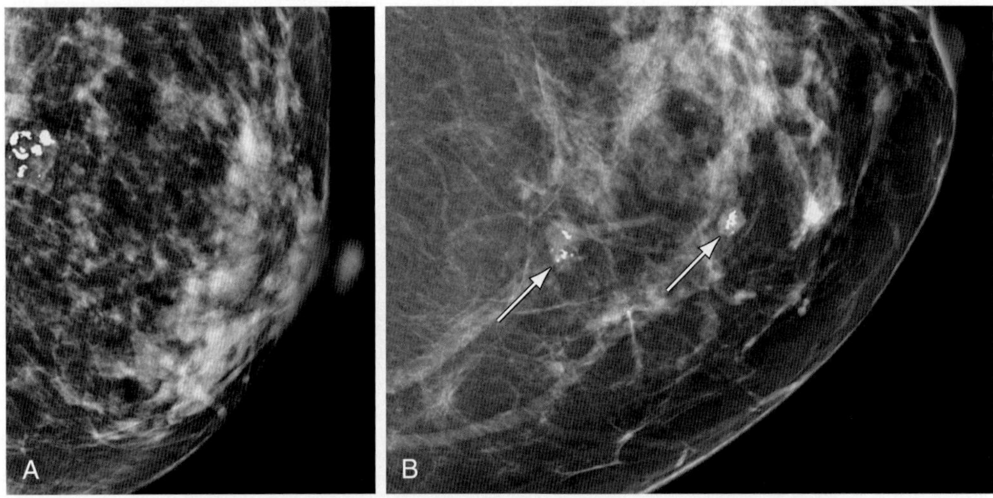

■ **FIGURE 18-23** Typical involuting fibroadenomas(**A, B**) (*arrows*).

and eosin stain (Figs. 18-36 to 18-38). Calcium phosphate microcalcifications are found in both benign and malignant lesions of the breast. Other mammographically detected calcifications are calcium oxalate crystals, which appear clear, birefringent, and nonbasophilic on light microscopy. Calcium oxalate crystals are often seen in association with benign microcysts and apocrine cysts and are located within the lumina of the cysts. Under the polarized microscope, these crystals are refractile and are much easier to visualize (Figs. 18-39 and 18-40). Although calcium oxalate crystals are seen more frequently in association with benign breast lesions, there are rare occasions when these crystals are seen with ductal carcinoma in situ (Figs. 18-41 and 18-42).

The increasing use of stereotactic core needle biopsies has made it possible to sample nonpalpable, mammographically detected microcalcifications. It is critical to correlate that the microcalcifications seen on the slide by pathologists are the same microcalcifications detected by radiologists on the mammogram. Other benign associated conditions with microcalcifications are common (Figs. 18-43 to 18-50). Regular meetings and/or conversations between radiologists and pathologists are necessary to correlate the findings. At times, the search for microcalcifications on the slides can be a tedious and arduous task. It is extremely helpful if radiologists document in their report the following features of microcalcifications in mammographically detected core needle biopsy samples:

1. The number of calcifications in a cluster (rare, few, many, etc.)
2. The number of clusters and the size dimensions
3. If multiple areas of calcifications are seen, the distance between the clusters
4. The characteristics of calcifications, such as pleomorphic, branching, linear

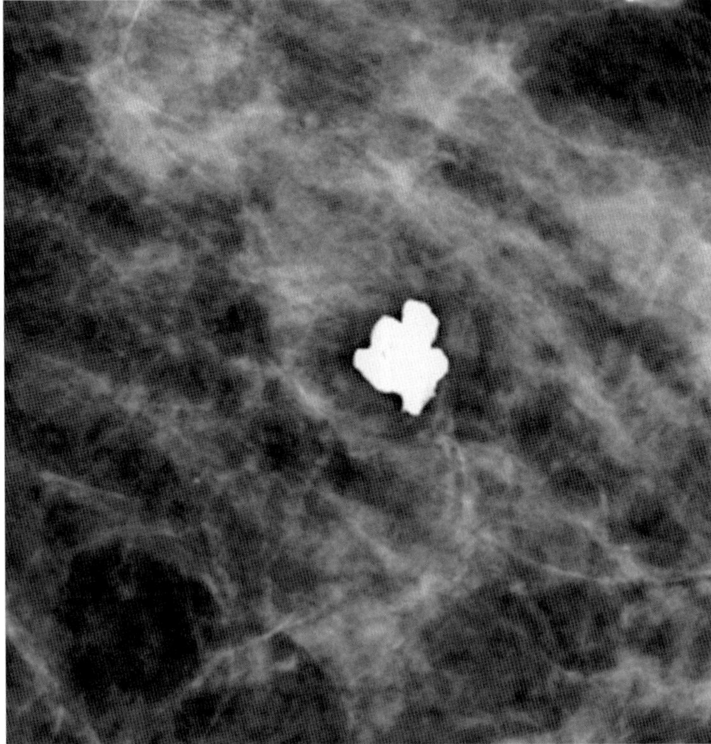

■ **FIGURE 18-24** *Popcorn*-shaped calcified fibroadenoma.

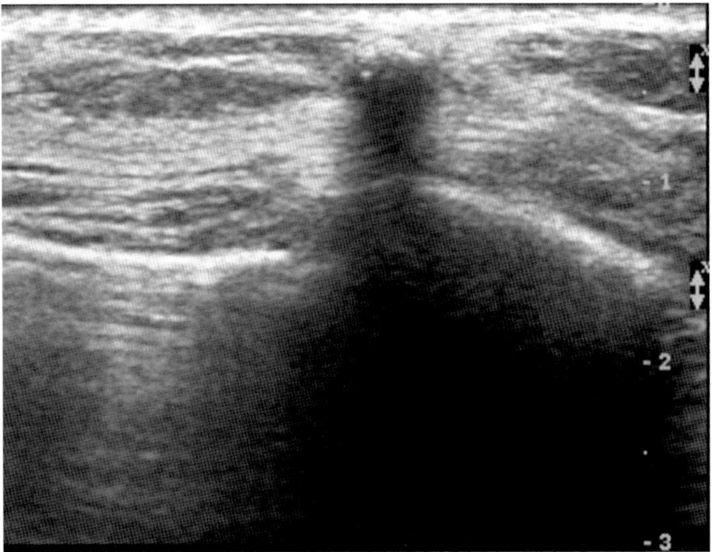

■ **FIGURE 18-25** Calcified fibroadenoma on ultrasound image appears as an irregular, hypoechoic mass with posterior shadowing due to the presence of the popcorn calcification.

5. Whether the area of microcalcifications is entirely or partially removed by core needle biopsy (post-biopsy mammogram findings)
6. Specimen radiograph documenting the presence or absence of the microcalcifications
7. The degree of suspicion using the BI-RADS classification
8. Placement of microclip after core needle biopsy
9. Any other relevant clinical information, such as previous cancer or ductal carcinoma in situ at the site, a history of radiation therapy, family history
10. Contact information including clinician's name and phone number

In some centers, the radiologists will select the cores with microcalcifications and place them in a separate container. This allows pathologists to focus attention on

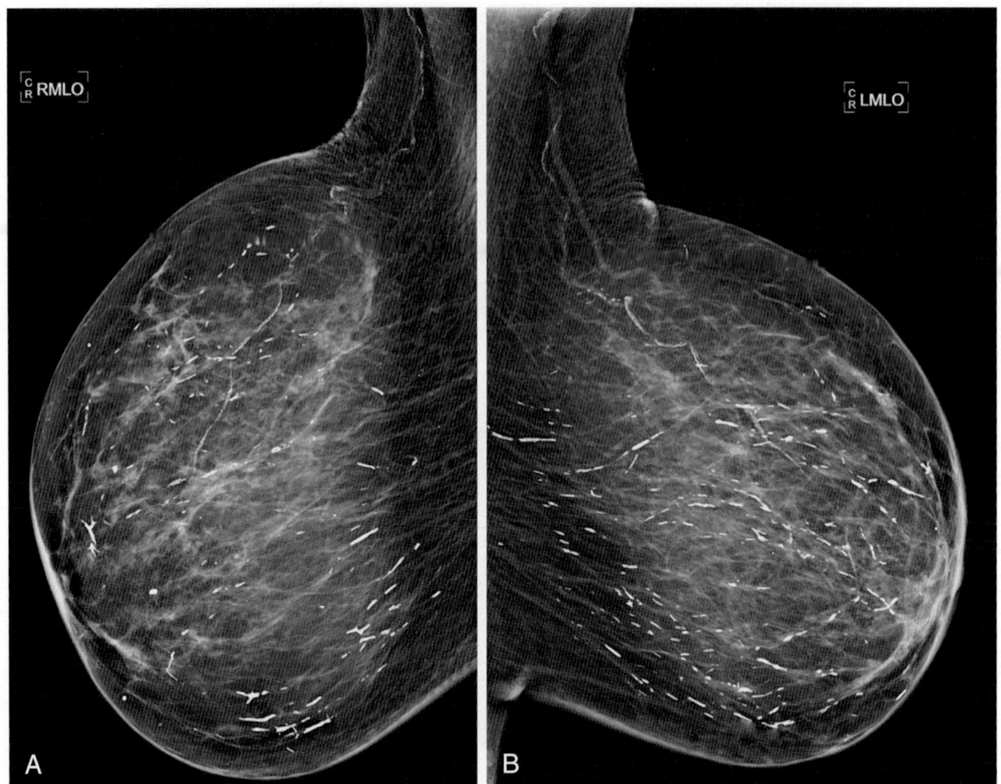

■ **FIGURE 18-26** Secretory calcifications. Right (**A**) and left (**B**) mediolateral oblique (MLO) views demonstrate typical bilateral symmetric and diffuse large rod like secretory calcifications.

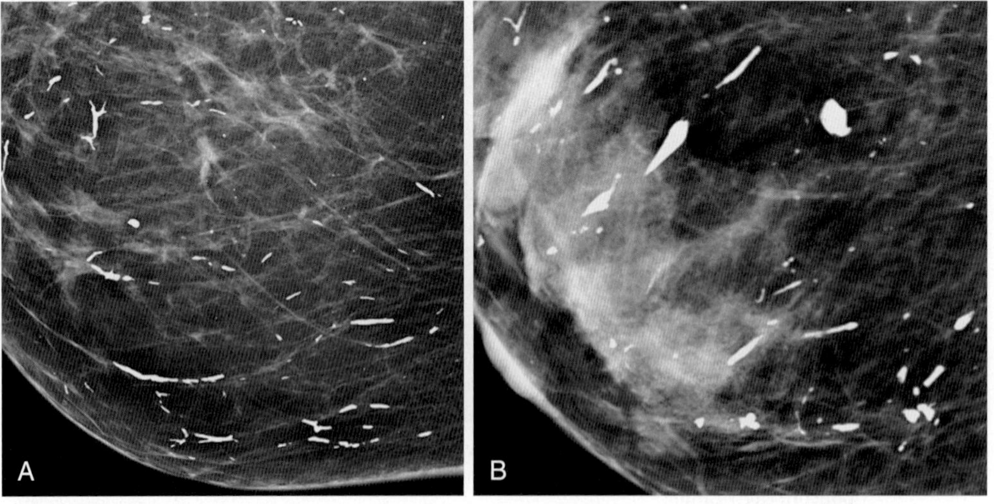

■ **FIGURE 18-27** Secretory calcifications. Typical dense, solid rodlike secretory calcifications (**A, B**).

this portion of the sample. Core needle biopsy samples routinely are examined by obtaining multiple deep levels to study the entire depth of the tissue removed. All slides are examined for the presence of microcalcifications and the precise microanatomic distribution of calcifications (benign ducts or ductal carcinoma in situ). If initial slides do not show microcalcifications, the polarizing lens will be used to find calcium oxalate crystals. If there are no microcalcifications found under a polarizing lens, radiographs of the tissue blocks are obtained. Radiographic examination of paraffin blocks is essential to find which block has calcifications when they are not evident in the histologic sections. The block that contains calcifications then will be selected and sequential deeper sections are

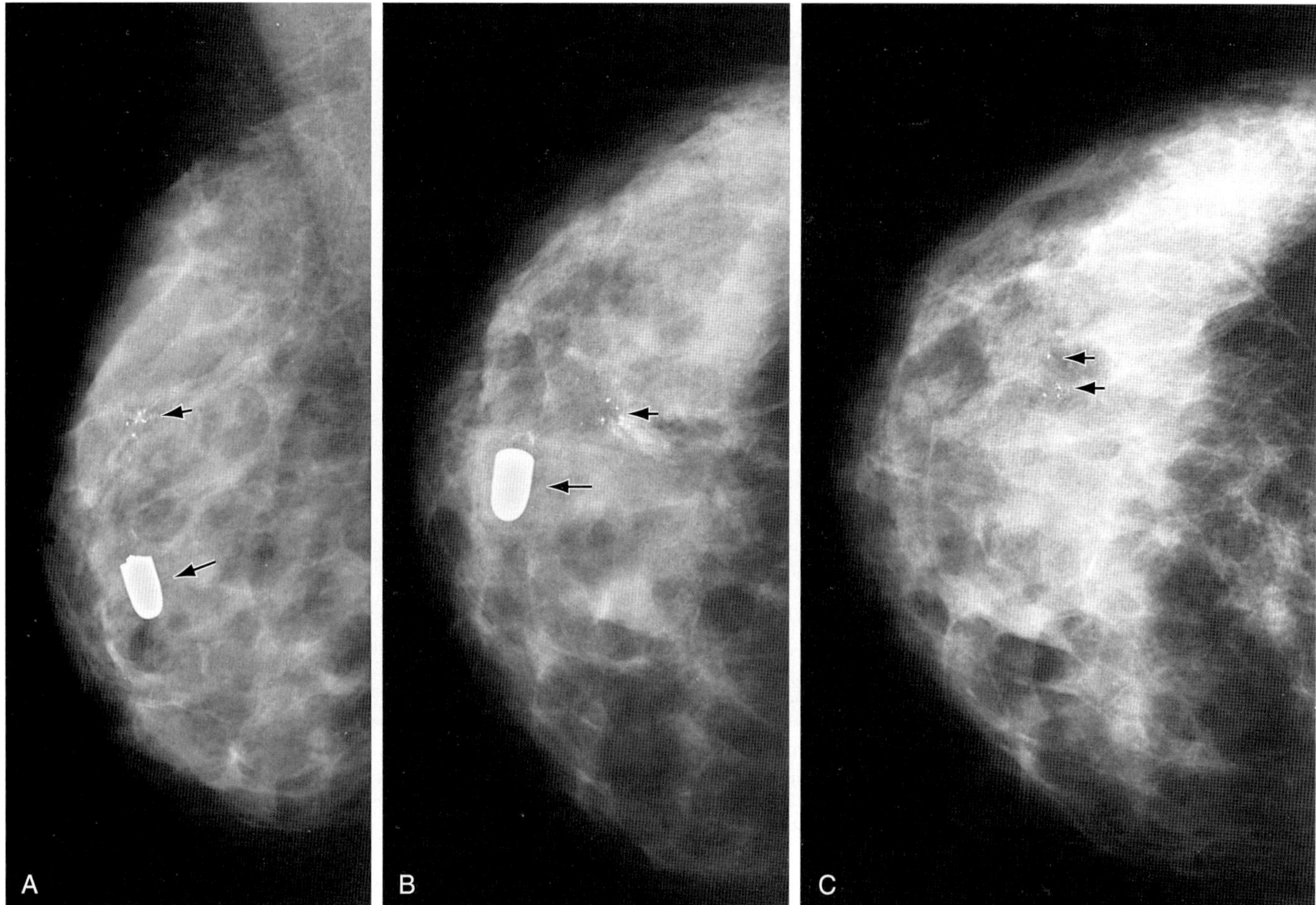

■ **FIGURE 18-28** Bullet in the breast after a gunshot wound. The right (**A**) mediolateral oblique (MLO) and (**B**) craniocaudal (CC) mammograms demonstrate a bullet (*large arrow*) in the subareolar region of the breast, with a cluster of small metallic bullet fragments at the 11-o'clock position of the breast (*small arrow*). On a routine screening mammogram 2 years after removal of the large bullet (**C**), the cluster of small metallic fragments (*arrows*) is more dispersed on this CC view because the woman has gained weight in the interval. The metallic fragments are too radiographically dense for their size to be calcifications.

cut and slides are produced until no tissue remains in the block. After such a workup, microcalcifications are usually found. However, on rare occasions, microcalcifications can be shattered or partially dissolved during tissue processing and calcifications can be lost in the course of trimming paraffin blocks with a microtome blade.

A high level of concordance between the mammographic and pathologic findings can be achieved in analysis of microcalcifications. If there is discordance between benign pathologic and mammographic features, surgical biopsy is warranted even if calcifications were obtained and documented in the core needle biopsy report. This is to avoid pitfalls because of the limited sampling that is inherent in the assessment of a core needle biopsy specimen.

The pathology report for the microcalcification core needle biopsy should have the following information:

1. Presence or absence of microcalcifications
2. Documentation of calcium oxalate via polarizing lens
3. What entity is seen in association with microcalcifications
4. Documentation for radiography of the blocks
5. Documentation for additional deeper sections of blocks and presence or absence of microcalcifications after exhaustive search for microcalcifications

The search for microcalcifications on the excisional biopsy is similar to that for the core needle biopsy sample. A microclip is placed after the core needle biopsy procedure by radiologists. Information regarding microclip placement is helpful for surgical specimen analysis. Microclips are seen from the lumpectomy specimen microscopically. The presence of a microclip indicates that the prior biopsy site is included within the excisional specimen. Specimen radiography is also helpful for identifying lesions with calcifications and to check for the presence of a microclip. Various types of microclip can be seen (Fig. 18-51).

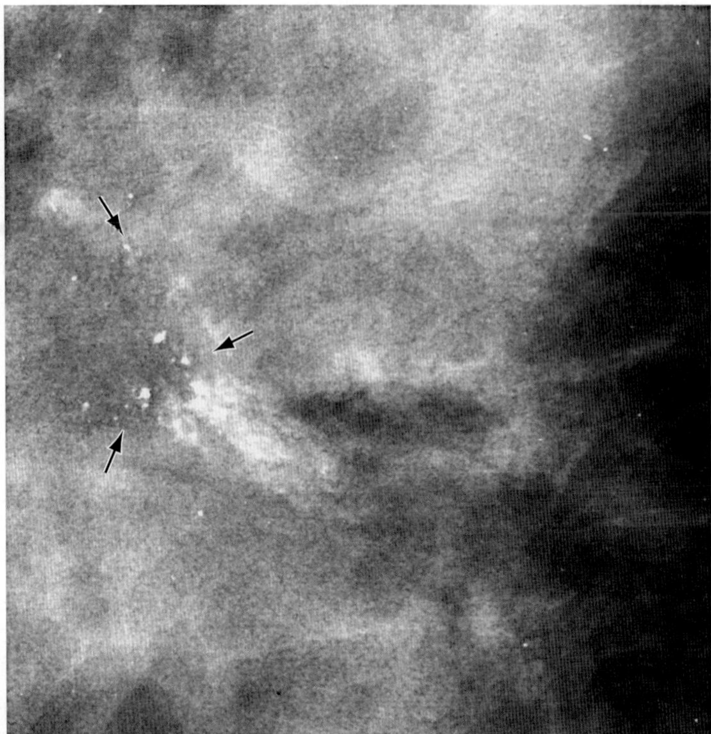

■ **FIGURE 18-29** Bullet fragments. Small metallic bullet fragments in the breast after a gunshot wound (*arrows*). In this case, the fragments range in size from approximately 0.5 to 2 mm. The fragments are too radiographically dense for their size to be calcifications.

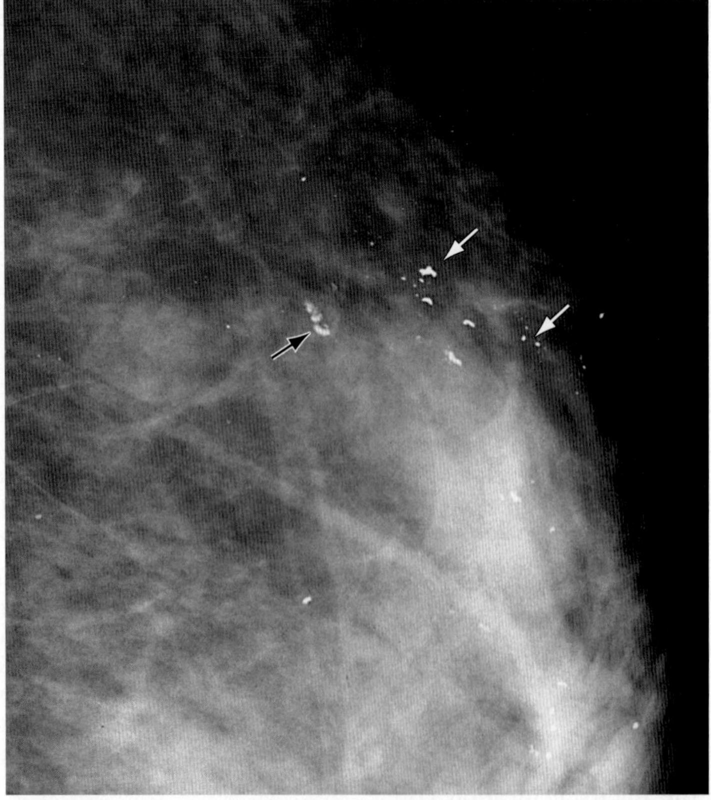

■ **FIGURE 18-30** Bullet fragments. Metallic bullet fragments (*white arrows*) and benign calcifications (*black arrow*) in the same region of the breast. Note the difference in radiographic density of the two materials.

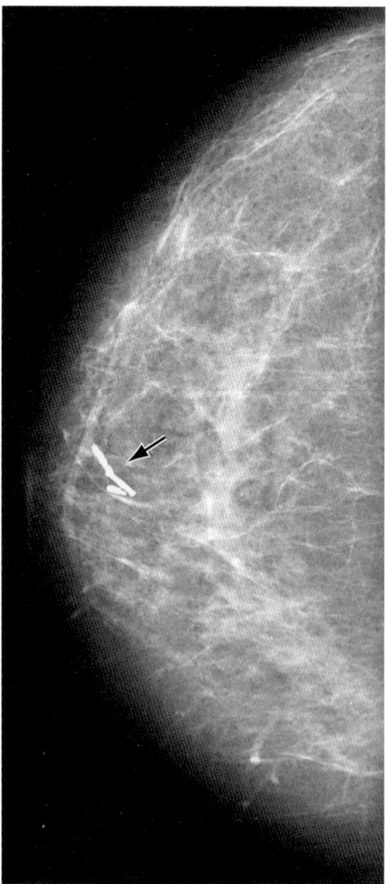

■ **FIGURE 18-31** Foreign body. Fragmented sewing needle (*arrow*) in the subareolar region of the right breast.

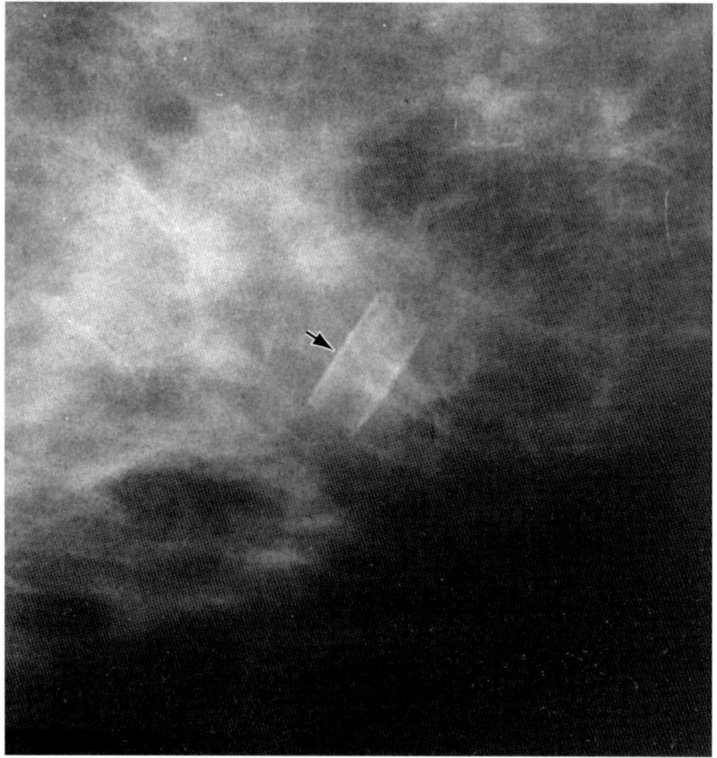

■ **FIGURE 18-32** Retained Hickman catheter Dacron cuff (*arrow*).

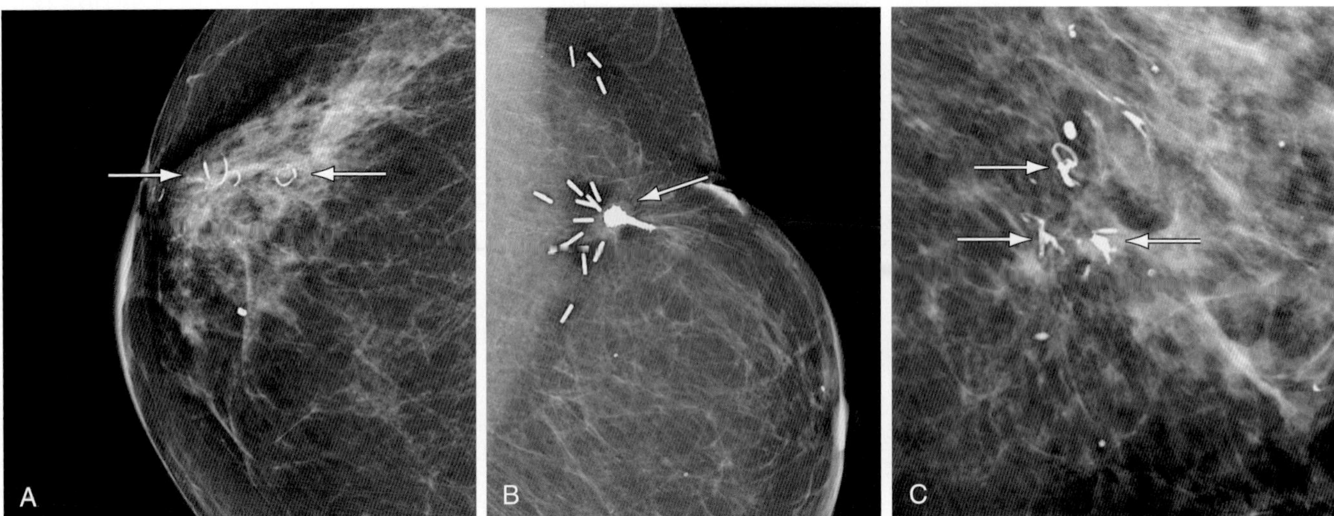

■ **FIGURE 18-33** **A,** Calcified sutures (*arrows*) status post lumpectomy. **B,** Left mediolateral oblique (MLO) views demonstrate calcified suture granuloma (arrow) in a patient status post lumpectomy and radiation treatment. **C,** Curvilinear calcified sutures (*arrows*) after lumpectomy.

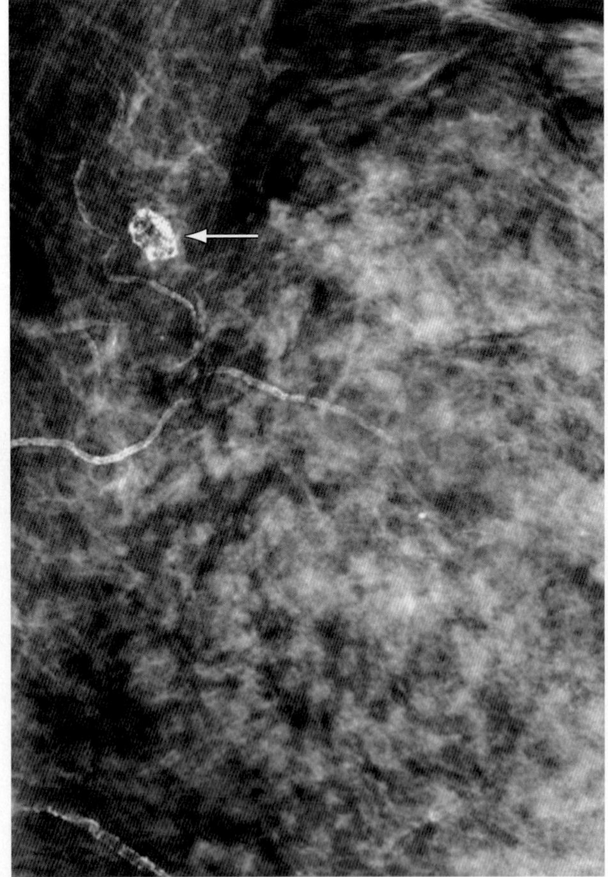

■ **FIGURE 18-34** Gold deposits (*arrow*) within axillary lymph node in a patient who was treated for rheumatoid arthritis with gold therapy.

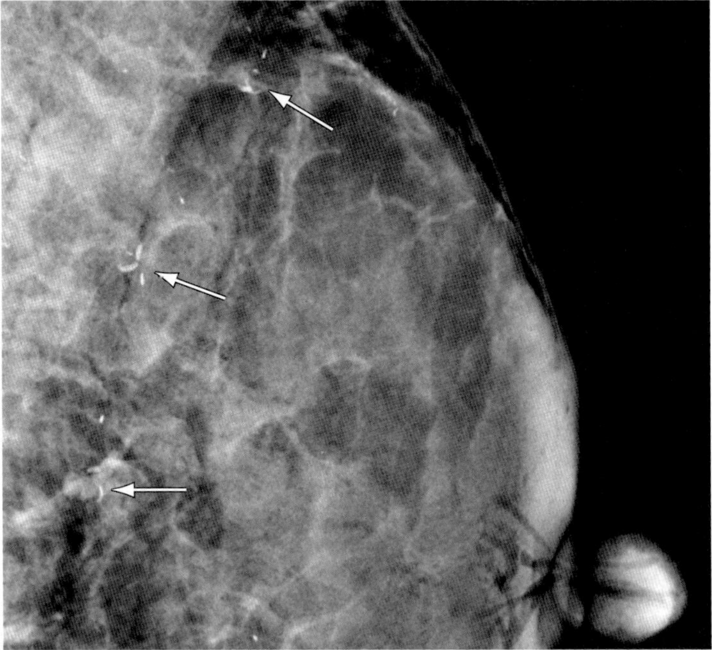

■ **FIGURE 18-35** Curvilinear benign-appearing parasitic calcifications (*arrows*).

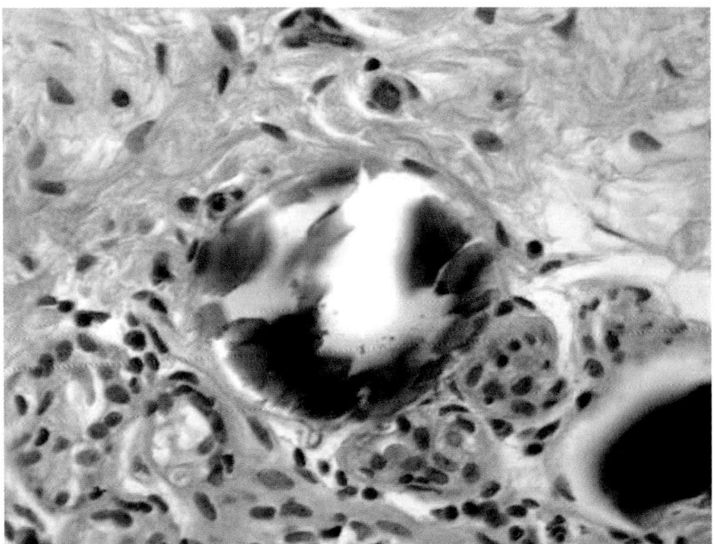

■ **FIGURE 18-36** Microcalcification seen with benign breast terminal ductal-lobular unit (H&E, ×400).

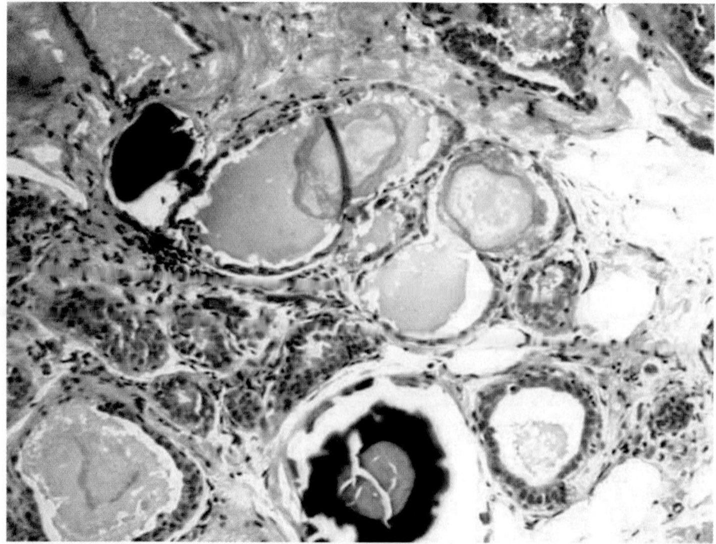

■ **FIGURE 18-37** Microcalcification seen with lactational changes in pregnancy (H&E, ×400).

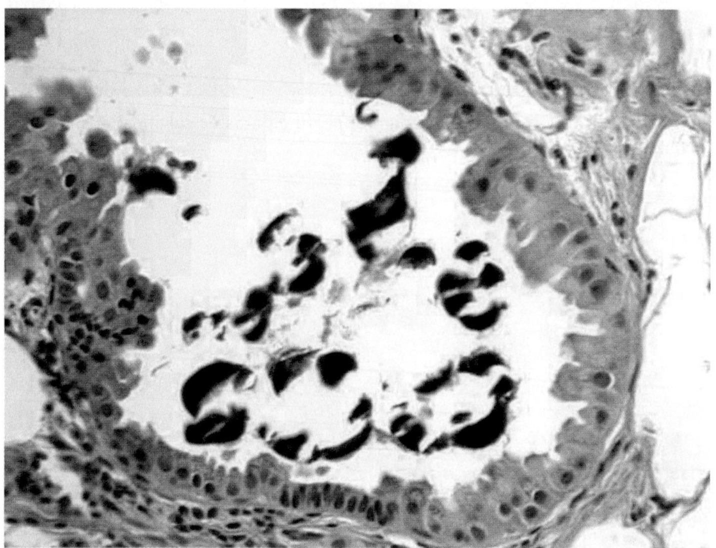

■ **FIGURE 18-38** Apocrine metaplasia with luminal microcalcifications (calcium phosphate type) (H&E, ×400).

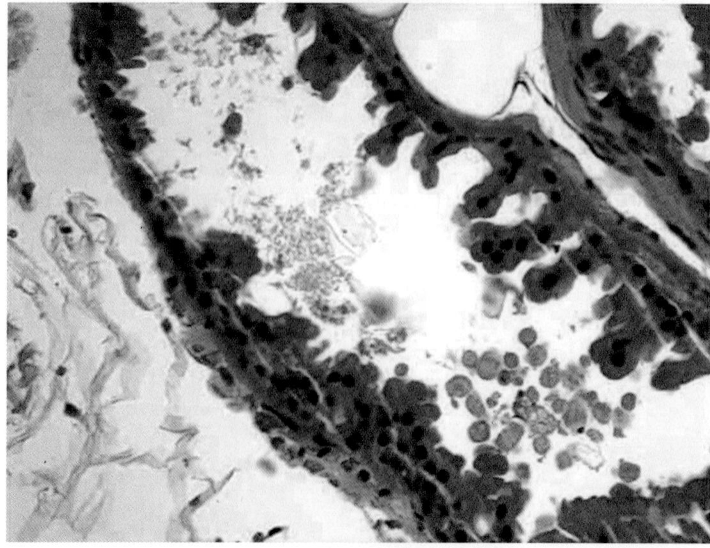

■ **FIGURE 18-39** Apocrine metaplasia with luminal refractile optically clear microcalcifications (calcium oxalate type) (H&E, ×400).

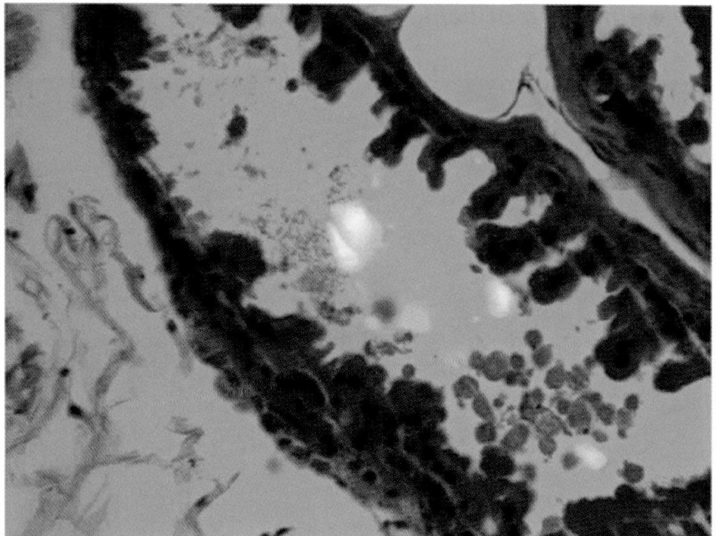

■ **FIGURE 18-40** Appearance under polarizing lens showing the same picture as in Figure 18-4 (H&E, ×400).

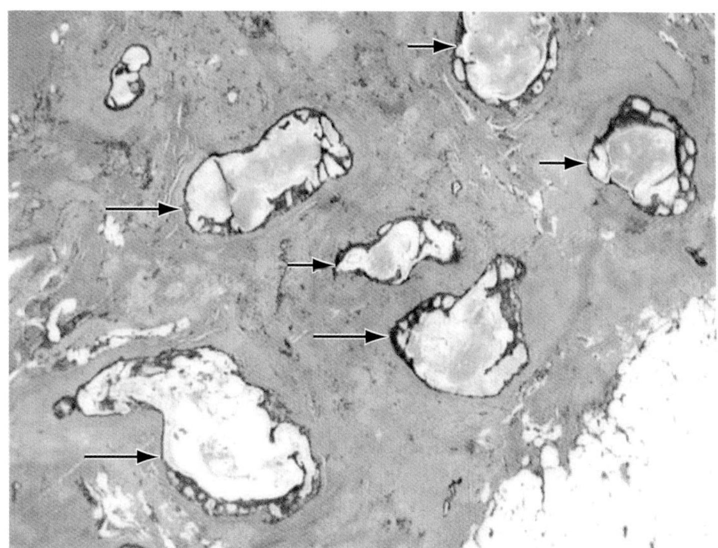

■ **FIGURE 18-41** Scatter ductal carcinoma in situ (DCIS). Excisional biopsy was done for abnormal microcalcifications (H&E, ×40). *Arrows* indicate DCIS.

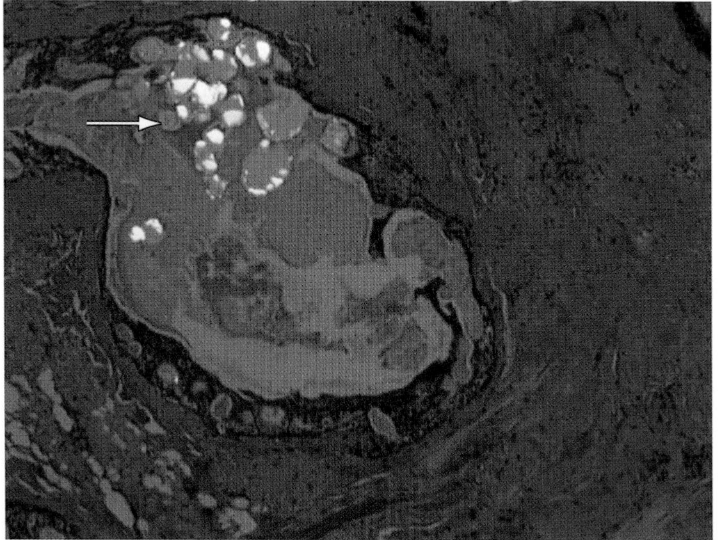

■ **FIGURE 18-42** Under the polarizing lens, calcium oxalate crystals are seen within the luminal area of the ductal carcinoma in situ (DCIS). *White arrow* points to calcium oxalate crystals ×200.

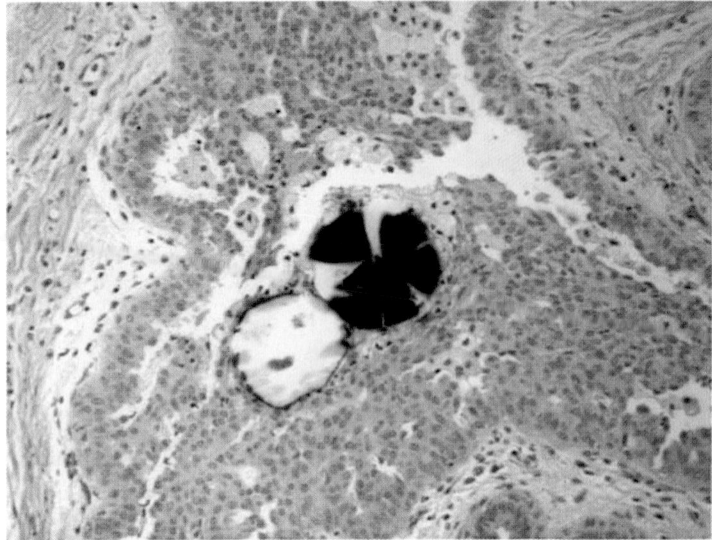

■ **FIGURE 18-43** Usual ductal hyperplasia with luminal microcalcifications (H&E, ×200).

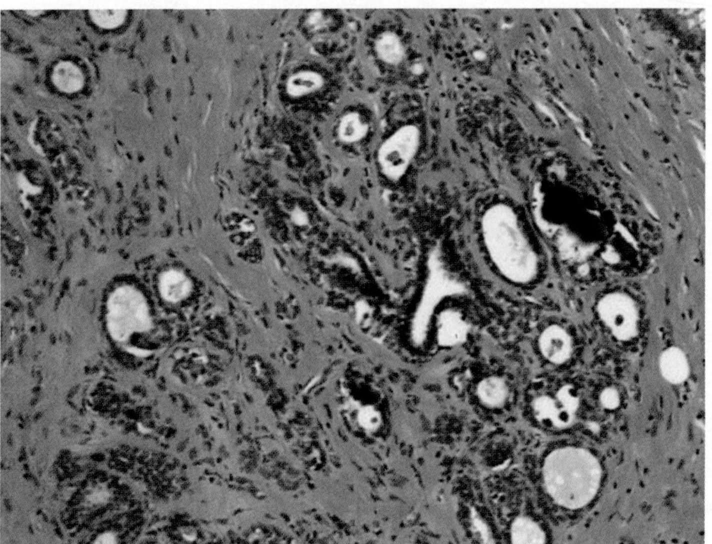

■ **FIGURE 18-44** Sclerosing adenosis with microcalcifications (H&E, ×200).

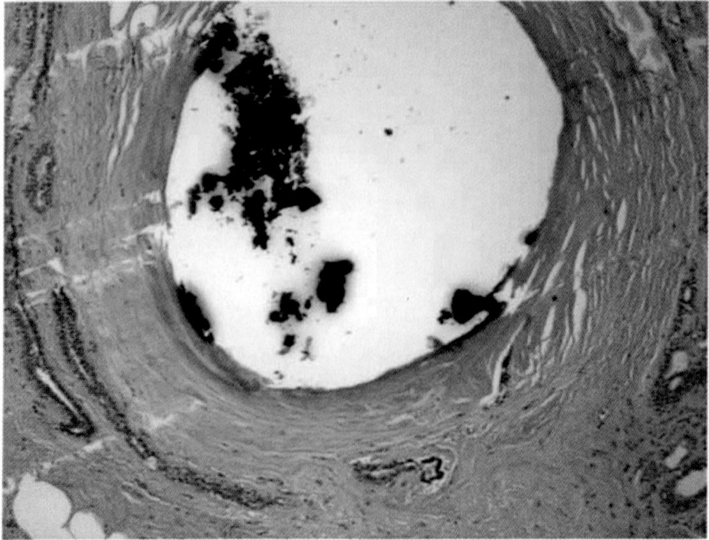

■ **FIGURE 18-45** Large calcification is seen with stroma. No epithelial cells are noted around the calcified area (H&E, ×400).

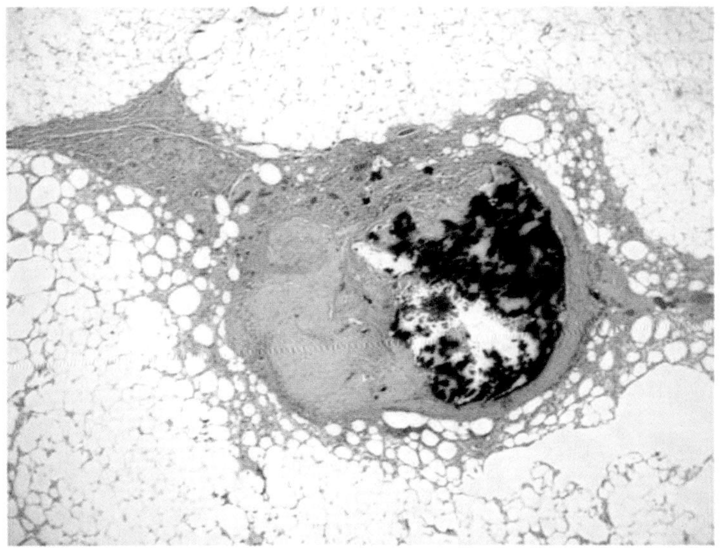

■ **FIGURE 18-46** Large calcification is seen with association with fat necrosis. This was an old surgical biopsy site (H&E, ×200).

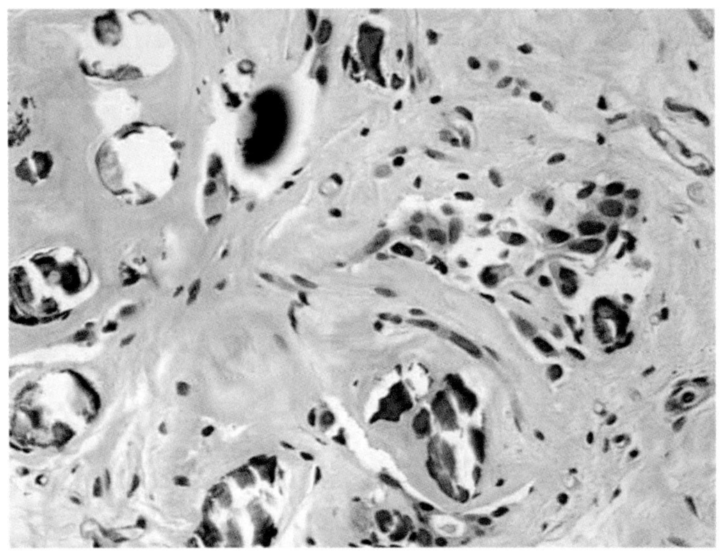

■ **FIGURE 18-47** Multiple small microcalcifications are seen with sclerotic changes with reactive epithelium associated with radiation changes (H&E, ×400).

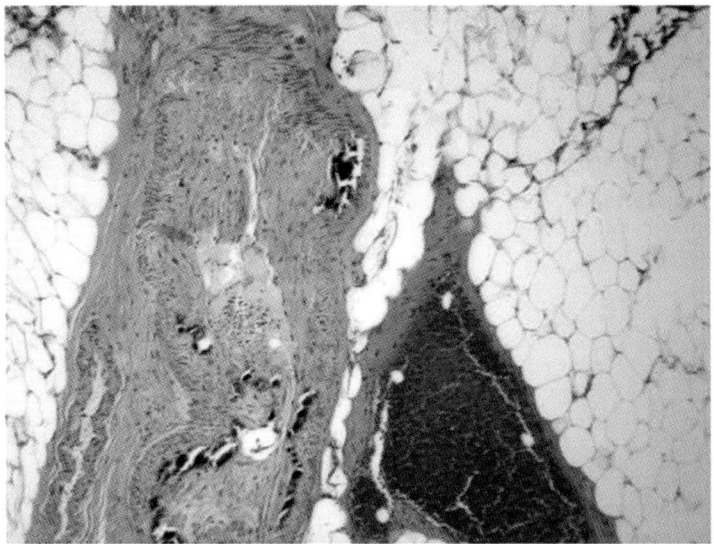

■ **FIGURE 18-48** Mönckeberg calcification is seen in the vessels in the breast tissue of an elderly woman (H&E, ×200).

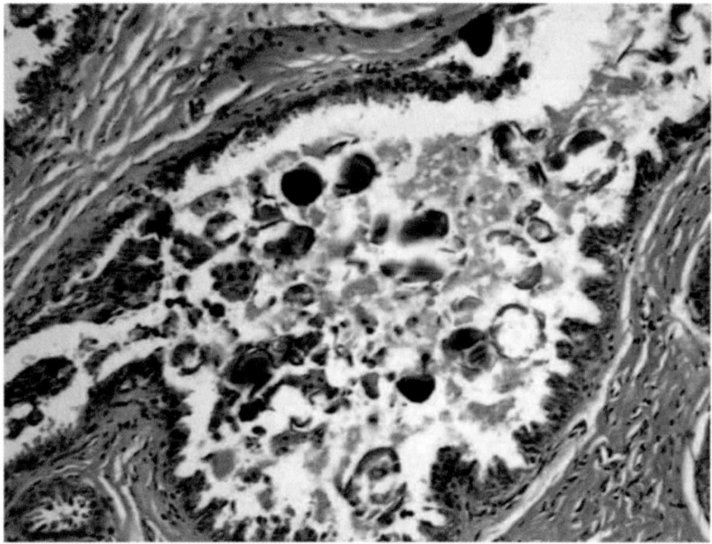

■ **FIGURE 18-49** Microcalcifications seen within columnar cell lesion (H&E, ×200).

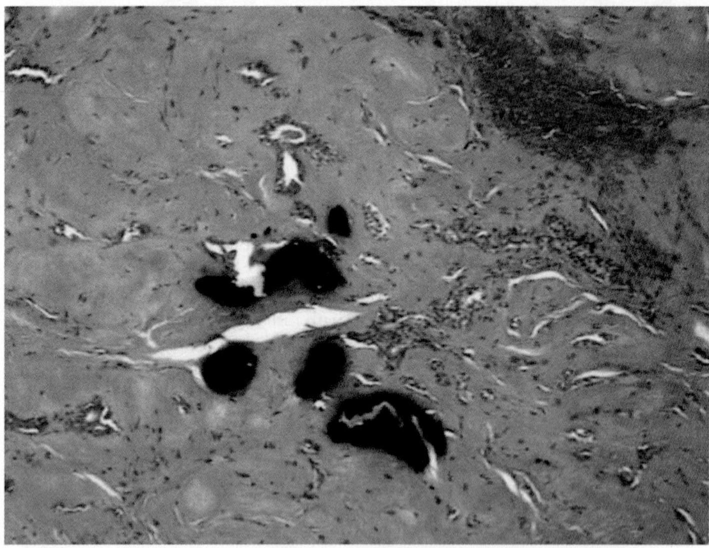

■ **FIGURE 18-50** Microcalcifications seen with involuted and hyalinized fibroadenoma (H&E, ×40).

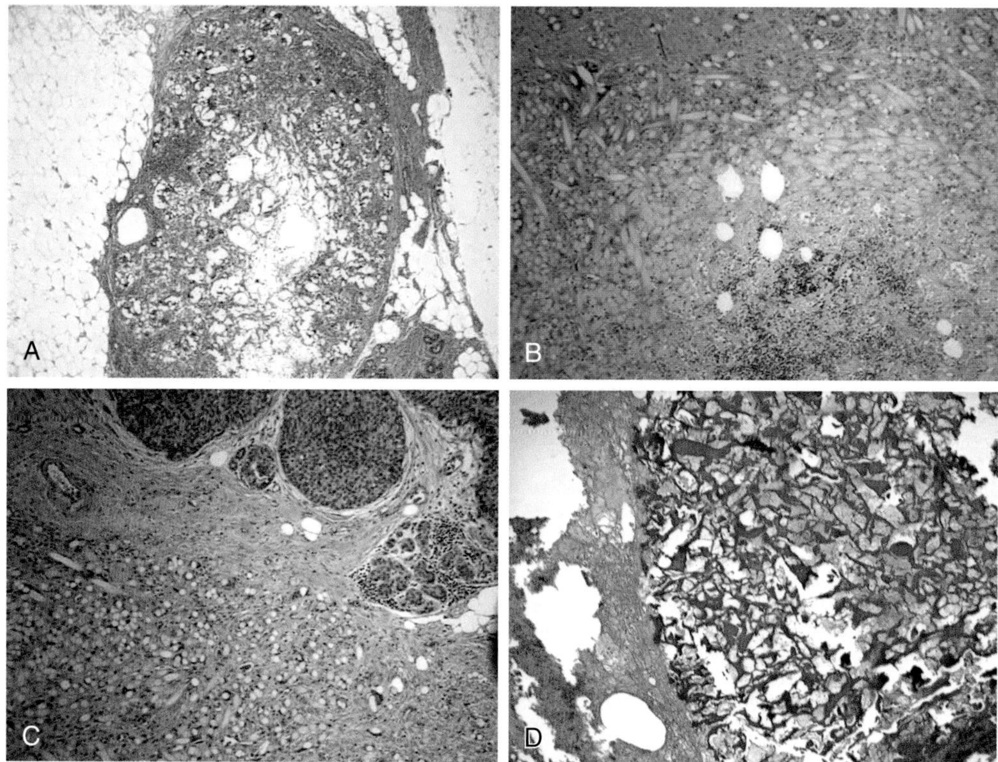

■ **FIGURE 18-51** Various types of microclips seen from lumpectomy specimen (H&E, ×100).

KEY POINTS

- Milk of calcium is best demonstrated as amorphous, rounded calcifications that are not visible on the CC projection that become linear or crescent shaped (teacup sign) on the mediolateral projection.
- Dermal calcifications are typically faint spherical or polygonal lucent-centered calcifications that are frequently clustered and occur most often in the inferior and medial aspects of the breasts. A tangential view may be obtained to best assess that these calcifications are truly in the skin.
- Vascular or Mönckeberg calcifications demonstrate the classic tram-track appearance of two parallel calcific lines on mammography.
- Fat necrosis may have a variety of mammographic appearances. One common and characteristic finding is a radiolucent or mixed fat and soft tissue circumscribed mass with a calcified or noncalcified rim, known as a lipid or oil cyst.
- Involuting fibroadenomas typically demonstrate popcorn-shaped coarse calcifications.
- Typical secretory calcifications are seen on mammography as dense, solid, rodlike calcifications, which are usually bilateral, symmetric, and diffuse.
- It is essential to ensure concordance between the mammographic calcification features and the pathology description. Regular meetings and conversation between the radiologists and pathologists are necessary to correlate the findings.
- There are two types of histologic calcifications. One type is basophilic concretions of calcium phosphates that appear lamellar and as concentric layers of dark purple color on hematoxylin and eosin stain. Another type is calcium oxalate crystals, which appear clear, birefringent, and nonbasophilic by light microscopy.

SUGGESTED READINGS

Bassett LW. Mammographic analysis of calcifications. *Radiol Clin North Am* 1992;**30**:93–105.

Castellanos MR, Paramanathan K, El-Sayegh S, Forte F, Buchbinder S, Kleiner M. Breast cancer screening in women with chronic kidney disease: the unrecognized effects of metastatic soft-tissue calcification. *Nat Clin Pract Nephrol* 2008;**4**:337–41.

Monda LA. Differentiation of breast calcifications. *Radiol Technol* 2001;**72**:532–44.

Sickles EA. Breast calcifications: mammographic evaluation. *Radiology* 1986;**160**:289–93.

Tse GM, Tan PH, Pang AL, Tang AP, Cheung HS. Calcification in breast lesions: pathologists' perspective. *J Clin Pathol* 2008;**61**:145–51.

REFERENCES

1. Sickles EA, Abele JS. Milk of calcium within tiny benign breast cysts. *Radiology* 1981;**141**:655-8.
2. Homer MJ, Cooper AG, Pile-Spellman ER. Milk of calcium in breast microcysts: manifestation as a solitary focal disease. *AJR Am J Roentgenol* 1988;**150**:789-90.
3. Linden SS, Sickles EA. Sedimented calcium in benign breast cysts: the full spectrum of mammographic presentations. *AJR Am J Roentgenol* 1989;**152**:967-71.
4. Pennes DR, Rebner M. Layering granular calcifications in macroscopic breast cysts. *Breast Dis* 1988;**1**:109-12.
5. Kopans DB, Meyer JE, Homer MJ, Grabbe J. Dermal deposits mistaken for breast calcifications. *Radiology* 1983;**149**:592-4.
6. Berkowitz JE, Gatewood OM, Donovan GB, Gayler BW. Dermal breast calcifications: localization with template-guided placement of skin marker. *Radiology* 1987;**163**:282.
7. Frenna TH, Meyer JE. Identification of atypical skin calcifications. *Radiology* 1993;**187**:584.
8. Gyves-Ray KM, Adler DD. Dermatomyositis: an unusual cause of breast calcifications. *Breast Dis* 1989;**2**:195-201.
9. Black KA, Zilko PJ, Dawkins RL, Armstrong BK, Mastaglia GL. Cancer in connective tissue disease. *Arthritis Rheum* 1982;**25**:1130-3.
10. Callen JP. Dermatomyositis. *Dermatol Clin* 1983;**1**:461-73.
11. Gold RH, Bassett LW, Coulson WF. Mammographic features of malignant and benign disease. In: Bassett LW, Gold RH, editors. *Breast cancer detection: mammography and other methods in breast imaging*. 2nd ed. Orlando, Fla: Grune & Stratton; 1987. p. 15-65.
12. Sickles EA, Galvin HB. Breast arterial calcification in association with diabetes mellitus: too weak a correlation to have clinical utility. *Radiology* 1985;**155**:577-9.
13. Van Noord PA, Beijerinck D, Kemmeren JM, van der Graaf Y. Mammograms may convey more than breast cancer risk: breast arterial calcification and arteriosclerotic related diseases in women of the DOM cohort. *Eur J Cancer Prev* 1996;**5**:483-7.
14. Evans AJ, Cohen ME, Cohen GF. Patterns of breast calcification in patients on renal dialysis. *Clin Radiol* 1992;**45**:343-4.
15. Sommer G, Kopsa H, Zazgornik J, Salomonowitz E. Breast calcifications in renal hyperparathyroidism. *AJR Am J Roentgenol* 1987;**148**:855-7.
16. Bassett LW, Gold RH, Cove HC. Mammographic spectrum of traumatic fat necrosis: the fallibility of "pathognomonic" signs of carcinoma. *AJR Am J Roentgenol* 1978;**130**:119-22.
17. Bassett LW, Gold RH, Mirra JM. Nonneoplastic breast calcifications in lipid cysts: development after excision and primary irradiation. *AJR Am J Roentgenol* 1982;**138**:335-8.
18. Evers K, Troupin RH. Lipid cyst: classic and atypical appearances. *AJR Am J Roentgenol* 1991;**157**:271-3.
19. Kopans DB. Pathologic, mammographic, and ultrasonographic correlation. In: Kopans DB, editor. *Breast imaging*. 2nd ed. Philadelphia: Lippincott-Raven; 1997. p. 511-615.
20. Huynh PT, Parellada JA, Shaw de Paredes E. Dilated duct pattern at mammography. *Radiology* 1997;**204**:137-41.
21. Beyer GA, Thorsen MK, Shaffer KA, Walker AP. Mammographic appearance of the retained Dacron cuff of a Hickman catheter. *AJR Am J Roentgenol* 1990;**155**:1203-4.
22. Wakabayashi M, Reid JD, Bhattacharjee M. Foreign body granuloma caused by prior gunshot wound mimicking malignant breast mass. *AJR Am J Roentgenol* 1999;**173**:321-2.
23. Stacey-Clear A, McCarthy KA, Hall DA, Pile-Spellman ER, Mrose HE, White G. Calcified suture material in the breast after radiation therapy. *Radiology* 1992;**183**:207-8.
24. Bruwer A, Nelson GW, Spark RP. Punctate intranodal gold deposits simulating microcalcifications on mammograms. *Radiology* 1987;**163**:87-8.
25. Radhi JM, Thavanathan MJ. Hydatid cyst presenting as a breast lump. *Can J Surg* 1990;**33**:29-30.
26. Vega A, Ortega E, Cavada A, Garijo F. Hydatid cyst of the breast: mammographic findings. *AJR Am J Roentgenol* 1994;**162**:825-6.
27. Gorman JD, Champaign JL, Sumida FK, Canavan L. Schistosomiasis involving the breast. *Radiology* 1992;**185**:423-4.
28. Britton CA, Sumkin J, Math M, Williams S. Mammographic appearance of loiasis. *AJR Am J Roentgenol* 1992;**159**:51-2.

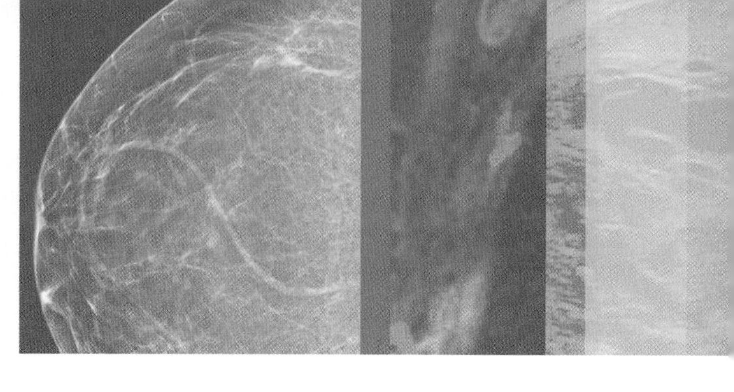

CHAPTER 19

High-Risk Breast Diseases

Sophia Kim Apple, Laura Doepke, and Lawrence W. Bassett

High-risk breast disease includes papillary lesions, flat epithelial atypia (FEA), atypical ductal hyperplasia (ADH), lobular neoplasia, including atypical lobular hyperplasia (ALH), lobular carcinoma in situ (LCIS), and benign phyllodes tumor.

PAPILLARY LESIONS

Definition

Papillary lesions of the breast are heterogeneous groups that are separated into three types: solitary central papillomas, multiple papillomas (papillomatosis), and juvenile papillomatosis. Benign solitary papillomas can also present as intracystic lesions. A *papilloma* is a lesion arising from and involving a central large lactiferous duct, and *papillomatosis* arises from and involves smaller terminal ductal lobular units (TDLUs). Papillomatosis is usually multifocal with peripheral lesions. Juvenile papillomatosis was described by Rosen and associates in 1980 in a group of "adolescents and young women with a striking constellation of changes usually described as components of fibrocystic disease."[1]

Prevalence and Epidemiology

Solitary papillomas are usually located within a major lactiferous duct in the subareolar or central region of the breast. Rarely, they involve the nipple.

Multiple papillomas develop within a group of ducts, are usually located peripherally in the breast, and involve TDLUs. Affected women tend to be younger, and the process is more often bilateral and less often associated with nipple discharge than in solitary papillomas.[2] Severe ductal papillomatosis is associated with changes usually seen in fibrocystic change in older women.

Juvenile papillomatosis usually presents in a young woman as a focal palpable mass that mimics fibroadenoma. Also called "Swiss cheese disease," this condition has been reported in women aged 10 to 48 years.[1]

Etiology and Pathophysiology

Papillomas are lesions of benign ductal epithelium that proliferates. The exact cause of this proliferation is unknown.

Manifestations of Disease

Clinical Presentation

Solitary papillomas usually present as bloody or serous nipple discharge and are frequently nonpalpable and nontender. Multiple papillomatosis is usually asymptomatic and nonpalpable. Juvenile papillomatosis can present as a palpable mass lesion.

Imaging Indications and Algorithm

When a patient presents with spontaneous, clear or bloody nipple discharge, the imaging algorithm should include diagnostic mammography (in woman older than 30 years of age), ultrasonography, and possibly ductography.

Imaging Findings by Modality

Mammography

Solitary papillomas are often mammographically occult because of their small size; however, they may be seen as a circumscribed subareolar mass or a cluster of calcifications on mammography (Fig. 19-1).[3,4] When the practitioner is unable to visualize with mammography or ultrasonography, galactography may be useful (Fig. 19-2).

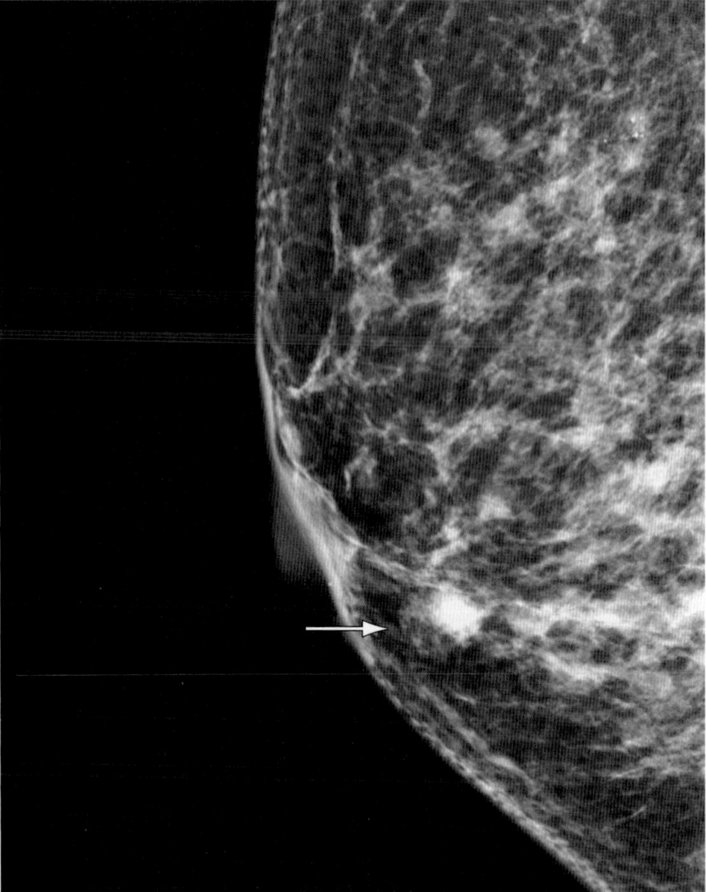

■ **FIGURE 19-1** Solitary papilloma on mammogram. An oval, indistinct, high density mass (*arrow*) in a patient with nipple discharge proved to be an intraductal papilloma at excision.

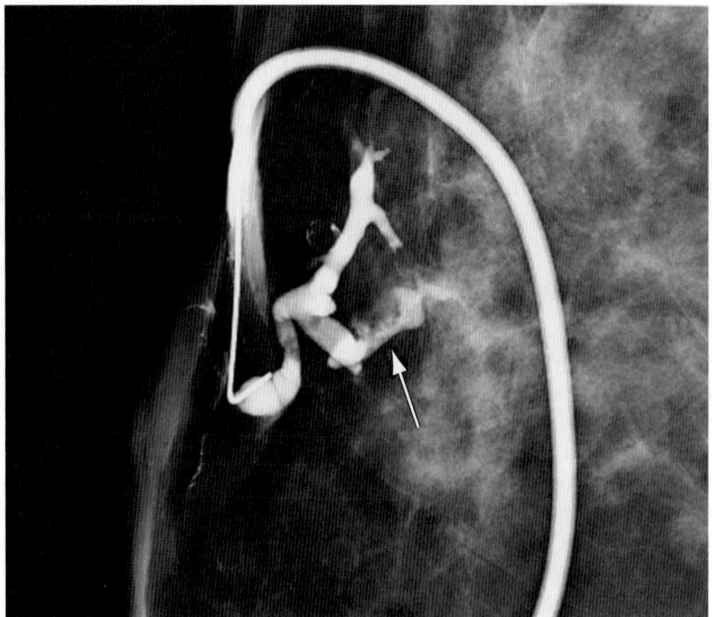

■ **FIGURE 19-2** Solitary papilloma on ductography. Magnification craniocaudal view demonstrates a filling defect (*arrow*) that was excised and found to be a solitary papilloma.

Multiple peripheral papillomas may be seen on mammographic examination as multiple masses, occasionally with microcalcifications (Fig. 19-3).[3] Because of the relatively young age of affected women, little in the literature addresses the mammographic findings of juvenile papillomatosis.

Ultrasonography

The ultrasonographic appearance of papillomas is variable. These lesions often appear as an intraductal filling defect that may or may not be associated with ductal dilatation. The mass may appear entirely solid or may appear as a complex mass with cystic and solid components. Papillomas can also appear as an intracystic mass. If the mass is very small, the only ultrasonographic abnormality may be isolated ductal dilatation (Fig. 19-4).[5]

Magnetic Resonance Imaging (MRI)

The MRI appearance is nonspecific and cannot be differentiated from malignancy based on imaging characteristics alone. Lesions can appear as small, smooth benign-appearing masses to irregular masses with rapid washout, mimicking invasive carcinomas (Fig. 19-5).[6]

Classic Signs

- Mammography may demonstrate a subareolar circumscribed mass.
- Ultrasonography often demonstrates an intraductal filling defect.
- Classic appearance on ductography is a filling defect, but this cannot be differentiated from malignancy or hematoma by imaging alone.

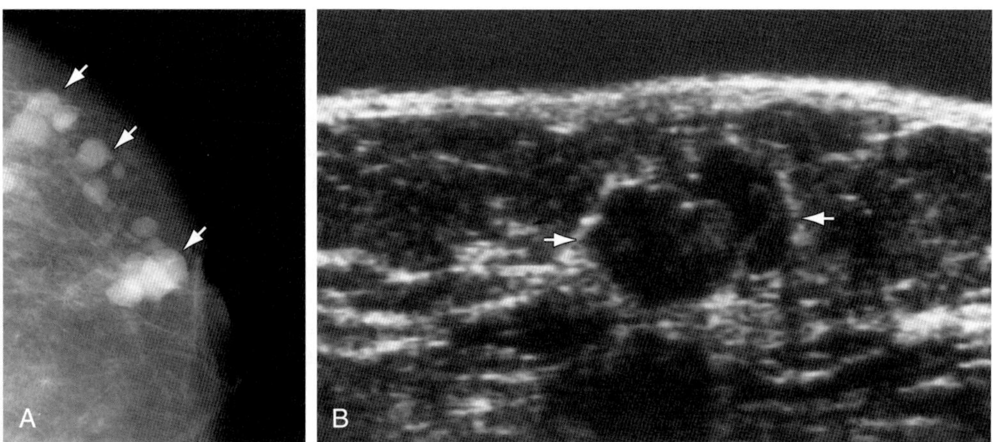

■ **FIGURE 19-3** Multiple peripheral papillomas. Craniocaudal mammogram demonstrating multiple round, circumscribed masses.

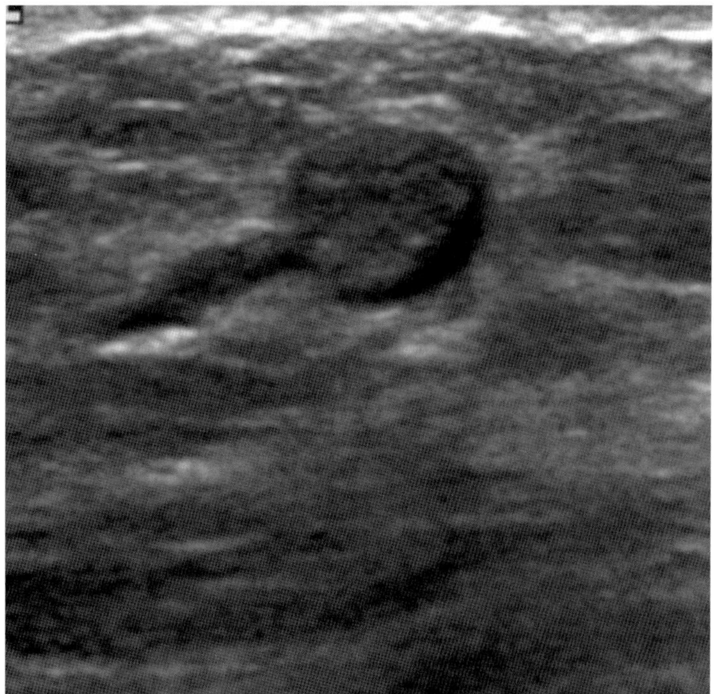

■ **FIGURE 19-4** Intraductal papilloma on ultrasound. Dilated duct in the subareolar region is partially occluded by an isoechoic, round mass representing a papilloma.

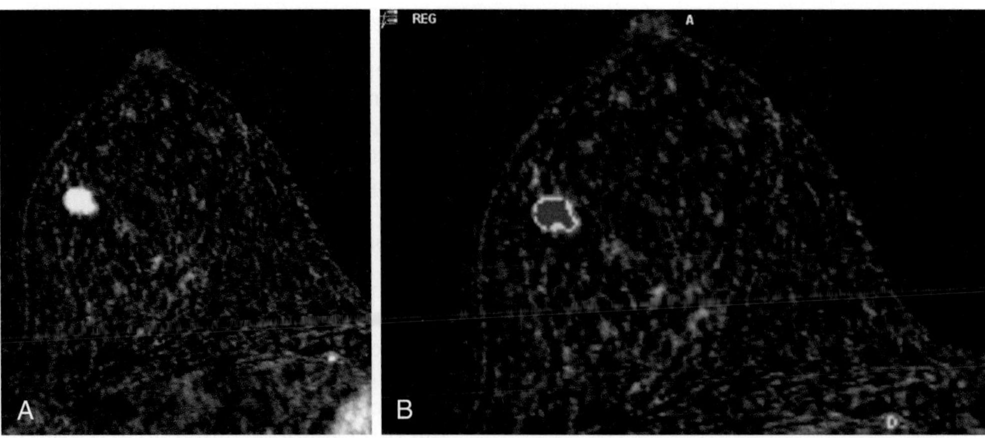

■ **FIGURE 19-5** A and B, Magnetic resonance image appearance of a papilloma. An oval, homogeneously enhancing mass with lobular margins is seen in the right breast with rapid washout. This was later sampled and found to be a papilloma.

Differential Diagnosis

From Clinical Presentation

The differential diagnosis from the clinical presentation would include malignancy, duct ectasia, and fibrocystic change.

From Imaging Findings

The differential diagnosis from the imaging findings would include malignancy and intraductal papilloma.

Pathology Findings

An intraductal papilloma is usually a cystically dilated duct with a solid component composed of arborescent fronds of fibrovascular stroma with a stalk that arises from the duct lumen (Figs. 19-6 and 19-7). The fronds are usually covered with a benign two-cell epithelial layer; however, the large volume of the epithelial lining may undergo hyperplasia at any location and evolve to ADH, ductal carcinoma in situ (DCIS) or invasive papillary carcinoma. Histologic evaluation of the proliferative epithelial lining determines whether the papilloma is benign, high risk, or malignant. Hemorrhagic infarct, dense sclerosis, squamous metaplasia, and apocrine metaplasia can occur within papillomas. The presence of entrapped ducts within sclerosis that mimic invasive carcinoma can be challenging. The presence of myoepithelial cells can aid the correct diagnosis. Papillomatosis is synonymous with multiple papillomas involving multiple TDLUs in the peripheral breast (Fig. 19-8). It can present as a palpable lesion, but more commonly is found incidentally by mammography. Nipple discharge or bleeding is not a common symptom of papillomatosis. In contrast to papilloma, papillomatosis involves several papillary lesions within multiple expanded TDLUs. Atypia can occur within papillomatosis. Papillomatosis is known to have a higher recurrence rate and malignant transformation than central papilloma.[7]

Atypical papilloma occurs when a sheet-like cellular proliferation of uniform luminal cells with well-defined cytoplasmic borders is admixed with the usual papilloma.

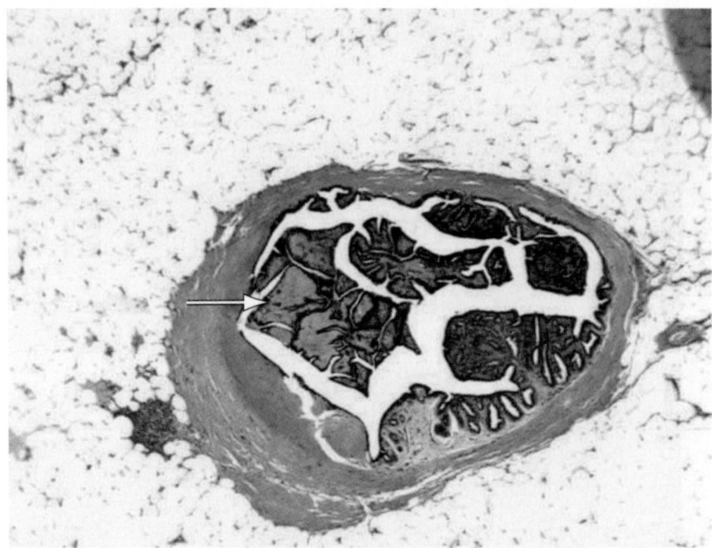

■ **FIGURE 19-6** Low power view of intraductal papilloma showing cystically dilated duct with luminal solid component. Epithelial cells are seen with arborizing central fibrovascular structures (*arrow*) (H&E, ×40).

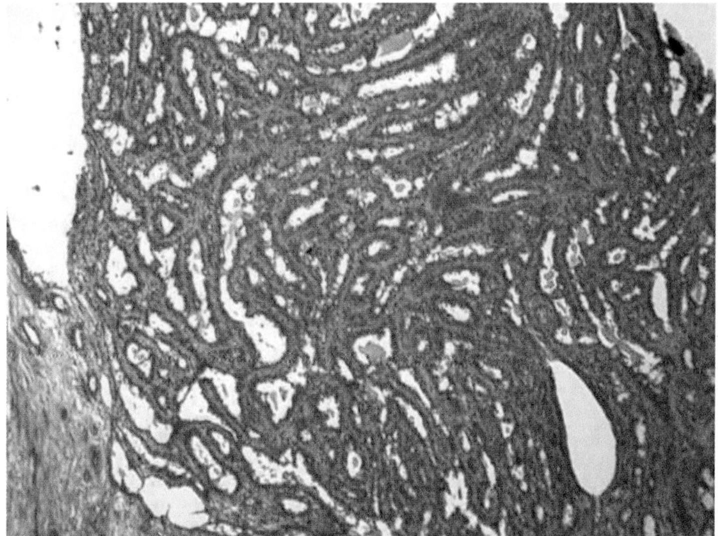

■ **FIGURE 19-7** Higher power view of intraductal papilloma. Proliferating cells are inner ductal cells and the outer myoepithelial cells with stroma are intervening in all glandular areas (H&E, ×200).

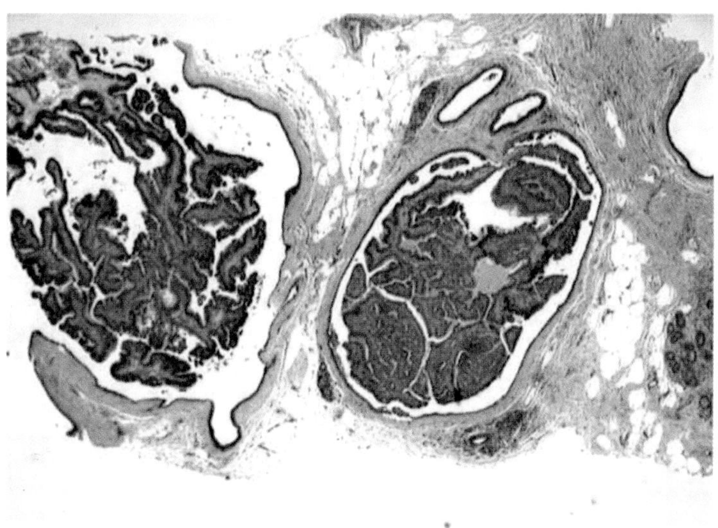

■ **FIGURE 19-8** Multiple papillomatosis. Peripheral papillary lesions involving many of terminal ductal lobular units (TDLUs) (H&E, ×40).

When these uniform populations of luminal cells predominate in a papilloma, DCIS within papilloma is an appropriate diagnosis (Figs. 19-9 and 19-10). The percentage of these proliferations required to diagnose ADH or DCIS within papilloma varies according to classification with a cutoff of 30%. This semiquantitative criterion is somewhat arbitrary.

Synopsis of Treatment Options

There are several concerns when papillary lesions are encountered in core needle biopsy (CNB) specimens. Firstly, there is the difficulty for the pathologist of differentiating between atypical and malignant papillary lesions based on limited, fragmented specimens. Secondly, it is uncertain whether the histologic features of the specimens are representative of the most worrisome areas of the papillary lesion. The presence of atypia in a papilloma implies a relative carcinoma risk 7.5 times that of a papilloma without atypia.[7] A papilloma diagnosed at CNB warrants open biopsy if ADH is present in the epithelium. However, routine open biopsy after a CNB diagnosis of papilloma without atypia is controversial. Again, one problem is the small number of papillomas encountered at biopsy. One study of seven cases of papillomas identified at CNB (0.65% of CNBs) provided evidence that 11-gauge vacuum-assisted devices adequately sampled papillomas, that no cancers were found at surgical excision or follow-up, and that open biopsy is not necessary unless atypia is identified or there is imaging/histologic discordance.[8] In a retrospective review, Mercado and colleagues[9] reported on 12 benign papillomas (1.6% of all

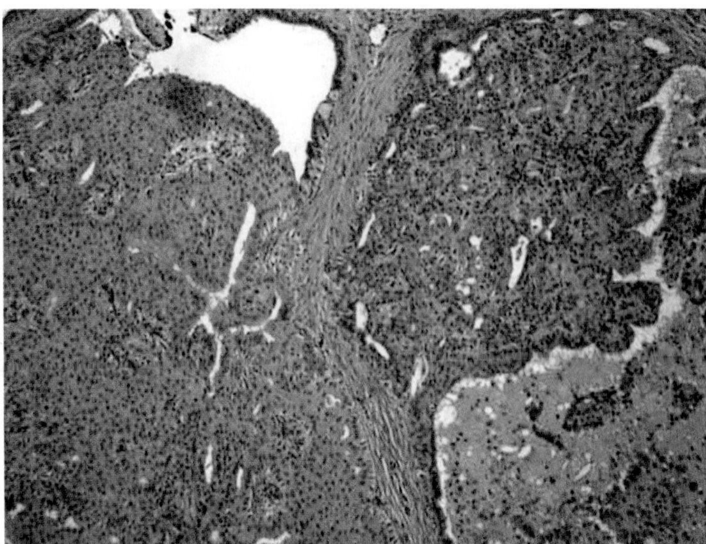

■ **FIGURE 19-9** Atypical papilloma. Solid sheets of monotonous epithelial proliferation with well-defined cytoplasmic borders without intervening fibrovascular cores (H&E, ×100).

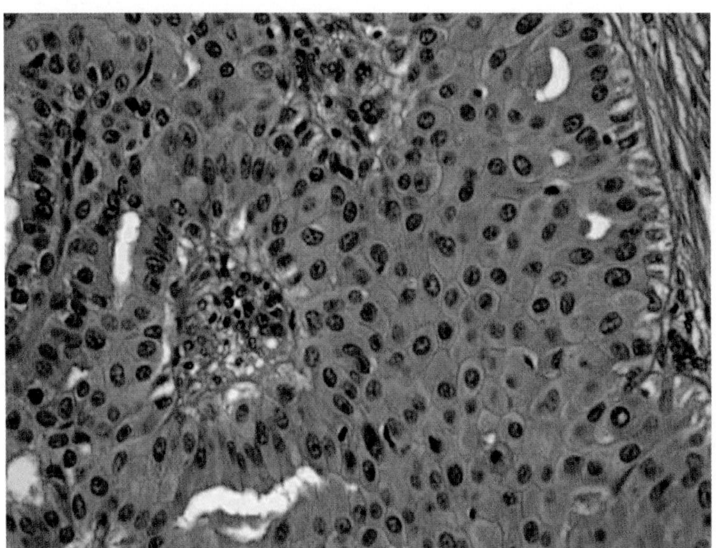

■ **FIGURE 19-10** Ductal carcinoma in situ (DCIS) within papilloma with monotonous epithelial proliferation. Note the loss of myoepithelial cells and inconspicuous arborizing fibrovascular stroma (H&E, ×400).

CNBs), of which six had surgical excision; one of these six cases revealed DCIS adjacent to a papilloma without atypia. However, the latter case had discordant imaging/pathology findings, with the mammogram showing calcifications in a linear distribution. Most authors concluded that when the histologic diagnosis is benign, the papillary lesions could be safely managed with imaging follow-up rather than with surgical excision. However, there are many articles that demonstrate that malignancy in papillomas read as benign can range from 4% to 25%. This could lead to a false sense of security for benign papillomas from a core needle biopsy. Atypical papillary lesions require surgical excision because histologic underestimation occurs at a frequency similar to that in other atypical lesions undergoing CNB. The limited data available suggest that diagnosis of a benign papilloma on CNB has a small, but definite chance of atypia or malignancy on surgical excision. Most recently, Jacobs and colleagues[10] recommended excisional biopsy in all papillary lesions of the breast. Complete excisional biopsy with a rim of normal breast tissue is recommended for atypical papillary lesions.

Multiple peripheral papillomas are associated with an increased risk for subsequent development of breast carcinoma, and a high tendency for recurrence after local excision exists. It used to be thought that multiple peripheral papillomas increased the risk of breast cancer but central solitary papillomas did not. However, a study by Page and coworkers[7] concluded that increased risk of breast cancer from a papilloma was related to the presence or absence of ADH rather than its location. The treatment of choice is wide local excisional biopsy.

Juvenile papillomatosis may be a marker for families at risk for breast cancer, because 28% to 33% of affected women have a family history of breast carcinoma, and it has been suggested that the woman herself may have an increased risk of developing breast cancer later in life.[2] Bazzocchi and colleagues[11] reported coexisting carcinoma in 15% of women and ADH in another 15% of cases.

The treatment of choice is wide local excision of the lesion, with careful surveillance of the affected woman and her family members.

FLAT EPITHELIAL ATYPIA

Definition

Columnar cell lesions are defined as a collection of dilated TDLUs with tall columnar epithelial cells. Columnar cell lesions (CCL) are separated into four different lesions: columnar cell change, columnar cell hyperplasia, columnar cell change with atypia, and columnar cell hyperplasia with atypia. Columnar cell change with atypia and columnar cell hyperplasia with atypia are now referred to as *flat epithelial atypia* (FEA).

Prevalence and Epidemiology

The exact prevalence of FEA is unknown; however, the number of diagnoses is increasing given advances in breast imaging and the increasing number of CNBs.

Etiology and Pathophysiology

The cellular origin of FEA is not completely understood.

Manifestations of Disease

Clinical Presentation

There is no specific clinical presentation of FEA because this is almost always a clinically silent entity that often appears as suspicious calcifications on mammography.

Imaging Indications and Algorithm

Because FEA is often discovered on mammography, the appropriate imaging algorithm would include a diagnostic exam, including magnification views. If the calcifications are deemed suspicious, tissue diagnosis with stereotactic CNB or excisional biopsy is indicated.

Imaging Technique and Findings

Mammography

Although no absolutely typical mammographic appearance has been described, FEA is often seen associated with microcalcifications (Fig. 19-11).

Ultrasonography

There is no ultrasonographic abnormality seen with FEA because the abnormality is limited to suspicious microcalcifications seen on mammography.

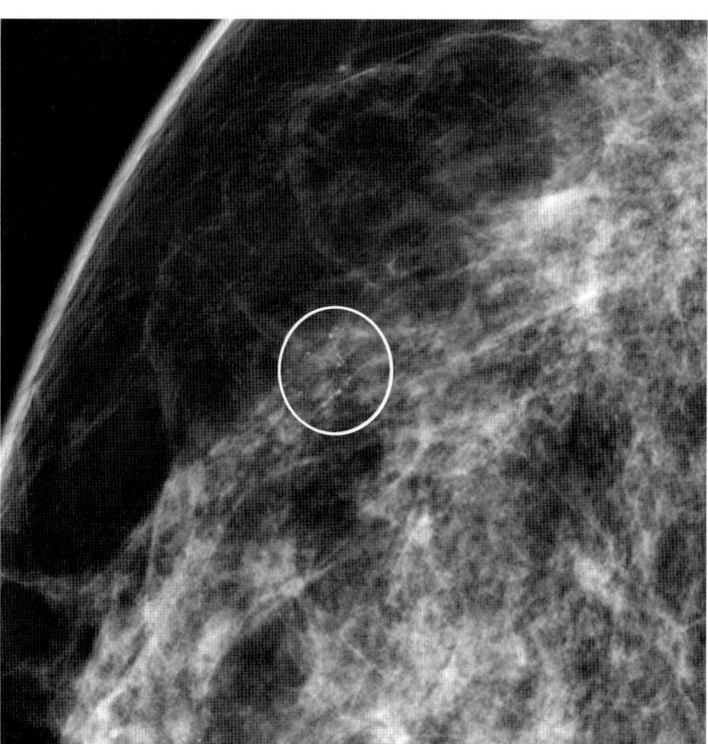

■ **FIGURE 19-11** A linear distribution of amorphous calcifications originally seen on screening mammogram (*circle*). Diagnostic workup confirmed their suspicious appearance. Stereotactic core needle biopsy (CNB) demonstrated flat epithelial atypia. Open biopsy was subsequently performed.

Magnetic Resonance Imaging

No MRI abnormality has been described in relation to FEA.

Classic Signs

There is no classic appearance to the microcalcifications associated with FEA and, for this reason, suspicious calcifications merit tissue diagnosis.

Differential Diagnosis

From Clinical Presentation

FEA is clinically silent.

From Imaging Findings

The differential diagnosis from the mammographic appearance would include usual ductal hyperplasia, ADH, and other CCLs (columnar cell change, columnar cell hyperplasia, and DCIS).

Pathology Findings

Technologic advances in mammography and the increasing use of CNB have increased the diagnosis of the CCL owing to its associated microcalcifications. This entity includes a wide range of pathologic findings distinguished by columnar (ovoid, elongated) epithelial cells lining the TDLU. CCLs have been described variously as columnar cell hyperplasia, blunt duct adenosis, hyperplastic terminal groupings, columnar metaplasia, and columnar alteration with prominent apical snouts and secretions (CAPSS). For practical purposes CCLs can be placed into two categories: columnar cell change and columnar cell hyperplasia (Figs. 19-12 and 19-13). *Columnar cell change* is defined as TDLUs with variably dilated acini lined by one or two layers of columnar epithelial cells. Flocculent secretions and apical snouts are often present. *Columnar cell hyperplasia* is characterized by cellular stratification of more than two cell layers but otherwise sharing many of the same features. Calcifications are reported to be present in 75% of columnar cell lesions. The calcifications are usually psammomatous, typically non-branching basophilic calcium phosphate and are often round on mammography (Fig. 19-14). Although CCL and apocrine metaplasia may have luminal projection of cytoplasmic "snouts," a CCL is morphologically different from apocrine metaplasia. Apocrine metaplasia is composed of larger cells with round nuclei that are centrally located with abundant granular eosinophilic cytoplasm (Fig. 19-15). More recently, the World Health Organization (WHO) classification has named CCL with atypia as FEA when there is atypia associated with columnar cell changes and/or hyperplasia.[12] The designation of *flat* refers to an absence of complex architectural patterns, such as *rigid micropapillary* and *cribriform* or *arcade* present in ADH or DCIS. Cytologic atypia is typically of low nuclear grade and characterized by loss of polarity, enlarged monotonous nuclei, and conspicuous large nucleoli (Fig. 19-16). High-grade cytologic atypia is not a feature of FEA.

CCLs with architectural and/or cytologic features of atypia can be associated with low-grade DCIS and invasive breast cancer, especially tubular carcinoma. (Fig. 19-17). CCL is reported to be associated with lobular neoplasia, including LCIS, invasive lobular carcinoma, low-grade DCIS, and invasive tubular carcinoma.[13] The association of CCL, tubular carcinoma, and lobular neoplasia is referred to as *Rosen's Triad*.[14] Reports in the medical literature on CCLs with atypia indicate that DCIS or invasive cancer was found at subsequent surgical excision in up to 14% to 21% of cases.[15-17] Based on current literature, surgical excision is recommended if a CNB demonstrates a CCL with atypia (FEA).[10] However, the level of cancer risk associated with lesions that do not fulfill established criteria for ADH or DCIS is unknown and requires evaluation in follow-up studies. There are limited clinical outcome studies on FEA;

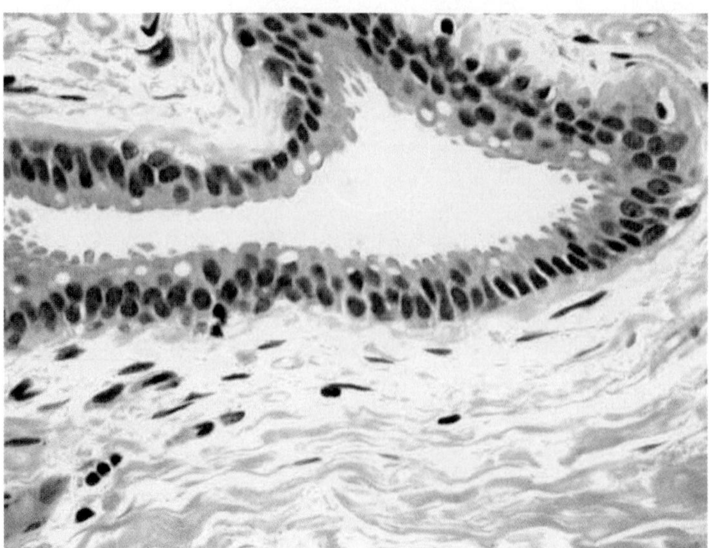

■ **FIGURE 19-12** Columnar cell change (CCL). Dilated lobular ductules lined by one to two layers of tall columnar cells with basally oriented nuclei and luminal cytoplasmic snouts (H&E, ×200).

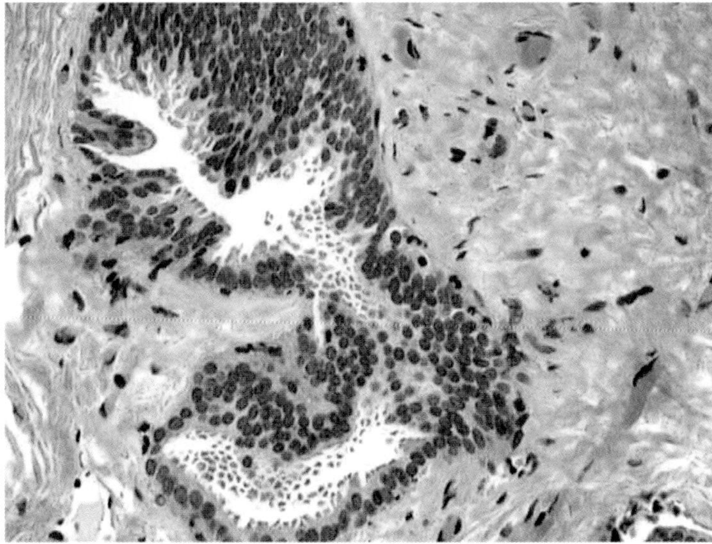

■ FIGURE 19-13 Columnar cell hyperplasia (CCH) is characterized by more than two cells layers of columnar cells with stratification and thickened epithelium. Transition between CCL and CCH is seen (H&E, ×200).

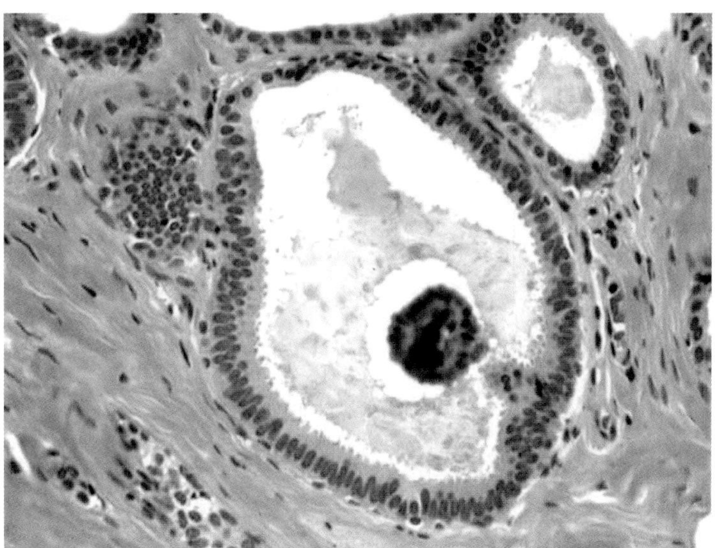

■ FIGURE 19-14 CCL is commonly sampled due to indeterminate microcalcifications seen with mammogram. Luminal area shows calcium phosphate calcification (H&E, ×200).

only two follow-up studies have directly addressed the clinical significance of FEA. Eusebi and coworkers[17] reported that 1 patient (4%) of 25 patients had a "local recurrence" after an average follow-up of 19.2 years with FEA.The other study was by the European Organization for Research and Treatment of Cancer trial 10835; none of 59 patients had a local recurrence of lesions similar to FEA for an average of 5.4 years follow-up.[18] The conclusion of these researchers is that the likelihood of local recurrence or progression to invasive breast cancer is exceedingly low.

Synopsis of Treatment Options

When a diagnosis of FEA is made on CNB, surgical excision is recommended. Although emerging data suggest that FEA may represent an early form of low-grade DCIS and is neoplastic, current management is to follow up with annual screening mammography. It is unknown at this time if closer follow-up after surgical excision is appropriate, and further clinical outcome studies are necessary.

ATYPICAL DUCTAL HYPERPLASIA

Definition

ADH is defined as a proliferative lesion that has some but not all the features of DCIS at both architecture and cytologic levels. Cytologic criterion of ADH is low nuclear grade, and the most common types of architecture of ADH are cribriform and micropapillary patterns.

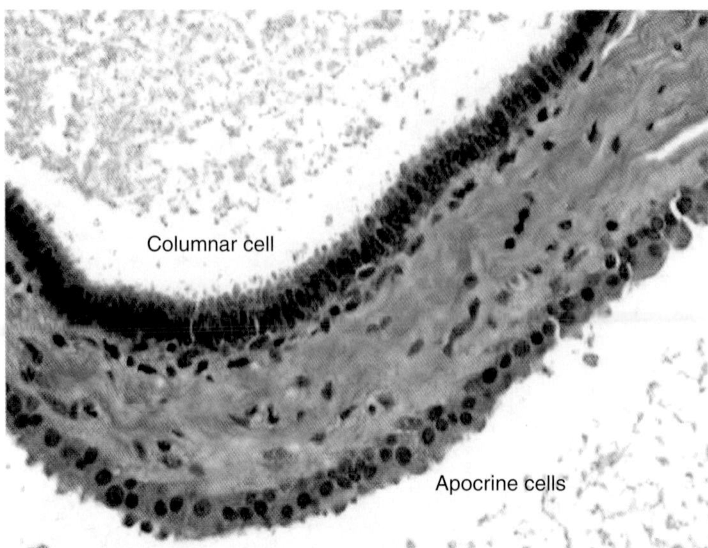

■ **FIGURE 19-15** CCL on top and apocrine metaplasia at the bottom. Both of these cells have luminal cytoplasmic snouts. Apocrine metaplasia is characterized by having round nuclei with central prominent nucleoli and prominent granular cytoplasm, whereas CCL shows tall cells without abundant eosinophilic granular cytoplasm (H&E, ×200).

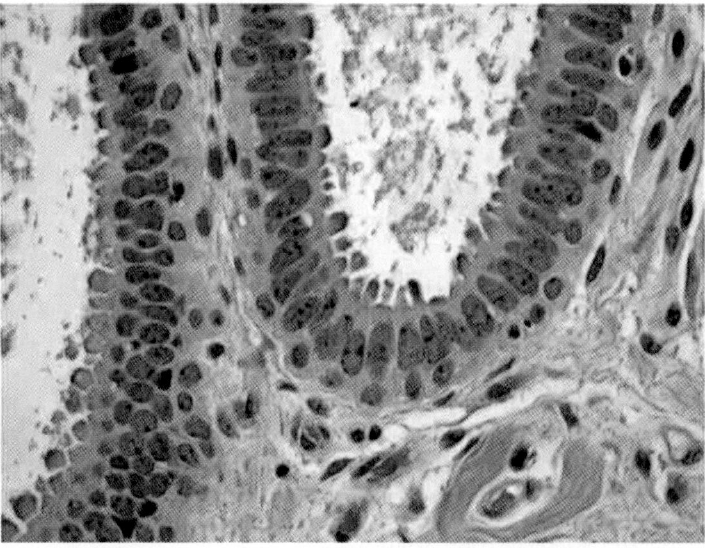

■ **FIGURE 19-16** Flat epithelial atypia (FEA) is characterized by having cytologic atypia: loss of nuclear polarity with large nuclear-to-cytoplasmic ratio and prominent nucleoli (H&E, ×400).

Prevalence and Epidemiology

Extensive use of screening mammography has led to a significant increase in diagnoses of ADH. It was reported that ADH diagnosis was estimated to be 2% to 5% in the premammographic period and increased to 22% to 28% after the introduction of mammography.

Etiology and Pathophysiology

ADH is atypical ductal proliferation. The etiology of this proliferation is not completely understood.

Manifestations of Disease

Clinical Presentation

ADH is usually clinically silent.

Imaging Indications and Algorithm

ADH usually appears as suspicious microcalcifications on screening mammography. Diagnostic mammography should be performed in this situation. If the patient presents with a palpable abnormality, ultrasonography should also be

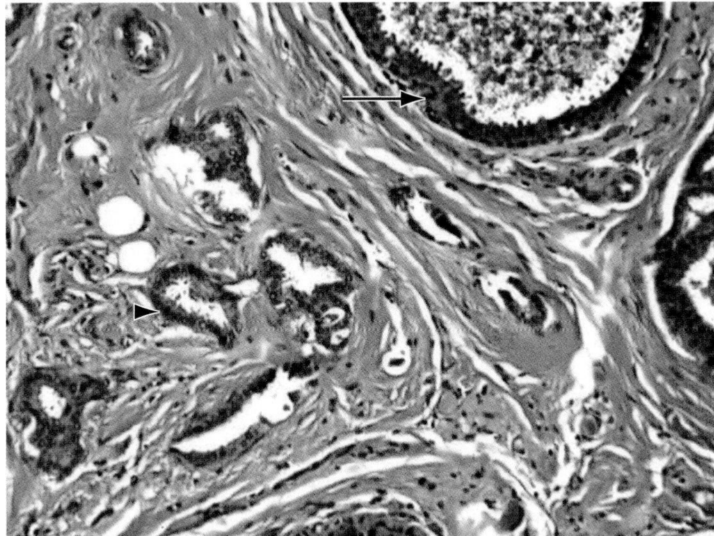

■ **FIGURE 19-17** Flat epithelial atypia (FEA) is seen (*arrow*) and invasive tubular carcinoma is seen (*arrowhead*). FEA is commonly seen with tubular carcinoma and lobular neoplasia (not shown) (H&E, ×200).

performed. If the microcalcifications are deemed suspicious or a mass is identified, then tissue diagnosis is warranted.

Imaging Technique and Findings

Mammography

Few studies have documented the mammographic findings of epithelial hyperplasia, and these have dealt with atypical hyperplasias. The lesion is often found within or adjacent to another benign or malignant mammographic abnormality. The most common mammographic presentation is suspicious microcalcifications, which may appear heterogeneous, pleomorphic, or amorphous. Masses, architectural distortion, and asymmetries are uncommon presentations of ADH (Fig. 19-18).

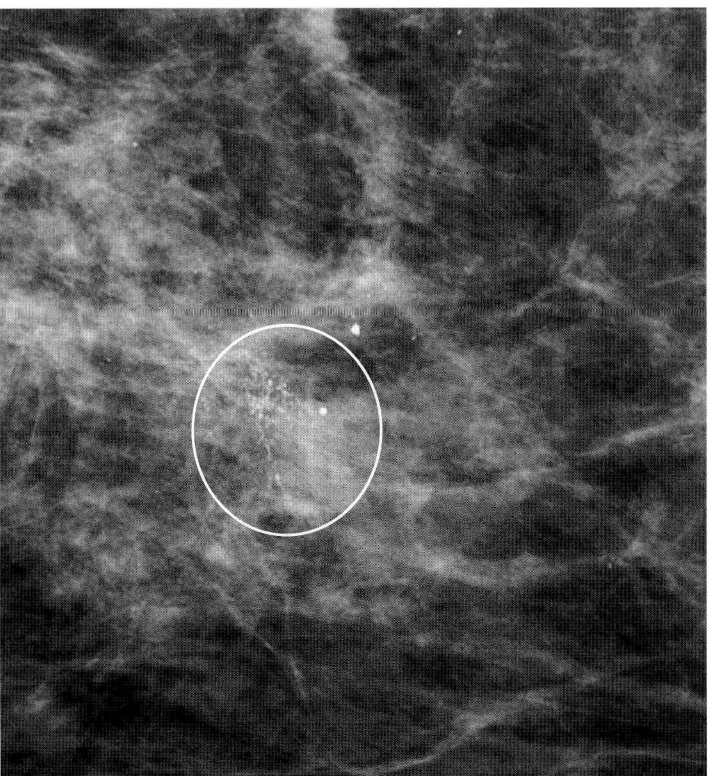

■ **FIGURE 19-18** Atypical ductal hyperplasia (ADH). A linear distribution of fine, linear calcifications adjacent to a cluster of fine pleomorphic calcifications reminiscent of a TDLU. Diagnostic workup confirmed their suspicious appearance. Stereotactic core needle biopsy revealed ADH.

Ultrasonography

There are no reported characteristic ultrasonographic features.

Magnetic Resonance Imaging

There are no reported characteristic features of ADH on MRI. There have been reports of enhancing masses and non-mass-like enhancement seen with ADH on MRI,[19] but these findings are nonspecific and tissue diagnosis is warranted if they are suspicious.

Differential Diagnosis

From Clinical Presentation

ADH is clinically silent.

From Imaging Findings

The differential diagnosis of suspicious microcalcifications would include usual ductal hyperplasia and CCLs, including FEA, and DCIS.

Pathology Findings

ADH is a proliferative lesion. Histologically, it has features that lie in the middle of the spectrum between usual ductal hyperplasia and DCIS of low nuclear grade. In diagnosing ADH, both architectural and cytologic atypia should be present but fall short of all criteria needed for DCIS. Architectural arrangements of usual ductal hyperplasia, ADH, and DCIS are illustrated by Page (Fig. 19-19).[20]-Qualitative criteria have been based on microscopic structure and cytologic details while quantitative criteria have been based on the number of duct cross sections that exhibit the abnormality: if a single duct is involved, then the designation is ADH; if two or more ducts are involved, then the designation is DCIS if the nuclear grade is low. Another scheme is based on the microscopic linear dimension of a lesion: a diagnosis of ADH is made when the atypical ductal proliferation is less than 2 mm, and a diagnosis of DCIS is made when these foci are greater than 2 mm in an aggregate cross-sectioned diameter. Two duct cross sections or 2 mm as criteria are both arbitrary cutoffs, and no scientific studies have been done to compare clinical outcome. Architectural complexity such as *rigid micropapillary*, *cribriform*, *arcades*, and *Roman-bridge* patterns are commonly seen with ADH and DCIS. Cytologic atypia is low grade and characterized by nuclear enlargement, a monotonous appearance, increased nuclear-to-cytoplasmic ratio, nuclear hyperchromasia, an irregular chromatin pattern, and the presence of nucleoli (Fig. 19-20). If the nuclear grade is intermediate or high, the diagnosis is DCIS regardless of the size or number of ductal proliferation.

Distinction between ADH and DCIS is even more challenging in CNB samples owing to the fragmented nature and the limited sample of the needle biopsy specimens. It has long been established that any CNB that reveals ADH necessitates open biopsy. There are several reasons surgical excision should be performed after a CNB diagnosis of ADH. Firstly, the distinction between advanced ADH and low-grade DCIS can be difficult as their features overlap. Secondly, DCIS may lie at the periphery of sites diagnosed as ADH on CNB. In a review of the literature, 25% to 26% of excisional biopsies after CNB diagnoses of ADH were found to have DCIS or invasive carcinomas, or both, even when large-needle (e.g., 11-gauge) vacuum-assisted devices are used.[21,22]

Therefore, there is consensus that ADH on CNB mandates open surgical biopsy.

Synopsis of Treatment Options

The diagnosis of ADH conveys a four to five times increased risk of development of malignancy when compared with the general population. Careful clinical follow-up with annual mammography is advised after excisional biopsy for ADH that was detected on CNB. It is unknown at this time if closer follow-up after surgical excision is appropriate, and further clinical outcome studies are necessary.

LOBULAR NEOPLASIA

Definition

Lobular neoplasia is separated into atypical lobular hyperplasia (ALH) and lobular carcinoma in situ (LCIS). No specific clinical signs or symptoms can be attributed to LCIS or ALH. ALH is used to describe hyperplasia of the TDLU that have some but not all of the features of LCIS. Its distinction from ductal hyperplasia, described in the previous section, is based on cytologic and architectural features rather than the site of origin. Differentiation between the two types of hyperplasia is important because of their different behavior, particularly with respect to multifocality, multicentricity, and discontinuous distributions. On cytologic examination, the atypical cells in ALH tend to be round or ovoid and exhibit marked uniformity with little variation in size or shape. Mitotic activity is rare. The proliferation tends to be polymorphic as with ductal hyperplasia, and contains mixtures of myoepithelial and epithelial cells. ALH, in its most severe form, merges with LCIS, and the distinction is mainly quantitative.

Prevalence and Epidemiology

The diagnosis of lobular neoplasia has increased owing to higher rates of biopsies after the introduction of CNB and is usually an incidental finding.

Etiology and Pathophysiology

Lobular neoplasia is a proliferation of the breast lobule that may or may not distend the lobule cause distension. The actually etiology of this proliferation is incompletely understood.

Manifestations of Disease

Clinical Presentation

Lobular neoplasia is a clinically silent disease and usually not tender or palpable.

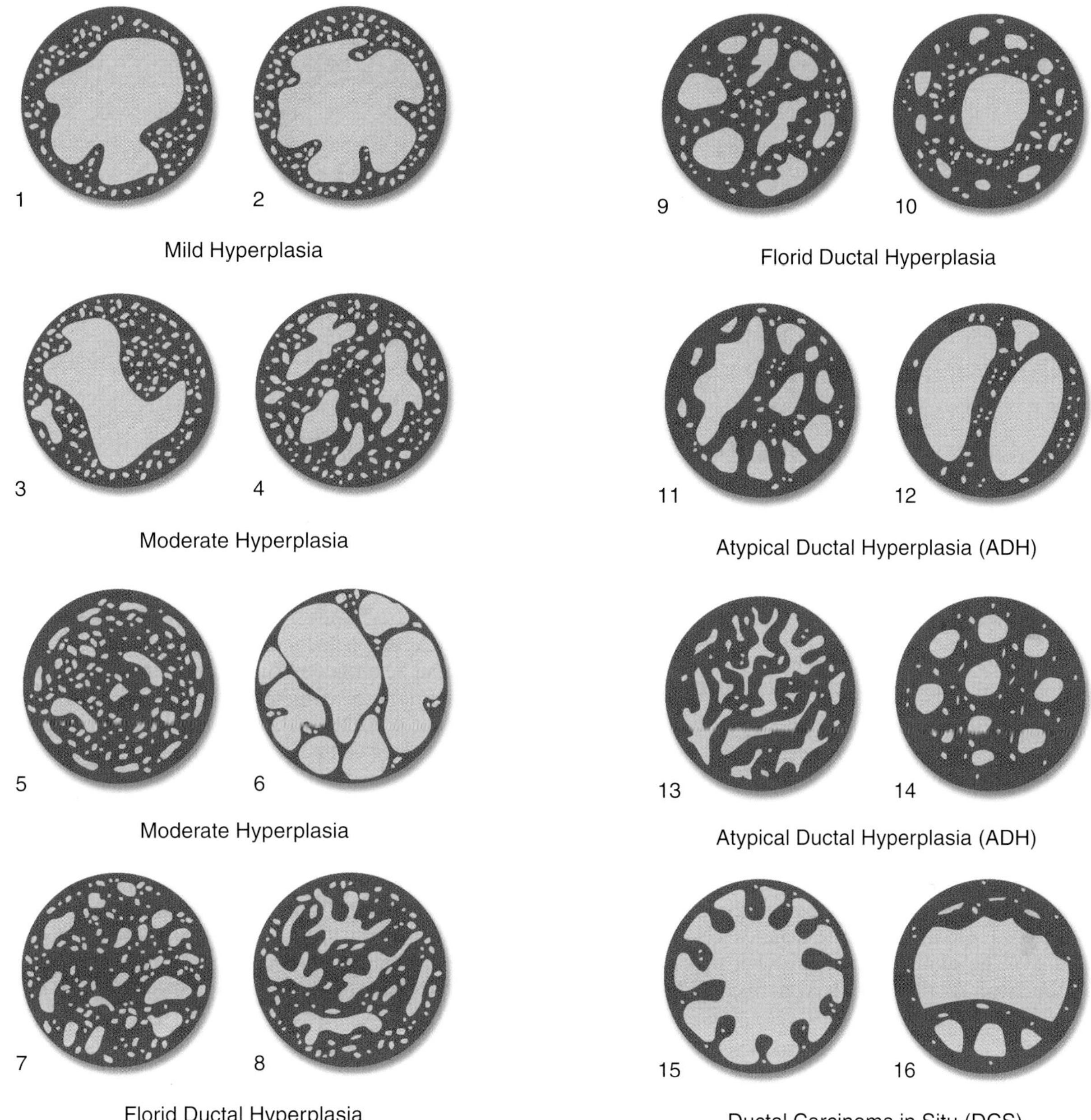

■ **FIGURE 19-19** Architectural patterns of ductal hyperplasia of usual type, atypical ductal hyperplasia and ductal carcinoma in situ. *(Adapted from Page DL, Anderson TJ. Diagnostic histopathology of the breast. Churchill Livingstone;1988.p. 170-171.)*

Imaging Technique and Findings

Mammography

Lobular neoplasia has no clinical or mammographic manifestations and is essentially incidentally found after biopsy for some other imaging finding. However, calcifications have been reported to occur in some LCIS lesions.

Ultrasonography

Lobular neoplasia has no specific ultrasonographic appearance.

Magnetic Resonance Imaging

Lobular neoplasia has no specific MRI appearance.

Classic Signs

There are no classic imaging signs for lobular neoplasia.

Differential Diagnosis

From Clinical Presentation

Lobular neoplasia is clinically silent.

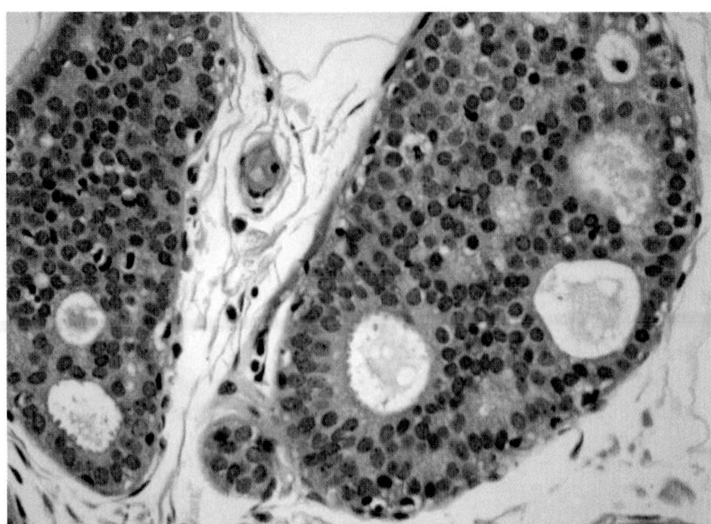

■ **FIGURE 19-20** Atypical ductal hyperplasia (ADH). The ducts have a lining of solid small, monotonous cells with cribriform microlumina. In the center, there are darker and smaller myoepithelial cells admixed with ductal cells, which is characteristic of ductal hyperplasia of usual type (H&E, ×200).

From Imaging Findings

Because the diagnosis of lobular neoplasia is usually an incidental finding, there is no specific differential diagnosis.

Pathology Findings

Lobular neoplasia is a spectrum of lesions including LCIS, ALH, and large ductal involvement with cells of ALH and LCIS. Histologically, LCIS is characterized by distention of the lobule with proliferating small, uniform cells. However, if the same small uniform cells proliferate but do not distend the lobule and if less than one half or three fourths of the acini in a TDLU are involved, the diagnosis is ALH (Figs. 19-21 to 19-23). The experts differ on what precise criteria should be used to distinguish ALH from LCIS. Again, qualitatively, when some, but not all, of the criteria for LCIS are present, ALH is usually diagnosed.

Traditional teaching is that lobular neoplasia is not a direct precursor to malignancy such as DCIS but rather a marker that identifies women with an increased risk of developing breast cancer.[23] It was thought that the risk for breast cancer was equal for either breast and could occur at any location. The risk for future breast cancer for ALH is three times higher and for LCIS up to ten times higher than that for the general population. Thus, it would not seem reasonable to recommend excisional biopsy when CNB biopsy reveals lobular neoplasia because eventual breast cancer could be anywhere in either breast. Also, lobular neoplasia has no mammographic manifestations and it would be difficult to localize the extent of the area

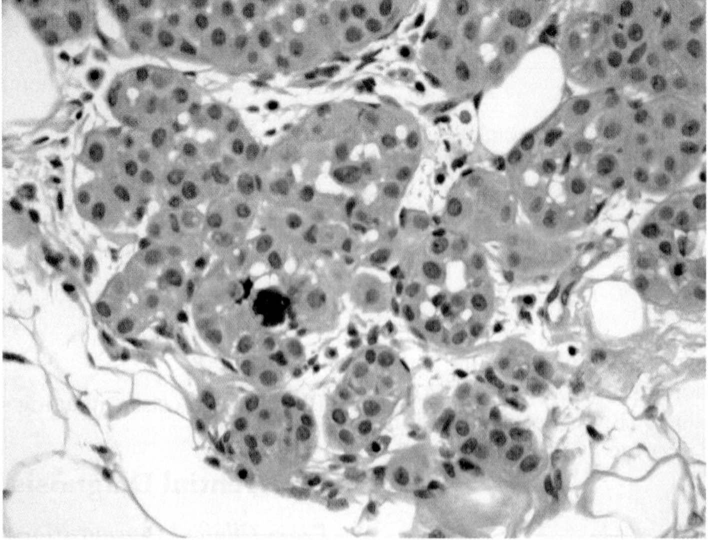

■ **FIGURE 19-21** Atypical lobular hyperplasia (ALH) with focal area of microcalcifications. Lobular neoplasia cells involved partial area of lobules and not expanding the terminal ductal lobular units (TDLUs) (H&E, ×400).

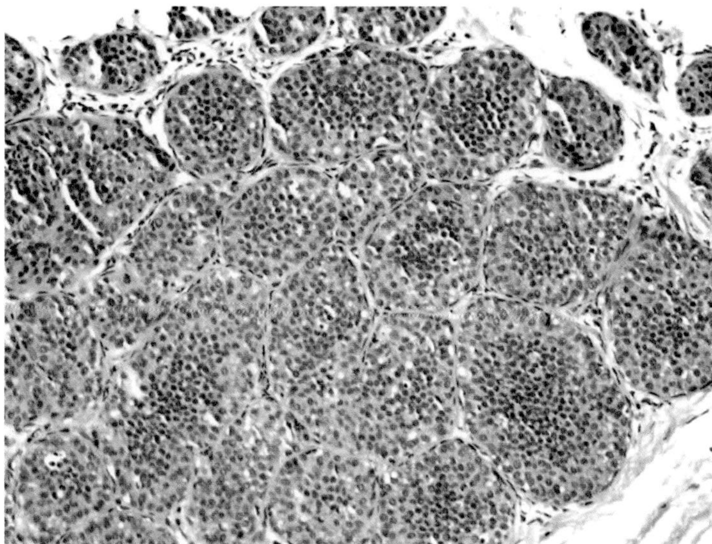

■ **FIGURE 19-22** Lobular carcinoma in situ (LCIS) showing expansion of lobular neoplasia cells which are dyshesive monotonous small cells (H&E, ×200).

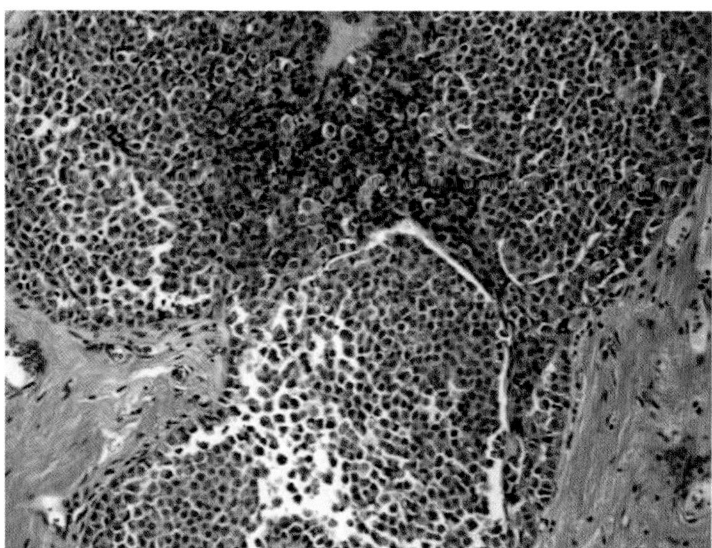

■ **FIGURE 19-23** Lobular carcinoma in situ (LCIS) involving large ducts. Marked distention of large ducts with central necrosis filled with monomorphic cells resembling ductal carcinoma in situ (DCIS). Neoplastic cells are dyshesive and not forming ducts (H&E, ×200).

to excise. The most recent literature indicates that lobular neoplasia is not only a risk factor but possibly a direct precursor to carcinoma in some situations. A retrospective study by Page and colleagues[24] found that breast cancers that developed after a biopsy showing lobular neoplasia were not equal bilaterally. In this retrospective study, when lobular neoplasia was diagnosed on biopsy, subsequent cancers were three times more likely to develop in the ipsilateral breast than the contralateral breast. This suggests that lobular neoplasia is intermediate between a local precursor and a generalized risk factor for breast cancer. The management of a CNB specimen showing lobular neoplasia has been controversial, and the data from various studies have not been consistent. There are two reasons it might be reasonable to recommend surgical excision after a CNB yielding lobular neoplasia alone (no other breast lesions seen). First, lobular neoplasia is usually mammographically occult. Thus, the mammographic lesion that prompted the biopsy may correctly be assumed to be undiagnosed. The second reason is that breast malignancy is frequently found to have areas of LCIS nearby. The malignant lesion can be ductal or lobular in origin. Thus, a CNB diagnosis of lobular neoplasia alone may represent a sampling error problem similar to that seen with ADH. Shin and coworkers[25] support using excisional biopsy after lobular neoplasia is suggested. They reported 14 cases of LCIS, or LCIS and ALH; and 6 cases with ALH alone found on CNB revealed 3 (21%) of 14 patients with a diagnosis of DCIS had invasive carcinoma at excisional biopsy. Among the six patients with ALH on CNB, one had infiltrating lobular carcinoma at excisional biopsy, two had LCIS, and the remaining were benign. The conclusion was that surgical biopsy should be considered after any CNB diagnosis of LCIS and any discordant biopsy with ALH. A more recent review of 6081 consecutive patients who underwent CNB identified 35 (0.58%) cases of LCIS or ALH. Of 15 patients with LCIS at CNB, 4 (27%) were upgraded to DCIS or invasive cancer; and in 20 patients with ALH, 2 were upgraded to DCIS (10%). The CNB upgrade of lobular neoplasia to malignancy (17%) after excisional biopsy was not significantly different than for ADH. As a result, biopsy was recommended when LCIS or ALH were identified at CNB.[26]

Variants of Lobular Carcinoma in Situ

There are a few variants of lobular neoplasia, namely, signet ring LCIS, pleomorphic LCIS, and massive acinar distention LCIS (Figs. 19-24 to 19-26). Some of the LCIS variants, especially those with nonclassic low- to intermediate-grade nuclear atypia and presence of central necrosis, have histologic features similar to the solid type of DCIS. This has been described as indeterminate type of carcinoma in situ, pleomorphic LCIS, or mixed ductal and lobular carcinoma in situ. Fortunately, this type of carcinoma in situ (CIS) is rare, but concordant with the theory that most cancer of the breast arises from the TDLU, which has both lobular and ductal components. Unlike the usual "bland" or "classic" LCIS composed of uniform small cells, in some cases the cells may have cytologic pleomorphism and central necrosis with microcalcifications and is similar in appearance to DCIS. When the diagnosis of LCIS versus DCIS is uncertain, an E-cadherin stain can be used to differentiate

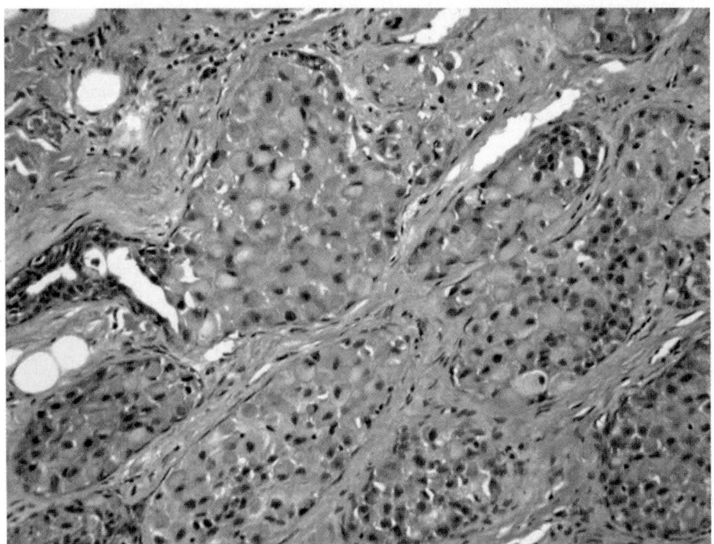

■ **FIGURE 19-24** Lobular carcinoma in situ (LCIS) signet ring cell type with abundant eccentrically located cytoplasm with nuclei pushed to one side (H&E, ×200).

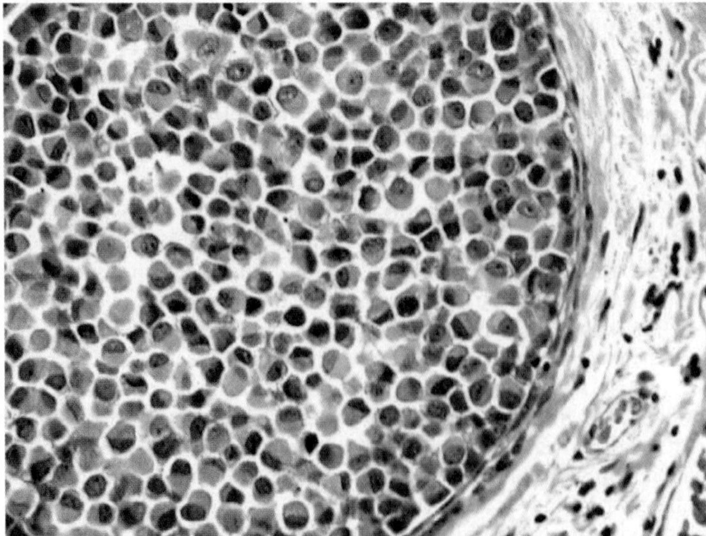

■ **FIGURE 19-25** Pleomorphic lobular carcinoma in situ (PLCIS) with large dyshesive cells and high nuclear to cytoplasm ratio (N : C). Nuclei are pushed to one side with abundant eosinophilic cytoplasm exhibiting plasmacytoid features. Prominent nucleoli are also noted (H&E, ×400).

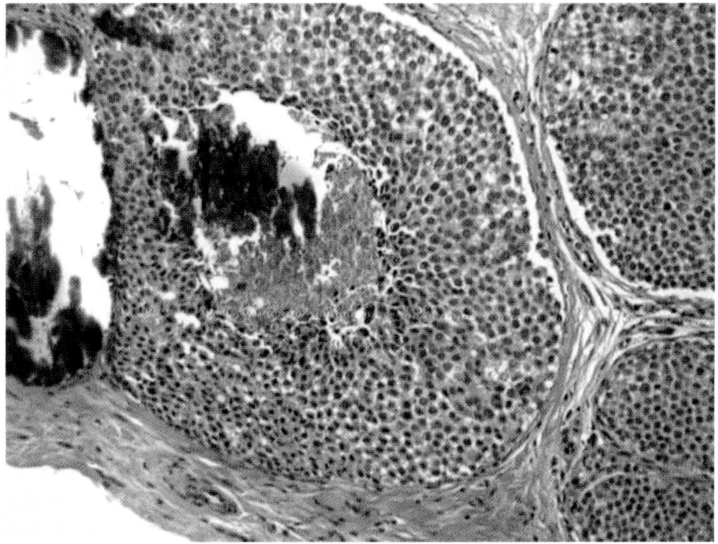

■ **FIGURE 19-26** Intermediate grade lobular carcinoma in situ with central necrosis and calcifications resembling histologic features of ductal carcinoma in situ (DCIS) (H&E, ×200).

between the two (Fig. 19-27). The E-cadherin stain is a membrane stain that is positive with most cases of DCIS but not LCIS, and this stain has been used to differentiate ductal from lobular phenotypes. The variants of LCIS, such as pleomorphic and indeterminate CIS, are often detected by mammography, are similar to DCIS, and are known to behave more aggressively; hence, recommendation is further surgery.[27-29] These variant carcinomas in situ were most likely to have been diagnosed as DCIS prior to the E-cadherin stain era if the surgical margins were positive re-excision and radiation therapy would have been recommended. In the post-E-cadherin era, the same lesion may have been referred to as distended LCIS, mixed ductal or lobular carcinoma, and indeterminate CIS. Whether radiation therapy is necessary in these variants of LCIS is unknown. Currently, patients with these lesions are recommended to have at least re-excision if the surgical margins are positive. Future studies to address unique clinical management strategies for variants of LCIS are needed.

Synopsis of Treatment Options

There are divergent views about the appropriate management of lobular neoplasia. Patients with the diagnosis of LCIS are known to have a higher risk of developing cancer in the future. Typically, women with LCIS simply increase their surveillance for breast cancer, having multiple physical examinations each year and mammograms once or twice a year. This allows early detection to identify breast cancer at the most treatable stage if it does occur. In the

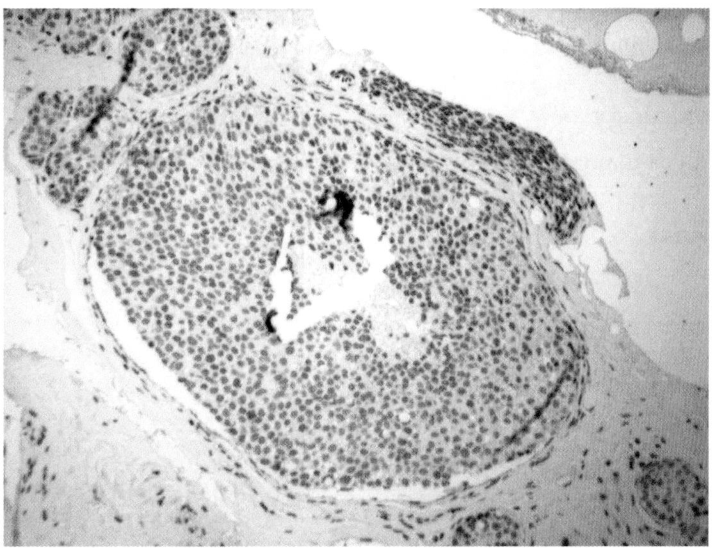

■ **FIGURE 19-27** The same carcinoma in situ (CIS) as seen in Figure 19-20 showing negative E-cadherin stain supporting the diagnosis of lobular phenotype (LCIS) (E-cadherin stain, ×100).

past, LCIS was commonly treated with bilateral mastectomy. This radical treatment option is usually reserved for women with a very strong family history of breast cancer or a known genetic mutation, such as *BRCA1* or *BRCA2*, or both, which dramatically increases the risk of developing breast cancer. Studies have also shown that hormonal therapy, such as tamoxifen, may reduce the risk of developing breast cancer in postmenopausal women with LCIS. A similar drug, raloxifene, may also reduce the risk of developing breast cancer and is used in premenopausal women with a diagnosis of LCIS. A clinical trial is underway comparing the effectiveness of raloxifene and tamoxifen to prevent development of breast cancer in high risk women (Study of Tamoxifen and Raloxifene [STAR]).

Although there is some controversy, an open biopsy is recommended when LCIS or ALH is identified at CNB, especially in the case of mammographically-detected lesions such as a mass, calcifications, or architectural distortion. Variants of LCIS, such as pleomorphic LCIS and indeterminate carcinoma in situ, are often mammographically similar to DCIS and are known to behave more aggressively; further surgery is recommended.

PHYLLODES TUMOR

Definition

Phyllodes tumor is an uncommon neoplasm and was, in the past, known as cystosarcoma phyllodes. Because of these neoplasms are benign, however, the term phyllodes tumor is used today. This tumor occasionally has been equated with a giant fibroadenoma because both contain epithelial and mesenchymal elements, but the stroma of the phyllodes tumor is much more cellular than in a fibroadenoma.

Prevalence and Epidemiology

Phyllodes tumors are uncommon and usually present in older patients (age 40-52 years) when compared with fibroadenoma. The incidence has been reported as low as 0.3% to 0.5% of all female breast tumors.[30]

Etiology and Pathophysiology

The specific etiology of phyllodes tumors is unknown.

Manifestations of Disease

Clinical Presentation

The average age at presentation is between 40 and 52 years, a decade or two older than the average age at presentation for fibroadenomas. Although small lesions are occasionally encountered, the most common clinical presentation is a large and rapidly growing mass. The clinical behavior of phyllodes tumor is unpredictable. The majority of phyllodes tumors are benign, but approximately 5% to 25% contain areas of malignancy. Less than 20% of malignant lesions metastasize via hematogenous spread, but when this occurs it is most commonly to the lung, pleura, and bone.

Imaging Indications and Algorithm

When a patient presents with a palpable abnormality, the imaging workup should include diagnostic mammography and ultrasonography. CNB should also be performed.

Imaging Technique and Findings

Mammography

On mammography, most phyllodes tumors are large, circumscribed, noncalcified masses that are round, oval, or lobulated. When small, the appearance is identical to a fibroadenoma. When large, the size may suggest the diagnosis. Calcifications are rare (Fig. 19-28).

Ultrasonography

Ultrasonography demonstrates a solid mass, often with inhomogeneous internal echoes and posterior acoustic enhancement, and sometimes containing small peripheral cystic spaces, and multilobulation (Fig. 19-29). It is not possible to reliably differentiate between phyllodes tumor, fibroadenoma, and a circumscribed carcinoma based on the imaging features.

Magnetic Resonance Imaging

The MRI appearance of phyllodes tumors is variable and nonspecific. Wurdinger and coworkers[31] found that a comparison of compared the MRI appearance of

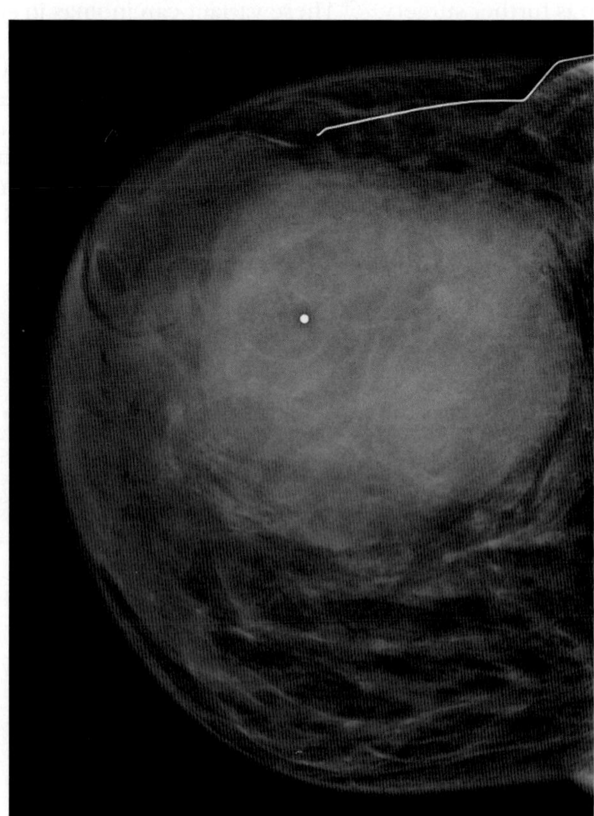

■ **FIGURE 19-28** Recurrent malignant phyllodes. Mammography in a patient with a palpable abnormality demonstrates a circumscribed round mass without associated calcifications. The patient previously had surgical excision of a malignant phyllodes, which has recurred.

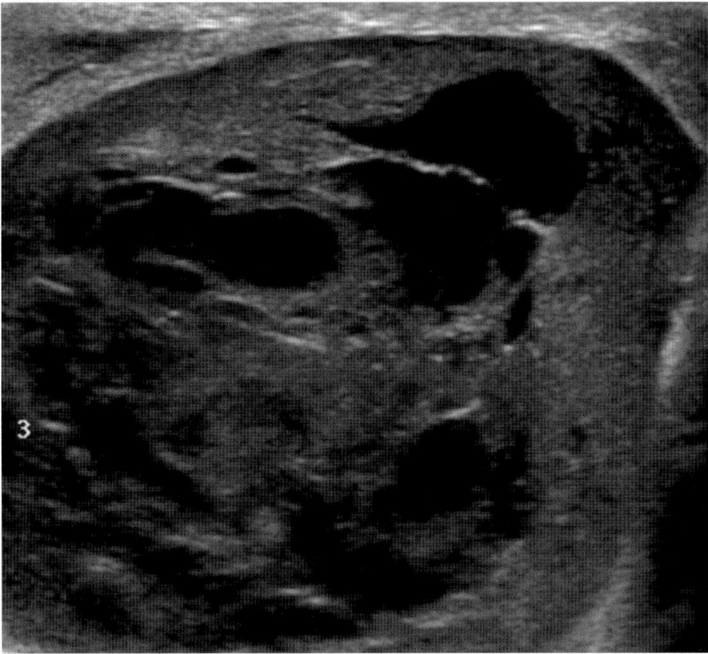

■ **FIGURE 19-29** Recurrent malignant phyllodes. Ultrasound image of the same patient in Figure 19-28 demonstrates a large, circumscribed complex mass with a hypoechoic solid component and internal cystic spaces.

fibroadenomas with phyllodes tumors and found that phyllodes tumors are usually circumscribed masses with a round or lobular shape and contain internal septations, internal cysts, and hemorrhage (especially in larger phyllodes tumors). Contrast enhancement is variable.[31] Yabuuchi and colleagues[32] performed a retrospective study to evaluate whether MRI signal characteristics and appearance can help in distinguishing between benign and malignant phyllodes. They found that a T1 signal higher than normal breast tissue, cystic change with irregular walls, and T2 signal lower than normal breast tissue are suggestive of a malignant histopathologic grade of phyllodes tumor.

Classic Signs

The classic presentation of a phyllodes tumor is a rapidly enlarging mass in a woman older than the typical age for fibroadenoma.

There is no classic radiographic appearance of a phyllodes tumor on imaging, and tissue diagnosis is needed to differentiate between phyllodes and fibroadenoma.

Differential Diagnosis

From Clinical Presentation

The differential diagnosis from the clinical presentation of a palpable abnormality would include fibroadenoma, invasive carcinoma, and, possibly, papilloma.

From Imaging Findings

When the lesion is small, the imaging appearance cannot be differentiated from fibroadenoma. Invasive carcinomas and papillomas are also considerations. The presence of calcifications would discourage the diagnosis of phyllodes tumor.

Pathology Findings

Phyllodes tumors are divided into three classifications; benign, borderline or low grade, and malignant, based on stromal cellularity, number of mitotic figures, characteristics of margins, stromal overgrowth, presence of heterologous components, and necrosis. The most common clinical presentation is a rapidly growing mass that may stretch the skin without causing skin ulceration. Phyllodes tumor is similar to fibroadenoma in that it is a fibroepithelial lesion with both stroma and epithelial proliferations. This type of tumor has increased stromal cellularity and a leaf-like pattern (Fig. 19-30). Intracanalicular fibroadenoma may have a leaf-like pattern and stromal cellularity and may be found in a cellular (juvenile) fibroadenoma. Therefore, the differential diagnosis of fibroadenoma and benign phyllodes tumor can be challenging in some cases. Grading of the phyllodes tumor is based on semiquantitative criteria. Malignant phyllodes tumors usually have infiltrative borders, marked stromal cellularity with nuclear pleomorphism, increased mitotic figures, stromal overgrowth (defined by having no glandular structure in low power view in at least in one field) (Figs. 19-31 and 19-32), and the presence of heterologous components such as liposarcoma or chondroid, or both, and skeletal or osteoid elements. They may be confused with pure sarcoma of the breast, such as osteogenic sarcoma in the case of bone formation. In such cases, a diligent search for a glandular component by submitting at least one block per 1 cm of tumor can help to confirm the diagnosis of malignant phyllodes tumor. Borderline phyllodes tumor has somewhat circumscribed margins and a lesser degree of the features just described. Benign phyllodes tumor has well-circumscribed pushing borders in relation to adjacent breast tissue, uniform stromal distribution, rare mitotic

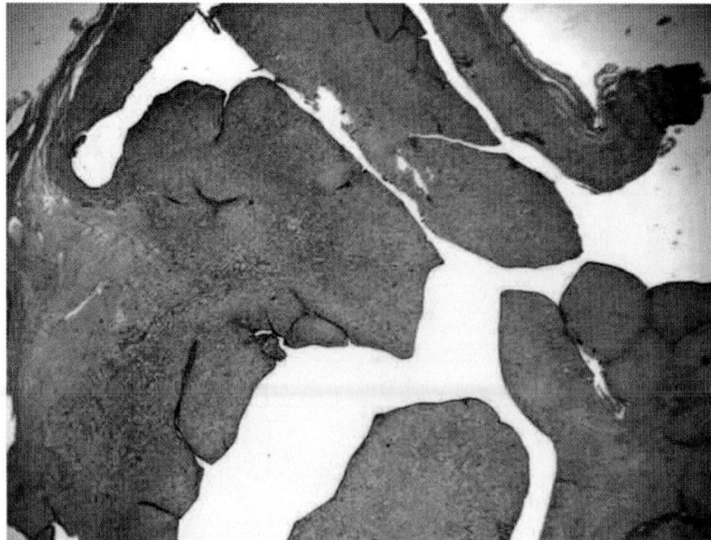

■ **FIGURE 19-30** Phyllodes tumor with large leaf-like papillary fronds projection into cystic spaces (H&E, ×40).

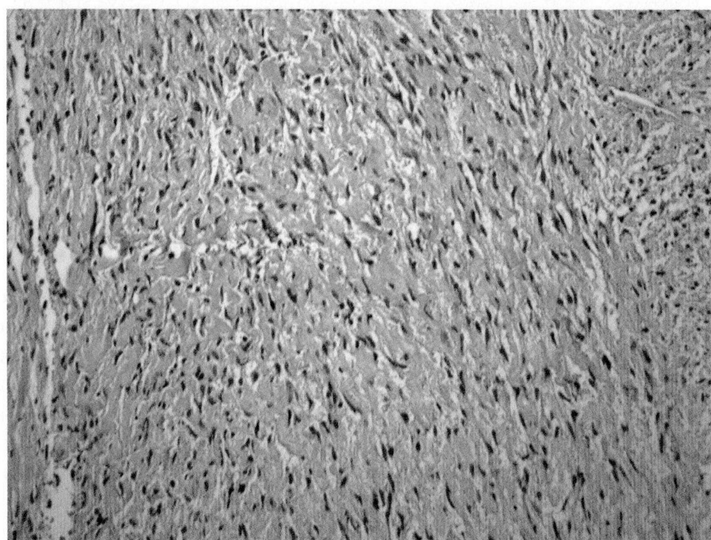

■ **FIGURE 19-31** Phyllodes tumor with stromal overgrowth; no glandular tissue is seen (H&E, ×40).

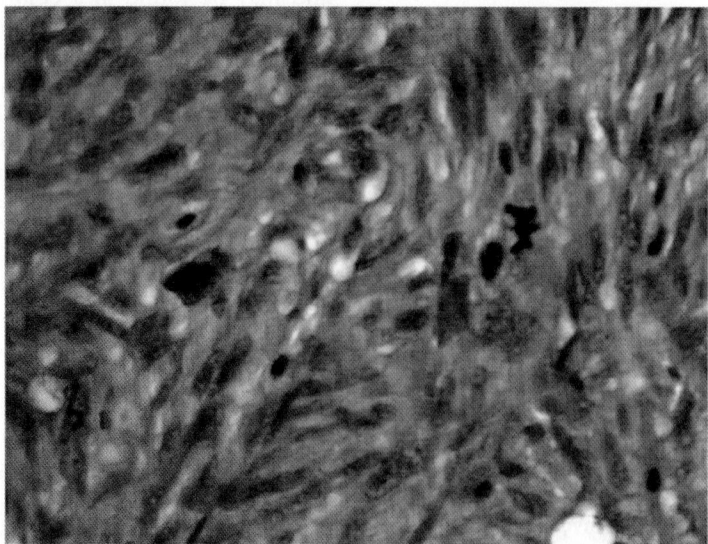

■ **FIGURE 19-32** Malignant phyllodes tumor with marked nuclear stromal pleomorphism and atypical mitotic figure (H&E, ×400).

figures (usually not more than 2 per 10 high-power fields), and modest stromal cellularity.

Synopsis of Treatment Options

Core needle biopsy with a diagnosis of phyllodes tumor or differential diagnosis of phyllodes should be excised generally indicates tumor excision. Margin assessment should be done on the excision of phyllodes tumor. It is difficult to predict the biologic behavior of phyllodes tumors. Even histologically benign tumors are capable of at least local recurrence and, rarely, malignant transformation, especially if not completely excised with a rim of normal breast tissue. The average majority of published data suggest a local recurrence of malignant phyllodes tumors of 27% and a rate of metastases of 22% to pulmonary areas. Local recurrence after surgery is dependent on the width of the excisional margins.[33]

KEY POINTS

- Papillary lesions of the breast are a heterogeneous group of lesions and include papilloma, papillomatosis, sclerosing papilloma, atypical papilloma, carcinoma arising within a papilloma that includes intraductal papillary carcinoma, and invasive papillary carcinoma.
- A papillary lesion diagnosed at CNB may warrant open biopsy to rule out atypia or malignancy, or both, arising within the background of papilloma, but this is still controversial.
- Technical advances with digital mammography and the increasing use of CNB have led to an increase in the diagnosis of columnar cell lesions associated with microcalcifications.
- Flat epithelial atypia is diagnosed when there is a low-grade cytologic atypia in a columnar cell lesion (not an architectural atypia as seen with ADH). FEA diagnosed at CNB probably warrants open biopsy to rule out commonly associated lesions such as ADH, low-grade DCIS, tubular carcinoma, and lobular neoplasia.
- Atypical ductal hyperplasia has features that lie in the middle of the spectrum between usual ductal hyperplasia and low-grade DCIS.
- Distinction between ADH and DCIS is by qualitative and quantitative analysis and can be difficult. This distinction is even more challenging in CNB samples owing to the fragmented nature and limited sample afforded by the needle biopsy procedure. It has long been established that any CNB that reveals ADH necessitates open biopsy.
- Lobular neoplasia is a spectrum of lesions including LCIS, ALH, and large ductal involvement with lobular neoplasia.
- Lobular neoplasia has traditionally been considered a risk factor only. The most recent literature supports indicates that lobular neoplasia is not only a risk factor but also may be a direct precursor to cancer. Thus surgical excision should be done when this diagnosis is returned from a CNB.
- Rare variants of LCIS, namely, signet ring LCIS, pleomorphic LCIS, and massive acinar distention LCIS, can mimic DCIS. E-cadherin immunohistochemistry stain may be helpful to delineate between them. The biological behavior of these variants is unknown and is probably more akin to DCIS rather than to classic LCIS.
- Phyllodes tumors are fibroepithelial tumors and based on histologic features are divided into three classifications: benign, borderline or low grade, and malignant.

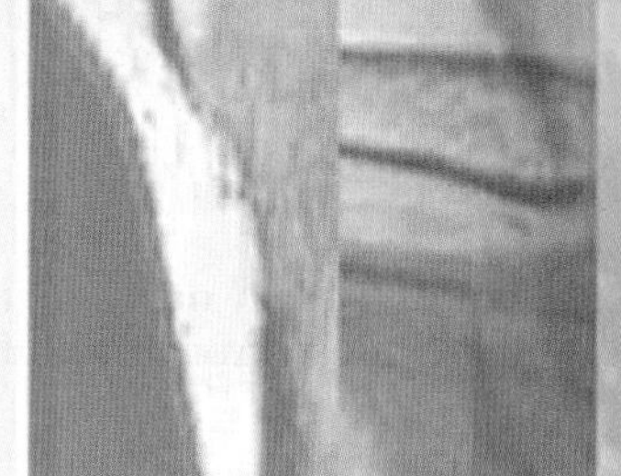

CASE STUDY

Chapter 19 High-Risk Breast Diseases

HISTORY

A 47-year-old woman presented with a history of spontaneous, clear nipple discharge from the left breast.

FINDINGS

Normal mammogram (Fig. 19-33) showed no evidence of subareolar mass. Mammography is a part of the imaging algorithm in a patient with spontaneous nipple discharge.

Ultrasound demonstrates a dilated duct and associated filling defect or mass within the duct (Fig. 19-34). Ductography demonstrates an abrupt cutoff of contrast and a partially visualized

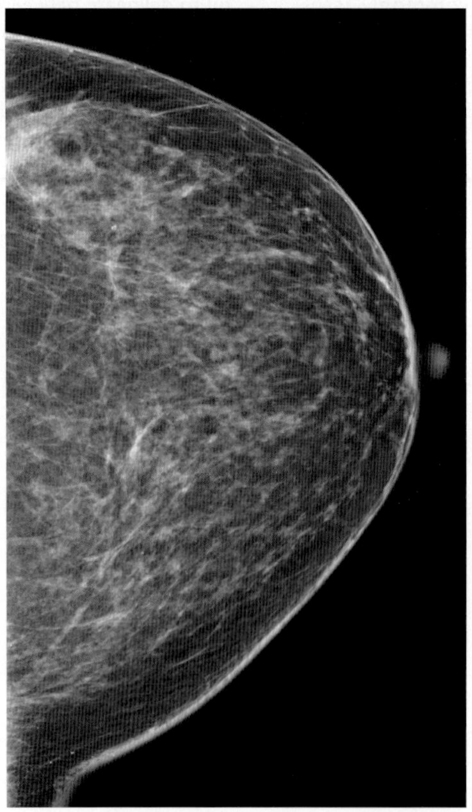

■ **FIGURE 19-33** Normal mammogram without evidence of subareolar mass. Mammography is a part of the imaging algorithm in a patient with spontaneous nipple discharge.

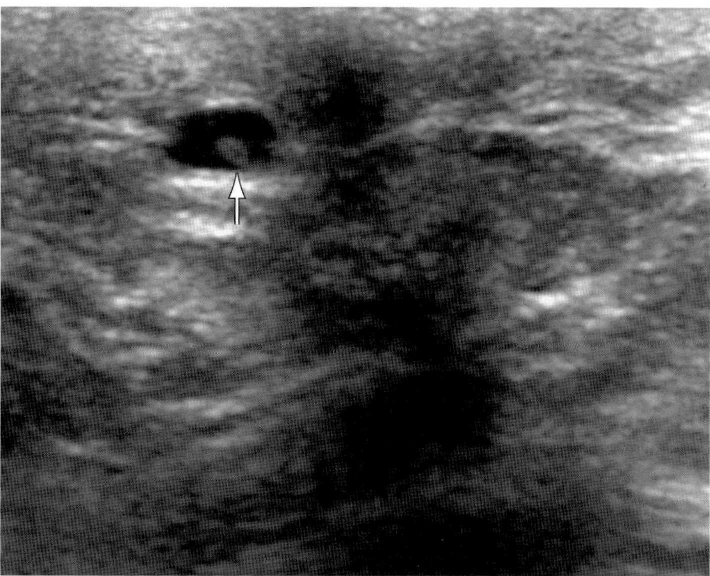

■ **FIGURE 19-34** Ultrasound image in the same patient as in Figure 19-33 demonstrates a portion of a dilated duct and associated filling defect or hypoechoic oval mass (*arrow*) within the duct.

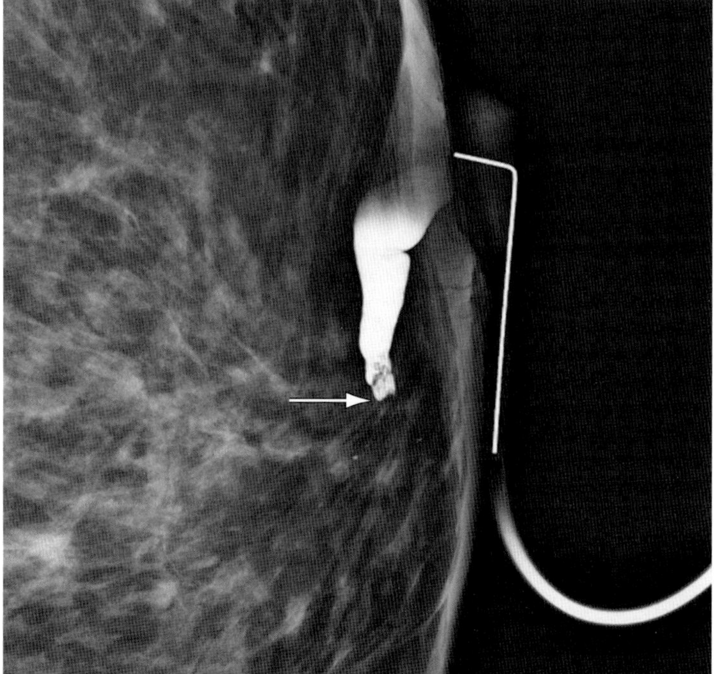

■ **FIGURE 19-35** Ductogram performed on the same patient in Figures 19-33 and 19-34 demonstrates an abrupt cutoff of contrast (*arrow*) and a partially visualized filling defect. An abrupt cutoff of contrast should raise suspicion for a mass even if the mass or filling defect is not directly visualized.

filling defect (Fig. 19-35). An abrupt cutoff of contrast should raise suspicion for a mass even if the mass or filling defect is not directly visualized.

DIFFERENTIAL DIAGNOSIS

Differential diagnosis includes intraductal papilloma or malignancy.

DIAGNOSIS

The diagnosis was intraductal papilloma. Fine-needle aspiration material yielded cellular material with papillary fronds and tufting of the epithelial cells. Delicate capillary proliferation is seen within papillary groups (Fig. 19-36). No nuclear atypia is noted.

CNB and excisional biopsy showed cystically dilated spaces with papillary fronds and central fibrovascular cores. Epithelial cells are not atypical and myoepithelial cells are seen within each frond (Figs. 19-37 and 19-38).

COMMENT

This mass was localized preoperatively with ultrasound-guided needle localization.

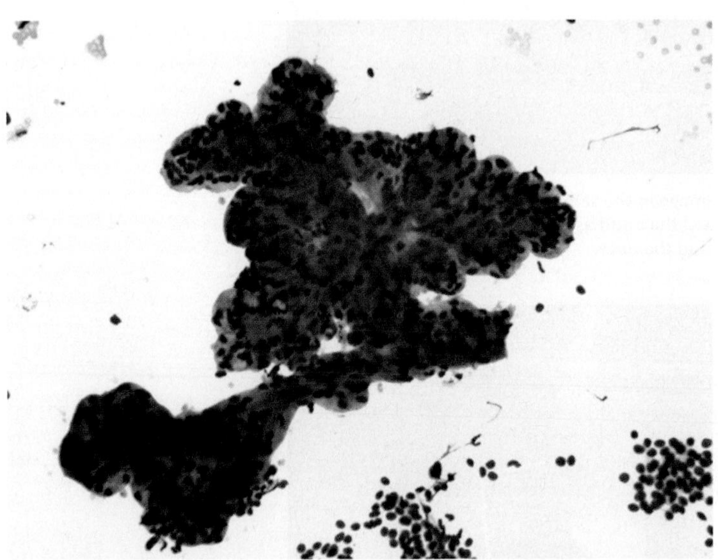

■ **FIGURE 19-36** Fine-needle aspiration specimen yielded cellular material with papillary fronds and tufting of the epithelial cells. Delicate capillary proliferation is seen within papillary groups. No nuclear atypia is noted (May-Grunewald Giemsa stain [MGG], ×200).

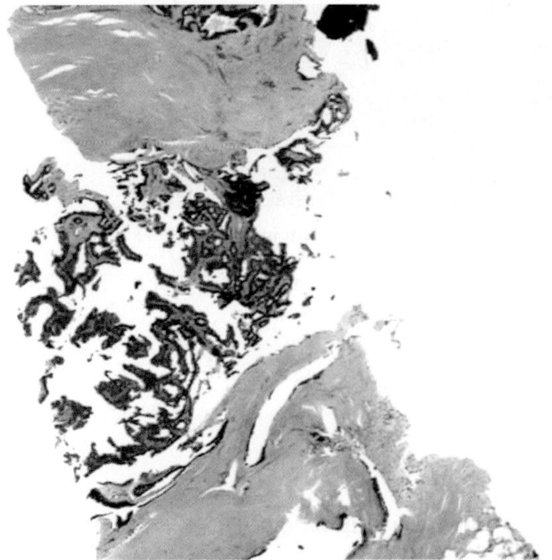

■ **FIGURE 19-37** Core needle biopsy shows cystically dilated spaces with papillary fronds and central fibrovascular cores. Epithelial cells are not atypical and myoepithelial cells are seen within each frond (H&E, ×40).

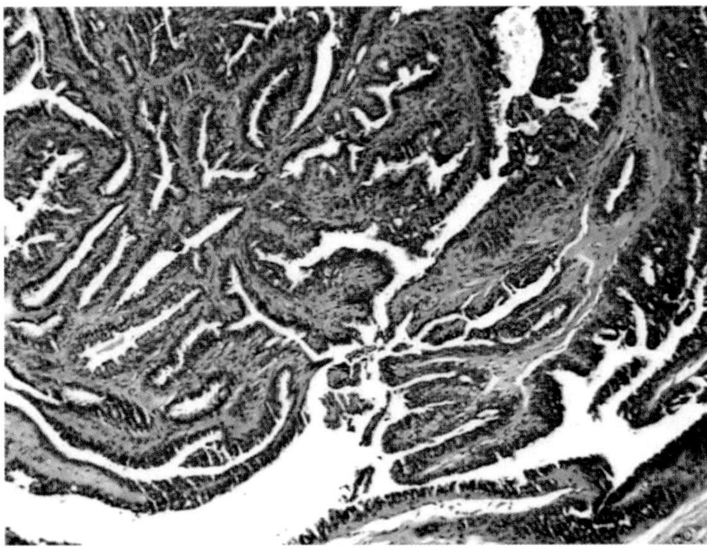

■ **FIGURE 19-38** Excisional biopsy showed cystically dilated spaces with papillary fronds and central fibrovascular cores. Epithelial cells are not atypical and myoepithelial cells are seen within each frond (H&E, ×100).

SUGGESTED READINGS

Bassett L, Winchester DP, Caplan RB, Dershaw DD, Dowlatshahi K, Evans WP 3rd, et al. Stereotactic core-needle biopsy of the breast: a report of the Joint Task Force of the American College of Radiology, American College of Surgeons, and College of American Pathologists. *CA Cancer J Clin* 1997;**47**:171-90.

Brookes MJ, Bourke AG. Radiological appearances of papillary breast lesions. *Clin Radiol* 2008;**63**:1265-73. Epub 2008 Jun 24.

Fitzgibbons PL, Henson DE, Hutter RV. Benign breast changes and the risk for subsequent breast cancer; an update of the 1985 consensus statement. Cancer Committee of the College of American Pathologists. *Arch Pathol Lab Med* 1998;**122**:1053-5.

Pandey S, Kornstein MJ, Shank W, de Paredes E. Columnar cell lesions the breast: mammographic findings with histopathologic correlation. *Radiographics* 2007;**27**:S79-89.

REFERENCES

1. Rosen PP, Cantrell B, Mullen DL, DePalo A. Juvenile papillomatosis (Swiss cheese disease) of the breast. *Am J Surg Pathol* 1980;**4**:3-12.
2. Rosen PP. Papilloma and related benign tumors. In: Rosen PP, editor. *Rosen's breast pathology*. 2nd ed. Philadelphia: Lippincott Williams & Wilkins; 2001. p. 77-119.
3. Cardenosa G, Eklund GW. Benign papillary neoplasms of the breast: mammographic findings. *Radiology* 1991;**181**:751-5.
4. Woods ER, Helvie MA, Ikeda DM, Mandell SH, Chapel KL, Adler DD. Solitary breast papilloma: comparison of mammographic, galactographic, and pathologic findings. *AJR Am J Roentgenol* 1992;**159**:487-91.
5. Ganesan S, Karthik G, Joshi M, Damodaran V. Ultrasound spectrum in intraductal papillary neoplasms of breast. *Br J Radiol* 2006;**79**:843-9.
6. Daniel BL, Gardner RW, Birdwell RL, Nowels KW, Johnson D. Magnetic resonance imaging of intraductal papilloma of the breast. *Magn Reson Imaging* 2003;**21**:887-92.
7. Page DL, Salhany KE, Jensen RA, Dupont WD. Subsequent breast carcinoma risk after biopsy with atypia in a breast papilloma. *Cancer* 1996;**78**:258-66.
8. Rosen EL, Bently RC, Baker JA, Soo MS. Imaging guided core needle biopsy of papillary lesions of the breast. *AJR Am J Roentgenol* 2002;**179**:1185-92.
9. Mercado CL, Hamele-Bena D, Singer C, Koenigsberg T, Pile-Spellman E, Higgins H, et al. Papillary lesions of the breast: evaluation with stereotactic directional vacuum-assisted biopsy. *Radiology* 2001;**221**:650-5.
10. Jacobs TW, Connolly JL, Schnitt SJ. Nonmalignant lesions in breast core needle biopsies: to excise or not to excise? *Am J Surg Pathol* 2002;**26**:1095-1110.
11. Bazzocchi F, Santini D, Martinelli G, Piccaluga A, Taffurelli M, Grassigli A, et al. Juvenile papillomatosis (epitheliosis) of the breast. A clinical and pathologic study of 13 cases. *Am J Clin Pathol* 1986;**86**:745-8.
12. Tavassoli FA, Devilee P. *World Health Organization Classification of Tumours. Pathology and genetics. Tumours of the breast and female genital organs*. Lyon: IARC Press; 2003.
13. Tarek MA, Abdel-Fatah MB, Desmond GP, Lee AH, Reis-Filho JS, Ellis IO. High frequency of coexistence of columnar cell lesions, lobular neoplasia and low grade ductal carcinoma in situ with invasive tubular carcinoma and invasive lobular carcinoma. *Am J Surg Pathol* 2007;**31**:417-26.
14. Brandt SM, Young GQ, Hoda SA. The "Rosen Triad": tubular carcinoma, lobular carcinoma in situ, and columnar cell lesions. *Adv Anatomical Pathol* 2008;**15**:140-6.
15. Kunju LP, Kleer CG. Significance of flat epithelial atypia on Mammotome core needle biopsy: should it be excised? *Hum Pathol* 2007;**38**:35-41.
16. Martel M, Barron-Rodrigues P, Ocal IT, Dotto J, Tavassoli FA. Flat DIN (Flat epithelial atypia) on core biopsy: 63 cases identified retrospectively among 1,751 core biopsies performed over an 8-year period (1992-1999). *Virchows Arch* 2007;**452**:883-91.
17. Eusebi V, Feudale E, Foschini MP, Micheli A, Conti A, Riva C, et al. Long term follow-up of in situ carcinoma of the breast. *Semin Diagn Pathol* 1994;**11**:223-35.
18. Bijker N, Peterse JL, Duchateau L, Julien JP, Fentiman IS, Duval C, et al. Risk factors for recurrence and metastasis after breast conserving therapy for ductal carcinoma in-situ: analysis of European Organization for Research and Treatment of Cancer Trial 10853. *J Clin Oncol* 2001;**19**:2263-71.

19. Liberman L, Holland AE, Marjan D, Murray MP, Bartella L, Morris EA, et al. Underestimation of atypical ductal hyperplasia at MRI-guided 9-gauge vacuum-assisted breast biopsy. *AJR Am J Roentgenol* 2007;**188**:684-90.
20. Page DL, Anderson TJ. *Diagnostic histopathology of the breast*. Churchill Livingstone; 1988. p. 170-1.
21. Brem RF, Behrndt VS, Sanow L, Gatewood OM. Atypical ductal hyperplasia: histologic underestimation of carcinoma in tissue harvested from impalpable breast lesions using 11-gauge stereotactically guided directional vacuum-assisted biopsy. *AJR Am J Roentgenol* 1999;**172**:1405-7.
22. Ioffe OB, Berg WA, Siverberg SG, Kumar D. Mammographic histopathologic correlation of large-core needle biopsies. *Mod Pathol* 1998;**11**:721-7.
23. Andersen JA. Lobular carcinoma in situ of the breast. An approach to rational treatment. *Cancer* 1977;**39**:2597-602.
24. Page DL, Schuyler PA, Dupont WD, Jensen RA, Plummer WD Jr, Simpson JF. Atypical lobular hyperplasia as a unilateral predictor of breast cancer risk: a retrospective cohort study. *Lancet* 2003;**361**:125-9.
25. Shin SJ, Rosen PP. Excisional biopsy should be performed if lobular carcinoma in situ is seen on needle core biopsy. *Arch Pathol Lab Med* 2002;**126**:697-701.
26. Foster MC, Helvie MA, Gregory NE, Rebner M, Nees AV, Paramagul C. Lobular carcinoma in situ or atypical lobular hyperplasia: Is excisional biopsy necessary? *Radiology* 2004;**231**:813-9.
27. Lakhani SR, Audretsch W, Cleton-Jensen AM, Cutuli B, Ellis I, Eusebi V, et al. The management of LCIS. Is LCIS the same as DCIS? *Eur J Cancer* 2006;**42**:2205-11.
28. Sapino A, Frigerio A, Peterse JL, Arisio R, Coluccia C, Bussolati G. Mammographically detected in situ lobular carcinomas of the breast. *Virchows Arch* 2000;**436**:421-30.
29. Sneige N, Wang J, Baker BA, Krishnamurthy S, Middleton LP. Clinical, histopathologic and biologic features of pleomorphic lobular (ductal-lobular) carcinoma in situ of the breast. *Mod Pathol* 2002;**15**:1044-50.
30. Sheen-Chen SM, Hsu W, Eng HL, Huang CC, Ko SF. Intratumoral hemorrhage of mammary phyllodes tumor after menstrual induction: a puzzling presentation. *Tumori* 2007;**93**:631-3.
31. Wurdinger S, Herzog AB, Fischer DR, Marx C, Raabe G, Schneider A, et al. Differentiation of phyllodes breast tumors from fibroadenomas on MRI. *AJR Am J Roentgenol* 2005;**185**:1317-21.
32. Yabuuchi H, Soeda H, Matsuo Y, Okafuji T, Eguchi T, Sakai S, et al. Phyllodes tumor of the breast: correlation between MR findings and histologic grade. *Radiology* 2006;**241**:702-9.
33. Asoglu O, Ugurlu MM, Blanchard K, Grant CS, Reynolds C, Cha SS, et al. Risk factors for recurrence and death after primary surgical treatment of malignancy phyllodes tumors. *Ann Surg Oncol* 2004;**11**:1011-7.

CHAPTER 20

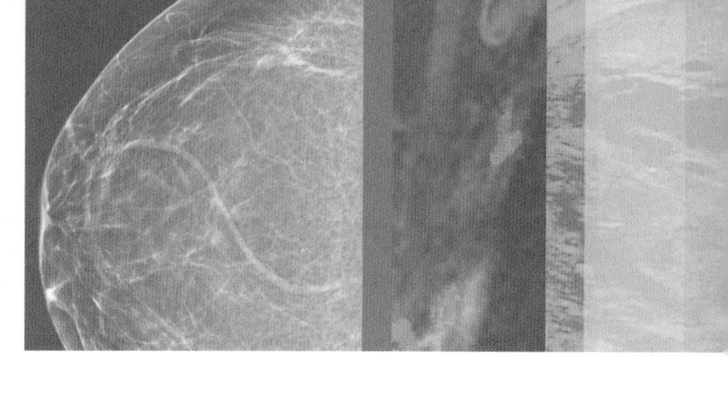

Infectious and Inflammatory Diseases of the Breast

Sophia Kim Apple, Jane M. Dascalos, and Lawrence W. Bassett

MASTITIS

Definition

Mastitis is defined as inflammation of the parenchyma of the breast and can be infectious or noninfectious. Infections can be caused by bacteria, fungi, or parasites. Noninfectious inflammatory processes involving the breast include plasma cell mastitis, granulomatous mastitis, and lymphocytic mastitis.

Prevalence and Epidemiology

Mastitis is not uncommon. Most cases of mastitis and breast abscess occur during lactation, in diabetic patients, and in heavy smokers.

Etiology and Pathophysiology

Most cases of mastitis occur during lactation, are pyogenic, and are caused by *Staphylococcus aureus* and *Streptococcus* species.[1] However, many infections are due to mixed flora. Infection results from disruption of the epithelial interface of the nipple-areolar complex with retrograde dissemination of the organisms. Women who are not lactating, particularly heavy smokers, without known etiology, may also develop pyogenic retrograde infections, often with the development of relatively superficial subareolar abscesses due to blockage of the subareolar ducts with subsequent infection. Rarely, the breast may become infected with echinococcosis,[2,3] blastomycosis,[4] schistosomiasis,[5] loiasis,[6] tuberculosis,[7] or other granulomatous and parasitic diseases.

Obtaining a complete history and ordering culture and sensitivity studies are necessary to make the diagnosis. In addition to infectious mastitis, a local inflammatory reaction may occur in response to inspissated secretions or an immune response with accumulation of plasma cells (plasma cell mastitis), granulomatous formation (granulomatous mastitis),[8] or lymphocytic infiltration (lymphocytic mastitis).

Manifestations of Disease

Clinical Presentation

At the early stage of acute mastitis, the breast may develop induration with localized tenderness and swelling, the skin may demonstrate erythema with diffuse cellulitis, and the patient may be febrile.

At the suppurative stage, the induration is increased and eventually a fluctuant abscess forms. At this stage, the skin erythema increases and the breast may be very tender. The patient may suffer from fever and chills.

Nonpyogenic and noninfectious mastitis have more subtle presentations that can involve pain or a lump or can present as an incidental finding on screening mammography.

Imaging Indications and Algorithm

If the patient presents with symptoms of infection and a palpable abnormality, the workup begins with mammography and ultrasonography. If erythema and swelling are present without an abscess, many physicians advocate prompt skin punch biopsy to differentiate between infection and malignancy, particularly for nonlactating women, whereas others prescribe a trial of antibiotics. If the classic findings of abscess are identified by ultrasonography, percutaneous drainage can be performed with the aspirate sent for culture and sensitivity.[9,10] This is followed by an oral course of antibiotics, close clinical follow-up, and possibly ultrasonography. If the abscess recurs, the patient will require surgical incision and drainage and possibly removal of the abscess wall. Inflammatory breast carcinoma is a diagnosis of exclusion in a patient who presents with breast edema, redness, and pain.

Imaging Findings by Modality

Mammography

When mammography is performed, the most common findings in pyogenic mastitis are skin and trabecular thickening from breast edema (Figs 20-1 and 20-2). These findings may be diffuse or focal. Pain and edema usually limit the compressibility of the breast; therefore, image quality is often compromised in these patients. When mammographically visible within the edema, abscesses usually appear as noncalcified oval masses with indistinct margins.(Fig. 20-3). Air is very rarely seen within an abscess. The differential diagnosis from the mammogram includes inflammatory carcinoma and other invasive breast carcinomas.

The mammographic findings in unusual granulomatous and parasitic infections are usually nonspecific (Fig. 20-4) and may include diffuse breast edema, masses, and calcifications. Trichinosis infection may be seen mammographically as diffuse punctate microcalcifications limited to the pectoralis muscles bilaterally (Fig. 20-5).[11]

Ultrasonography

Ultrasonography is an ideal imaging method for the detection of focal breast abscesses.[12] Most women easily tolerate the gentle compression of the ultrasound transducer. Ultrasonography depicts abscess cavities within the area of infection and inflammation. The skin thickening and breast edema are easily seen on ultrasonographic examination (Fig. 20-6). Abscesses are

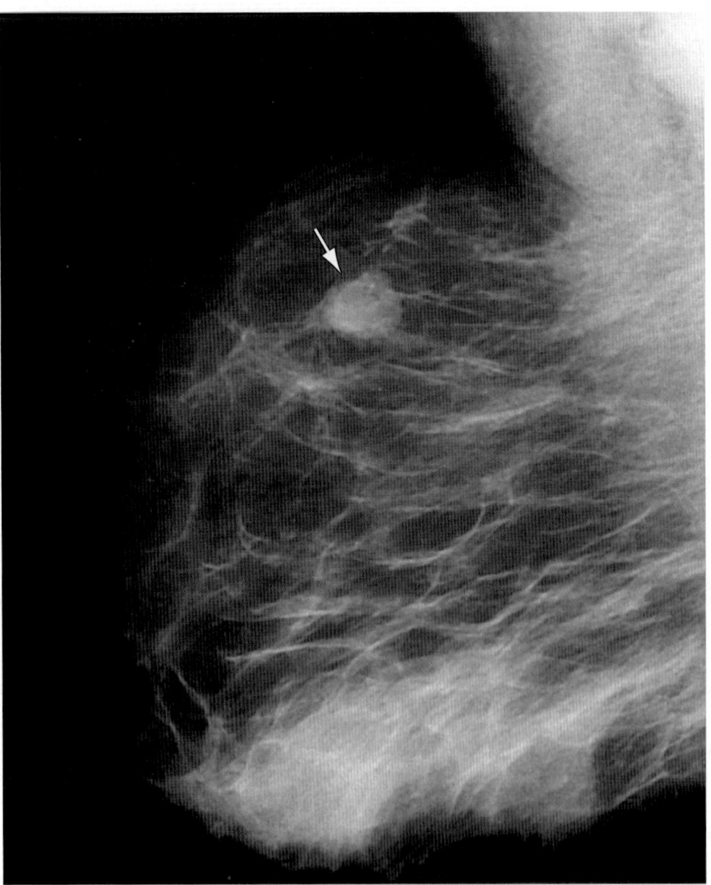

■ **FIGURE 20-1** Mastitis with a reactive lymph node. The right mediolateral oblique mammogram demonstrates trabecular thickening and inferior asymmetry. The round, circumscribed mass (*arrow*) in the upper outer quadrant was ultrasonographically shown to be a lymph node. The node returned to normal size after antibiotic therapy.

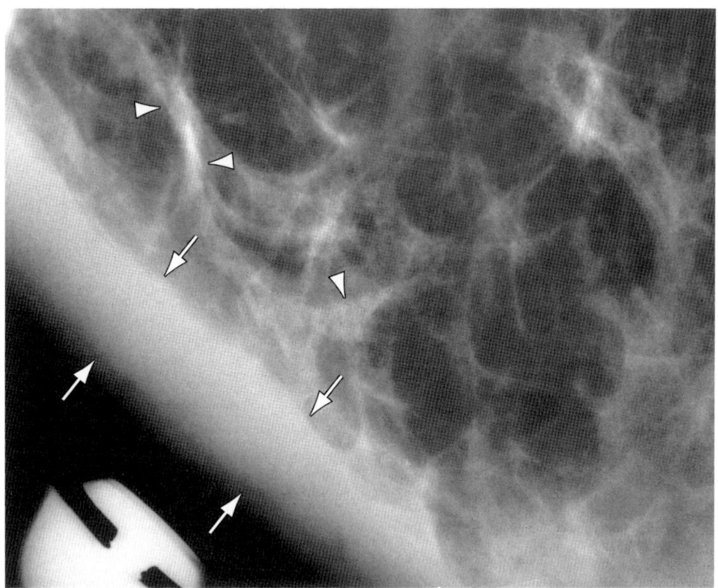

■ **FIGURE 20-2** Mastitis with massive skin (*arrows*) and trabecular (*arrowheads*) thickening.

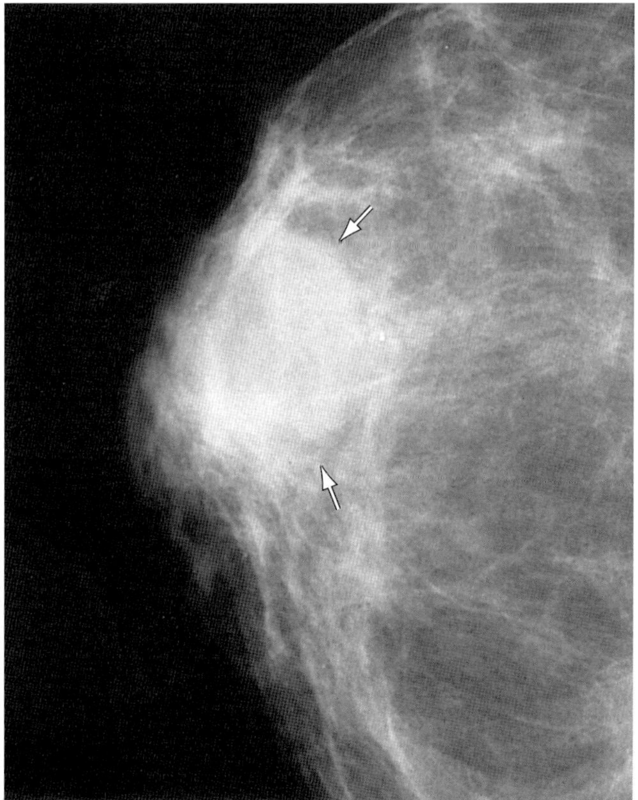

■ **FIGURE 20-3** Subareolar abscess (*arrows*) presenting as an oval partially obscured and partially indistinct mass.

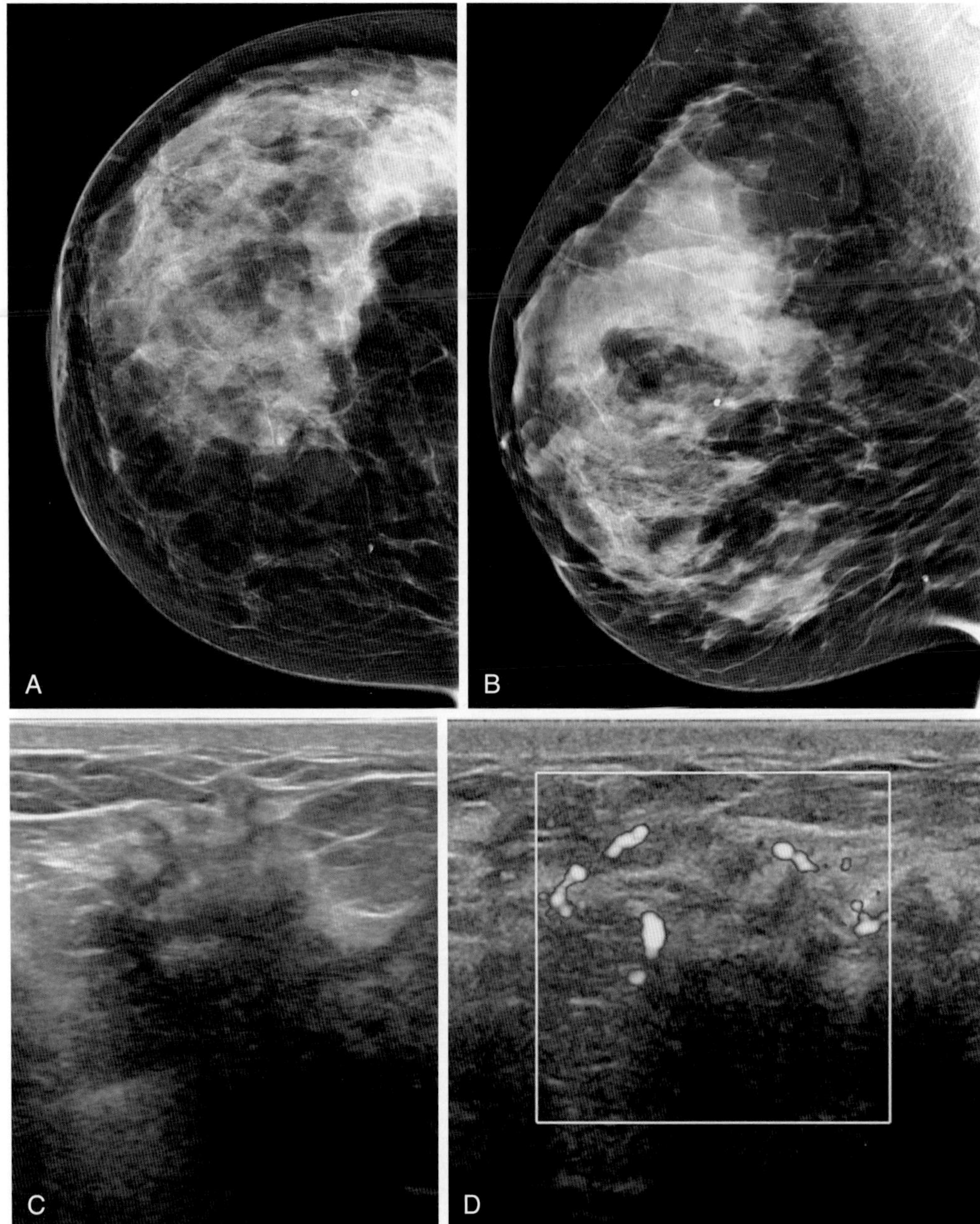

■ **FIGURE 20-4** Granulomatous mastitis. A 39-year old woman presented with a 1-week history of right breast pain and swelling in the lower outer quadrant. The craniocaudal (**A**) and mediolateral oblique (**B**) mammograms show dense tissue in the area of pain. Ultrasound evaluation shows heterogeneous echotexture, architectural distortion, ultrasonographic shadowing, and skin thickening (**C**). Targeted power Doppler ultrasound imaging demonstrates that the vascularity is diffusely increased (**D**).

usually irregular hypoechoic or anechoic masses with indistinct margins, sometimes with fluid or debris levels and usually with posterior acoustic enhancement (Fig. 20-7). Rarely, air within an abscess may produce bright specular reflections (Fig. 20-8). The size and exact location of the abscess are visible, allowing for accurate localization for treatment and therapy monitoring. Unusual granulomatous infections can present as architectural distortion and attenuation of the ultrasound beam (see Fig. 20-4).

Sometimes it is not clear if the lesion is a necrotic mass or an abscess. In this case an attempt can be made at percutaneous drainage with consent also obtained for core biopsy if the lesion proves to represent a complex mass (Fig. 20-9).

Magnetic Resonance Imaging

On T2 weighted imaging an abscess appears as a high signal collection with the degree of signal intensity corresponding to the water content of the abscess.The surrounding tissue and skin can also demonstrate high T2 signal intensity depending on the degree of surrounding edema.T1-weighted imaging shows intermediate signal

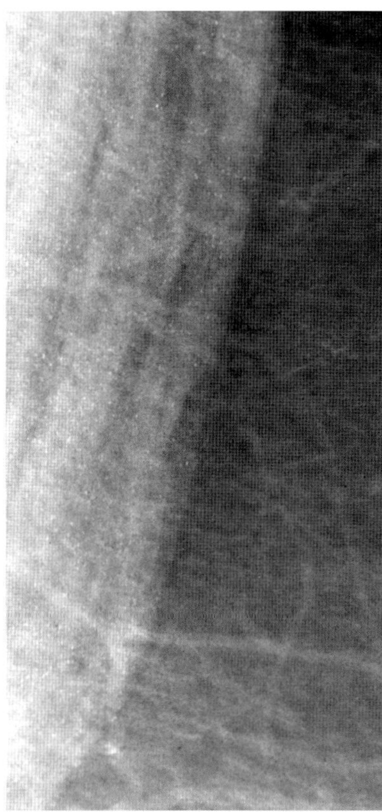

■ **FIGURE 20-5** Trichinosis. Diffuse punctate microcalcifications are seen throughout the pectoralis muscle. These are bilateral, and no calcifications are present within the breast parenchyma. *(Courtesy of Jan Patterson, San Francisco, Calif.)*

of the abscess mass with the surrounding capsule of lower signal intensity compared with the abscess itself. Postcontrast T1-weighted images show no enhancement of the main component of the abscess, with peripheral enhancement of the rim and sometimes the surrounding tissue.

Classic Signs

The classic appearance ultrasonographically is a hypoechoic mass without vascular flow in a patient with symptoms of infection.

Differential Diagnosis

From Clinical Presentation

A patient with breast abscess does not always present with the classic symptoms of abrupt onset of fever and pain. Smoldering infections can present as asymptomatic masses, in which case it is difficult to differentiate clinically between an abscess and malignant mass.

From Imaging Findings

The differential diagnosis from an imaging standpoint includes a complicated cyst, complex mass (including necrotic malignant neoplasm), and phyllodes tumor.

From Pathology Findings

Breast abscesses are commonly seen during the lactational period due to obstruction to the flow in one or more lactiferous ducts. The etiology of breast abscess is usually bacterial and most commonly *S. aureus* and *Streptococcus* species, which are skin inhabitants. Histologically, skin ulceration, tissue necrosis, and numerous neutrophils are seen, most often obscuring existing large lactiferous ducts. If drainage by needle aspiration and antibiotic therapy cannot control the disease process, surgical excision may be necessary (Figs. 20-10 and 20-11).

Subareolar abscess occurs both in lactating and nonlactating women predominately in the reproductive age group, but it can occur in postmenopausal women. Most cases of subareolar and periareolar abscesses are caused by anaerobic infections, but other microorganisms, including *Staphylococcus, Proteus, Bacteroides,*

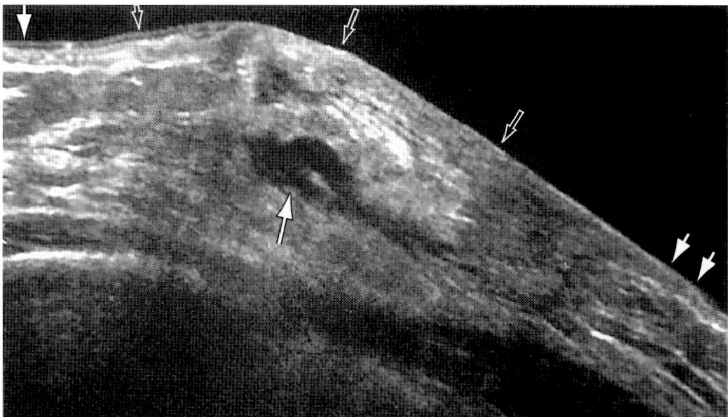

■ **FIGURE 20-6** Mastitis with small abscess. Panoramic ultrasound image demonstrates the transition between normal (*small white arrows*) and inflamed breast tissue (*open arrows*). The fat is abnormally echogenic, and there is loss of the normal architecture within the area of inflammation. A small oval, circumscribed abscess cavity with mixed echogenicity is visible within the area of mastitis (*black arrow*).

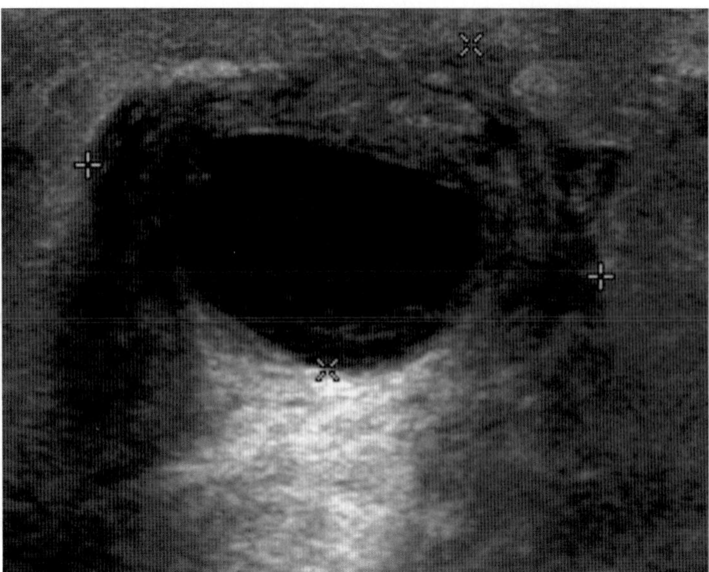

■ **FIGURE 20-7** Abscess. Ultrasonogram of a breast abscess. An oval partially circumscribed and partially indistinct mass, anechoic with hypoechoic debris, is noted. The overlying skin is thickened. Note the prominent posterior acoustic enhancement.

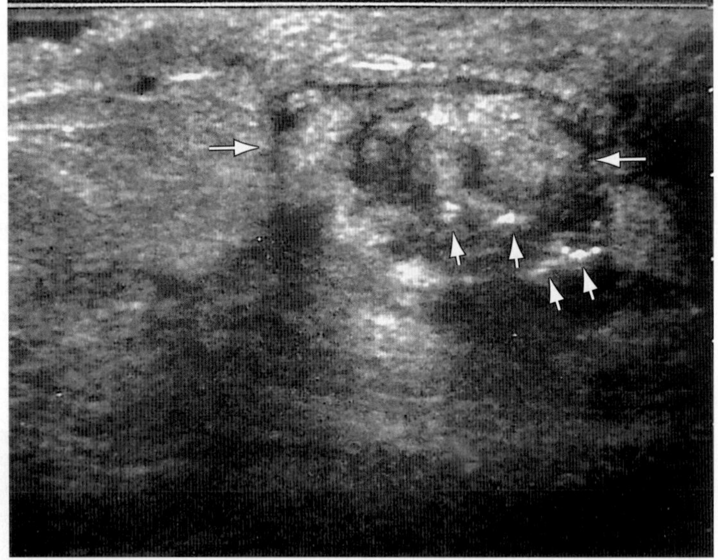

■ **FIGURE 20-8** Abscess (*left single white black arrow*) containing air. There is an oval, indistinct mass with heterogeneous echogenicity. Bright specular reflections (*right white arrows*) within the 2.5-cm mass are from air within the lesion.

and *Streptococcus,* have been reported. Microscopically, the abscess involves the large ducts, and squamous metaplasia is commonly seen with central acute inflammatory infiltrates distending the lactiferous duct. A sinus tract may develop from the abscess to overlying skin causing ulceration. Treatment requires drainage and antibiotic therapy.

Granulomatous mastitis is a rare benign inflammatory condition with unknown etiology and is sometimes called *granulomatous lobular mastitis*. The lesion can be related to the nonlactating breast as well as a lactating condition even many years after pregnancy. Granulomas are composed of aggregates of epithelioid histiocytes, Langerhans giant cells, lymphocytes, and plasma cells

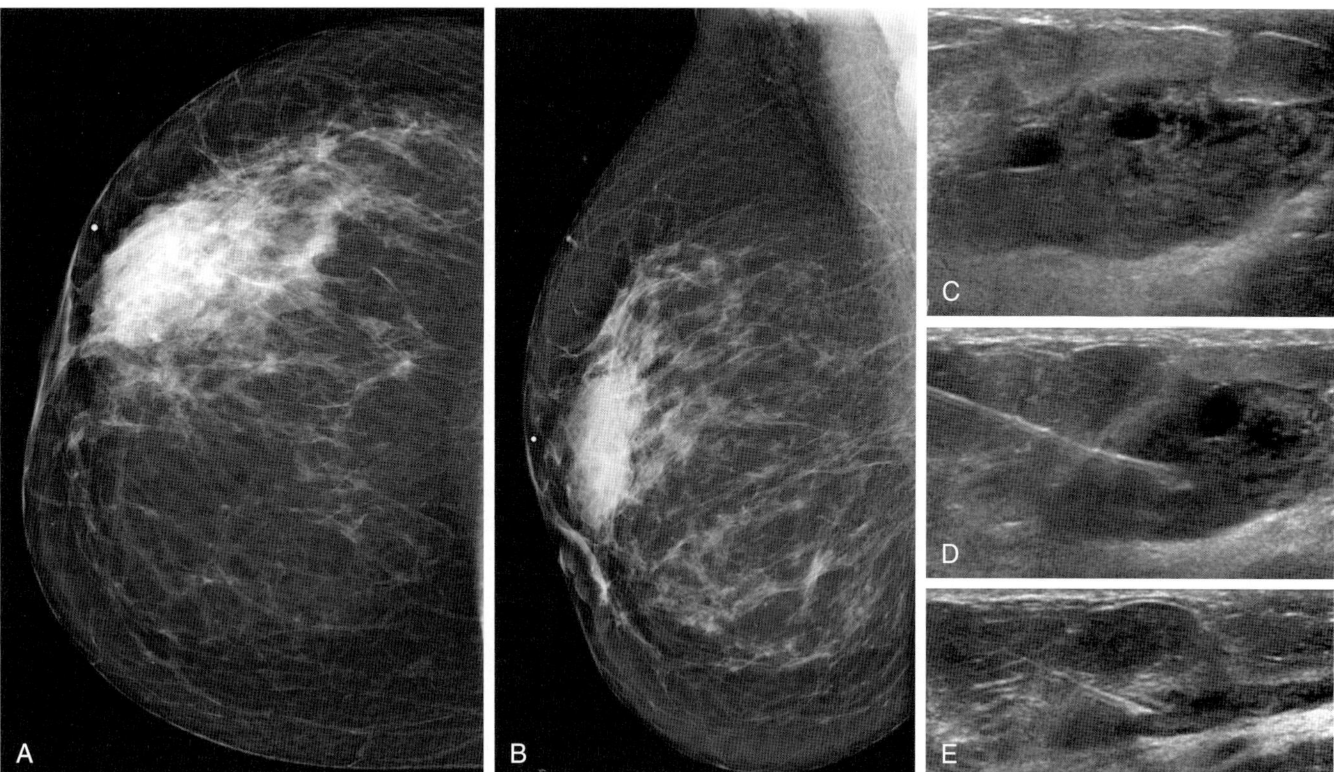

■ **FIGURE 20-9** Abscess. A 39-year-old patient presented with a mildly painful lump in the right breast at the 11 o'clock position that had rapidly increased in size over past 2 months. Craniocaudal (**A**) and mediolateral (**B**) mammograms demonstrate an oval mass with indistinct margins. An oval partially circumscribed and partially indistinct complex mass was seen ultrasonographically (**C**). An attempt was made at needle aspiration (**D**), which demonstrated purulent material, and nearly completely drained (**E**). The patient was placed on antibiotics with follow-up. The abscess subsequently recurred and necessitated surgical removal of the abscess wall.

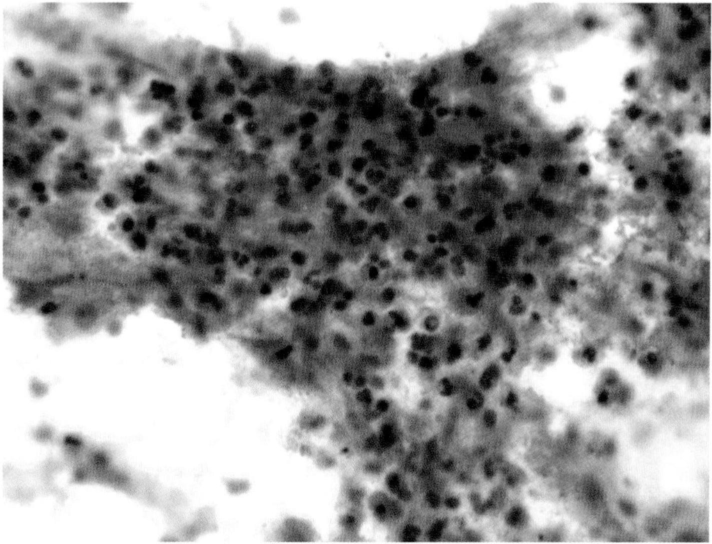

■ **FIGURE 20-10** Collection of acute inflammatory cells composed of neutrophils (Papanicolaou [PAP] stain, ×400).

within the breast tissue. Confluent inflammatory processes can obscure the lobulocentric distribution. Complete resection, corticosteroid therapy, or both, are recommended. The condition can recur in 38% if not excised completely (Figs 20-12 and 20-13).[13] Other extremely rare types of infectious granulomatous mastitis are caused by infections such as echinococcosis and coccidiomycosis (Figs 20-14 to 20-17).

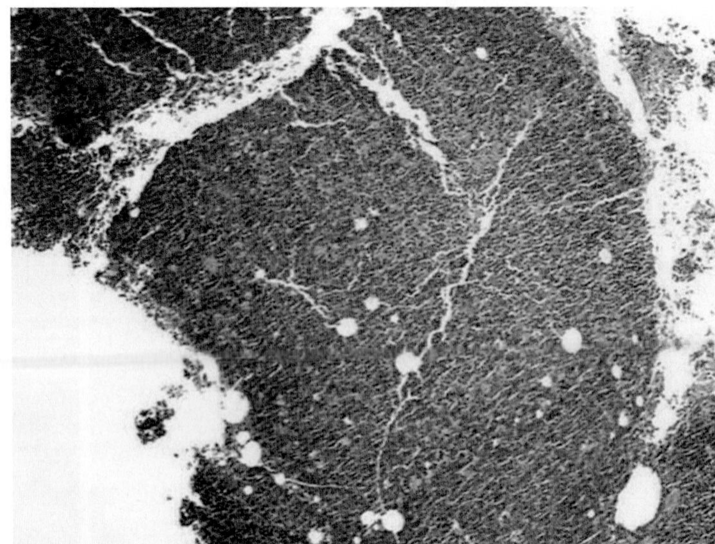

■ **FIGURE 20-11** An intense infiltrate of lymphocytes, plasma cells, histiocytes, and multinucleated giant cells within fibrotic background (H&E, ×200).

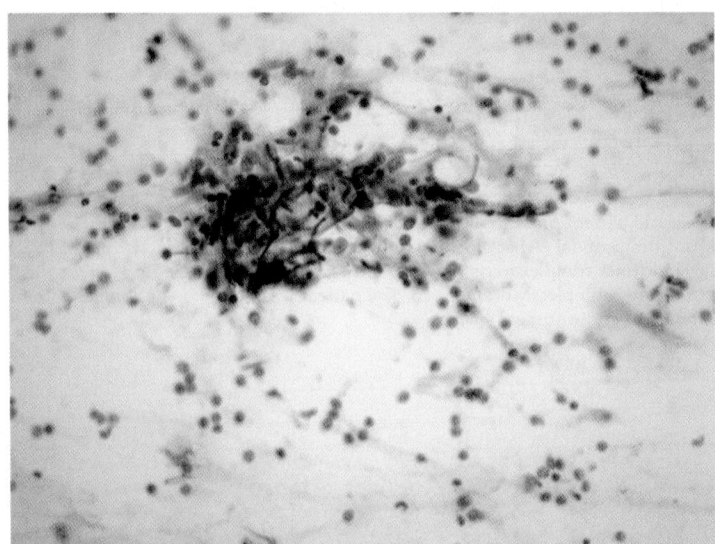

■ **FIGURE 20-12** An aggregate of granulomatous inflammation characterized by spindle shapes of histiocytes (Papanicolaou [PAP] stain, × 40).

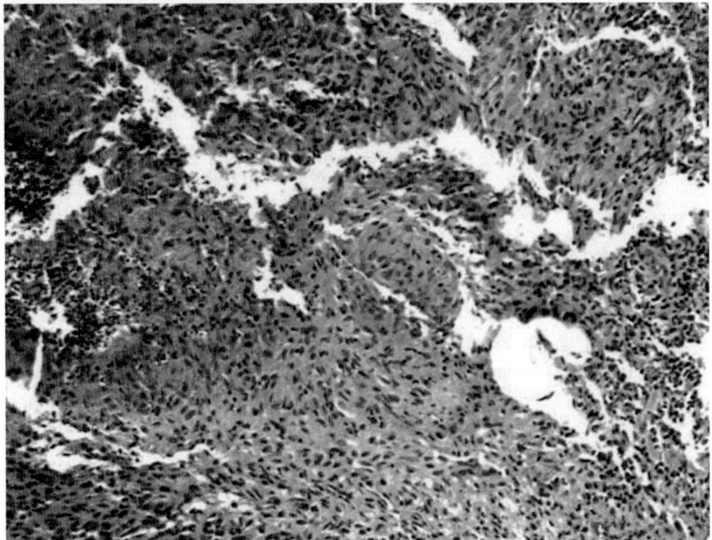

■ **FIGURE 20-13** Core needle biopsy of acute subareolar abscess with numerous acute inflammatory cells (H&E, ×200).

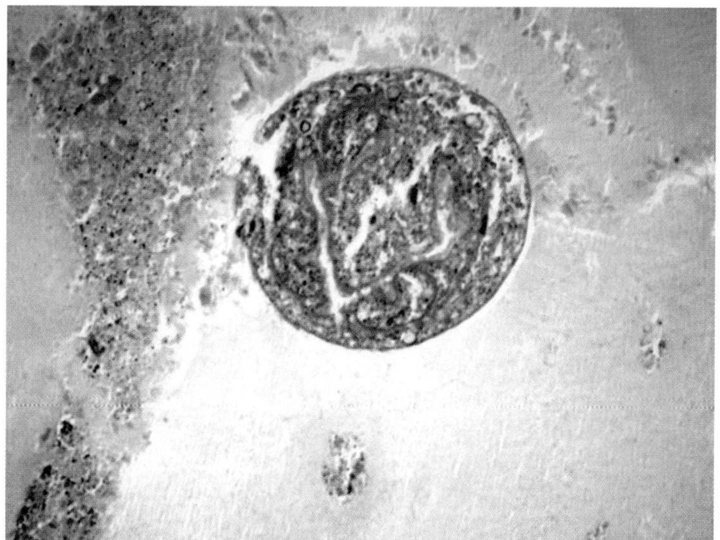

■ **FIGURE 20-14** Echinococcosis (hydatid disease). The inner lining of the cyst is a germinal membrane from which numerous daughter embryos develop (H&E, ×400).

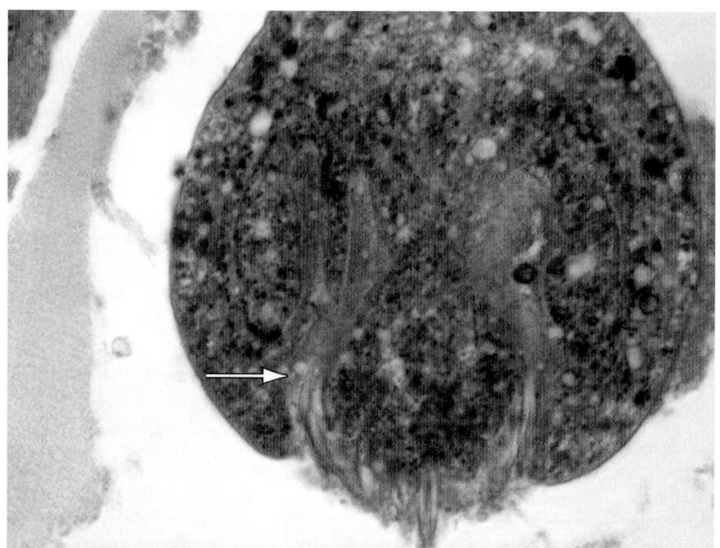

■ **FIGURE 20-15** Note the hooklets of Echinococcosis (arrow) (hydatid disease) (H&E × oil magnification).

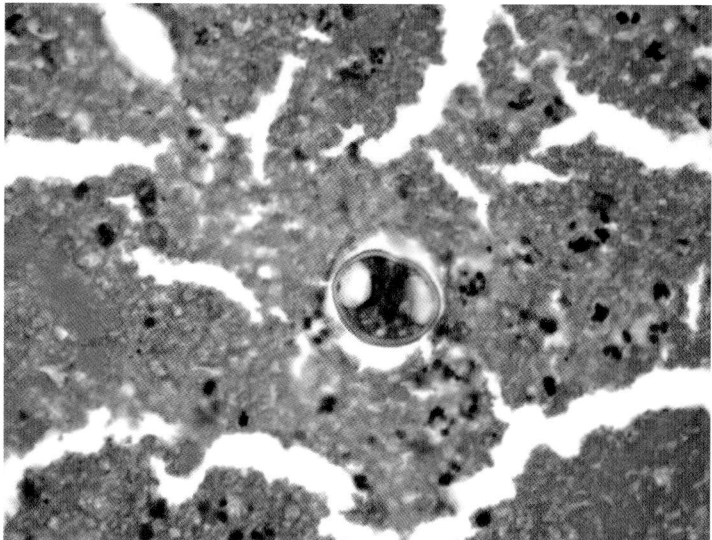

■ **FIGURE 20-16** Coccidiomycosis. Smooth-walled spherule with endospores inside (H&E, ×600).

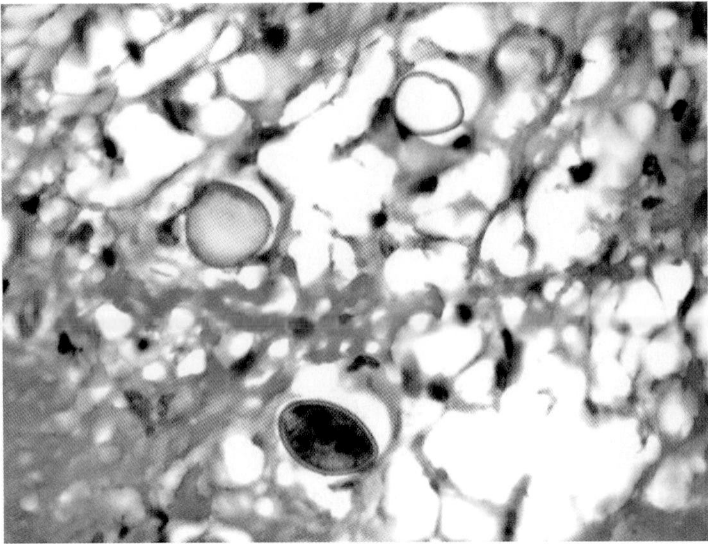

■ **FIGURE 20-17** Coccidiomycosis with several spherules; some of them are empty shells (H&E, ×600).

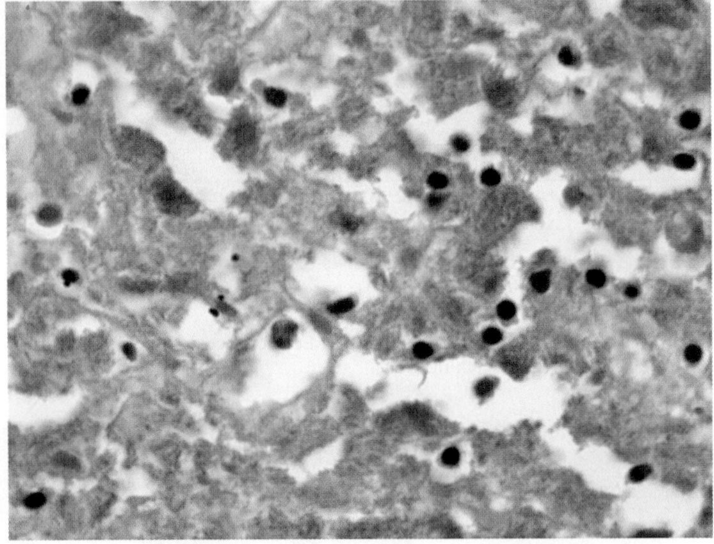

■ **FIGURE 20-18** Numerous rod-shaped organisms staining red with Fite stain.

KEY POINTS

- Mastitis can be infectious or noninfectious. Infections can be caused by bacteria, fungi, or parasites. Most infections are pyogenic and caused by *Streptococcus* and *Staphylococcus* species. Mastitis most commonly occurs in lactating females. Abscess formation can occur and should be treated with percutaneous or surgical drainage.
- Mammographic findings of mastitis include skin and trabecular thickening and indistinct or spiculated masses if an abscess is present. On ultrasonography an abscess is usually hypoechoic with indistinct margins.
- Many infections are due to mixed flora. Most of the cases of subareolar and periareolar abscess are caused by anaerobic infections, but other microorganisms including *Staphylococcus, Proteus, Bacteroides*, and *Streptococcus* have been reported.
- Granulomatous mastitis is a rare benign inflammatory condition most commonly of unknown etiology.
- When considering mastitis in the differential diagnosis, the diagnosis of exclusion is inflammatory breast carcinoma.

Tuberculous mastitis is extremely rare in the United States. Histologic features are similar to those of granulomatous mastitis, except caseating necrosis is more commonly observed in tuberculosis. Tuberculous mastitis more commonly involves the ducts than lobules. Acid-fast mycobacteria (AFB) are not visible on routine hematoxylin and eosin (H&E) stain, but special stains (Fite, AFB stains) can enhance visualization of the mycobacterial organism (Fig. 20-18). Surgical biopsy with microbial culture may be necessary to establish the diagnosis.

Synopsis of Treatment Options

For pyogenic infections of the breast, conservative treatment options include percutaneous drainage with antibiotics and close clinical follow-up or surgical incision and drainage. Corticosteroid therapy, complete resection, or both, are recommended for granulomatous mastitis if the etiology is unknown. If the etiology is known, the appropriate antifungal, antimycobacterial, or antiparasitic treatment should be given. Inflammatory breast carcinoma is the diagnosis of exclusion in a patient who presents with breast edema, redness, and pain.

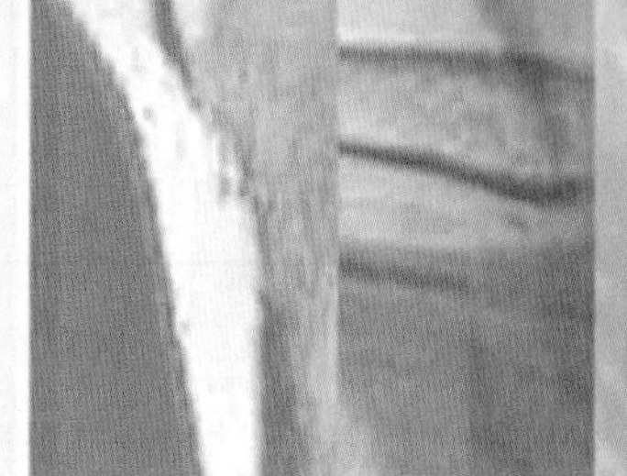

CASE STUDY

Chapter 20 Infectious and Inflammatory Diseases of the Breast

HISTORY

A 55-year-old woman presented with a breast lump. She complained that the area is palpable, red, warm to the touch, and swollen. Additional pertinent history was elicited: the patient is a native of India who recently immigrated to the United States.

FINDINGS

Clinical examination showed a tender mass with erythema of the overlying skin in the outer right breast and ipsilateral axillary lymphadenopathy and right arm lymphedema. Mammography showed a band-like opacity in the outer hemisphere of the breast extending into the axilla. Ultrasonography revealed multiple oval hypoechoic masses with the *filarial dance* sign which is movement of worms in real time. Core needle biopsy (CNB) was performed that contained chylous cystic material.

The specimens demonstrated the presence of worms with surrounding breast parenchyma and chronic inflammatory reaction (Fig. 20-18). A female worm demonstrated developing microfilariae and coiled form of larvae (Figs 20-19 to 20-22). Both the larvae and the adult worm were surrounded by dense fibrosis and chronic inflammation rich in histiocytes, eosinophils, plasma cells, and lymphocytes.

DIFFERENTIAL DIAGNOSIS

Differential diagnosis included granulomatous inflammation, acute abscess, and mammary filariasis.

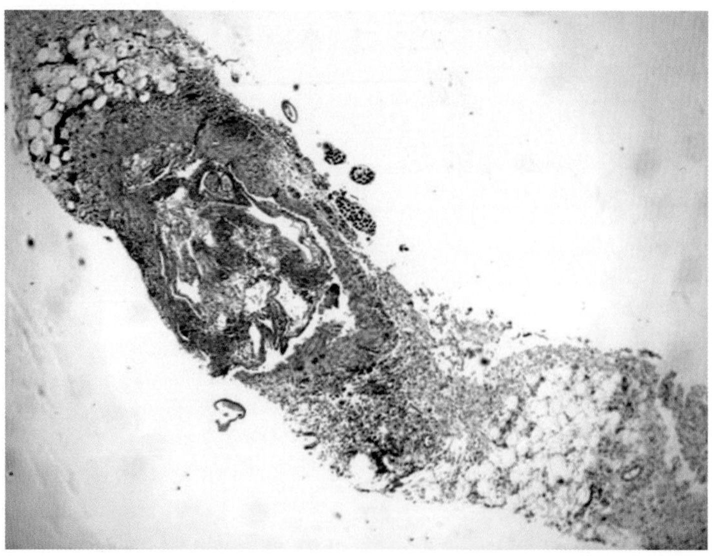

■ **FIGURE 20-19** Core needle biopsy of mammary filariasis. Note the surrounding dense fibrosis and inflammatory infiltrates (H&E, ×40).

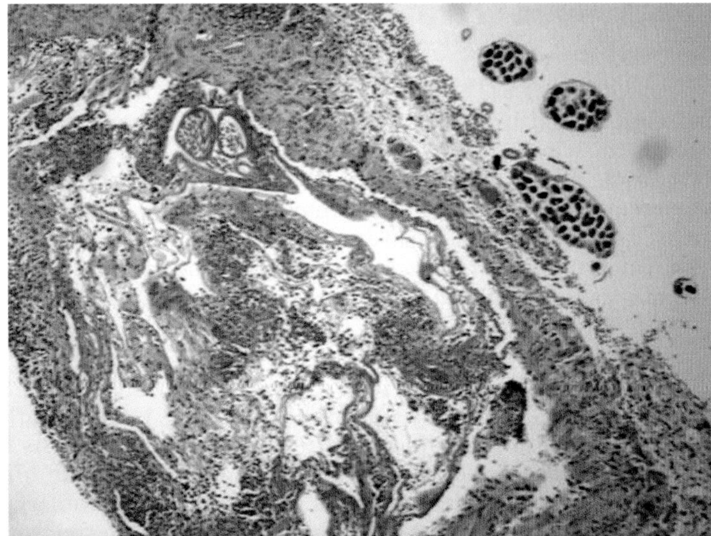

■ **FIGURE 20-20** Adult worm of *Wuchereria bancrofti.* A female worm is shown here filled with developing microfilariae. (H&E, ×200).

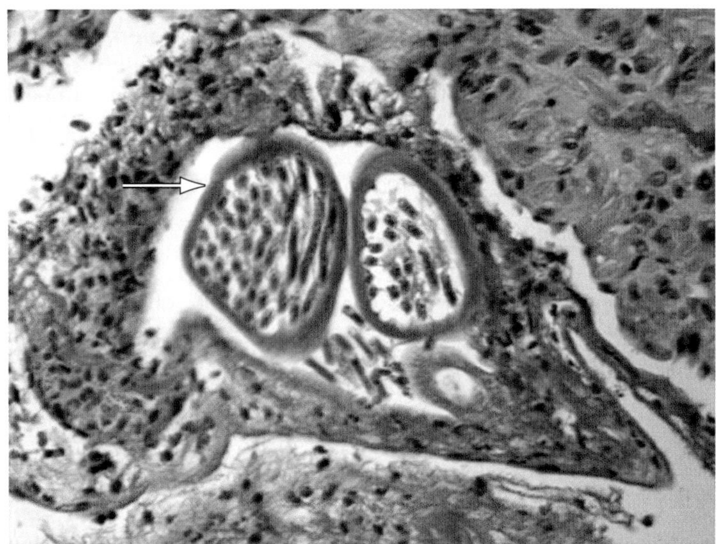

■ **FIGURE 20-21** Adult worm of *Wuchereria bancrofti* in higher power. A female worm is shown here filled with developing microfilariae in the uterus (H&E, ×400).

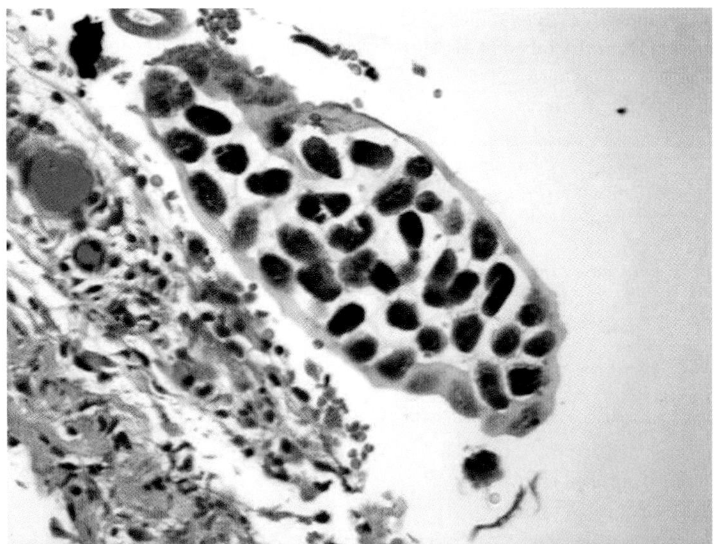

■ **FIGURE 20-22** Gravid adult worm with coiled forms of larvae *Wuchereria bancrofti* (H&E, ×600).

DIAGNOSIS

Mammary filariasis is most often caused by *Wuchereria bancrofti.* This condition has been reported in the Indian subcontinent, where the organism is endemic. Involvement of the breast is rare and can occur in the chronic phase of the infection. The patient usually presents with a unilateral painless solitary nontender breast mass, most commonly located in the upper outer quadrant. The adult worm moves vigorously in the human body. This movement can be detected by ultrasonography and is known as the *filarial dance,* a classic diagnostic feature of live adult worms.[14] Mammary filariasis may cause calcifications and an associated mass.

COMMENTARY

Mammary filariasis is a rare condition. Lymphatic filariasis affects many people worldwide and is found throughout the tropics and subtropics. The filarial life cycle consists of five developmental or larval stages in a vertebral host and an arthropod intermediate host and vector. Adult female worms produce thousands of first-stage larvae or microfilariae that are ingested by a feeding insect vector, usually mosquitoes and flies. Some microfilariae have a unique circadian periodicity in the peripheral circulation over a 24-hour period. The best detection of microfilariae occurs at night and can be seen in the peripheral blood. Microfilariae then undergo two developmental changes in the insect. In the third stage, larvae then are inoculated back into the vertebral host during the act of feeding for the final two stages of development. The treatment of choice is single-dose regimens of ivermectin or albendazole. The treatment goals are to eradicate the infestation, reduce morbidity, and prevent complications. Significant regression of the breast mass is expected clinically after 6 weeks of antifilarial treatment.

REFERENCES

1. Meguid MM, Kort KC, Numann PJ, Oler A. Subareolar breast abscess: the penultimate stage of the mammary duct associated disease sequence. In: Bland KI, Copeland EM, editors. *The breast: comprehensive management of benign and malignant disorders*. Philadelphia: Saunders; 2004. p. 93-131.
2. Radhi JM, Thavanathan MJ. Hydatid cyst presenting as a breast lump. *Can J Surg* 1990;**33**:29-30.
3. Vega A, Ortega E, Cavada A, Garijo F. Hydatid cyst of the breast: mammographic findings. *AJR Am J Roentgenol* 1994; **162**:825-6.
4. Seymour EQ. Blastomycosis of the breast. *AJR Am J Roentgenol* 1982;**139**:822-3.
5. Gorman JD, Champaign JL, Sumida FK, Canavan L. Schistosomiasis involving the breast. *Radiology* 1992;**185**:423-4.
6. Britton CA, Sumkin J, Math M, Williams S. Mammographic appearance of loiasis. *AJR Am J Roentgenol* 1992;**159**:51-2.
7. Aguirrezabalaga J, Sogo C, Parajo A. Mammary tuberculosis. Three case reports. *Breast Dis* 1994;**7**:377-82.
8. Han BK, Choe YH, Park JM, Moon WK, Ko YH, Yang JH, et al. Granulomatous mastitis: Mammographic and sonographic appearances. *AJR Am J Roentgenol* 1999;**173**:317-20.
9. Karstrup S, Solvig J, Nolsoe CP, Nilsson P, Khattar S, Loren I, et al. Acute puerperal breast abscesses: US-guided drainage. *Radiology* 1993;**188**:807-9.
10. Garg P, Rathee SK, Lal A. Ultrasonically guided percutaneous drainage of breast abscess. *J Indian Med Assoc* 1997;**95**:584-5.
11. Ikeda DM, Sickles EA. Mammographic demonstration of pectoral muscle microcalcifications. *AJR Am J Roentgenol* 1988;**151**:475-6.
12. Hayes R, Michell M, Nunnerley HB. Acute inflammation of the breast-The role of breast ultrasound in diagnosis and management. *Clin Radiol* 1991;**44**:253-6.
13. Imoto S, Kitaya T, Kodama T, Hasebe T, Mukai K. Idiopathic granulomatous mastitis. case report and review of the literature. *Jpn J Clin Oncol* 1997;**27**:274-7.
14. Jungmann P, Dreyer G. Detection by ultrasound of living adult *W. bancrofti* in female breast. *J Trop Med Hyg* 1992;**95**:1425-6.

SECTION

FIVE

Imaging of the Breast Malignancies

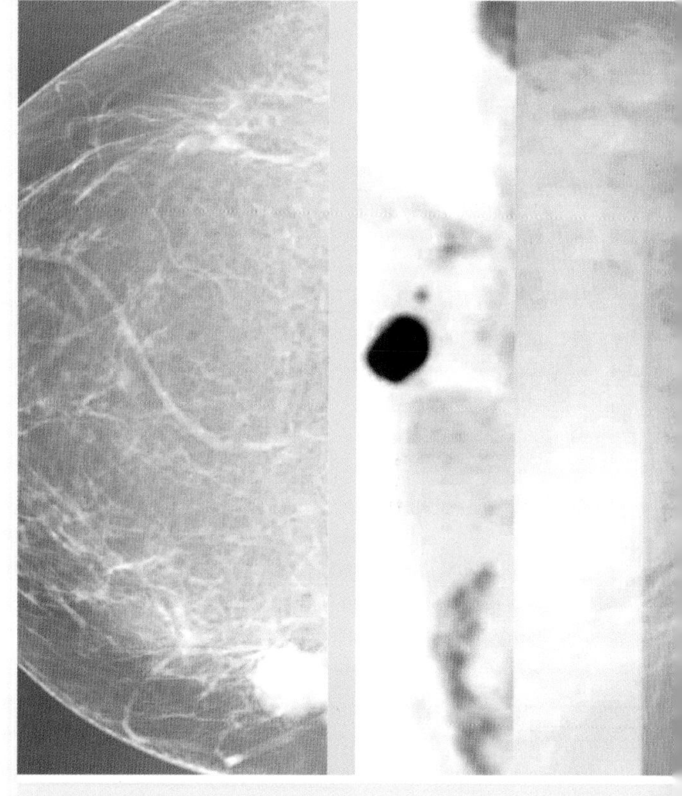

CHAPTER 21

Ductal Carcinoma in Situ and Paget's Disease

Sophia Kim Apple, Jennifer M. J. Overstreet, and Lawrence W. Bassett

Carcinoma in situ (CIS, or noninvasive carcinoma) is a distinct lesion of the breast that has potential to become invasive cancer. CIS lesions cannot metastasize because they are, by definition, restricted to the glandular lumen surrounded by myoepithelial cells and basement membrane material and have no access to lymphatics or blood vessels. CIS can be divided into two major types: ductal carcinoma in situ (DCIS, or intraductal carcinoma) and lobular carcinoma in situ (LCIS). LCIS is discussed in Chapter 19. The most important difference is that traditionally DCIS is considered a true preinvasive lesion whereas LCIS is considered a risk factor for breast carcinoma. New data are supportive of LCIS being more than just a risk factor, however.

DCIS may also be associated with invasive carcinoma. Of particular interest to radiologists are those cases of invasive cancer with an extensive intraductal component (EIC-positive, or EIC+). EIC is defined as the presence of DCIS in greater than or equal to 25% within the area of invasive carcinoma, outside the area of invasive carcinoma, or both. In EIC+ cases, successful treatment often depends on knowledge of the complete extent of the nonpalpable, noninvasive portion. Also of interest are those cases in which extensive DCIS is associated with microinvasion. EIC is discussed in more detail later.

Paget's disease of the nipple and noninvasive papillary carcinoma are subtypes of intraductal carcinoma that are also discussed in this chapter.

DUCTAL CARCINOMA IN SITU

Definition

The terms *intraductal carcinoma* and *ductal carcinoma in situ* (DCIS) are synonymous. DCIS is a preinvasive lesion. It is defined as malignant cells that are confined within the ductal structures and basement membranes that replace normal ductal epithelium. When these malignant cells replace ducts and lobules, we called them DCIS and cancerization of lobules (COL), respectively. Paget's disease of nipple is defined by having DCIS cells within the epidermis of the nipple, mammary areolar skin, or both. Because all cases of DCIS do not confer the same likelihood for eventual invasion and metastasis, it is important to understand that DCIS comprises a spectrum of lesions.

Prevalence and Epidemiology

Before the widespread use of screening mammography, DCIS was thought to be a relatively uncommon lesion, accounting for less than 5% of all breast carcinomas.[1] Today, DCIS makes up about 30% of breast malignancies detected in screening programs, and the majority of cases of DCIS are detected on mammography.[2] A major breakthrough in knowledge about DCIS occurred when Holland and Hendriks described their findings in mastectomy specimens containing DCIS.[3] They concluded that DCIS typically is distributed within a single segment of the duct system and is unicentric and segmental rather than multifocal or multicentric. This finding is consistent with the observation that breast cancer recurrences are usually in the region of the original tumor.[4]

Etiology and Pathophysiology

DCIS is defined as malignant ductal cells that proliferate within the ducts and basement membranes and eventually replace the benign cells within the ducts proximally and the lobules distally. DCIS comprises a spectrum of lesions. Several classification systems have been developed on the basis of the extent of the lesion, clinical findings, and histologic features. The most commonly used classification divides DCIS into two major types: the more aggressive comedocarcinoma and the more indolent noncomedo carcinoma During examination of excised specimens containing comedocarcinoma, the involved ducts may extrude a thick material resembling that of a comedo—thus the name *comedocarcinoma*.[5] Comedocarcinoma is characterized by more aggressive malignant cytologic features and behavior. The noncomedo carcinoma subtypes are less aggressive clinically. In reality, the histologic subtypes of DCIS are often intermediate and intermixed, and the prognosis probably depends on the nuclear grade as well as other factors summarized later in this chapter in the section on pathology. In general, morphologically extensive, fine linear and fine linear branching calcifications (like those seen in comedocarcinoma [see later]) are associated with more aggressive DCIS and greater extent of disease.[6]

Manifestations of Disease

Clinical Presentation

The majority of intraductal carcinomas do not have clinical signs or symptoms. When present, the most common clinical manifestations are palpable masses, nipple discharge, and Paget's disease.[5] Comedo-type DCIS is more likely than noncomedo-type DCIS to manifest as a palpable mass. Several studies have suggested that comedo-type DCIS is also more commonly associated with microinvasion and lymph node involvement, reflections of its more aggressive behavior. A periductal, inflammatory reaction also can occur, at times leading to a mammographically visible or clinically palpable mass.[6]

Imaging Indications and Algorithm

DCIS is almost always detected on screening mammography. Diagnostic mammography, including magnification views, and ultrasonography to identify a possible invasive component may follow. If, on the other hand, DCIS presents as a palpable mass or Paget's disease, diagnostic mammography and ultrasonography should follow.

Imaging Findings by Modality

Mammography

Ductal Carcinoma In Situ

Mammography plays a key role in the detection of DCIS, in which calcifications are the mammographic hallmark. The typical appearance is fine, linear, discontinuous, and branching calcifications with a diameter of usually less than 0.5 mm (Figs 21-1 through 21-5). Their appearance suggests filling of the duct lumen involved irregularly by breast cancer (fine linear or casting).

Mammographically, microcalcifications of noncomedo DCIS are granular, hazy, amorphous, or indistinct particles characterized by variable size and shape. In contrast, the individual calcifications of comedo DCIS are likely to be larger and more coarse as well as discontinuous, linear, and branching. However, these radiographic features are not always reliable in differentiation among the histologic subtypes of lesions.[3,7]

Another important feature of DCIS is the distribution of the calcifications. They are usually found in a linear, branching, or segmental distribution. The distribution of

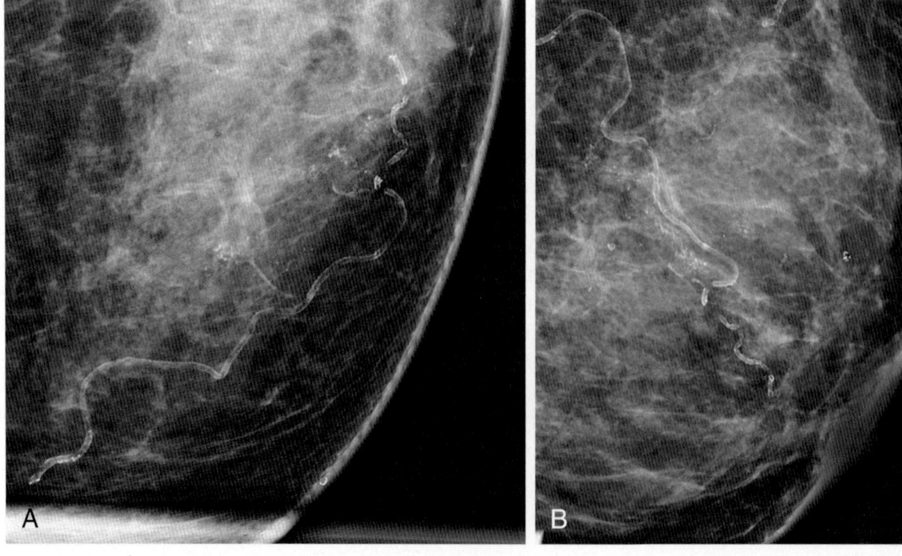

■ **FIGURE 21-1** Ductal carcinoma in situ. Craniocaudal (**A**) and mediolateral (**B**) digital magnification views of the left breast show amorphous calcifications in a segmental distribution within the upper inner quadrant.

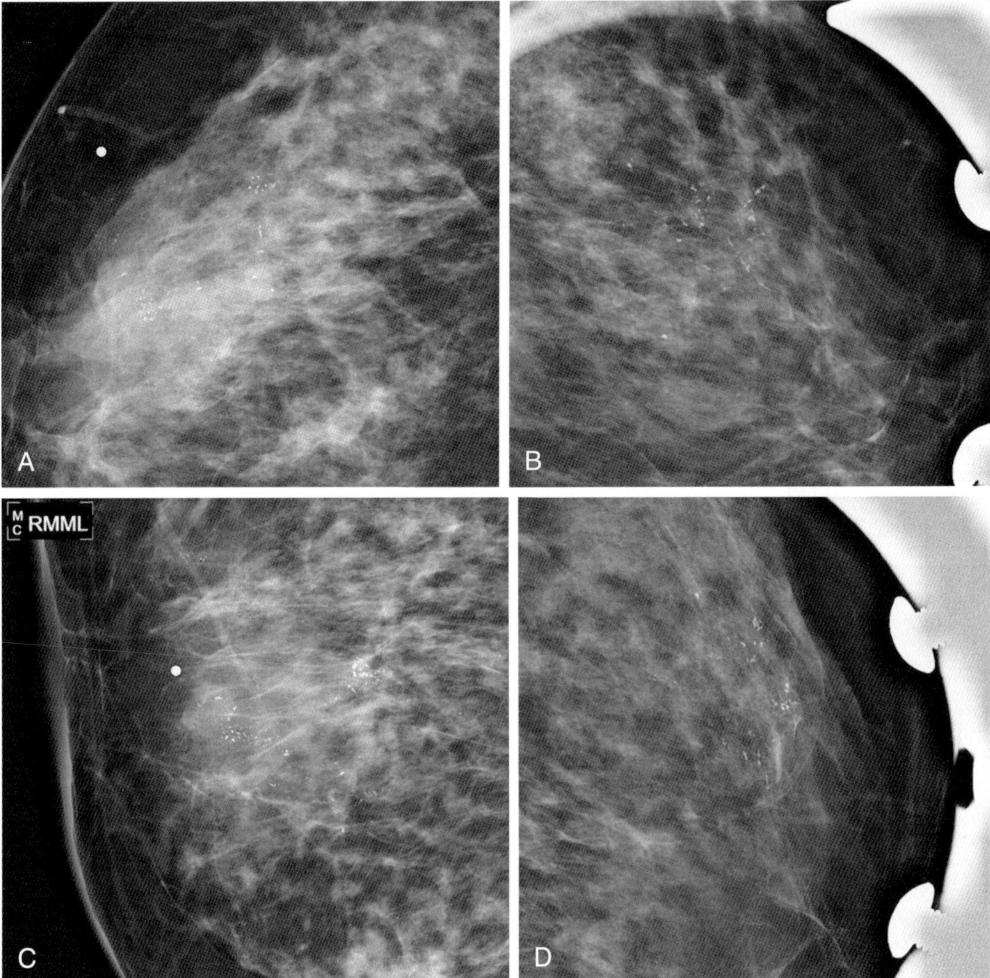

■ **FIGURE 21-2** Bilateral ductal carcinoma in situ. Bilateral craniocaudal (**A**, **B**) and mediolateral (**C**, **D**) digital magnification views show linear, branching, pleomorphic calcifications distributed segmentally in the upper outer quadrants of the breasts bilaterally. The right nipple appears somewhat retracted. This patient presented with symptoms of bloody nipple discharge in the right breast.

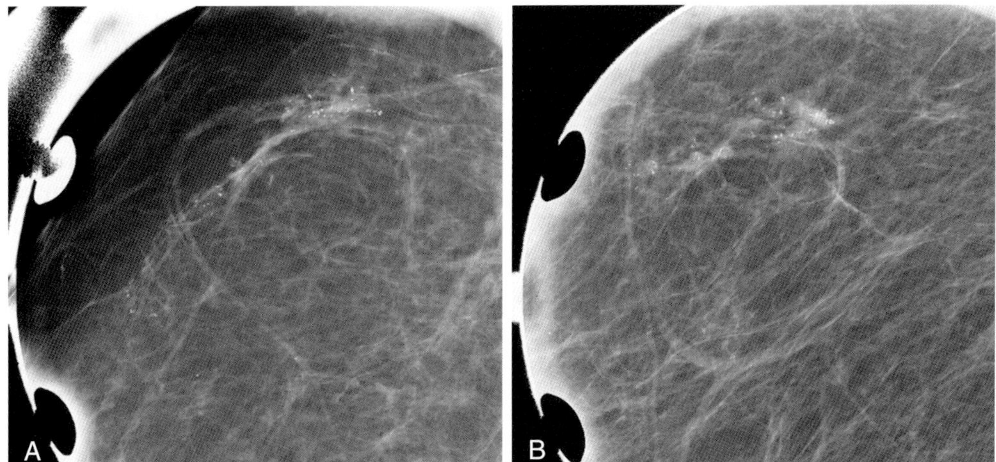

■ **FIGURE 21-3** Ductal carcinoma in situ. Craniocaudal (**A**) and mediolateral (**B**) digital magnification views of the right breast show a cluster of pleomorphic calcifications in a ductal distribution in the upper outer quadrant. Cluster and ductal are distribution modifiers and are mutually exclusive. This appears more of a linear distribution.

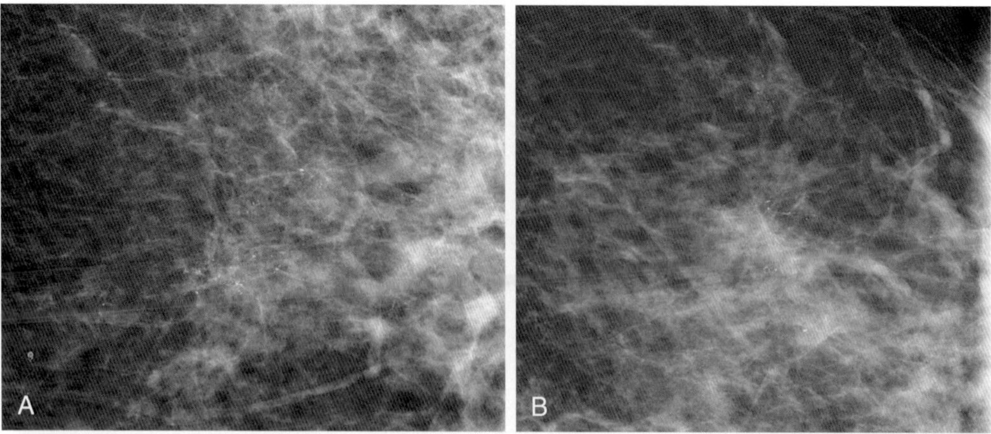

■ **FIGURE 21-4** Ductal carcinoma in situ. Craniocaudal (**A**) and mediolateral (**B**) digital magnification views of the left breast show clustered amorphous and fine, linear, branching calcifications in the upper inner quadrant.

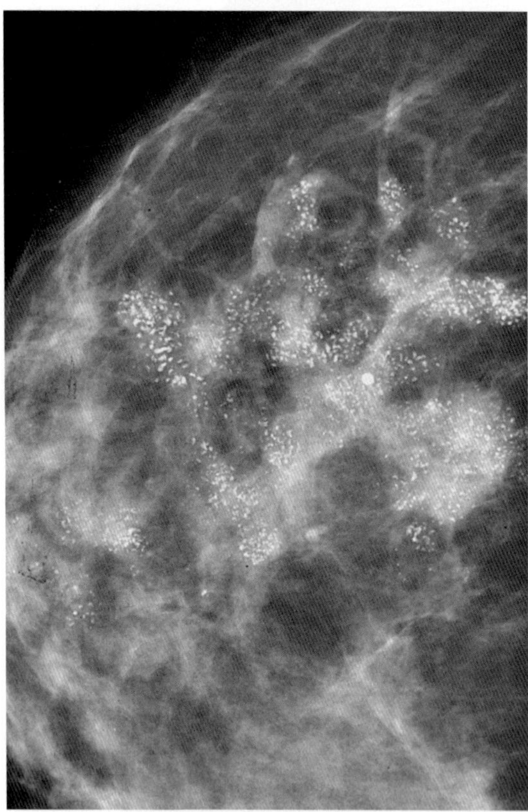

■ **FIGURE 21-5** Extensive ductal carcinoma in situ manifesting as fine pleomorphic and coarse, heterogeneous calcifications in a segmental distribution. The tumor is in the terminal branches of the ductal system and extends into the lobules. The associated soft tissue density seen represents malignancy dilating the terminal ducts and lobules.

calcifications in an individual case depends on the lesion's anatomic location. Those in major ducts are likely to be distributed in a line toward the nipple, whereas those in smaller subdivisions of the ductal system may be distributed like the branches of the interlobular and intralobular ducts. Interestingly, it has been observed that the visible calcifications of comedo DCIS closely match the actual extent of the lesion but noncomedo DCIS may be more extensive than suggested by its calcifications. In general, the discrepancy is less than 2 cm in 80% to 85% of cases.[3]

In a little more than 10% of cases, only a soft tissue mass can be appreciated in mammograms.[7,8] These changes are the manifestation of a solid mass of tumor cells or associated inflammation, edema, and fibrosis at the periphery of the involved ducts.[8] DCIS can occur within preexisting sclerosing adenosis or radial scar and can be palpable or present as a mass lesion on a mammogram (Figs 21-6 and 21-7).

Other unusual manifestations of DCIS are asymmetry, focal asymmetry, mass with ill-defined margins, dilated retroareolar ducts, and architectural distortion (Fig. 21-8).

Invasive Cancer with Extensive Intraductal Component

Tumors are classified as being EIC+ if they are predominantly intraductal with small areas of invasion or if they are primarily invasive with the following: (1) DCIS filling nonobliterated ducts within the invasive cancer; or (2) DCIS in the tissue adjacent to the invasive tumor.[9] The significance of the EIC+ designation is the greater incidence of local recurrence of breast cancer after surgical excision and radiotherapy: the incidence of recurrence for EIC+ cases is approximately 25% at 5 years, compared with 6% for cases without an EIC (EIC-negative).[10] These findings verify observations of others that the presence of EIC+ in DCIS is a marker for widespread residual tumor after excision.[11] However, if all of the DCIS is successfully removed, the local recurrence rate is similar to that for EIC-negative tumors.

Mammography plays an important role in the management of EIC+ cases. Firstly, mammographic wire localization is essential prior to surgical excision. The purpose of the localization procedure is to excise all demonstrable lesions before radiotherapy, and as such, multiple wires are often used to identify the full extent of the lesion to facilitate complete surgical excision.[12] We refer to this procedure as "bracketing of the lesion" (Figs 21-9 to 21-12). At the time of surgical excision of DCIS, a specimen radiograph should always be obtained. However, it should be remembered that the specimen radiograph is not an adequate tool by which to ensure that all malignant calcifications have been removed.[13]

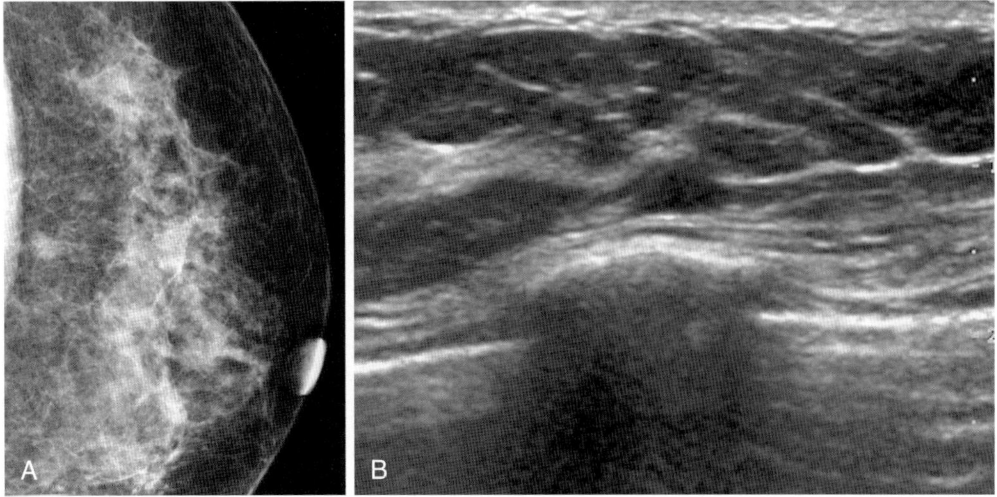

■ **FIGURE 21-6** Ductal carcinoma in situ presenting as a mammographic mass. Craniocaudal digital mammogram (**A**) of the left breast shows an oval indistinct mass with measuring 4 mm at the 6-o'clock position. Correlative ultrasound image (**B**) shows a 4 × 4 × 3-mm oval hypoechoic mass with partially indistinct margins next to the chest wall that corresponds to the mammographic findings.

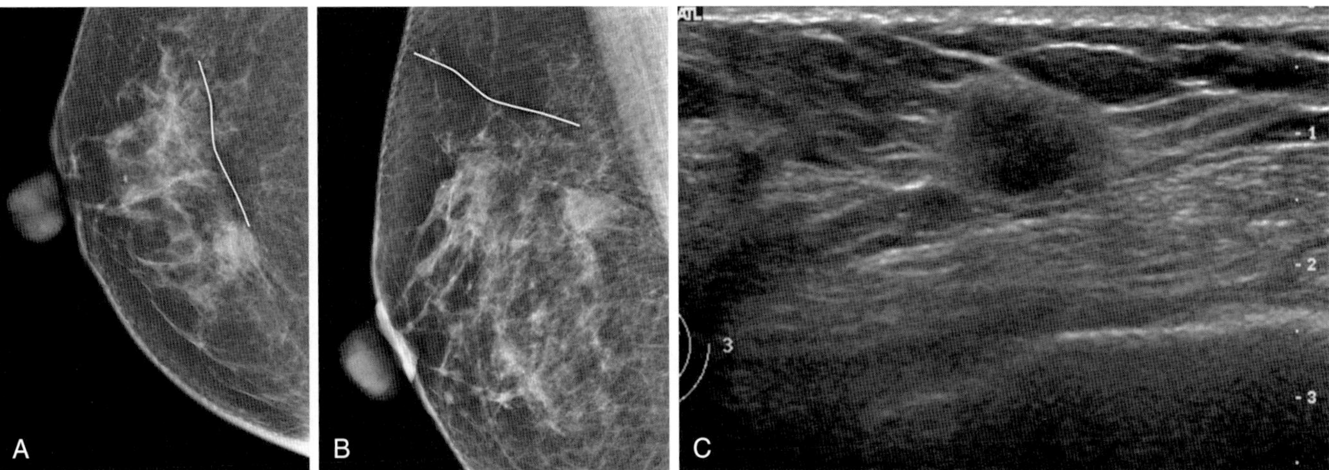

■ **FIGURE 21-7** Ductal carcinoma in situ with sclerosing adenosis presenting as a mammographic mass. Craniocaudal (**A**) and mediolateral (**B**) digital magnification views of the right breast demonstrate an equal density round mass with obscured margins in the upper inner quadrant at the 2-o'clock position at a middle depth. Correlative ultrasound image (**C**) demonstrates an 11 × 9 × 9-mm oval hypoechoic mass with indistinct margins and a thick echogenic halo consistent that corresponds to the mammographic mass.

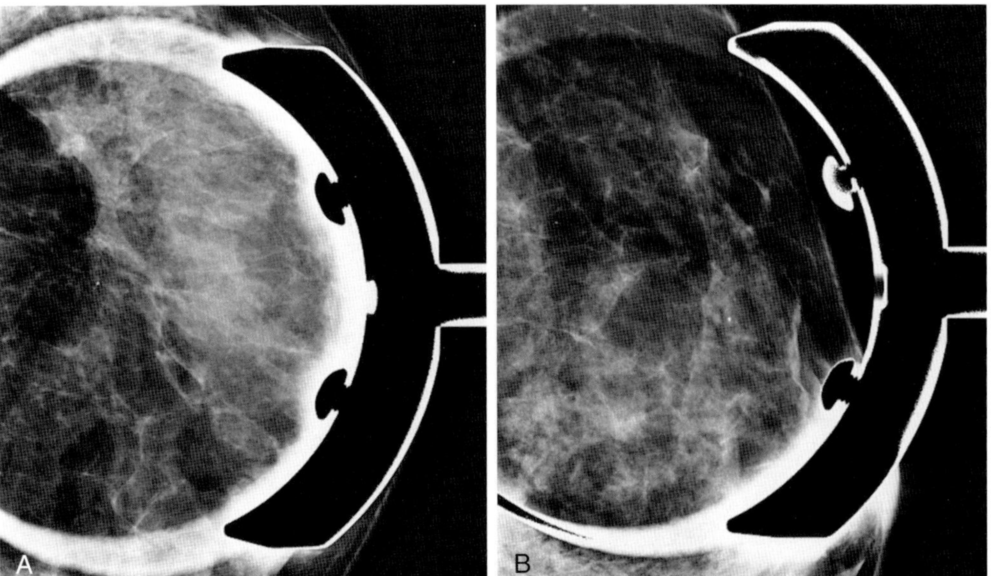

■ **FIGURE 21-8** Ductal carcinoma in situ with radial scar and sclerosing adenosis presenting as architectural distortion. Craniocaudal (**A**) and mediolateral (**B**) digital magnification view of the left breast show an area of architectural distortion at 12 o'clock.

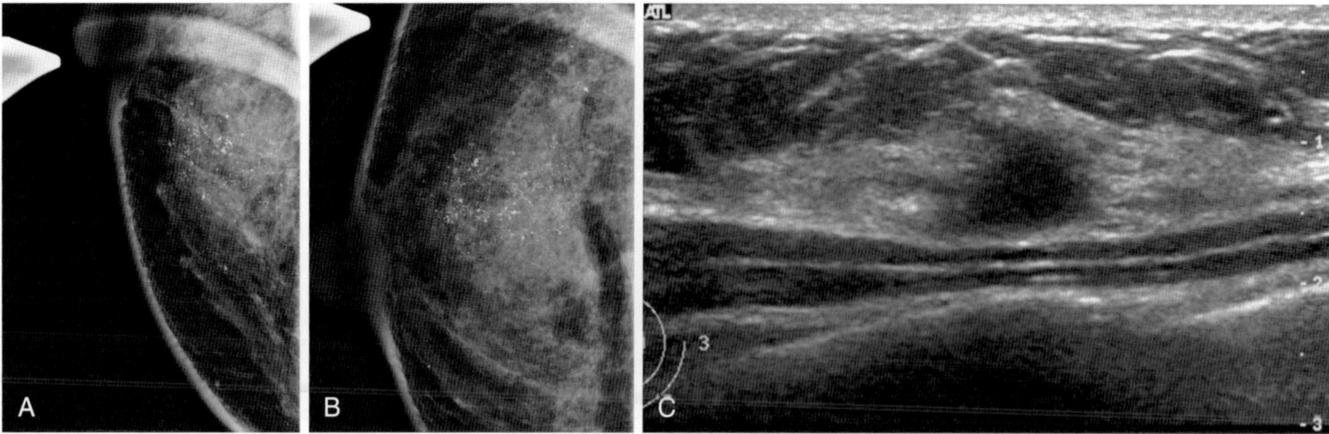

■ **FIGURE 21-9** Extensive intraductal component. Craniocaudal (**A**) and mediolateral (**B**) digital magnification views of the right breast show pleomorphic and fine, linear calcifications in a segmental distribution that measure approximately 2.3 × 2.6 cm in the retroareolar, central breast. The invasive carcinoma corresponded on ultrasound (**C**) to an irregular hypoechoic mass with indistinct and spiculated margins measuring 0.8 × 0.7 × 0.8 cm at the 1-o'clock position 3 to 4 cm from the nipple.

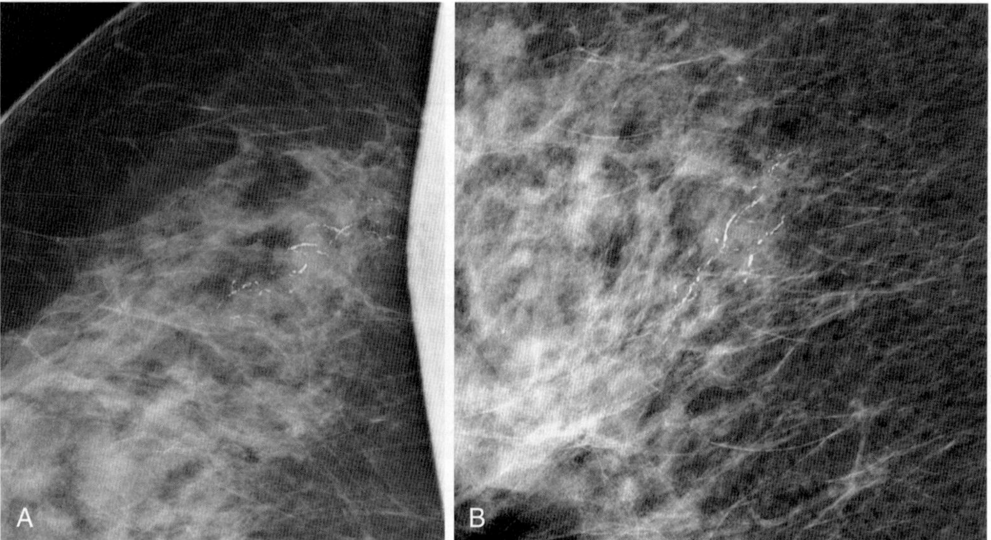

■ **FIGURE 21-10** Extensive intraductal component. Craniocaudal (**A**) and mediolateral (**B**) digital magnification views of the right breast show fine linear and fine linear branching calcifications distributed segmentally at the 9-o'clock position, middle depth.

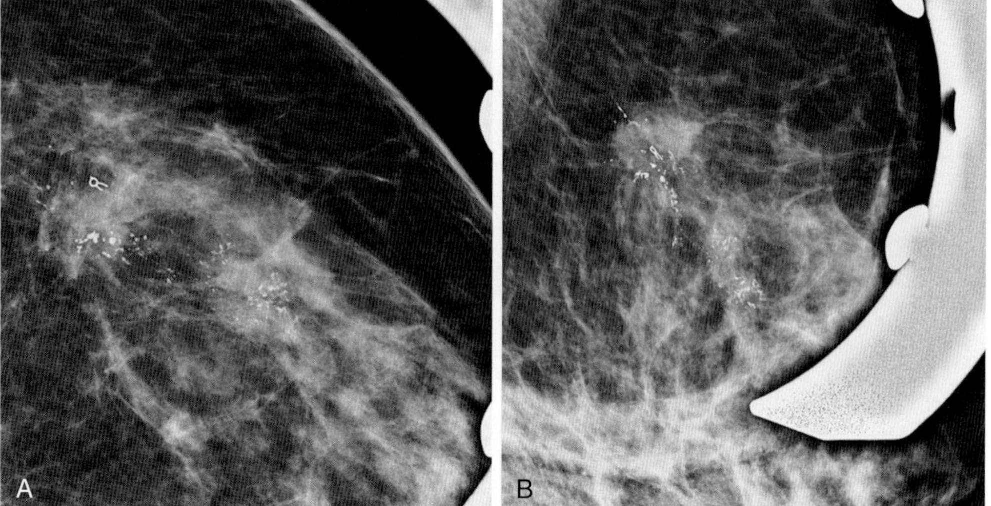

■ **FIGURE 12-11** Extensive intraductal component (EIC). Craniocaudal (**A**) and mediolateral (**B**) digital magnification views of the left breast show a 12 × 13-mm high-density irregular mass with spiculated margins in the upper outer quadrant, consistent with the biopsy-proven invasive ductal carcinoma. A microclip is identified. Pleomorphic calcifications extending anteriorly beyond the mass in a segmental distribution represent the EIC.

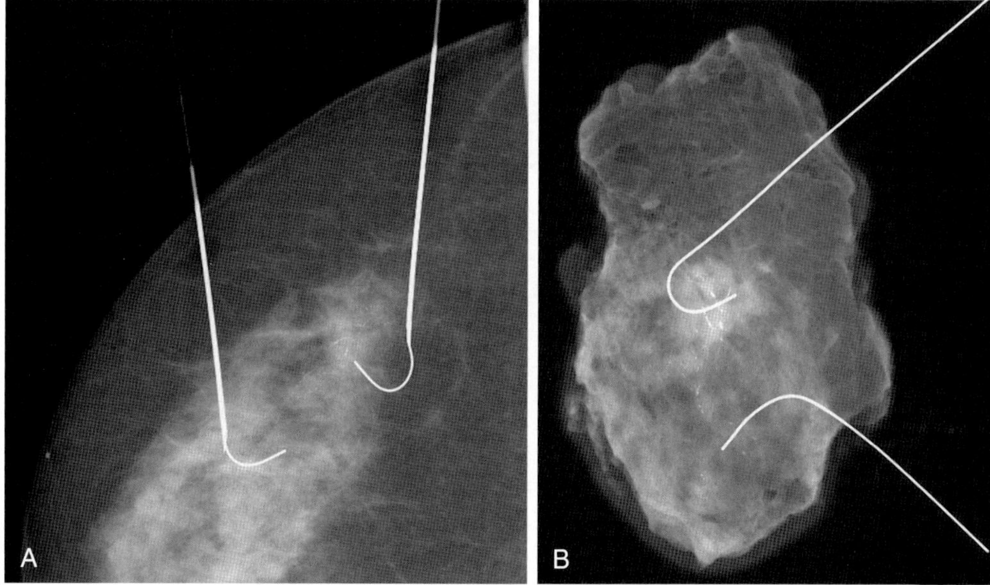

■ FIGURE 21-12 Same patient as in Figure 21-10. Craniocaudal digital mammogram (**A**) demonstrating how two needles are used to bracket the fine, linear calcifications in this patient with biopsy-proven infiltrating ductal carcinoma prior to surgical excision. Specimen radiograph (**B**) after lumpectomy verifies the presence of the extensive calcifications.

It is usually the responsibility of the pathologist to determine whether the margins of the resected tissue are free of tumor. However, the complex branching of the breast ductal system may lead to errors as to whether intraductal tumor has been completely removed. In other words, although the margins of the surgical specimen may appear to be clear of tumor in the histologic sections, DCIS can still be present in the breast. Therefore, after surgery and before radiotherapy in women with DCIS manifested as calcifications, it is important that mammography be performed to enable a search for residual malignant calcifications. The preradiotherapy mammograms are usually obtained 3 to 4 weeks after surgery to allow as much time as possible to reduce the discomfort associated with mammographic compression. We perform the postoperative preradiotherapy examination with a wire placed over the surgical site. In addition to standard views, magnification views are obtained over the region of the wire. If soft tissue edema obscures the surgical site, a magnification view tangential to the wire is performed to move overlying edematous skin and subcutaneous tissues away from the area of interest.

Noninvasive Papillary Carcinoma

Papillary carcinoma should be categorized as noninvasive or invasive. Noninvasive papillary carcinoma can occur either as a malignancy in which the epithelium proliferates as villous projections into the duct lumen or as an intracystic lesion. Bloody nipple discharge is seen in about 20% of cases. Correlation between histologic type and mammographic appearance has been reported.[14] Papillary carcinoma growing within a large duct usually manifests on mammograms as clustered calcifications. Noninvasive intracystic papillary carcinomas appear on mammograms as circumscribed masses that on ultrasonography are complex masses with echogenic tissue projecting from the wall of the cyst into the lumen (Fig. 21-13).

Ultrasonography

Occasionally, DCIS may be seen on ultrasound examination when it is accompanied by inflammation, edema, or surrounding desmoplastic reaction or fibrosis. It may present as a hypoechoic mass with partially circumscribed or indistinct margins. Ultrasound may also demonstrate associated calcification (see Figs. 21-6, 21-7, and 21-14).

Magnetic Resonance Imaging

The literature suggests that magnetic resonance imaging (MRI) can detect mammographically occult DCIS.[15] The appearance of DCIS is variable on MRI. Non-mass-like clumped or heterogeneous enhancement in a linear, segmental, or ductal distribution is the most common appearance (Figs. 21-15 and 21-16). However, focal or regional enhancement can also be seen. Occasionally, DCIS may appear as an enhancing mass (Fig. 21-17).

Classic signs

Fine, linear, discontinuous, and branching calcifications in a linear or segmental distribution on mammograms are highly suggestive of DCIS.

Differential Diagnosis

From Clinical Presentation

DCIS may present as a palpable breast mass. The differential diagnosis includes benign versus malignant causes.

From Imaging Findings

When a mammogram demonstrates fine, linear, discontinuous, and branching calcifications in a linear or segmental distribution, the appearance is typical of DCIS.

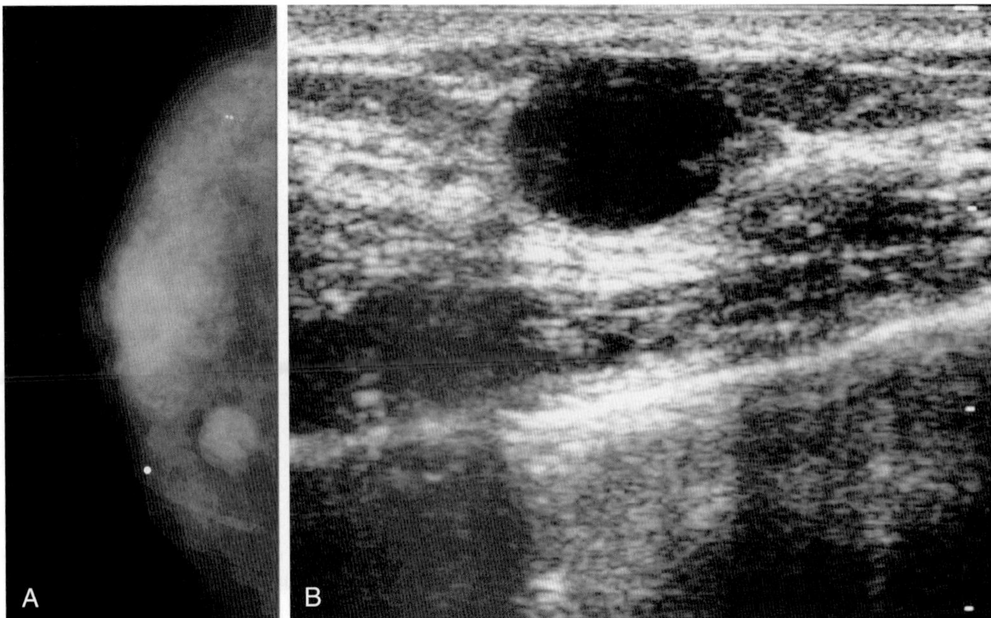

■ **FIGURE 21-13** Intracystic papillary carcinoma. A large palpable mass was present. Mammography (**A**) shows a high-density round mass with circumscribed margins. Correlative ultrasound image (**B**) demonstrates a round, complex mass with hypoechoic masses protruding from the wall of the cyst into the lumen.

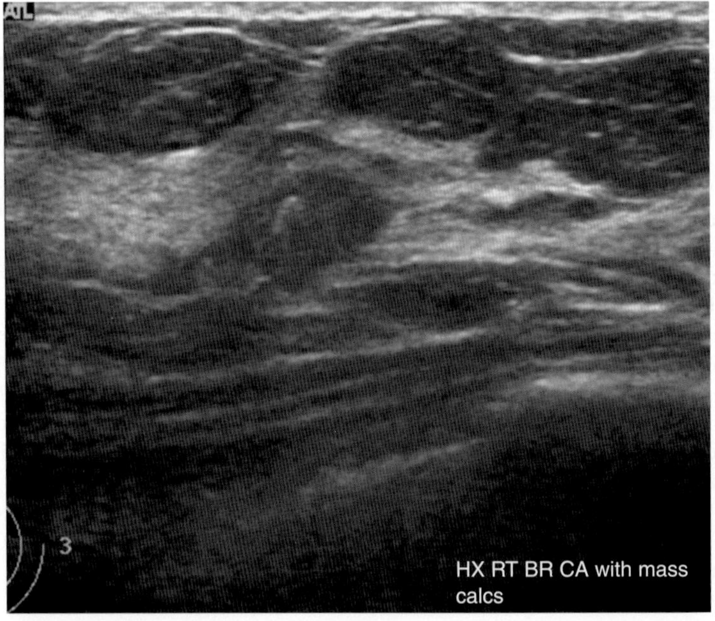

■ **FIGURE 21-14** Ductal carcinoma in situ. Ultrasound image of the upper inner quadrant of the right breast shows a hypoechoic oval mass with indistinct margins measuring 20 × 7 × 11 mm at approximately the 3-o'clock position, 2 to 3 cm from the nipple. The echogenic focus represents a microclip placed during prior biopsy of calcifications.

However, invasive carcinoma cannot be excluded by imaging. When DCIS presents as clustered calcifications, the differential diagnosis also includes benign lesions such as sclerosing adenosis and high-risk lesions such as atypical ductal hyperplasia (ADH) and flat epithelial atypia (FEA).

Pathology Findings

Gross Pathology

Mammographically detected suspicious DCIS with pleomorphic microcalcifications does not have a distinct gross appearance. In fact, most of DCIS is not palpable, except

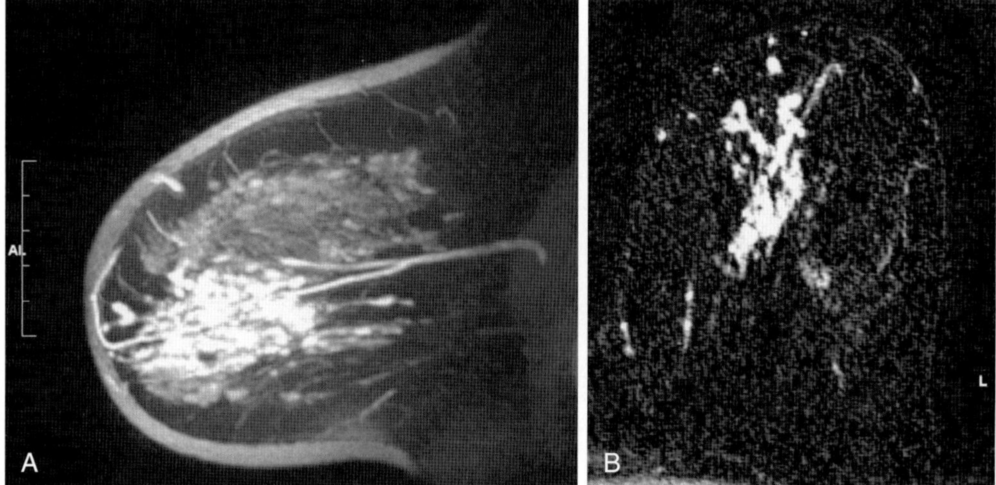

■ **FIGURE 21-15** Ductal carcinoma in situ on magnetic resonance imaging (MRI). Sagittal MIP (maximum intensity projection) (**A**) and axial subtraction (**B**) magnetic resonance (MR) images of the left breast show non–mass-like clumped enhancement in a segmental distribution in the lower inner quadrant.

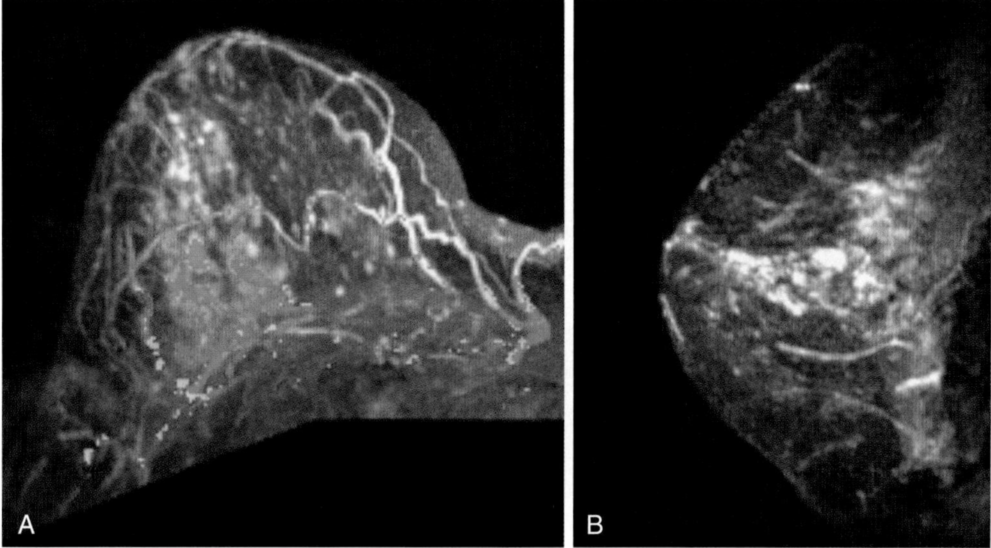

■ **FIGURE 21-16** Ductal carcinoma in situ on magnetic resonance imaging (MRI). Axial MIP (maximum intensity projection) (**A**) and sagittal MIP (**B**) views of the right breast show non–mass-like clumped, heterogeneous enhancement in a segmental distribution noted in the upper outer quadrant that extends from the nipple laterally toward the pectoralis. Kinetics demonstrate a rapid initial phase with a persistent delayed phase (*blue color*).

intracystic papillary carcinoma and some papillary DCIS with cystic and hemorrhagic areas. Comedo-type DCIS often shows white to pale yellow flecks composed of necrotic material extruding from the cut surface and hence called *comedo*. Occasionally, DCIS can present as a mass lesion, in which case it may be palpable grossly. Clinical presentation of DCIS within a mass is due to DCIS involving either sclerosing adenosis or comedo-type DCIS with fibrotic and desmoplastic stromal background. Because most DCIS is nonpalpable and not visible grossly, it is critical that pathologists handle specimens carefully to determine the extent of DCIS and the margin status (see Chapter 31).

Microscopic Findings

In contrast to most beliefs, DCIS is not a single disease entity but rather a spectrum of diseases. DCIS is a heterogeneous group of lesions both biologically and morphologically. All DCIS is malignant cell proliferation within the duct spaces surrounded by myoepithelial cells and basement material (Fig. 21-18). Traditionally, DCIS was separated into comedo type and noncomedo type as discussed earlier. More recent systems divide DCIS into three classifications composed of architecture, nuclear grade, and presence or absence of central coagulative (comedo) necrosis. An accurate classification of DCIS is important because of the difference in prognostic factors and outcome. The nuclear grade is the most important one to classify. A lesion with a higher nuclear grade and necrosis (comedo-type DCIS) is at much higher risk of short-term local recurrence and invasive transformation.

Architecture classification refers to the microscopic arrangement forming particular shapes of tumor cells, which can be solid, cribriform, papillary, and micropapillary.

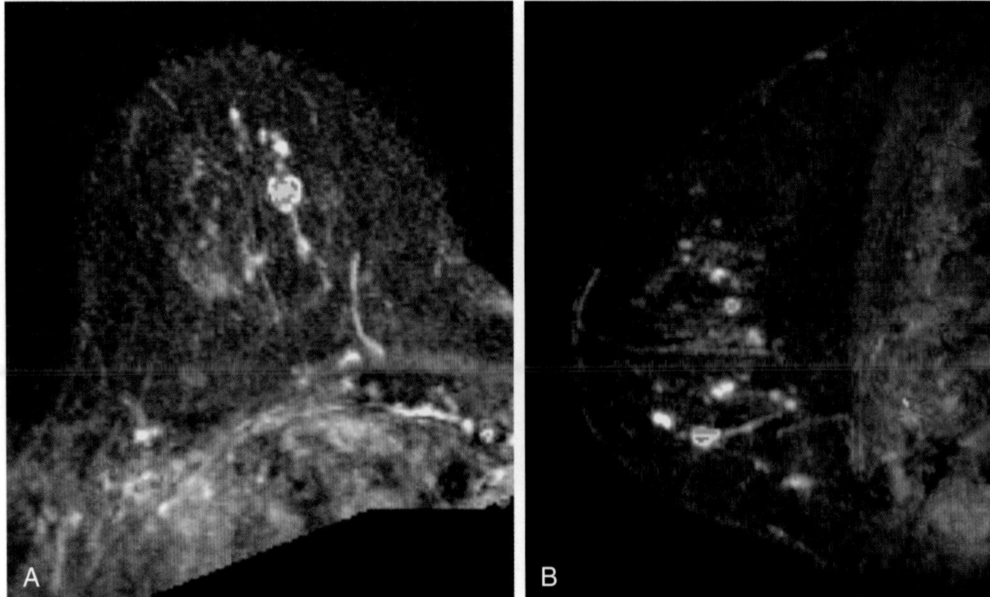

■ **FIGURE 21-17** Ductal carcinoma in situ presenting as a mass on magnetic resonance imaging (MRI). Axial (**A**) and sagittal (**B**) subtraction images demonstrate a homogeneously enhancing round mass with smooth margins that measures 0.7 cm TR × 0.7 cm AP × 0.6 cm SI at the 6-o'clock position, 4 cm from the nipple. Color overlay shows kinetic data with a worse curve demonstrating rapid washout.

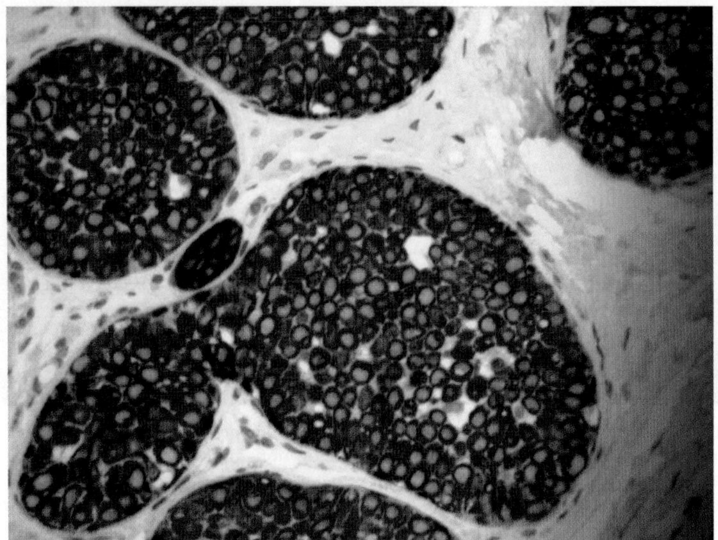

■ **FIGURE 21-18** Ductal carcinoma in situ with double immunohistochemical stains: epithelial component of DCIS is red (cytokeratin 7 [CK 7]) stained and myoepithelial cells are brown (smooth-muscle myosin heavy-chain [SMMHC]) stained. Myoepithelial cells surround the entire ductal proliferation (×200).

There are also special types of DCIS, such as apocrine, neuroendocrine, hypersecretory, or clear cell. Intracystic papillary carcinoma and solid-papillary DCIS are special variants of DCIS as well (see Chapter 22 under Specialized Carcinoma). Most DCIS shows a mixture of architectural patterns. Most commonly, mixed patterns are solid, micropapillary, and cribriform types within the same breast. In fact, it is rather unusual to see a pure population of one architectural type of DCIS. The architectural pattern of DCIS is least important in terms of biological prognostic value. For this reason, some pathologists may not report it. One important aspect of the architectural pattern occurs in micropapillary DCIS, which is reported to have a frequent multifocal and diffuse involvement of the breast tissue.[16]

Although microscopic variants of architectural and cytologic pattern may not correlate well with biological prognosis, the morphologic features are readily identifiable and should be recorded in the pathology report.

Comedo-type DCIS has central coagulative necrosis and high-grade nuclear pleomorphism with often loosely cohesive cells. COL is also commonly seen with comedo-type DCIS (Figs 21-19 and 21-20). Mitotic figures are easily seen. Comedo necrosis is characterized by having pyknosis (nuclear shrinkage), karyorrhectic debris

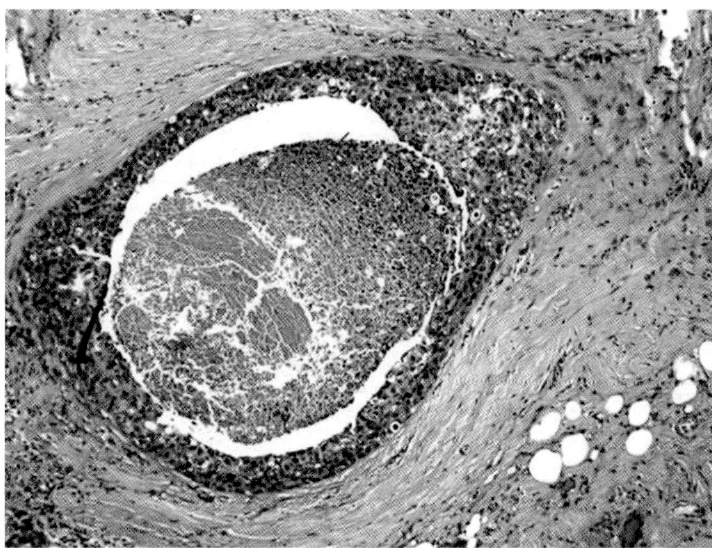

■ **FIGURE 21-19** Ductal carcinoma in situ comedo type showing central necrosis with high nuclear grade (H&E, ×200).

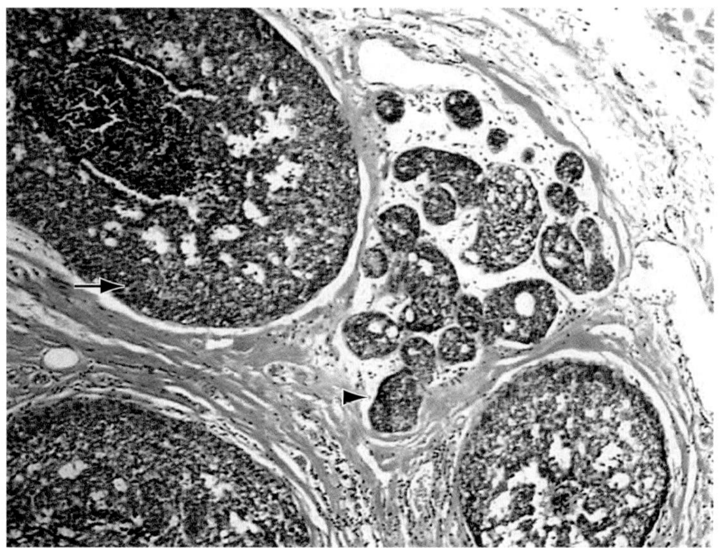

■ **FIGURE 21-20** Ductal carcinoma in situ (*arrow*) and cancerization of lobules (COL; *arrowhead*). Malignant epithelial cells are seen within the terminal ductal lobular unit and expanding acini (H&E, ×100).

(nuclear fragmentation), and apoptosis (programmed cell death). The necrotic center often has calcium phosphate microcalcifications. Comedo necrosis can be seen focally or diffusely involving DCIS. Proteinaceous luminal secretion, apoptotic cells, and foamy histiocytes are insufficient to be regarded as comedo necrosis. Comedo-type DCIS is defined by having comedo tumor necrosis and high nuclear grade. Hence, comedo-type DCIS can be seen regardless of the architectural pattern, whether the DICS is micropapillary or solid as long as the high nuclear grade and central necrosis are present. Central comedo necrosis with intermediate- or low-grade nuclear grade is not considered comedo-type DCIS. Periductal fibrosis, desmoplasia, and the presence of lymphoplasmacytic infiltrates are commonly seen with comedo-type DCIS. At times the periductal fibrosis with stromal desmoplasia is prominent, mimicking invasive carcinoma, and areas of microinvasive carcinoma can be seen more frequently with this type of DCIS.

Cribriform-type DCIS is characterized by having round, rigid secondary lumens with sieve-like arrangement. Nuclei of the epithelial cells are polarized toward the basement membrane with a luminal area formed by cytoplasm (Fig. 21-21). Microcalcifications are not commonly seen with low-grade cribriform-type DCIS. When present, calcifications are found within the lumen. The differential diagnosis of cribriform DCIS includes invasive cribriform carcinoma, adenoid cystic carcinoma, and a benign entity known as *collagenous spherulosis* (CP) (Figs 21-22 and 21-23). CP is rare and usually an incidental finding on excisional biopsy. Microcalcifications may be seen with CP. CP is characterized by having hyperplastic and not

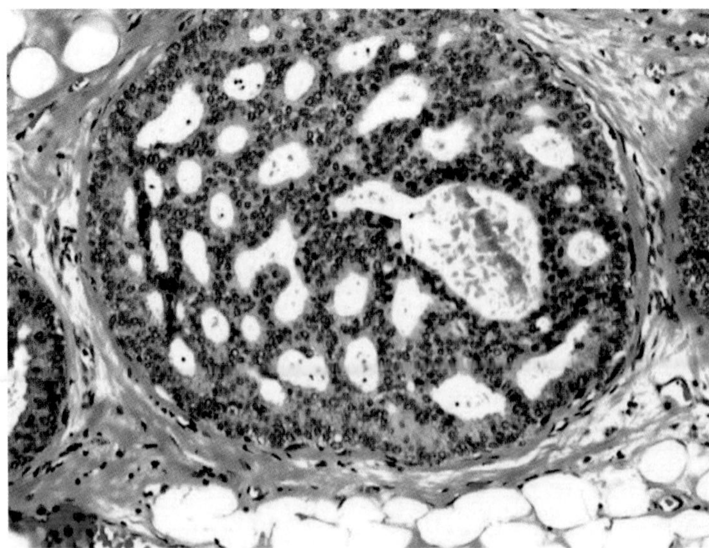

■ **FIGURE 21-21** Ductal carcinoma in situ cribriform type with punched-out round to oval lumens filling the entire ductal structure (H&E, ×200).

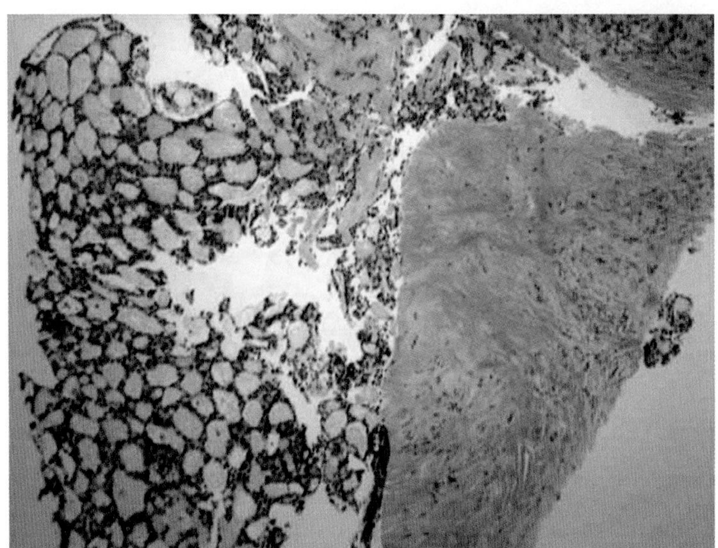

■ **FIGURE 21-22** Adenoid cystic carcinoma on core biopsy. Invasive tumor with conspicuous hyaline, cylindromatous, basement membrane material in glandular proliferation (H&E, ×100).

neoplastic glandular proliferation with a rigid lumen that resembles a cribriform pattern. The lumens are filled by spherule-shaped ground substance and basement membrane materials forming stellate fibrils radiating from a central nidus toward the periphery of the spherule. Spherules are often positive for periodic acid-Schiff and other basement membrane stains, including type IV collagen and laminin. Lobular carcinoma in situ (LCIS) can occur with CP. Cribriform DCIS can be distinguished from CP because spherules of CP are outlined by myoepithelial cells whereas DCIS cells are not. The presence of myoepithelial cells encircling lumen can be verified by immunohistochemical stains.

Micropapillary DCIS is characterized by having uniform population of cells forming occasional epithelial tufts projecting into the lumen without fibrovascular cores. The papillae are variable in sizes and shapes; some are long and slender and others are short, forming bumps or mounds. The similar lesions supported by fibrovascular cores are papillary DCIS (Figs 21-24 and 21-25).

Solid-type DCIS is characterized by having uniform sheets of epithelial cells filling most or all of the duct space (Fig. 21-26).

Apocrine-type DCIS is characterized by having abundant granular, eosinophilic cytoplasm with round nuclei with prominent central nucleoli. Apical cytoplasmic protrusion into the lumen can be seen but at times is absent (Fig. 21-27). Apocrine DCIS is often designated as having moderate to severe nuclear pleomorphism and is often estrogen receptor (ER), progesterone receptor (PR), and HER-2/neu (human epidermal growth factor receptor 2) negative. Androgen receptor has been reported to be positive with apocrine-type DCIS and carcinoma cells.

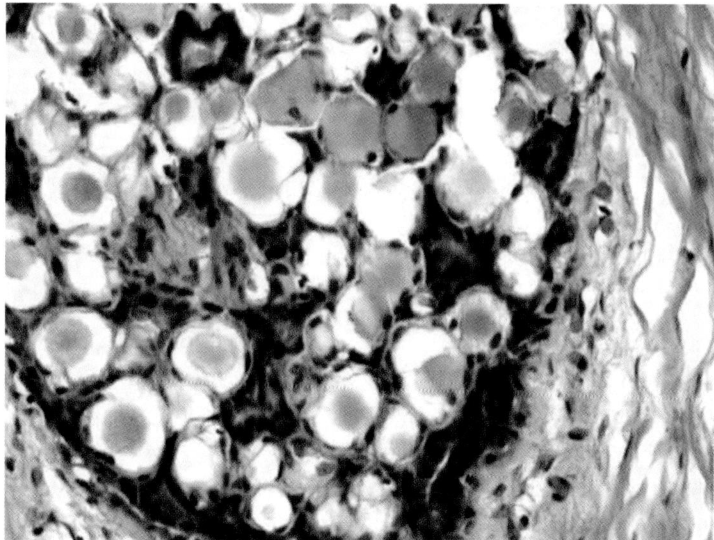

■ **FIGURE 21-23** Collagenous spherulosis (CP) mimicking cribriform ductal carcinoma in situ. Hyperplastic glandular proliferation with lumens filled with spherule-shaped ground substance and basement membrane materials forming stellate fibrils. CP is an incidental finding (H&E, ×400).

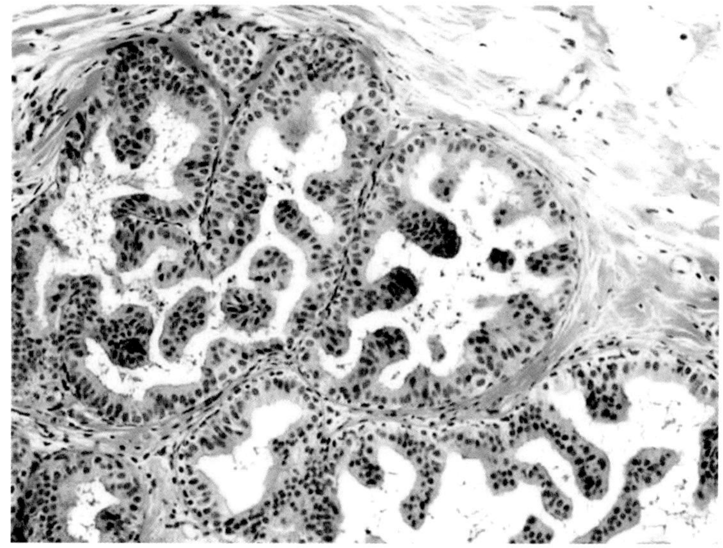

■ **FIGURE 21-24** Ductal carcinoma in situ micropapillary type showing long papillary fronds projection into the lumen duct without fibrovascular cores within the fronds (H&E, ×100).

Clinging-type DCIS is characterized by having a single or several flat layers of highly atypical cells around the ductal profile with empty lumens (Fig. 21-28).

Clear cell intraductal carcinoma is a rare variant of DCIS with cytoplasm showing abundant and clear appearance. Cytoplasmic membranes are often distinct (Fig. 21-29).

Spindle cell intraductal carcinoma is characterized by having proliferation of spindle cells in a mostly solid pattern. Nuclei are spindle shaped with scant cytoplasm that has ill-defined cytoplasmic borders (Fig. 21-30).

Other rare variants: There are other rare variants of DCIS, such as secretory type, cystic hypersecretory type (Fig 21-31), mucinous type (Fig. 21-32), and neuroendocrine type.The dimorphic variant of DCIS consists of two distinctly different populations of cells and is often seen in association with papillary carcinoma.

Ductal Carcinoma in Situ Mimicking Invasive Carcinoma

DCIS can be seen in association with sclerosing adenosis, radial scar, adenosis, and within fibroadenoma. When DCIS is seen with sclerosing adenosis, the lesion can be palpable and visible with imaging studies. These lesions may mimic invasive carcinoma microscopically and can be extremely challenging. Immunohistochemical (IHC) stains can be useful to distinguish between invasive carcinoma and DCIS involving sclerosing adenosis (Figs 21-33 to 21-35). A newly described entity of DCIS is a basal-like phenotype based on DNA microarray profiling studies. These studies have resulted in the identification and classification of breast cancers based on gene expression signatures and clinical outcome. Basal-like DCIS is

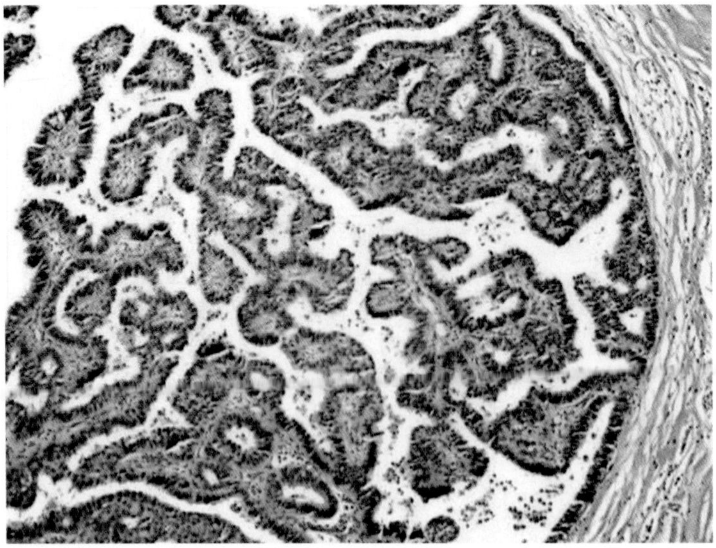

■ **FIGURE 21-25** Ductal carcinoma in situ papillary type showing papillary fronds with fibrovascular cores within each projection (H&E, ×100).

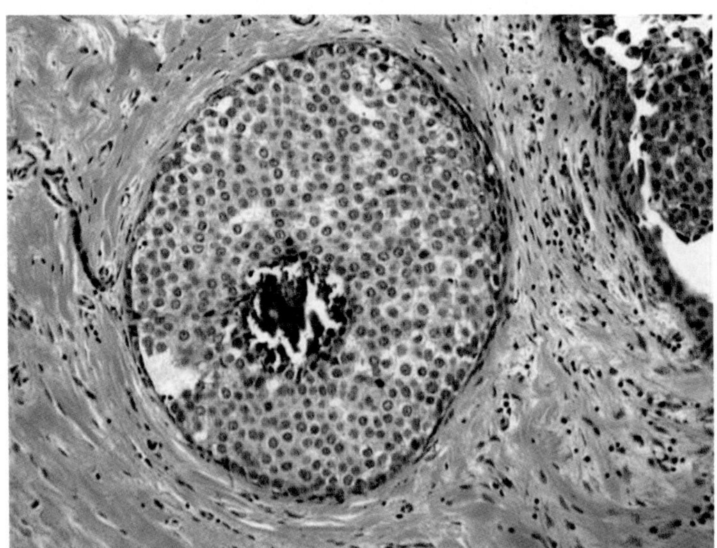

■ **FIGURE 21-26** Ductal carcinoma in situ solid type showing monotonous population of epithelial cells filling the entire duct with central microcalcification (H&E, ×200).

typically ER, PR, and HER-2/neu negative (triple-negative) and shows some characteristics of breast myoepithelial cell origin with a high proliferation index. Basal-like DCIS and invasive carcinoma have been described as the prevalent types in *BRCA1 (breast cancer 1, early onset gene)*-related breast carcinoma and are known to have a poor prognosis.[17]

PAGET'S DISEASE OF THE NIPPLE

In 1874, Sir James Paget's described the findings of nipple and areolar eruption. Grossly, Paget's disease has the appearance of eczema, with scaly inflamed areas involving the nipple and areola. A wedge biopsy of nipple can successfully establish the diagnosis of Paget's disease because the epidermis is adequately represented and lactiferous ducts can also be seen. Punch biopsy is also acceptable, although it usually does not contain a large area of epidermis. A superficial "shaved" biopsy is usually inadequate to diagnose Paget's disease because it does not contain a dermal-epidermal junctional area. Microscopically, Paget's disease is characterized by adenocarcinoma cells within the epidermis in single cells or in clusters in the basal portion of the epidermis (Figs 21-36 and 21-37). Nuclei tend to be large and have prominent nucleoli, as seen in adenocarcinoma cells. The cytoplasm is abundant, is clear to pale with vacuoles, and may contain mucin secretion. The superficial dermis is usually seen with a moderate amount of lymphohistiocytic infiltrates. An ulcerated epidermal surface can be seen with Paget's disease, which may further hinder the diagnosis due to a lack of sufficient epidermis to examine and the associated obscuring granulation tissue beneath. Immunohistochemical stains that

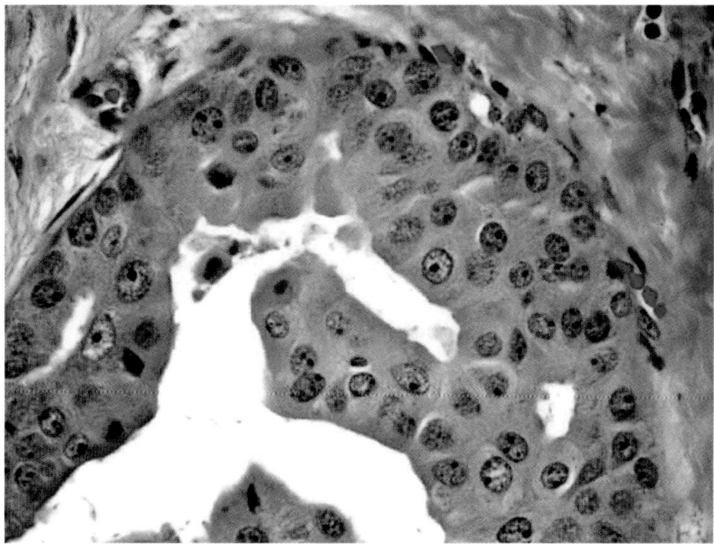

■ **FIGURE 21-27** Ductal carcinoma in situ apocrine type. Nuclei are located at the center with prominent nucleoli, and cytoplasm is abundant, eosinophilic, and granular (H&E, ×400).

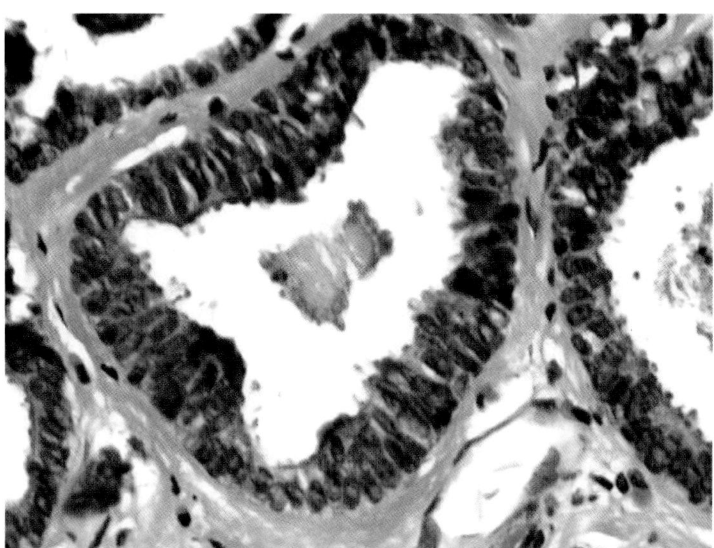

■ **FIGURE 21-28** Ductal carcinoma in situ clinging or flat type. Flat refers to the devoid of pattern such as papillae or cribriform. Nuclear are highly atypical and pseudostratified. Flat epithelial atypia (FEA) is a differential diagnosis, but FEA should have low nuclear grade (H&E, ×400).

are helpful for Paget's disease are cytokeratin 7 (CK 7), polyclonal carcino embryonic antigen (pCEA), and epithelial membrane antigen (EMA). ER is positive only in 50% because the underlying adenocarcinoma tends to be poorly differentiated. HER-2/neu may be positive, and mucicarmine is usually positive, for Paget's disease.

An associated carcinoma, either DCIS or invasive ductal carcinoma in the breast or nipple, has been reported to occur in more than 95% when Paget's disease is present in the nipple. The presence of Paget's cells in the epidermis within a biopsy specimen that contains a benign florid papillomatosis/nipple adenoma is indicative of underlying adenocarcinoma of breast; therefore, appropriate further study is necessary. LCIS cells can spread upward (pagetoid spread) into large lactiferous ducts of the nipple; however, it is rare to see Paget's disease near LCIS. The differential diagnosis of Paget's disease includes melanoma in situ, bowenoid squamous cell carcinoma in situ, florid papillomatosis/nipple adenoma, syringomatous adenoma, clear cell changes in epidermis, and Toker cell hyperplasia. Malignant melanoma is usually positive for S-100, HMB-45, Mart-1, and tyrosinase, whereas Paget's disease is usually negative for all these markers. Bowen disease (squamous cell carcinoma) is usually positive for cytokeratin 34bE13 (CK 903) but negative for CK 7, pCEA, EMA, and ER. Toker cell hyperplasia is a subset of benign clear cells found in the nipple epidermis either singly or in small groups. These cells are also positive with CK 7, as in

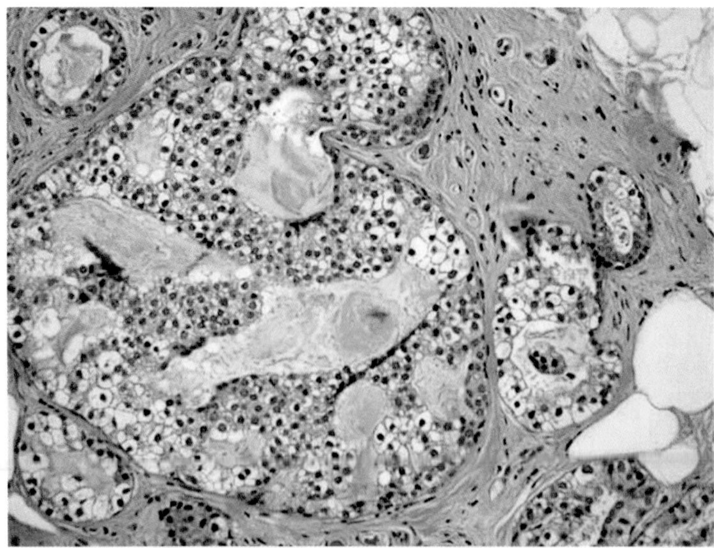

■ **FIGURE 21-29** Ductal carcinoma in situ clear cell type. Cytoplasm is clear and vacuolated and shows well-defined cell borders (H&E, ×200).

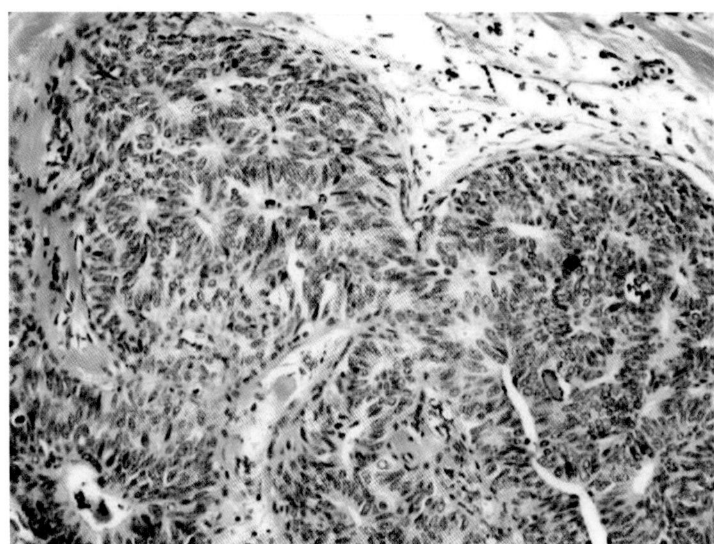

■ **FIGURE 21-30** Ductal carcinoma in situ spindle cell type. The carcinoma cells have spindle-shaped nuclei with a hint of palisading, and rosette-like microlumens are seen (H&E, ×200).

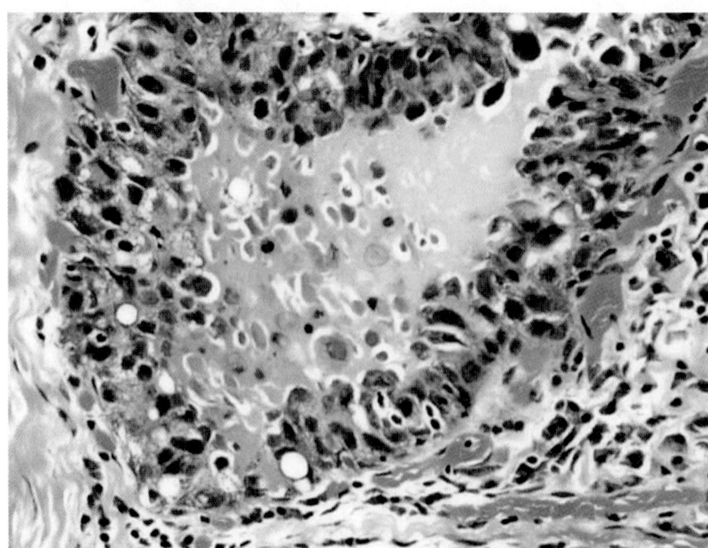

■ **FIGURE 21-31** Ductal carcinoma in situ cystic hypersecretory type. Note flat to focal micropapillary proliferation with significant nuclear atypia. Secretion within cytoplasm with apical cytoplasmic bleb is filling the luminal contents (H&E, ×400).

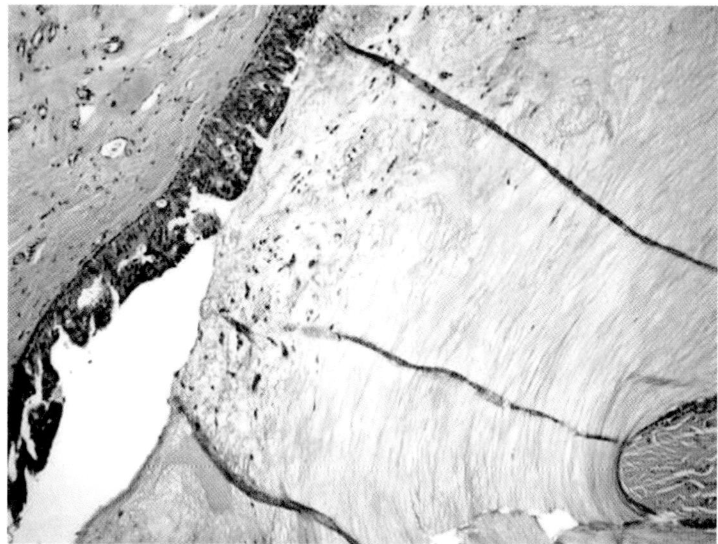

■ **FIGURE 21-32** Ductal carcinoma in situ mucinous type. Luminal area shows mucin lined by atypical ductal proliferation. Without the atypical lining cells, the entity would be called a mucocele-like lesion (H&E, ×400).

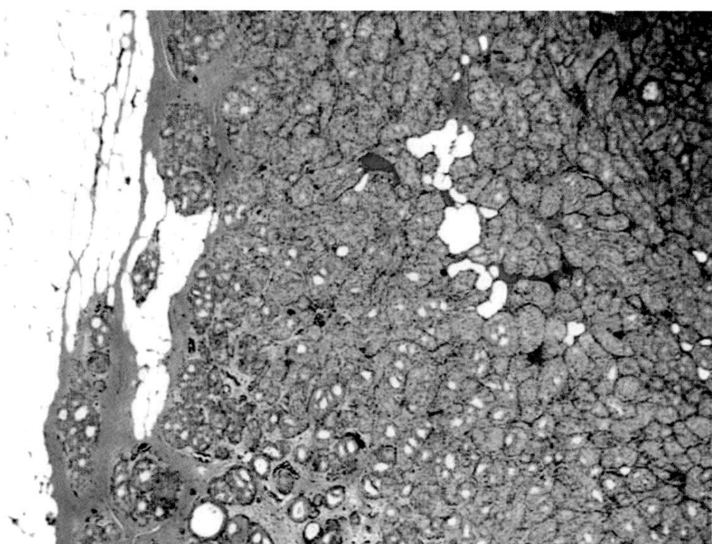

■ **FIGURE 21-33** Ductal carcinoma in situ involving sclerosing adenosis mimicking invasive ductal carcinoma (H&E, ×40).

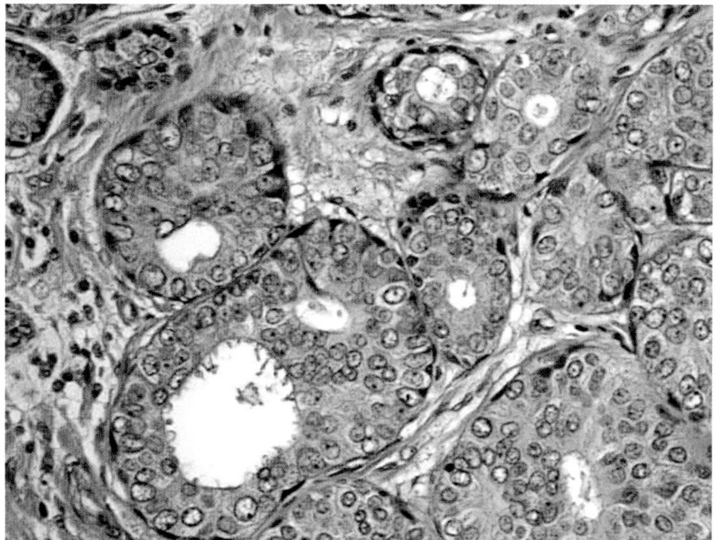

■ **FIGURE 21-34** Ductal carcinoma in situ involving sclerosing adenosis. In high power view, the presence of myoepithelial cells is visible (H&E, ×400).

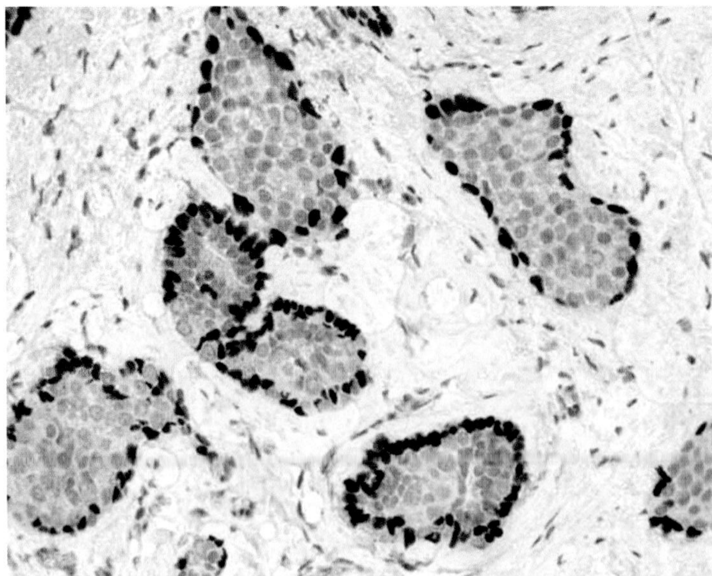

■ **FIGURE 21-35** Ductal carcinoma in situ arising in sclerosing adenosis. The nuclei of myoepithelial cells are highlighted surrounding each glandular proliferation associated with sclerosing adenosis (P63 immunohistochemical stain, ×100).

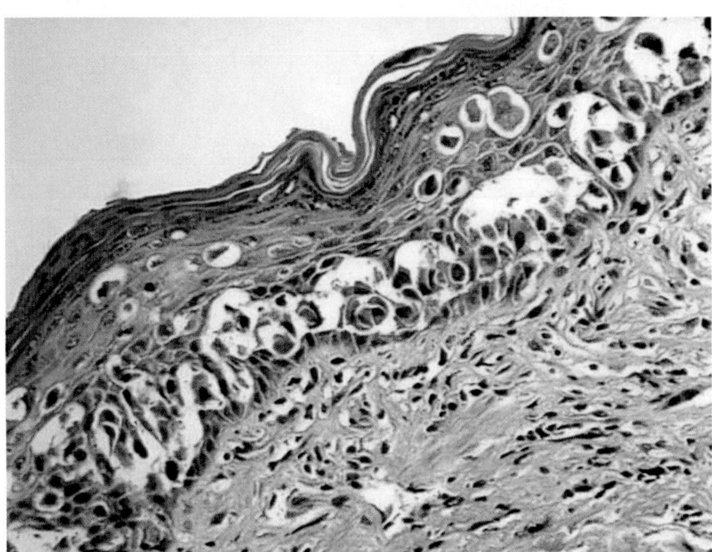

■ **FIGURE 21-36** Paget's disease. Carcinoma cells forming bands and clusters in the base of the epidermis and upward spread into superficial dermis. The tumor cells show abundant pale cytoplasm and pleomorphic nuclei (H&E, ×200).

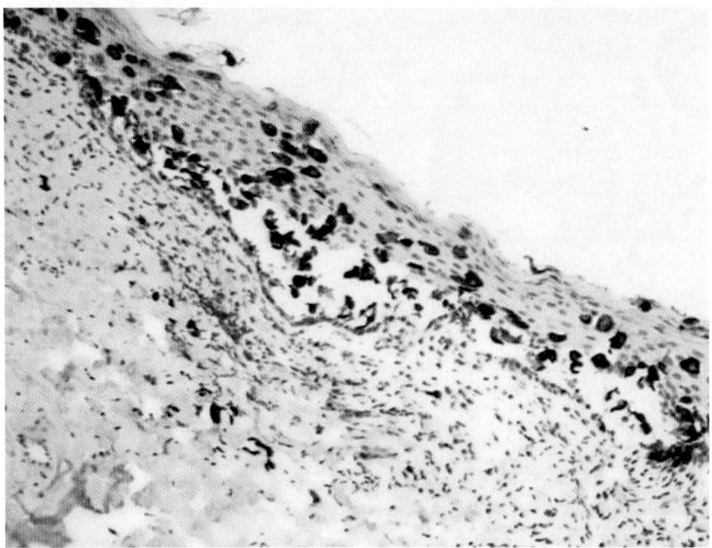

■ **FIGURE 21-37** Paget's disease highlighting the Paget's cells. Cytokeratin 7 stain positivity excludes melanoma cells (CK 7 IHC stain, ×200).

Paget's disease, but other immunohistochemical markers should be negative, such as pCEA, ER, and HER2/neu. Toker cells are negative for mucicarmine.

NIPPLE ADENOMA/FLORID PAPILLOMATOSIS OF THE NIPPLE

Nipple adenoma is also referred to as erosive adenoma, erosive adenomatosis, papillary adenoma, florid papillomatosis, and nipple duct adenoma. Nipple discharge or bleeding is the most common symptom, followed by enlargement and induration of the nipple associated with ulceration. Clinically, Paget's disease is the most common differential diagnosis. Microscopically, cystic and solid areas of an expanded lactiferous duct with epithelial proliferation are seen under the nipple epidermis (Figs 21-38 and 21-39). Ulceration can be seen when the nipple adenoma erodes into the surface. Epithelial hyperplasia is seen mostly in tubule, papillary, and sclerotic patterns with apocrine and squamous metaplasia. Myoepithelial cells are present within and surrounding the ductal hyperplasia. Malignant transformation of a nipple adenoma and coexistence of carcinoma with a nipple adenoma have been reported to occur but are rare. Complete excision with a narrow rim of normal breast tissue is recommended for nipple adenoma, which often requires removal of the nipple. Local recurrences of nipple adenoma may occur after subtotal excision.

DUCTAL CARCINOMA IN SITU NUCLEAR GRADE

Nuclear grade is separated into low, intermediate, and high based on the classification of Lagios (Table 21-1).[18] The size, variation and shape of nuclei, presence or absence of nucleoli, and mitotic activities are the determining factors.

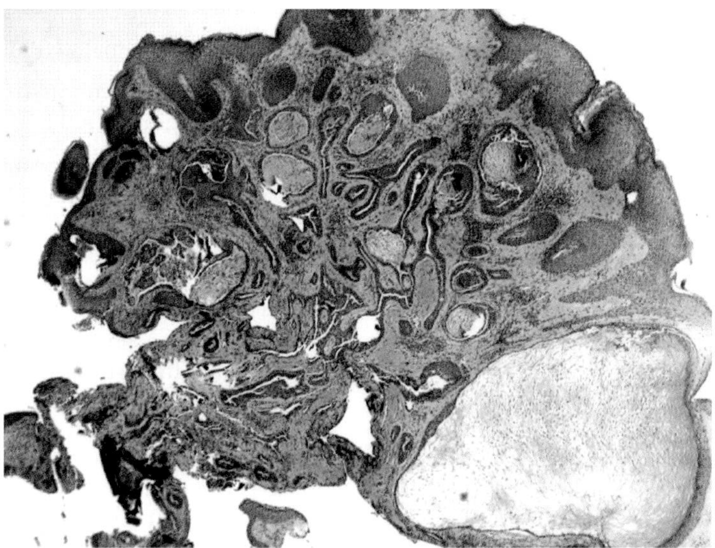

■ **FIGURE 21-38** Nipple adenoma. Low-power view showing florid ductal proliferation with areas of central necrosis under the epidermis with cyst formation (H&E, ×40).

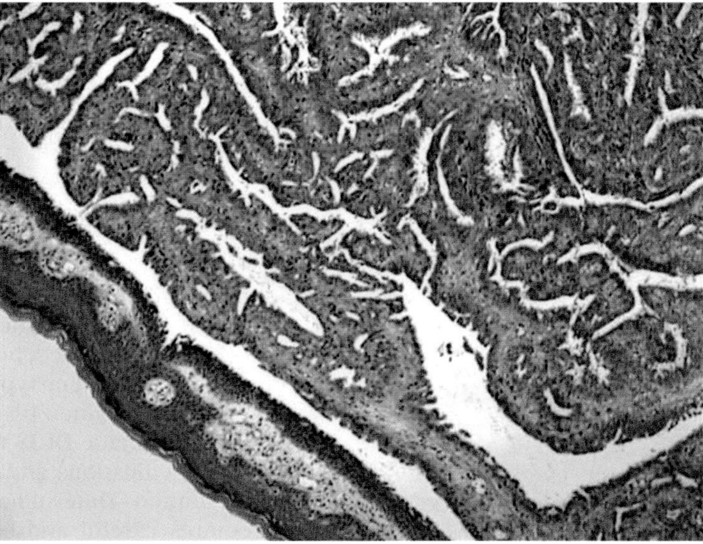

■ **FIGURE 21-39** Nipple adenoma with papillary pattern with florid epithelial hyperplasia and myoepithelial cells (H&E, ×200).

TABLE 21-1. Summary of Nuclear Grade According to Lagios

Criteria	Low Grade	Intermediate Grade	High Grade
Nuclear diameter*	1.0-1.5	1.5-2.0	>2.0
Nuclear diameter (mm)	10-12	13-16	>16
Nuclear variation in size and shape	Mild	Moderate	Marked
Chromatin	Fine, even	Coarse, even	Coarse, uneven
Nucleoli	Rare to absent, small, indistinct	Some, small	Large, many
Mitotic activity	Low	Intermediate	High

*Compared with diameter of a red blood cell.

TABLE 21-2. Modified Lagios Classification System

Architecture	Nuclear Grade	Necrosis	Final Grade
Comedo	High	Extensive	High
Noncomedo*	Intermediate	Focal/absent	Intermediate
Noncomedo†	Low	Absent	Low

* Often a mixture of noncomedo patterns.
† Solid, cribriform, papillary, or focal micropapillary ductal carcinoma in situ.
From Mack L, Kerkvliet N, Doig G, O'Malley FP. Relationship of a new histological categorization of ductal carcinoma in situ of the breast with size and the immunohistochemical expression of p53, c-erb B2, bcl-2, and ki-67. *Hum Pathol* 1997;**28**:97479.

The final DCIS grade is based on the modified Lagios classification (Table 21-2). Low-grade DCIS has nuclei that are small with a regular, uniform appearance and without a variation in shapes and sizes that have inconspicuous nucleoli and are often without comedo necrosis. Intermediate-grade DCIS has nuclei that are moderately increased in sizes and of variable shapes with or without focal comedo necrosis. High-grade DCIS has nuclei that are markedly variable in sizes and shapes with vesiculated open nuclear chromatin, prominent nucleoli, and irregular nuclear membrane, often with comedo necrosis. Within the same specimen, it is not unusual to find a mixed nuclear grade (low and intermediate, intermediate to high grade) in DCIS. Assigning the nuclear grade can be challenging at times; however, it is prudent to report a higher nuclear grade when reporting the final DCIS grade.

The Van Nuys Prognostic Index (VNPI) on Ductal Carcinoma in Situ

The Van-Nuys system also uses three grading methods that correspond to a prognostic index based on three factors: nuclear grade, size of DCIS, and the margin status. These three prognostic factors are important in breast conservational therapy for DCIS. The Van Nuys Prognostic Index (VNPI) was developed to aid in the complex selection process for choice of treatment. Based on the total VNPI scores, the treatment modality between lumpectomy only, lumpectomy plus irradiation, or mastectomy is determined.

Nuclear grade is based on the modified Bloom and Richardson score: low grade, 1; intermediate grade, 2; and high grade, 3. The largest maximum dimension of DCIS is measured and scored as follows:

DCIS size $\leq$ 1.5 cm = 1 point
DCIS size from 1.6 to 4.0 cm = 2 points
DCIS size of $\geq$ 4.1 cm = 3 points

The margins status with DCIS is measured microscopically on the slides:

DCIS measuring $\geq$ 1.0 cm to the margin = 1 point
DCIS measuring 0.1 to 0.9 cm to the margin = 2 points
DCIS measuring < 0.1 cm = 3 points

The combined final VNPI is calculated as the follows:

VNPI SCORE = tumor-size pts $\times$ 0.749 + nuclear pts $\times$ 0.869 + margin pts $\times$ 0.864

The new University of Southern California (USC)/VNPI combines four significant predictors of local recurrence[19]: overall tumor size (largest single-direction size measure), closest clear surgical margin width (thinnest width), pathologic nuclear grade classification, and patient age. Scores of 1 (best) to 3 (worst) are assigned for each of the four predictor parameters and then totaled to give an overall VNPI score ranging from 4 to 12. Based on VNPI score, the recurrence rate and 8-year disease-free survival rate were studied. VNPI score is usually not provided by pathologists; however, all information necessary to calculate this score should be available from pathology reports on all DCIS cases, which include type of DCIS, grade of DCIS, presence or absence of comedo necrosis, extent/size of DCIS, status of the margin specifying distance from margin to DCIS, and presence of microcalcifications. Because a substantial number of DCIS biopsies or excisions, or both, are performed after detection of microcalcifications on mammography, it is essential that the pathologist document the presence of microcalcifications with associated disease, such as benign ducts, DCIS, or invasive carcinoma. Correlation of pattern and quantity of microcalcifications between mammographic and pathologic findings is important.

Size of Ductal Carcinoma in Situ: Extent of Disease

DCIS is expected to be involved in a segmental distribution radially, which may involve one or multiple quadrants based on the anatomy of the ductal system. Holland and colleagues[20] demonstrated, however, different distribution patterns among different types of DCIS: high-grade DCIS was more closely defined by mammographic microcalcifications, and low-grade DCIS was more likely unassociated with microcalcifications and often exhibited a discontinuous distribution. Determination of an accurate size of DCIS requires careful and sequential method of pathologic processing of the whole specimen. Representative sections or nonsequential sections of pathologic sampling will not only limit estimating the extent of the DCIS but also compromise the margin status on breast conservation specimens. Even for mastectomy it is important to have a sequential method of pathologic sampling because one cannot submit the entire specimen (see Chapter 31, Specimen Processing)

Margin Assessment

Complete excision of DCIS is the ultimate goal of surgical treatment. Breast conservation therapy is an acceptable treatment modality for DCIS unless there is multicentric or multifocal disease. The three-dimensional structure of each duct system originating from a major lactiferous duct is complex and may cross into the different quadrants of the breast. There is no proof that each segment is encased in a fibrous or facial capsule. It is important not to sample representative section of the margins on a breast conservation specimen. Sampling of the margin may be sufficient in invasive carcinoma where tumor is quiet visible and palpable, but most DCIS is not visible and palpable. A positive margin occurs when DCIS is transected at the inked and often cauterized edge of the breast tissue. A consensus is needed regarding what is an acceptable negative margin. Due to the controversy in definition of negative margins, it is necessary to convey in the pathology report the distance between the edge of DCIS and the closest resection margin in millimeters (e.g., "DCIS is within 1 mm of the inked margin or 5 mm of the inked margin") in all six specimen surfaces (anterior, posterior, lateral, medial, superior, and inferior). Silverstein and coworkers[21] analyzed the residual DCIS in re-excisional biopsies or mastectomy specimens after the initial breast conservation therapy in relationship with margin status and found that the size of the free margin was directly related to local recurrence-free survival rate. A multivariate analysis showed that early age at diagnosis, positive margin status, and high nuclear grade were independently associated with local recurrence.

Multifocality and Multicentricity

The definition of multifocal and multicentric breast disease is not uniform in various studies. Some studies use the terms *multifocal and multicentric* interchangeably. Others use *multicentricity* as two different extents of distribution: as either noncontiguous DCIS (two different quadrants) or as two foci of DCIS separated by 5 cm of uninvolved breast tissue. *Multifocality* is defined as the presence of a *skip* area (gaps) of DCIS or discontinuous growth of DCIS within a single ductal unit. Comedo-type DCIS is frequently seen as unifocal, contiguous, and involving one quadrant, whereas micropapillary DCIS is more often multifocal and multicentric and involving multiple quadrants. Low-grade DCIS lesions are more frequently involved by discontinuous growth and therefore truly multifocal. Multifocal disease within the same quadrant is common, but multicentric disease is uncommon.

Local Recurrence of Ductal Carcinoma in Situ after Breast Conserving Surgery

Breast-conserving surgery after a diagnosis of DCIS is an acceptable and desirable option for most women, potentially leading to a better cosmetic result. An increasing number of women with DCIS have been treated with breast-conserving surgery, with or without irradiation and with or without tamoxifen therapy. The local recurrence rate of DCIS after mastectomy is 1% to 2%, but for breast-conserving surgery ranges from 5% to 40%, depending on a variety of factors, which include, but are not limited to, tumor size, age at presentation, nuclear grade, presence or absence of necrosis, margin status, and hormone receptor status. Approximately 50% of all local recurrences are invasive carcinoma that are potentially life threatening. DCIS lacks stromal invasion and does not have the ability to metastasize, whereas invasive carcinoma expresses the full malignant phenotype—the ability to metastasize. However, much of the prospective and retrospective data have not documented a significant difference in breast cancer-specific survival for patients with DCIS regardless of treatment.

The probability of recurrence is higher in excision-only patients when compared with excision followed by radiation therapy. After radiation therapy, a diagnosis of recurrent disease may be difficult due to the histologic changes of radiation atypia and fibrosis. In particular, the distinction between cancerization of lobules by malignant carcinoma cells versus radiation atypia can be challenging, especially on the small core needle biopsy specimen. Radiation also induces marked fibrosis, atrophy and distortion of lobules and ducts with obscuration of myoepithelial cells. The cells within the ducts and lobules may show loss of polarity, enlarged nuclei with nucleoli, and multivacuolated nuclei and cytoplasm. Features favoring radiation atypia are reduction of lobular size without epithelial proliferations, lack of mitosis, a thickened basement membrane, and interlobular and intralobular fibrosis (Fig. 21-40).

Metastatic Disease to Axillary Lymph Node in Ductal Carcinoma in Situ

DCIS is a preinvasive disease with malignant epithelial cells still contained within the duct surrounded by myoepithelial cells and basement membrane, and as such does not have the capability to metastasize to axillary lymph nodes. Thus, the presence of axillary nodal metastases should not occur. However, this is not the case. In an American College of Surgeons study, the incidence of axillary involvement associated with DCIS was reported from 1% to 4% after using routine hematoxylin and eosin (H&E) stains. When an IHC stain for cytokeratins was used with routine H&E stains, the detection of axillary nodal metastases increased to 12% to 13% in sentinel lymph node biopsy of patients with DCIS without histologic evidence of microinvasion.[22] Lymph node metastasis in patients with DCIS may be explained in several ways. Firstly, small foci of microinvasion can be missed on pathologic examination of the breast specimens even when the entire specimen is submitted for microscopic examination, because each block thickness is 2 to 3 mm and only one slide from the

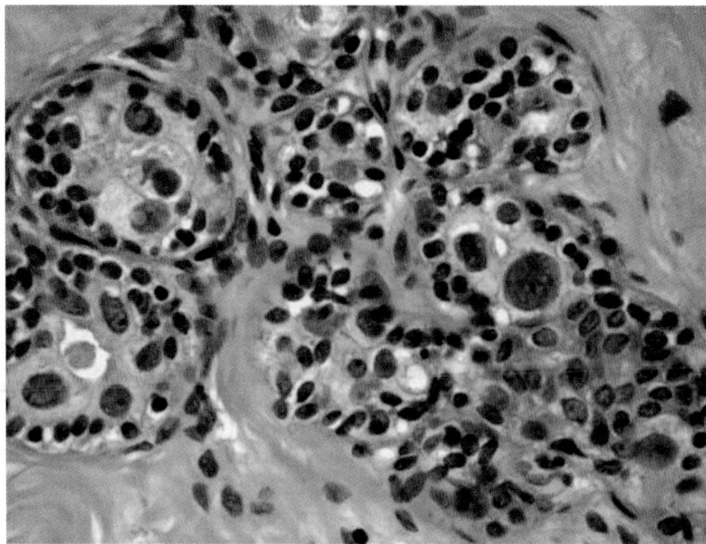

■ **FIGURE 21-40** Radiation atypia mimicking cancerization of lobules. Marked variation of nuclear size and shapes with atypia is noted (H&E, ×400).

block is cut and stained with H&E for pathologic examination. Secondly, not all IHC cytokeratin stain detected cells are metastatic tumor cells. Cytokeratin-positive benign cells in a subcapsular area of lymph node include benign epithelial inclusion, ectopic breast tissue, macrophages, or histiocytic cells with granular keratin debris (Figs 21-41 to 21-44) and passive epithelial transport, so-called displaced epithelial cells. Intracapsular nevus can mimic metastatic carcinoma cells. Benign epithelial inclusion and ectopic breast tissue within the subcapsular area of lymph nodes have a benign epithelial morphologic appearance and myoepithelial cells are present. Metastatic cells do not have myoepithelial cells. Confirmatory IHC stains such as p63 and smooth-muscle myosin heavy-chain (SMMHC) can also be done (Figs 21-45 and 21-46). The concept of displaced epithelial cells is more controversial; some believe that not all cytokeratin positive cells are metastatic carcinoma cells to lymph nodes. Some of these cells may be benign or represent tumor cells that are artificially transported to the node during the sentinel lymph node procedure or after breast biopsy, and never develop into clinically significant tumors. Displaced epithelial cells are commonly associated with hemosiderin-laden or foamy macrophages, foreign body giant cells, and damaged red blood cells, which favor mechanical displacement. They may also display different tumor morphology and IHC stain characteristics.[23] The issue is how to separate what is true metastasis from what is artifactual. Therefore, many authors advocate not doing sentinel lymph node biopsy for DCIS. Others, however, strongly advocate performing sentinel lymph node biopsy, especially when DCIS is of the high-grade comedo type and is extensive as demonstrated on imaging exams (>2.5 cm). Currently, based on American Joint Committee on Cancer (AJCC) 2003 staging of lymph nodes, metastatic lesions not greater than 0.2 mm, whether detected by H&E staining or by IHC

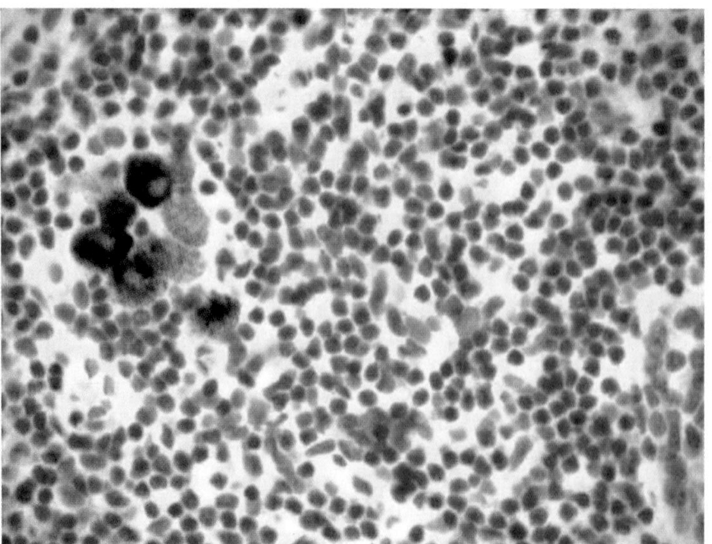

■ **FIGURE 21-41** Sentinel lymph node showing aggregates of histiocytes with dusty and granular stain (cytokeratin stain, ×400).

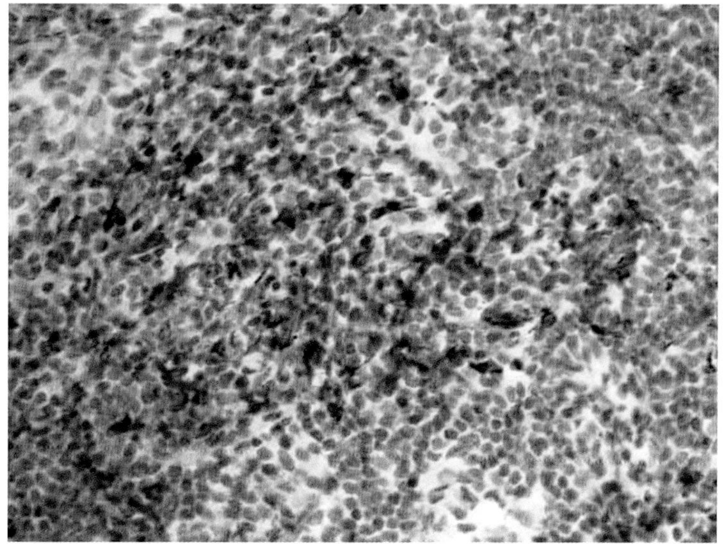

■ **FIGURE 21-42** Sentinel lymph node. Dendritic cells picking up cytokeratin stain (×200).

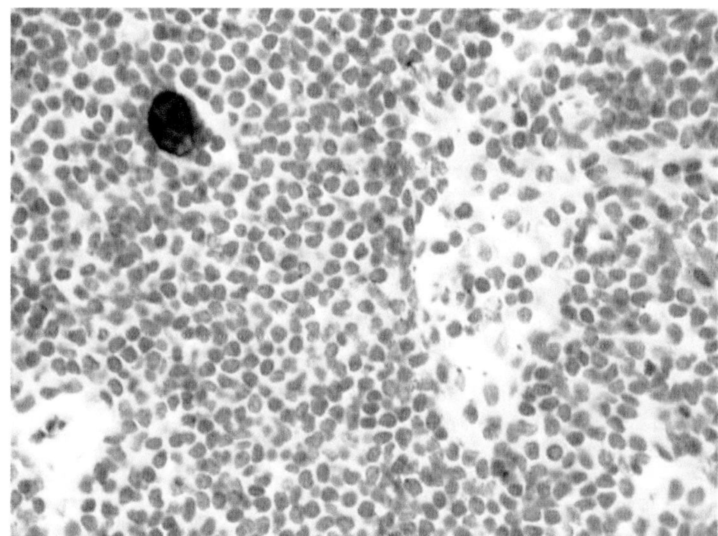

■ **FIGURE 21-43** Sentinel lymph node showing nonspecific debris. The plane of focus is not at the same level as the lymph node (cytokeratin stain, ×400).

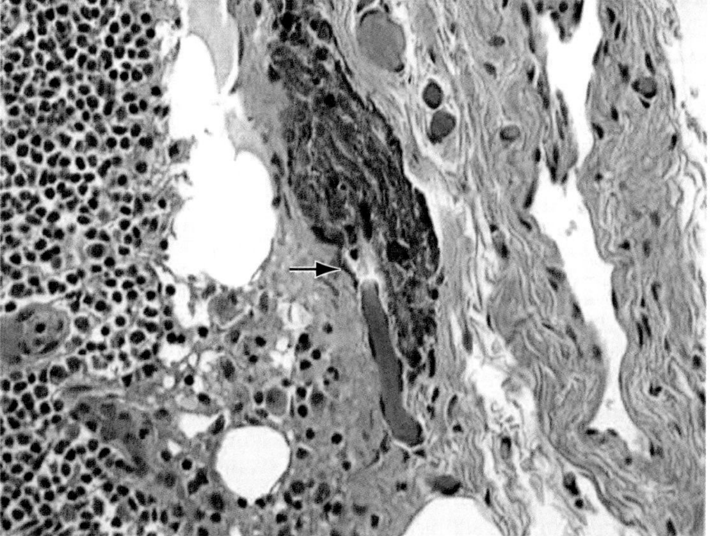

■ **FIGURE 21-44** Lymph node with intracapsular nevus (*arrow*). Melanin pigments are noted within the clusters of benign nevus (H&E, ×200).

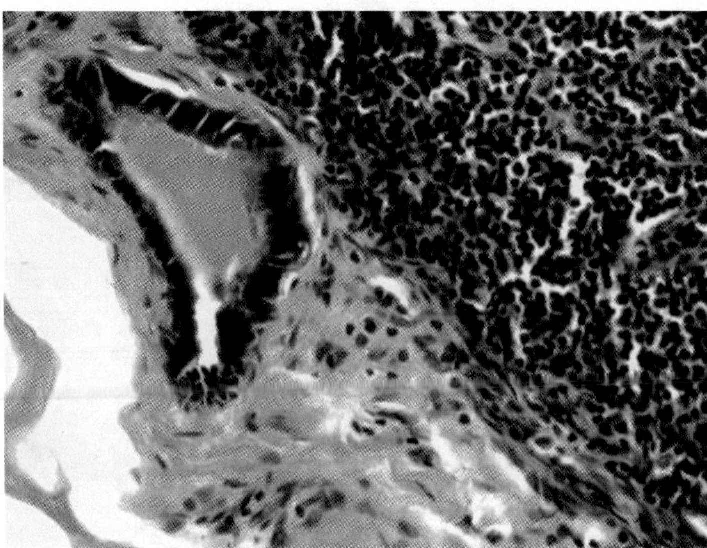

■ **FIGURE 21-45** Benign inclusion in sentinel lymph node. Glandular cells seen within the intracapsular lymph node show no nuclear atypia (H&E, ×400).

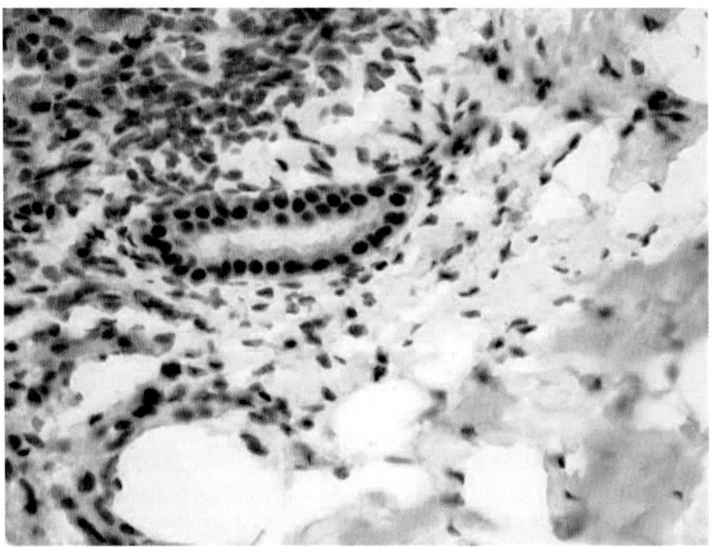

■ **FIGURE 21-46** Benign inclusion in sentinel lymph node. Positive stain with myoepithelial cells around the benign inclusion (P63 stain, ×400).

staining, are classified as isolated tumor cells pN0(i+). A classification of pN0(i-) is used to indicate no detectable tumor cells by either H&E and/or IHC staining methods. *Micrometastases* are defined as tumor deposits greater than 0.2 mm but not greater than 2.0 mm in largest dimension and are classified as pN1mi.

Metastatic lesions identified only through the use of real time reverse transcript polymerase chain reaction (RT-PCR) are currently classified as pN0 (mol), because there are as yet insufficient data to determine whether such lesions are clinically significant. In cases where there are multiple metastatic lesions in a lymph node and deeper cuts of the node do not show a junction between two or more foci, classification is made according to the size of the largest lesion. It is not clear whether isolated tumor cells or micrometastatic tumors detected by H&E stains or IHC stains are clinically significant. The College of American Pathologists (CAP) does not support routinely performing IHC stains on sentinel lymph nodes due to a lack of data on what to do with the information. However, many institutions perform IHC stains routinely on sentinel lymph nodes. Further studies with thorough long-term clinicopathologic correlative and follow-up evaluation are needed to determine several questions:

1. What characteristics define a positive sentinel lymph node?
2. When is it appropriate to do full axillary dissection after sentinel lymph node?
3. What is clinically relevant metastatic disease to lymph node?
4. What should be the standard of care in terms of how to process the sentinel lymph node—whether to do IHC for cytokeratins routinely or not and how many sections to cut and examine with H&E stains on sentinel lymph nodes?

It is possible that our ability to detect metastatic disease has exceeded our understanding of its clinical relevance at this point. The American College of Surgeons Oncology group (ACSOG) Z0010 study and NSABP B-32 trials are under way to evaluate the significant of IHC-detected metastases in patients with early invasive breast cancer. If IHC stains detect significant metastases in these early breast cancers, perhaps this data can be extrapolated to DCIS. Until the results from the ACSOG Z0010 and NSABP B-32 studies are established, the clinical significance and indication for the full axillary lymph node dissection is not known with IHC-detected tumor on sentinel lymph node(s).

Ductal Carcinoma in Situ Diagnosis Reproducibility

The reproducibility of diagnosing low grade DCIS versus atypical ductal hyperplasia among pathologists is known to be poor, although the criteria for DCIS are widely accepted. There are at least two reports on this discrepancy rate among breast pathologists. The first was reported by Rosai[24] in which he selected five pathologists and sent the same 17 slides with a small circle to ensure that each pathologist examined the same ducts/lobules with diagnostic choices of included ductal hyperplasia of usual type, ADH, and DCIS. There was disagreement among the pathologists on all cases and, in fact, 35% of the cases had diagnoses varying from usual ductal hyperplasia to ADH to DCIS. The second study was performed by Schnitt et al[25] in which 24 tissue slides of ductal proliferations with a visible single small area were examined by six pathologists specializing in breast disease but this time narrative and diagrammatic information and criteria by Page and colleagues were given. In this study, there was 58% agreement on the 24 cases. Five of six pathologists agreed in 71%, and four of six pathologists agreed in 92%. Most of the discrepancies were between ADH and DCIS. The cases sent by Schnitt and coworkers were intentionally difficult and ambiguous cases and not classic or routine specimens. The distinction between advanced ADH and low-grade DCIS can be difficult because their features overlap. The effort to clarify the criteria by giving strict quantitative or qualitative measures may enhance reproducibility for some and confuse others. There are other factors such as cauterized artifact of ductal proliferation at the surgical margin (Fig. 21-47) that may inhibit the diagnosis further. The management of DCIS at the margin usually leads to re-excision, whereas ADH at the margin requires no further surgery. The distinction between these two different lesions leads to drastically different management.

It is inevitable that numerous factors will lead to differences in opinion among pathologists. For this reason, there is a tradition of seeking a second opinion from expert breast pathologists by community-based pathologists, albeit expert breast pathologists may also not agree with each other. Although there appears to be lack of reproducibility among pathologists, DCIS seen in everyday practice has a classic appearance and is easily recognizable and should lead to an accurate diagnosis and appropriate management.

Ductal Carcinoma in Situ Biological Factors

All breast cancers are thought to arise from stem cells in normal terminal ductal lobular units (TDLUs). ERs and PRs play an important role in regulating the growth, differentiation, and proliferation of normal breast epithelium. Many studies have demonstrated that normal breast epithelium, DCIS, and invasive carcinoma cells express ER and PR. Usually, PR expression parallels ER expression. Approximately 75% of DCIS express ER, depending on histologic differentiation; ER is most positive in low-grade and well-differentiated DCIS. Only 25% of high-grade DCIS is known to express ER. Commonly, high-grade DCIS such as comedo type of DCIS and basal-like DCIS lack both ER and PR expression. There is a reduced incidence of both contralateral and ipsilateral DCIS in patients who received both tamoxifen and breast-conserving surgery. The NSABP B-24 trial of lumpectomy and radiation therapy for DCIS with patients randomized to receive or not receive tamoxifen

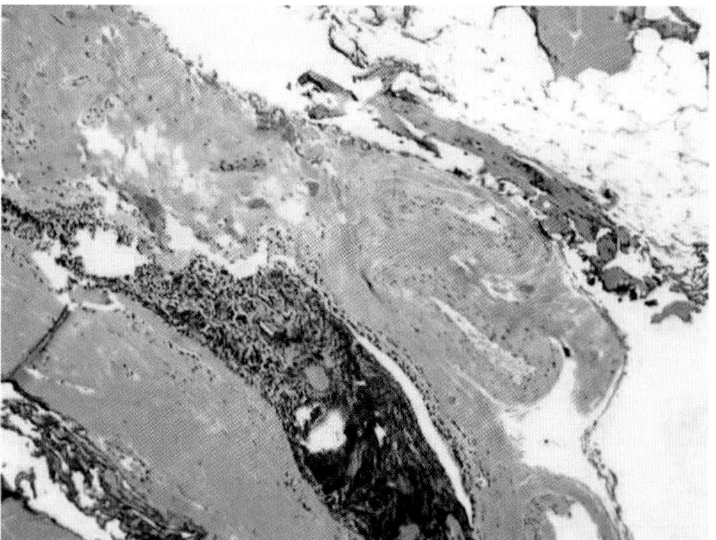

■ **FIGURE 21-47** Ductal proliferation with severe crushed cauterized artifact at the margin of the resection. Due to thermal injury, ductal cells are stretched and burned, precluding an accurate interpretation (H&E, ×200).

demonstrated 37% fewer breast cancer events for the tamoxifen-treated arm of the study with a median follow-up of 74 months.[26] A subsequent analysis of ER status for DCIS in a subset of patients in this study showed that the reduction in breast cancers was greatest for women with ER-positive DCIS who were treated with tamoxifen. There was no significant benefit with tamoxifen in women with ER-negative DCIS. However the small number of these events precluded determination of significance in this population. The Update Committee of the American Society of Clinical Oncology concluded that current data are insufficient to make a general recommendation for the use of ER status of DCIS to make decisions about tamoxifen treatment. Nonetheless, individual clinicians may find this information helpful for advising patients about hormonal treatment. For this reason, some of the oncologists are asking pathologists to study ER and PR status in DCIS cases. Ongoing studies are evaluating whether these biomarkers will be helpful in determining the best treatment for DCIS. Because ER, PR, and HER-2/neu status in DCIS is used for investigational protocols and not for diagnosis, determination of ER, PR, and HER-2/neu for DCIS is not routinely required for all patients at this time. The decision to perform these biomarkers on cases of DCIS should be made in conjunction with the clinicians who will use this information to treat the patient with tamoxifen or other antiestrogenic selective estrogen receptor modulators (SERMS) therapy, which usually continues over 5 years. The adverse side effects of SERMS include hot flashes, endometrial hyperplasia and cancer, blood clots, and pulmonary embolism, to name a few. Some are minor side effects, and others are life-threatening. The risks and benefits of SERMS should be carefully considered by each individual patient.

Ductal Carcinoma in Situ in Male Breast

Breast carcinomas are rare in males. Most of the tumors occur in the retroareolar region. The growth pattern of DCIS is similar to that in the female breast, including cribriform, papillary, solid, and comedo types, but in males, papillary carcinoma is relatively more common. The majority of papillary carcinomas are intracystic and noninvasive. ADH and Paget's disease have been reported in the male breast. Male breasts lack acini, unlike the female breast, and, thus, lobular differentiation is extremely rare in males. LCIS and invasive lobular carcinoma have reportedly been found in rare cases. Cosmetic aspects of treatment are less of concern for males, and thus most men undergo a simple mastectomy for DCIS.

Fine-Needle Aspiration Findings

A fine-needle aspiration (FNA) procedure is usually done on a palpable mass; however, DCIS is often a nonpalpable lesion. Rarely, DCIS can present as a palpable mass, in particular when it is associated with sclerosing adenosis or a preexisting radial scar lesion. The FNA specimen often yields cellular materials (Figs 21-48 to 21-51). Cells are in aggregates, sheets, and a single cell pattern with a necrotic background especially when DCIS is of the comedo type. When compared with normal breast epithelium, the malignant cells have nuclei that are three to four times larger, with irregular nuclear chromatin, a nuclear membrane, and prominent nucleoli. Single cells with retained cytoplasm are a characteristic of malignant epithelial cells. The limitation of FNA is the inability to determine in situ disease from invasive carcinoma. However, the invasive nature can be detected on core needle biopsy or excisional biopsy.

Synopsis of Treatment Options

The optimal treatment option for DCIS includes individualized care with a multidisciplinary approach. Excision alone, excision with radiation, tamoxifen, or both, and mastectomy are all potentially appropriate and acceptable treatment options for DCIS. All apparent DCIS should be excised with a sufficient rim (margin) of normal breast tissue around it. The type of surgical procedure includes lumpectomy or mastectomy and is influenced by patient preferences, age, breast size, extent and grade of lesion, margin width, and mammographic and pathologic findings.

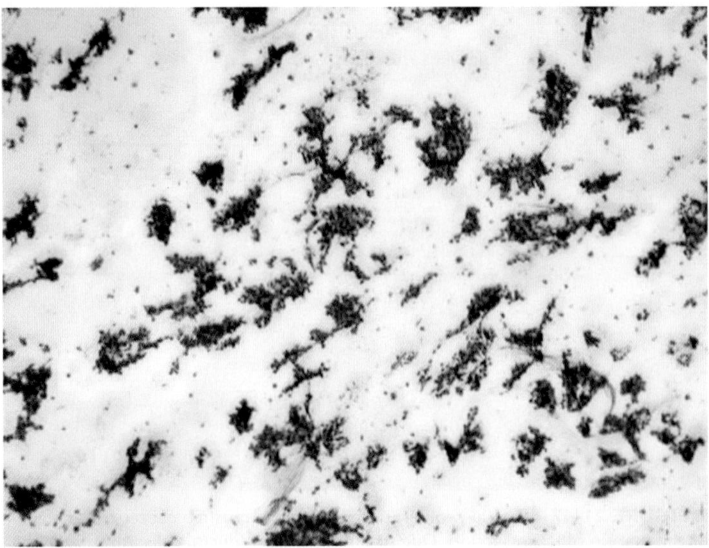

■ FIGURE 21-48 Fine-needle aspiration showing hypercellular material (Papanicolaou [PAP] stain, ×40).

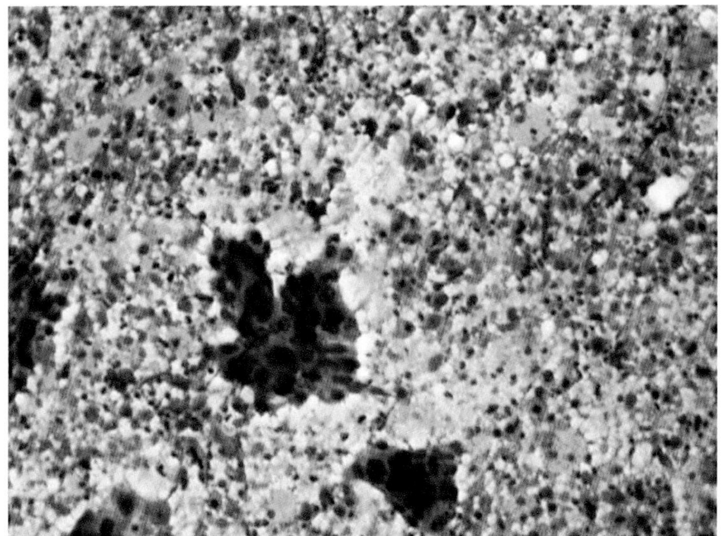

■ **FIGURE 21-49** The background material shows necrosis and a few aggregates of highly atypical cells (Papanicolaou [PAP] stain, ×400).

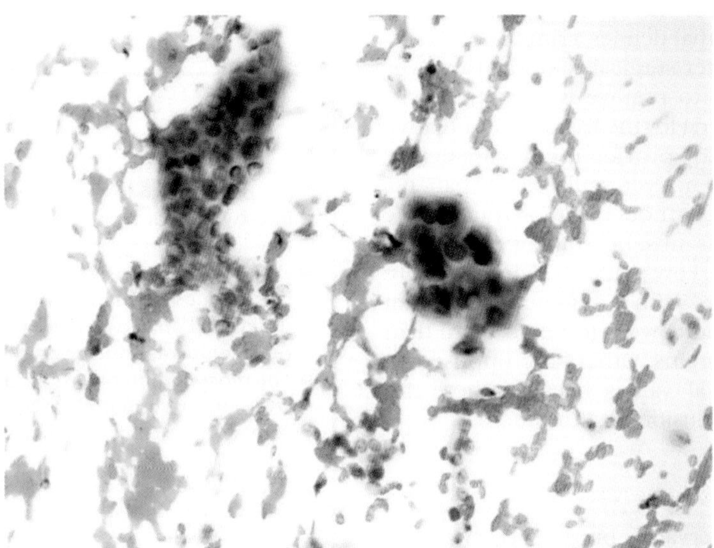

■ **FIGURE 21-50** Left side is a benign ductal epithelium. Right side is malignant epithelial cells (Papanicolaou [PAP] stain, ×200).

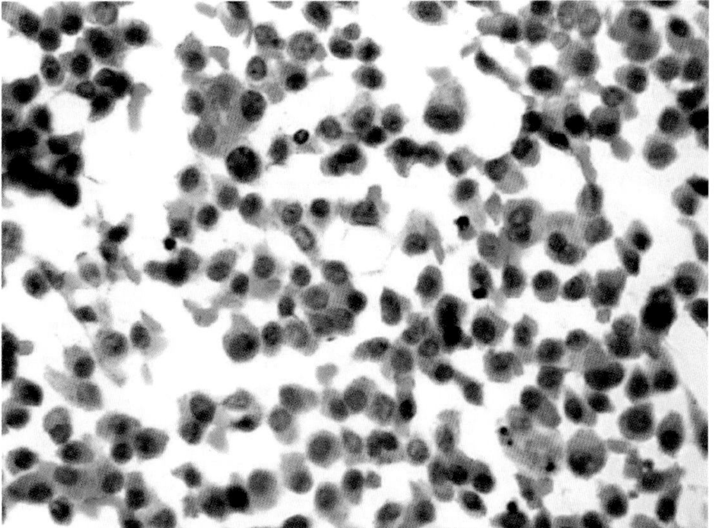

■ **FIGURE 21-51** Numerous single cells with retained cytoplasm are a characteristic feature of malignant epithelium (Papanicolaou [PAP] stain, ×400).

The goal of surgery is complete excision, but this may not be accomplished if the size of the lesion is large in comparison with the size of the breast, in which case mastectomy may be the only option. Mastectomy is not necessarily superior to lumpectomy regarding risk of mortality or long-term survival, and the loss of a breast can be traumatic. Mastectomy is indicated when a lesion is large or multicentric and lumpectomy would distort the shape of the breast, causing a suboptimal cosmetic result. If there is persistent margin involvement after one or more attempts at conservative excision and in *BRCA1*- or *BRCA2*-related breast cancer patients, mastectomy is the best treatment option. Mastectomy also is performed if the patient so chooses after an informed discussion regarding advantages and disadvantages of both surgical options. Bilateral mastectomy is not recommended based on a diagnosis of unilateral DCIS unless the individual patient desires to have such treatment. Radiation therapy is not recommended after mastectomy.

For conservative lumpectomy, the goal is to remove all of the DCIS with a clear margin that defines a rim of normal tissue surrounding the DCIS after surgical removal. However, how much tissue or margin to remove is a controversial issue. The 1994 selection criteria for the Eastern Cooperative Oncology Group (ECOG) study provide useful parameters, although the study results are not yet available. For patients who are considering excision without radiation therapy, the criteria suggested that margins must be 3 mm or greater and clear in all specimen surfaces. Low-grade DCIS lesions were to be no more than 2.5 in size with a minimum of 3.0 mm margins. High-grade DCIS lesions were to be no more than 1 cm with 3 mm of clear margins. Others are opposed to assigning definitive numerical values because there are insufficient data to draw conclusions at this time.

Radiation Therapy

Radiation therapy after conservative breast surgery generally reduces the risk of recurrence by at least 50%. Because the survival rate for DCIS is extremely high regardless of type of treatment received, radiation therapy may be unnecessary for many DCIS patients. However, there are no standard criteria as to which patients need radiation therapy and which do not. Some strongly believe that it would be unwise to use radiation therapy if the parameter dictates a low risk of local recurrence with wide margins whereas others believe that most patients with breast conservative therapy should get radiation therapy to reduce the recurrence rate. Most women receive radiation therapy after breast conservation therapy in the United States. Clean margins are required for a patient to receive radiation therapy.

Tamoxifen Therapy

ER and PR studies on DCIS are necessary to assess who may benefit from hormonal therapy. Hormonal therapy is currently given to patients who had DCIS that was ER positive, PR positive, or both. Tamoxifen decreases the future risk of recurrence after breast-sparing surgery and irradiation. The future risk of cancer in the contralateral breast is also known to be decreased. It is unknown whether tamoxifen improves long-term survival, since DCIS is not a life-threatening disease and most patients survive for a long time whether or not they take tamoxifen. Other hormonal agents such as raloxifene and aromatase inhibitors also are available and likely to benefit patients. Clinical studies for these agents are ongoing.

KEY POINTS

- Carcinoma in situ is a distinct lesion of the breast that has the potential to become invasive cancer. It can be divided into two major types: ductal carcinoma in situ (DCIS) and lobular carcinoma in situ (LCIS).
- DCIS is a preinvasive lesion to invasive breast cancer. It is defined as malignant cells that are confined within the ductal structures and basement membranes that replace normal ductal epithelium.
- The most commonly used classification divides DCIS into two major types: the more aggressive comedo-type carcinoma and the more indolent noncomedo-type carcinoma.
- Paget's disease of the nipple is defined as having DCIS cells within the skin of the nipple, the mammary areolar skin, or both.
- DCIS makes up approximately 30% of breast malignancies detected by screening mammography, and the majority of cases of DCIS are detected on mammography.
- Fine, linear, discontinuous, and branching calcifications on a mammogram are typical of DCIS.
- DCIS may present as an ill-defined hypoechoic mass on ultrasonography.
- Non–mass-like clumped or heterogeneous enhancement in a linear or segmental or ductal distribution is the most common appearance of DCIS on MRI.

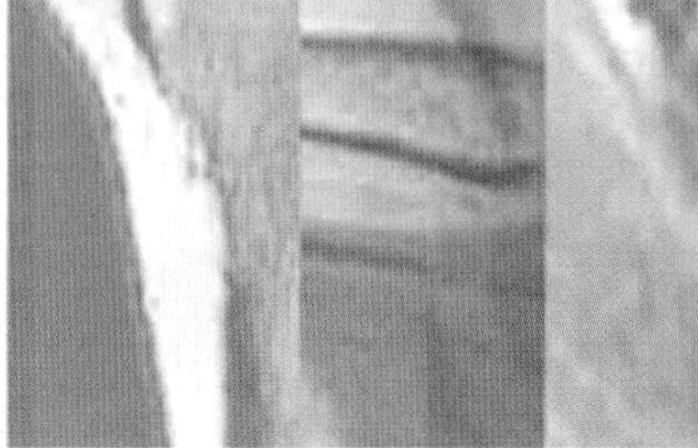

CASE STUDY

Chapter 21 Ductal Carcinoma in Situ and Paget's Disease

HISTORY

A 71-year-old woman presented for a screening mammogram. No films are available for comparison.

FINDINGS

Bilateral screening mammogram (craniocaudal [CC] and mediolateral oblique [MLO] digital views) shows that the breast is almost entirely fat. Within the left breast there are heterogeneous calcifications distributed segmentally in the lower outer quadrant (Fig. 21-52). This was rated an American College of Radiology (ACR) Breast Imaging Reporting and Data System (BI-RADS) 0 for additional imaging evaluation. The right breast was negative.

The patient returned for a diagnostic mammogram that included mediolateral and magnification digital views. These show heterogeneous calcifications distributed segmentally spanning from the 3-o'clock to 5-o'clock positions extending from the nipple to the posterior depth (Fig. 21-53). Correlative ultrasonography of the outer hemisphere did not demonstrate any abnormality. The left breast was given a BI-RADS 4 rating, with the recommendation for stereotactic core needle biopsy.

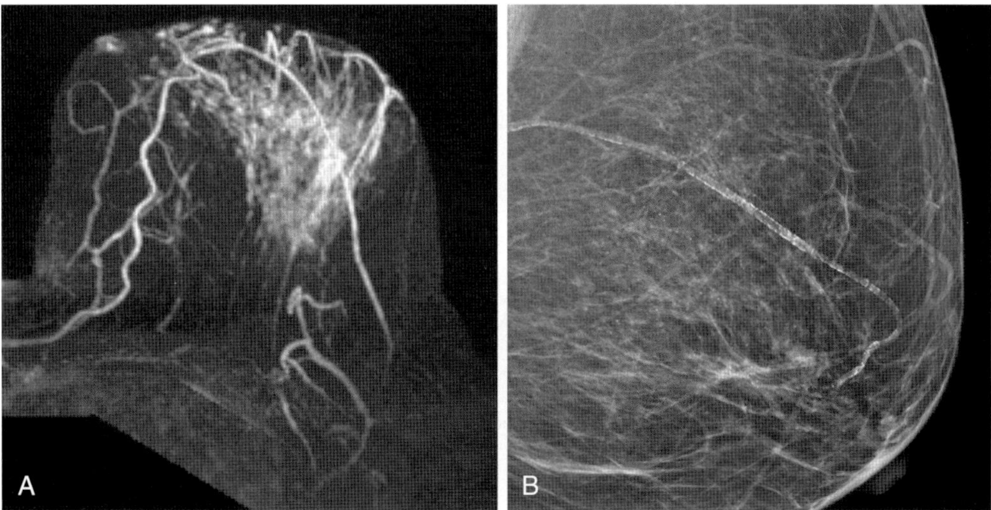

■ **FIGURE 21-52** Craniocaudal (**A**) and mediolateral (**B**) digital views of the right breast show heterogeneous calcifications distributed segmentally in the lower outer quadrant.

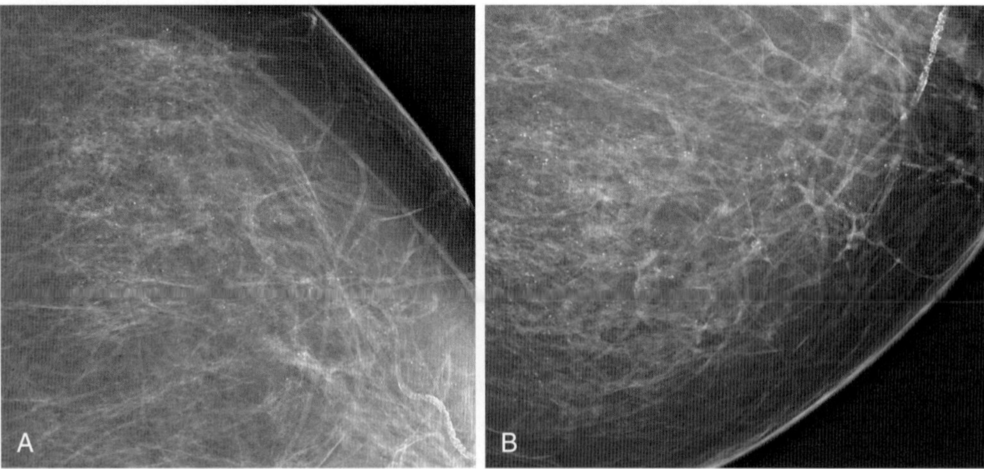

■ **FIGURE 21-53** Craniocaudal (**A**) and mediolateral (**B**) digital magnification views of the left breast show fine, pleomorphic calcifications distributed segmentally spanning from the 3-o'clock to 5-o'clock positions extending from the nipple to the posterior depth.

DIFFERENTIAL DIAGNOSIS

This appearance of segmentally distributed heterogeneous calcifications is highly suggestive of DCIS on mammography. The primary consideration is the extent of disease and the presence or absence of invasive carcinoma.

DIAGNOSIS

Stereotactic core needle biopsy was performed showing DCIS (cribriform and solid types with central necrosis) without evidence of invasive carcinoma. This diagnosis was confirmed at excision (Fig. 21-54).

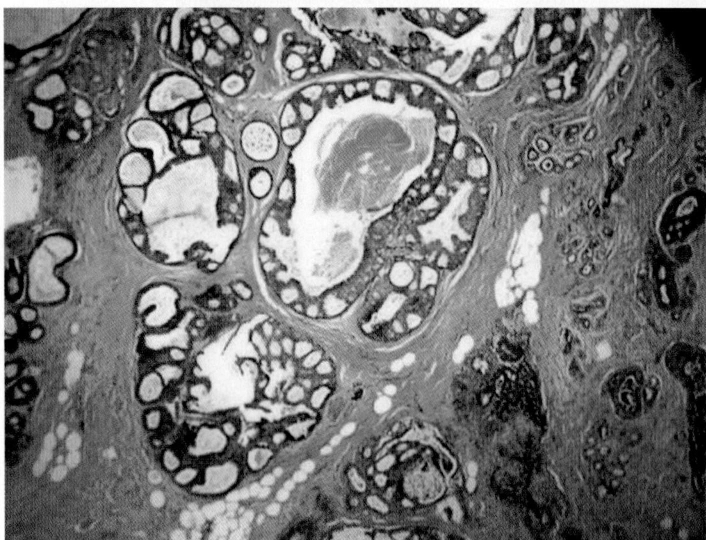

■ **FIGURE 21-54** Excisional biopsy showing cribriform ductal carcinoma in situ with central necrosis (H&E, ×100).

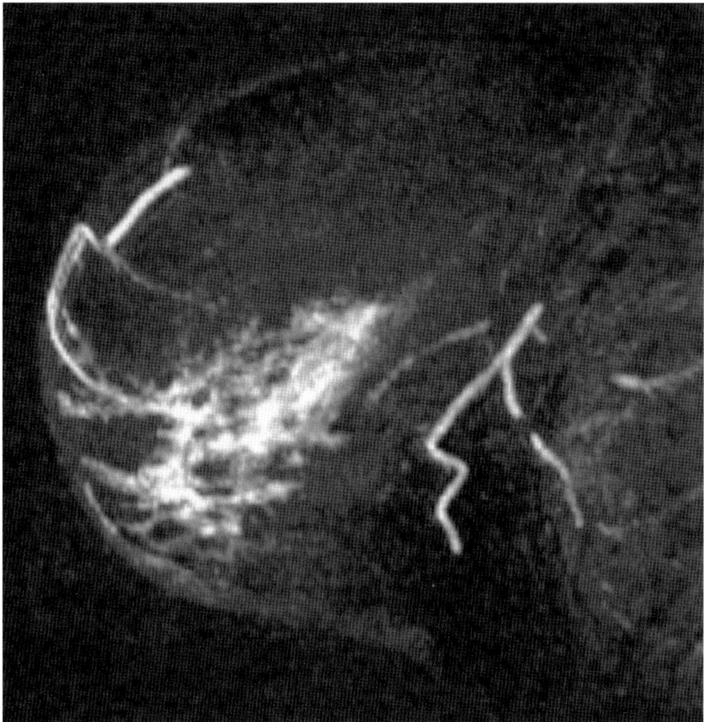

■ **FIGURE 21-55** Sagittal maximum intensity projection (MIP) magnetic resonance (MR) images of the left breast show an area of heterogeneous non–mass-like enhancement in a segmental distribution extending from the nipple to the mid third of the breast in the lower outer quadrant.

COMMENTARY

In this patient with such a large extent of calcification, MRI was ordered before excision. MRI demonstrated a 7.7 × 6.6 × 4.5-cm area of heterogeneous non–mass-like enhancement in a segmental distribution extending from the nipple to the mid third of the breast in the lower outer quadrant, correlating with the area of calcification seen on the mammogram (Fig. 21-55). Kinetic analysis showed a medium initial phase and a persistent delayed phase.

SUGGESTED READINGS

Giuliano AE. *Z0010: a prognostic study of sentinel node and bone marrow micrometastases in women with clinical T1 or T2 N0 M0 breast cancer.* Available at www.acosog.org/studies/synopes/Z0010_Synopsis.pdf.

Krag DN. *Protocol B-32: a randomized phase III clinical trial to compare sentinel node resection to conventional axillary dissection in clinically node-negative breast cancer patients.* 2003. Available at www.nsabp.pitt.edu/B-32.asp.

Solin LJ, Fourquet A, Vicini FA, Haffty B, Taylor M, McCormick B, et al. Mammographically detected ductal carcinoma in situ of the breast treated with breast conserving surgery and definitive breast irradiation: long term outcome and prognostic significance of patient age and margin status. *Int J Radiat Oncol Biol Phys* 2001;**50**:991-1002.

REFERENCES

1. Rosner D, Bedwani RN, Vana J, Baker HW, Murphy GP, et al. Noninvasive breast carcinoma: results of a national survey by the American College of Surgeons. *Ann Surg* 1980;**192**:139–47.
2. Bassett LW, Liu TH, Giuliano A, Gold RH. Prevalence of carcinoma in palpable vs. impalpable mammographically-detected lesions. *AJR Am J Roentgenol* 1991;**157**:21–4.
3. Holland R, Hendriks JH. Microcalcifications associated with ductal carcinoma in situ: mammographic-pathologic correlation. *Semin Diagn Pathol* 1994;**11**:181–92.
4. Paulus DD. Malignant masses in the therapeutically irradiated breast. *AJR Am J Roentgenol* 1994;**135**:789–95.
5. World Health Organization. *Histological Typing of Breast Tumors*. 2nd ed. (International Histological Classification of Tumors. No 2, p. 19.) Geneva: World Health Organization; 1981.
6. Zunzunegui RG, Chung MA, Oruwari J, Golding D, Marchant DJ, Cady B. Casting-type calcifications with invasion and high-grade ductal carcinoma in situ: a more aggressive disease? *Arch Surg* 2003;**138**:537–40.
7. Stomper PC, Connolly JL, Meyer JE, Harris JR. Clinically occult ductal carcinoma in situ detected with radiologic-pathologic correlation. *Radiology* 1989;**172**:235–41.
8. Kinkel K, Gilles R, Feger C, Guinebretiere JM, Tardivon AA, Masselot J, et al. Focal areas of increased opacity in ductal carcinoma in situ of the comedo type: Mammographic-pathologic correlation. *Radiology* 1994;**192**:443–6.
9. Schnitt SJ, Connolly JL, Khettry U, Mazoujian G, Brenner M, Silver B, et al. Pathologic findings on re-excision of the primary site in breast cancer patients considered for treatment by primary radiation therapy. *Cancer* 1987;**59**:675–81.
10. Boyages J, Recht A, Connolly J, Schnitt S, Rose MA, Silver B, et al. Factors associated with local recurrence as a first site of failure following the conservative treatment of early breast cancer. *Recent Results Cancer Res* 1989;**115**:92–102.
11. Holland R, Connolly JL, Gelman R, Mravunac M, Hendriks JH, Verbeek AL, et al. The presence of an extensive intraductal component following a limited excision correlates with prominent residual disease in the remainder of the breast. *J Clin Oncol* 1990;**8**:113–8.
12. Stomper PC, Margolin FR. Ductal carcinoma in situ: the mammographer's perspective. *AJR AM J Roentgenol* 1994;**162**:585–91.
13. Graham RA, Homer MJ, Sigler CJ, Safaii H, Schmid CH, Marchant DJ, et al. The efficacy of specimen radiography in evaluating the surgical margins of impalpable breast carcinoma. *AJR Am J Roentgenol* 1994;**162**:33–6.
14. Soo MS, Williford ME, Walsh R, Bentley RC, Kornguth, et al. Papillary carcinoma of the breast: imaging findings. *AJR Am J Roentgenol* 1995;**164**:321–6.
15. Kuhl CK, Schrading S, Bieling HB, Wardelmann E, Leutner CC, Koenig R, et al. MRI for diagnosis of pure ductal carcinoma in situ: a prospective observational study. *Lancet* 2007;**370**:485–92.
16. Bellamy CO, McDonald C, Salter DM, Chetty U, Anderson TJ. Noninvasive ductal carcinoma of the breast: the relevance of histologic categorization. *Hum Pathol* 1993;**24**:16–23.
17. Livasy CA, Perou CM, Karaca G, Cowan DW, Maia D, Jackson S, et al. Identification of a basal-like subtype of breast ductal carcinoma in situ. *Hum Pathol* 2007;**38**:197–204.
18. Lagios MD, Margolin E, Wesgahl PR, Rose MR. Mammographically detected duct carcinoma in situ. Frequency of local recurrence following tylectomy and prognostic effect of nuclear grade on local recurrence. *Cancer* 1989;**63**:618–24.
19. Silverstein MJ, Lagios MD, Craig PH, Waisman JR, Lewinsky BS, Colburn WJ, et al. A prognostic index for ductal carcinoma in situ of the breast. *Cancer* 1996;**77**:2267–74.
20. Holland R, Veling SH, Marvunac M, Hendriks JH. Histologic multiplicity of Tis, T1–2 breast carcinomas. Implications for clinical trials of breast-conserving surgery. *Cancer* 1985;**56**:979–90.
21. Silverstein MJ, Lagios MD, Groshen S, Waisman JR, Lewinsky BS, Martino S, et al. The influence of margin width on local control of ductal carcinoma in situ of the breast. *N Engl J Med* 1999;**340**:1455–61.
22. Cox CE, Nguyen K, Gray RJ, Salud C, Ku NN, Dupont E, et al. Importance of lymphatic mapping in ductal carcinoma in situ (DCIS): why map DCIS? *Am Surg* 2001;**67**:513–9.
23. Bleiweiss IJ, Nagi CS, Jaffer S. Axillary lymph nodes can be falsely positive due to iatrogenic displacement and transport of benign epithelial cells in patients with breast carcinoma. *J Clin Oncol* 2006;**24**:2013–8.
24. Rosai J. Borderline epithelial lesions of the breast. *Am J Surg Pathol* 1991;**15**:209–21.
25. Schnitt SJ, Connelly JL, Tavassoli FA, Fechner RE, Kempson RL, Gelman R, et al. Interobserver reproducibility in the diagnosis of ductal proliferative breast lesions using standardized criteria. *Am J Surg Pathol* 1992;**16**:1133–43.
26. Fisher B, Dignam J, Wolmark N, Wickerham DL, Fisher ER, Mamounas E, et al. Tamoxifen in treatment of intraductal breast cancer: National Surgical Adjuvant Breast and Bowel Project B-24 randomised controlled trial. *Lancet* 1999;**353**:1993–2000.

CHAPTER 22

Invasive Ductal Carcinomas

Sophia Kim Apple, Lawrence W. Bassett, and Cheryce M. Poon

Invasive cancer is believed to evolve from an intraductal noninvasive precursor. The majority of invasive breast cancers are believed to arise in the terminal ductal-lobular unit. Approximately three fourths of invasive breast cancers are classified as the *not otherwise specified* (NOS) type. The NOS group has heterogeneous histologic patterns. Special types of invasive breast carcinomas show distinctive pathologic features, which in some instances have different prognostic significance when compared with the NOS type.[1] Although some clinical and mammographic findings may suggest a specific type of invasive cancer, considerable overlap occurs, and a specific diagnosis requires histologic evaluation. In this chapter we discuss the general clinical and mammographic features of invasive breast cancers, specific histologic types of invasive breast cancer, metastases to the breast, biomarkers, and treatment.

INVASIVE DUCTAL CARCINOMA IN WOMEN

Definition

Invasive or infiltrating ductal carcinoma (IDC) is the most common type of invasive breast cancer, accounting for 80% of invasive breast cancers. IDC begins in the milk duct, as does ductal carcinoma in situ (DCIS), but spreads outside the duct into the surrounding breast with the ability to metastasize to distant sites (most commonly to bone, brain, liver, and/or lungs). The most common clinical presentation of an IDC is as a hard, nonmobile and usually painless mass. Mammographically, the most common presentation is as an irregular spiculated high-density mass with indistinct or spiculated margins.[2] Associated pleomorphic calcifications occur in 40% of cases.

Prevalence and Epidemiology

Breast cancer is the most common invasive cancer in women in the Western world, with the highest incidence rates occurring in the United States, Australia, and countries in Western Europe. The lifetime risk of developing breast cancer in a woman is 12% (1 in 8); and beginning at ages 30 to 39, it is the most commonly diagnosed cancer in women in the United States.[3] For 2008, the American Cancer Society estimated 184,450 new cases of breast cancer and 40,480 deaths due to breast cancer for women in the United States.[4] The estimated number of new cases of invasive breast cancer in men in the United States for 2007 was 2030 (1% of all breast cancers), with 450 expected deaths.[5]

Since broad surveillance of breast cancer began in 1975, there are four significant phases regarding the incidence rates of invasive breast cancer in women reported by the American Cancer Society. The first of these is between 1975 and 1980, which showed a constant incidence rate of invasive carcinoma. However, between 1980 and 1987, incidence rates increased by 3.7% per year, attributed mostly to the introduction of mammography, although other factors such as delayed childbearing and having fewer children were believed to be important. Between 1987 and 2001, incidence rates increased by 0.5% per year due to continued mammography screening, obesity, and the introduction of hormone replacement therapy (HRT). Between 2001 and 2004, there was a decreased incidence rate of 3.5% per year, attributable to a decrease in screening mammography and decreased use of HRT after the publication of the results of the Women's Health Initiative randomized trial in 2002.[6] Overall, the incidence of breast cancer rates in women of all races since the early 1980s has increased. The increased rate of detection in white women is mostly due to the detection of smaller tumors (≤2 cm) and localized-stage tumors likely due to screening mammography. However, African-American women and other minorities are more likely to be diagnosed with larger tumor size and advanced stage when compared with white women.

Incidence rates vary across racial and ethnic groups with the following figures reported from 1996 to 2000: 141 cases per 100,000 among white women, 122 per 100,000 among African-Americans, 97 per 100,000 among Asian-American/Pacific Islanders, 90 among Hispanics, and 58 in Native Americans/Alaskan Natives.[7] Suspected reasons for the higher incidence rates in white women include an older age at first birth, use of HRT, and greater access to screening mammography.[8]

Since 1990, death rates decreased by 2.5% per year in white women and by 1% per year in African-American women. However, between 1980 and 2000 there has been a growing disparity in the death rates observed between white and African-American women, with the age-standardized death rate 32% higher in African-Americans.

Most importantly, 63% and 29% of breast cancers are diagnosed at local and regional-stage disease, corresponding to a 5-year survival rate of 97% and 79%, respectively. Therefore, as physicians, we should encourage and motivate women to have regular mammograms, self breast examinations, and clinical breast examinations (CBEs).[8]

Etiology and Pathophysiology

Understanding and knowing the risk factors for breast cancer are important to continue to reduce the incidence rates of breast cancer. Risk factors can be classified into those that cannot be modified, those that can be modified, and those that are potentially modifiable.

Risks factors that cannot be modified include genetics and family history, age, race/ethnicity, height, age at menarche, breast density on mammograms, and medical history. Mutations involving the breast cancer 1, early onset (*BRCA1*) and breast cancer 2, early onset (*BRCA2*) tumor suppressing genes confer a lifetime risk of breast cancer between 40% and 80%. Although this mutation is found predominantly in Ashkenazi Jews (1%-2%), it is also present in the white population (0.24%).[9] The relative risk (RR) for a positive family history are 1.8 given a first-degree relative aged 50 years or older with postmenopausal breast cancer; 3.3 given a first-degree relative with premenopausal breast cancer; 1.5 given a second-degree relative with breast cancer; and 3.6 given two first-degree relatives with breast cancer.[10] The incidence rate of breast cancer increases dramatically at the age of 40 years, with a peak incidence occurring at 75 to 79 years of age and a median age of 61 years.[11,12] Early menarche (2-5 years earlier than the average age of 16) confers a RR of 1.3 and late menopause (55 or older) confers a RR of 1.2 to 1.5.[10,13] Medical history would include women who have been treated with chest wall irradiation during childhood or adolescence for Hodgkin lymphoma. The risk increases with increasing dosage of radiation to the breasts and the younger the patient is at the time of treatment. For this subgroup of patients, the surveillance guidelines suggest annual mammograms starting 8 years after treatment or beginning at the age of 25 years.[14]

Risk factors considered modifiable include diet, body mass index, physical activity, smoking, exogenous estrogen use, alcohol consumption, and reproductive history. An increased body mass index (80th percentile vs. 20th percentile) confers a RR of 1.2 to 1.9. For postmenopausal women there is a risk reduction ranging between 20% to 80% for physical activity, although no clear relationship has been established for premenopausal women at this time. The use of HRT for at least 5 years confers a RR of 1.2. Alcohol consumption of two drinks daily versus none confers a RR of 1.2. Pregnancy before the age of 20 markedly reduces the incidence of breast cancer whereas nulliparity and a late age of a first live birth (>30 years) increases the incidence with a RR of 1.7 to 1.9.[10,13]

Risk factors considered potentially modifiable include age at first birth, age at menopause, and breast feeding. There is a reported 4.3% risk reduction of breast cancer for each year of breastfeeding.[15]

Manifestations of Disease

Clinical Presentation

CBE and mammography are complementary for breast cancer detection. Although mammography is more sensitive, CBE detects some cancers not evident on mammograms. In the Breast Cancer Detection Demonstration Projects of the 1970s, the proportion of cancers detected by mammography alone was 42% whereas the proportion detected by physical examination alone was 9%.[16] Clinical signs of breast carcinoma are a palpable mass, palpable asymmetry, skin changes, nipple discharge, and pain. Several factors influence when these clinical signs become apparent.[17] For example, palpation of a mass is more likely to be delayed in a woman with large breasts than in a woman with small breasts. The location of the mass is another factor. A superficial mass is usually more readily palpated than one deep within the breast. Skin changes, such as retraction, also are evident sooner in women with a superficial tumor. Tumors located directly under the nipple can lead to nipple retraction or spontaneous nipple discharge, but the same findings would take much longer to manifest if the tumor were deeper in the breast.

Mass

A palpable mass is the most common physical sign of breast cancer.[18] The mass of invasive breast cancer is typically, but not necessarily, hard and fixed rather than soft and freely movable. However, carcinomas are occasionally freely movable and may in this way mimic benign masses. The invasive breast cancer mass may be tender, but it is usually painless. If a cyst is suspected, it can be verified by needle aspiration or ultrasonography. Cancers are usually first noticed by the woman herself. Sometimes, the discovery occurs after trauma to the breast and is therefore incorrectly attributed to the traumatic event. Malignant breast masses often seem to be larger on palpation than measured on the mammogram or by ultrasonography. This size disparity is due to the associated edema and cicatrization incited by malignant tumors and manifested on palpation.

The most likely etiology of a palpable breast mass depends to some extent on the age of the patient. In women younger than age 30 years, fibroadenomas are the most common source of a palpable breast mass. In women between 30 and 50 years, cysts are more common. In women older than 50 years, the etiology of a palpable breast mass is more likely to be breast cancer. Considerable overlap is seen in the kind of lesions that occur in different age groups, and breast cancer cannot be excluded on the basis of the patient's age alone.

Asymmetry

A localized nodularity or thickening may represent breast cancer. Breast cancer can be found in up to 5% of people with palpable breast thickening.[19] However, when these findings are bilateral and symmetric, cancer is unlikely. Therefore, clinical examination of the breast should always include a comparison of findings in the same location in the other breast.

Physiologic nodularity, which can be defined as multiple tiny localized benign nodules confined to an area of the breast, is one of the most common findings at palpation and also one of the most difficult clinical diagnoses.[20] The correct diagnosis of physiologic nodularity depends on the experience of the examiner. When an area of suspected physiologic nodularity is identified, it must be compared with the same area of the other breast. Bilaterally symmetric nodularity is strong evidence for benignity. Physiologic nodularity is particularly likely to occur in the upper outer quadrants.

Skin Changes

Invasive breast cancer can also cause changes in the overlying skin. Breast cancer may become attached to a suspensory ligament, and the cicatrization process associated with many breast cancers can lead to thickening and shortening of the ligament, leading to skin retraction. The skin retraction, also referred to as skin dimpling or flattening, may be difficult to see in the early stages of development. Therefore, visual inspection of the breast should be made under good light. Observing the breast in various dependent positions and having the woman raise her arms over her head are also helpful in bringing out the phenomenon of skin retraction. The breasts should be inspected with the woman upright, leaning forward, and supine. Like palpation, visual inspection should include a comparison of the two breasts, observing for asymmetry in the skin contour. Symmetric skin changes can represent "false dimpling," reflecting attachment of the normal suspensory ligaments to the skin.[17] The latter phenomenon is more likely to occur in the axillary area, where the skin is closely attached to the extensions of the tail of the breast.

Paget's disease of the nipple and areola is an uncommon condition associated with underlying carcinoma in which the nipple has a chronic, moist, scaly, or erythematous eruption. Symptoms include itching, burning, oozing, and bleeding. The associated carcinoma is intraductal or invasive carcinoma that has spread through the subareolar ducts to the nipple skin.

Inflammatory carcinoma makes up less than 4% of total cases of invasive breast carcinoma.[21] The diagnosis is based on clinical detection of redness, heat, and edema of the skin.[22] This type of breast carcinoma has a grave prognosis.

Nipple Retraction

The nipple is often involved in invasive cancer, and a gradual flattening or retraction of the nipple is an important sign.[17] Nipple retraction should be differentiated from benign nipple inversion, which can usually be reversed by application of manual pressure around the margins of the nipple. Clinical history also is important. Therefore, if nipple retraction is observed, it is important to determine whether it is congenital, of long standing, progressive, or of recent onset. If the nipple changes are progressive or of recent onset, it is more likely related to underlying breast cancer. Nipple retraction can also be associated with fat necrosis, plasma cell mastitis, and Mondor disease.

Nipple Discharge

Discharge from the nipple is usually of benign origin. However, if the nipple discharge is bloody or serous, coming from only one or two ducts, and spontaneous and persistent, carcinoma should be considered. Breast cancer is present in only about 2% of women with nipple discharge.[23] Discharge associated with breast cancer should test positive for hemoglobin.[24] Bloody nipple discharge can also be caused by trauma and a solitary papilloma. The likelihood that a nipple discharge is due to cancer increases with age.[25] When invasive cancer is associated with a nipple discharge, a careful clinical examination frequently uncovers an associated palpable mass.[23]

Axillary Adenopathy

Rarely, enlarged axillary lymph nodes are the first clinical evidence of invasive breast carcinoma.[26] The involved nodes are often hard or tender. Fixed nodes are particularly likely to harbor malignancy. Mammography reveals an ipsilateral carcinoma in up to 50% of women with metastatic adenocarcinoma in axillary lymph nodes.[27] Other causes of metastatic adenocarcinoma in axillary nodes are contralateral breast carcinoma, lung carcinoma, and gastrointestinal carcinoma.

Breast Pain

Pain is the only subjective symptom of breast cancer. Although breast pain is a relatively uncommon presentation, its presence does not exclude the diagnosis of cancer. Women so frequently have breast pain that the presence of this symptom is usually interpreted to mean that malignancy does not exist. In a like manner, the frequency of breast pain may be the reason that a woman does not mention it when she presents with a palpable cancer. However, the very fact that breast pain is so common is another reason that its presence does not rule out the possibility of cancer. Although generalized breast pain is usually not an indication of malignancy, a complaint of localized breast pain should be taken seriously. It has been estimated that about 15% of palpable malignant breast lumps are painful.[18]

Imaging Indications and Algorithm

The mammographic signs of invasive breast cancer are often divided into primary, secondary, and indirect signs.

Imaging Findings by Modality

Mammography Primary Signs

Mass

The most common mammographic sign of an invasive breast cancer is a mass. A *mass* has been defined as a space-occupying lesion that is seen in at least two mammographic projections.[28] In about 40% of cases, the mass is associated with malignant calcifications. Typically, the mass of an invasive breast cancer has an irregular shape, ill-defined or spiculated margins, and high radiographic density (Figs. 22-1 and 22-2). A spiculated or ill-defined margin is probably the most significant mammographic feature differentiating malignancies from benign masses. Occasionally an invasive breast cancer has a circumscribed margin (Fig. 22-3), but this feature occurs in less than 10% of cases. Furthermore, when spot compression and magnification mammography techniques are employed, a malignant lesion usually manifests with partially ill-defined margins (Fig. 22-4).[29]

Radiographic density is another feature distinguishing malignant from benign masses. The term *density* is used to define the radiographic attenuation of the lesion relative to the expected attenuation of an equal volume of normal fibroglandular tissue.[28] Although this feature is not always reliable, malignant masses usually show higher radiographic density than do normal tissues or benign masses.[30]

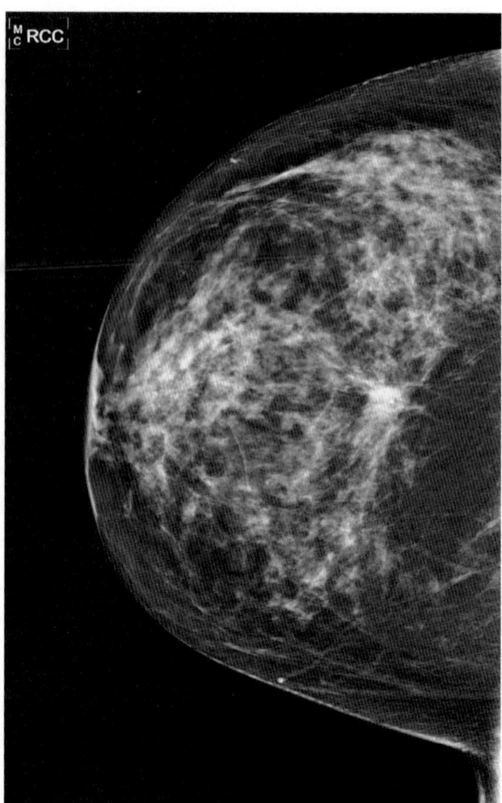

■ **FIGURE 22-1** Invasive ductal carcinoma, not otherwise specified (IDC, NOS). The mass has an irregular shape, spiculated margins, and high radiographic density.

Microcalcifications

Invasive breast cancers are commonly associated with microcalcifications, either within the tumor or adjacent to it (Fig. 22-5). The calcifications outside a malignant

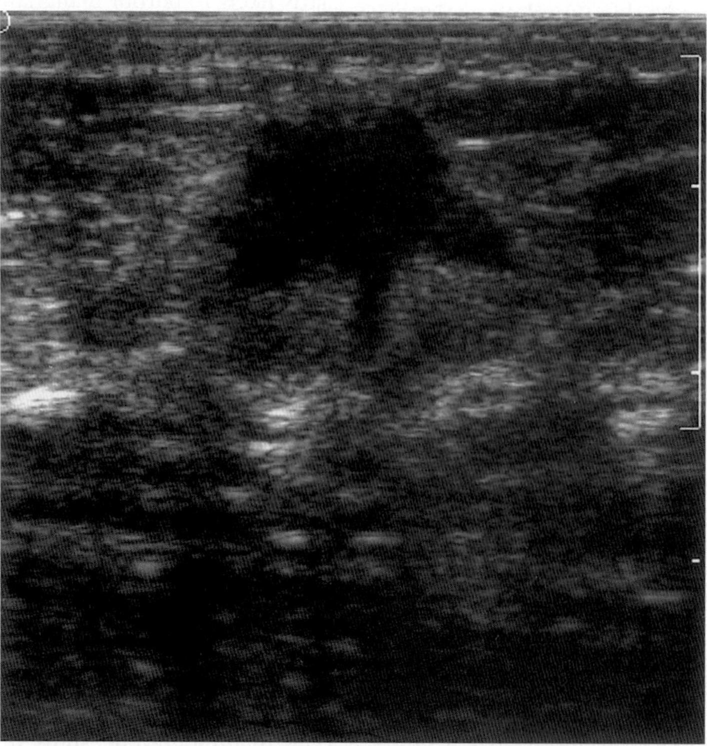

■ **FIGURE 22-2** Invasive ductal carcinoma, not otherwise specified (IDC, NOS). Ultrasonography demonstrates a hypoechoic, irregular mass with angular, spiculated margins and an echogenic halo.

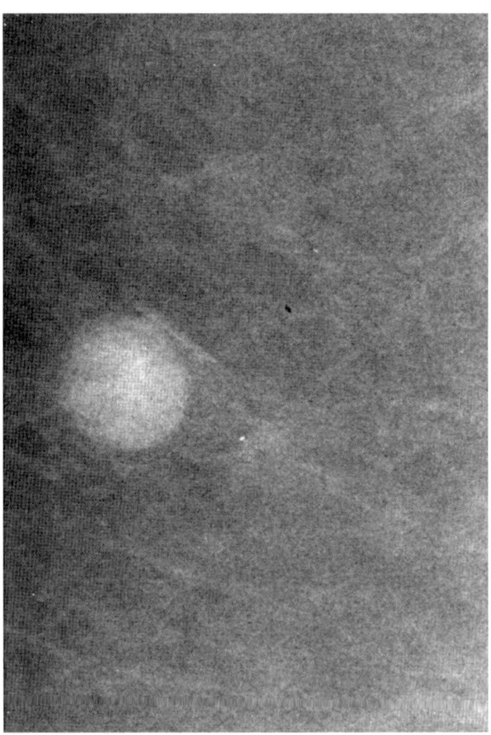

■ **FIGURE 22-3** Invasive ductal carcinoma, not otherwise specified (IDC, NOS). The mass is round and has primarily circumscribed margins, suggesting benignity.

mass usually represent an intraductal component of the tumor. It is important that all of the calcifications are identified before excisional biopsy so that they can be completely excised (Fig. 22-6). If an extensive intraductal component (EIC) is present, the tumor is regarded as EIC-positive and the prognosis for successful breast-conserving surgery diminishes. Rarely, benign-appearing solitary or coarse calcifications may be found within an invasive breast tumor, and the latter finding should not defer the decision for a biopsy if the mass is suggestive of cancer (Fig. 22-7).

Mammography Secondary Signs

Secondary signs of malignancy are usually associated with advanced cancers that are readily detected on CBE or mammography. These secondary signs are skin thickening or retraction, nipple retraction, and axillary node enlargement. When evident mammographically, these manifestations suggest a poor prognosis.

Skin Thickening

The skin is usually 0.5 to 2 mm in thickness, except at the inframammary crease, near the cleavage, and in the periareolar region, where it is normally thicker. Invasive carcinomas may be associated with localized adjacent skin thickening, which suggests infiltration of the skin by the

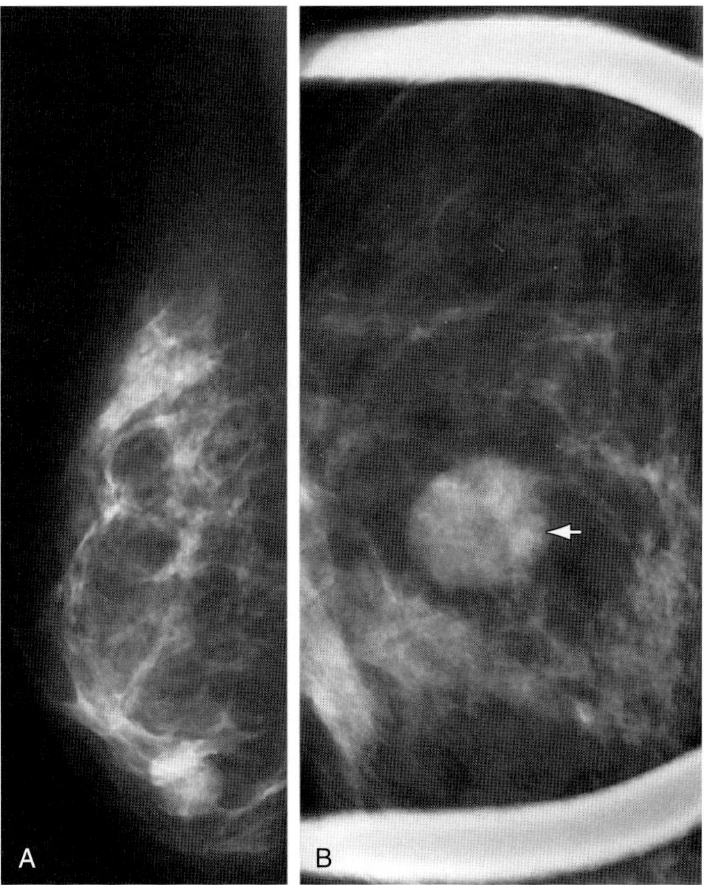

■ **FIGURE 22-4** Invasive ductal carcinoma, not otherwise specified (IDC, NOS). **A,** Right mediolateral (ML) view shows a round partially circumscribed and partially obscured mass in the inferior aspect of the breast. **B,** Spot compression view with magnification reveals that the posterior margin (*arrow*) of the mass is ill defined. Biopsy revealed ductal carcinoma, not otherwise specified.

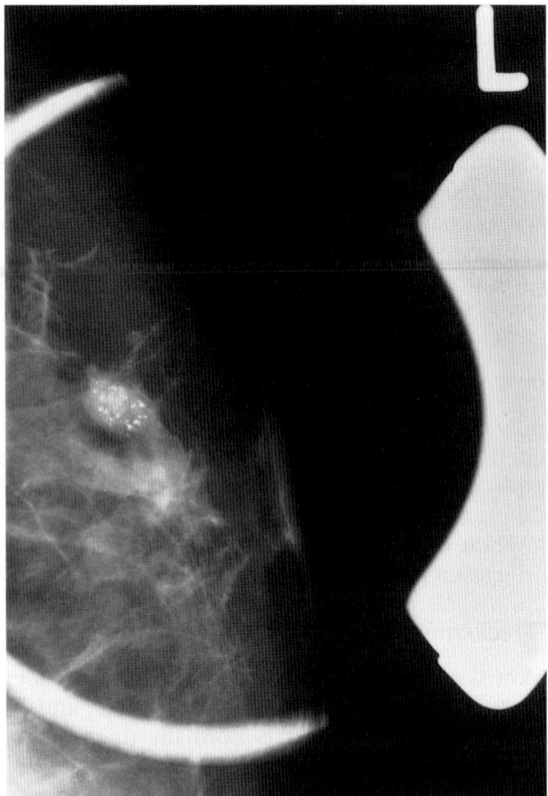

■ **FIGURE 22-5** Invasive ductal carcinoma, not otherwise specified (IDC, NOS). Spot compression view with magnification shows oval partially obscured and partially circumscribed mass containing clustered, coarse heterogeneous microcalcifications highly suggestive of malignancy.

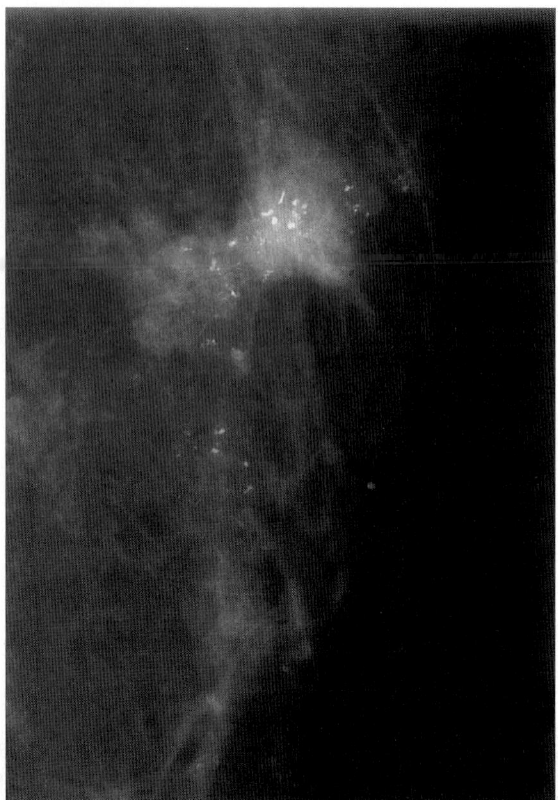

■ **FIGURE 22-6** Invasive ductal carcinoma, not otherwise specified (IDC, NOS). There is a lobular, spiculated mass containing fine linear, coarse heterogeneous and fine pleomorphic calcifications. Additional microcalcifications are located adjacent to the mass. Biopsy showed IDC with an extensive intraductal component (EIC).

tumor. Diffuse skin thickening may be associated with lymphatic obstruction secondary to underlying carcinoma or with metastases to axillary nodes.

Inflammatory carcinoma is a clinical diagnosis that is based on the features of an inflamed breast, which may feel hot and heavy to the patient. Skin biopsy may reveal extensive permeation of the dermal lymphatics by tumor cells. Inflammatory carcinoma is associated with diffuse skin thickening and increased radiographic density of the breast (Fig. 22-8). The differentiation between mastitis and carcinoma with lymphangitic spread (inflammatory carcinoma) may be difficult. In both conditions, the primary lesion may be completely obscured by edema. In this situation, abscess may be excluded mammographically only if typical branching malignant calcifications are present. In general, the diagnosis of inflammatory carcinoma is made clinically and through biopsy unless the mammogram reveals an obvious malignancy.

Generalized skin thickening also may be associated with an abscess, progressive systemic sclerosis, obstruction of the superior vena cava, pemphigus, nephrotic syndrome, congestive heart failure, lymphoma, lymphatic extension from a contralateral breast carcinoma, and changes secondary to radiotherapy.

Skin Retraction

Skin retraction associated with carcinoma comprises a spectrum of changes from a small local dimpling of the skin overlying a small tumor to shrinkage of the entire breast associated with a large, deeply located tumor. Skin retraction and nipple retraction are usually first observed on visual inspection of the breast. Skin retraction may be exaggerated or noticed for the first time as a result of the application of mammographic compression. When the x-ray beam is tangential to the involved breast surface, flattening of the breast contour or retraction can be seen on the mammogram (Fig. 22-9).

Skin retraction associated with breast cancer is attributed to the proliferation of fibrous tissue, or *cicatrization*, not only within the tumor itself but also in the surrounding breast tissue. In time, the cicatrization process results in contraction of the ligaments of Cooper, with the suspensory ligaments of the breast pulling the skin toward the lesion. Occasionally, skin retraction may occur with inflammation from bacterial infection or fat necrosis.

Nipple Retraction

Cicatrization associated with an adjacent breast cancer can lead to changes in subareolar ducts, causing them to thicken and shorten. Eventually, flattening and retraction of the nipple area occurs, which can be observed on mammograms (Fig. 22-10). As mentioned previously, nipple retraction should be differentiated from nipple inversion. The latter condition is usually a long-standing process that is often bilateral and may occur in healthy women.

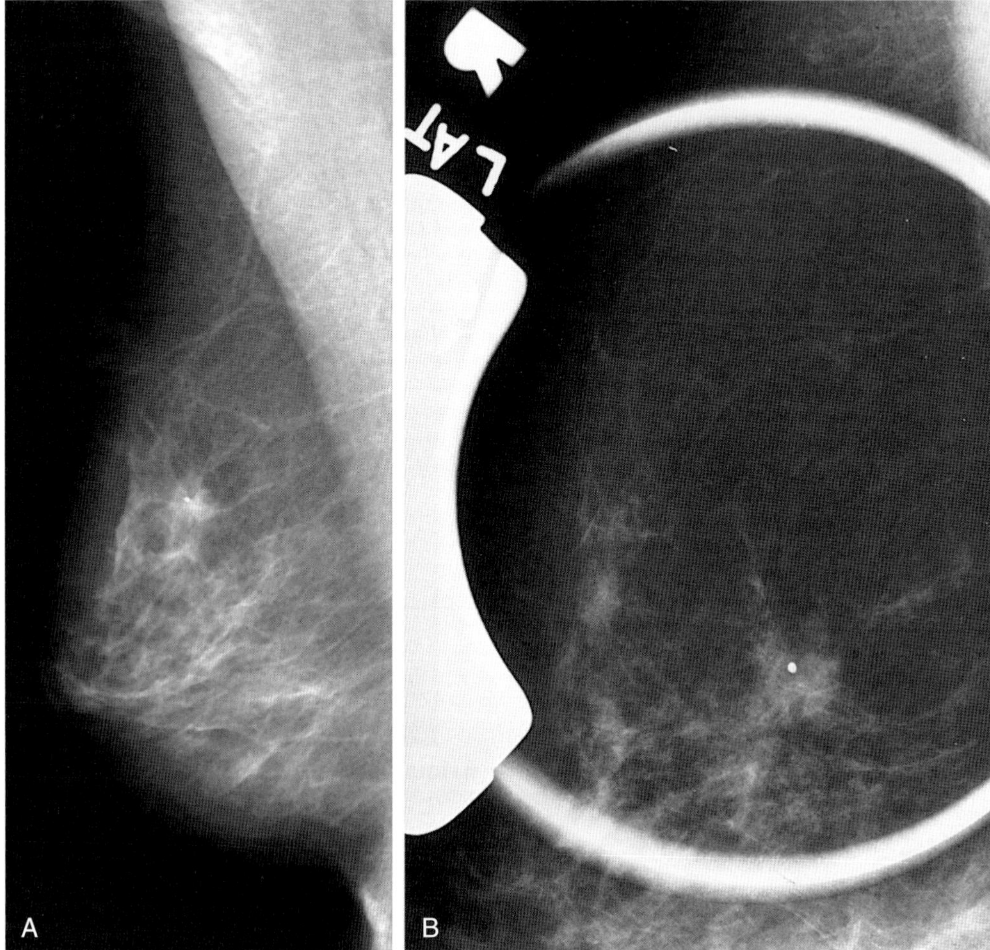

■ **FIGURE 22-7** Invasive ductal carcinoma, not otherwise specified (IDC, NOS), containing a benign calcification. **A,** Right mediolateral oblique (MLO) view shows a solitary, round, dense calcification within an irregular mass. **B,** Spot compression magnification view shows that the mass has an irregular shape and indistinct margins. No additional calcifications were found. Biopsy demonstrated invasive ductal carcinoma.

Retraction of the skin or nipple may also occur secondary to scarring from a previous surgical procedure or secondary to an abscess (Fig. 22-11). Thus, it is important to be aware of the exact site of any previous biopsies when viewing the mammograms. This information is usually reported by the woman on a history questionnaire and recorded on a diagram by the radiologic technologist. Often, a thin radiopaque wire is placed directly over the site of a biopsy scar to expedite the correlation of mammographic findings.

Axillary Lymph Node Metastases

Involvement of the axillary lymph nodes is one of the most important factors in the prognosis of an individual case of breast cancer. Routine use of the mediolateral oblique (MLO) projection ensures that at least the lower axilla can be visualized on a screening examination. The axillary tail view shows a greater amount of axillary tissue than does the MLO view. However, radiographic evaluation of the axillary nodes has proved to be of limited clinical value.[31] Absence of radiolucent fat within a node larger than 2 cm suggests axillary node metastases (Figs. 22-12A,B and 22-13).

The lymph node involved by metastasis may be small and the metastasis detectable only with microscopic examination. Malignant cells first enter the lymph node through afferent lymphatics and become entrapped in the subcapsular sinusoidal spaces (Fig. 22-12C), where the tumor emboli proliferate and eventually destroy the sinusoidal spaces and the adjacent lymphoid tissue. This process often is associated with a desmoplastic response (Fig. 22-12D), resulting in the increased density of the lymph node seen on mammograms. Sometimes the entire lymph node is replaced by tumor, leaving no identifiable nodal structure. The number and the size of lymph nodes with metastasis are directly related to the prognosis. The presence of extranodal spread in the form of lymphatic and vascular space involvement or tumor mass in the perinodal fibroadipose tissue also adversely affects the prognosis (Figs. 22-12E and 22-12F).

Enlarged axillary nodes may be seen in several benign diseases, such as sarcoidosis, tuberculosis, and rheumatoid arthritis.[32] Malignant conditions other than breast carcinoma that may result in enlarged nodes include lymphoma, leukemia, and metastases from extramammary malignancies. Furthermore, no reliable radiographic criteria exist to exclude early nodal involvement with metastases. Surgical

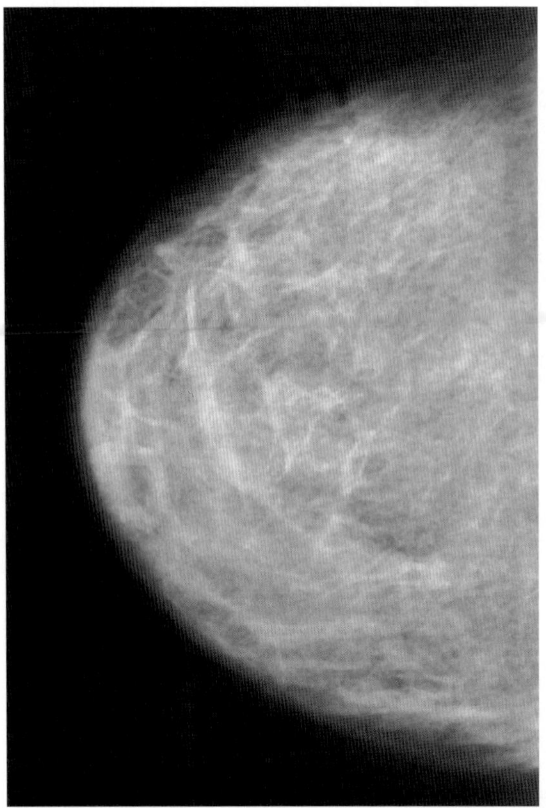

■ **FIGURE 22-8** Inflammatory carcinoma. Mammogram shows diffuse skin thickening and diffusely increased radiographic density.

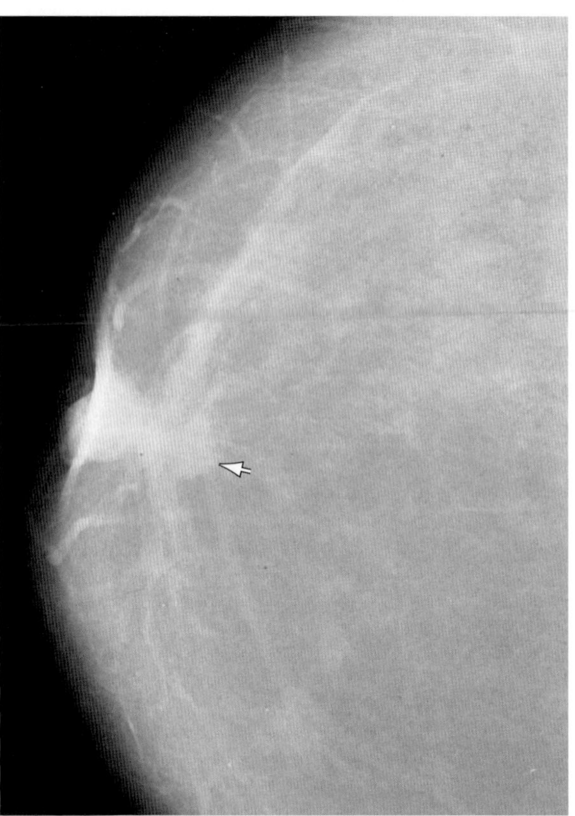

■ **FIGURE 22-10** Invasive ductal carcinoma, not otherwise specified (IDC, NOS). The nipple is retracted due to underlying spiculated carcinoma (*arrow*).

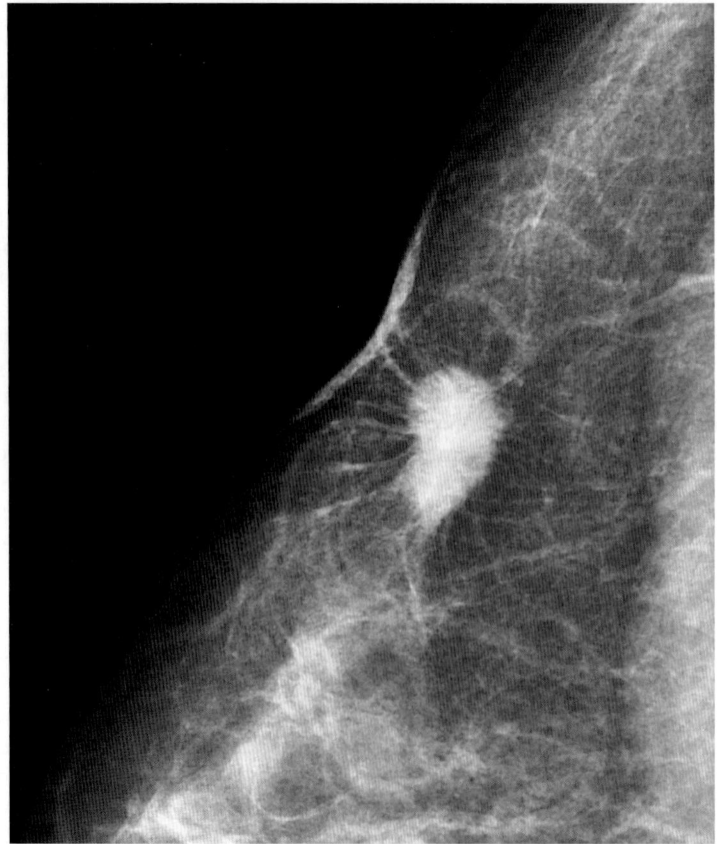

■ **FIGURE 22-9** Invasive ductal carcinoma, not otherwise specified (IDC, NOS). Close-up of mammogram with x-ray beam tangential to the area of skin retraction shows the underlying oval, spiculated, high density mass representing carcinoma with attachment to Cooper ligaments. Skin thickening can be seen.

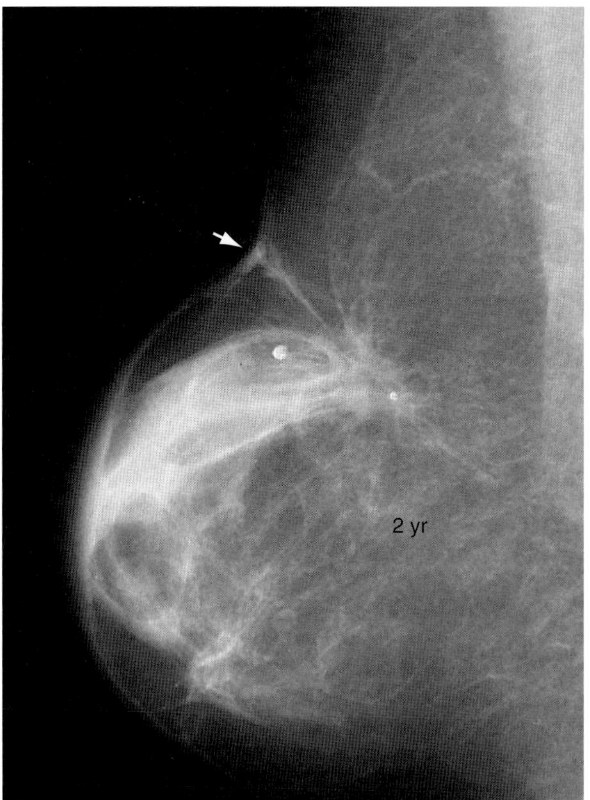

■ **FIGURE 22-11** Scar, 2 years after biopsy. An architectural distortion is seen, associated with retraction and thickening of the overlying skin (*arrow*). Benign calcifications are also present. The findings are typical of a postoperative scar: The abnormality changed shape from one view to another, was not palpable, and was smaller than on the examination performed 1 year earlier.

exploration with histologic evaluation is currently the only reliable way to exclude lymph node metastases due to invasive breast carcinoma.

Mammography Indirect Signs

Although the majority of invasive breast cancers are identified as irregular masses with ill-defined or spiculated margins, some carcinomas are identifiable only from indirect mammographic signs. The indirect signs of malignancy include a developing asymmetry, architectural distortion, focal asymmetry and a unilateral single dilated duct.[33]

Developing Asymmetry

Because the breasts of postmenopausal women are expected to undergo involution, the appearance of a new or growing asymmetry in mammograms should be considered a possible sign of early breast cancer. To identify a developing asymmetry the radiologist must have access to previous mammograms.[34] The developing asymmetry may be classified as an asymmetry if it cannot be recognized in previous studies (Figs. 22-14 and 22-15), or it may be an evolving asymmetry, which was present at the previous examination but was smaller and was not recognized as significant (Fig. 22-16). If the asymmetry has mammographic features that might indicate a cyst, ultrasonography or aspiration should be done. If a simple cyst is disclosed and it matches the site of the mammographic abnormality, no further evaluation is necessary. The presence of a cyst in a postmenopausal woman who is not receiving HRT is unusual, however, and the surrounding

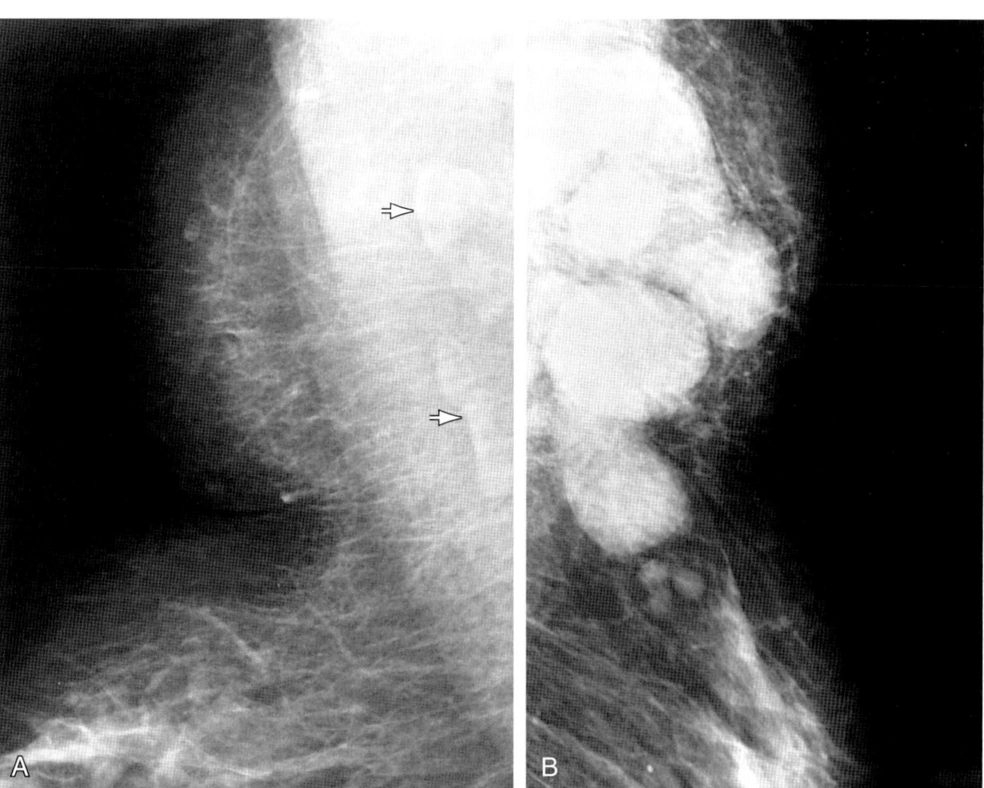

■ **FIGURE 22-12** Axillary lymph node metastases from breast carcinoma. **A,** Right mediolateral oblique (MLO) view shows normal nodes (*arrows*) with radiolucent fat in hilum of nodes. **B,** Left MLO view multiple, large, oval circumscribed, high density masses compatible with axillary adenopathy. Biopsy showed adenocarcinoma, consistent with a primary breast tumor. **C** to **F,** Progression of lymph node metastasis:

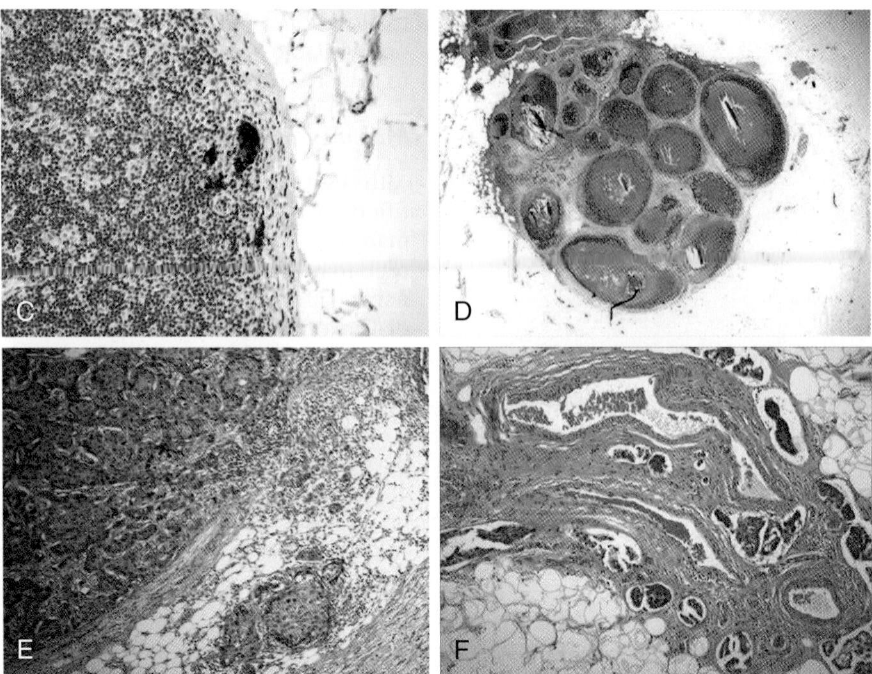

■ FIGURE 22-12—cont'd **C,** Cytokeratin stain x of early metastasis in the subcapsular region of the lymph node; **D,** massive replacement of lymph node with desmoplastic stromal reaction; **E,** extracapsular soft tissue extension; **F,** extracapsular vascular invasion.

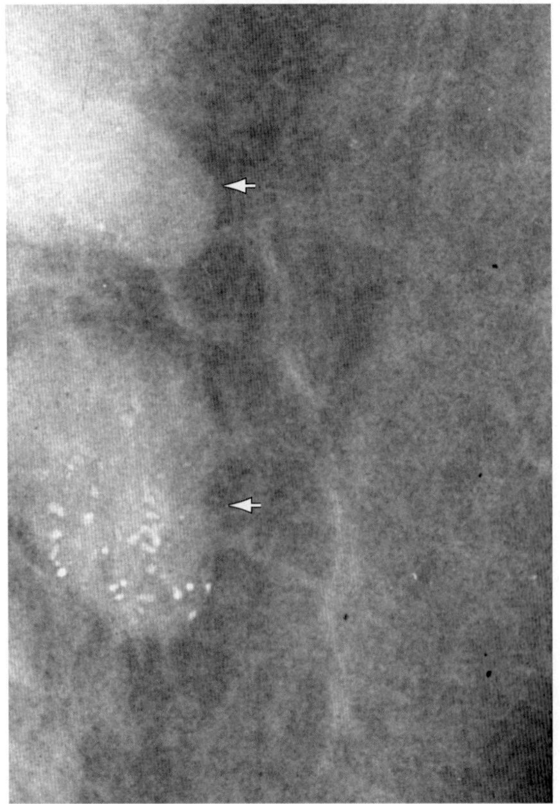

■ FIGURE 22-13 Calcified axillary node metastases from breast carcinoma. Close-up of nodes shows characteristic fine, pleomorphic malignant calcifications (*arrows*) that were present in the primary breast carcinoma. The presence of calcification in metastatic nodes is uncommon.

tissue should be carefully scrutinized. Asymmetric tissue is not uncommon in women undergoing HRT. The mammographic tissue asymmetries due to HRT can usually be differentiated from an asymmetry associated with breast cancer. The asymmetries associated with exogenous hormone therapy usually are present in several areas of the same breast and are bilateral. If a solitary asymmetry is present in a woman receiving HRT, it may be difficult to rule out breast cancer. In the latter situation, it may be useful for the HRT to be stopped for 2 months; if the asymmetry persists after suspension of HRT, biopsy should be considered.

Architectural Distortion

Architectural distortion may be the earliest sign of breast carcinoma (Fig. 22-17). *Architectural distortion* is a focal abnormal arrangement of the parenchymal tissues, including the ducts and ligaments. The normal architecture is distorted with no definite mass visible.[28] The term *architectural distortion* includes spiculations radiating from a point and focal retraction or distortion of the edge of the parenchyma. When associated with invasive carcinoma, this finding is usually due to fibrosis. An architectural distortion may be the only indicator of a large cancer located within dense breast tissue (Fig. 22-18). Spot compression or rolled views can be helpful in verification of a suspected architectural distortion (Fig. 22-19). In addition, ultrasonography is a useful imaging modality to confirm mammographic findings.

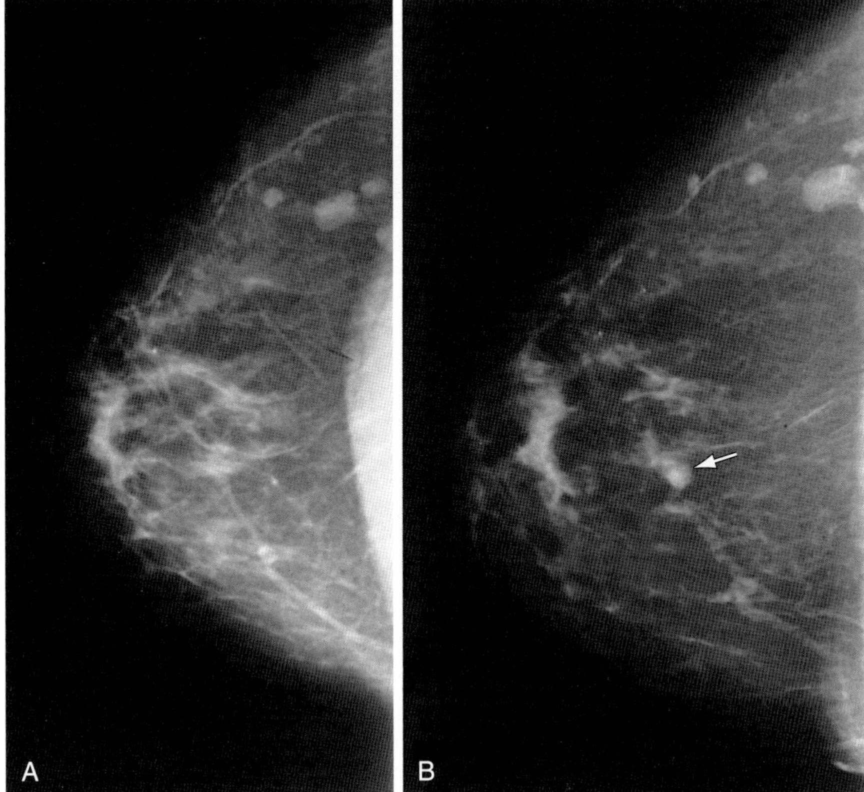

■ **FIGURE 22-14** Invasive ductal carcinoma, not otherwise specified (IDC, NOS), manifested as an asymmetry. **A,** Baseline mammogram showed only several benign oval, circumscribed masses representing intramammary lymph nodes. **B,** Mammogram obtained 1 year later shows a small asymmetry (*arrow*). Biopsy demonstrated IDC.

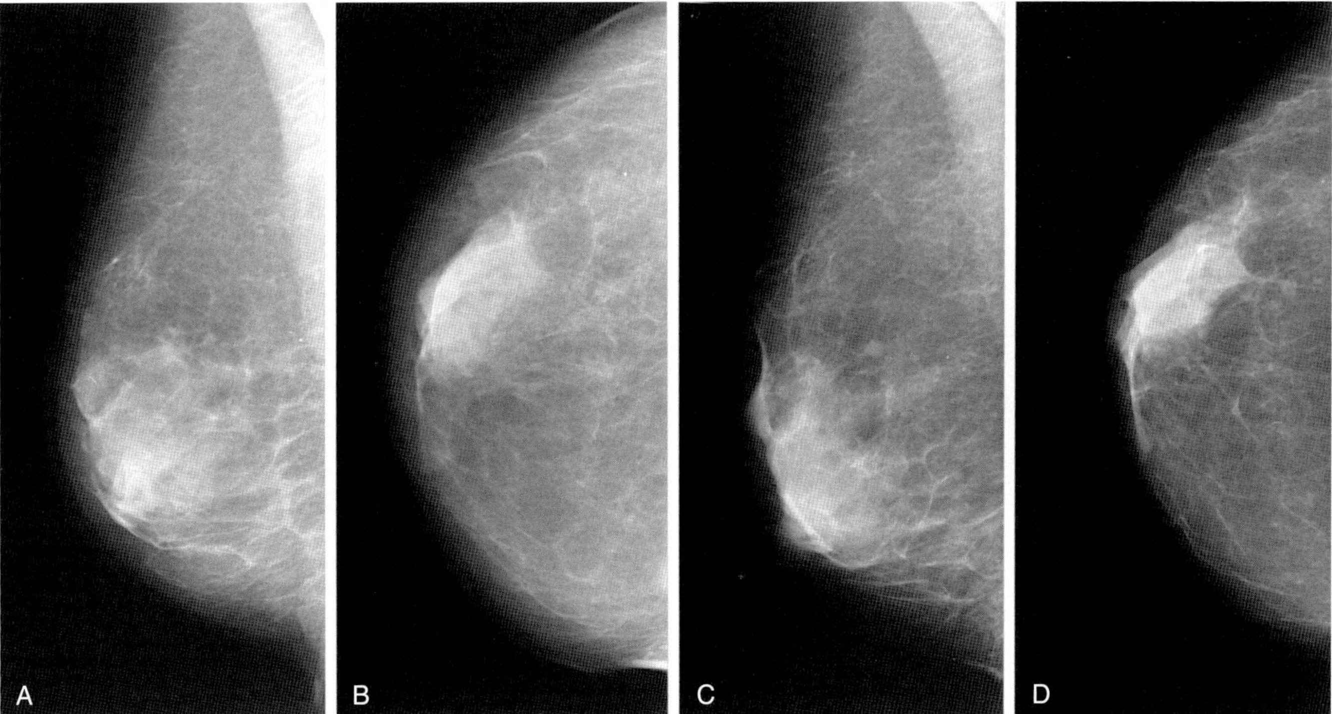

■ **FIGURE 22-15** Invasive ductal carcinoma, not otherwise specified (IDC, NOS), manifested as an asymmetry. Baseline mediolateral oblique (MLO) (**A**) and craniocaudal (CC) (**B**) mammograms showed no abnormalities. Screening MLO (**C**) and CC (**D**) mammograms obtained 1 year later show a new 5-mm asymmetry.

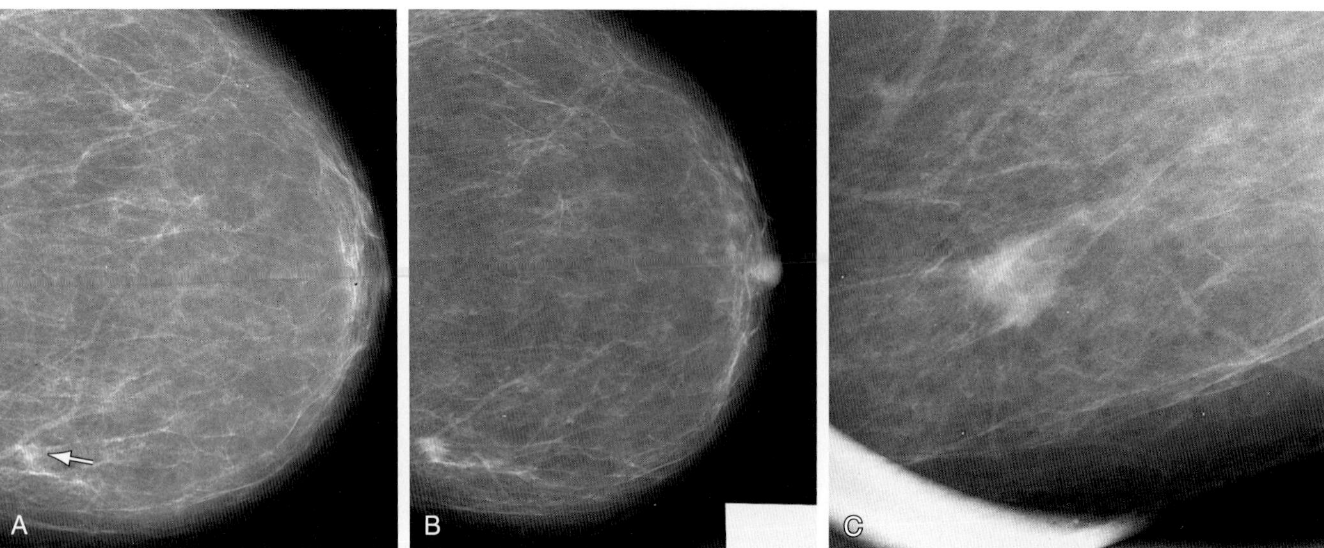

■ **FIGURE 22-16** Invasive ductal carcinoma, not otherwise specified (IDC, NOS), manifested by an evolving asymmetry. **A,** Left craniocaudal (CC) mammogram. A small asymmetry (*arrow*) in the medial aspect of the breast was not considered to be significant. Left CC (**B**) and spot compression magnification (**C**) views performed 1 year later reveal increased size and density of the asymmetry.

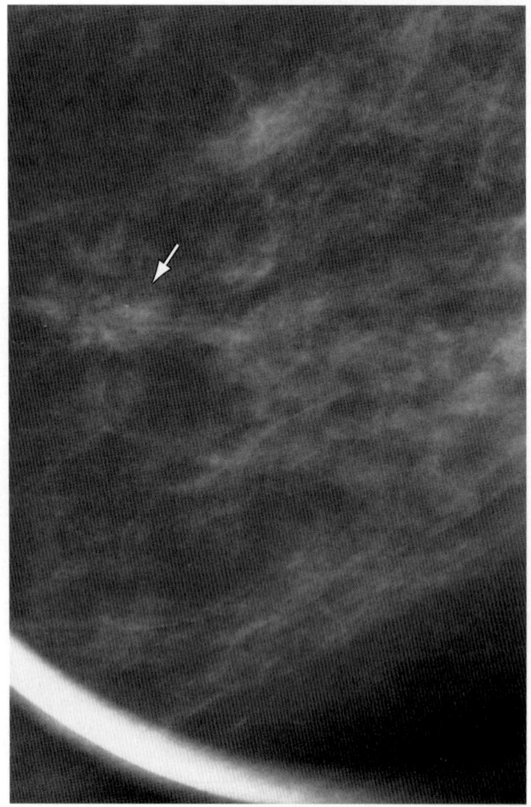

■ **FIGURE 22-17** Invasive ductal carcinoma, not otherwise specified (IDC, NOS), identified by architectural distortion. Spot compression magnification view demonstrates the architectural distortion (*arrow*) with no central mass.

Architectural distortions can also be associated with surgical and radial scars. Because postoperative scarring results in distortions of the parenchyma, it is important to be aware of the location of any previous operations.[35] The radiologic technologist should enter the location of visible scars on a diagram of the breast. Some radiologists find it useful for the radiologic technologist to place a wire directly over surgical scars before performing mammograms so that the exact site of the scar is indicated in the images.[36]

A radial scar, or radial sclerosing lesion (RSL), can also manifest mammographically as an architectural distortion or mass-like density. Typically, a radial scar can have a radiolucent center with radiating long, thin spicules. However, exceptions to these general rules are common, and it is not possible to differentiate radial scars from breast cancers mammographically.[37]

Asymmetry

Asymmetry refers to a relative increase in the volume of fibroglandular tissue compared with the contralateral breast. If this asymmetry occupies more than a quadrant of the breast the term *global asymmetry* can be applied and usually represents a normal variation in distribution of fibroglandular tissue. However, an asymmetry that is confined to an area no larger than a quadrant, is identifiable on orthogonal views and does not have the features of a mass (i.e., convex outward borders) may be termed a *focal asymmetry* and could represent a breast cancer. However this usually indicates an island of normal glandular tissue, especially if interspersed fat is present. To appreciate a parenchymal asymmetry, one must view the mammograms of the two breasts side by side and back to back. Because variations in the distribution of the parenchymal tissue occur normally, an unacceptably high rate of unnecessary false-negative biopsy findings would result if biopsy were performed for all asymmetric densities.

A biopsy is not indicated unless suspicious clinical or mammographic features are associated with the asymmetric density or is developing. Association of an asymmetric density with a palpable abnormality is of greater concern, and a biopsy should be considered in such cases (Fig. 22-20).

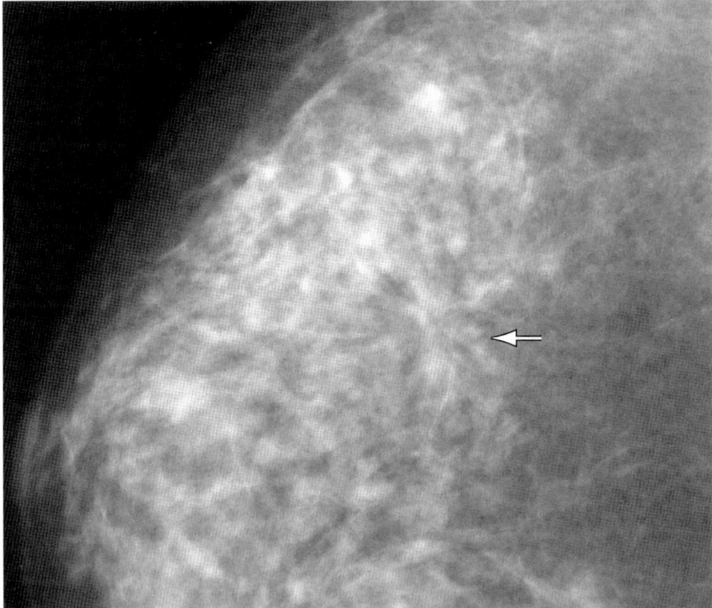

■ **FIGURE 22-18** Invasive ductal carcinoma, not otherwise specified (IDC, NOS), signified by architectural distortion (*arrow*).

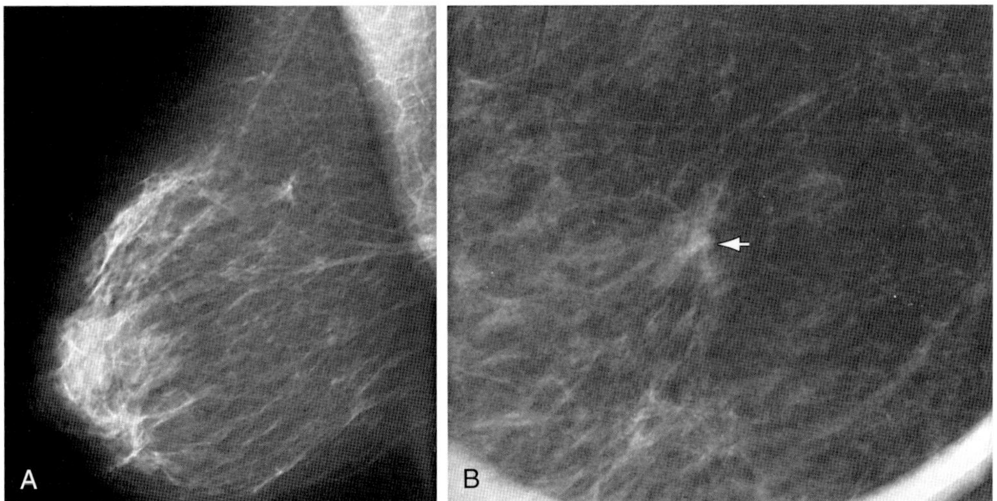

■ **FIGURE 22-19** Small invasive ductal carcinoma, not otherwise specified (IDC, NOS), signified by architectural distortion. **A,** Mediolateral oblique (MLO) mammogram shows an architectural distortion 8 mm in diameter (*arrow*). **B,** Close-up of spot compression view over the area of concern confirms the architectural distortion (*arrow*).

When a question exists as to the nature of a focal asymmetry, additional evaluation is warranted. Spot compression views usually show whether the area of increased asymmetric tissue is normal compressible tissue. Accessory breast tissue in the axilla is a common normal variant that should not be mistaken for a significant asymmetric density (Fig. 22-21). In addition, ultrasonography is a useful imaging modality to confirm benignity or detect an underlying lesion such as an ultrasonographic mass or architectural distortion.

Single Dilated Duct

Dilatation of a unilateral single subareolar duct has also been reported to be an indirect sign of an early carcinoma (Fig. 22-22).[33] However, this finding is rarely the presenting sign of malignancy. More often, a single dilated duct is due to duct ectasia or an intraductal papilloma. If mammography discloses suspicious calcifications or a spiculated mass at the site of the dilated duct, a biopsy should be considered. If a persistent, spontaneous, hemoglobin-positive nipple discharge is present, ductography, aspiration cytology, or biopsy is performed.

Ultrasonography

On ultrasonography, an IDC presents as a mass that is usually irregular in shape with indistinct (poorly defined) or spiculated margins. However, it can be seen as a round mass

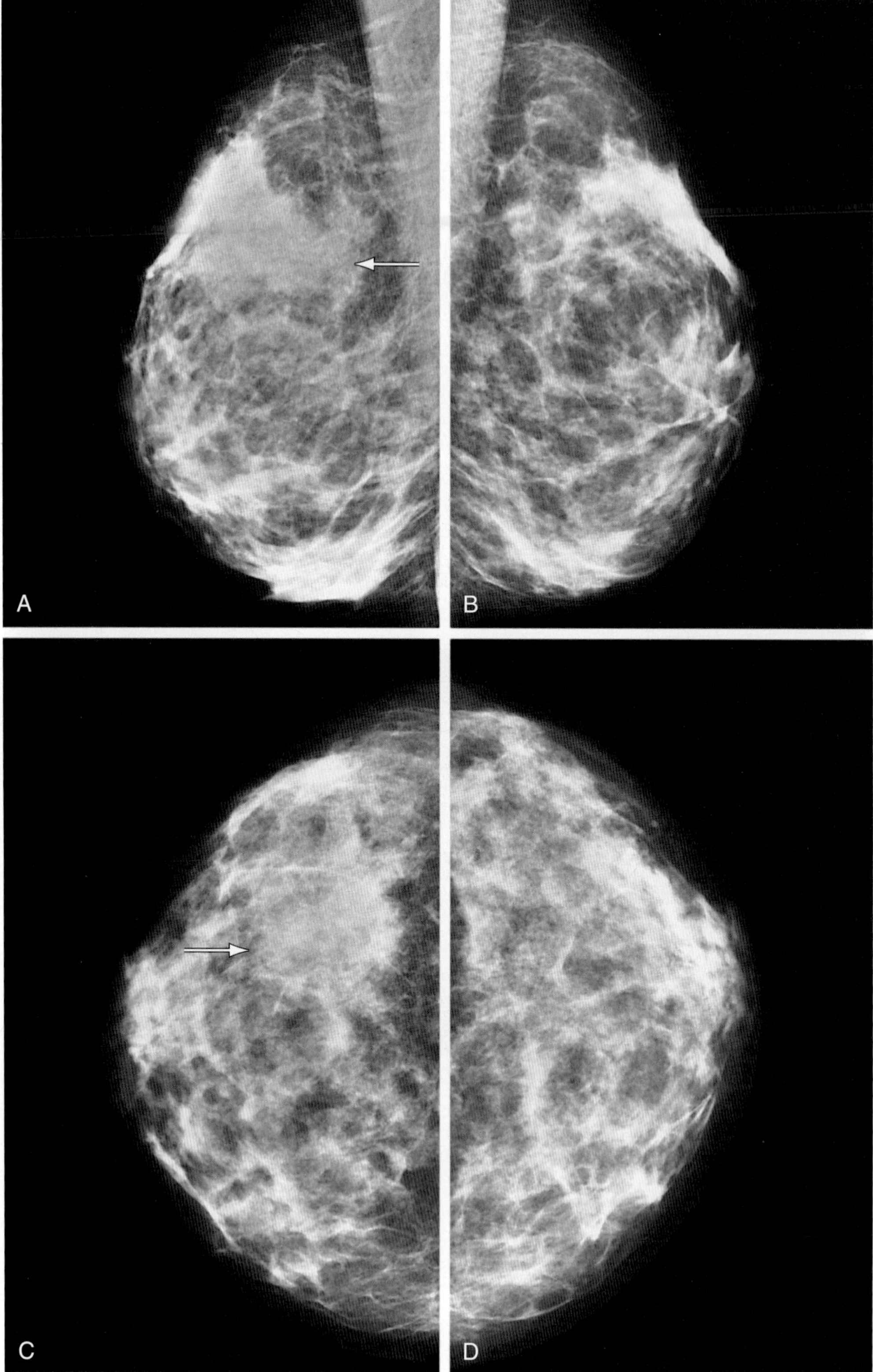

■ **FIGURE 22-20** Invasive ductal carcinoma, not otherwise specified (IDC, NOS), signified by asymmetric breast tissue. Right (**A**) and left (**B**) mediolateral oblique (MLO) views show global asymmetry with increased breast tissue (*arrow*) in the upper hemisphere. **C** and **D,** The asymmetric tissue (*arrow*) is confirmed on the craniocaudal (CC) views. A clinical breast examination was performed after the mammogram demonstrated discrete "thickening" in the right upper outer quadrant. A biopsy showed invasive carcinoma.

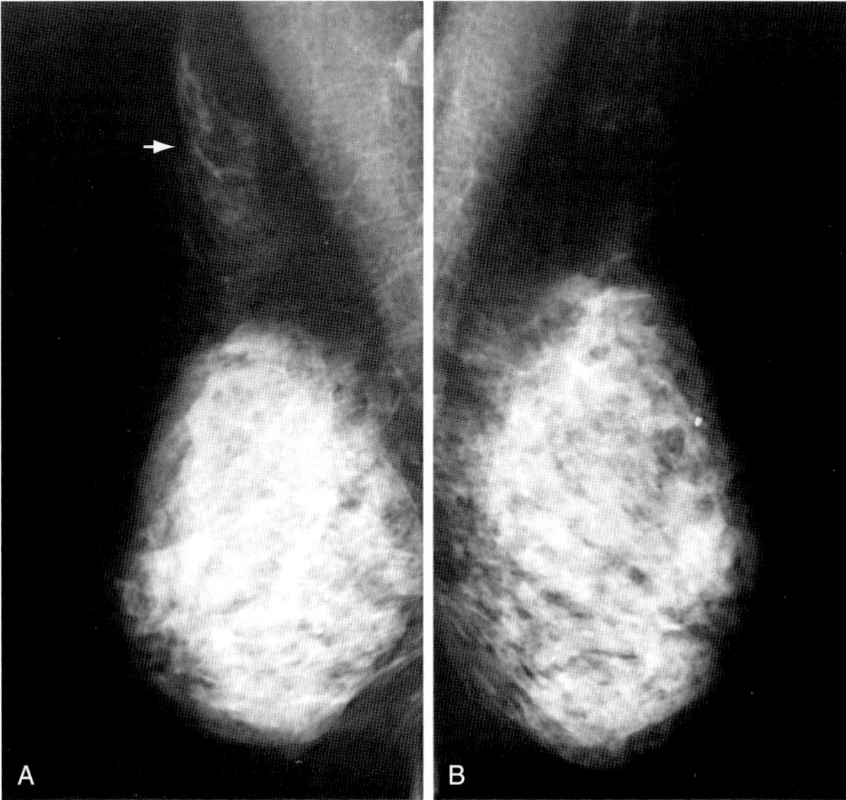

■ **FIGURE 22-21** Asymmetrical breast tissue in axilla. Right (**A**) and left (**B**) mediolateral oblique (MLO) views show an area of asymmetry (*arrow*) in the right axilla compatible with ectopic breast tissue. This asymmetric tissue is a normal variant.

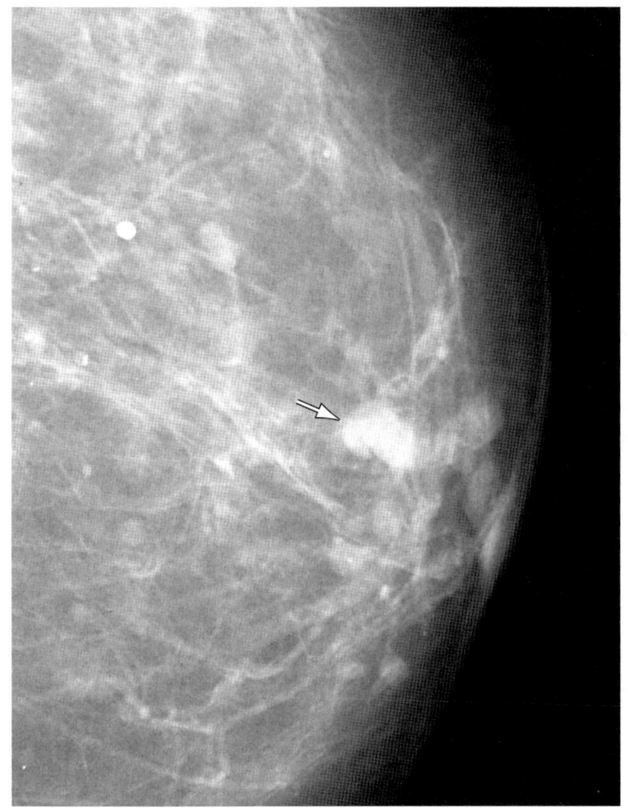

■ **FIGURE 22-22** Invasive ductal carcinoma manifesting as a unilateral, solitary, dilated duct. The dilated subareolar duct (*arrow*) was tortuous and not related to nipple discharge. (*Courtesy of R.J. Brenner, Los Angeles, Calif.*)

in some cases. Other common features include posterior acoustic shadowing due to fibrosis or tumor shadowing and a vertically oriented axis (an orientation that is not parallel to the skin line).

Magnetic resonance imaging

The typical magnetic resonance imaging (MRI) finding of IDC is an irregularly shaped mass with irregular or spiculated margins. Typical enhancement patterns include heterogeneous internal enhancement or rim enhancement, and the kinetic curve usually will demonstrate rapid and strong enhancement followed by rapid washout.

Differential Diagnosis

Clinical Presentation

The differential diagnosis includes benign breast process and malignancy depending on the clinical presentation, such as palpable mass or ill-defined skin thickening. Most of the clinical presentation with the differential diagnosis is discussed under the manifestations of disease in this chapter.

Imaging Findings

Most of the findings of mammographic and other modalities are discussed under the manifestations of disease in this chapter with differential diagnosis.

Pathology Findings

Gross Pathology

IDC usually forms a solid mass lesion with a firm, gray to white, stellate appearance on cut surface. Chalky white streaks can be seen, which usually implies necrosis. Fat necrosis also shows a similar gross appearance as IDC. Fat necrosis, however, shows more fatty and yellow color with a greasy cut surface. Peau d'orange appearance is seen in the inflammatory carcinoma (Fig. 22-23). Ulcerated mass is also seen in a neglected inflammatory breast carcinoma (Fig. 22-24). The gross measurement of IDC is more accurately determined than that for invasive lobular carcinoma. However, macroscopic gross examination of tumor size and microscopic tumor size were similar only 21% of the time.[38] Gross tumor size is an estimation of actual tumor size of invasive carcinoma. Underestimation occurs when the tumor cells are spreading into fat tissue without stromal fibrosis, and overestimation occurs when there is extensive intraductal component associated with periductal fibrosis. Also, sclerosing or fibrotic lesions can be palpable and mistaken for an invasive carcinoma grossly. Tumor configurations can be described at the time of gross examination as stellate, circumscribed, rounded, smooth, or encapsulated. In general, the gross examination of tumor parallels mammographic descriptions and size. The most accurate tumor size, and therefore final tumor size for staging, should be determined by the microscopic examination. The TNM classification is used for staging the breast carcinomas. The American Joint Committee on Cancer (AJCC) 2003 6th edition revised version and new AJCC 2009 version which is the most current staging classification is most commonly used for TNM stage. TNM staging is based on the primary tumor size (T), extent of regional axillary lymph node metastases (N), and extent of distant metastases (M) (Tables 22-1 and 22-2). Stage grouping is listed in Table 22-3.

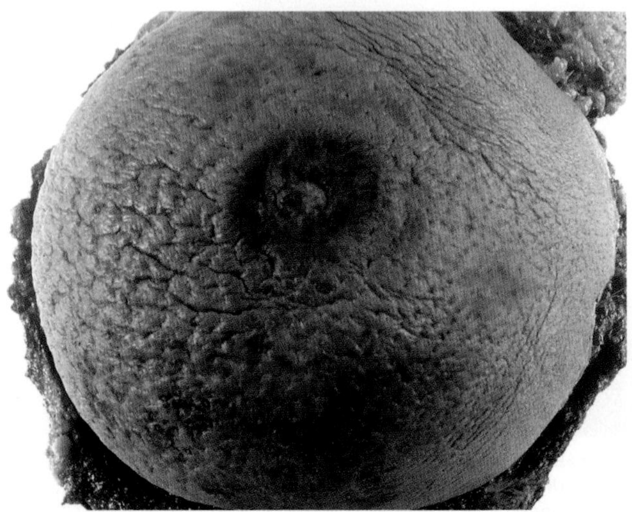

■ **FIGURE 22-23** Gross image of breast showing peau d'orange characteristic features of inflammatory carcinoma.

Histologic Grade

Invasive ductal carcinoma, not otherwise specified (IDC, NOS) type is the most common type of ductal carcinoma

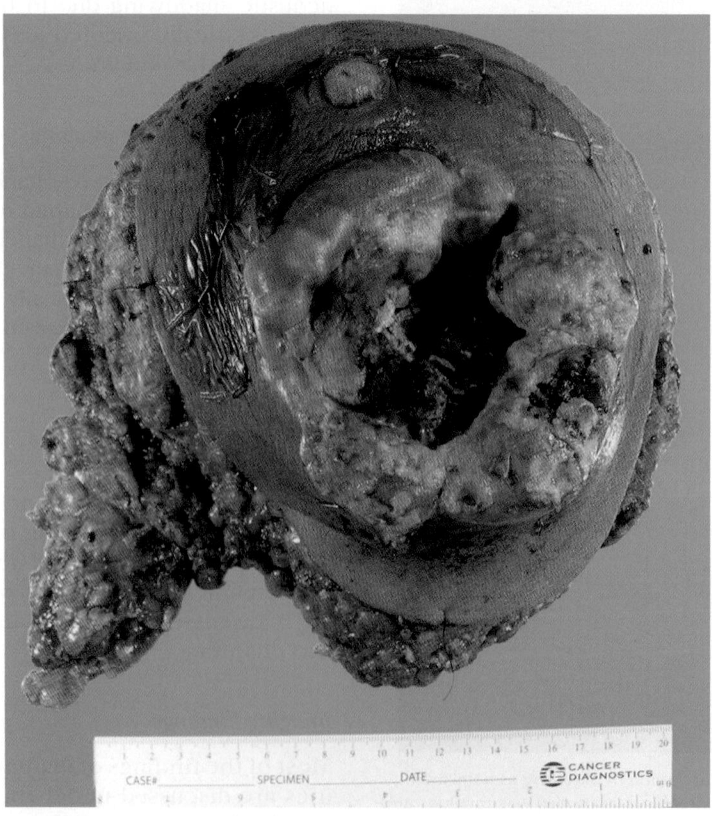

■ **FIGURE 22-24** Gross image of breast with skin ulceration and necrotic tumor, other features of advanced stage inflammatory carcinoma.

TABLE 22-1. Tumor, Node, Metastasis Staging System for Breast Cancer

Primary tumor (T)		
TX		Primary tumor cannot be assessed
T0		No evidence of primary tumor
Tis		Carcinoma in situ
	Tis (DCIS)	Ductal carcinoma in situ
	Tis (LCIS)	Lobular carcinoma in situ
	Tis (Paget)	Paget's disease of the nipple with no tumor. Note: Paget's disease associated with a tumor is classified according to the size of the tumor.
T1		Tumor ≤ 2 cm in greatest dimension
	T1mic	Microinvasion ≤ 0.1 cm in greatest dimension
	T1a	Tumor > 0.1 cm but not > 0.5 cm in greatest dimension
	T1b	Tumor > 0.5 cm but not > 1 cm in greatest dimension
	T1c	Tumor > 1 cm but not > 2 cm in greatest dimension
T2		Tumor > 2 cm but not >5 cm in greatest dimension
T3		Tumor > 5 cm in greatest dimension
T4		Tumor of any size with direct extension to
		(a) chest wall or
		(b) skin, only as described below
	T4a	Extension to chest wall, not including pectoralis muscle
	T4b	Edema (including peau d'orange) or ulceration of the skin of the breast, or satellite skin nodules confined to the same breast
	T4c	Both T4a and T4b
	T4d	Inflammatory carcinoma
Regional lymph nodes (N)		
pNX		Regional lymph nodes cannot be assessed (e.g., previously removed or not removed for pathologic study)
pN0		No regional lymph node metastasis histologically, no additional examination for isolated tumor cells
	pN0(i–)	No regional lymph node metastasis histologically, negative IHC finding for ITCs
	pN0(i+)	No regional lymph node metastasis histologically, positive morphologic and IHC findings for ITCs, no ITC cluster > 0.2 mm
	pN0(mol–)	No regional lymph node metastasis histologically, negative molecular findings (RT-PCR)
	pN0(mol+)	No regional lymph node metastasis histologically, positive molecular findings (RT-PCR)
	pN1mi	Micrometastasis (> 0.2 mm, none > 2.0 mm)
	pN1	Metastasis in one to three axillary lymph nodes and/or in internal mammary nodes with microscopic disease detected by sentinel lymph node dissection but not clinically apparent*
	pN1a	Metastasis in one to three axillary lymph nodes (at least 1 tumor deposit > 2.0 mm)
	pN1b	Metastasis in internal mammary nodes with microscopic disease detected by sentinel lymph node dissection but not clinically apparent
	pN1c	Metastasis in one to three axillary lymph nodes and in internal mammary lymph nodes with microscopic disease detected by sentinel lymph node dissection but not clinically apparent
pN2		Metastasis in four to nine lymph nodes, or in clinically apparent internal mammary lymph nodes in the absence of axillary lymph node metastasis
	pN2a	Metastasis in four to nine axillary lymph nodes (at least one tumor deposit > 2.0 mm)
	pN2b	Metastasis in clinically apparent internal mammary lymph nodes in the absence of axillary lymph node metastasis
pN3		Metastasis in 10 or more axillary lymph nodes, or in infraclavicular lymph nodes, or in clinically apparent ipsilateral internal mammary lymph nodes in the presence of one or more positive axillary lymph nodes, or in more than three axillary lymph nodes with clinically negative microscopic metastasis in internal mammary lymph nodes; or in ipsilateral supraclavicular lymph nodes

(Continued)

TABLE 22-1. Tumor, Node, Metastasis Staging System for Breast Cancer—Cont'd

Regional lymph nodes (N)	
pN3a	Metastasis in 10 or more axillary lymph nodes (at least one tumor deposit > 2.0 mm), or metastasis to the infraclavicular lymph nodes
pN3b	Metastasis in clinically apparent ipsilateral internal mammary lymph nodes in the presence of one or more positive axillary lymph nodes; or in more than three axillary lymph nodes and in internal mammary lymph nodes with microscopic disease detected by sentinel lymph node dissection but not clinically apparent
pN3c	Metastasis in ipsilateral supraclavicular lymph nodes
Distant metastasis (M)	
MX	Distant metastasis cannot be assessed
M0	No distant metastasis
M1	Distant metastasis

IHC, immunohistochemistry; ITC, isolated tumor cell; RT-PCR, reverse transcriptase polymerase chain reaction.
* "Clinically apparent" is defined as detected by imaging studies (excluding lymphoscintigraphy) or by clinical examination.
From The American Joint Committee on Cancer (AJCC) and the International Union Against Cancer (UICC): Cancer Staging Manual, 6th ed. New York: Springer, 2003.

TABLE 22-2. Pathologic Staging for Invasive Ductal Carcinoma (pT-NM)

TNM Descriptors (required only if applicable) (select all that apply)

___ m (multiple foci of invasive carcinoma)

___ r (recurrent)

___ y (post-treatment)

Primary Tumor (Invasive Carcinoma) (pT)

___ pTX: Primary tumor cannot be assessed

___ pT0: No evidence of primary tumor*

___ pTis (DCIS): Ductal carcinoma in situ*
___ pTis (LCIS): Lobular carcinoma in situ*

___ pTis (Paget): Paget's disease of the nipple *not* associated with invasive carcinoma and/or carcinoma in situ (DCIS and/or LCIS) in the underlying breast parenchyma*

pT1: Tumor ≤20 mm in greatest dimension

___ pT1mi: Tumor ≤1 mm in greatest dimension (microinvasion)

___ pT1a: Tumor >1 mm but ≤5 mm in greatest dimension

___ pT1b: Tumor >5 mm but ≤10 mm in greatest dimension

___ pT1c: Tumor >10 mm but ≤20 mm in greatest dimension

___ pT2: Tumor >20 mm but ≤50 mm in greatest dimension

___ pT3: Tumor >50 mm in greatest dimension

pT4: Tumor of any size with direct extension to the chest wall and/or to the skin (ulceration or skin nodules). ***Note:*** **Invasion of the dermis alone does not qualify as pT4.**

___ pT4a: Extension to chest wall, not including only pectoralis muscle adherence/invasion

___ pT4b: Ulceration and/or ipsilateral satellite nodules and/or edema (including peau d'orange) of the skin which do not meet the criteria for inflammatory carcinoma

___ pT4c: Both T4a and T4b

___ pT4d: Inflammatory carcinoma†

CAP Approved Breast – Invasive Carcinoma of the Breast

*Data elements with asterisks are not required. However, these elements may be clinically important but are not yet validated or regularly used in patient management.

(Continued)

TABLE 22-2. Pathologic Staging for Invasive Ductal Carcinoma (pT-NM)—Cont'd

Regional Lymph Nodes (pN) (choose a category based on lymph nodes received with the specimen; immunohistochemistry and/or molecular studies are not required) If internal mammary lymph nodes, infraclavicular nodes, or supraclavicular lymph nodes are included in the specimen, consult the *AJCC Cancer Staging Manual* for additional lymph node categories.

***Modifier* (required only if applicable)**

___ (sn): Only sentinel node(s) evaluated. If six or more sentinel nodes and/or nonsentinel nodes are removed, this modifier should not be used.

Category (pN)‡

___ pNX: Regional lymph nodes cannot be assessed (e.g., previously removed, or not removed for pathologic study)

___ pN0: No regional lymph node metastasis identified histologically

___ pN0 (i-): No regional lymph node metastases histologically, negative IHC

___ pN0 (i+): Malignant cells in regional lymph node(s) no greater than 0.2 mm and no more than 200 cells (detected by H&E or IHC including ITC)

___ pN0 (mol-): No regional lymph node metastases histologically, negative molecular findings (reverse transcriptase polymerase chain reaction [RT-PCR])

___ pN0 (mol+): Positive molecular findings (RT-PCR), but no regional lymph node metastases detected by histology or IHC

___ pN1mi: Micrometastases (greater than 0.2 mm and/or more than 200 cells, but none greater than 2.0 mm)

___ pN1a: Metastases in one to three axillary lymph nodes, at least 1 metastasis > 2.0 mm

___ pN2a: Metastases in four to nine axillary lymph nodes (at least 1 tumor deposit > 2.0 mm)

___ pN3a: Metastases in 10 or more axillary lymph nodes (at least 1 tumor deposit > 2.0 mm)

CAP Approved Breast – Invasive Carcinoma of the Breast

*Data elements with asterisks are not required. However, these elements may be clinically important but are not yet validated or regularly used in patient management.

The pathologist should use judgment regarding whether it is likely that the cluster of cells represents a true micrometastasis or is simply a small group of isolated tumor cells.

Distant Metastasis (M)

___ Not applicable

___ cM0(i+): No clinical or radiographic evidence of distant metastasis, but deposits of molecularly or microscopically detected tumor cells in circulating blood, bone marrow, or other nonregional nodal tissue that are ≤0.2 mm in a patient without symptoms or signs of metastasis

___ pMI: Distant detectable meatastasis as determined by classic clinical and radiographic means and/or histologically proven > 0.2mm

---

*For the purposes of this checklist, these categories should only be used in the setting of preoperative (neoadjuvant) therapy for which a previously diagnosed invasive carcinoma is no longer present after treatment.

†Inflammatory carcinoma is a clinical-pathologic entity characterized by diffuse erythema and edema (peau d'orange) involving one third or more of the skin of the breast. The skin changes are due to lymphedema caused by tumor emboli within dermal lymphatics, which may or may not be obvious in a small skin biopsy. However, a tissue diagnosis is still necessary to demonstrate an invasive carcinoma in the underlying breast parenchyma or at least in the dermal lymphatics, as well as to determine biological markers, such as estrogen receptor, progesterone receptor, and HER-2 status. Tumor emboli in dermal lymphatics without the clinical skin changes described above do not qualify as inflammatory carcinoma. Locally advanced breast cancers directly invading the dermis or ulcerating the skin without the clinical skin changes and tumor emboli in dermal lymphatics also do not qualify as inflammatory carcinoma. Thus the term inflammatory carcinoma should not be applied to neglected locally advanced cancer of the breast presenting late in the course of a patient's disease. The rare case that exhibits all the features of inflammatory carcinoma, but in which skin changes involve less than one third of the skin, should be classified by the size and extent of the underlying carcinoma.

‡For category pN, Isolated tumor cell (ITC) clusters are defined as small clusters of cells not greater than 0.2 mm or single tumor cells, or a cluster of fewer than 200 cells in a single histologic cross-section§. ITCs may be detected by routine histology or by immunohistochemical (IHC) methods. Nodes containing only ITCs are excluded from the total positive node count for purposes of N classification but should be included in the total number of nodes evaluated.

§Approximately 1000 tumor cells are contained in a 3-dimensional 0.2 mm cluster. Thus, if more than 200 individual tumor cells are identified as single dispersed tumor cells or as a nearly confluent elliptical or spherical focus in a single histologic section of a lymph node, there is a high probability that more than 1000 cells are present in the node. In these situations, the node should be classified as containing a micrometastasis (pN1mi). Cells in different lymph node cross sections or longitudinal sections or levels of the block are not added together; the 200 cells must be in a single node profile even if the node has been thinly sectioned into multiple slices. It is recognized that there is substantial overlap between the upper limit of the ITC and the lower limit of the micrometastasis categories because of inherent limitations in pathologic nodal evaluation and detection of minimal tumor burden in lymph nodes. Thus, the threshold of 200 cells in a single cross-section is a guideline to help pathologists distinguish between these two categories.

From The American Joint Committee on Cancer (AJCC) and the International Union Against Cancer (UICC): Cancer Staging Manual, 7th ed. New York: Springer, 2009.

TABLE 22-3. Tumor, Node, Metastasis Stage Grouping for Breast Cancer

Stage	Grouping		
0	Tis	N0	M0
I			
1A	T1mic	N0	M0
1B	T0	N1mi	M0
	T1mic	N1mi	M0
IIA	T0	N1mi	M0
	T1mic	N1mi	M0
	T2	N0	M0
IIB	T2	N1	M0
	T3	N0	M0
IIIA	T0	N2	M0
	T1mic	N2	M0
	T2	N2	M0
	T3	N1	M0
	T3	N2	M0
IIIB	T4	N0	M0
	T4	N1	M0
	T4	N2	M0
IIIC	Any T	N3	M0
IV	Any T	Any N	M1

TABLE 22-4. Mitotic Count Score Categories Based on Field Diameter of Microscope

Field diameter (mm)	Area (mm²)	Number of mitoses per 10 fields corresponding to: Score 1	Score 2	Score 3
0.40	0.125	≤4	5 to 9	≥10
0.41	0.132	≤4	5 to 9	≥10
0.42	0.139	≤5	6 to 10	≥11
0.43	0.145	≤5	6 to 10	≥11
0.44	0.152	≤5	6 to 11	≥12
0.45	0.159	≤5	6 to 11	≥12
0.46	0.166	≤6	7 to 12	≥13
0.47	0.173	≤6	7 to 12	≥13
0.48	0.181	≤6	7 to 13	≥14
0.49	0.189	≤6	7 to 13	≥14
0.50	0.196	≤7	8 to 14	≥15
0.51	0.204	≤7	8 to 14	≥15
0.52	0.212	≤7	8 to 15	≥16
0.53	0.221	≤8	9 to 16	≥17
0.54	0.229	≤8	9 to 16	≥17
0.55	0.238	≤8	9 to 17	≥18
0.56	0.246	≤8	9 to 17	≥18
0.57	0.255	≤9	10 to 18	≥19
0.58	0.264	≤9	10 to 19	≥20
0.59	0.273	≤9	10 to 19	≥20
0.60	0.283	≤10	11 to 20	≥21
0.61	0.292	≤10	11 to 21	≥22
0.62	0.302	≤11	12 to 22	≥23
0.63	0.312	≤11	12 to 22	≥23
0.64	0.322	≤11	12 to 23	≥24
0.65	0.332	≤12	13 to 24	≥25
0.66	0.342	≤12	13 to 24	≥25
0.67	0.353	≤12	13 to 25	≥26
0.68	0.363	≤13	14 to 26	≥27
0.69	0.374	≤13	14 to 27	≥28

Adapted from Pathology Reporting of Breast Disease. Copyright 2005 National Health Service Cancer Screening Programme and The Royal College of Pathologists.

(~80% of all breast cancer). The terms "infiltrative" and "invasive" are synonymous. The histologic appearance of IDC, NOS type is heterogeneous depending on nuclear grades, tubule formations, and the number of mitotic figures. The grading system is known as Modified Scarff-Bloom and Richardson grade and score (SBR).

Tubule formation:
- >75% of the tumor 1
- 10%-75% 2
- <10 % 3

Nuclear pleomorphism:
- Small regular, uniform cells 1
- Moderate increase in size with variability 2
- Marked variation 3

Mitotic counts of tumor:
- Score 1: (see Table 3)
- Score 2:
- Score 3:
- (Using 10 high power fields (HPF) with 40× objective: Table 22-4)

All the scores are added together and when the points are between 3 and 5, 6 and 7, or greater than 8, they are designated as well differentiated (Grade 1), moderately differentiated (Grade 2), and poorly differentiated (Grade 3) IDC, respectively (Figs. 22-25 to 22-27). The nuclear grade is the same as DCIS nuclear grade (Figs. 22-28 to 22-30). There is a substantial level of interobserver and even intraobserver differences in histologic grades. The subjectivity is induced by variable factors, such as areas of counting mitotic figures and technical variability such as fixation. Most pathologists count 10 HPFs; some use consecutive 10 HPFs and others use selected fields that will induce the highest mitotic figures. The exact method of counting mitotic figures has not been well established or standardized. It is recommended to count mitotic figures in most cellular tumor foci and at the periphery of the tumor where tumor cells are actively proliferating. The Bloom and Richardson study showed that the most common grade of tumor is moderately differentiated (Grade 2) IDC, comprising 45%, followed by 29% of poorly differentiated (Grade 3), and 26% of well-differentiated (Grade 1) IDC in their 1409 patients. They found that the tumor grade and frequency of axillary metastasis correlated well,

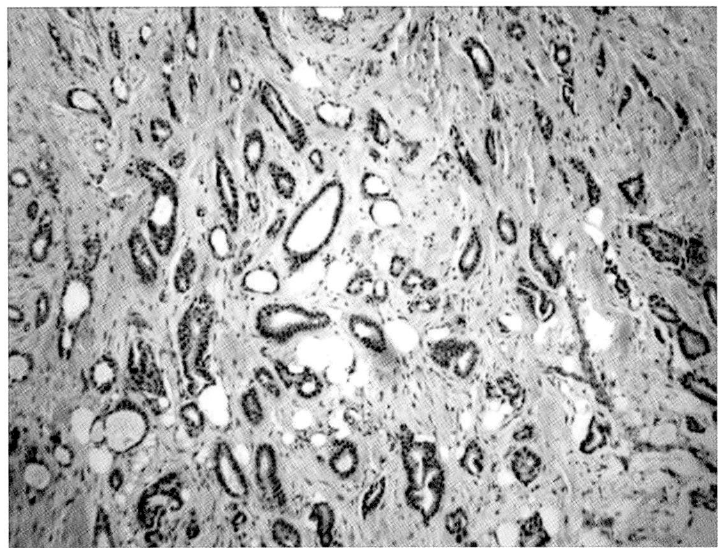

■ **FIGURE 22-25** Well-differentiated invasive ductal carcinoma (IDC). Most of the tumor cells are forming a glandular or tubular pattern (H&E, ×100).

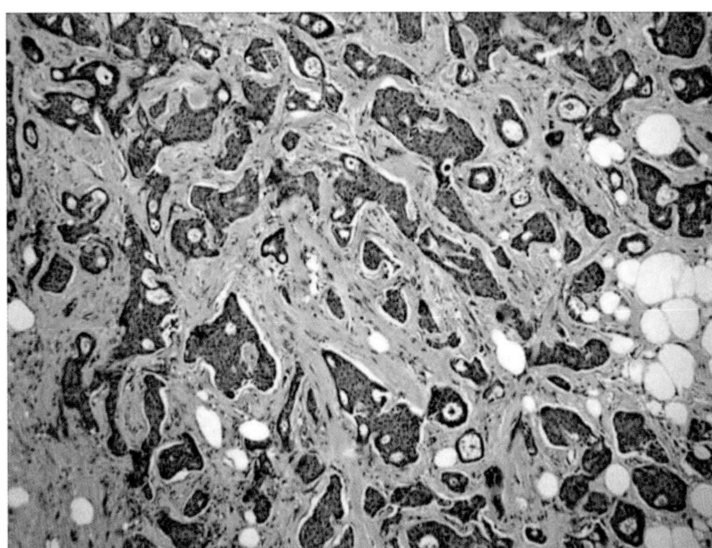

■ **FIGURE 22-26** Moderately differentiated invasive ductal carcinoma (IDC). Tubule formation is greater than 10% but less than 75% (H&E, ×100).

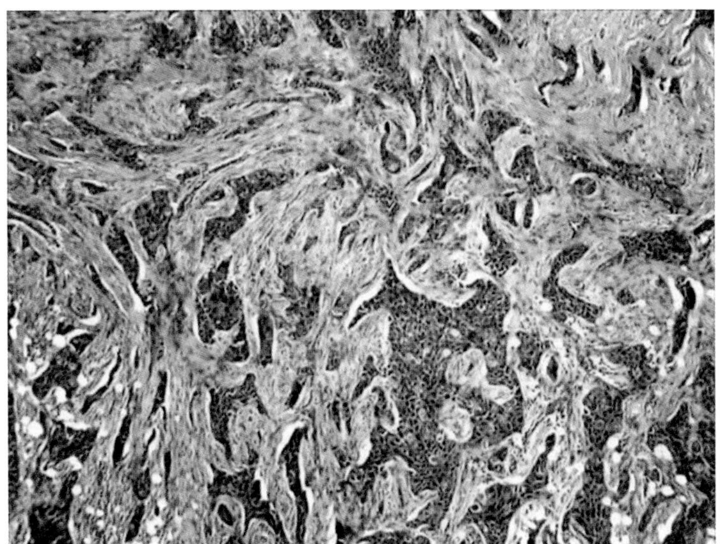

■ **FIGURE 22-27** Poorly differentiated invasive ductal carcinoma (IDC). No tubular formation is noted (H&E, ×100).

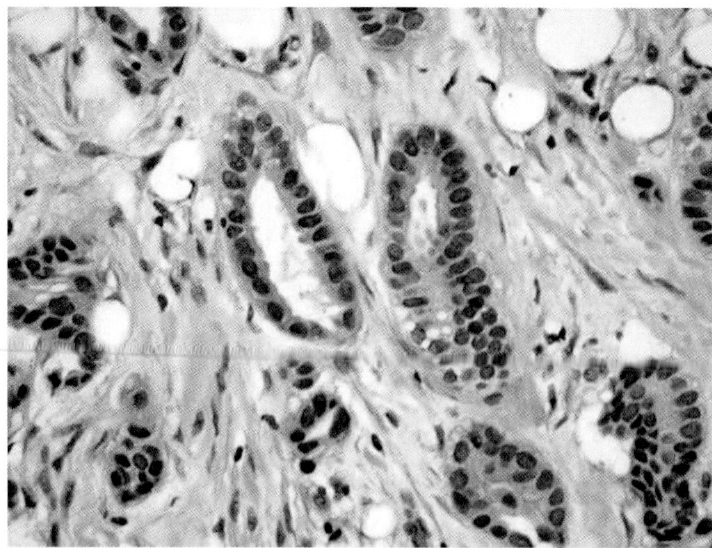

■ **FIGURE 22-28** Low nuclear grade with small, regular and uniform nuclear size without variability (H&E, ×400).

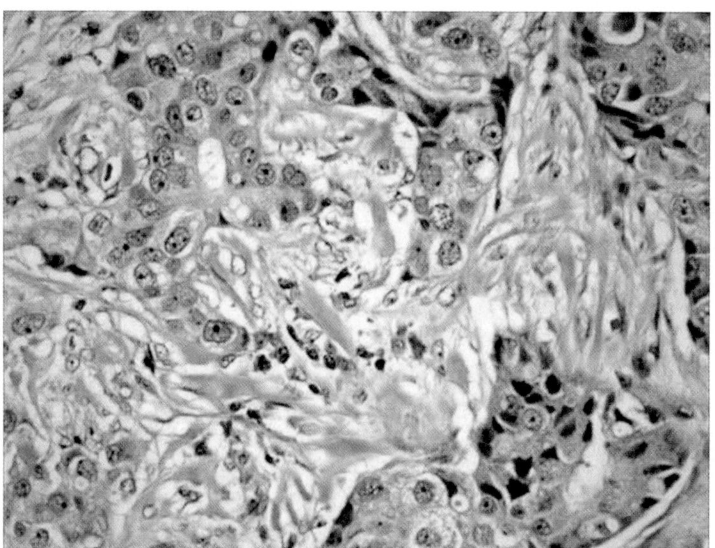

■ **FIGURE 22-29** Intermediate nuclear grade. Moderate increase in nuclear size with variable shapes (H&E, ×400).

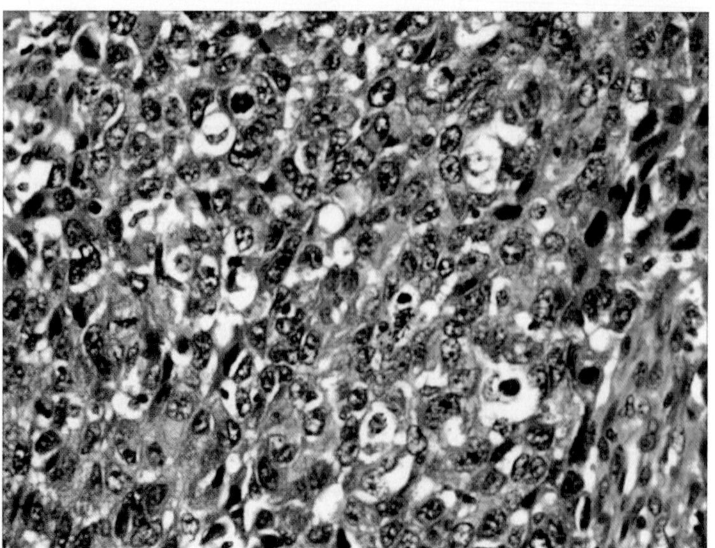

■ **FIGURE 22-30** High nuclear grade with marked variation in nuclear sizes and shapes with vesiculated nuclei (open chromatin) (H&E, ×400).

TABLE 22-5. Survival Rate with Grade of Tumor Based on Lymph Node Status

Grade	Node-negative	Node-positive
5-Year Survival Rate		
1	86%	66%
2	66%	33%
3	64%	19%
10-Year survival rate		
1	61%	51%
2	47%	14%
3	42%	9%
15-Year Survival rate		
1	49%	15%
2	29%	11%
3	25%	7%

and the survival rate is directly associated with axillary lymph node metastatic rate (Table 22-5).

Numerous other studies have been validating the survival rate related to lymph node metastasis which correlates with tumor grading. SBR grading should be a part of the routine pathology report of an IDC. Other descriptions in the pathology microscopic examination sections should contain the following items:

1. Tumor type
2. Tumor grade (SBR score)
3. Presence or absence of DCIS with types, necrosis and nuclear grade
4. Extensive intraductal component: present or absent
5. Size of invasive tumor
6. Margins status
7. Microcalcifications: absent or present associated with type of lesions
8. Lymph-vascular invasion: present or absent
9. Benign breast tissue characteristics including documentation of prior biopsy site and other significant findings (i.e., fibroadenoma, papilloma)
10. Skin/nipple: presence or absence of Paget's disease; presence or absence of dermal lymphatic invasion
11. Lymph node status:
    a. number of lymph nodes
    b. positive metastatic lymph nodes
    c. size of metastatic tumor (macrometastasis, micrometastasis, or isolated tumor cells)
    d. Extracapsular invasion: present or absent
12. Breast biomarkers studies
13. TNM stage (see Tables 22-1 and 22-2)

Microinvasive Carcinoma

Microinvasion (T1 mic) is defined as an invasive focus of 0.1 cm or less in greatest dimension (Fig. 22-31). Diagnosing microinvasion is one of the most challenging areas in pathology and hence often resulting in uncertainty in the report with such caveats as "cannot rule out microinvasion, highly suspicious for microinvasion, etc." Microinvasion is suspected when the tumor cells are separated from the DCIS or protruding from the DCIS, breaking through the myoepithelial cells and basement membrane, and often eliciting lymphohistiocytic and stromal desmoplastic responses. Tangentially cut DCIS can mimic microinvasive carcinoma. Isolated individual tumor cells or rare small clusters of tumor cells located in periductal and perilobular stroma can be seen. Microinvasive carcinoma should have no myoepithelial cells, and hence immunohistochemical (IHC) stains can be helpful to confirm invasion. Microinvasive carcinoma is often associated with high-grade comedo-type DCIS. There is no consensus as to the amount or extent of invasive carcinoma to qualify as microinvasion. The definition of microinvasion varies

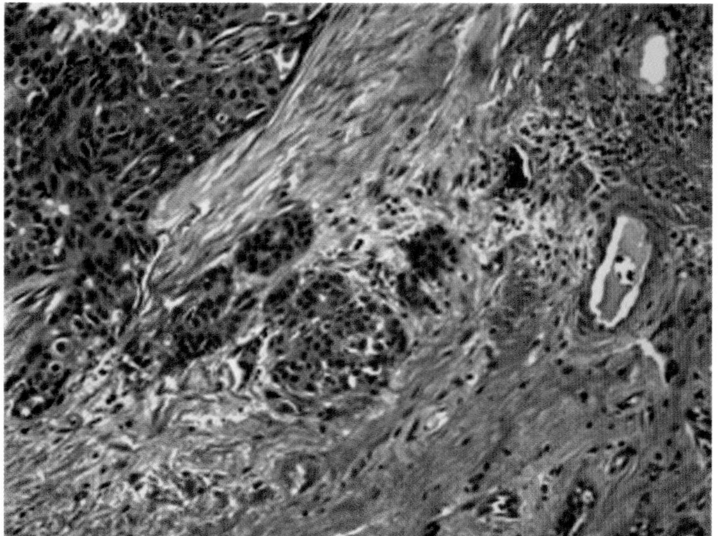

■ **FIGURE 22-31** Microinvasive ductal carcinoma. Small islands of invasive carcinoma cells are seen adjacent to large area of ductal carcinoma in situ (DCIS). Stroma shows mild degree of desmoplasia and inflammatory cells (H&E, ×100).

from no qualifying amount of invasive cells, microscopic focus of malignant cells, maximum extent of invasion of less than 2 mm or invasive carcinoma comprising less than 10% of the tumor, one or two microscopic foci of possible invasion no more than 1 mm in maximum diameter, and single focus of invasive carcinoma less than 2 mm or up to three foci of invasion each 1 mm or less in greatest dimension from various authors in the literature.

A false-positive finding for microinvasion is due to misinterpreting cancerization of lobules (COL), radial scar, or sclerosing adenosis associated with DCIS. A false-negative finding for microinvasion occurs when the invasive area is masked by heavy lymphohistiocytic infiltrates. Sentinel lymph node procurement is recommended with microinvasive carcinoma. Foci of microinvasive carcinoma should not be added together for the final size. For cases in which there are multiple areas of microinvasive tumors within one slide, or multiple slides, the largest linear dimension of one focus of microinvasive tumor is the final size for the T stage. Overall grade or modified Bloom and Richardson score is not given for microinvasive carcinoma.

Extensive Intraductal Components

The term *extensive intraductal component* (EIC) is used when DCIS is present in substantial amount in association with invasive carcinoma. The definition of substantial amount differs with each author but, in general, EIC-positive tumor is defined when DCIS is present in more than or equal to 25% of tumor volume within the area of the invasive tumor and/or beyond the edges of the invasive tumor. EIC also applies to predominant DCIS seen with multiple or single areas of invasive tumor. An accurate size of invasive tumor can be difficult to assess when there is a minimal amount of invasive tumor within the entire bed of EIC. Although the invasive tumor is measured from one end to another as the maximum linear dimension, the volume or tumor burden of invasive tumor is not equivalent to a situation in which the invasive tumor is nodular, involving the entire length of the area without skip areas (Fig. 22-32). The pathology report should clearly indicate the amount of the invasive tumor in this situation. The presence of EIC is associated with a higher risk of local recurrence than tumors that lack an EIC. Also, significant residual DCIS is found on re-excision when EIC is present on the initial lumpectomy.[39] Others have found that the presence of EIC was not associated with increased risk of local recurrence.[40] In this particular study, however, patients with positive margins of excision were excluded and some of these patients may have had EIC-positive cases. EIC-positive tumors are frequently associated with positive margins on breast-conserving surgery. Several other data suggest that the presence of EIC is not an independent predictor of local recurrence when the microscopic margins are taken into consideration. Despite the conflicting data, the majority of the EIC-positive tumors can be suspected on imaging studies, and this may serve to guide the surgical treatment as the extent of excision.

Perineural Invasion

Perineural invasion can be seen in approximately 10% of invasive carcinoma, more commonly with invasive lobular carcinoma than IDC. Perineural invasion has not been proven to be of independent prognostic significance. It is when the clusters of tumor cells are seen around the perineurium. Neural invasion is defined as clusters of tumor cells actually within the neural tissue itself (Fig. 22-33).

Lymph-Vascular Invasion

Lymph-vascular invasion (LVI) is defined as tumor cells found within lymphatic vessels. Lymphatic vessels are often seen juxtaposed and adjacent to arterioles and venules. The superficial dermis also contains many

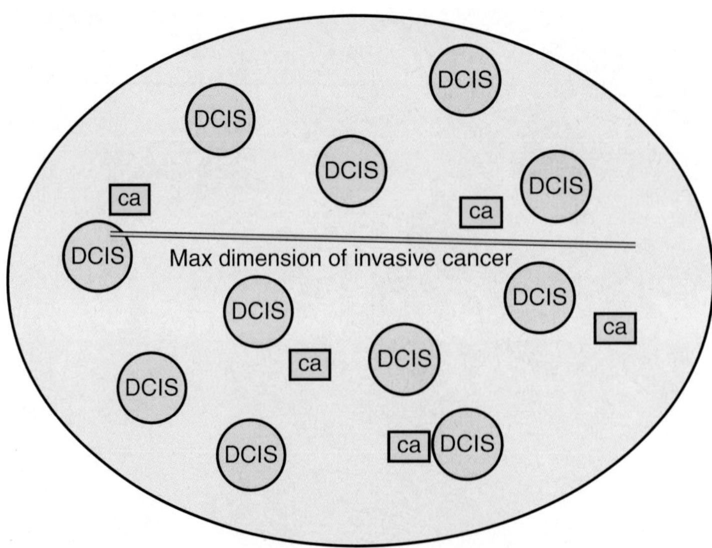

■ **FIGURE 22-32** Diagram showing extensive intraductal component as *circles* and invasive carcinoma as *squares*. Maximum linear dimension of the invasive carcinoma is artificially larger than the actual tumor volume.

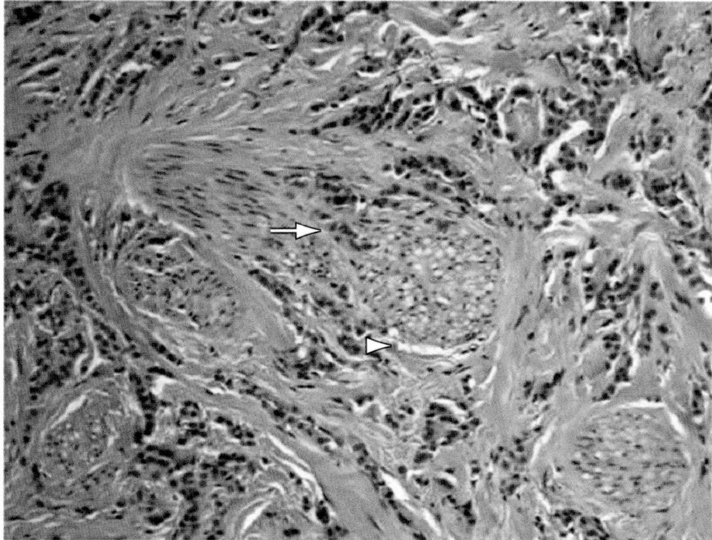

■ **FIGURE 22-33** Perineural invasion by tumor cells (H&E, ×200). Peripheral nerve with area of perineurium (*arrowhead*) with tumor cell infiltrating (*arrow*).

lymph-vascular spaces, and tumor emboli can be seen (Figs. 22-34 and 22-35). Lymphatic vessels are lined by flattened endothelial cells and devoid of red blood cells within the lymphatic spaces. Reproducibility of LVI among pathologists is poor owing to many other situations mimicking LVI, such as shrinkage artifact in which artifactual spaces are formed around nests of tumor cells (DCIS) most likely caused by tissue processing (Fig. 22-36). Micropapillary type invasive mammary carcinoma has a significant amount of clefting artifact that mimics LVI (Fig. 22-37). A reliable way to confirm LVI is by using IHC stains, such as factor VIII, CD 34, CD 31, and, more recently, D2-40 which highlights the endothelial cells around the lymph-vascular spaces. However, difficulty lies when the small area suspicious for LVI is no longer present in the deeper sections when IHC stain studies are performed. The best area to look for LVI is the extratumoral area to avoid shrinkage artifact. Extratumoral LVI occurs in approximately 15% of IDC, and 5% to 10% of the time LVI is seen without lymph node metastasis. LVI is an unfavorable prognostic indicator even when pathologically negative axillary lymph nodes are found. Vascular invasion by tumor emboli can be seen, and death due to metastatic carcinoma is reported with significantly greater frequency. Vascular invasion is a predictor of local recurrence and a lower survival rate. The distinction between LVI and vascular invasion, especially small capillary size vessels, is not clear cut.

Breast Biomarkers

Estrogen receptor (ER), progesterone receptor (PR), human epidermal growth factor receptor 2 (HER-2/neu), and Ki-67 are most commonly evaluated as breast

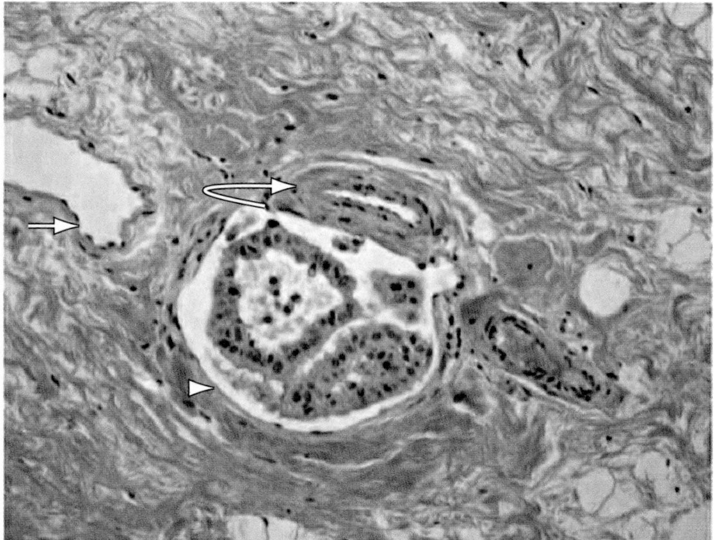

■ **FIGURE 22-34** Lymph-vascular invasion (LVI) is seen. Note the adjacent arteriole (*curved arrow*) and venule (*arrow*) and dilated lymphatic space filled with tumor cells (*arrowhead*) (H&E, × 400).

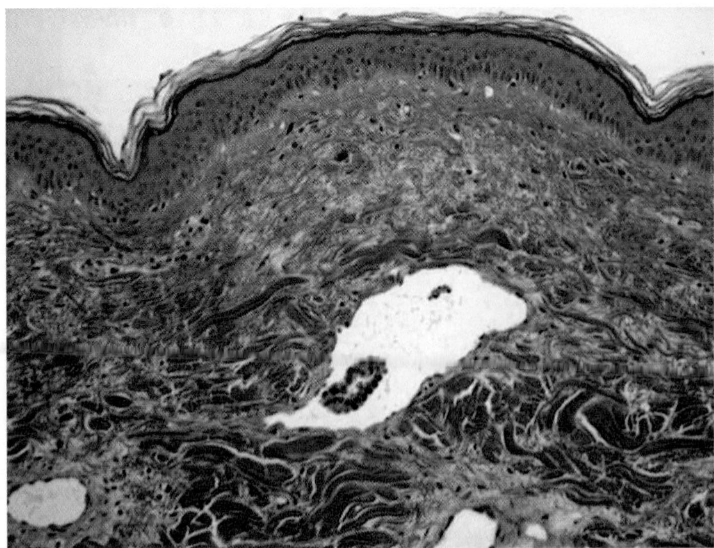

■ FIGURE 22-35 Skin epidermis and underlying superficial dermis with lymph-vascular invasion (LVI) (H&E, ×200).

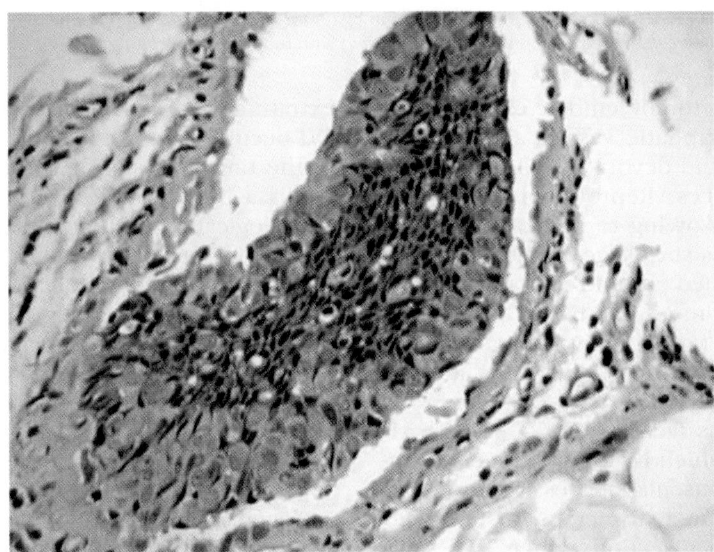

■ FIGURE 22-36 Ductal carcinoma in situ (DCIS) with significant degree of clefting artifact due to tissue processing. This can mimic lymph-vascular invasion (LVI) (H&E, ×200).

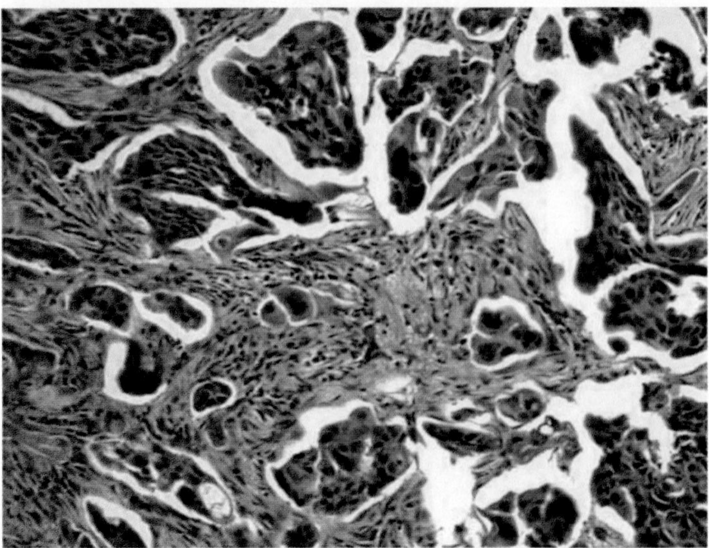

■ FIGURE 22-37 Micropapillary invasive carcinoma showing significant degree of clefting around the tumor cell nests. This is also a mimicker of lymph-vascular invasion (LVI) (H&E, ×200).

biomarkers for invasive mammary carcinoma. Other biomarkers, such as TP53, DNA ploidy studies, and epidermal growth factor receptor (EGFR) are done at some institutions but have limited predictive function at this time.

ER and PR studies by IHC analysis are strong predictive markers of response to tamoxifen-based therapy. The receptors are weak prognostic markers of clinical outcome such as probability of recurrence and disease-free and overall survival. IHC analysis of endocrine receptors has replaced ligand-binding assays in most pathology laboratories. Ligand-binding assay requires fresh frozen tissue, whereas IHC assays can be done in formalin-fixed paraffin-embedded tissue blocks. All IHC studies are affected by preanalytical factors such as type of fixative used, prolonged time before fixation, "ischemic time," duration of fixation, antigen retrieval techniques, and choice of antibodies used. IHC assays for ER and PR are not consistent among pathology laboratories. Also, the discordant rate of ER and PR biomarkers between the core needle biopsy (CNB) and excisional biopsy ranges from 0% to 38% in the current published studies within the same laboratory. One of the reasons for discrepancy is because of difference in fixation time. The ideal fixation time is reported to be 6 to 8 hours as minimum and not longer than 72 hours as maximum in 10% buffer formalin for both core needle and excisional biopsies by Goldstein and coworkers.[41] For core needle biopsy specimens, radiologists who perform the procedure need to document when the core specimens are placed in 10% buffered formalin to track how long tissue is fixed. For excisional biopsy specimens, pathologists need to document when specimens are placed in 10% buffered formalin. For excisional specimen, the largest invasive carcinoma block should be used to test for biomarker studies. If smaller invasive carcinomas are of different histologic type or of higher grade, additional biomarkers should be also done. At the present time, it is not known whether CNB or excisional breast biomarkers results are more reliable; however, based on the report of Mann and coworkers,[42] CNB may have better sensitivity and, hence, receptor studies should be performed on CNB samples rather than on excisional biopsies. Most common ER antibodies used in U.S. laboratories are 6F11, ID5, and SP1. SP1 is a rabbit monoclonal antibody, and it is known to have higher affinity and be more robust when compared with other antibodies. Most breast cancers are either strongly and diffusely ER positive or clearly ER negative (Fig. 22-38). The definitions of what is ER positive and ER negative are not standardized and vary from laboratory to laboratory. A study by Viale and colleagues[43] reported that there is a significant discrepancy in interpretation of ER and PR from 6549 patient samples from 25 different countries between local and central laboratories. Local laboratories reported an ER-positive cutoff as 10% of tumor cells staining independent of intensity. A central laboratory reported an ER-positive cutoff as 1% of tumor cells staining. This study showed that a central laboratory confirmed 97% of ER-positive results from local laboratories. Approximately 1% of tumors assessed locally as ER positive were reclassified as ER-negative tumors after review at a central laboratory, and about 1% of tumors assessed locally as ER-negative tumors were reclassified as ER-positive tumors. Discordance was even more prevalent in PR.

It is reported that 75% to 85% of invasive breast cancers are positive and 15% to 25% of carcinomas are negative for ER, PR, or both. To avoid false negative results, appropriate internal controls and external controls should be in place and practitioners should consider repeating ER and PR on excisional specimen when CNB results are negative.

The HER-2/neu discrepancy rate is higher than that of ER and PR between central and local laboratories. The concordance rate is estimated to be 81.6% with the U.S. Food and Drug Administration (FDA)-approved Hercep kit and 75% when other IHC stains are used. Accurate analysis of hormonal receptor studies is critical for hormonal adjuvant therapy. Accurate analysis of HER-2/neu is critical for trastuzumab (Herceptin) therapy. There are two different methodologies in evaluation of HER-2/neu:

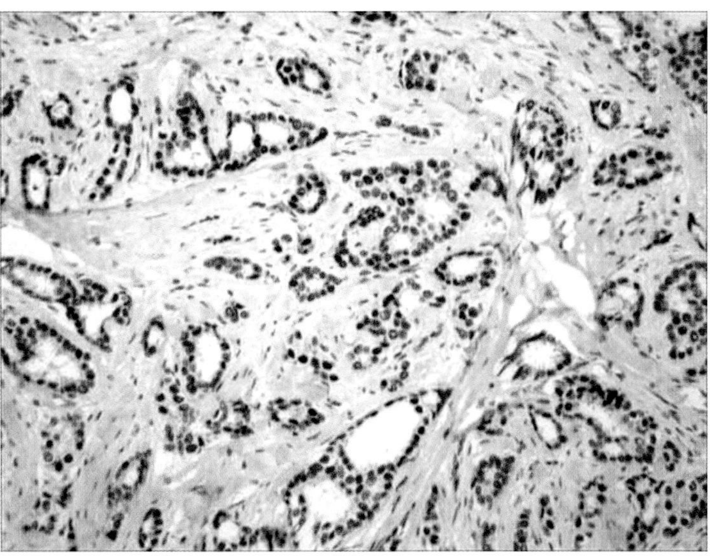

■ FIGURE 22-38 Estrogen receptor (ER) stain is nuclear stain showing brown staining over most of the tumor cell nuclei (ER by IHC stain ×200).

immunohistochemistry assay (DAKO HercepTest) and fluorescence in situ hybridization (FISH) assay (Vysis PathVysion HER2 DNA Probe).

IHC stain for HER-2/neu is a semi-quantitative IHC assay that determines HER-2 protein overexpression and utilizes breast cancer tissues routinely processed for histologic evaluation. The FISH HER-2/neu test is designed to detect amplification of the *HER-2* gene and utilizes FISH by using formalin-fixed, paraffin-embedded breast cancer tissue specimens. When HER-2/neu is positive either by IHC stain or FISH test, it is indicated as an aid in the assessment of patients for whom trastuzumab treatment is being considered. IHC stain is scored on a 0 to 3+ scale based on staining intensity and completeness of membrane staining:

Score 0 No staining is observed or membrane staining is observed in less than 10% of tumor cells.

Score 1+ A faint to barely perceptive membrane staining is detected in more than 10% of tumor cells. The cells are stained in only part of their membrane.

Score 2+ A weak to moderate complete membrane staining is detected in more than 10% of tumor cells.

Score 3+ A strong complete membrane staining is observed in more than 10% of tumor cells.

However, owing to poor reproducibility in interpretation of the HER-2/neu IHC stain, a new standard protocol and guideline has been published as a part of recommendation of quality assurance programs.[44] The new ASCO/CAP guideline in 2007 recommends all tissue to be fixed at least 6 hours to a maximum of 48 hours in formalin for IHC test for HER-2/neu. In addition, the score 0 to 3+ is altered as follows:

Score 0 No staining is observed in invasive tumor cells.

Score 1 Weak, incomplete membrane staining in any proportion of invasive tumor cells, or weak, complete membrane staining in less than 10% of cells.

Score 2 Complete membrane staining that is non-uniform or weak but with obvious circumferential distribution in at least 10% of cells, or intense complete membrane staining in 30% or less of tumor cells.

Score 3 Uniform intense membrane staining of more than 30% of invasive tumor cells (Figs. 22-39 to 22-42).

Interpretation of FISH analysis has also changed under this new guideline. FISH analysis of *HER-2/neu* gene amplification was positive when the ratio was greater than or equal to 2.0 and not amplified when the ratio was less than 2.0. Under this new guideline, positive *HER-2/neu* gene amplification is when the FISH ratio is greater than 2.2 and HER-2 gene copy is greater than 6.0, negative *HER-2/neu* is defined as a FISH ratio less than 1.8 or HER-2 gene copy is less than 4.0. A FISH ratio of 1.8 to 2.2 or HER-2 gene copy of 4.0 to 6.0 is considered equivocal for *HER-2* gene amplification. If the FISH result is equivocal, then counting additional cells for FISH is recommended or performing repeat FISH and/or an IHC test. If additional tests are still equivocal for *HER-2* gene amplification, patients with a ratio of greater than or equal to 2.0 are eligible for the adjuvant trastuzumab trials (Fig. 22-43).

It is critical that only the invasive component of the tumor is tested for FISH analysis for *HER*-2 gene. A FISH analysis is done on a darkfield fluorescent microscope without architectural correlation with a light microscope. The HER-2/neu test for DCIS is known to be more frequently positive for overexpression by IHC and also amplified with FISH (Figs. 22-44 and 22-45).[45] The case illustrated from Figures 22-44 and 22-45 shows discrepancy between IHC stain and FISH HER-2/neu analysis. The HER-2/neu test by IHC was given a score of 0 for invasive tumor, but the FISH test came back as highly amplified for the *HER-2* gene. Further evaluation and correlation revealed that DCIS overexpressed with HER-2/neu IHC stain and amplified with FISH. The invasive component was not overexpressed by IHC stain and not amplified by FISH when a repeated FISH test was performed.

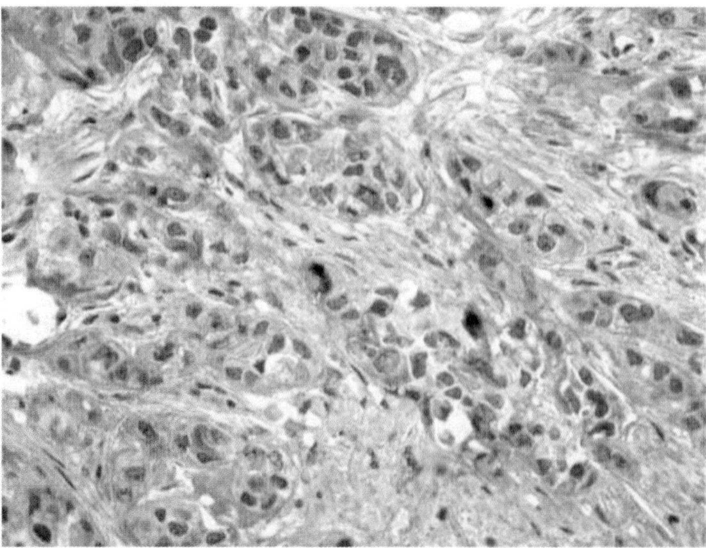

■ **FIGURE 22-39** HER-2/neu immunohistochemical (IHC) stain with score of zero. No membrane staining is observed around the tumor cell cytoplasm.

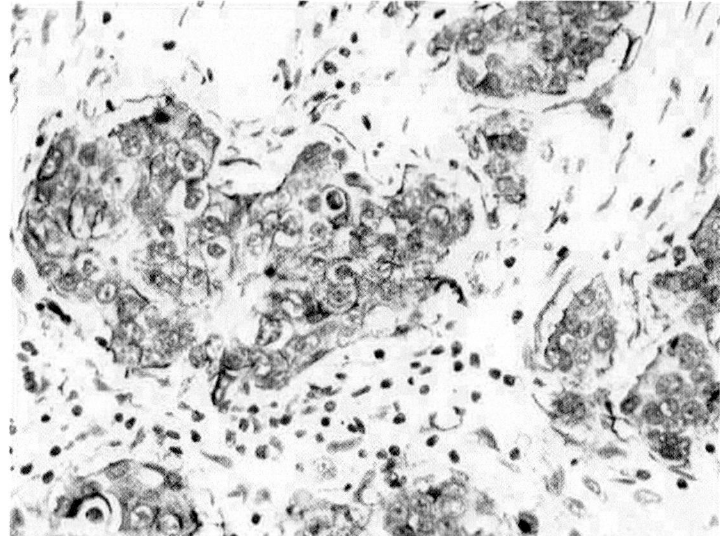

■ **FIGURE 22-40** HER-2/neu immunohistochemical (IHC) stain with score of 1+. Partial and weak membrane staining is observed around the tumor cell cytoplasm.

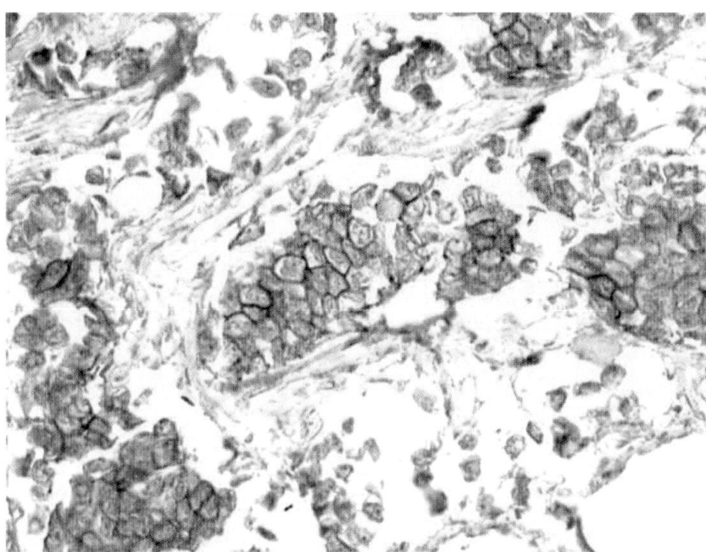

■ **FIGURE 22-41** HER-2/neu immunohistochemical (IHC) stain with score of 2+. Partial to complete membrane staining is observed around some of the tumor cell cytoplasm.

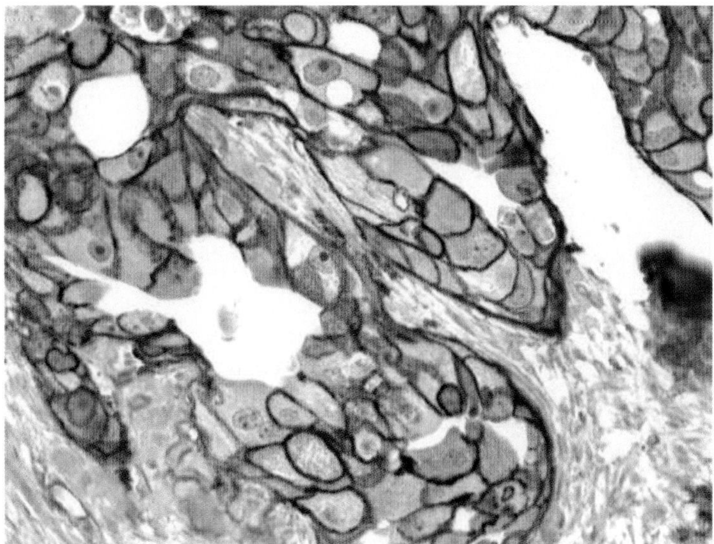

■ **FIGURE 22-42** HER-2/neu immunohistochemical (IHC) stain with score of 3+. Complete membrane staining is observed around all of the tumor cell cytoplasm.

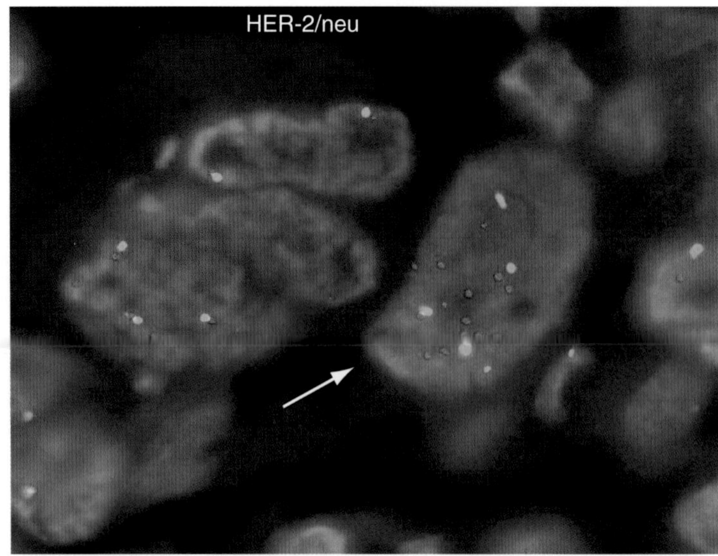

■ **FIGURE 22-43** HER-2/neu testing done by fluorescence in situ hybridization (FISH) analysis.

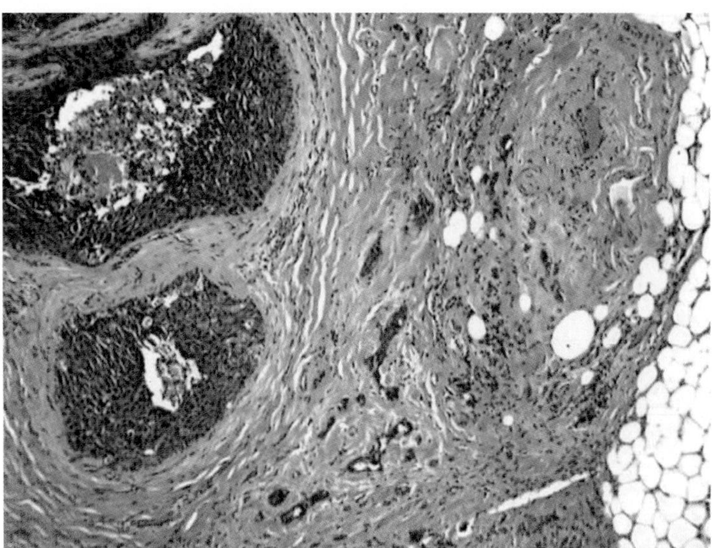

■ **FIGURE 22-44** Ductal carcinoma in situ (DCIS) is seen on the left and invasive ductal carcinoma (IDC) is seen on the right side of the slide (H&E, ×200).

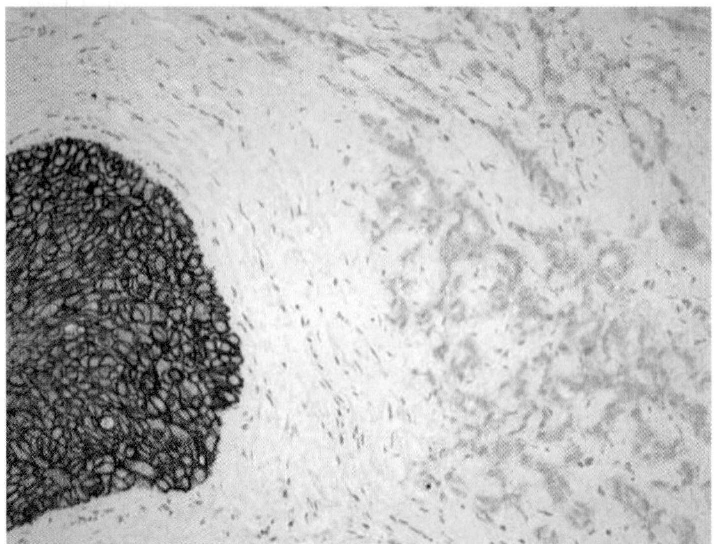

■ **FIGURE 22-45** HER-2/neu immunohistochemical (IHC) stain showing the score of 3+ for ductal carcinoma in situ (DCIS) and 0 for invasive ductal carcinoma (IDC). Fluorescence in situ hybridization (FISH) test for HER-2/neu should be performed on only the invasive cells.

PR is also associated with prognostic factor. Banerjee and colleagues described that patients with PR-positive tumors had better prognosis in 5-year survival than PR-negative tumors in the subgroups of at least four positive lymph nodes.[46]

Ki-67 is a monoclonal antibody to nuclear component and is expressed in proliferating cells throughout the cell cycle and not just active mitosis. Ki-67 expression is higher for the cells in S-phase. Ki-67 expression is also directly related to the grade of the mammary carcinoma; poorly differentiated and high nuclear grade IDC has higher percentage of Ki-67 expression. The mean value of Ki-67-positive cells in normal breast tissue ranges from 3% to 4%. ER- and PR-negative tumors are more likely to have a higher Ki-67 expression. There is a significant inverse relationship between Ki-67 expression and disease-free and overall survival rate.

SPECIAL TYPES OF INVASIVE MAMMARY CARCINOMA

Tubular Carcinoma

Tubular carcinoma is a distinct type of mammary carcinoma that is characterized by a haphazard arrangement of angulated tubule proliferations often with a hyaline and elastic background. Tubular carcinoma is known to have a good prognosis. To qualify for the diagnosis of tubular carcinoma, the angulated tubule proliferations should make up more than 90% of the lesion. Some authors claim 100% and others state that more than 75% of tubule formation is necessary to establish this diagnosis. A cribriform pattern may be admixed with tubular carcinoma. The nuclei are of low to intermediate grade, with prominent nucleoli, and cytoplasmic apical snouts projecting into the lumen are commonly present. Tubular carcinoma is often seen with lobular carcinoma in situ (LCIS) and flat epithelial atypia (FEA). Low-grade cribriform type DCIS is also commonly seen within or adjacent to haphazardly arranged, single-layered tubular carcinoma. Due to subtle nuclear atypia, the tubular carcinoma can be mistaken for sclerosing adenosis, microglandular adenosis, tubular adenosis, and radial scar. These lesions show lobular distribution with the presence of myoepithelial cells surrounding each tubule, whereas tubular carcinomas show an irregular distribution of tubules without myoepithelial cells (Fig. 22-46). Almost all tubular carcinomas are positive for ER and PR.

Tubulolobular Carcinomas

Tubulolobular carcinoma has both tubular and lobular elements. It has a low nuclear grade, and some authors designate this tumor as mixed ductal and lobular carcinoma. Tubulolobular carcinoma is known to have a higher local recurrence rate (17%) than tubular carcinoma (1%) and more likely to have axillary lymph node metastases. Almost all tubulolobular carcinomas are positive for ER and PR (Fig. 22-47).

Cribriform Carcinoma

Cribriform carcinomas are unusual variants of invasive mammary carcinoma with a sieve-like growth pattern that resembles cribriform DCIS. However, patients with cribriform carcinoma usually present with a mass lesion, unlike what is seen with cribriform DCIS. Cribriform carcinoma has irregular and more angular glands with fibrous stroma traversing through. The glands form fenestrations with uniform nuclei (Fig. 22-48).

A minor component of tubular carcinoma can be admixed. When mixed with IDC, NOS, the prognosis is worse than that for pure cribriform carcinoma. The differential diagnosis includes adenoid cystic carcinoma.

Adenoid Cystic Carcinoma

Adenoid cystic carcinoma has well-defined borders and presents as a mass lesion. Microscopically, it can have multiple well-circumscribed nodules. Adenoid cystic carcinoma shows cylindromatous components composed of basement membrane materials (Figs. 22-49 and 22-50). Perineural and neural invasion is frequently seen with this tumor. There is no in-situ component of this tumor. Three-tier grades are applied to the adenoid cystic carcinoma: grade 1 is absence of a solid component, grade 2 has less

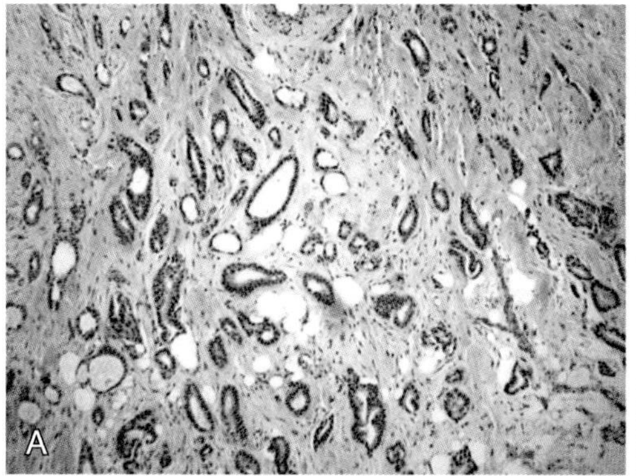

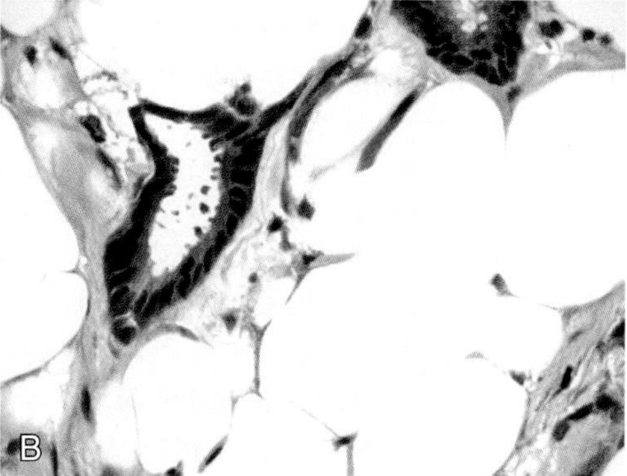

■ **FIGURE 22-46** **A**, Tubular carcinoma showing most of the tumor cells forming tubules (>90%) (H&E, ×100). **B**, Tubular carcinoma in high-power view showing apical luminal snouts and no myoepithelial cells (H&E, ×400).

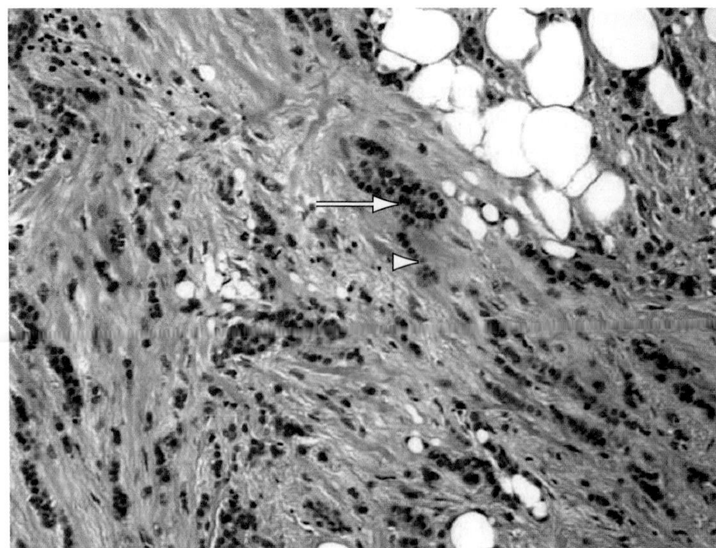

■ **FIGURE 22-47** Tubulolobular carcinoma. Some tumor cells are forming tubular pattern (*arrow*) and others are forming linear pattern (*arrowhead*) as seen in invasive lobular carcinoma (H&E, ×200).

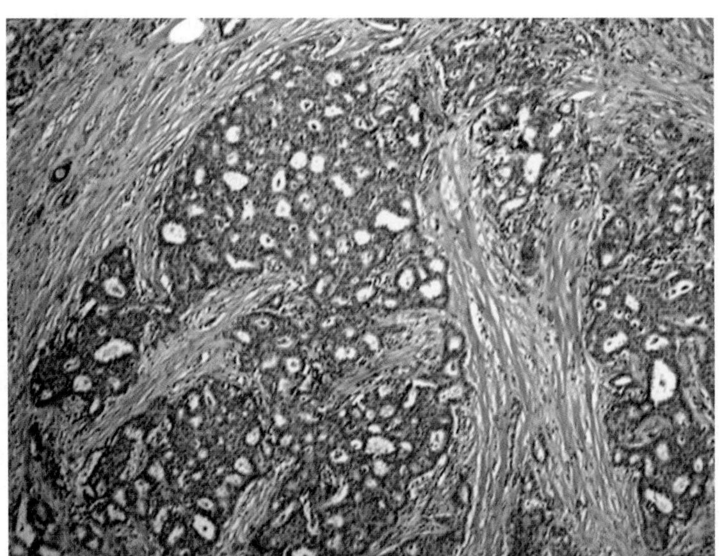

■ **FIGURE 22-48** Cribriform carcinoma. In low power view, the differential diagnosis includes ductal carcinoma in situ (DCIS) of cribriform type (H&E, ×200).

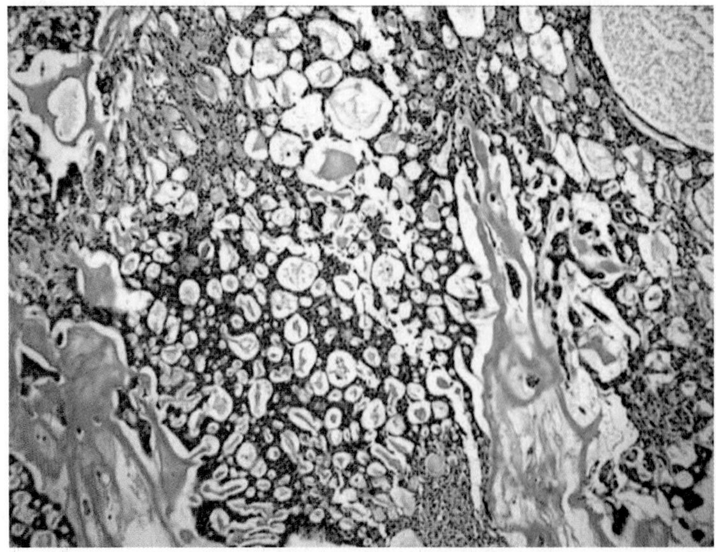

■ **FIGURE 22-49** Adenoid cystic carcinoma (H&E, ×200).

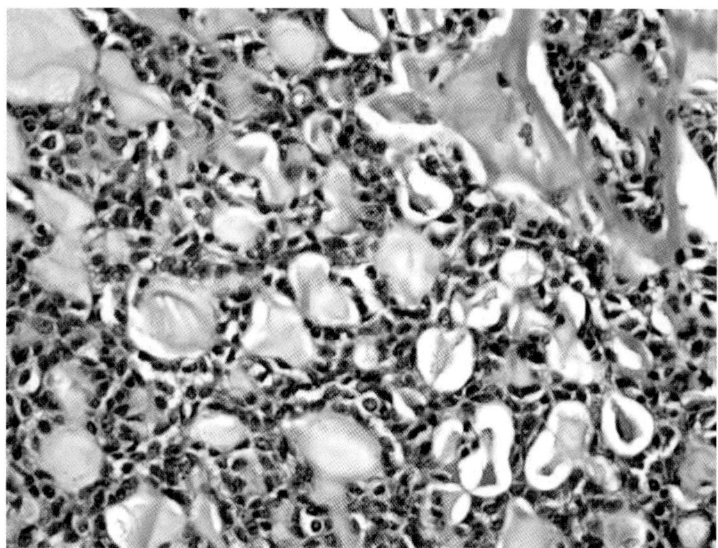

■ **FIGURE 22-50** Adenoid cystic carcinoma showing cylindromatous basement membrane materials (H&E, ×400).

than 30% solid component, and grade 3 is defined as more than 30% solid component. High-grade (grade 3) tumors show poorly differentiated nuclei and sparse cytoplasm often resembling small cell carcinoma (see below). Low-grade adenoid cystic carcinoma resembles cribriform DCIS and collagenous spherulosis.

Small Cell Carcinoma

Small cell carcinoma is one of the most uncommon variants of mammary carcinoma. The diagnosis of small cell carcinoma should be made when metastatic disease from other sites, such as lung or Merkel cell carcinoma from skin, are excluded. Fine needle aspiration of small cell carcinoma shows a clustered and linear pattern (coin-stacking) of small cells with nuclear molding and "salt-and-pepper" chromatin (Fig. 22-51). Marked nuclear pleomorphism with prominent nucleoli is not the feature of small cell carcinoma. Numerous apoptosis and mitotic figures are commonly present. Small cell carcinoma is known to have a poor prognosis.

Colloid (Mucinous) Carcinoma

The names colloid carcinoma and mucinous carcinoma are used interchangeably. Colloid carcinoma is generally well circumscribed with a gelatinous cut surface on gross examination. Microscopically, colloid carcinoma shows abundant extracellular mucus with floating tumor cells. In rare circumstances, the tumor is entirely composed of extracellular mucus without epithelial cells. It may require multiple sections at different levels to detect carcinoma cells (Fig. 22-52). Pure colloid carcinoma is known to have a good prognosis. Criteria for the diagnosis of colloid carcinoma are strict. Greater than 90% of the tumor should be of the mucinous type with well to moderately

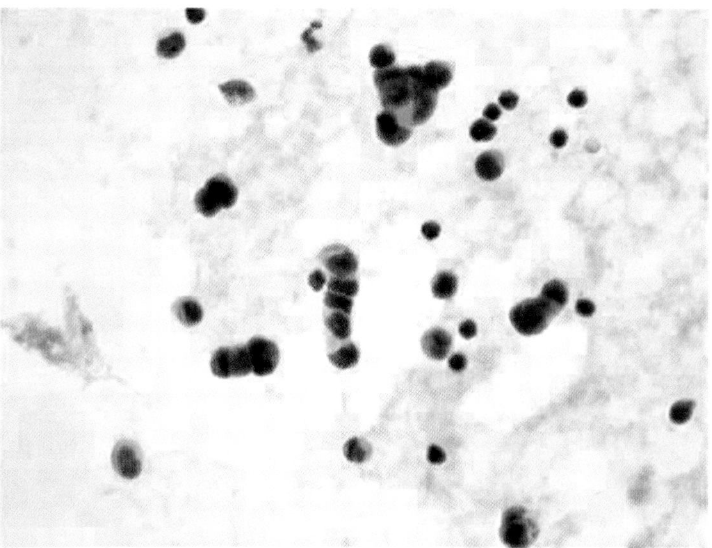

■ **FIGURE 22-51** Fine-needle aspiration (FNA) of breast small cell carcinoma showing tumor cells in linear (coin-stacking) pattern with nuclear molding.

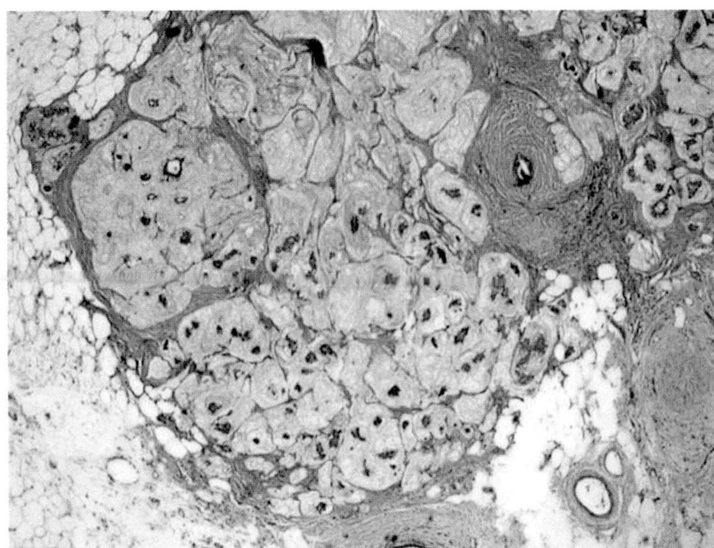

■ **FIGURE 22-52** Low power view of colloid (mucinous) carcinoma with abundant mucinous material and floating tumor cells (H&E, ×40).

differentiated nuclei. An intraductal component, usually of the mucinous type DCIS, is common with colloid carcinoma (Fig. 22-53). Other types of DCIS, such as cribriform, papillary and solid types, can be also present. The tumor size and margin assessment can be difficult when there is only extravasated mucin dissecting into stroma by either DCIS or invasive colloid carcinoma. Early invasive colloid carcinoma is also difficult to diagnose. The differential diagnosis includes stripped mucinous DCIS cells into the extracellular mucin. The margin of colloid carcinoma is determined by the extent of mucinous components even without the floating epithelial cells.

Papillary Carcinoma

Papillary carcinoma is estimated to be only 1% to 2% of breast carcinoma in women. Nearly 50% of papillary carcinomas arise in the central breast, and the other 50% in the peripheral breast. Central papillary carcinoma is frequently associated with nipple discharge or bleeding. It is known as intracystic papillary carcinoma with and without invasion. Peripheral papillary carcinoma is known as solid papillary DCIS with or without invasion. The invasive component is frequently IDC, NOS and is suspected when part of the tumor is lacking circumscription (Fig. 22-54). Intracystic papillary carcinoma is usually well circumscribed with cystic and solid features. The cut surface frequently demonstrates a hemorrhagic and friable appearance. Intracystic papillary carcinoma is also known as encapsulated papillary carcinoma. Microscopically, intracystic papillary carcinoma shows epithelial proliferations with supporting fibrovascular cores of the stroma, as seen in intraductal papilloma. However, the cells of intracystic papillary carcinoma are more regular and uniform without

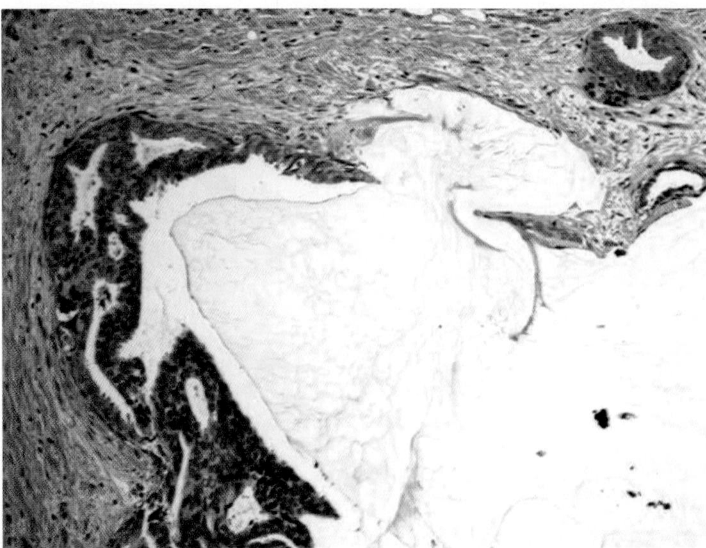

■ **FIGURE 22-53** Mucinous ductal carcinoma in situ (DCIS) with mucus dissecting into the stroma. These features can be seen adjacent to colloid carcinoma (H&E, ×400).

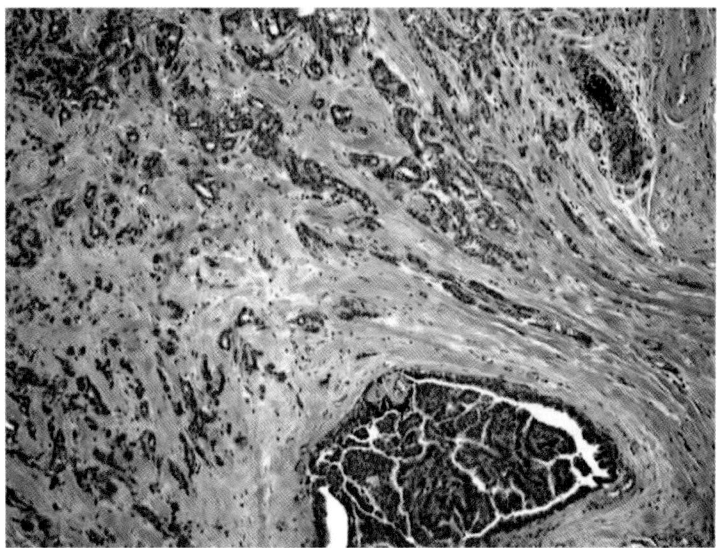

■ **FIGURE 22-54** Papillary ductal carcinoma in situ (DCIS) with invasive ductal carcinoma, not otherwise specified (IDC, NOS) type (H&E, ×200).

the presence of myoepithelial cells as in the proliferative epithelial component. The presence of myoepithelial cells within the papillary lesion is inconsistent with intracystic papillary carcinoma. Mitotic figures are conspicuous. The expanded borders of intracystic papillary carcinoma often show attenuation of myoepithelial cells. Lack of myoepithelial cells at the periphery of the cystically dilated wall is shown by multiple IHC stains, and some authors claim that intracystic papillary carcinomas are invasive but behave as DCIS and thus prefer the terminology of encysted papillary carcinoma (Figs. 22-55 and 22-56). Solid papillary DCIS is well circumscribed and multinodular and more commonly seen in the peripheral breast. A delicate network of fibrovascular stroma is distributed in an arborizing pattern throughout the compact solid papillary epithelial proliferation and is typically ovoid to spindle-shaped and of low nuclear grade. Neuroendocrine features with positive immunoreactive chromogranin and synaptophysin are common. Chromogranin and synaptophysin are peptide hormones in the cytoplasm, which makes a granular appearance in many neuroendocrine tumors. Histologically, an organoid growth pattern—solid growth with peripheral palisading and rosette-like or glandular luminal structure—is seen (Figs. 22-57 and 22-58). Extracellular and intracellular mucin is also a common feature, and if invasive carcinoma is seen, it is usually colloid carcinoma adjacent to the solid papillary DCIS. Axillary nodal metastases have been documented with noninvasive papillary carcinoma in about 1% of patients. The frequency of lymph node metastases in invasive papillary carcinoma is higher and depends on the size of the invasive component as well as the nuclear grade. Still, the prognosis of invasive papillary carcinoma is favorable even in women who have axillary lymph node metastases.

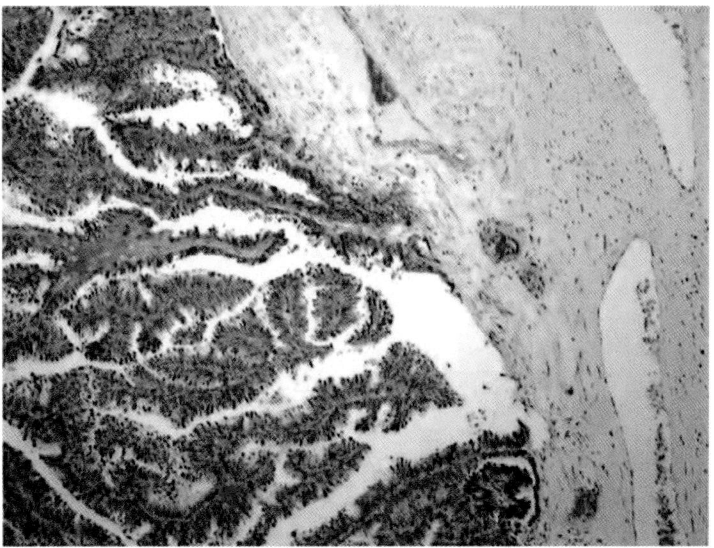

■ **FIGURE 22-55** Intracystic papillary carcinoma, noninvasive type (H&E, ×200).

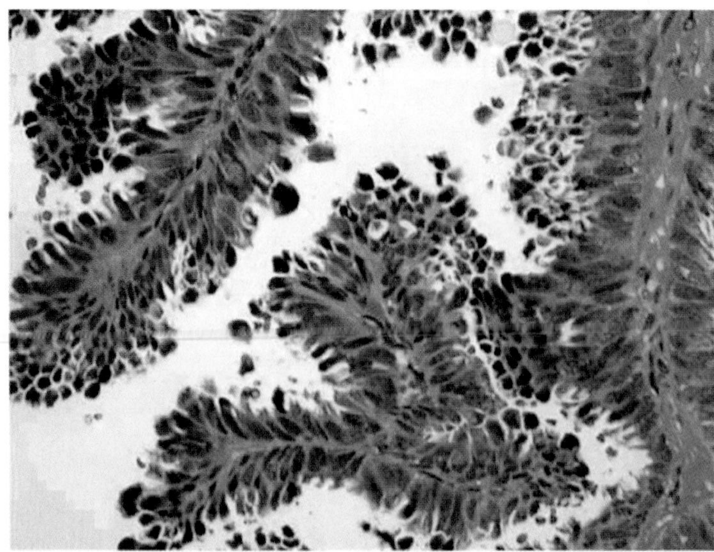

■ **FIGURE 22-56** Intracystic papillary carcinoma, non-invasive type showing papillary fronds with atypical cells and fibrovascular cores (H&E, ×400).

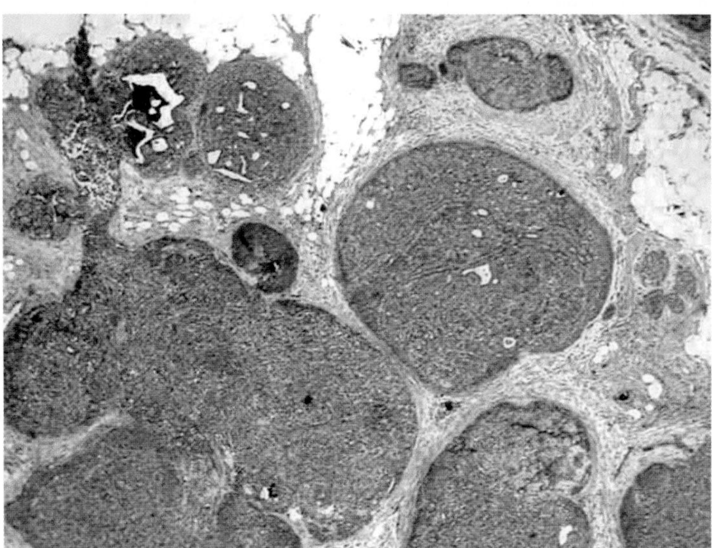

■ **FIGURE 22-57** Solid cystic papillary ductal carcinoma in situ (DCIS) with multinodular pattern located at the periphery of the breast (H&E, ×200).

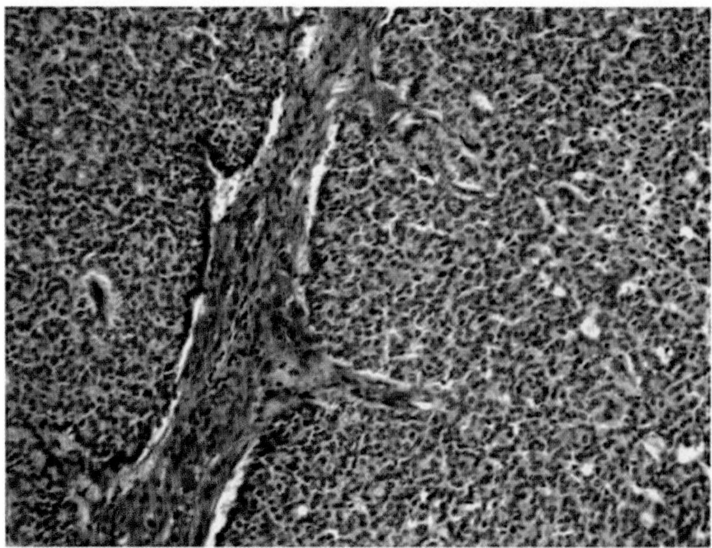

■ **FIGURE 22-58** Solid cystic papillary ductal carcinoma in situ (DCIS) showing organoid pattern (H&E, ×400).

Invasive Micropapillary Carcinoma

Invasive micropapillary carcinoma is a morphologically distinctive form of mammary carcinoma with clefts or spaces around tumor cells with a network of loose fibrocollagenous or delicate reticular stroma. Microlumens are present at the central portion of tumor cells. Nuclear grade is mostly intermediate to high with higher mitotic rates. Psammomatous calcifications may be seen. The spaces appear empty, resembling lymph-vascular invasion but without endothelial cells. The tumor cells are immunoreactive to epithelial membrane antigen (EMA) with the cell membranes at the periphery referred to as an *inside-out growth pattern* (Figs. 22-59 and 22-60). Invasive micropapillary carcinoma sometimes shows a mucinous extracellular background. Interestingly, micropapillary carcinoma has been reported to have a higher incidence of lymph node metastasis. When micropapillary carcinoma is seen within the axillary lymph node, it maintains the similar morphologic appearance of inside-out tumor clusters as seen from the breast parenchymal tumor. Micropapillary carcinoma of the breast has been reported to have a higher recurrence rate, high metastatic disease to lymph nodes, higher HER-2/neu positive tumors, and a significantly shorter disease-free and overall survival rate. The differential diagnosis includes metastatic ovarian serous papillary tumors (Figs. 22-61 and 22-62). The presence of DCIS with micropapillary carcinoma helps to exclude metastatic disease from ovarian tumor. When DCIS is not present, clinical and imaging studies to rule out other possible primary sites may be necessary.

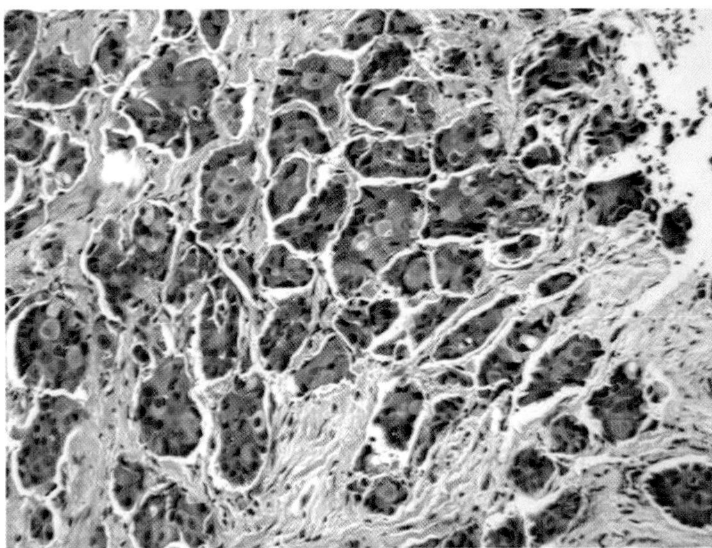

■ **FIGURE 22-59** Micropapillary carcinoma (H&E, ×400)

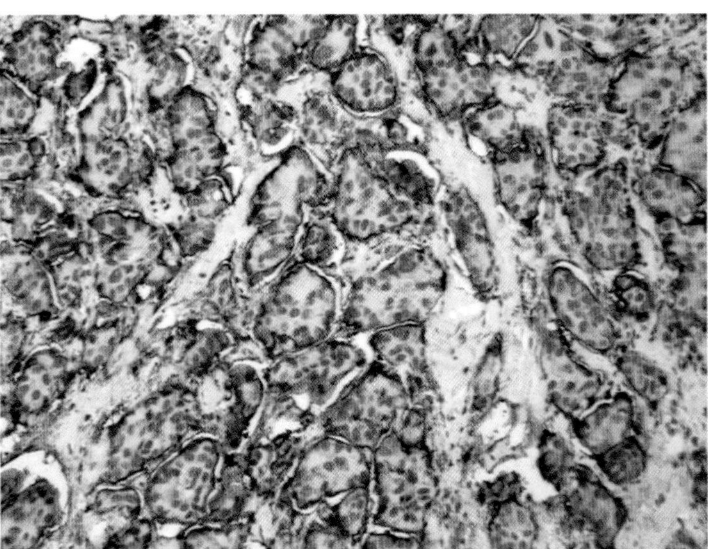

■ **FIGURE 22-60** Epithelial membrane antigen (EMA) stain showing the cell membrane at the periphery, a classic feature of *inside out*.

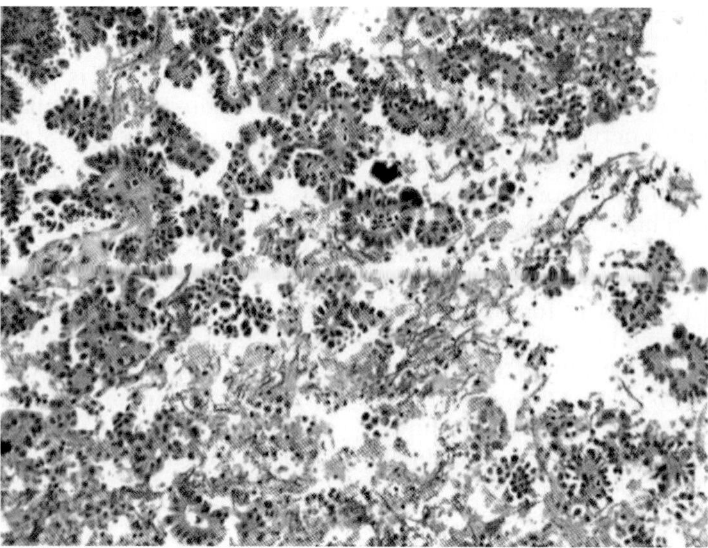

■ **FIGURE 22-61** Ovarian metastatic carcinoma to breast simulating micropapillary carcinoma of the breast (H&E, ×100).

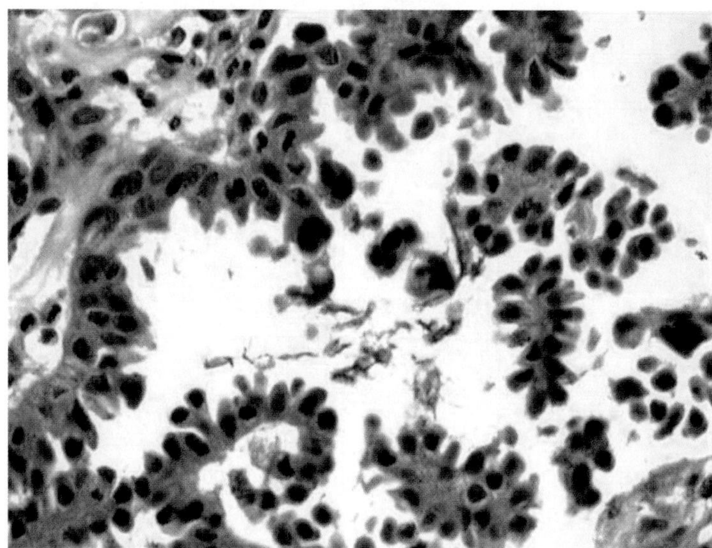

■ **FIGURE 22-62** Ovarian metastatic carcinoma to breast showing papillary tufting without clefting artifact (H&E, ×400).

Medullary Carcinoma

Medullary carcinoma is a distinct entity of mammary carcinoma. Grossly, it shows a well-circumscribed margin and may be confused with a fibroadenoma. The cut surface is tan to gray. Microscopically, medullary carcinoma is a well-delineated mass with an expansile and "pushing" border into the adjacent breast tissue. The tumor cells show high nuclear grade and are clustered in a syncytial pattern with a pronounced amount of lymphoplasmacytic infiltrates. Syncytial pattern is defined as tumor cells forming anastomosing cords and sheets separated by minimal to no connective tissue. The syncytial growth pattern is usually greater than 75% of tumor without any glandular pattern (Figs. 22-63 and 22-64). Medullary carcinoma is known to have a favorable prognosis despite the poorly differentiated and high nuclear grade. Underdiagnosing poorly differentiated IDC as medullary carcinoma is dangerous; thus, some authors emphasize strict criteria for a diagnosis of medullary carcinoma. The presence of dense collagenous stroma, DCIS, or any tumor cells in a glandular pattern is not a feature of medullary carcinoma. When any of these features are present, the diagnosis of atypical medullary carcinoma can be made and this type has a similar prognosis as poorly differentiated IDC, NOS type. Most medullary carcinoma tumor cells are "triple-negative" tumors, namely, ER, PR, and HER-2/neu negative. Classic medullary and atypical medullary carcinomas have been reported to be more common among younger patients and *BRCA1*-related hereditary breast cancer. In 1990, a National Surgical Adjuvant Breast and Bowel Project (NSABP) review of 8-year survival for node-negative patients reported a favorable prognosis of medullary carcinoma.[47] However, the 10-year survival rate in a Nottingham series shows no substantial difference in survival rate between medullary carcinoma and atypical

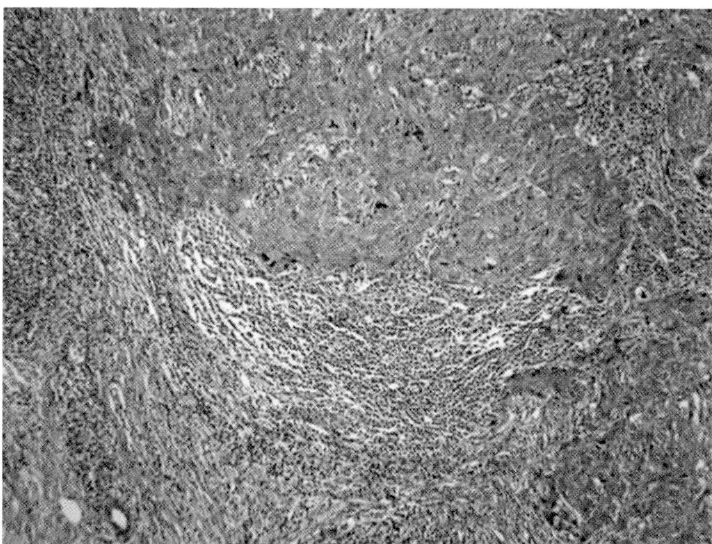

■ **FIGURE 22-63** Low power view of invasive ductal carcinoma (IDC) with medullary features (H&E, ×40).

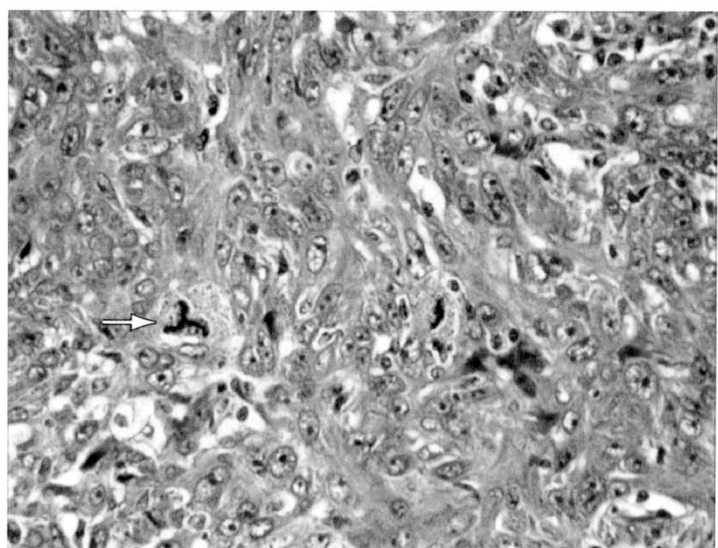

■ **FIGURE 22-64** Medullary carcinoma features are syncytial aggregates of high nuclear grade tumor cells with prominent lymphohistiocytic and plasma cells (H&E, ×400). Tripolar mitotic figure is shown (*arrow*).

medullary and IDC, NOS type.[48] Patients with *BRCA1*-related breast cancers commonly present at a lower stage and an earlier age (mean age, 42.8 years) than medullary or atypical medullary carcinomas. *BRCA1*-related breast cancers also have a higher proliferation index (high Ki-67) and higher grade with lower recurrence rates than sporadic breast carcinomas. It is possible that *BRCA1*-related medullary carcinoma of the breast has a better prognosis than sporadic breast carcinoma with medullary and atypical medullary features.

Apocrine Carcinoma

Apocrine carcinoma has a morphologically and histologically distinct appearance, but is clinically and prognostically no different from other IDCs. Some authors suggest that apocrine carcinoma has a better prognosis, and others claim that the overall survival rate is similar to that of nonapocrine carcinomas. Grossly, apocrine carcinoma is not distinguishable from other IDC, NOS types. Microscopically, the tumor cells show abundant granular cytoplasm that is positive for diastase-resistant periodic acid-Schiff (PAS) stain. The nuclei are centrally located and have prominent nucleoli (Fig. 22-65). A vast majority of intraductal and invasive apocrine carcinoma is high grade with comedo-type necrosis. Immunoreactivity of gross cystic disease fluid protein-15 (GCDFP-15) (Fig. 22-66) is commonly positive, with apocrine carcinoma in about 75% of cases. Gross cystic disease fluid protein-15 (GCDFP-15) is also positive with nonapocrine carcinoma in about 23%. Apocrine carcinoma is usually ER, PR, and HER-2/neu negative but commonly positive with androgen receptor (AR) and carcinoembryonic antigen (CEA). The origin of apocrine carcinoma has been postulated to arise from apocrine metaplastic cells, which are commonly

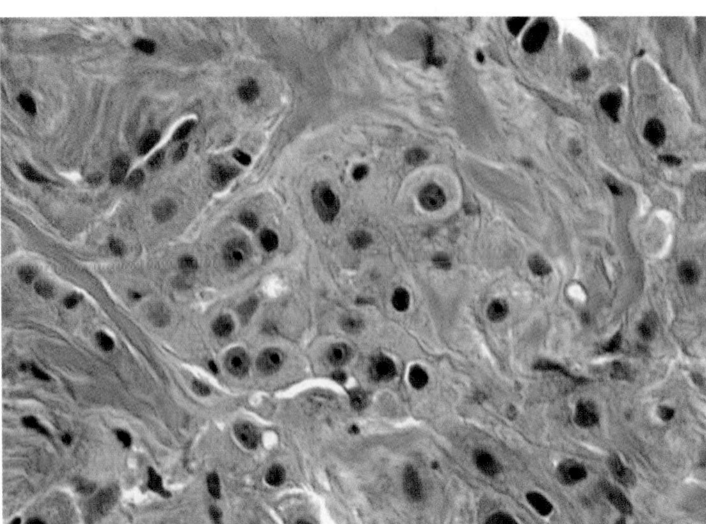

■ **FIGURE 22-65** Apocrine carcinoma with abundant granular cytoplasm, nuclei with prominent central nucleoli (H&E, ×400).

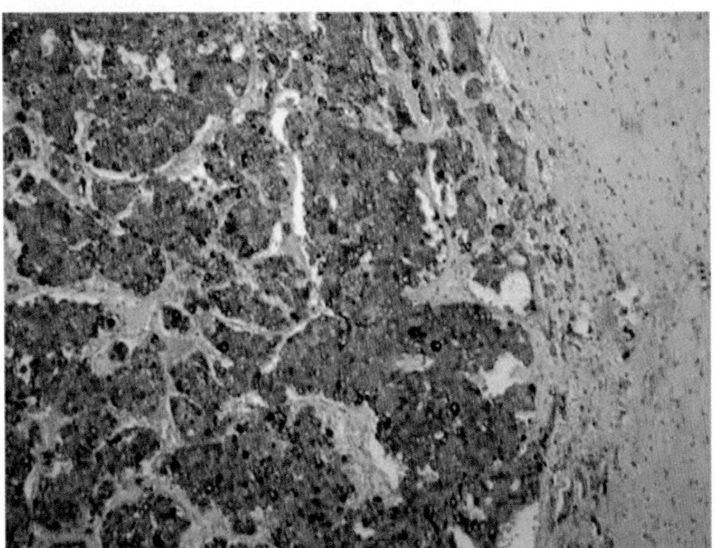

■ **FIGURE 22-66** Gross cystic disease fluid protein 15 (GCDFP-15) stain for apocrine carcinoma is often positive.

seen in fibrocystic changes of the breast. Others have shown that the presence of apocrine metaplasia, even hyperplasia or atypical intraductal hyperplasia of apocrine cells, did not increase the chances of subsequent development of invasive apocrine carcinoma.

Secretory Carcinoma

Secretory carcinoma is an unusual tumor and occurs in a younger age group of women with a median age of 25. Microscopically, secretory carcinoma is characterized by having abundant intracellular and extracellular secretory material, which is intensely eosinophilic. The neoplastic cells lack pleomorphism and can be deceptively bland. Cytoplasm shows vacuolated secretory contents, and luminal content shows secretory droplets and condensation of proteinaceous material (Fig. 22-67). The secretory material is positive with diastase-resistant PAS and also with Alcian blue and mucicarmine. Secretory material is positive for a-lactalbumin and CEA, and nuclei are ER and PR positive by IHC stains. Because of the rarity of this type of tumor, the long-term prognosis is not well documented except for a few case reports. In general, the prognosis depends on lymph node status and tumor size. Long-term follow-up may be necessary owing to patient with the tumor presenting at a younger age.

Glycogen-Rich Carcinoma

Glycogen-rich carcinoma is an unusual mammary tumor, accounting for less than 1% of all breast carcinomas. Microscopically, it is a unique carcinoma owing to its clear cells that form cords, solid nests, and papillary patterns. The tumor cells are polygonal and tend to have sharply defined

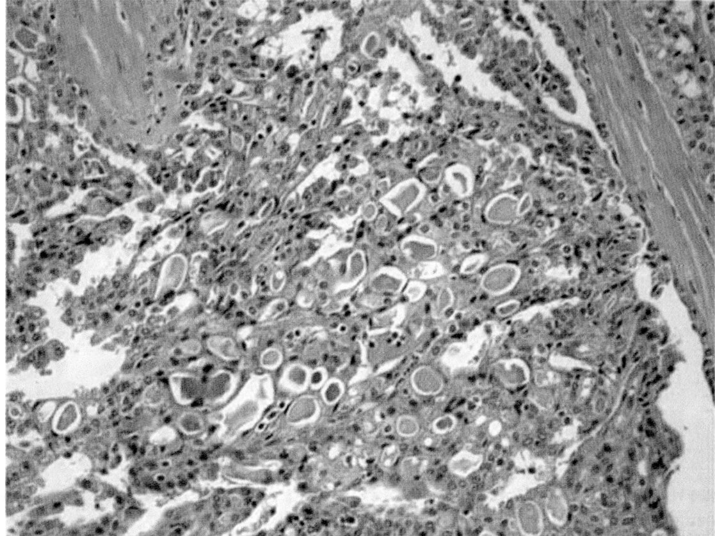

■ **FIGURE 22-67** Secretory carcinoma showing abundant intraluminal secretory proteinaceous material (H&E, ×400).

cytoplasmic borders. The cytoplasm is clear and not granular due to high glycogen content and stains positive with diastase-sensitive PAS (Figs. 22-68 and 22-69). Many glycogen-rich carcinomas are ER positive. An intraductal component, when present, can be clear cell DCIS, but other mixed types, such as solid, cribriform, and comedo DCIS, can be seen. The differential diagnosis includes metastatic renal cell carcinoma, lipid-rich carcinoma, and apocrine carcinoma. Apocrine carcinomas are ER negative, and lipid-rich carcinomas are oil-O-red positive. Patients with metastatic renal cell carcinoma usually present with a compatible clinical history and the metastases are much more vascular than glycogen-rich carcinoma of the breast.

Metaplastic Carcinoma

Metaplastic carcinoma consists of heterogeneous groups of neoplasms. The term *metaplastic carcinoma* is synonymous with matrix-producing carcinoma, carcinosarcoma, and spindle cell carcinoma. In 2003, new World Health Organization (WHO) classifications of metaplastic carcinoma were subdivided into pure epithelial and mixed epithelial and mesenchymal groups. The pure epithelial group consists of squamous cell carcinoma, adenocarcinoma with spindle cells differentiation, and adenosquamous carcinoma, including mucoepidermoid carcinoma. The mixed epithelial and mesenchymal group consists of carcinoma with chondroid metaplasia, carcinoma with osseous metaplasia, and carcinosarcoma. The common denominator of mixed metaplastic carcinoma is the presence of mesenchymal cell populations such as chondroid and osteoid in addition to an epithelial component (Fig. 22-70). Pure squamous cell carcinoma of the breast is rare. Neoplastic squamous cells can be keratinizing, nonkeratinizing, spindle, and acantholytic types, often exhibiting intercellular bridges, keratin pearls, and keratohyaline granules in variable amounts

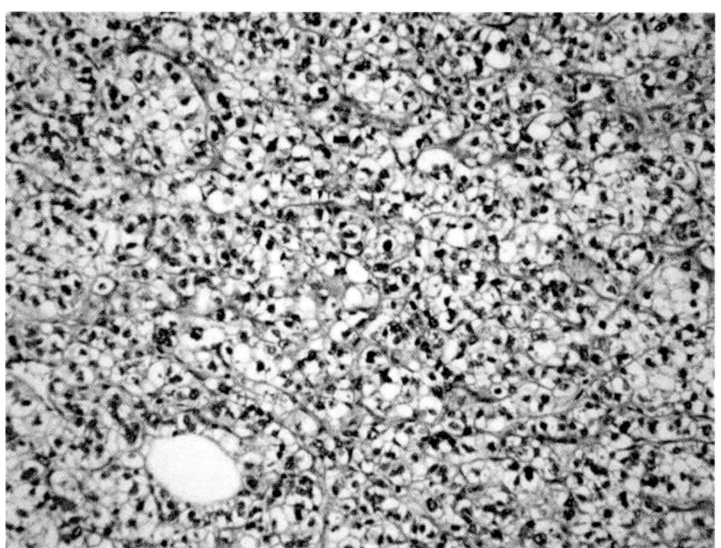

■ **FIGURE 22-68** Glycogen rich carcinoma showing abundant clear cells in polygonal shapes (H&E, ×400).

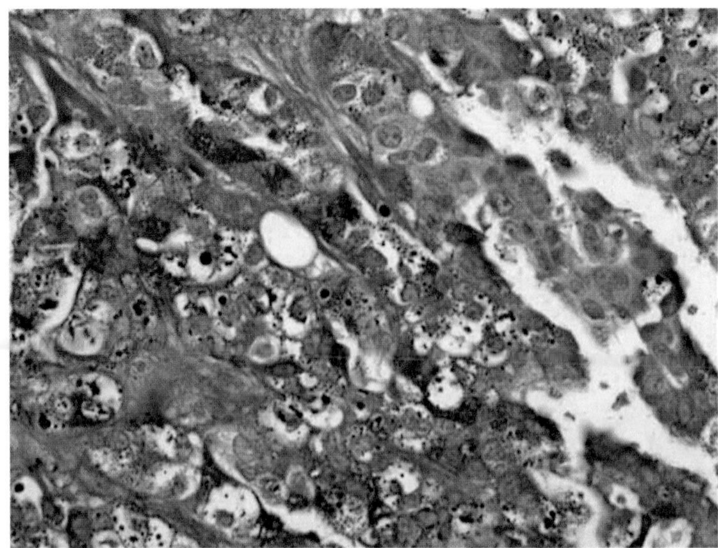

■ **FIGURE 22-69** Periodic acid-Schiff (PAS) stain is positive for glycogen rich carcinoma supporting the presence of glycogen contents.

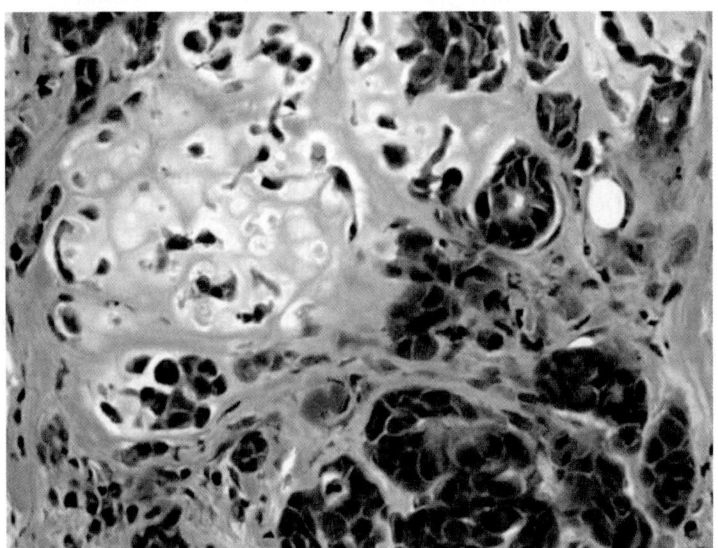

■ **FIGURE 22-70** Metaplastic carcinoma with chondroid element (H&E, ×200).

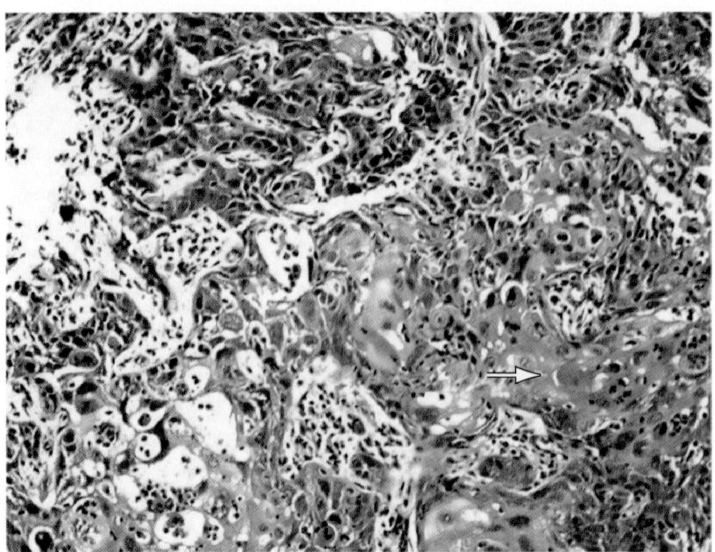

■ **FIGURE 22-71** Metaplastic carcinoma with pure squamous cell carcinoma of the breast (H&E, ×400). Keratinization is shown with *arrow*.

(Fig. 22-71). Necrosis and cystic formation is commonly seen with squamous cell carcinoma. Squamous cell carcinoma is positive for high molecular weight keratin such as CK5/6 and 34ßE12 and often negative for ER, PR and HER-2/neu by IHC stains.

Spindle cell carcinoma is probably the most common epithelial cell type of metaplastic carcinoma. The tumor cells are deceptively bland appearing and often misdiagnosed as benign lesions, especially with a limited sample from core needle biopsy. Spindle cell carcinomas may have a few islands of squamous cells or adenocarcinoma cells. Spindle cell proliferation is seen to infiltrate into preexisting terminal ductal-lobular units in the fibrotic stromal background (Figs. 22-72 and 22-73). To aid the diagnosis of spindle cell carcinoma, multiple cytokeratin stains should be applied, such as high molecular weight cytokeratin (34ßE12, p63, CK5/6, CK7) (Fig. 22-74). The origin of metaplastic carcinoma has been postulated as myoepithelial cells. Spindle cell carcinomas are known to be positive for p63 and smooth muscle myosin heavy chain (SMMHC), which are myoepithelial cell markers. Other IHC stains such as desmin, vimentin, and actin can be positive with spindle cell carcinoma, which further may lead to an erroneous diagnosis, such as myoepithelioma, myofibroblastoma, and smooth muscle tumor.

Among the mixed metaplastic carcinomas, chondroid and osseous differentiation is the most common. Other uncommon types of mesenchymal components include adipose tissue and fibrous, angiomatous, and skeletal muscle. The matrix can be benign or frankly malignant sarcoma, such as chondrosarcoma, osteogenic sarcoma, rhabdomyosarcoma, liposarcoma, and fibrosarcoma. Primary sarcomas are exceedingly rare in the breast. Metaplastic carcinoma or malignant phyllodes tumor with

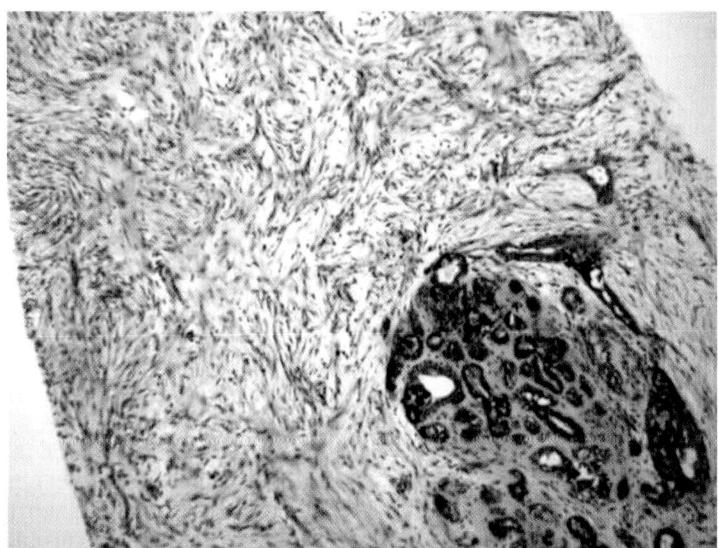

■ **FIGURE 22-72** Core needle biopsy of spindle cell carcinoma. Spindle cells are infiltrating into terminal-ductal lobular unit (H&E, ×100).

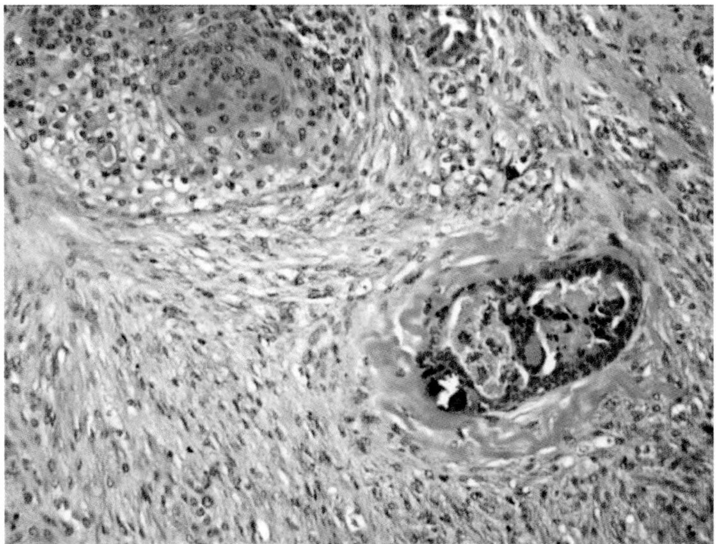

■ **FIGURE 22-73** Spindle cell carcinoma with focal areas of squamous and osteoid differentiation (H&E, ×400).

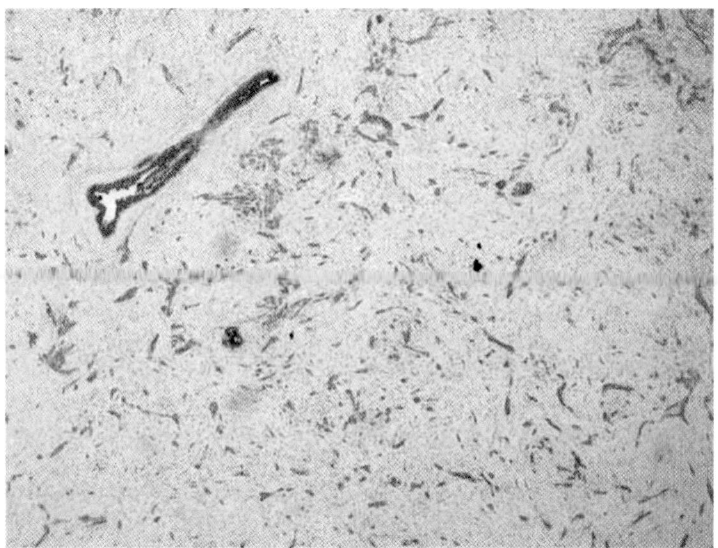

■ **FIGURE 22-74** Spindle cell carcinoma. Scattered positive cells are noted (cytokeratin, ×200).

chondroid, osseous or adipose metaplasia should be ruled out before diagnosing primary sarcomas of the breast, especially without a history of radiation therapy. Various keratin stains are negative in matrix-producing metaplastic carcinoma, but focal positive staining can be seen with spindle cells or other epithelial cells in matrix-producing metaplastic carcinoma.

Metaplastic carcinomas often metastasize to lung or liver via a hematogenous route. Metastases to axillary lymph nodes are relatively uncommon, especially with matrix-producing metaplastic carcinomas. The prognosis of patients with metaplastic carcinoma depends on the tumor stage at the time of diagnosis.

Inflammatory Carcinoma

The original definition of inflammatory carcinoma referred to the clinical appearance of breast carcinoma. Some authors include histologic changes such as dermal lymphatic emboli or direct involvement of tumor in the papillary and reticular dermis as a clinicopathologic definition of inflammatory breast cancer (Fig. 22-75). Dilation of lymphatic vessels in papillary and reticular dermis may be associated. Clinically, inflammatory breast carcinoma is characterized by erythema and thickening with *peau d'orange* changes of the skin. Patients with inflammatory carcinoma tend to have higher-grade and poorly differentiated IDC. The skin of inflammatory carcinoma displays a striking appearance, and hence many clinicians perform punch biopsy of different areas of skin to prove histologic changes of inflammatory carcinoma. However, even with the classic clinical appearance of inflammatory carcinoma, skin biopsy specimens often fail to show evidence of lymphatic tumor emboli. The skin biopsy is reportedly negative in 50% of patients. On the other hand, patients who have cutaneous lym-

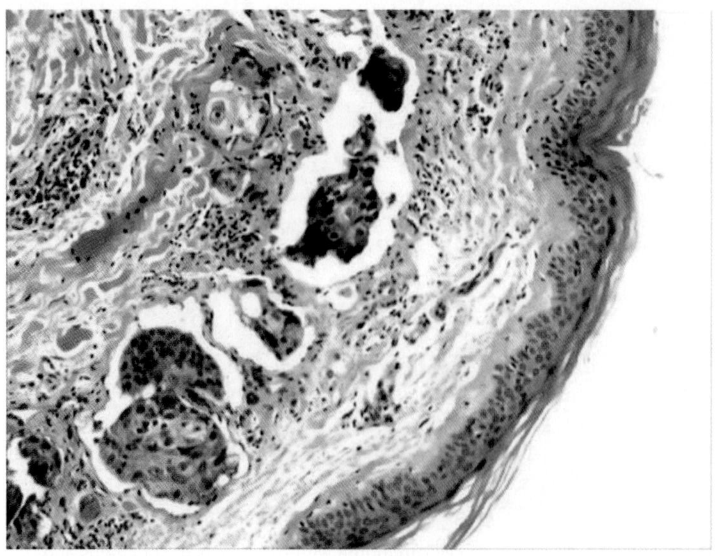

■ **FIGURE 22-75** Dermal lymphatic invasion with tumor plugs (H&E, ×200).

phatic emboli without clinical manifestation of inflammatory carcinoma have been described as having "occult inflammatory carcinoma." In occult inflammatory carcinoma, the primary breast parenchymal tumor tends to be larger and more multicentric. When compared with clinical inflammatory carcinoma, patients with occult inflammatory carcinoma tend to have a better prognosis. Historically, patients with inflammatory carcinoma had less than a 5% survival rate in 5 years. But with neoadjuvant chemotherapy followed by surgery and radiation therapy, the 5-year survival rate is now greater than 50%.

Other Unusual Carcinomas and Metastatic Carcinomas

Other unusual subtypes of mammary carcinoma, which include histiocytoid carcinoma, lipid-rich carcinoma, and carcinomas with osteoclastic giant cells, are extremely rare. Metastatic carcinomas are discussed in Chapter 24.

UNUSUAL PRESENTATIONS OF BREAST CARCINOMA

Less than 1% of patients can present with metastatic breast carcinoma in the axillary lymph node as the first manifestation of the disease. This is defined as *occult carcinoma.* The location of the primary tumor is usually the ipsilateral breast, and a clinical and imaging workup is necessary to find the primary tumor. Retrospective mammography review has detected abnormalities in the breast in 12% to 35% of these patients in the literature. However MRI has proven to be the most effective method for detecting occult carcinomas. Occasionally, axillary metastatic carcinoma occurs in the contralateral axilla; it is seen in 3.6% of patients, most of who had previous mammary carcinoma. Management of occult carcinoma presenting as axillary lymph node metastasis is either observation or ipsilateral mastectomy. Studies have shown that the frequency of finding a primary tumor in the ipsilateral mastectomy varies from 55% to 82%, with an average of 75%. Most of the tumors from the mastectomy specimens were visible during the gross examination. Twenty-five percent to 30% of the clinically occult primary carcinomas were not seen grossly. Thorough sampling is necessary in this scenario, but there are rare cases where, despite the most careful and extensive sampling of a mastectomy specimen, no primary breast tumor is found. The possible explanation is that the axillary tail contains breast tissue that can be the source of the primary site. It has been reported that a high proportion of the primary mammary carcinoma had apocrine cytology in both metastases and the primary tumor. Other primary sites such as the lung also may be a possibility.

Bilateral Carcinomas

Bilateral carcinoma is uncommon. It is usually divided into two types: synchronous and metachronous. *Synchronous carcinoma* refers to detection of simultaneous bilateral carcinomas at the same examination. *Metachronous* carcinomas are non-simultaneous carcinomas of the contralateral breast; they are found during follow-up, sometimes many years later. The exact incidence of bilateral breast carcinoma is difficult to determine because contralateral lesions can sometimes be metastases. It is known, however, that the likelihood of bilaterality depends on the histologic type of the cancer. Invasive lobular carcinoma has a higher likelihood of bilaterality than other cancers, with reported rates up to 30%. IDC has a lower reported incidence of bilaterality, the contralateral focus of cancer usually being intraductal carcinoma. Overall, the risk of development of cancer in the other breast after mastectomy is reported to be 1% per year, about six times higher than in the general population.

Axillary Lymph Node Metastases

Axillary lymph nodes determine the N status of the TNM stage. Intramammary lymph nodes also are coded as axillary lymph nodes. Metastatic carcinoma in any other lymph nodes such as supraclavicular, cervical, and contralateral internal mammary sites are all considered metastases and reported as M1. Axillary lymph nodes are divided into level I, II, and III. Level I lymph nodes are located at the lateral border of the pectoralis minor muscle, level II lymph nodes are located in the mid region, and level III lymph nodes are located at the apex near the medial area of the pectoralis minor muscle. Internal mammary lymph nodes are located in the intercostal spaces along the edge of the sternum, and some medially located breast tumors may drain into this area first. Tumor size is associated with the probability of lymph node metastasis. One of the largest studies published regarding the relationship of tumor size, lymph node status, and survival was done from a data base of 24,740 breast cancer cases by the Surveillance, Epidemiology and End Results (SEER) program of the National Cancer Institute (See Table 22-5). In this study, 5-year survival rate was decreased as the tumor size and probability of axillary lymph node metastases increased. Another study by Roger and associates showed the frequency of axillary lymph nodal involvement for stages T1a, T1b, and T1c with a tumor size between 1.1 and 1.5 cm, and T1c with a size 1.6 to 2.0 cm, as 3%, 10%, 21%, and 35%, respectively.[49] Currently, the best documented prognostic survival factor for breast cancer is the presence or absence of metastatic axillary lymph nodes. The overall survival of breast carcinoma is also directly related to the number of axillary lymph node metastases. Osborne studied 5-year survival rates by the number of involved axillary lymph nodes in 505 patients with breast cancer (Tables 22-6 and 22-7). The data were collected before the sentinel lymph node era without IHC stains for cytokeratin. Adding cytokeratin IHC stain to conventional hematoxylin and eosin (H&E) stain for examining lymph nodes resulted in an increasing number of axillary lymph node micrometastases or isolated tumor cells. Clinical significance of both micrometastasis and isolated tumor cells in the sentinel lymph nodes are discussed in Chapter 21 under DCIS and in this chapter under "Invasive Lobular Carcinoma".

TABLE 22-6. Distribution of Breast Cancer Cases by Size and Lymph Node Status

Tumor Size Diameter (cm)	1-3 Positive Lymph Nodes	4+ Positive Lymph Nodes
<0.5	15.6%	5.0%
0.5-0.9	14.1%	6.5%
1.0-1.9	22.5%	10.6%
2.0-2.9	26.1%	18.9%
3.0-3.9	27.4%	24.8%
4.0-4.9	25.6%	34.4%
>5.0	23.4%	46.7%

Data from the 1989 Cancer SEER Registry. National Cancer Institute, National Institutes of Health, Bethesda, Md.

TABLE 22-7. Summary of 5-year survival by the Number of Axillary Lymph Node Involvement in 505 Patients

No. Positive Axillary Lymph Nodes	Overall Survival
0	82.8%
1	80.15%
2	64.6%
3	70.0%
4	47.1%
4-6	54.1%
7-12	50.0%
Summary Based on AJCC N stage	
0	82.8%
1-3	73.0%
≥4	45.7%
≥13	28.4%

From Osborne CK. Prognostics factors in breast cancer. Principles Pract Oncol 1990;4:11.

BREAST CANCER IN THE MALE

Definition

Male breast cancer is a rare disease, accounting for less than 1% of all cases of breast carcinoma in Western countries. Association with a family history of breast cancer in first- or second-degree relatives, or both, is difficult to assess in males, mainly owing to lack of information and underestimation in the earlier years of these studies.

Because of the very low incidence of breast cancers in men, the great majority of mammographic diagnoses should be benign, with most of these being gynecomastia. Therefore, it is important to recognize the features of benign conditions such as gynecomastia to reduce the number of unnecessary surgical biopsies performed in men. By the same token, suspicious lesions should be recognized and thoroughly evaluated. Indications for mammography in men include evaluation of a palpable mass, recent onset of breast enlargement or tenderness, nipple-areolar skin changes or discharge, and a history of previous breast cancer. Screening mammography is not generally indicated for men. However, mammographically detected nonpalpable cancers have been reported in the contralateral breast of men with a history of breast cancer, suggesting that such men are in a high-risk category, thus justifying screening. Nonetheless, the incidence of either synchronous or metachronous bilateral breast carcinoma in men is reported to be less than 2%.

Prevalence and Epidemiology

Breast cancer in men accounts for 0.2% to 0.9% of all reported breast cancers and less than 1.0% of all cancers in men in the United States. Male breast cancer is rare before the age of 40 years, but thereafter the risk increases exponentially with time. The mean age of men with breast cancer is 59 years, which is 6 to 11 years older than the mean age in women. Bilateral breast cancer is seen in only 1.4% of cases. Incidence rates around the world are less than 1 case per 100,000 man-years and have largely remained stable in the United States and Europe in the past few decades. In the United States, approximately 1500 new cases are diagnosed annually, about 400 of which result in death. The relationship of breast cancer to gynecomastia is controversial, but most evidence suggests that the two conditions are not related. The reported coexistence of gynecomastia with breast cancer varies in different series from 2% to 35%, probably reflecting the differences in the patient populations studied. Fifty percent of male breast cancer patients have ipsilateral axillary adenopathy at the time of first presentation.

Etiology and Pathophysiology

Although most cases of male breast cancer are sporadic, a number of risk factors have been identified. Klinefelter's syndrome is the strongest risk factor (50-fold increase) for male breast cancer. In addition to a higher risk of cancer, patients with this syndrome commonly have coexistent gynecomastia.

In the patient undergoing estrogenic treatment for prostate cancer, determining whether a malignancy in the breast is a primary breast carcinoma or a metastasis from prostatic carcinoma can be difficult. For this reason, it is recommended that prostate specific antigen (PSA) IHC staining be performed on the histologic sections of male breast tumors.

Male-to-female transsexuals who are receiving long-term estrogen therapy could be at increased risk for development of breast cancer, although several studies have not shown exogenous estrogen to be a causal factor. Full acinar and lobular formation will occur in these patients, who are treated with progestative chemical castration combined with feminizing estrogen therapy. Transsexuals should be followed closely for the possible development of breast cancer. Baseline mammograms have been recommended, with additional studies performed when clinical indications are present. However, only four cases of breast cancer have been reported in transsexuals. The precise role of estrogen as an etiologic factor in breast cancer in men is still unknown.

Several cases of early-onset female breast cancer seem to occur with most cases of familial disease, which include male breast cancer. This is seen most often with *BRCA2* mutations and, to a lesser degree, with *BRCA1* mutations. Although women with the *BRCA2* mutation have an 80% chance of experiencing breast cancer, men with this mutation have only a 5% chance. The carrier risk of germline *BRCA2* mutations is higher in Jewish and Icelandic populations. Because daughters of men with breast cancer are at increased risk for development of breast cancer, *BRCA* gene mutation screening may be indicated.

Manifestations of Disease

Clinical Presentation

Breast cancer in the male typically manifests as a firm, painless mass in the subareolar region, eccentric to the nipple. Nipple retraction or inversion, skin thickening, encrustation, and ulceration are the presenting symptoms in approximately one third of patients. Nipple discharge can be due to benign conditions such as papilloma, duct ectasia, and gynecomastia. Amoroso and coworkers reported that in about 2% of benign male breast diseases, nipple discharge was a symptom. About half of the benign lesions manifesting as nipple discharge are papillomas, and nearly all instances of bloody discharge are caused by papillomas. However, nipple discharge occurs in 14% of men with breast cancers, and this discharge is likely to be serosanguineous. In fact, bloody nipple discharge has a stronger association with underlying carcinoma in men than in women. Ipsilateral axillary adenopathy at presentation is common in male breast carcinoma, and its presence as the only sign has been reported. In 5% of cases, male breast cancer manifests as Paget's disease, with erythema, inflammation, skin nodules, and satellite lesions.

Imaging Technique and Findings

Mammography

In younger men, mammography is reserved for those with compelling clinical indications, such as skin changes and nipple discharge. Although mammography is not a replacement for clinical examination, Evans and colleagues[50] found that the modality was able to accurately distinguish between malignant and benign male breast disease. In the absence of overt clinical signs of cancer, a mammographic diagnosis of gynecomastia does not warrant a tissue diagnosis.

Male breast cancer can present as a spiculated, ill-defined or circumscribed mass. Eccentric masses are highly suspicious for carcinoma. Gynecomastia may show some adherence of the skin but never causes ulceration or encrustation. Skin retraction and ulceration are helpful secondary signs and poor prognostic signs. In addition, skin thickening, nipple retraction, and axillary adenopathy may be present. Calcifications are uncommon in male breast carcinoma. If calcifications are seen, however, they can appear pleomorphic, large, round, and scattered.

Ultrasonography

Very few reports detail the ultrasonographic features of male breast cancer, which are similar to those found in female breast cancer. Lesions appear as hypoechoic with irregular margins, and sound transmission may vary from dense distal acoustic shadowing to acoustic enhancement. Complex cystic masses are also suggestive of malignancy, particularly papillary DCIS. Secondary signs of malignancy may be important and can include architectural distortion of normal breast tissue and disruption of the subcutaneous fat layer. Although nonspecific, the presence of axillary lymph nodes, especially those without normal fatty hilum, can also indicate malignancy.

Classic Signs

Pathology Findings

Most male patients with breast cancer present with a painless mass usually located at the subareolar area and, rarely, the upper outer quadrant. Gynecomastia is the most common cause of mass lesion in male breast. The definition of gynecomastia is proliferations of glandular and stroma causing hypertrophy of the breast. The term *gynecomastia* should be used strictly within this context and separated from pseudogynecomastia due to excess fat in obese patients causing bilateral breast enlargement. There is no direct relationship between gynecomastia and male breast cancers. Carcinoma of the male breast appears identical to female breast ductal carcinomas as in DCIS. Invasive lobular carcinoma and LCIS are rare in male breast cancer. When bona fide lobular carcinoma is seen in the male breast, karyotype and E-cadherin IHC studies may be recommended. Papillary carcinoma, usually the intracystic and noninvasive form, is more common in males (3%-5%) compared with females (1%-2%). Metastatic carcinoma from another primary site should be in the differential diagnosis of breast tumors in males, including prostatic adenocarcinoma, especially when the DCIS component is lacking. Using IHC stains, such as PSA, may be helpful in these circumstances. Immunoreactivity of ER and PR is associated with the degree of differentiation of breast cancers. Low- to intermediate-grade carcinoma is ER and PR positive, whereas high-grade and poorly differentiated breast cancer may be negative for ER and PR. HER-2/neu has been reported to be positive in 17% of male breast cancer by IHC stains. Most patients have been treated with total mastectomy and axillary dissection. Prognosis is related to the stage of disease at the time of diagnosis. Some reported that male and female patients with the same stage of disease have a similar prognosis, and others have reported a less favorable outcome in males.

Synopsis of Treatment Options

The treatment options for IDC are similar to those for DCIS (see Chapter 21). The best course of treatment for IDC is individualized care with a multipronged approach. Excision alone, excision with irradiation or tamoxifen, or both, and band mastectomy are all potentially appropriate and acceptable treatment options for IDC. All apparent IDC and DCIS should be excised with a sufficient rim (margin) of normal breast tissue. The type of surgical procedure includes lumpectomy or mastectomy and is influenced by patient preference, age, breast size, extent and grade of lesion, margin width, and the mammographic and pathologic findings. Irradiation and endocrine therapy should also be considered on an individual basis according to the tumor biology and biomarker studies.

Not all breast cancers of the same type, size, and stage behave in a similar fashion or have identical survival rates. We know that even at smaller tumor sizes (T1), some tumors behave worse than others with distant metastasis. As we begin to understand the biology of breast cancers, it is evident that breast cancers are truly heterogeneous groups of tumors with different prognosis. Microarray profiling has, unquestionably, been established as a powerful tool in unraveling mechanistic insights into tumor biology. The variations in gene expression patterns by cDNA microarrays and hierarchical clustering provided a distinctive "molecular portrait" of each tumor and make it possible to classify these tumors into subtypes based solely on differences in these patterns. With this method, there are five different subclassifications of breast cancer types: HER-2 positive, luminal A, luminal B, luminal C, and triple negative (basal-like). Luminal A breast tumors have the best prognosis and are ER and PR positive and HER-2/neu negative. Luminal B tumors are ER, PR, and HER-2/neu positive. When the breast tumor is ER- and PR-negative and HER-2/neu-positive it is designated as a luminal C tumor. Basal-like tumors are so-called triple-negative (ER, PR, HER-2/neu) tumors and have the worst prognosis due to the lack of Herceptin as a treatment option and no hormone manipulation feasible. Biologically, a HER-2/neu negative is better than a HER-2/neu positive tumor. Trials to subclassify the triple-negative tumor by the IHC stains are under way. Many reports have identified that the triple-negative tumors, so-called basal-like tumors, express high molecular weight cytokeratins such as CK5, CK6, CK14, and CK17. Others have identified epidermal growth factor receptor (EGFR) in basal-like tumors. Basal-like breast cancer is defined when the tumor is ER, PR, and HER-2/neu negative, but not all triple-negative tumors are basal-like tumors. Basal-like tumors are known to have earlier recurrence and reduced survival with a shorter disease-free rate.

Currently, the treatment recommendations for luminal A and luminal B subtypes of tumors are tamoxifen and aromatase inhibitors, respectively. Basal-like tumors are difficult to treat with a traditional chemotherapy regimen. Studies are being done on treatment with a platinum-based chemoreagent as well as a poly (ADP-ribose) polymerase (PARP) inhibitor, which is related to the DNA repair process.

Although microarray profiling has been a powerful tool in unraveling mechanistic insights into tumor biology, this new classification is too early to be useful in pathology reporting at this time. The great danger of using new technology with newer problems is that the older and more traditional prognostic factors and scientific lessons are quickly forgotten.[51] In terms of male breast cancers, owing to the rarity of male disease, most treatment regimens follow those already established for female breast cancer. Most authorities believe that modified radical mastectomy is the best means to achieve locoregional control unless there is chest wall extension, in which case more radical resection, radiation therapy, or both, can be used. Thus far, no studies have demonstrated the efficacy of systemic adjuvant treatment in male breast cancer. Generally, however, men with node-positive cancers or with node-negative cancers and a significant risk of recurrence undergo adjuvant treatment.

Metastatic spread of male breast cancer parallels that seen in women, with the majority of lesions occurring in the lung and bone. Liver lesions tend to occur less commonly in men. Metastases to the breast from extramammary malignancies can occur, and most arise from prostatic carcinoma. In addition, metastases arising from melanoma, renal adenocarcinoma, leukemia, lymphoma, urothelial carcinoma, and lung carcinoma also occur.

There are also two primary lesions in male breast cancer patients, with a disproportionately high percentage (41%) of colon and rectal carcinomas occurring simultaneously with breast carcinoma. In contrast, the overall incidence of two primary lesions is only 3% in female breast cancer patients.

Stage for stage, the survival rate of male breast carcinoma is similar to that of women. The overall prognosis for men with breast cancer is worse than for women and has been attributed to a number of factors: delayed diagnosis, anatomic factors, inappropriate staging, later stage of disease at presentation, and older age at diagnosis. The prognosis largely depends on lymph node status and tumor size, although histologic grade and duration of symptoms also appear to be significant. The presence of a family history of breast cancer does not seem to affect outcome. The overall 5-year survival for male breast cancer is approximately 50%. The 5-year survival rate is approximately 53% for men with carcinomas smaller than 2 cm, 44% for those with tumors 2 to 5 cm, and only 25% for those with tumors larger than 5 cm. Furthermore, associated comorbid medical conditions also result in worse outcomes.

KEY POINTS

- Invasive or infiltrating ductal carcinoma (IDC) is the most common type of invasive breast cancer, accounting for 80% of invasive breast cancers.
- The mammographic signs of invasive breast cancer are often divided into primary, secondary, and indirect signs.
- Most important prognostic factor for breast cancer is the status of lymph node metastasis.
- Breast biomarker studies are an important aspect of predictive value for breast cancer.

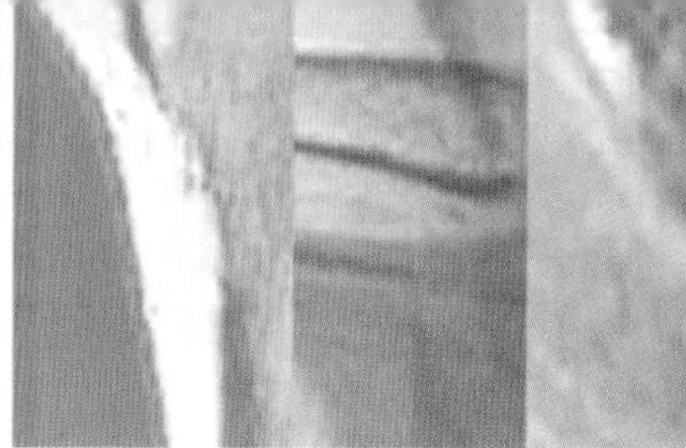

CASE STUDIES

Chapter 22 Invasive Ductal Carcinomas

CASE 1

HISTORY

An 81-year-old woman presented for a screening mammogram without any significant complaints.

FINDINGS

This mass is an American College of Radiology Breast Imaging Reporting and Data System (BI-RADS) category 5, which is highly suggestive of malignancy. See Figures 22-76A through 22-76E.

DIAGNOSIS

The tumor is a moderately differentiated invasive ductal carcinoma, measuring 1.2 cm (Fig. 22-76F):

Modified Bloom-Richardson score: 6 of 9 (6/9),
Tubule formation: 3
Nuclear grade: 2
Mitosis: 1

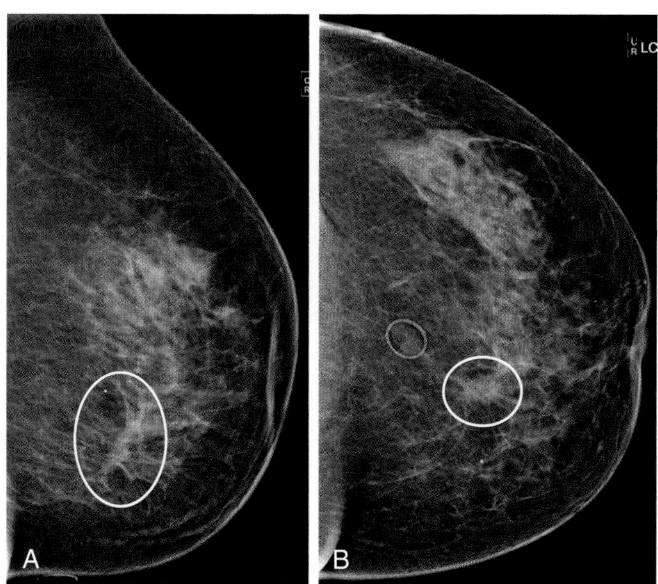

■ **FIGURE 22-76** **A,** Left lateral medial view of 12 mm isodense irregular mass with spiculated margins at 7 o'clock in the lower inner quadrant mid third breast. **B,** Left craniocaudal (CC) view of 12 mm isodense irregular shaped mass with spiculated margins at 7 o'clock in the lower inner quadrant mid third breast. There is a mole marker (*smaller circle*) on the left CC view.

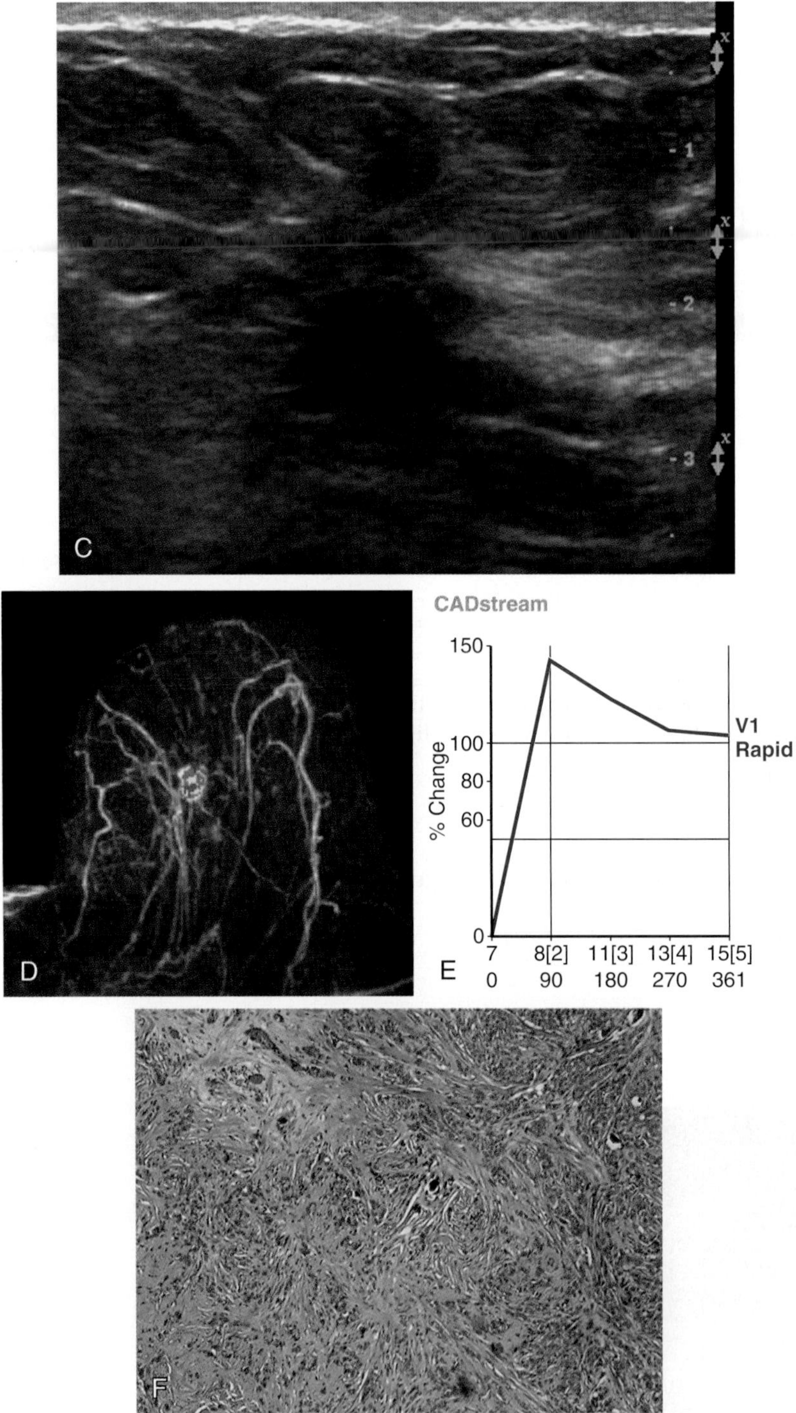

■ FIGURE 22-76—cont'd C, Ultrasound image in the lower inner quadrant demonstrates a 2 cm mass corresponding to the mammographic abnormality. Ultrasound characteristics of the finding include spiculation, an orientation that is not parallel to the skin line, posterior acoustic shadowing, and an irregular shape. **D,** Magnetic resonance imaging (MRI; axial maximum intensity projection image). An irregular enhancing mass in the left breast with spiculated margins at the 7-o'clock position measuring 16 × 14 × 11 mm is shown. **E,** The kinetic curve demonstrates rapid enhancement and washout. **F,** Invasive ductal carcinoma is seen with microcalcifications (H&E, ×100).

CASE 2

HISTORY

A 58-year-old woman presented with a palpable right breast mass. She initially reported a palpable mass in her right breast 1 year earlier but did not follow up with her clinicians until today when she presented with the same but enlarging palpable mass in her right breast. Her most recent mammograms are from 8 years ago.

FINDINGS

This mass is a BI-RADS category 5 tumor, which is highly suggestive of malignancy. See Figures 22-77A through 22-77E.

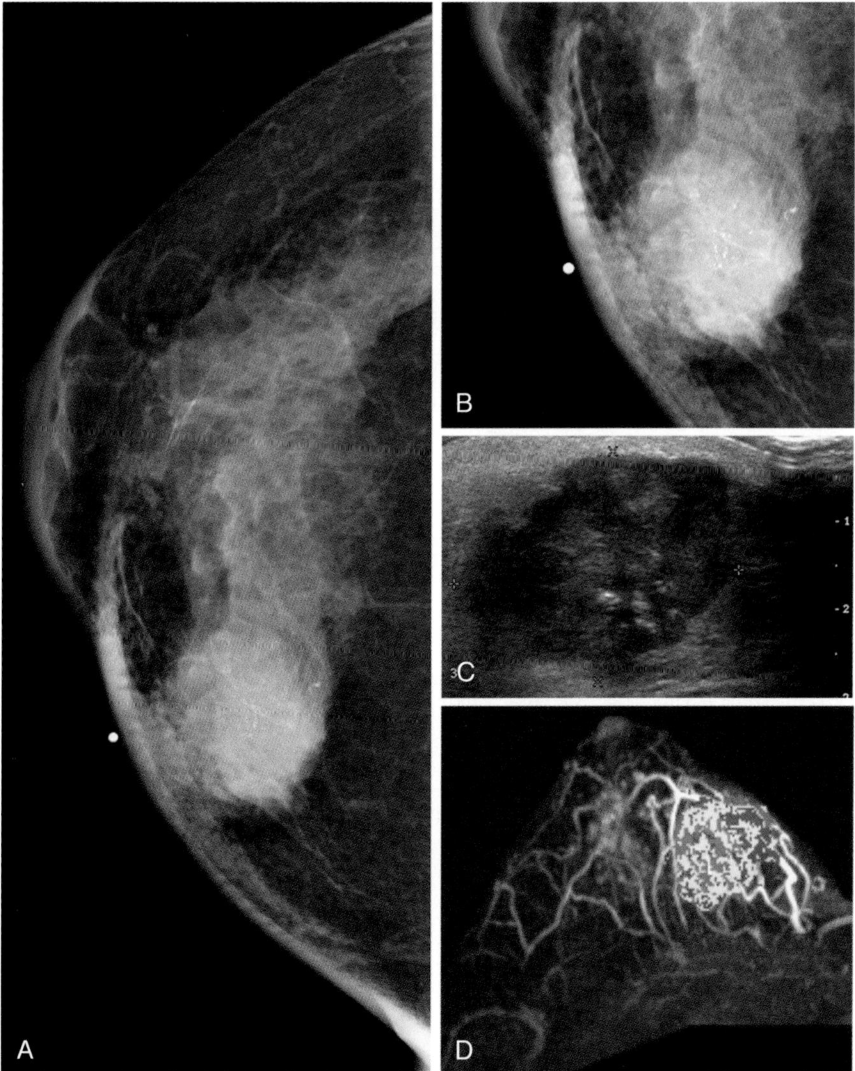

■ FIGURE 22-77 **A,** Right craniocaudal (CC) view. BB marker placed over the palpable mass at about 2 o'clock of the right breast. Beneath the marker is a 4.0-cm high-density oval mass with indistinct margins. **B,** Right magnified CC view. There are associated fine, pleomorphic calcifications measuring about 2 cm and overlying skin thickening. **C,** Ultrasound image demonstrates a 4.2 × 3.3 × 2.6 cm oval, circumscribed mass with mixed echogenicity that spans from the 1-o'clock to 3-o'clock positions in the right breast. There are punctate hyperechoic areas representing the pleomorphic calcifications. **D,** Magnetic resonance image (MRI; axial maximum intensity projection image). The primary tumor is seen in the upper inner quadrant.

DIAGNOSIS

The diagnosis is invasive ductal carcinoma, poorly differentiated, modified (Figs. 22-77F and 22-77G):

Bloom-Richardson score: 8 of 9
Tubule formation: 3
Nuclear atypia: 2
Mitoses: 3
Size of invasive tumor: 3.5 cm
Tumor involves superficial dermis of skin

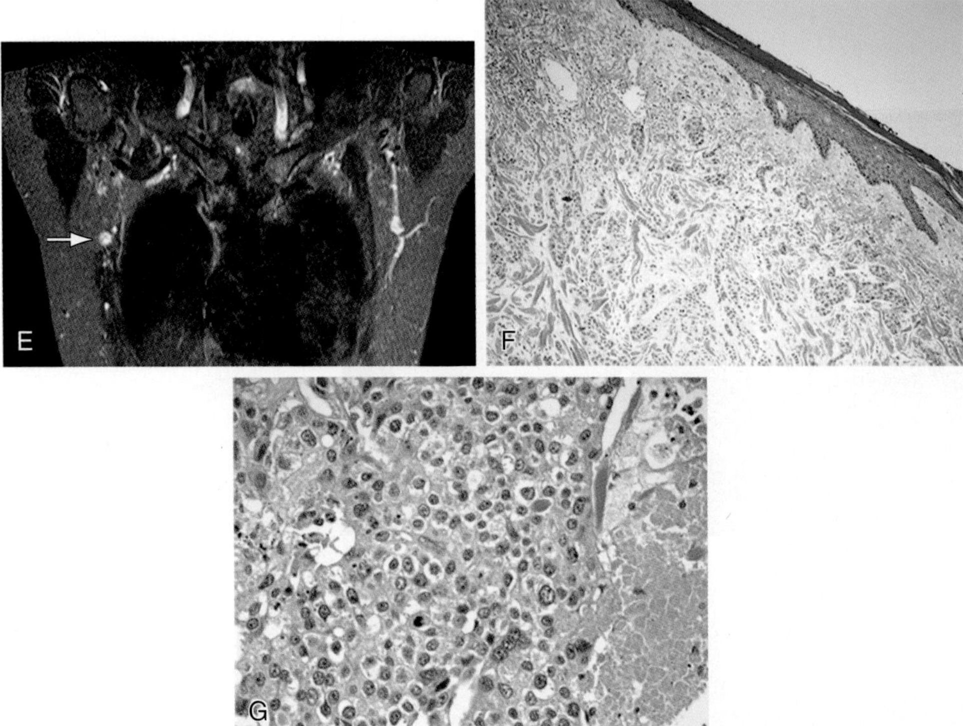

■ **FIGURE 22-77—cont'd** **E,** MRI (coronal T2 image). There is a suspicious right axillary lymph node measuring 1.3 × 1.0 cm that is suggestive of metastasis. **F,** Invasive ductal carcinoma (IDC) is present at the superficial dermis of the skin (H&E, ×200). **G,** High-grade IDC with mitosis and tumor necrosis (H&E, ×400).

CASE 3

HISTORY

A 56-year-old woman presented with a palpable mass in the left breast associated with skin thickening, erythema, and pain.

FINDINGS

This mass is a BI-RADS Category 5 which is highly suggestive of malignancy. See Figures 22-78A through 22-78E.

DIAGNOSIS

The tumor is an IDC, moderately differentiated, with an extensive intraductal component (Fig. 22-78F).

Modified Bloom-Richardson score: 7 of 9
Tubule formation: 3
Nuclear pleomorphism: 2
Mitoses: 2

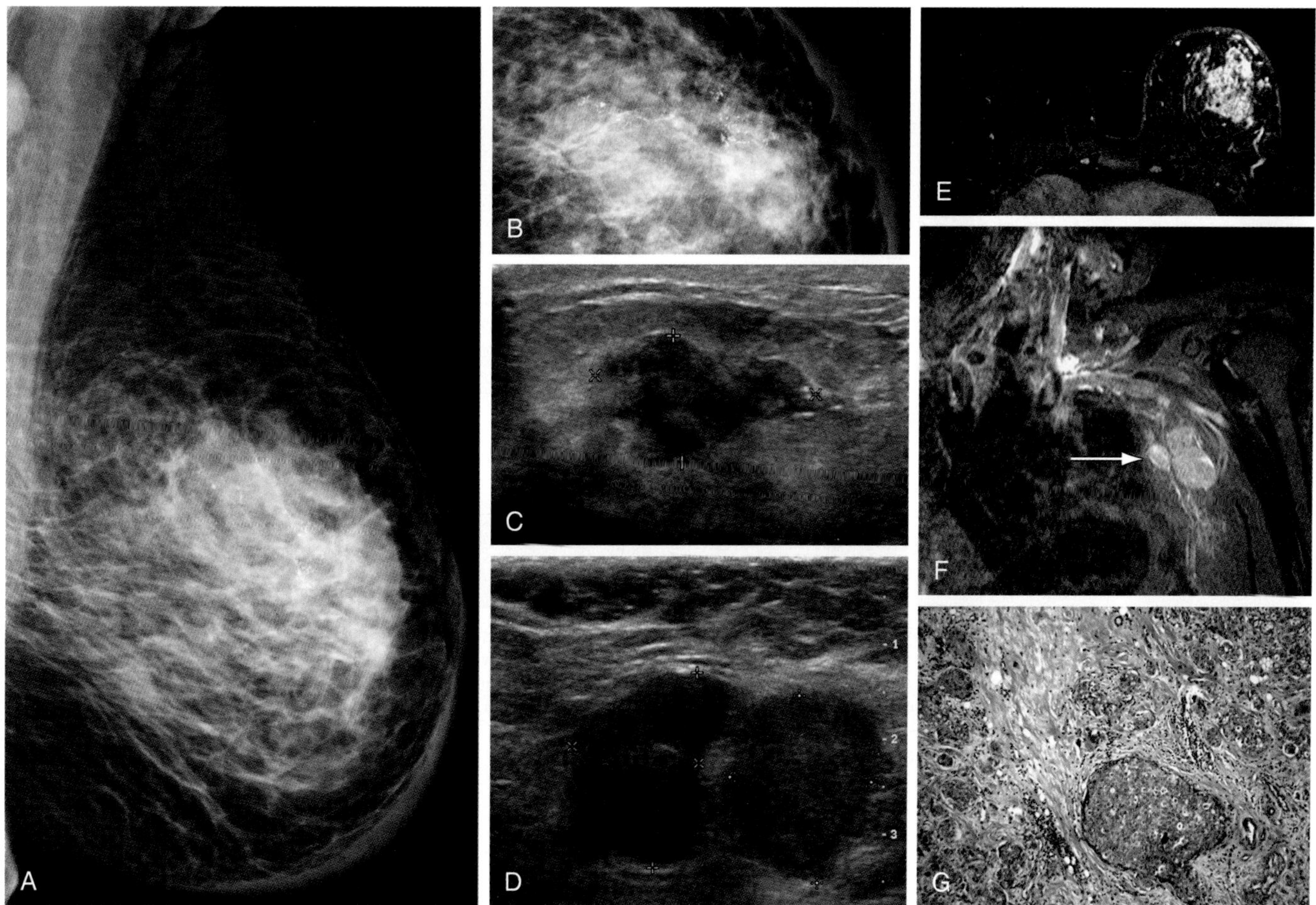

■ **FIGURE 22-78** **A,** Left mediolateral oblique (MLO) view. Asymmetry in the upper hemisphere between the 11-o'clock and 2:30-o'clock positions measuring 7.8 cm AP × 7.2 cm ML × 7.0 cm SI. There is diffuse trabecular and skin thickening. The visualized left axillary area shows a partially seen dense lymph node. **B,** Magnified left craniocaudal (CC) view. This area contains pleomorphic microcalcifications with a segmental distribution. **C,** Ultrasound image of the left upper hemisphere demonstrates multiple lobular and circumscribed hypoechoic solid lesions (only one lesion shown) containing calcifications. In addition, there is skin thickening and edema involving the breast. **D,** Ultrasound image of the left axilla shows at least two large abnormal lymph nodes measuring 2 cm and 2.2 cm. **E,** Magnetic resonance imaging (MRI; axial subtraction image) demonstrates regional, homogeneous enhancement in the left breast in the upper outer quadrant. The kinetic curve demonstrates rapid enhancement and washout. In addition, there is diffuse skin and trabecular thickening. **F,** Magnetic resonance imaging (MRI; coronal T2-weighted image). Extensive, bulky left axillary lymphadenopathy. **G,** Invasive ductal carcinoma (IDC) with ductal carcinoma in situ (H&E, × 200).

CASE 4

HISTORY

A 72-year-old man with bilateral gynecomastia presents with a subareolar lump in the right breast.

FINDINGS

This mass is a BI-RADS category 5, which is highly suggestive of malignancy. See Figures 22-79A through 22-79 C.

DIAGNOSIS

Diagnosis is IDC (Figs. 22-79D and 22-79E).

Fine-needle aspiration (FNA) was performed on this mass, and it was confirmed to be an adenocarcinoma.

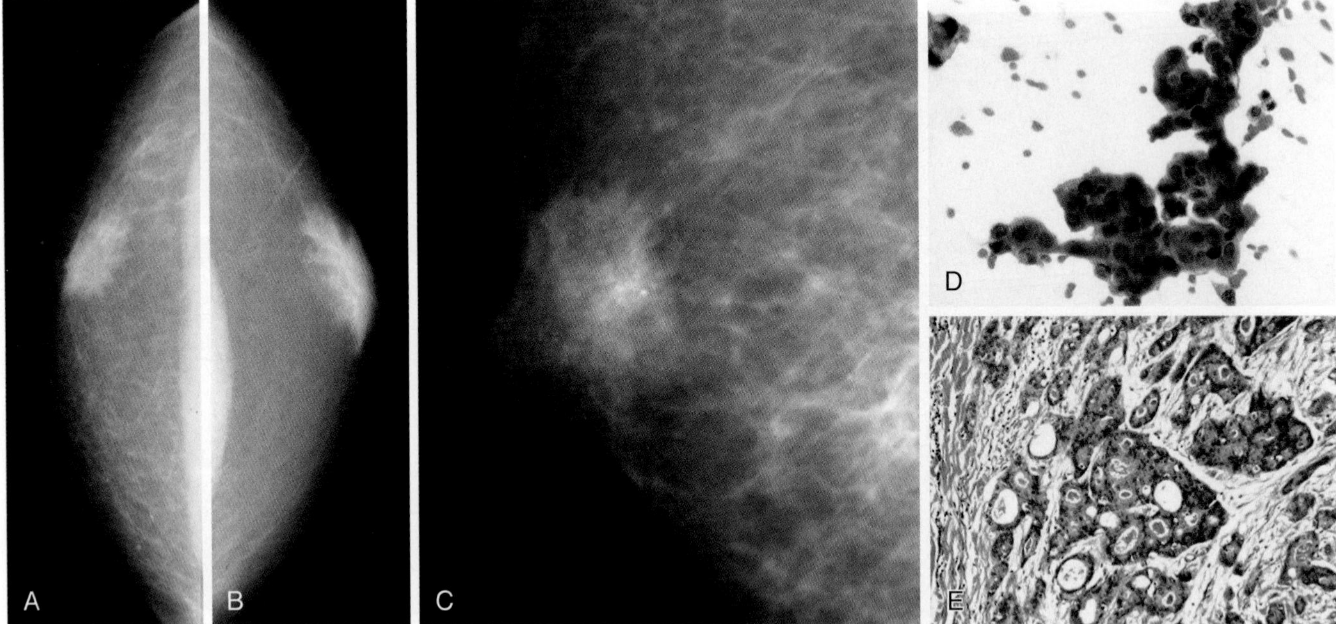

■ **FIGURE 22-79** **A,** Right craniocaudal (CC) view. Gynecomastia. **B,** Left CC view. Gynecomastia. **C,** Magnified right mediolateral oblique (MLO) view. Beneath the area of gynecomastia is a subareolar mass that has an irregular shape with obscured and spiculated margins. There are associated pleomorphic calcifications and skin and trabecular thickening. **D,** Aggregates of malignant cells with high nuclear to cytoplasmic ratio and hyperchromatic nuclei. Glandular structure is seen (fine-needle aspiration [FNA] image PAP stain, ×400). **E,** Excisional biopsy shows invasive ductal carcinoma (IDC) with many tubular formations (H&E, ×200).

CASE 5

HISTORY

A 65-year-old woman without any significant complaints presented for a screening mammogram.

FINDINGS

This mass is a BI-RADS category 4C, which is moderately suggestive of malignancy. See Figures 22-80A and 22-80B.

DIAGNOSIS

This lesion is an 8-mm well-differentiated IDC (Fig. 22-80C):

Modified Bloom-Richardson score: 5 of 9
Tubule formation: 2
Nuclear pleomorphism: 1 to 2
Mitoses: 1

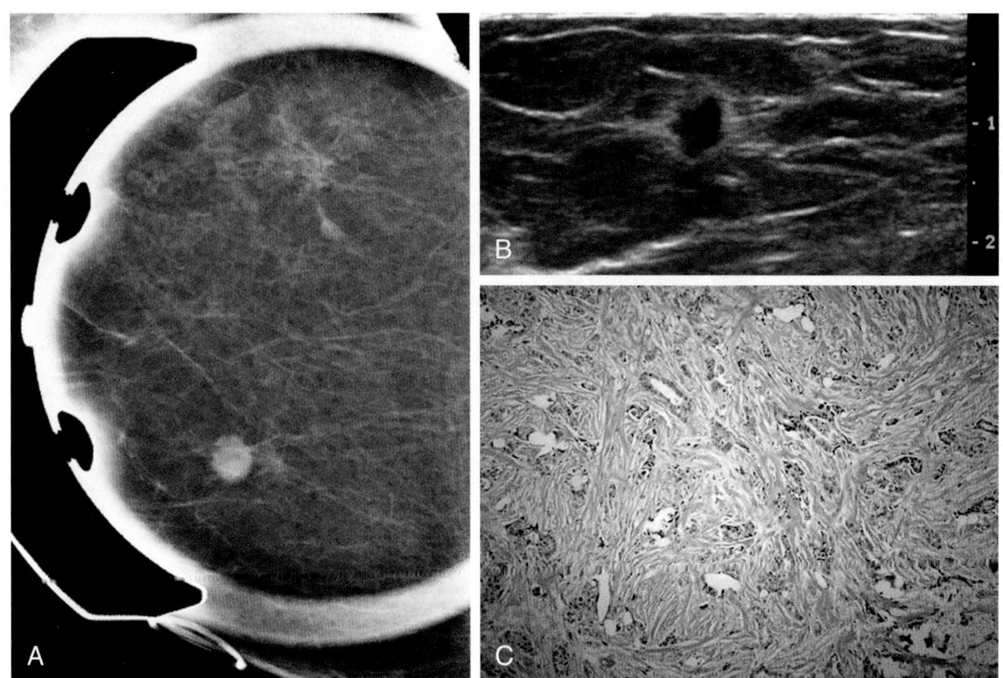

■ **FIGURE 22-80** **A,** Spot compression right craniocaudal (CC) view of 6 × 8 mm dense round mass with spiculated margins at 3 o'clock middle depth. **B,** Ultrasound image demonstrates a 7 mm hypoechoic, anti-parallel mass with angulated margins and an echogenic rim at 3 o'clock, corresponding to the spiculated mass seen on mammography. **C,** Well-differentiated invasive ductal carcinoma (IDC) (H&E, ×100).

CASE 6

HISTORY

An 80-year-old woman without any significant complaints presented for a screening mammogram.

FINDINGS

This mass is a BI-RADS Category 4C which is moderately suggestive of malignancy. See Figures 22-81A through 22-81 C.

DIAGNOSIS

This was a 10-mm, moderately differentiated IDC (Figs. 22-81D and 22-81E):

Modified Bloom-Richardson score: 6 of 9
Tubule formation: 3
Nuclear pleomorphism: 1 to 2
Mitoses: 1

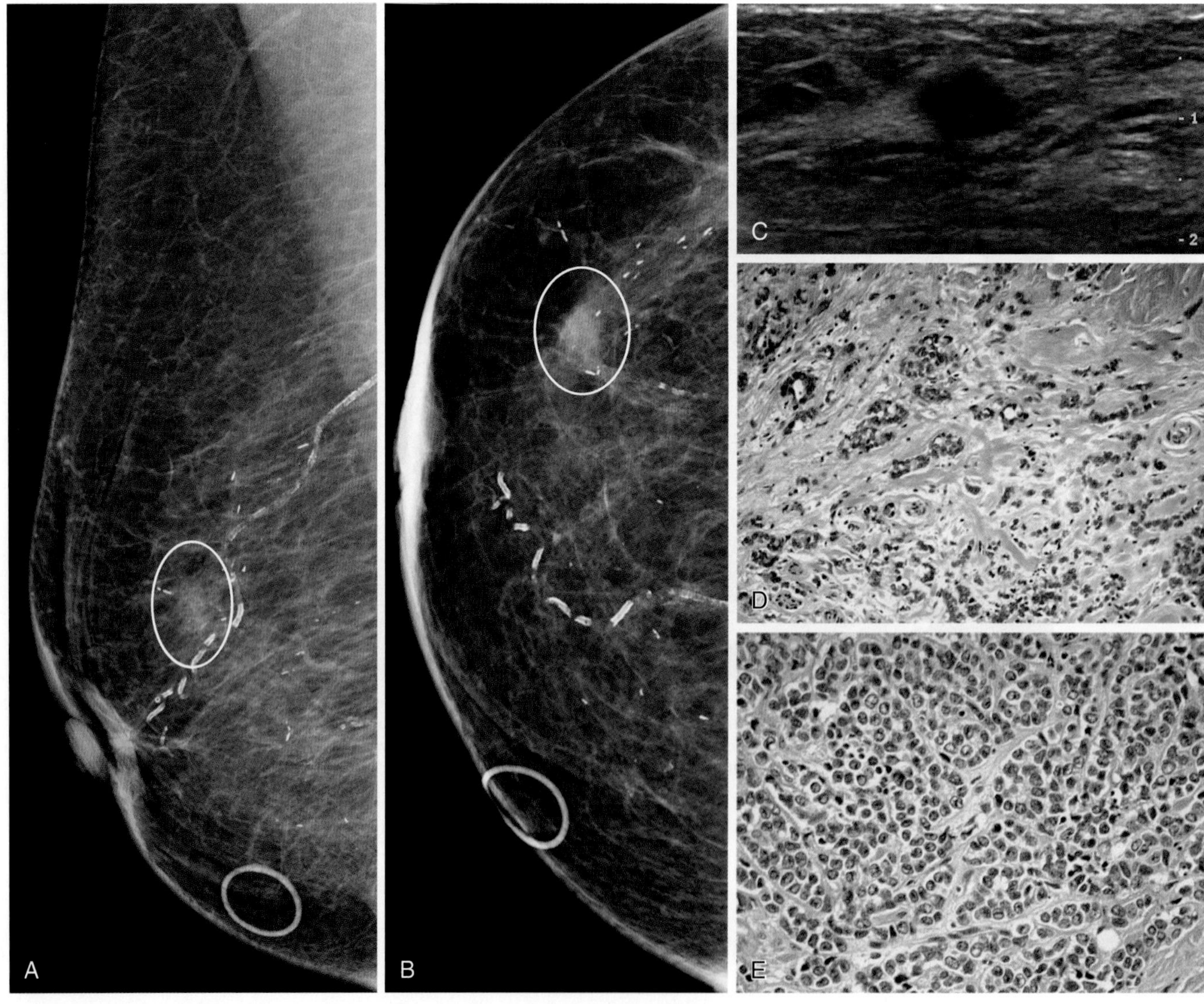

■ **FIGURE 22-81** **A,** Right mediolateral oblique (MLO) view. There is a focal asymmetry (*circled*) measuring 9 mm at the 9-o'clock position in the middle third of the breast. **B,** Right craniocaudal (CC) view. There is a focal asymmetry (*circled*) measuring 9 mm at the 9-o'clock position in the middle third of the breast. **C,** Ultrasound image demonstrates an 8 mm solid mass in the subareolar region at the 9-o'clock position. Characteristics of the finding include a hypoechoic echo pattern, oval shape, echogenic rim, and indistinct margins. **D,** Invasive carcinoma showing both tubule formations, features of ductal and linear pattern, and features of lobular carcinoma (H&E, ×200). **E,** The same case as Fig. 22-81D in high-power view showing open nuclear chromatin (H&E, ×400).

CASE 7

HISTORY

A 43-year-old woman without any significant complaints presented for a baseline screening mammogram.

FINDINGS

This mass is a BI-RADS category 5, which is highly suggestive of malignancy. See Figures 22-82A through 22-82C.

DIAGNOSIS

The tumor is a 25-mm moderately differentiated IDC that was confirmed to be DCIS, comedo type, with a high nuclear grade with central necrosis (Fig. 22-82D):

Modified Bloom-Richardson score: 6 of 9
Tubule formation: 3
Nuclear pleomorphism: 2
Mitoses: 1

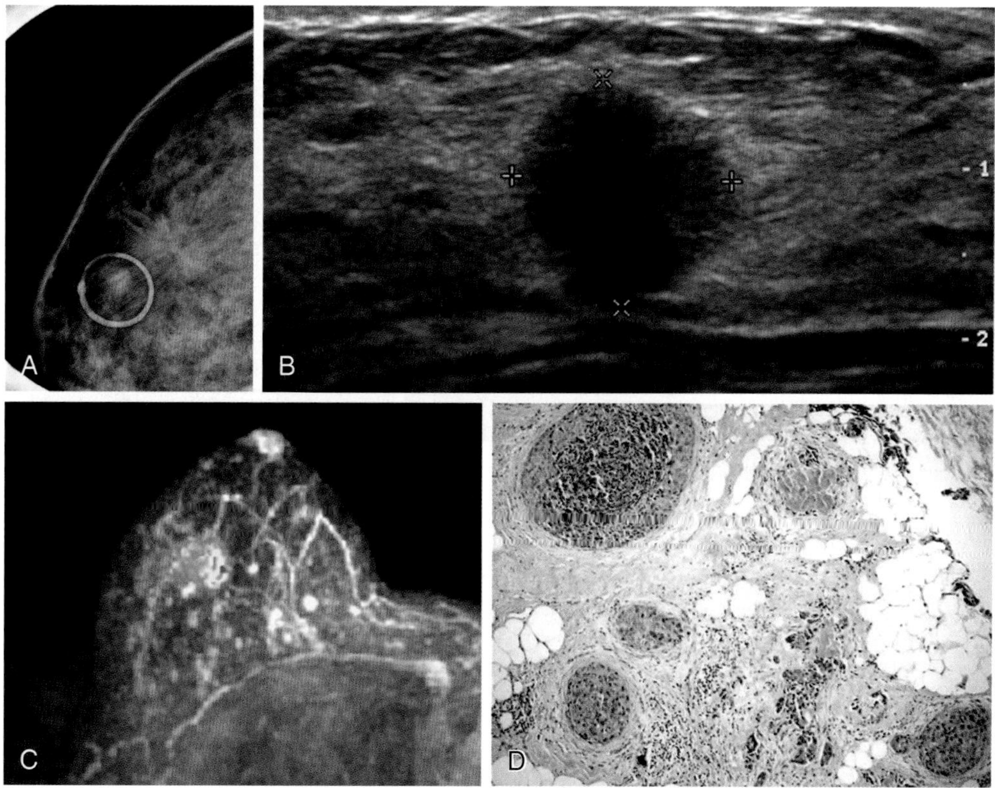

■ **FIGURE 22-82** **A,** Spot compression right craniocaudal (CC) view. There is a dense irregular shaped mass with spiculated margins and a few associated central microcalcifications. Mole marker (*circle*) is seen adjacent to the mass. **B,** Ultrasound image demonstrates a 1.6 cm solid mass with microcalcifications at the site of the mammographic and clinically palpable mass. The characteristics of the finding include an oval, taller than wide shape, echogenic rim, and indistinct and spiculated margins. **C,** Magnetic resonance imaging (MRI; axial MIP image) demonstrates a 2.3 cm lobulated mass with smooth margins at the 10-o'clock position in the right breast. The kinetic curve shows rapid enhancement and washout. There are no other significant findings. **D,** Invasive ductal carcinoma (IDC) with ductal carcinoma in situ (DCIS) (H&E).

CASE 8

HISTORY

A 67-year-old woman without any significant complaints presented for a screening mammogram.

FINDINGS

This mass is a BI-RADS category 5, which is highly suggestive of malignancy. See Figures 22-83A and 22-83B.

DIAGNOSIS

This IDC was 8 mm and well differentiated with an extensive intraductal component spanning 13 mm (Fig. 22-83C):

Modified Bloom-Richardson score: 5 of 9
Tubule formation: 2
Nuclear pleomorphism: 1 to 2
Mitoses: 1

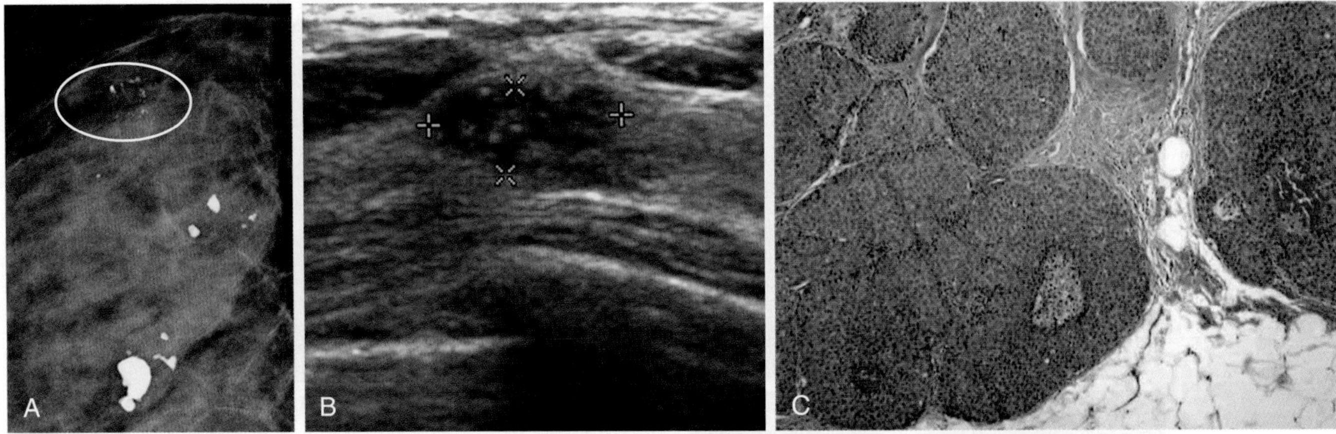

■ **FIGURE 22-83** **A,** Magnified right craniocaudal (CC) view. There is a 10 mm cluster of pleomorphic microcalcifications (*circled*) in the upper outer quadrant at the 10-o'clock position in the posterior third of the breast. There are two adjacent hyalinized benign fibroadenomas. **B,** Ultrasound image at the 10-o'clock position far laterally demonstrates a 1.0 cm solid hypoechoic oval shaped mass with indistinct margins containing internal hyperechoic, punctate foci that correspond to the pleomorphic microcalcifications seen on mammography. **C,** Ductal carcinoma in situ (DCIS), solid type with focal area of central necrosis is seen. Invasive carcinoma is not shown from this image (H&E, ×100).

SUGGESTED READINGS

Page DL, Fleming ID, Fritz A, Balch CM, Haller DG, Morrow M. In: Greene FL, editor. *AJCC cancer staging manual*. 6th ed. New York: Springer-Verlag; 2002. Available at: *www.springer-ny.com*.

Appelbaum AH, Evans GF, Levy KR, Amirkhan RH, Schumpert TD. Mammographic appearances of male breast disease. *Radiographics* 1999;**19**:559-68.

Carter CL, Allen C, Henson DE. Relation of tumor size, lymph node status, and survival in 24,740 breast cancers cases. *Cancer* 1989;**63**:181-7.

Mahoney MC, Bevers T, Linos E, Willett WC. Opportunities and strategies for breast cancer prevention through risk reduction. *CA Cancer J Clin* 2008;**58**:347-71.

Morrow M, Strom EA, Bassett LW, Dershaw DD, Fowble B, Giuliano A, et al. Standard for breast conservation therapy in the management of invasive breast carcinoma. *CA Cancer J Clin* 2002;**52**:277-300.

Rosen PP. *Rosen's Breast pathology*. 2nd ed. 2001.

Smith RA, Cokkinides V, Brawley OW. Cancer screening in the United States, 2009: a review of current American Cancer Society guidelines and issues in cancer screening. *CA Cancer J Clin* 2009;**59**:27-41.

Tavassoli FA. *Pathology of breast disease*. 2nd ed. 1999.

Vogel VG. Breast cancer prevention: a review of current evidence. *CA Cancer J Clin* 2000;**50**:156-70.

REFERENCES

1. Page DL, Anderson TJ, Connelly JL, Schnitt SF. Miscellaneous features of carcinoma. In: Page DL, Anderson TJ, editors. *Diagnostic histopathology of the breast*. Edinburgh: Churchill Livingstone; 1987.
2. Newstead GM, Baute PB, Toth HK. Invasive lobular and ductal carcinoma: mammographic findings and stage at diagnosis. *Radiology* 1992;**184**:623-7.
3. Surveillance, Epidemiology and End Results (SEER) Program (www.seer.cancer.gov). SEER*Stat Database: Incidence-SEER 9 Regs Public Use, Nov. 2002 Sub (1973-2000) 18 Age Groups, National Cancer Institute, DCCPS, Surveillance Research Program, Cancer Statistics Branch, released April 2003, based on the November 2002 submission.
4. American Cancer Society. *Cancer Facts & Figures*. Atlanta: American Cancer Society; 2008.
5. Jemal A, Siegel R, Ward E, Murray T, Xu J, Thun MJ. Cancer statistics, 2007. *CA Cancer J Clin* 2007;**57**:43-66.
6. American Cancer Society. *Breast Cancer Facts & Figures*. Atlanta: American Cancer Society; 2007-2008.
7. Ries LAG, Eisner MP, Kosary CL, et al. *SEER Cancer Statistics Review, 1975-2000*. Bethesda, MD: National Cancer Institute; 2003.
8. Ghafoor A, Jemal A, Ward E, Cokkinides V, Smith R, Thun M. Trends in breast cancer by race and ethnicity. *CA Cancer J Clin* 2003;**53**:342-55.
9. Levy-Lahad E, Friedman E. Cancer risks among BRCA1 and BRCA2 mutation carriers. *Br J Cancer* 2007;**96**:11-5.
10. Singletary SE. Rating the risk factors for breast cancer. *Ann Surg* 2003;**237**:474-82.
11. National Cancer Institute, US National Institutes of Health. *Surveillance, Epidemiology, and End Results (SEER) Program (www.seer.cancer.gov)*. SEER*Stat Database: Incidence-SEER 17 Regs Limited-Use, Nov 2006 Sub (1973-2004 varying), Linked to County Attributes, Total US, 1969-2004 Counties, National Cancer Institute, DCCPS, Surveillance Research Program, Cancer Statistics Branch, released April 2007, based on the November 2006 submission.
12. National Cancer Institute, US National Institutes of Health. *Surveillance, Epidemiology, and End Results (SEER) Program (www.seer.cancer.gov) DevCan Database: SEER 17 Incidence and Mortality*. National Cancer Institute, DCCPS, Surveillance Research Program, Cancer Statistics Branch, released April 2006, based on the November 2005 submission. 2000-2003.
13. Vogel VG. Breast cancer prevention: a review of current evidence. *CA Cancer J clin* 2000;**50**:156-70.
14. Children's Oncology Group. *Long-term follow-up guidelines for survivors of childhood, adolescent, and young adult cancers*. Bethesda, MD: Children's Oncology Group; 2006.
15. Collaborative Group on Hormonal Factors in Breast Cancer. Breast cancer and breastfeeding: collaborative reanalysis of individual data from 47 epidemiological studies in 30 countries, including 50302 women with breast cancer and 96973 women without the disease. *Lancet* 2002;**360**:187-95.
16. Bearhs OH, Shapiro S, Smart C, et al. Report of the working group to review the National Cancer Institute-American Cancer Society breast cancer detection demonstration projects. *J Natl Cancer Inst* 1979;**62**:639-98.
17. Cutler M. Diagnosis and differential diagnosis. In: Cutler M, editor. *Tumors of the breast*. Philadelphia: JB Lippincott; 1962. p. 168-76.
18. Donegan WL, Spratt JS, editors. *Cancer of the breast*. 4th ed. Philadelphia: WB Saunders; 1995.
19. Kaiser JS, Helvie MA, Blacklaw RL, Roubidoux MA. Palpable breast thickening: role of mammography and US in cancer detection. *Radiology* 2002;**223**:839-44.
20. Haagaensen CD. Diseases of the breast. 3rd ed. Philadelphia: WB Saunders; 1986.
21. Taylor GW, Meltzer A. Inflammatory carcinoma of the breast. *Am J Cancer* 1938;**33**:33-49.
22. Lee BJ, Tannenbaum NE. Inflammatory carcinoma of the breast. *Surg Gynecol Obstet* 1924;**29**:580-95.
23. Devitt JE. Management of nipple discharge by clinical findings. *Am J Surg* 1985;**149**:789-92.
24. Chaudary MA, Millis RR, Davies GC, Hayward JL. Nipple discharge: The diagnostic value of testing for occult blood. *Ann Surg* 1982;**196**:651-5.
25. Copeland MM, Higgins TG. Significance of discharge from the nipple in nonpuerperal mammary conditions. *Ann Surg* 1960;**151**:638.
26. Halsted WS. A clinical and histologic study of certain adenocarcinomas of the breast. *Ann Surg* 1898;**28**:557-76.
27. Ashikari R, Rosen PP, Urban JA, Senoo T. Breast cancer presenting as an axillary mass. *Ann Surg* 1976;**183**:415-7.
28. American College of Radiology. *Breast imaging reporting and data system (BI-RADS)*. Reston, VA: American College of Radiology; 1995.
29. Sickles EA. Nonpalpable, circumscribed, noncalcified solid breast masses: likelihood of malignancy based on lesion size and age of patient. *Radiology* 1994;**192**:439-42.
30. Jackson VP, Dines KA, Bassett LW, Gold RH, Reynolds HE. Diagnostic importance of radiographic density of noncalcified breast masses: Analysis of 91 lesions. *AJR Am J Roentgenol* 1991;**157**:25-8.
31. Kalisher L, Chu AM, Peyster RG. Clinicopathological correlations of xeroradiography in determining involvement of metastatic axillary nodes in female breast cancer. *Radiology* 1976;**121**:333-5.
32. Andersson I, Marsal L, Nilsson B, et al. Abnormal axillary lymph nodes in rheumatoid arthritis. *Acta Radiol Diagn (Stockh)* 1980;**21**:645-9.
33. Sickles EA. Mammographic features of "early" breast cancer. *AJR Am J Roentgenol* 1984;**143**:461-4.
34. Bassett LW, Shayestehfar B, Hirbawi I. Obtaining previous mammograms for comparison: Usefulness and costs. *AJR Am J Roentgenol* 1994;**163**:1083-6.
35. Bassett LW, Hendrick RE, Bassford TL. *Quality Determinants of Mammography*. (Clinical Practice Guideline, N. 13. AHCPR Publication No. 95-0632.) Rockville, MD: Agency for Health Care Policy and Research, Public Health Service, U.S. Department of Health and Human Services; October 1994.
36. Mendelson E. Evaluation of the postoperative breast. *Radiol Clin North Am* 1992;**30**:107-38.
37. Hassell P, Klein-Parker H, Worth A, Poon P. Radial sclerosing lesions of the breast: mammographic and pathologic correlation. *Can Assoc Radiol J* 1999;**50**:370-5.
38. Abner AL, Colllins L, Peiro, Recht A, Come S, Shulman LN, et al. Correlation of tumor size and axillary involvement with prognosis in patients. *Cancer* 1998;**83**:2502-8.
39. Holland R, Connolly JL, Gelman R, Mravunac M, Hendriks JH, Verbeek AL, et al. The presence of an extensive intraductal component following a limited excision correlates with prominent residual disease in the remainder of the breast. *J Clin Oncol* 1990;**8**:113-8.

40. Fisher ER, Sass R, Fisher B, Gregorio R, Brown R, Wickerham L. Pathologic findings from the National Surgical Adjuvant Breast Project (Protocol 6). II. Relation of local breast recurrence to multicentricity. *Cancer* 1986;**57**:1717-24.
41. Goldstein NS, Ferkowicz M, Odish E, Mani A, et al. Miminum formalin fixation time for consistent estrogen receptor immunohistochemical staining of invasive breast carcinoma. *Am J Clin Pathol* 2003;**120**:86-92.
42. Mann GB, Fahey VD, Feleppa F, Buchanan MR. Reliance on hormone receptor assays of surgical specimens may compromise outcome in patients with breast cancer. *J Clin Oncol* 2005;**23**:5148-54.
43. Viale G, Regan MM, Maiorano E, Mastropasqua MG, Dell'Orto P, Rasmussen BB, et al. Prognostic and predictive value of centrally reviewed expression of estrogen and progesterone receptors in a randomized trial comparing letrozole and tamoxifen adjuvant therapy for postmenopausal early breast cancer BIG 1-98. *J Clin Oncol* 2007;**25**:3846-52.
44. Wolff AC, Hammond EH, Schwartz JN, Hagerty KL, Allred DC, Cote RJ, et al. American Society of Clinical Oncology/College of American Pathologists guideline recommendations for human epidermal growth factor receptor 2 testing in breast cancer. *J Clin Oncol* 2007;**25**:118-45.
45. Allred DC, Clark GM, Molina R, Tandon AK, Schnitt SJ, Gilchrist KW, et al. Overexpression of Her-2/neu and its relationship with other prognostic factors change during the progression of in situ to invasive breast cancer. *Human Pathol* 1992;**23**:974-9.
46. Banerjee M, George J, Song EY, Roy A, Hryniuk W, et al. Tree-based model for breast cancer prognostication. *J Clin Oncol* 2004;**22**:2567-75.
47. Fisher ER, Redmond C, Fisher B, Bass G. Pathologic findings from the national surgical adjuvant breast and bowel projects (NSABP). Prognosis discriminant for 8-year survival for node-negative invasive breast cancer patients. *Cancer* 1990;**65**:2121-8.
48. Maier WP, Rosemon GP, Goldman LI, Kaplan GF, Tyson RR. A ten year study of medullary carcinoma of the breast. *Surg Obstet Gynecol* 1977;**144**:695-8.
49. Roger V, Beito G, Jolly PC. Factors affecting the incidence of lymph node metastases in small cancers of the breast. *Am J Surg Pathol* 1989;**157**:501-2.
50. Evans GF, Anthony T, Turnage RH, Schumpert TD, Levy KR, Amirkhan RH, et al. The diagnostic accuracy of mammography in the evaluation of male breast disease. *Am J Surg* 2001;**181**:96-100.
51. Sorlie T, Perou CM, Tibshirani R, Aas T, Geisler S, Johnsen H, et al. Gene expression patterns of breast carcinomas distinguish tumor subclasses with clinical implications. *Proc Natl Acad Sci USA* 2001;**98**:10869-74.

CHAPTER 23

Invasive Lobular Carcinoma

Sophia Kim Apple, January K. Lopez, and Lawrence W. Bassett

Invasive lobular carcinoma (ILC) is the second most common type of mammary carcinoma and accounts for approximately 10% of breast carcinomas. Compared with other types of breast carcinomas, ILC can be difficult to palpate and to visualize mammographically, posing unique challenges with regard to diagnosis and management owing to its elusive nature.

Although ILC and invasive ductal carcinoma (IDC) are often clinically and radiographically indistinguishable, several characteristic features help to differentiate ILC from its more familiar counterpart. Histologically, however, ILC is easily distinguishable from IDC. In this chapter we discuss the clinical, imaging, and histopathologic features of ILC.

Definition

Invasive lobular carcinoma is breast cancer that forms single cells and a targetoid pattern around terminal ductal lobular units, often without stromal desmoplasia.

Prevalence and Epidemiology

Although the reported incidence of ILC is variable, literature indicates that ILC comprises about 10% of invasive breast carcinomas.[1-6] The variation in reported incidence may reflect the fact that 55% of ILCs are found in combination with other histologic subtypes, most commonly ductal carcinoma not otherwise specified (NOS), which makes the determination of the precise incidence difficult.[7]

Owing to its diffuse nature and lack of stromal desmoplastic response, ILC tends to be insidious at onset. It is more likely than IDC to present in older patients and tends to present as a larger tumor, with a greater likelihood of stage III or IV disease (10% to 13% vs. 6% to 9% for IDC).[1,2] Positive surgical margins are more often found with ILC after conservative excisional biopsy (59% vs. 43%).[2] ILC also has a higher rate of multicentricity and bilaterality than other types of breast tumors, with a reported incidence ranging from 20% to 29%.[3] Although varying statistics have been reported, there is no convincing evidence that ILC is associated with a higher rate of lymph node positivity than IDC.[1,2]

The classic type of ILC tends to present as low nuclear grade and as estrogen and progesterone receptor (ER/PR)-positive tumors with better overall mortality rates than IDC NOS.[1,2]

Etiology and Pathophysiology

It is a common misconception that lobular carcinoma arises from acini and that ductal carcinoma arises from ducts of the breast. Both lobular and ductal carcinomas occur from the terminal ductal lobular unit (TDLU). ILCs and IDCs are distinguished by the morphologic appearance of the tumor cells and not by the origin of the cells within the TDLU.

Manifestations of Disease

Clinical Presentation

Although patients with ILC most commonly present with physical findings, it can be difficult to detect on clinical grounds and tends to be poorly defined, rubbery, and difficult to palpate on clinical breast examination (CBE).[2]

It has been suggested that the elusive nature of the tumor may be due to its failure to elicit a desmoplastic reaction.[2,3] ILC also has been reported as difficult to diagnose with fine-needle aspiration (FNA) cytology.

Imaging Indications and Algorithm

Mammography

Although most of the time ILC is detectable on mammography, the false-negative rate is higher compared with other invasive breast carcinomas, with reported rates of up to 32%.[4,8] The reported sensitivity of mammography for ILC ranges from 57% to 81%.[4,5]

Compared with IDC NOS, ILC has a greater tendency to form lesions with density equal to or less than that of normal fibroglandular tissue, particularly with spiculated masses. Additionally, ILC presents as a principal mammographic abnormality that is only detectable on one of the standard craniocaudal (CC) and mediolateral oblique (MLO) views, usually the craniocaudal projection (Figs. 23-1 and 23-2).[6,9] This is thought to be due to the failure of ILC to elicit a desmoplastic response.

In the dense breast, these tumors may be more difficult to detect, even when they are large (Figs. 23-3 and 23-4). As a result, ILCs are considered among the most difficult cancers to detect with mammography.[10]

Similar to IDC, the most common mammographic presentation is that of a mass, usually with spiculated or indistinct margins (Fig. 23-5).[5,6] Round and circumscribed masses are uncommon, comprising 1% to 3% of ILC cases.

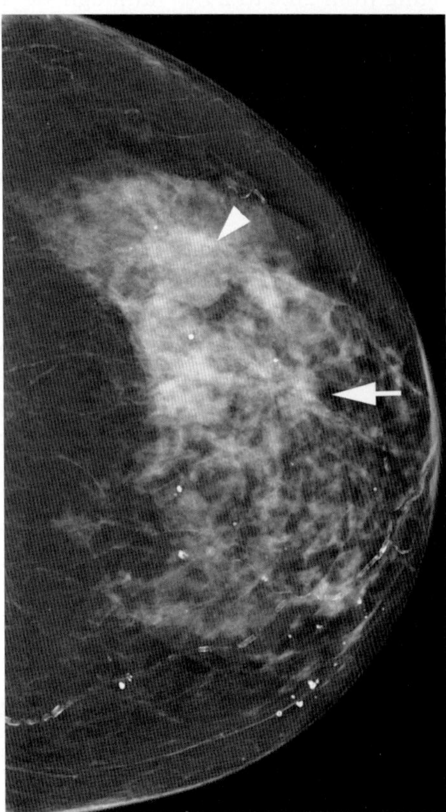

■ **FIGURE 23-1** Invasive lobular carcinoma (ILC) findings from screening mammogram. Craniocaudal view of the left breast shows heterogeneously dense fibroglandular tissue with a subtle architectural distortion in the retroareolar region (*arrow*), which demonstrates density equal to that of the surrounding normal parenchyma. A partially circumscribed, partially obscured oval mass in the 3-o'clock position was found to be a cyst on a subsequent ultrasound study (*arrowhead*).

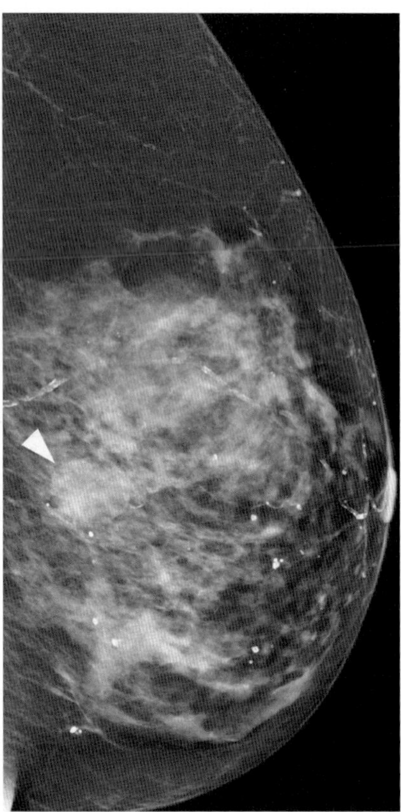

■ **FIGURE 23-2** Invasive lobular carcinoma (ILC) findings from screening mammography. Mediolateral view of the left breast demonstrates no definite abnormality corresponding to the architectural distortion seen on the craniocaudal view. The mass, shown to be a, cyst is denoted by an arrowhead (same case as Figure 23-1).

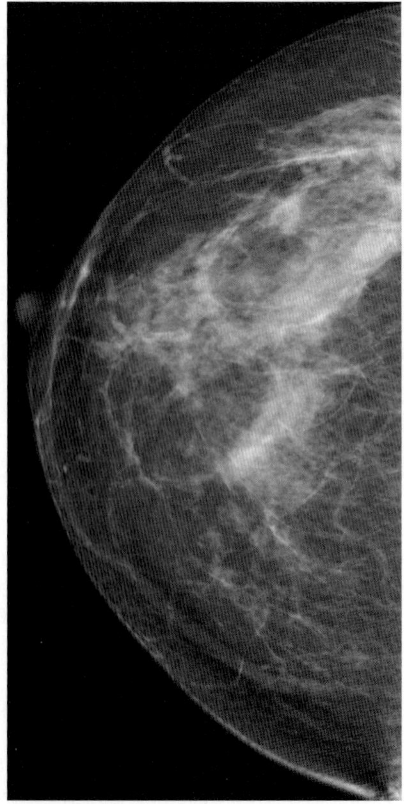

■ **FIGURE 23-3** Right craniocaudal mammography view demonstrates heterogeneously dense breast parenchyma without suspicious radiographic signs of malignancy. Subsequent ultrasound study (not shown) in the area of a palpable abnormality was also normal.

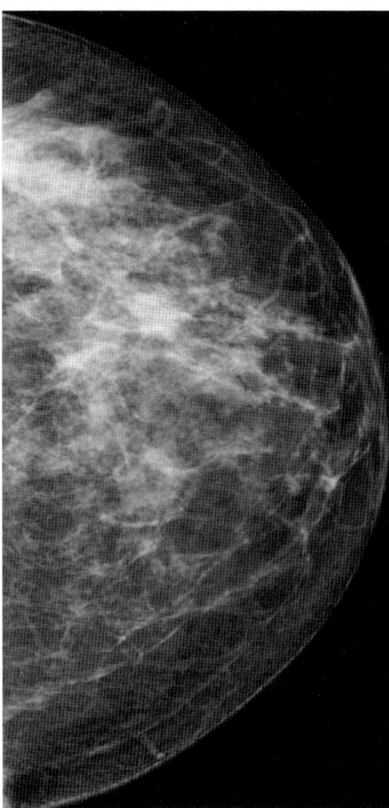

■ **FIGURE 23-4** Same case as Figure 23-3. Left craniocaudal mammography view demonstrates heterogeneously dense breast parenchyma without suspicious radiographic signs of malignancy. Subsequent ultrasound study (not shown) in the area of a palpable abnormality was also normal.

Architectural distortion is the second most common principal mammographic abnormality in ILC, followed by mammographic asymmetries (Figs. 23-6 and 23-7). Benign or normal findings are seen in 8% to 16% of ILC cases.[4-6,9,11,12]

Unlike the IDC of NOS type, microcalcifications are uncommonly seen in ILC, although older reported statistics may be an underestimation in today's era of digital mammography and computer-aided detection. Reported incidence ranges from 0% to 24% (Fig. 23-8).[4-6,9,11,12]

In addition to the detection of ILC, mammography may also be useful in predicting the likelihood of residual carcinoma in patients after initial excisional biopsy. White and colleagues found that patients with mammographic findings of architectural distortion, focal asymmetry or no abnormality had a higher rate of residual invasive carcinoma after excisional biopsy compared with those presenting with spiculated masses.[13]

Ultrasonography

Because of its superior sensitivity for identifying multicentricity or multifocality, and greater accuracy in delineating the size of a mass than mammography or CBE, ultrasonography has proven to be a valuable adjunct in the detection and workup of ILC.[12] Reported sensitivity of ultrasonography for the detection of ILC ranges from 68% to 98%.[12,14]

In addition to its diagnostic utility, ultrasonography plays a vital role in biopsy and localization procedures for ILC. This modality is particularly useful for ILC

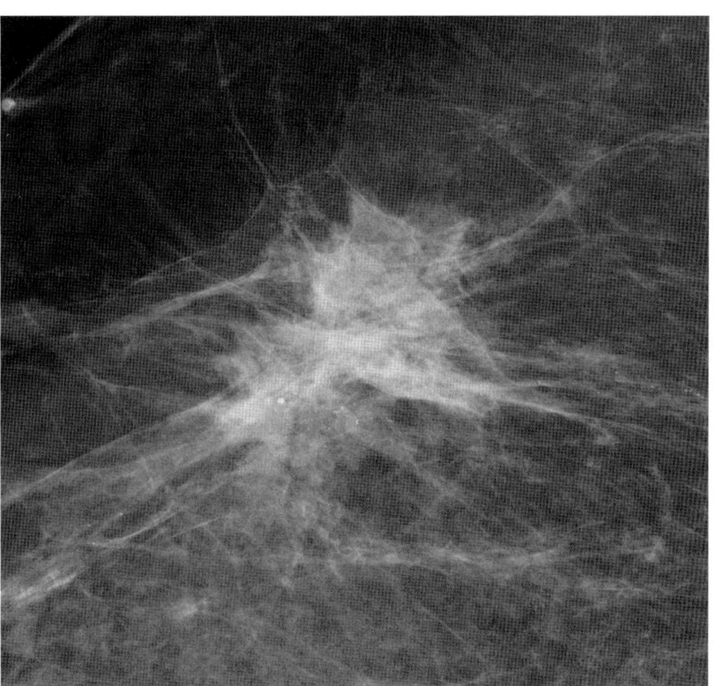

■ **FIGURE 23-5** Magnified spot compression craniocaudal mammography view shows an irregular mass with spiculated margins and associated amorphous calcifications.

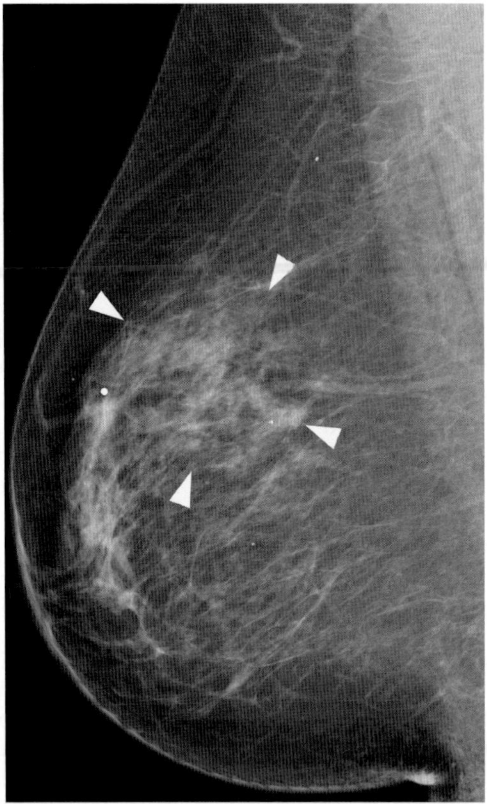

■ **FIGURE 23-6** Right mediolateral oblique mammography view demonstrates an ill-defined, low-density asymmetry in the right superior breast (*arrowheads*). This could not be identified on the craniocaudal view (not shown). *(From Lopez JK, Bassett LW. Invasive lobular carcinoma of the breast: spectrum of mammographic, US and MR imaging findings. RadioGraphics 2008;29:165-76.)*

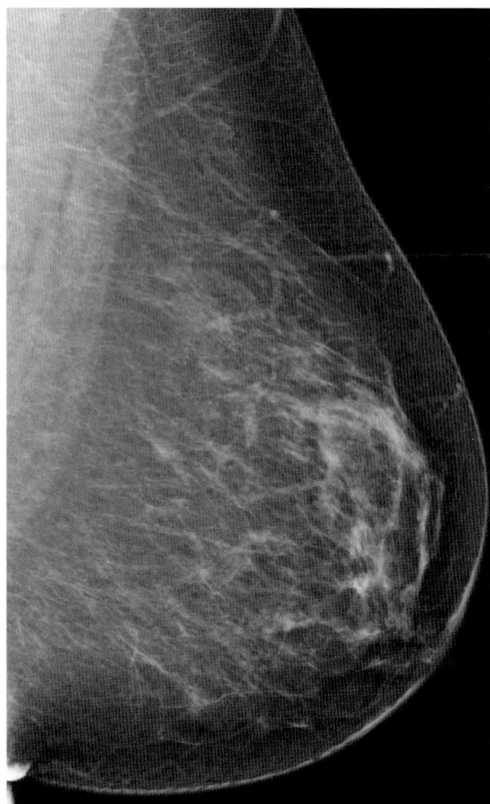

■ **FIGURE 23-7** Same case as Figure 23-6. Left mediolateral oblique mammography view demonstrates no suspicious abnormality. *(From Lopez JK, Bassett LW. invasive lobular carcinoma of the breast: spectrum of mammographic, US and MR imaging findings. RadioGraphics 2008;29: 165-76.)*

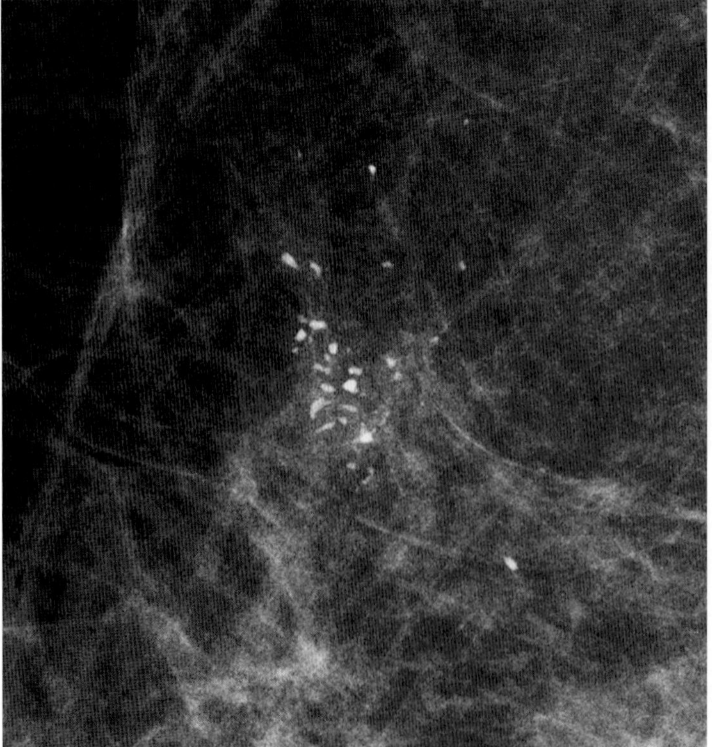

■ **FIGURE 23-8** Magnified mediolateral mammography view shows clustered coarse heterogeneous and fine pleomorphic calcifications without associated mass, distortion, or other principal abnormality.

lesions that are identified on a single mammographic view. A reported 54% to 61% of ILC cases manifest ultrasonographically as a heterogeneous, hypoechoic mass with angular or ill-defined margins and posterior acoustic shadowing (Figs. 23-9 and 23-10). Circumscribed masses, focal shadowing without a discrete mass (Figs. 23-11 and 23-12), and ultrasonographically invisible lesions (see Figs. 23-3 and 23-4) are less common ultrasonographic presentations.[12,14]

There is considerable overlap in ultrasonographic appearance of the various ILC subtypes, with classic ILC tending to show as focal shadowing without a discrete mass and pleomorphic ILC more typically seen as a shadowing mass. Signet-ring and alveolar subtypes are more likely to manifest as a lobulated, well-circumscribed mass.[14] Various types of ILC will be described under the pathology section of this chapter.

Magnetic Resonance Imaging

Dynamic contrast enhanced magnetic resonance imaging (MRI) is a useful adjunct to mammography and ultrasonography in the diagnosis and management of ILC, with a reported sensitivity of 95%.[15] Up to a third of ILCs are bilateral. Therefore, special attention should be paid to the contralateral breast when ILC is diagnosed. MRI is particularly useful in the surgical staging of ILC, owing to its superior accuracy compared with conventional imaging in delineating multifocal and multicentric disease and in estimating tumor size (Fig. 23-13).[15,16] Similar to mammography, the most common MRI manifestation of ILC is a solitary mass with spiculated or irregular margins (Fig. 23-14).[16-18]

Less common MRI presentations include a dominant lesion surrounded by multiple small enhancing foci, multiple small enhancing foci with interconnecting enhancing

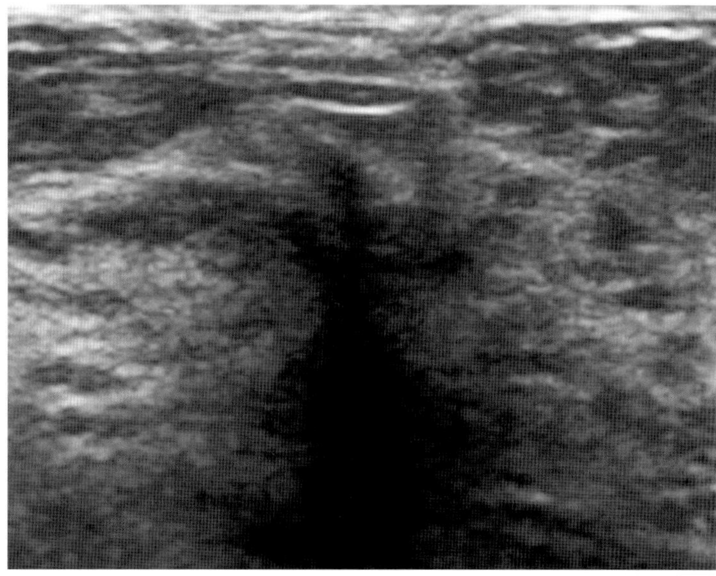

■ **FIGURE 23-9** Targeted ultrasound evaluation of the same patient as in Figure 23-1 shows an irregular, microlobulated hypoechoic mass and posterior acoustic shadowing.

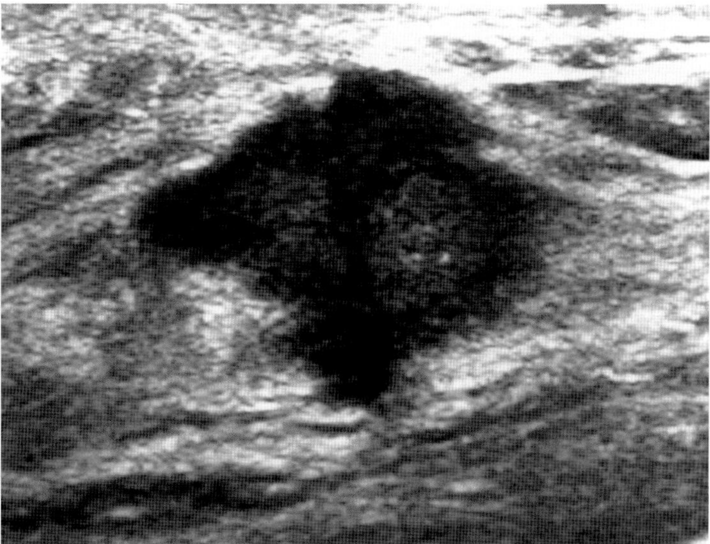

■ **FIGURE 23-10** Ultrasound image demonstrates an irregular hypoechoic mass with indistinct and angular margins.

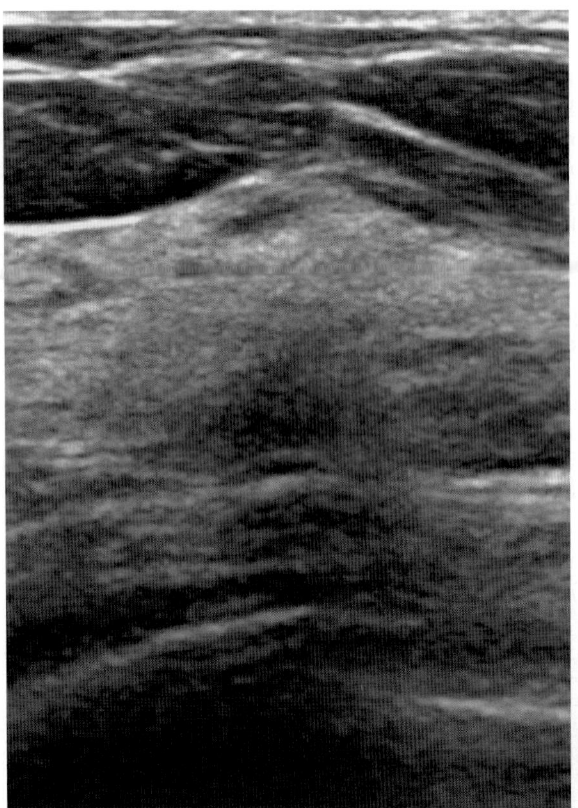

■ **FIGURE 23-11** Ultrasound image demonstrates an indistinct hypoechoic mass with posterior shadowing.

strands, architectural distortion, regional or focal inhomogeneous enhancement (Figs 23-15 and 23-16), enhancing septa, and normal findings.[16-18]

Qayyum and colleagues reported correlation of the enhancing strands and septa on MRI with the histopathologic appearance of tumor cells streaming within the breast stroma.[18] Although data examining the dynamic contrast behavior of ILC on breast MRI are very limited, available studies suggest that ILC has a tendency to dem onstrate delayed maximum enhancement, with the classic pattern of rapid enhancement and washout seen in most invasive breast carcinomas exhibited by only a minority of ILC lesions.[19]

Classic Signs

Although the most common imaging presentations of ILC are similar to those of IDC, classic features of ILC include mammographic density equal to or less than that of the surrounding fibroglandular tissue and principal abnormalities that are detectable only on a single mammographic projection, most commonly the CC view [6,9]

Differential Diagnosis

From Clinical Presentation

The typical clinical features of ILC are nonspecific and overlap considerably with those of other breast conditions, both benign and malignant. Although the ILCs are

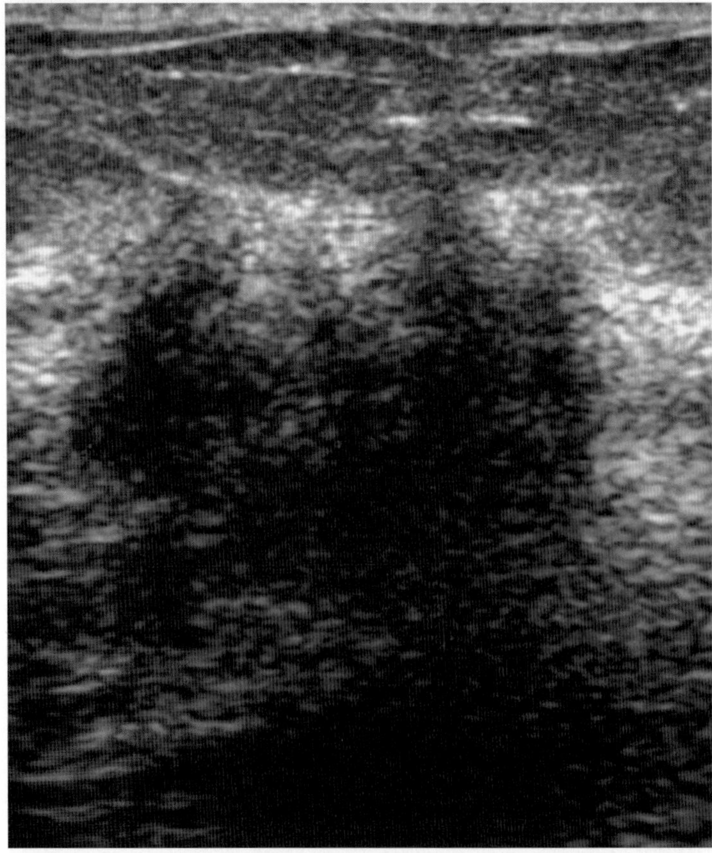

■ **FIGURE 23-12** Ultrasound image shows an irregular, hypoechoic mass with angular margins and posterior shadowing.

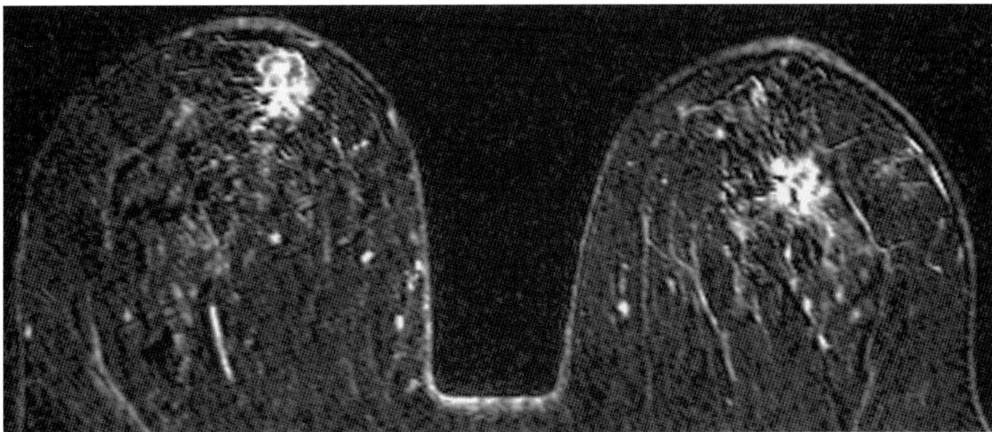

■ **FIGURE 23-13** Magnetic resonance imaging of the same patient as in Figures 23-1 and 23-9 demonstrates irregular, spiculated heterogeneously enhancing masses in the left and right breast corresponding to the mammographic and sonographic abnormalities on the left and an unsuspected irregular mass (IDC) in the right breast.

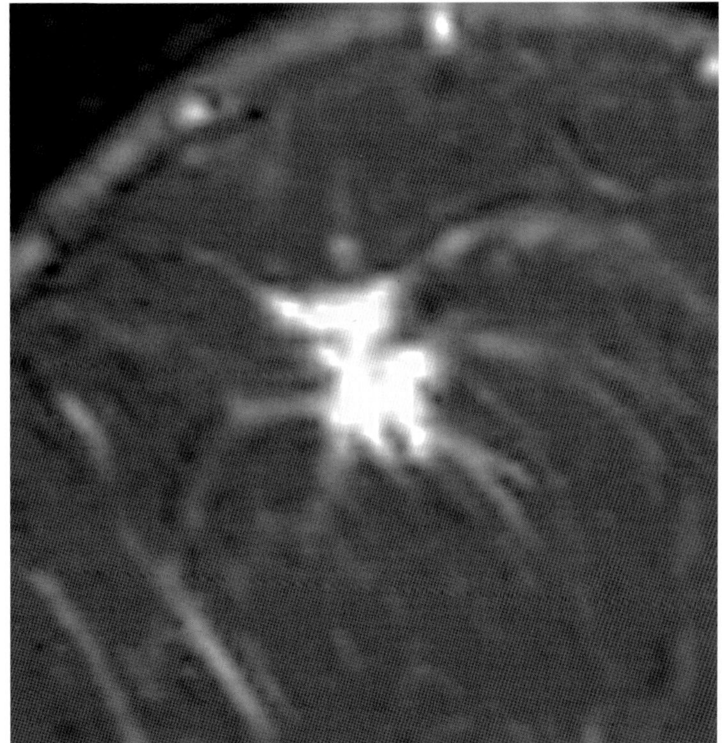

■ **FIGURE 23-14** Dynamic contrast-enhanced subtraction magnetic resonance imaging (MRI) demonstrates an irregular, spiculated homogeneously enhancing mass.

more often nonpalpable than other malignancies, the most common clinical presentation is still a palpable mass. Twenty-five (68.5%) of the 37 patients with ILC and 161 (70.3%) of the 229 patients with invasive ductal carcinoma (IDC) presented with clinically palpable masses.[9]

From Imaging Findings

The imaging features of ILC are nonspecific and can been seen with any of the other histologic types of invasive breast carcinoma, especially IDC.

From Pathology Findings

Gross Pathology

ILC is not prone to form calcifications or stromal desmoplasia and therefore is often difficult to palpate or visualize as IDC grossly. IDC often forms stromal desmoplasia that is edematous. Histologically, findings can vary from being predominantly cellular (fibroblasts/myofibroblasts) with little collagen to a dense acellular tissue (Fig. 23-17). ILC, however, does not elicit stromal desmoplasia but the tumor cells invades into fat and TDLU without any destruction of normal breast tissue (Fig. 23-18). Because

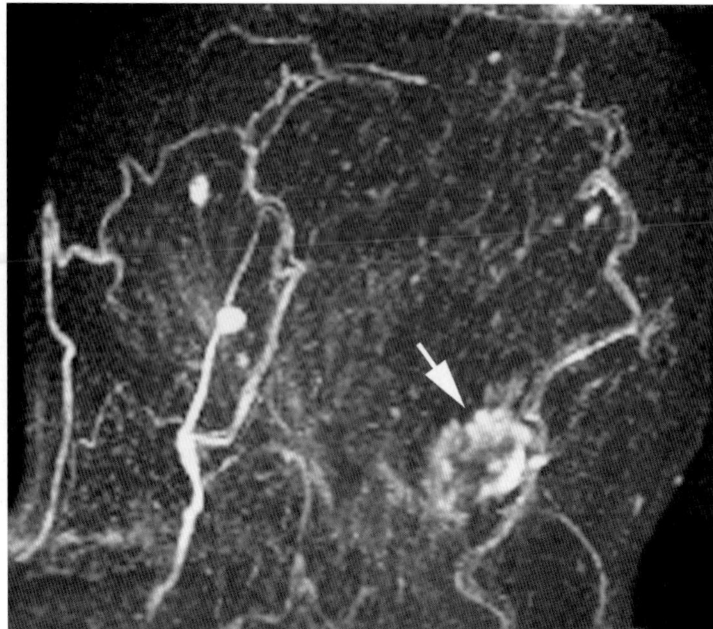

■ FIGURE 23-15 Maximum intensity projection (MIP) magnetic resonance (MR) image demonstrates a non–mass-like area of focal clumped enhancement in the posterior left breast (*arrow*).

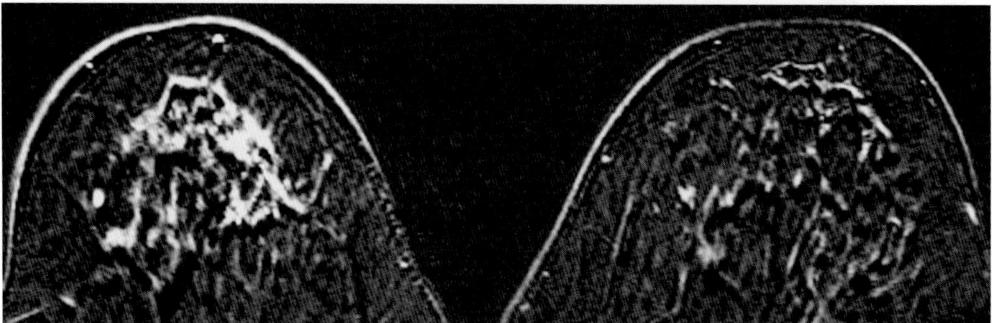

■ FIGURE 23-16 Fat-saturated subtraction magnetic resonance (MR) image of the same patient as in Figures 23-6 and 23-7 shows heterogeneous regional enhancement.

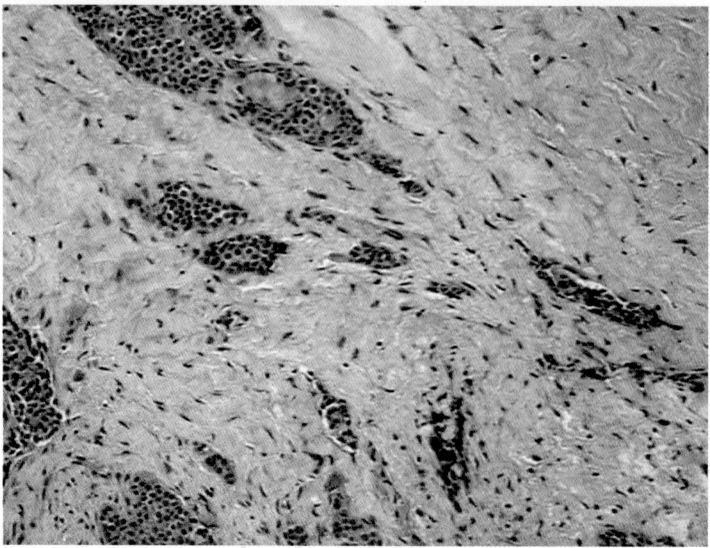

■ FIGURE 23-17 Invasive ductal carcinoma (IDC) with nesting pattern and stromal desmoplasia with blue hues (H&E, ×200).

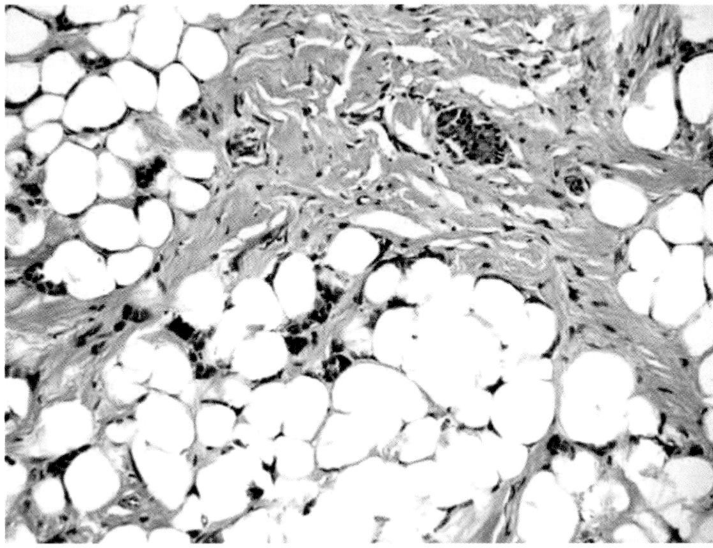

■ **FIGURE 23-18** Invasive lobular carcinoma (ILC) infiltrating into fat without eliciting stromal desmoplasia or lymphocytic response (H&E ×200).

of this rather insidious invasion, gross examination often underestimates the size of ILC. Unlike IDC, margins of the ILC are indistinct and the appearance of scirrhous tissue is often not appreciated at gross pathological examination. Some ILC can be nodular, palpable or slightly more firm than normal breast tissue on palpation. ILC is also more frequently seen in a multicentric and multifocal distribution.

Microscopic Pathology

Invasive lobular carcinoma is generally composed of single (CD) small cells arrayed in a linear pattern with a targetoid pattern invading into stroma, TDLU, and adipose tissue of the breast. Neoplastic cells display round nuclei often eccentrically placed with occasional intracytoplasmic vacuoles. There are mainly four variants of ILC: classic, signet ring, alveolar, and pleomorphic. The most common type is classic type of ILC, which has small to intermediate-sized nuclei with linear pattern and targetoid patterns of invasion (Figs. 23-19 and 23-20). The linear pattern is formed by slender strands of cells arranged in a straight line, and the targetoid pattern represents a concentric infiltration of tumor cells around TDLUs. The alveolar cell variant of ILC demonstrates solid round nests and irregular islands composed of small to medium-sized nuclei that are dyshesive and often mixed with the classic linear pattern (Fig. 23-21). The signet ring cell variant shows eccentrically placed nuclei with intracytoplasmic mucin and vacuoles containing a targetoid secretion (Fig. 23-22). Signet ring cell ILC is often indistinguishable from signet ring cell carcinoma of stomach or gastrointestinal tract cytomorphologically. Immunohistochemical (IHC) stains and clinical presentation may be helpful to delineate the primary source of a signet ring cell tumor. Most ILC cells are positive for ER and PR, whereas gastrointestinal

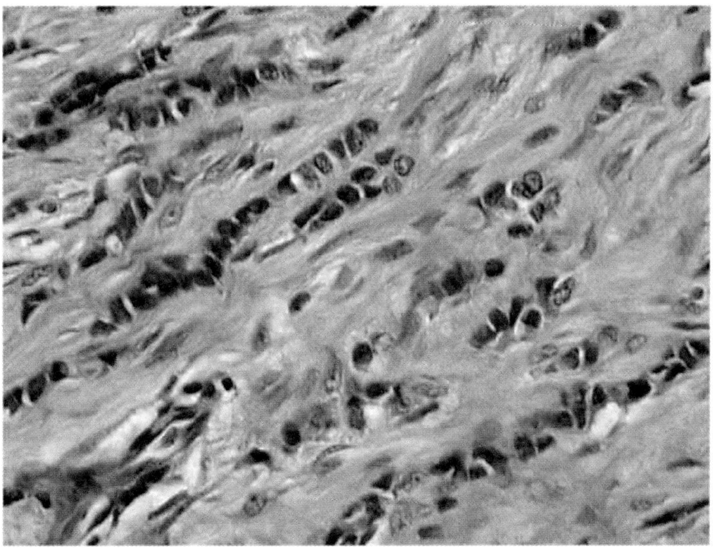

■ **FIGURE 23-19** Linear pattern with coin-stacking appearance of invasive lobular carcinoma (ILC). The tumor cells are small and uniform (H&E, ×400).

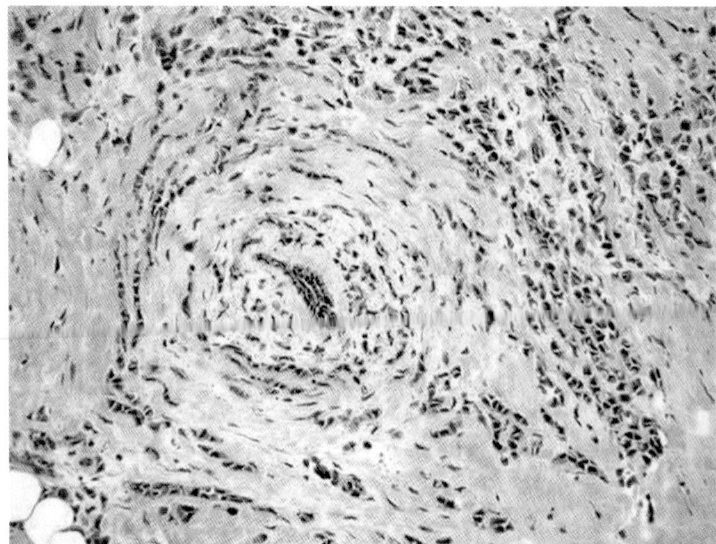

■ **FIGURE 23-20** Invasive lobular carcinoma (ILC) cells are encircling a normal duct forming targetoid pattern (H&E, ×200).

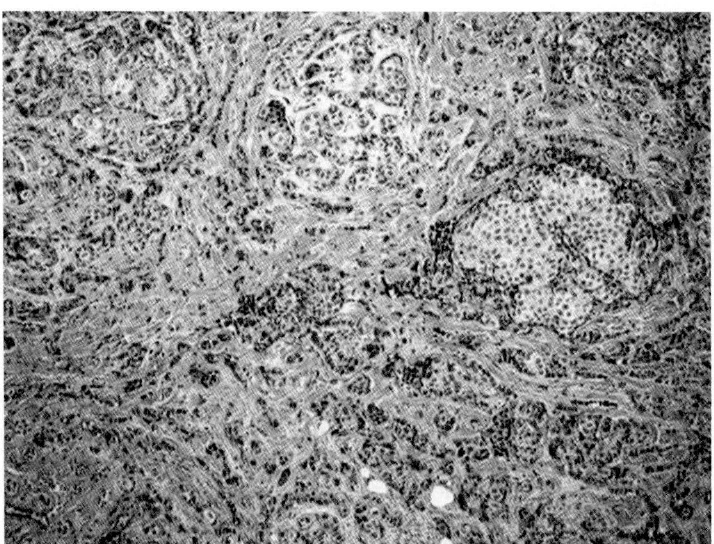

■ **FIGURE 23-21** Invasive lobular carcinoma (ILC), alveolar type with distended and discrete pockets of tumor cells. Classic type ILC is also seen adjacent to the alveolar pattern (H&E, ×200).

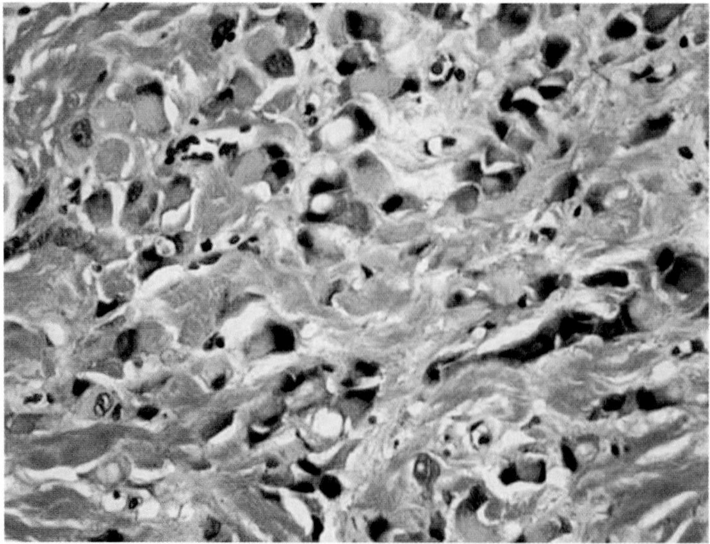

■ **FIGURE 23-22** Invasive lobular carcinoma (ILC), signet-ring cell type with intracytoplasmic mucin vacuoles (H&E, ×400).

tumors are not. Also, differential cytokeratin stains can be useful to distinguish the primary tumor site; breast carcinomas are often positive for cytokeratin-7 and negative for cytokeratin-20, whereas gastrointestinal carcinomas are positive for cytokeratin-20 and negative for cytokeratin-7. Breast carcinomas are also known to be positive for gross cystic disease fluid protein (GCDFP)-15 and mammaglobin IHC stains. Gastrointestinal tumors are not positive for those stains. The pleomorphic variant of ILC shows significant nuclear atypia with nuclear grade 2 to 3 and abundant eosinophilic cytoplasm (Fig. 23-23). It often mimics IDC except that cells are dyshesive (Fig. 23-24) and E-cadherin stain is usually negative. E-cadherin is a cell-cell adhesion molecule, and ILC is known to have lost E-cadherin expression.

Grading ILC is encouraged by using the modified Scarff-Bloom-Richardson (SBR) grading system. When the SBR grading system is applied, tubule formation of ILC is almost always scored a 3 and the score of mitotic figures is generally low (score of 1) for classic ILC.

Fine-Needle Aspiration Findings of ILC

FNA biopsy sample of ILC varies from hypercellular to hypocellular material, containing only fibrofatty tissue with rare atypical epithelial cells. Because of the hypocellular nature, the false-negative smears are the cause of a relatively frequent error in sampling. The scarce epithelial component may show honeycomb-flat sheets, loose clusters, small and tight clusters with irregular limits, isolated

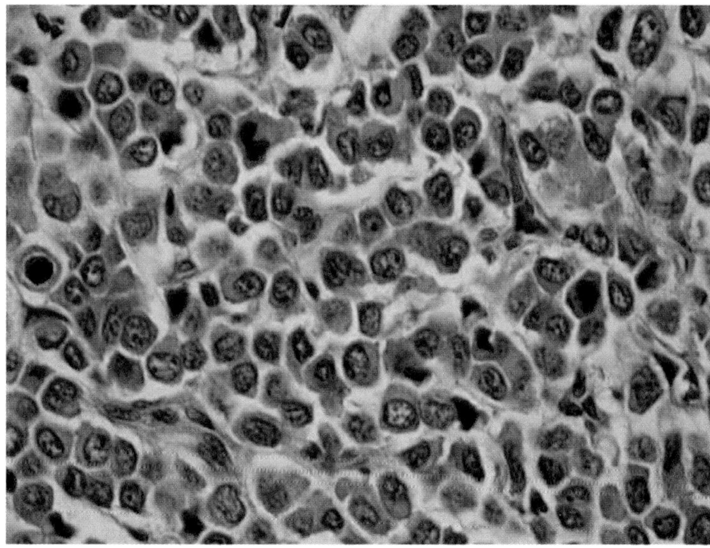

■ **FIGURE 23-23** Invasive lobular carcinoma (ILC), pleomorphic type with plasmacytoid features. The tumor cells are larger than those of classic type ILC (H&E, ×400).

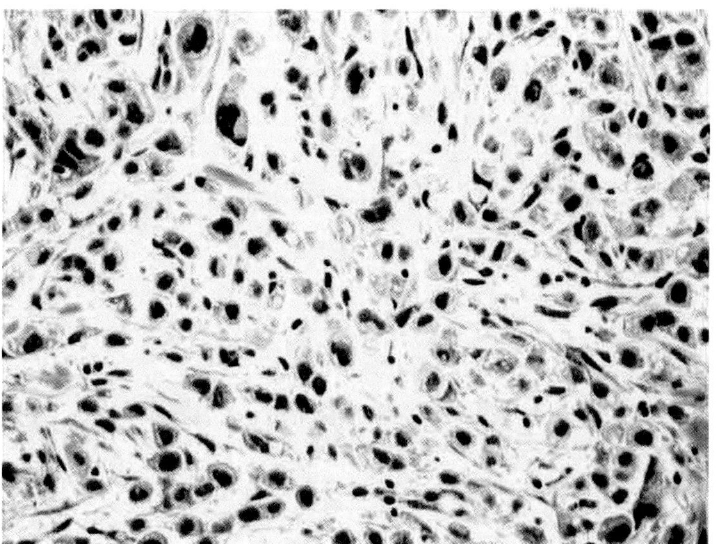

■ **FIGURE 23-24** Metastatic lobular carcinoma to axillary lymph node. Sheets of lobular carcinoma cells are seen close to sinusoid and invading into the lymph node parenchyma. The metastatic cells are more eosinophilic than lymphoid cells (H&E, ×40).

epithelial cells (dyshesive cells), and, rarely, a linear pattern (Figs 23-25 and 23-26). Nuclei are enlarged with angulated nuclear contour and nuclear crowding. Most of the classic ILC shows homogeneous chromatin, without prominent nucleoli. Cytoplasmic vacuolization with occasional signet-ring features and targetoid mucin droplets can be seen.

Metastatic Lobular Carcinoma to Lymph Nodes

The metastatic rate of ILC to axillary lymph nodes is similar to that of IDC and is directly related to tumor size (Table 23-1). Identification of metastatic tumor within axillary lymph nodes and sentinel lymph nodes can be challenging in ILC cases more than IDC cases when using routine hematoxylin and eosin (H&E) stains. Diagnosing metastatic lobular carcinoma to lymph nodes is difficult because the lobular carcinoma cells are often singly and diffusely scattered throughout the lymph node, and the tumor cells resemble histiocytes or intermediate-sized to large lymphocytes. Intraoperative assessment of a sentinel lymph node is even more difficult, especially when the tumor is either micrometastasis or isolated tumor cell deposits. As in IDC cases, sentinel lymph node assessment is usually done for ILC cases. When a sentinel lymph node is negative for metastatic carcinoma, no axillary lymph node dissection is

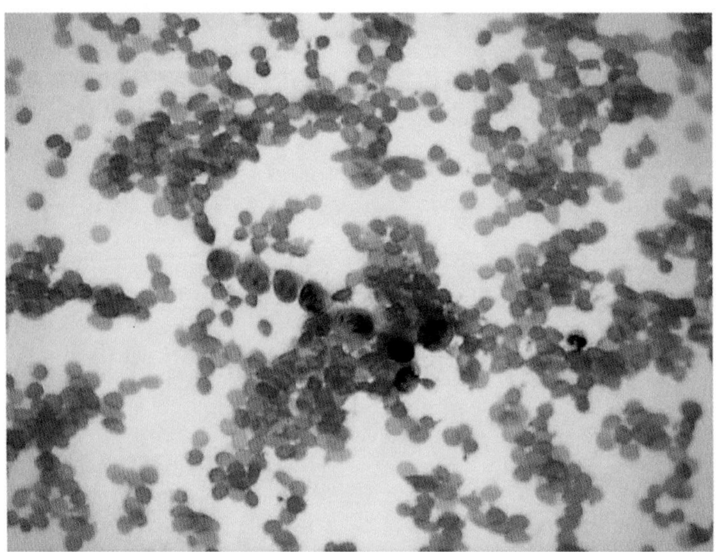

■ **FIGURE 23-25** Papanicolaou (PAP)-stained fine-needle aspiration smear of invasive lobular carcinoma (ILC) showing linear pattern of ILC cells. Mildly atypical cells are lined up in a coin-stacking appearance as seen in the tissue section (×400).

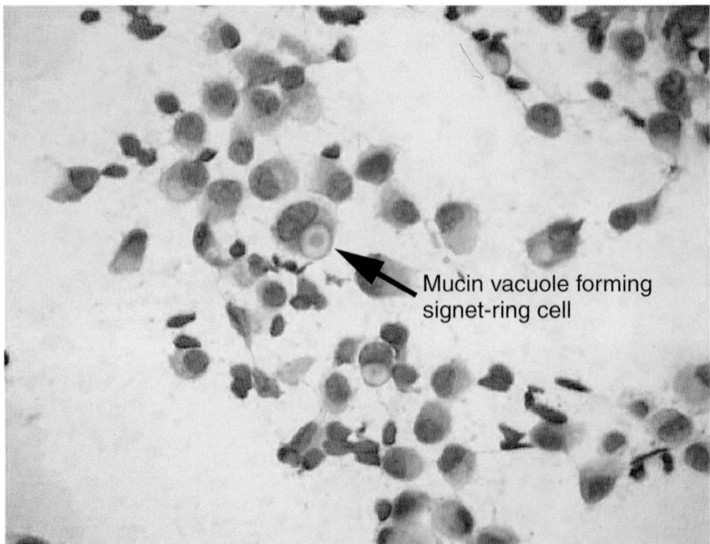

■ **FIGURE 23-26** May-Grunewald Giemsa (MGG) stained fine-needle aspiration smear of invasive lobular carcinoma (ILC) showing dyshesive signet ring cells with mucin droplet (*arrow*) in the cytoplasm that is characteristic of ILC (×400).

TABLE 23-1. Metastatic Nodal Frequency

Tumor Size	Frequency of Lymph Node Metastasis
< 1.0 cm	17%
1.1-2.0 cm	33%
2.1-3.0 cm	60%
3.1-4.0 cm	74%

performed. The presence of macrometastatic and micrometastatic disease in the sentinel lymph node will lead to an ipsilateral axillary dissection. However, when the sentinel lymph node shows only the isolated tumor cell (ITC) positive pN0 (i+), surgeons usually do not perform a full axillary dissection. Adjuvant chemotherapy also is not recommended with ITC in a sentinel lymph node.

The American Joint Commission on Cancer (AJCC) 2003 definition of macrometastasis, micrometastasis, and the isolated tumor cells for ILC is the same as for IDC.[20] However, ILC cells lack intercellular adhesion molecule E-cadherin and thus tumor cells have the ability to infiltrate and metastasize as single cells and deposit randomly within the lymph node, as seen in the breast parenchymal tumor. Although macrometastatic lobular carcinoma may have large clusters of tumor deposits in the lymph node, lobular carcinoma cells often have single cells or small clusters of tumor cells each measuring less than 0.2 mm throughout the lymph node, filling nodal parenchyma, nodal sinus, and subcapsular areas (see Figs. 23-27 and 23-28). This dispersed metastatic pattern is a natural occurrence of ILC; therefore, many pathologists will interpret it as macrometastasis, whereas a strict adherence to the criteria of the AJCC 2003 definition dictates that this pattern will be defined as ITC, pN0 (i+). There is no consistent rule for the definition of ITC, micrometastasis, or macrometastasis in ILC; some consider diffuse and scattered single cells to be macrometastasis in the case of lobular carcinoma, and some consider it to be ITC with "multiple clusters of isolated tumor cells" and provide estimated number of cells and or estimated total volume with a comment in the pathology report. The location of the tumor deposit may be important in determination of the ITC or micrometastasis; the study done by Cserni and colleagues reported micrometastases even if the tumor cells are less than 0.2 mm if the tumor cells are seen in the intraparenchyma of the lymph node.[21] The AJCC 2003 definition by Singletary does not mention the location of tumor deposit as a part of the definition of ITC versus micrometastasis.[20] Low reproducibility in interpretation of ITC and micrometastasis among pathologists is a problem in ILC metastatic disease. The clinical significance of ITC and micrometastasis in a sentinel lymph node is also not known. Many clinicians and pathologists alike tend to ignore and dismiss ITCs in the sentinel lymph node; however, further long-term studies are necessary. A few reported studies addressed the question of how many additional lymph nodes are positive when a sentinel lymph node was positive by macrometastatic, micrometastatic, and isolated tumor cells with metastatic ILC. Patil and associates found that 32% of patients who had macrometastasis or micrometastasis from the sentinel lymph node had additional positive ipsilateral axillary lymph nodes,[22] which is similar to the findings of Cserni and coworkers, who reported 38%.[21] Isolated tumor cells in a sentinel lymph node are reportedly associated with positive axillary lymph nodes in the range of 4% to 13% with ILC. Despite this rather high percentage of positive nonsentinel lymph nodes, when ITC is found in sentinel lymph node, it is generally not recommended to perform axillary dissection. The usage of cytokeratin IHC stain for axillary lymph node dissections other than a sentinel lymph node is not recommended, but a case-by-case basis is used by many pathologists. De Mascarel and colleagues[23] studied survival data on axillary lymph nodes from 89 patients with ILC with a median follow-up of 18 years. They found no significant difference in metastasis-free period between patients who had true node-negative and IHC-detected metastases. A new guideline with a long-term clinical follow-up study is necessary in the near future to understand the biologic significance of ILC metastatic tumor.

Non-Nodal Metastatic Pattern of ILC

The metastatic pattern of ILC is different from IDC in that ILC metastasize to serosal lining of the peritoneal area, retroperitoneal area, ovary, uterine cavity and serosa, gastrointestinal tract, and genitourinary tract. Metastatic IDC is more commonly found in lungs, pleura, and parenchymal central nervous system (CNS). The gynecologic and peritoneal-retroperitoneal metastases are common with ILC so that the primary presentation may be thought as an ovarian or peritoneal tumor. Bone marrow metastases are also common, as well as meningeal spread to the CNS.[3,24]

Biomarkers and Prognosis

Seventy percent to 92% of ILC tumor cells are ER and PR positive. ILC tumor cells are rarely Her-2/neu positive. Other tumor markers such as tumor protein p53 (TP53) and epidermal growth factor receptor (EGFR) are also known to be less positive in ILC when compared with IDC. The classic type of ILC is known to have a better prognosis than IDC. Although ILC has substantially fewer aggressive biologic predictive factors, recurrence and overall survival are known to be similar to that in IDC in a large multivariate analysis.[3] ER- and PR-negative and Her-2/neu-positive ILC is usually a pleomorphic variant of ILC. TP53 and EFGR are also more frequently seen with pleomorphic ILC. Pleomorphic ILC has been reported to have different biologic characteristics and clinical behavior compared with the classic ILC.[25] The pleomorphic variant of ILC is known to be an aggressive type, with 60% of women dying within 42 months of diagnosis.[26]

At the present time, both IDC and ILC are managed similarly in terms of surgical treatment. Adjuvant chemotherapy and hormonal therapy are dependent on the stage of the tumor and ER/PR status, similar to IDC. Routine biopsy of the contralateral breast is not indicated unless MRI or other imaging studies show abnormality.[27]

Invasive Lobular Carcinoma in Males

ILC in males is extremely rare. The normal male breast consists of only ducts and stroma. Hence, male breast carcinoma is usually of the invasive ductal type. Papillary carcinoma is also commonly seen in males. There are only a handful of reported cases of ILC in the male breast. Some cases of ILC in males were associated with exogenous hormonal therapy and endogenous estrogens, such as liver disease and cirrhotic conditions. Many of the reported ILC cases did not report lack of E-cadherin IHC stain to confirm ILC, perhaps owing to the unavailability of E-cadherin stain until recently. When morphologically compatible ILC is found in a male, genetic karyotyping is recommended to prove the male genotype. A few patients with reported cases of ILC had Klinefelter syndrome and breast cancer, early onset gene *(BRCA1)* mutation.[28,29]

Synopsis of Treatment Options

Despite its insidious presentation, the overall survival with ILC, when detected at the same size and stage, is believed to be slightly better than that of the NOS invasive ductal type. This may be because most ILCs are not triple-negative "basal-like" carcinoma but rather luminal A or luminal B types of breast cancers.

Because of its infiltrative growth pattern and tendency for skip lesions, initial trends for the treatment of ILC were biased toward more aggressive surgery, including mastectomy and standard axillary lymph node dissection. However, current data strongly support the idea that breast conservation treatment is effective in the treatment of early stage ILC, with similar rates of long-term recurrence and survival compared with IDC. Sentinel lymph node biopsy has also been shown to have equivalent accuracy and predictive value in ILC compared with IDC.[27,30]

KEY POINTS

- Invasive lobular carcinoma (ILC) is the second most common type of breast malignancy, accounting for about 10% of invasive breast carcinomas.
- Because of its lack of desmoplastic stromal reaction, ILC is insidious in its presentation and often difficult to detect both clinically and on conventional imaging.
- ILC most commonly presents as a spiculated or ill-defined mass on mammography, ultrasonography, and MRI.
- ILC has a tendency to form mammographic lesions with opacity density equal to or less than that of the surrounding fibroglandular tissue.
- Principal mammographic abnormalities are more often detectable on only a single mammographic (usually the craniocaudal) view.
- There are mainly four variants of ILC: classic, signet ring, alveolar, and pleomorphic. The most common type is the classic type of ILC.
- The classic type ILC shows two types of histologic patterns: the linear pattern is formed by slender strands of cells arranged in a straight line, and the targetoid pattern is concentric infiltration around TDLU by the tumor cells.

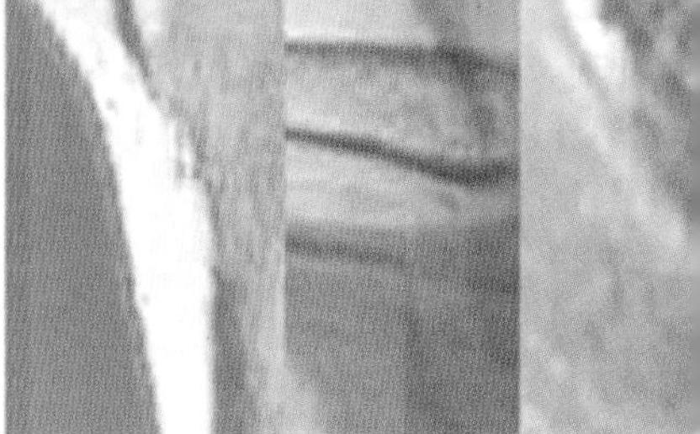

CASE STUDY

Chapter 23 Invasive Lobular Carcinoma

HISTORY

A 50-year-old woman presented with a 2-week history of palpable mass and skin dimpling in the right breast at the 10-o'clock position. The patient had a normal CBE and screening mammogram 1 month prior to the discovery of the findings. Ultrasonography performed at the time of symptomatic presentation demonstrated no abnormalities. The patient subsequently underwent FNA core needle biopsy, and excisional biopsy, followed by dynamic contrast-enhanced breast MRI (Figs 23-29 through 23-33).

FINDINGS

Fine-Needle Aspiration Findings

The smears show moderately cellular material composed of a dyshesive pattern of single atypical cells with retained cytoplasm. Many of the cells show plasmacytoid features with nuclei pushed to the periphery and abundant cytoplasm, some of which exhibits signet-ring mucinous cytoplasm.

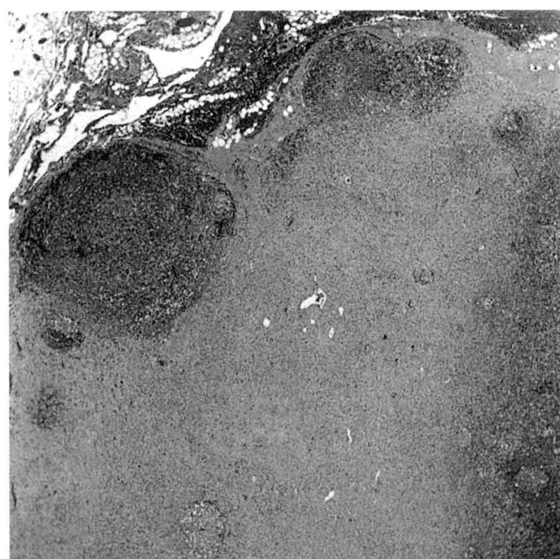

■ FIGURE 23-27 Macrometastatic lobular carcinoma in lymph node. Invasive lobular carcinoma is seen effacing the entire lymph node and involving subcapsular area. H&E stain × 40.

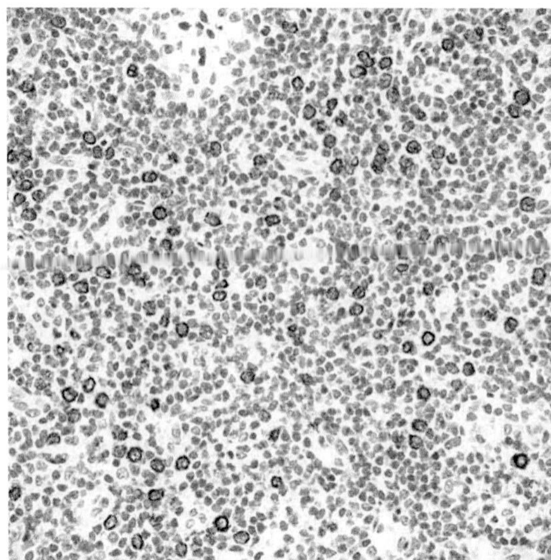

■ **FIGURE 23-28** Immunohistochemical cytokeratin stain x400 showing metastatic carcinoma cells involving the entire lymph node but arranged in small clusters or singly. Each aggregate is smaller than 0.2 mm which defines isolated tumor cells (ITC).

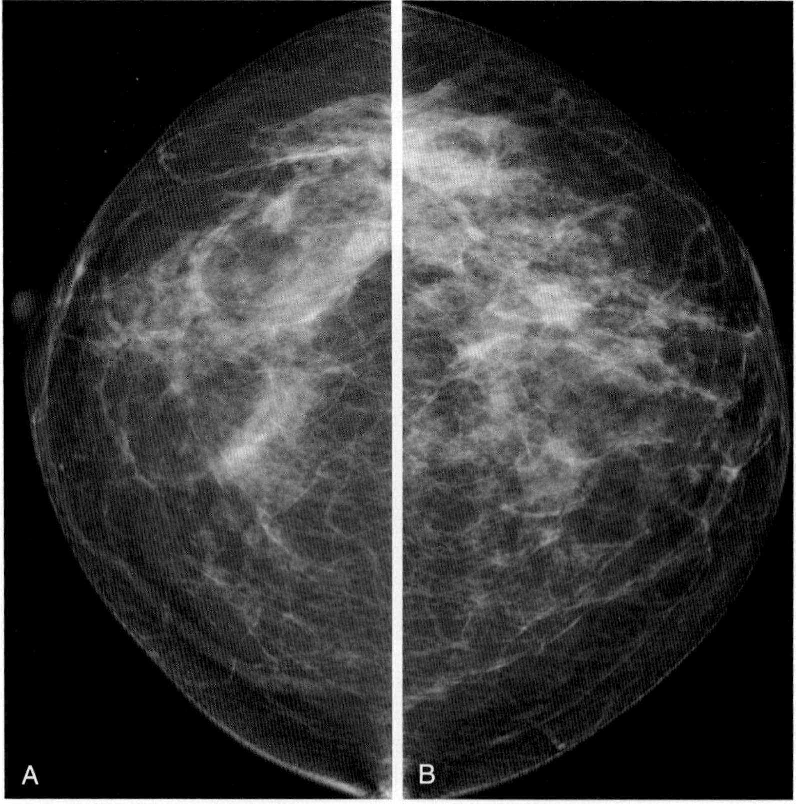

■ **FIGURES 23-29** Bilateral craniocaudal views (**A**, **B**) obtained at screening mammography demonstrate heterogeneously dense breast parenchyma without suspicious radiographic signs of malignancy. Directed ultrasound image (not shown) in the area of palpable abnormality was also normal.

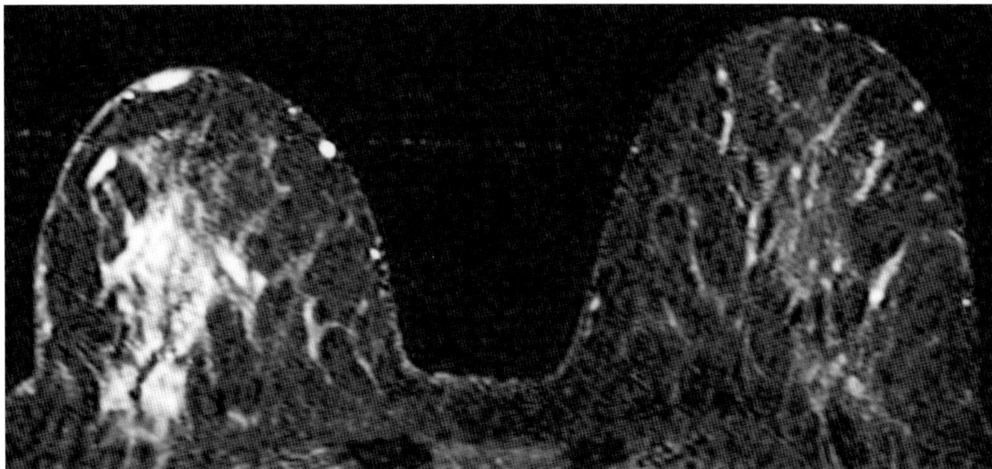

■ **FIGURES 23-30** Magnetic resonance imaging (MRI) demonstrates regional homogeneous enhancement in the right breast.

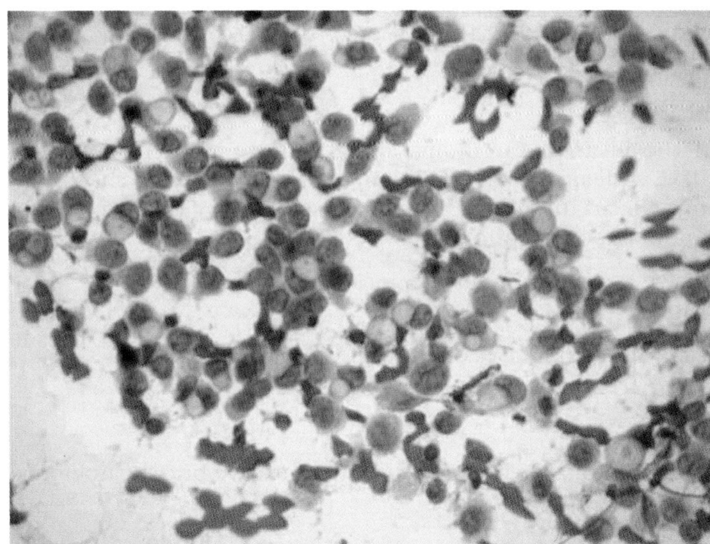

■ **FIGURE 23-31** Fine-needle aspiration of the case study: pleomorphic invasive lobular carcinoma (ILC) (Papanicolaou [PAP] stain, ×400).

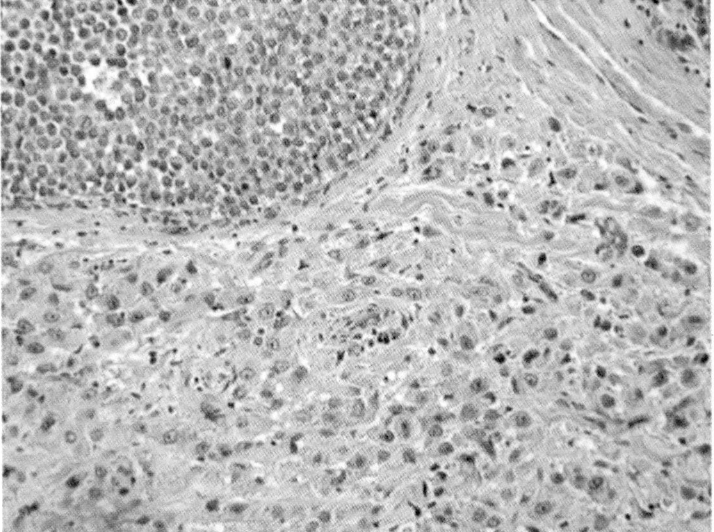

■ **FIGURE 23-32** Core needle biopsy of the case study: pleomorphic invasive lobular carcinoma (ILC) (H&E, ×200).

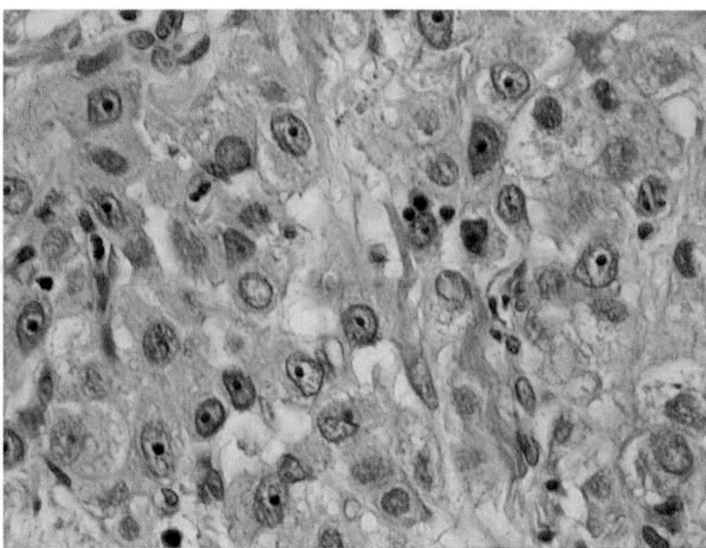

■ **FIGURE 23-33** Excisional biopsy of the case study in high power view: pleomorphic invasive lobular carcinoma (ILC) (H&E, ×600).

Core Needle Biopsy Findings

Cytomorphologic features of the invasive carcinoma and in-situ components are similar. Nuclei are larger than classic ILC, with a plasmacytoid arrangement. Nuclei also show central prominent nucleoli. Malignant cells are dyshesive, single, and in a linear pattern without a stromal response such as desmoplasia or lymphohistiocytic infiltrates.

Excisional Biopsy Findings

A large tumor was found with similar features as seen from the core needle biopsy.

DIFFERENTIAL DIAGNOSIS

The differential diagnosis includes IDC of NOS type, ILC, or other invasive breast carcinomas.

DIAGNOSIS

Pleomorphic invasive lobular carcinoma.

SUGGESTED READINGS

Fisher ER, Fisher B. Lobular carcinoma of the breast: an overview. *Ann Surg* 1977;**185**:377-85.

Harake MD, Maxwell AJ, Sukumar SA. Primary and metastatic lobular carcinoma of the breast. *Clin Radiol* 2001;**56**:621-30.

Harvey JA. Unusual breast cancers: useful clues to expanding the differential diagnosis. *Radiology* 2007;**242**:683-94.

Lopez JK, Bassett LW. Invasive lobular carcinoma of the breast: spectrum of mammographic, US and MR imaging findings. *Radiographics* 2008;**29**:165-76.

Mann RM, Hoogeveen YL, Blickman JG, Boetes C. MRI compared to conventional diagnostic work-up in the detection and evaluation of invasive lobular carcinoma of the breast: a review of existing literature. *Breast Cancer Res Treat* 2008;**107**:1-14.

Sickles EA. The subtle and atypical mammographic features of invasive lobular carcinoma. *Radiology* 1991;**178**:25-6.

REFERENCES

1. Li CI, Uribe DJ, Daling JR. Clinical Characteristics of different histologic types of breast cancer. *Br J Cancer* 2005;**93**:1046-52.
2. Silverstein MJ, Lewinsky BS, Waisman JR, et al. Infiltrating lobular carcinoma. Is it different from infiltrating duct carcinoma? *Cancer* 1994;**73**:1673-7.
3. Arpino G, Bardou VJ, Clark GM, Elledge RM. Infiltrating lobular carcinoma of the breast: tumor characteristics and clinical outcome. *Breast Cancer Res* 2004;**6**:R149-56.
4. Krecke KN, Gisvold JJ. Invasive lobular carcinoma of the breast: mammographic findings and extent of disease at diagnosis in 184 patients. *AJR Am J Roentgenol* 1993;**161**:957-60.
5. Le Gal M, Ollivier L, Asselain B, Meunier M, Laurent M, Vielh P, et al. Mammographic features of 455 invasive lobular carcinomas. *Radiology* 1992;**185**:705-8.
6. Hilleren DJ, Andersson IT, Lindholm K, Linnell FS. Invasive lobular carcinoma: mammographic findings in a 10-year experience. *Radiology* 1991;**178**:149-54.

7. Fisher ER, Gregorio RM, Fisher B, Redmond C, Vellios F, Sommers SC. The pathology of invasive breast cancer. A syllabus derived from findings of the national surgical adjuvant breast project (Protocol No. 4). *Cancer* 1975;**36**:1-85.
8. Berg WA, Gutierrez L, NessAiver MS, Carter WB, Bhargavan M, Lewis RS, et al. Diagnostic accuracy of mammography, clinical examination, US, and MR imaging in preoperative assessment of breast cancer. *Radiology* 2004;**233**:830-49.
9. Newstead GM, Baute PB, Toth HK. Invasive lobular and ductal carcinoma: mammographic findings and stage at diagnosis. *Radiology* 1992;**184**:623-7.
10. Mendelson E, Harris KM, Doshi N, Tobon H. Infiltrating lobular carcinoma: mammographic patterns with pathologic correlation. *AJR Am J Roentgenol* 1989;**153**:265-71.
11. Evans WP, Warren Burhenne LJ, Laurie L, O'Shaughnessy KF, Castellino RA. Invasive lobular carcinoma of the breast: mammographic characteristics and computer-aided detection. *Radiology* 2002;**225**:182-9.
12. Selinko VL, Middleton LP, Dempsey PJ. Role of sonography in diagnosing and staging invasive lobular carcinoma. *J Clin Ultrasound* 2004;**32**:323-32.
13. White JR, Gustafson GS, Wimbish K, Ingold JA, Lucas RJ, Levine AJ, et al. Conservative surgery and radiation therapy for infiltrating lobular carcinoma of the breast: the role of preoperative mammograms in guiding treatment. *Cancer* 1994;**74**:640-7.
14. Butler RS, Venta LA, Wiley EL, Ellis RL, Dempsey PJ, Rubin E. Sonographic evaluation of infiltrating lobular carcinoma. *AJR Am J Roentgenol* 1999;**172**:325-30.
15. Kneeshaw PJ, Turnbull LW, Smith A, Drew PJ. Dynamic contrast enhanced magnetic resonance imaging aids the surgical management of invasive lobular breast cancer. *Eur J Surg Oncol* 2003;**29**:32-7.
16. Schelfout K, Van Goethem M, Kersschot E, Verslegers I, Biltjes I, Leyman P, et al. Preoperative breast MRI in patients with invasive lobular breast cancer. *Eur Radiol* 2004;**14**:1209-16.
17. Weinstein SP, Orel SG, Heller R, Reynolds C, Czerniecki B, Solin LJ, et al. MR Imaging of the breast in patients with invasive lobular carcinoma. *AJR Am J Roentgenol* 2001;**176**:399-406.
18. Qayyum A, Birdwell RL, Daniel BL, Nowels KW, Jeffrey SS, Agoston TA, et al. MR imaging features of infiltrating lobular carcinoma of the breast: histopathologic correlation. *AJR Am J Roentgenol* 2002;**178**:1227-32.
19. Mann RM, Hoogeveen YL, Blickman JG, Boetes C. MRI compared to conventional diagnostic work-up in the detection and evaluation of invasive lobular carcinoma of the breast: a review of existing literature. *Breast Cancer Res Treat* 2008;**107**:1-14.
20. Singletary SE, Green FL, Breast Task Force. Revision of breast cancer staging: the 6th edition of the TNM classifications. *Semin Surg Oncol* 2003;**21**:53-9.
21. Cserni G, Bianchi S, Vezzosi V, Peterse H, Sapino A, Arisio R, et al. The value of cytokeratin immunohistochemistry in the evaluation of axillary sentinel lymph nodes in patients with lobular breast carcinoma. *J Clin Pathol* 2006;**59**:518-22.
22. Patil D, Susnik B. Keratin immunohistochemistry does not contribute to correct lymph node staging in patients with invasive lobular carcinoma. *Hum Pathol* 2008;**39**:1011-7.
23. De Mascarel I, Bonichon F, Coindre JM, Trojani M. Prognostic significance of breast cancer axillary lymph node micrometastases assessed by two special techniques: reevaluation with longer follow-up. *Br J Cancer* 1992;**66**:523-7.
24. Lamovec J, Bracko M. Metastatic pattern of infiltrating lobular carcinoma of the breast: an autopsy study. *J Surg Oncol* 1991;**48**:28-33.
25. Middleton LP, Palacios DM, Bryant BR, Krebs P, Otis CN, Merino MJ. Pleomorphic lobular carcinoma: morphology, immunohistochemistry, and molecular analysis. *Am J Surg Pathol* 2000;**24**:1650-6.
26. Eusebi V, Magalhales F, Azzopardi JG. Pleomorphic lobular carcinoma of the breast: an aggressive tumor showing apocrine differentiation. *Hum Pathol* 1992;**23**:655-62.
27. Chung MA, Cole B, Wanebo HJ, Bland KI, Chang HR. Optimal surgical treatment of invasive lobular carcinoma of the breast. *Ann Surg Oncol* 1997;**4**:545-50.
28. Rudan I, Rudan N, Basic N, Basic V, Rudan D. Differences between male and female breast cancer. II. Clinicopathologic features. *Acta Med Croatica* 1997;**51**:129-33.
29. Scheidbach H, Dworak O, Schmucker B, Hohenberger W. Lobular carcinoma of breast in an 85-year-old man. *Eur J Surg Oncol* 2000;**26**:319-21.
30. Singletary SE, Patel-Parekh L, Bland KI. Treatment trends in early-stage invasive lobular carcinoma. A report from the national cancer data base. *Ann Surg* 2005;**242**:281-9.

CHAPTER 24

Other Malignant Breast Diseases

Sophia Kim Apple, Christopher P. Hsu, and Lawrence W. Bassett

Most tumors arising from the breast are epithelial cells from a terminal ductal lobular unit (TDLU) exhibiting either ductal or lobular carcinoma. Malignant lesions arising from the stroma or adipose, lymphoid and vascular tissue of the breast are rare. However, primary lymphomas and various sarcomas do occur within breast parenchyma. The focus of this chapter is on primary lymphoma, malignant phyllodes tumor, primary angiosarcoma, metastatic sarcomas, and other metastatic diseases to the breast.

HEMATOPOIETIC DISEASES OF THE BREAST

Definition

Immune system neoplasms of the breast include lymphoma and leukemia (also known as chloromas).

Non-Hodgkin's lymphomas, specifically B-cell lymphomas, are the most common primary hematopoietic tumors of the breast. In contrast, T-cell lymphomas are rarely seen in breast. The diagnosis of primary breast lymphoma is limited to patients with no evidence of systemic lymphoma or leukemia at the time the breast lesion is detected. The secondary lymphoma of the breast is defined when the patient presents with lymphoma of the breast with concurrent or a history of systemic lymphoma or leukemia.

Granulocytic sarcoma, also known as chloroma, is an acute leukemia presenting in a solid organ such as the breast. These conditions are exceedingly rare.

Prevalence and Epidemiology

Primary lymphomas in the breast are extremely rare and account for 1.7% to 2.2% of breast malignancies.[1] Primary breast lymphoma can occur between the ages of 13 and 90 years, with a median age at diagnosis of approximately 55 years.

Manifestations of Disease

Clinical Presentation

Primary breast lymphoma usually presents as a rapidly growing mass lesion. The tumor is usually solitary; however, a diffuse pattern with multiple masses can also occur. Skin fixation and color alteration can be seen with cutaneous involvement and can resemble inflammatory breast carcinoma presenting as retraction, erythema, and/or a peau d'orange appearance. Enlarged lymph nodes have been described both in the axilla and the intramammary lymph nodes, with axillary lymph nodes involved in 30% to 40% of cases.[2] Bilateral disease is present in approximately 13% of cases.

Imaging Technique and Findings

Mammography

The majority of primary breast lymphomas present as solitary uncalcified masses on mammography.[3] Almost 30% are circumscribed, the remaining showing incompletely circumscribed margins (Fig. 24-1). Primary lymphoma may manifest as multiple masses (<10% of cases), making it impossible to distinguish primary from metastatic lymphoma on a mammogram (Fig. 24-2).

Pathology

The diagnosis of primary breast lymphoma should be limited to patients without any evidence of other systemic

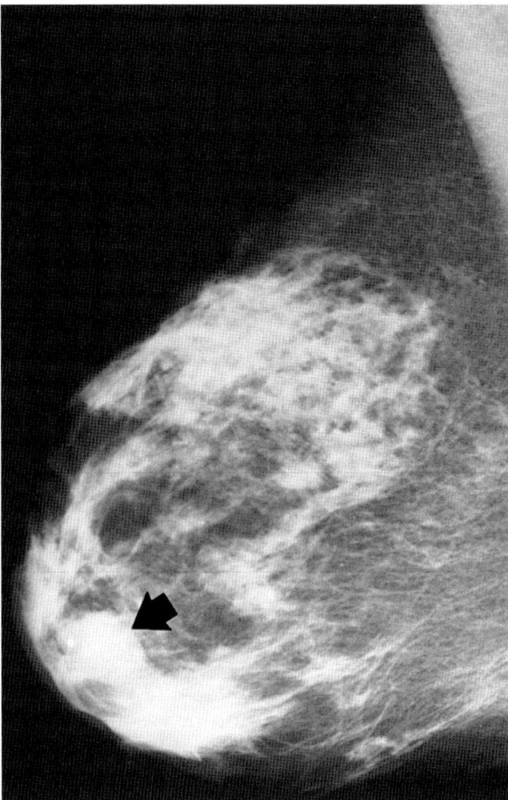

■ **FIGURE 24-1** Primary non-Hodgkin lymphoma of the breast. A 72-year-old woman felt a lump under the nipple. Right mediolateral oblique mammogram shows a partially circumscribed mass (*arrow*) at the site of the palpable abnormality. A radiopaque lead marker (BB) was placed on the skin over the palpable abnormality. Ultrasonography showed a solid mass.

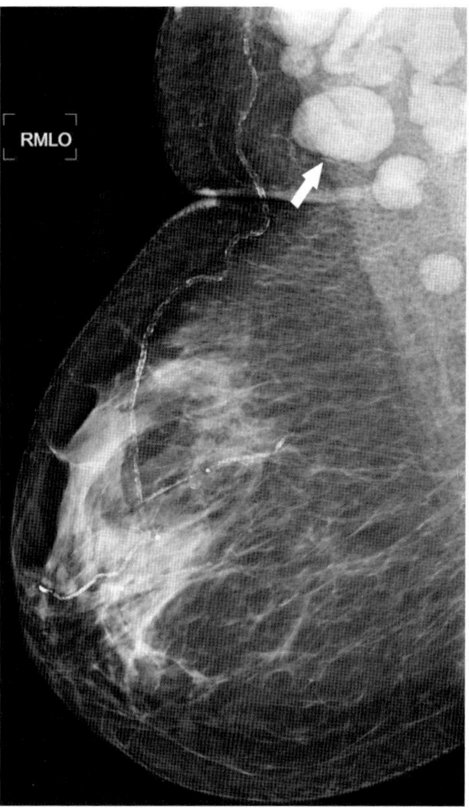

■ **FIGURE 24-2** Multiple round, circumscribed, high density masses seen in the axilla (*arrow*) on mammography compatible with axillary adenopathy. This patient had lymphoma.

hematopoietic malignancy. Since metastatic or secondary lymphomas are more common than the primary lymphoma of the breast, careful clinical and physical examination should be performed to exclude systemic hematopoietic malignancy. Primary breast lymphoma usually manifests as a palpable mass. Microscopically it is composed of a uniform population of tumor cells that diffusely infiltrates the breast parenchyma and obliterates the TDLU. Diffuse large B-cell lymphoma can be difficult to distinguish from poorly differentiated invasive ductal carcinoma and epithelioid angiosarcoma. Often, the limited tissue samples provided by core needle biopsy make it even more difficult to distinguish among all the differential diagnoses, thus compounding the problem (Figs 24-3 and 24-4).

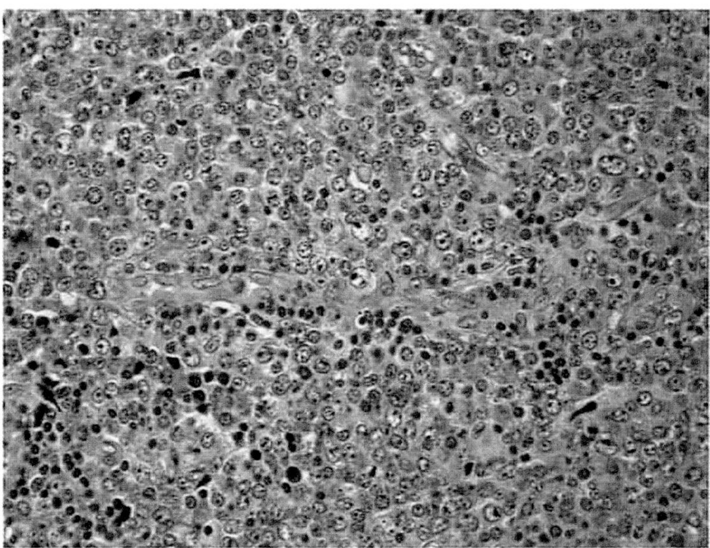

■ **FIGURE 24-3** Primary diffuse large B-cell lymphoma in breast. Tumor cells are diffusely infiltrating with uniform population of large cells with amphophilic cytoplasm (H&E, ×400).

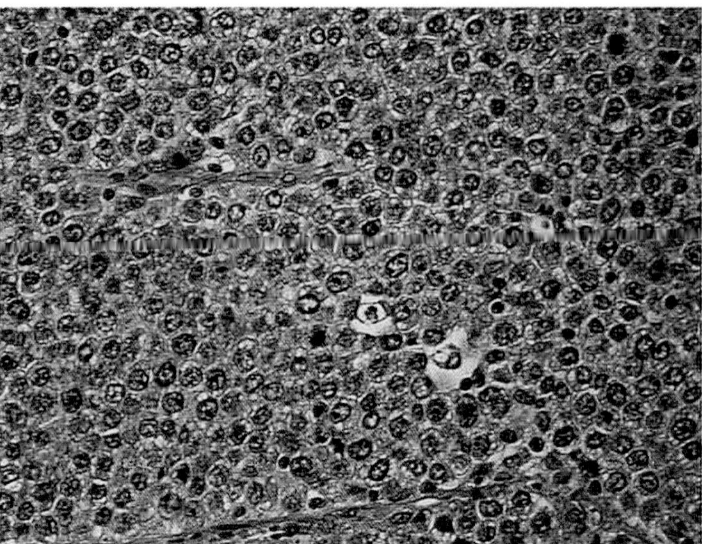

■ **FIGURE 24-4** Invasive high-grade ductal carcinoma showing aggregates and sheets of cells with uniform population of tumor cells (H&E, ×400).

A panel of immunohistochemical (IHC) stains is often helpful to distinguish among these entities. The common leukocyte antigen stain, also known as CD45, is usually positive for lymphoma but negative in carcinoma and epithelioid angiosarcoma. CD31 and CD34 are positive for epithelioid angiosarcoma but negative for lymphoma and carcinoma. Pancytokeratin stain is positive for carcinoma but negative for lymphoma and epithelioid angiosarcoma.

Peripheral T-cell lymphomas are exceedingly rare, representing less than 0.5% of all breast malignancies.[4] T-cell lymphomas have the clinical and pathologic features of inflammatory carcinoma, mainly due to subcutaneous involvement of skin. Peripheral T-cell lymphoma involves a subcutaneous nodular panniculitis, which is composed of chronic inflammatory infiltrates with lymphocytes, plasma cells, and occasional neutrophils surrounding adipose cells. At low power, the differential diagnosis includes fat necrosis as well as benign lymphohistiocytic cells (Figs. 24-5 and 24-6). At higher power, the lymphocytes are slightly atypical and focally surrounding adipocytes in a rim without granulomatous inflammation or vasculitis. Diagnosing peripheral T-cell lymphoma can be difficult especially when the biopsy material is superficial. Deep punch biopsies or excisional biopsies are most helpful in diagnosing peripheral T-cell lymphoma because the superficial papillary dermal tissue samples provided by more superficial biopsy techniques may not show any atypical lymphoma cells. Deep subcutaneous fat tissue biopsy is often necessary to see the panniculitis-like process.[5]

As stated earlier, granulocytic sarcoma (chloroma) is an acute leukemia presenting in a solid organ such as the breast. The most common type of chloroma is myeloblastic leukemia. Chloromas very rarely involve the breast. Microscopically, they present as diffuse infiltrates of granulocyte precursor cells. They may also occur as a complication in the course of chronic myeloid leukemia or other

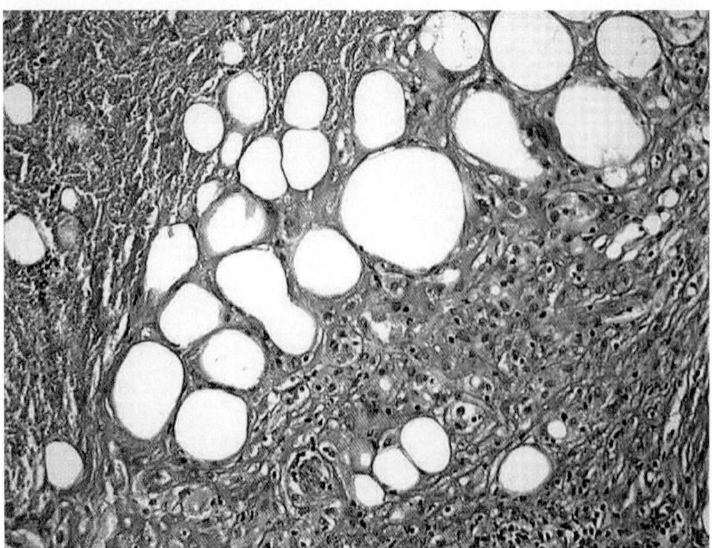

■ **FIGURE 24-5** Rare malignant T cell seen with panniculitis pattern mimicking fat necrosis (H&E, ×200).

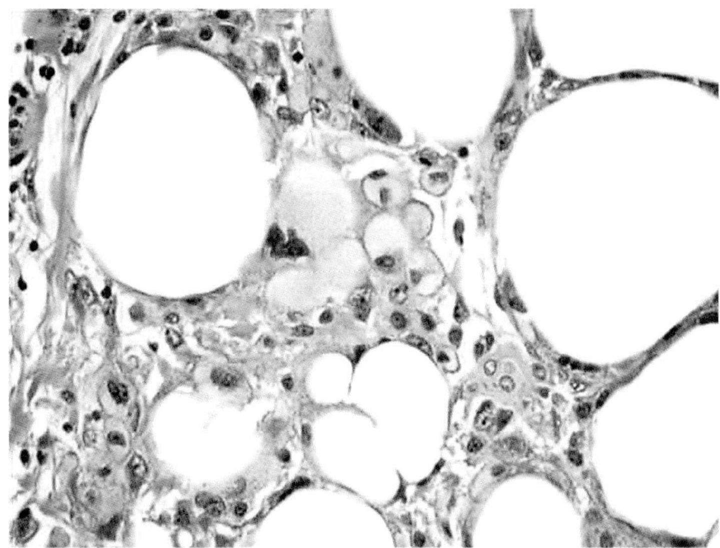

■ **FIGURE 24-6** Fat necrosis after excisional biopsy with foamy histiocytes and multinucleated giant cells (H&E, ×400).

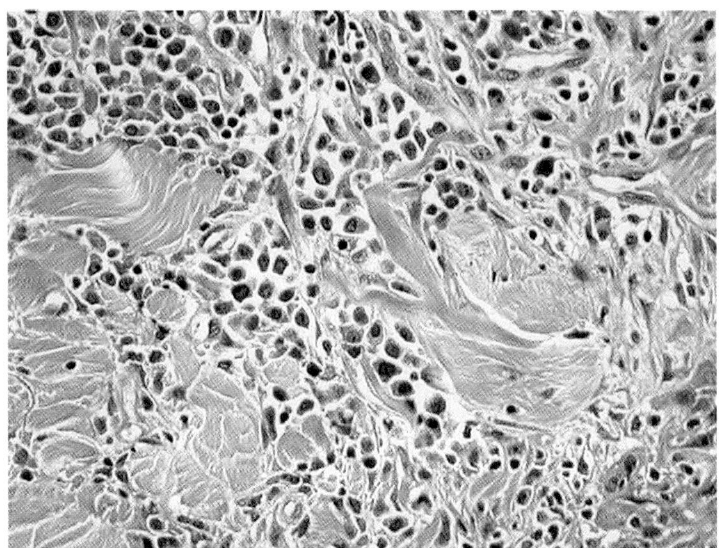

■ **FIGURE 24-7** Undifferentiated granulocytic cells are seen in the breast parenchyma mimicking carcinoma (H&E, ×400).

myeloproliferative disorders as well as during leukemic relapse or remission. Because of its rarity, this lesion can be easily misdiagnosed as carcinoma or lymphoma (Fig. 24-7).

MALIGNANT PHYLLODES TUMOR

Definition

Phyllodes tumors are fibroepithelial neoplasms. These were formally called *cystosarcoma phyllodes*; however, because not all phyllodes tumors behave in a malignant fashion, the term is no longer used. Although phyllodes tumors most commonly occur in women in their fifth decade, they have been seen in women of all ages.

Prevalence and Epidemiology

Phyllodes tumors usually occur in women from 30 to 70 years of age.[6] One study found that the mean age at presentation was 52 years.[7] Phyllodes tumors often resemble fibroadenomas; however, women with phyllodes tumors often present at ages 20 years or older than the median age of patients with fibroadenomas. A population-based study reported that the incidence of phyllodes tumor is higher in Asian and Latina patients than whites.[8]

Etiology and Pathophysiology

Phyllodes tumors are found with coexisting fibroadenoma or fibroadenomatoid nodules in about 40% of cases.

Whether the preexisting fibroadenoma is the cause or the origin of malignant transformation is not well documented in the literature. One study reported the preexisting fibroadenoma transforming into phyllodes tumor in three cases by clonal analysis.[9]

Manifestations of Disease

Clinical Presentation

Malignant phyllodes tumors are firm large masses (usually 4 cm or larger) that grow rapidly. Approximately 10% of all phyllodes tumors are malignant and metastasize.

Imaging Technique and Findings

Mammography

Malignant phyllodes tumors are usually noncalcified, round or lobular with circumscribed margins.(Fig. 24-8). They cannot be distinguished mammographically from benign phyllodes tumors.

Ultrasonography

On ultrasonography, malignant phyllodes tumors are hypoechoic masses with circumscribed margins (Fig. 24-9). Occasionally, they have cystic regions as well.

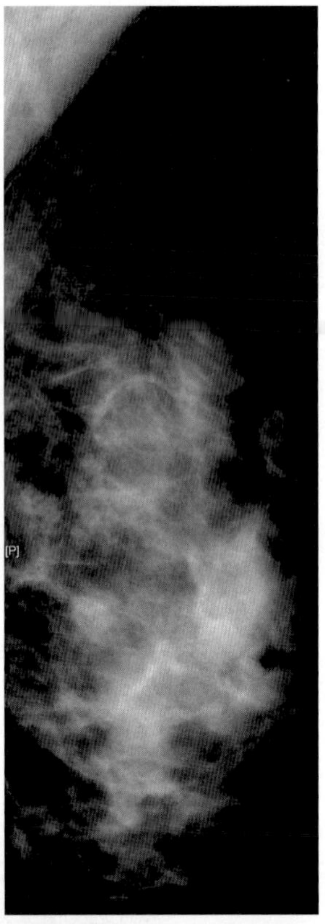

■ FIGURE 24-8 Mediolateral and mediolateral oblique (MLO) views of the left breast demonstrate a nodular density with partially obscured margins in the left upper hemisphere. This lesion was not seen on the craniocaudal projection. The density on the MLO projection was larger when compared with the results of the comparison examination.

Pathology

Grossly, malignant phyllodes tumors show a well-circumscribed and nonencapsulated tumor with a bulging cut surface. These tumors can also present as cystic formation or with numerous papillary nodules. Foci of degenerative changes, necrosis, hemorrhages, and infarction also have been seen.

Microscopically, malignant phyllodes tumors are biphasic tumors with both malignant stroma and benign intervening glands. This is basically analogous to fibroadenomas. The subclassification of phyllodes tumors is divided into three categories: benign, low-grade (borderline), and malignant. The criteria depend on stromal cellularity, presence of stromal overgrowth, cellular pleomorphism, mitotic counts per 10 high-power fields (HPF), margin analysis, stromal pattern, and heterogeneous stromal differentiation. Malignant phyllodes tumors have an infiltrative border rather than a pushing margin as seen in the benign counterpart. The stroma is highly cellular with marked degree of overgrowth and nuclear pleomorphism (Fig. 24-10). *Stromal overgrowth* is defined as stromal proliferation without intervening epithelial elements in at least one low power field (4×). Mitotic figures are typically greater than 5 per 10 HPF. Criteria for mitotic counts vary substantially from author to author with some breast pathologists requiring greater than 10 per 10 HPF before diagnosis of malignant subclassification. Often, heterologous components can be seen with liposarcoma, osteogenic sarcoma, chondrosarcoma, or rhabdomyosarcoma (Fig. 24-11). When overgrowth of

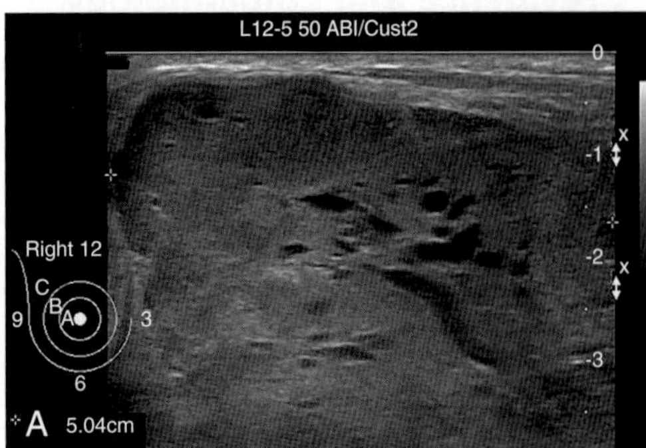

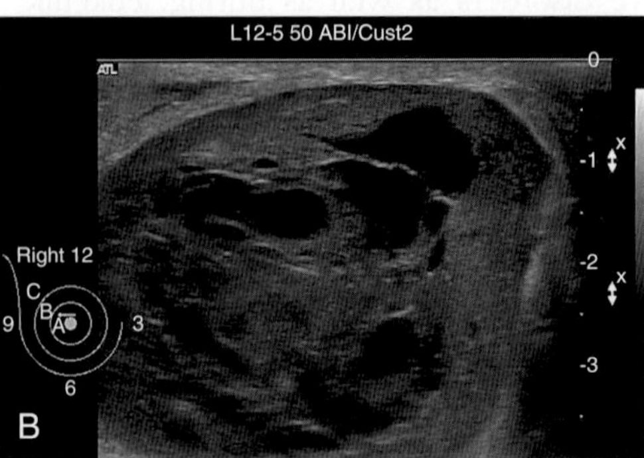

■ FIGURE 24-9 Ultrasound images (**A, B**) of a right breast show a well-circumscribed oval, complex mass. Excisional biopsy was consistent with a malignant phyllodes tumor.

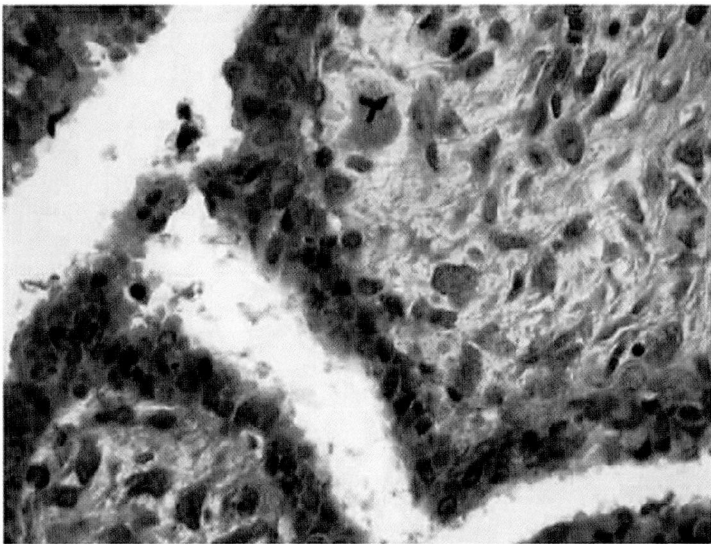

■ **FIGURE 24-10** Malignant phyllodes tumor showing highly cellular pleomorphic stromal cells with atypical tripolar mitotic figure (H&E, ×400).

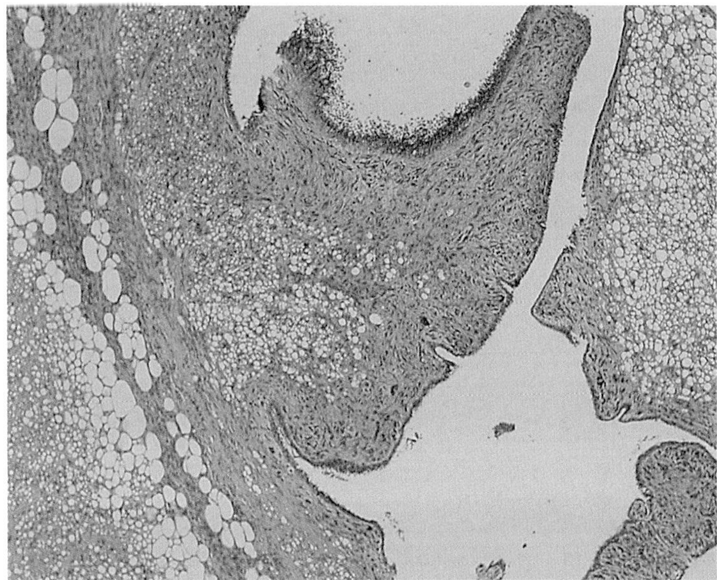

■ **FIGURE 24-11** Malignant phyllodes tumor with liposarcomatous heterologous element (H&E, ×400).

sarcomatous components without the epithelial component is seen, the differential diagnosis includes primary metastatic fibrosarcoma or other sarcomas. If the diagnosis of sarcoma is entertained, multiple sections (at least 1 block per 1 cm of tumor) should be taken and submitted to search for any epithelial components to eliminate any possibility of a malignant phyllodes tumor, because primary sarcomas are exceedingly rare. In phyllodes tumors, glands typically exhibit an enhanced intracanalicular growth pattern with leaf-like projections into dilated lumens, creating cysts (Figs 24-12 and 24-13). The epithelial component consists of luminal cells and outer myoepithelial cells. Florid ductal hyperplasia is commonly seen. Rarely, ductal or lobular carcinoma in situ (LCIS) can be seen associated with phyllodes tumor.

Low-grade malignant phyllodes tumors are also called borderline phyllodes tumors. They exhibit intermediate features between malignant and benign phyllodes and low-grade fibrosarcomas. The stroma is modestly cellular and exhibits mild to moderate nuclear atypia. Mitotic figures are infrequent, ranging from 2 to 5 per 10 HPF. Benign phyllodes tumors are the most common among all phyllodes tumors, representing about 60%. Of the remaining 40% of phyllodes tumors, half are low-grade malignant phyllodes and half are malignant phyllodes tumor. The classic features of benign phyllodes tumors are discussed in Chapter 19.

It is often difficult to predict the biological behavior of phyllodes tumors because even histologically benign phyllodes tumors are minimally capable of local recurrence.

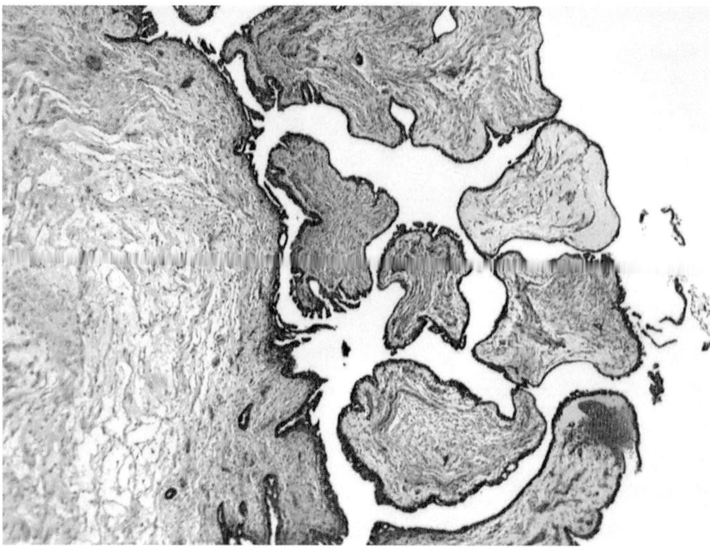

■ **FIGURE 24-12** Phyllodes tumor with leaf-like pattern, which is the pseudopapillary structure (H&E, ×400).

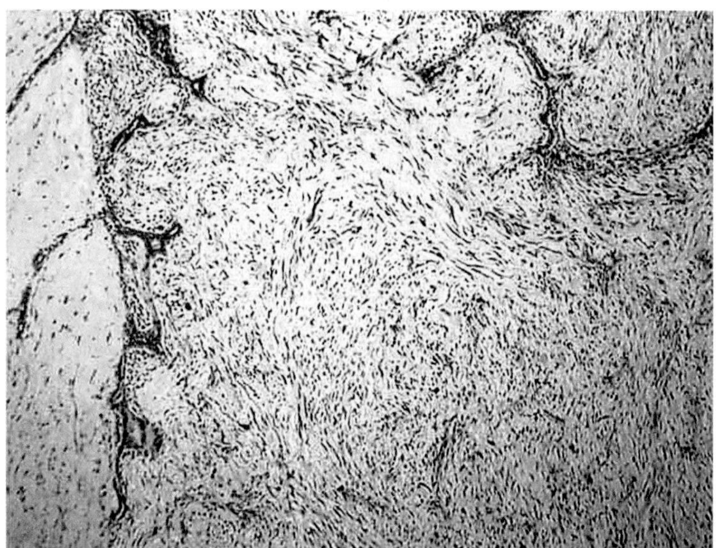

■ **FIGURE 24-13** Low-grade malignant (borderline) phyllodes tumor showing periglandular stromal cell condensation (H&E, ×100).

Rarely, malignant transformation can occur, especially in phyllodes tumors that were not completely excised with the inclusion of a rim of normal breast tissue. The average published data suggest a local recurrence of 27% for malignant phyllodes tumors and a rate of metastases of 22% to pulmonary and skeletal areas. Local recurrence rate of low-grade malignant and benign phyllodes tumors is 25% and 17%, respectively. Local recurrence after surgery is strongly dependent on the width of excisional margins. The most powerful indicator for local recurrence is completeness of excisional biopsy with a rim of uninvolved normal breast tissue. Local recurrence often occurs within 2 years, and most deaths from tumor occur within 5 years of diagnosis in malignant cases.[10] The literature has assessed a number of ancillary IHC studies to distinguish between various fibroepithelial lesions, However markers such as Ki-67, tumor protein p53 (TP53), vascular endothelial growth factor (VEGF), topoisomerase IIa, and CD10; have not been found helpful for diagnostic use. Furthermore, DNA ploidy studies and S-phase fractions did not add significantly to predict the outcome of these lesions.

MAMMARY SARCOMAS

Definition

Mammary sarcomas are a heterogeneous group of tumors arising from stromal cells. The diagnosis of primary sarcoma should only be made when stromal overgrowth from other malignant phyllodes tumor or metaplastic breast carcinoma is excluded by thorough sampling. This distinction is critical not only in terms of prognosis but also for the treatment.

Prevalence and Epidemiology

Pure primary sarcomas of the breast are exceedingly rare, with a small number of case reports in the literature. Various types of sarcomas have been reported to arise from the stromal tissues of the breast. These rare stromal lesions include phyllodes tumors (see earlier), liposarcomas, osteosarcomas, and angiosarcomas.

Manifestations of Disease

Clinical Presentation

Patients with primary breast liposarcoma commonly present with a slowly enlarging, nontender and solitary mass. These tumors are rarely fixed to the deep fascia or overlying skin, and thus are freely movable in the surrounding tissue. These tumors can show different rates of growth; the same tumor grows rapidly at one time and slowly at another. Liposarcomas vary markedly in their consistency to palpation, depending on the amount of fibrous and myxomatous tissue present. Most often they are firm, circumscribed, bulky tumors with a well-defined but delicate capsule. Local recurrence is common after inadequate resection with recurrent tumor with frequent invasion of the skin and pectoral muscles. Unlike most sarcomas of the breast, axillary metastasis can occur occasionally. The most common method of dissemination is via the bloodstream, with metastasis often occurring in the lungs, mediastinum, and joints. Death in these patients is frequently due to pulmonary metastases.[11]

Imaging Technique and Findings

Mammography

Osteosarcoma: On mammography, osteosarcomas vary in appearance. Most tumors present as large masses with relatively well-defined margins and lobulated borders (Fig. 24-14). Coarse and dense calcifications sometimes resembling bone are usually present. Masses with irregular margins have also been reported. When present, large areas of necrosis often correlate with a poor prognosis. On nuclear imaging studies, ^{99m}Tc-diphosphonate is a specific radionuclide marker for osteoid tumoral tissue, and uptake of this radionuclide marker is strongly suggestive of bone-forming neoplasms. Clinically, the alkaline phosphatase level has been found to be elevated in patients with osteoid-forming neoplasms.[12]

Primary angiosarcoma: On mammography, the appearance of a primary angiosarcoma is nonspecific. The most common finding is an ill-defined, noncalcified mass or focal asymmetry.[13] Because many women with primary breast angiosarcomas are young patients with dense breast parenchyma, angiosarcomas may be obscured and not detectable mammographically. Indeed, one study of 24 patients reported that up to 19% of patients had tumors not visible mammographically and only visible on ultrasonography and magnetic resonance imaging (MRI).[14]

Secondary angiosarcoma: On mammography, secondary angiosarcomas show postoperative and post-treatment changes. Skin thickening can be seen and misinterpreted as postirradiation skin changes.[15]

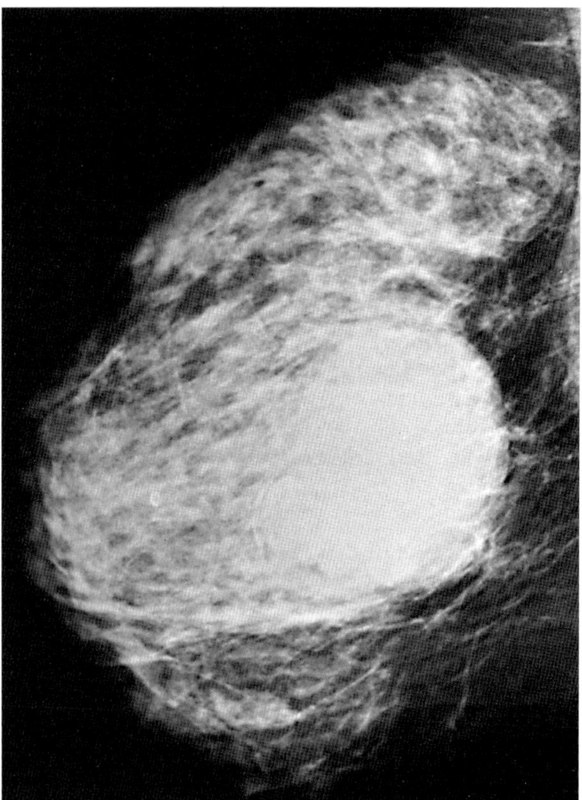

■ **FIGURE 24-14** Primary osteosarcoma of the breast. Right mediolateral oblique mammography view shows large, oval, circumscribed dense mass.

Ultrasonography

Angiosarcoma: On ultrasonography, breast angiosarcomas can appear circumscribed or ill-defined. They also have been reported as abnormal areas of mixed echogenicity. Rarely, color Doppler imaging can show tubular structures adjacent that are consistent with vasculatures.[16]

Magnetic Resonance Imaging

Primary liposarcoma: The imaging appearance of primary breast liposarcomas is variable, depending on the proportion of soft tissue to fatty component as well as the histologic subtype. Well-differentiated subtypes of liposarcoma will demonstrate a fat signal on MRI. However, many liposarcomas will demonstrate little to no fat signal; this occurs in more than 50% of myxoid subtype and the majority of pleomorphic and round-cell subtypes of liposarcoma.[17]

Primary angiosarcoma: On MRI, primary angiosarcomas appear as a heterogeneous mass of low signal intensity on T1-weighted images and of high signal intensity on T2-weighted images. Of note, higher grade lesions sometimes demonstrate irregular high T1-weighted signal within the mass, and these are believed to represent areas of hemorrhage or venous lakes within the mass. These tumors show variable enhancement depending on tumor grade. Low-grade angiosarcomas show progressive enhancement whereas high-grade angiosarcomas show rapid enhancement and washout. Often, large draining vessels may be visualized.

Secondary angiosarcoma: On MRI, secondary angiosarcomas appear similar to primary high-grade angiosarcomas with rapid enhancement with plateau or washout.[14]

Pathology

Grossly, sarcomas are large, fleshy, and firm with hemorrhage and necrosis. Many primary sarcomas of the breast likely represent either matrix-producing stromal overgrowth of metaplastic carcinoma or malignant phyllodes tumors with heterologous differentiation where the epithelial components have been undersampled and missed. Thus, extensive sampling is necessary to observe in-situ lesions or coexisting invasive carcinoma not otherwise specified. Rare cases of primary sarcomas have been reported in the literature, including liposarcomas, chondrosarcomas, osteogenic sarcomas, rhabdomyosarcomas, and leiomyosarcomas.

Primary breast liposarcomas are often large masses with necrosis and hemorrhage on the cut surface. Morphologically, liposarcomas show atypical lipoblasts. Myxoid and dedifferentiated/pleomorphic variants are the most common types of liposarcomas. Myxoid variant liposarcomas show a delicate arborizing vascular network with a myxoid background. Dedifferentiated/pleomorphic liposarcomas show bizarre large cells with atypical mitotic figures and resemble malignant fibrous histiocytomas (Fig. 24-15).

Primary osteogenic sarcomas in the breast are exceedingly rare. The tumor presents as a large hard firm mass due to bone formation. Morphologic features are similar to those of extraosseous osteogenic sarcomas. The tumor cells are composed of a mixture of fibroblasts, osteoblasts, and osteoclasts with an osteoid matrix (Fig. 24-16). Chondrosarcomas have atypical chondrocytes with a chondroid matrix. Metaplastic carcinomas with chondroid differentiation are the most likely diagnosis in the breast, rather than primary mammary chondrosarcoma.

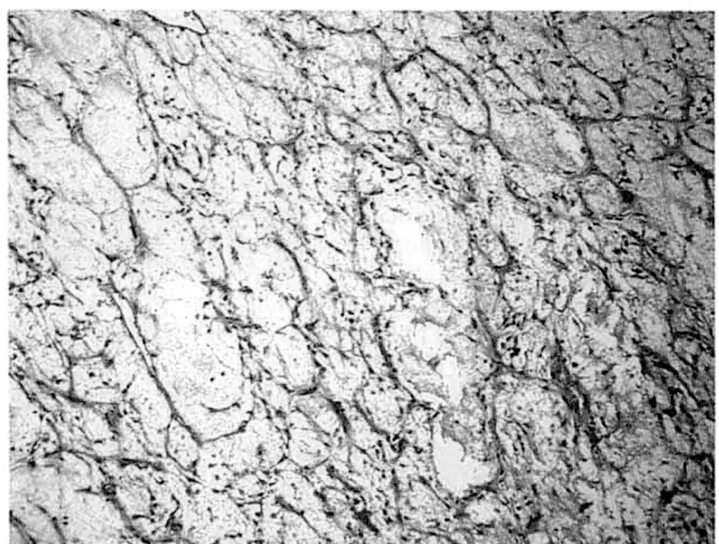

■ **FIGURE 24-15** Metastatic myxoid liposarcoma to the breast. The primary myxoid liposarcoma was located in the retroperitoneal area. One year later, a breast mass was noted. Vasculature network shows chicken-wire pattern with myxoid material (H&E, ×400).

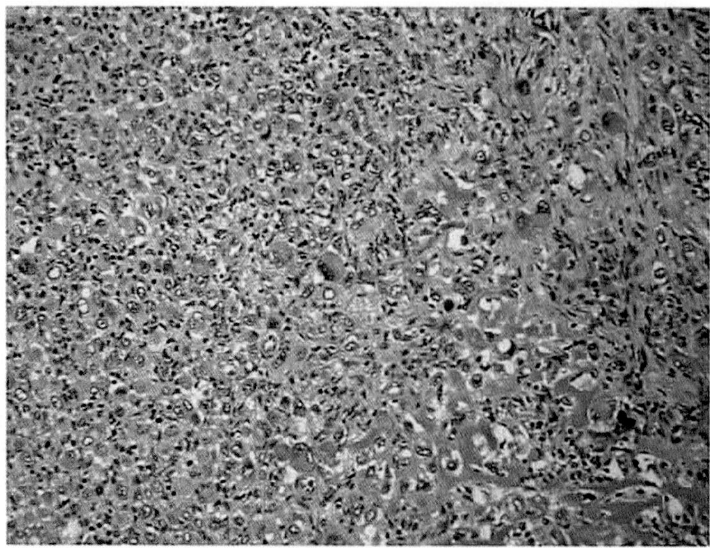

■ **FIGURE 24-16** Osteogenic sarcoma of the breast. Hyalinized osteoid formation is seen admixed with osteoclast giant cells, and osteoblasts (H&E, ×100).

Primary rhabdomyosarcomas are also extremely rare. Excluding rhabdoid differentiation from other more common breast tumors such as metaplastic carcinomas and phyllodes tumors, the most common rhabdomyosarcomas are metastatic tumors from soft tissues in young patients. Benign and malignant smooth muscle tumors are rare in breast tissue, representing less than 1% of primary breast neoplasms.

Leiomyosarcomas can occur in the breast as primary tumors originating from blood vessels or smooth muscle in the nipple areolar complex. In leiomyosarcomas, nuclear atypia, cellularity, coagulative tumor necrosis, and mitotic figures are seen with infiltrative borders. The diagnosis of primary breast leiomyosarcoma should be made only after other clinical studies and workup have excluded metastatic leiomyosarcomas from other body sites (Fig. 24-17).

Angiosarcomas of breast are more common than other primary breast sarcomas. Angiosarcomas are subdivided into two types: primary (de novo) and secondary (after mastectomy and radiation therapy). Stewart-Treves syndrome is a condition in which angiosarcoma arises in the lymphedematous upper extremity after mastectomy. This condition is unrelated to mammary carcinoma and is not seen within breast parenchyma. Postirradiation angiosarcomas have been reported even after 12 years post-treatment and are seen anywhere from 30 to 156 months after radiation therapy.[15] The risk of developing postirradiation angiosarcoma has not been correlated with dosage or duration of radiation therapy.

Grossly, angiosarcomas can appear anywhere from spongy hemorrhagic areas to firm masses with vascular engorgements. Microscopically, angiosarcomas are subdivided into grades I (well differentiated), II (intermediately differentiated), and III (poorly differentiated). Angiosarcomas must be sampled extensively to search for any areas of poorly differentiated foci. Microscopically, they can appear anywhere from solid, anastomosing branches to sieve-like growth patterns lined by a single layer of plump, hyperchromatic endothelial cells. Epithelioid angiosarcomas are usually found within grade III angiosarcomas and may mimic high-grade invasive ductal carcinoma (Figs 24-18 and 24-19). IHC stains for CD31, CD34, and factor VIII are positive for endothelial lining cells in epithelioid angiosarcomas. A new stain, FLI-1, is reported to be a sensitive marker for vascular origin. Well-differentiated low-grade angiosarcomas can appear as benign hemangiomas. However, even low-grade angiosarcomas should have some infiltration to the breast parenchyma, including the TDLU. A high index of suspicion is necessary to rule out low-grade angiosarcomas.

The prognosis of angiosarcomas is generally poor, depending on the tumor grade. High-grade angiosarcomas tend to metastasize to lungs and the contralateral breast. Lymph node metastases are rare. Most of the primary sarcomas are treated with total mastectomy to decrease the incidence of recurrence. Because the axillary lymph nodes are rarely involved by sarcomas, axillary dissection and/or sentinel lymph node sampling is usually not indicated.

METASTATIC DISEASES TO THE BREAST

Definition

Metastatic diseases to the breast from extramammary primary lesions are unusual. Metastatic lesions found in the breast from nonmammary malignant neoplasms are defined by tumor cells that originated from other body sites and that have no primary tumor within the breast parenchyma.

Prevalence and Epidemiology

A metastatic mass in the breast is rarely the initial sign of an extramammary malignancy. Usually lesions in other body locations are identified first. The largest reported single source of metastatic lesions to the breast is

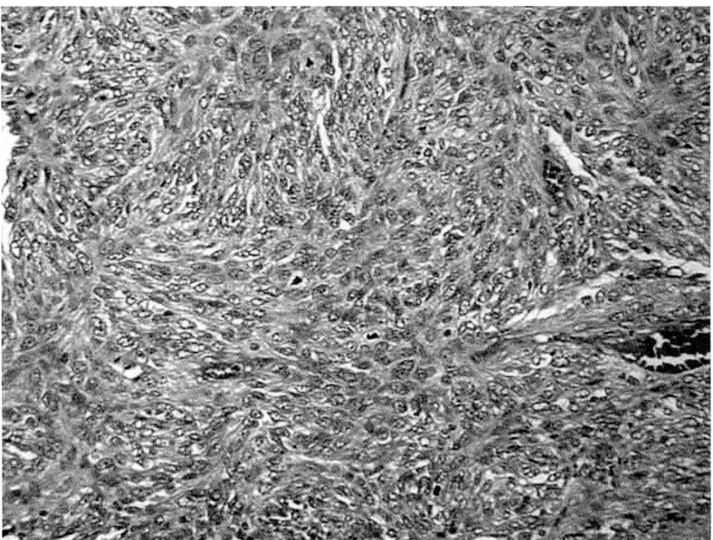

■ **FIGURE 24-17** Metastatic leiomyosarcoma from uterine primary tumor. Malignant spindle cells are seen with mitotic figures (H&E, ×400).

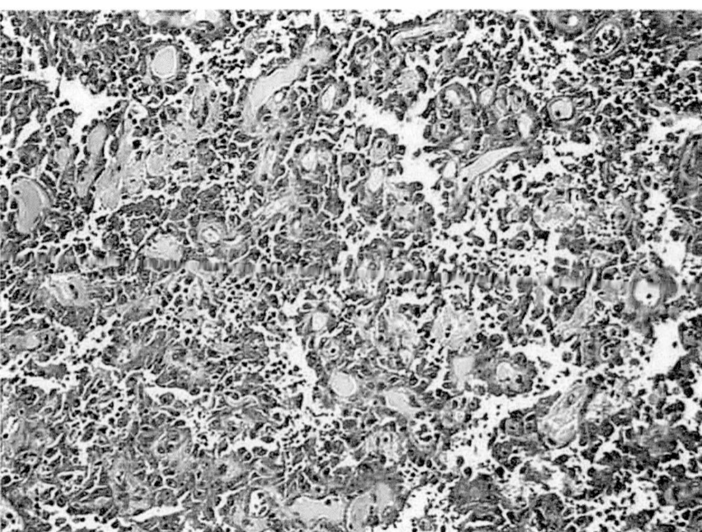

■ **FIGURE 24-18** High-grade epithelioid angiosarcoma with anastomosing pattern with papillary configuration (H&E, ×200).

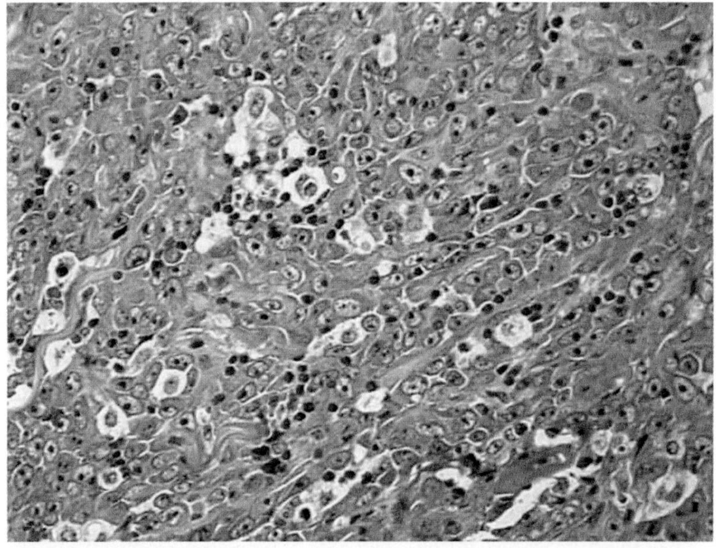

■ **FIGURE 24-19** Radiation-induced high-grade epithelioid angiosarcoma mistakenly diagnosed as high grade invasive ductal carcinoma (H&E, ×400).

melanoma, but a wide variety of other tumors may secondarily involve the breast.[16] On autopsy, the incidence of metastasis to the breast from other primary malignant neoplasms varies from 1.7% to 6.6%[18,19] In contrast, the rate observed clinically ranges from only 0.5% to 1.3%.[20] Metastatic lesions tend to have the same size on palpation as they appear on mammography. In contrast, the far more common infiltrating ductal carcinoma usually shows a discrepancy, feeling larger on clinical examination than is seen on mammography. This discrepancy reflects the proliferation of fibrous connective tissue associated with invasive ductal carcinomas as opposed to metastatic lesions. In addition, metastatic lesions do not cause thickening or retraction of the skin or nipple. Because metastatic lesions are not intraductal, they are not generally associated with nipple discharge.

Manifestations of Disease

Clinical Presentation

Metastases to the breast tend to be round, with a circumscribed to ill-defined mass that may be palpable or detected by mammography. They usually range from 1 to 3 cm at the time of detection. Although such metastases are usually solitary, multiple lesions may be seen.

Imaging Technique and Findings

Mammography

Mammographically, metastases to the breast tend to be round with circumscribed to ill-defined margins and lack the spiculation characteristic of the usual infiltrating

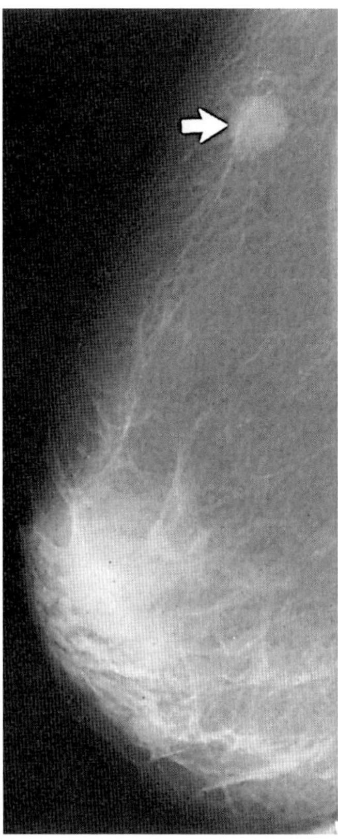

■ **FIGURE 24-20** Lung carcinoma metastatic to the breast. A 54-year-old woman with a known history of lung carcinoma noticed a mass (*arrow*) in the superior aspect of her right breast. Mammograms revealed a solitary, round, circumscribed mass at the site of the palpable abnormality. Biopsy revealed metastatic carcinoma.

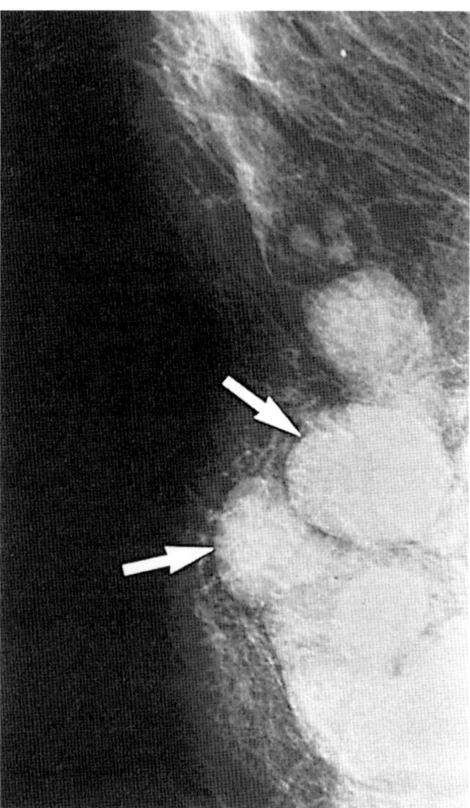

■ **FIGURE 24-21** Abnormal lymph nodes. Close-up of mediolateral oblique mammogram shows multiple large, round, dense circumscribed masses compatible with axillary adenopathy (*arrows*). Biopsy revealed metastatic adenocarcinoma from an unknown primary tumor.

ductal carcinoma (Fig. 24-20). They usually range from 1 to 3 cm at the time of detection. Although such metastases are usually solitary, multiple lesions may be seen (Fig. 24-21).

Pathology Findings

Metastatic malignant tumors to the breast are rare. The most common primary tumor sources for breast metastases in order of decreasing frequency are lymphomas, melanomas, lung tumors, and ovarian tumors.[21] Other reported primary malignancies that metastasize to the breast include small cell carcinoma, adenocarcinoma from the lung, renal cell carcinoma, intestinal carcinoid tumor, ovarian serous papillary carcinoma, adenocarcinoma and squamous cell carcinoma of uterine cervix, melanoma from skin and internal organs, adenocarcinoma of the gastrointestinal tract, thyroid carcinomas, minor salivary gland adenocarcinoma, and hematopoietic malignancy. Other reported sites include transitional cell carcinoma of the urinary bladder, alveolar soft part sarcoma, soft tissue sarcomas, and choriocarcinoma in the postpartum uterus. Most metastatic tumors to the breast have an underlying clinical history of primary tumor; however, treating clinicians may not have information about previously treated malignant tumors. Also, on rare occasion, metastatic tumor to the breast may be the initial presentation of a clinically occult neoplasm. In the absence of previous clinical history, an unusual histologic pattern with absence of an in-situ lesion may be the only clue to metastatic tumors to breast. The absence of in-situ carcinoma is not conclusive evidence that the tumor is metastatic from another site. Many mammary carcinomas do not show in-situ carcinoma especially when the tumor is rapidly growing with an aggressive pattern, such as triple negative, basal-like mammary carcinomas. Metastatic tumors to the breast tend to be multinodular without any of the atypia seen in atypical ductal hyperplasia, atypical lobular hyperplasia or in-situ carcinomas. However, the presence of atypical ductal proliferation does not necessarily indicate a breast origin. A high index of suspicion and good clinical correlation is especially vital in these cases.

Metastatic melanoma presenting clinically as a breast tumor may be difficult to recognize, especially if the primary melanoma is occult. Melanoma is considered a great mimicker and appears with any cytologic pattern, including epithelioid, sarcomatoid, clear cell type, and spindle cell shape. Melanin pigments may or may not be within the cytoplasm. Epithelioid melanoma can mimic a poorly differentiated invasive ductal carcinoma (Fig. 24-22). IHC stains may not be helpful in epithelioid cell type because estrogen receptor (ER), progesterone receptor (PR), and HER2/neu are commonly negative in poorly differentiated invasive ductal carcinoma and will be classified as triple-negative high-grade carcinoma. Keratin stains are most helpful to distinguish between invasive ductal carcinoma and melanoma. Other melanoma markers such as S-100, HMB-45, tyrosinase, and Mart-1 will be helpful to diagnose

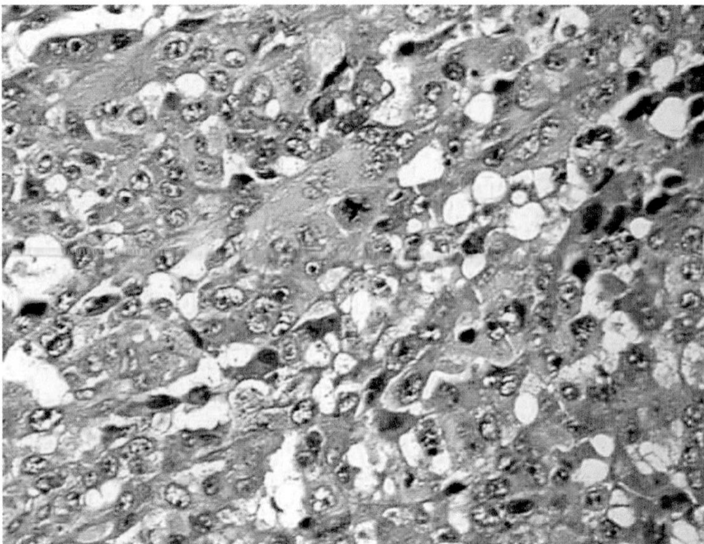

■ **FIGURE 24-22** Metastatic melanoma, epithelioid type, showing clusters of pleomorphic nuclei, prominent nucleoli, and abundant cytoplasm. A tetraploid mitotic figure is seen (H&E, ×400).

melanoma. Spindle cell melanoma can mimic spindle cell metaplastic carcinoma (Figs. 24-23 to 24-25). High-molecular-weight cytokeratins will be positive with spindle cell metaplastic carcinoma, whereas spindle cell melanoma will be negative with all cytokeratin markers. It is important to perform many high molecular cytokeratin stains when ruling-in spindle cell metaplastic carcinoma. The most helpful cytokeratin markers include 34*B*E13, cytokeratin 5/6, p63, and pancytokeratin cocktails. The differential diagnosis includes sarcomas such as leiomyosarcomas which can be distinguished by desmin, smooth muscle actin, and muscle-specific actin. When ordering IHC stains to rule-in or rule-out unknown primary tumor, it is helpful to order entire panels.

Metastatic renal cell carcinoma with clear cells is difficult to distinguish from primary breast carcinoma with clear cell features (Fig. 24-26). Clinical history and absence of ductal carcinoma in situ (DCIS) with clear cell features are helpful to delineate between these two conditions. IHC stains are not very helpful because both carcinomas will stain positive with cytokeratin. Metastatic carcinoid from the gastrointestinal tract resembles primary breast neuroendocrine type invasive ductal carcinoma (Figs 24-27 and 24-28).

Patients with metastatic ovarian carcinoma and serous papillary carcinoma can present with breast masses. In some cases, breast metastases are the first clinical finding and may be mistaken for micropapillary carcinoma of the breast. Metastatic ovarian serous papillary carcinomas

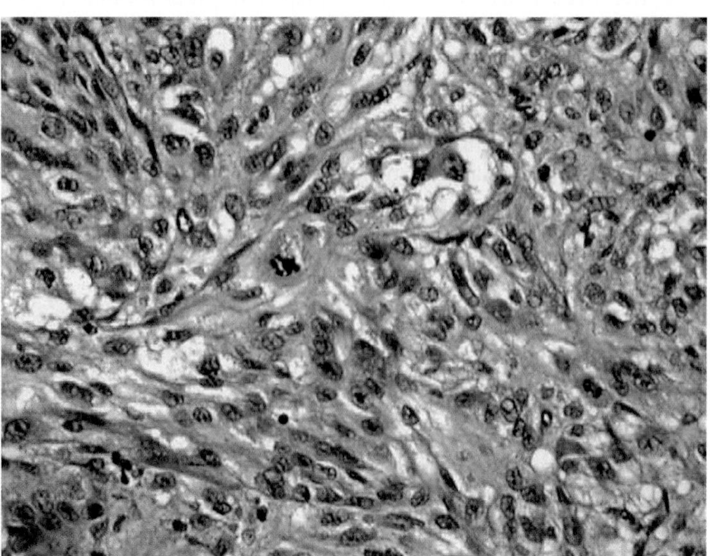

■ **FIGURE 24-23** Desmoplastic melanoma neurotrophic type resembles spindle cell metaplastic carcinoma (H&E, ×400).

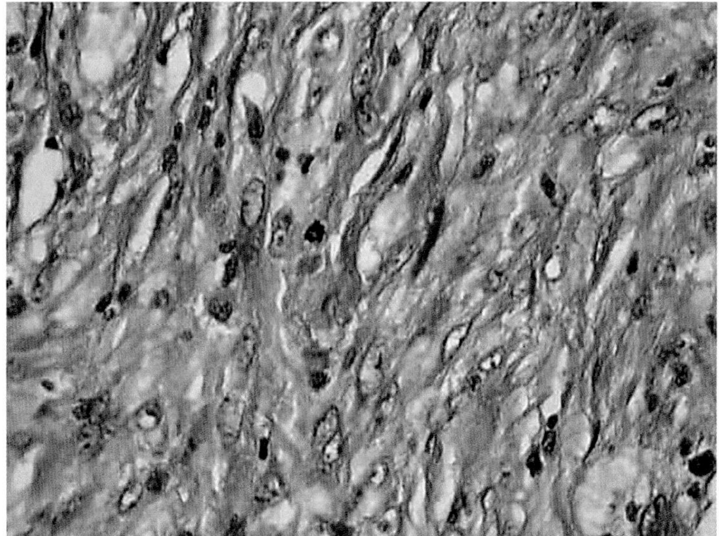

■ **FIGURE 24-24** Spindle cell metaplastic carcinoma. Note the mitotic figure (H&E, ×400).

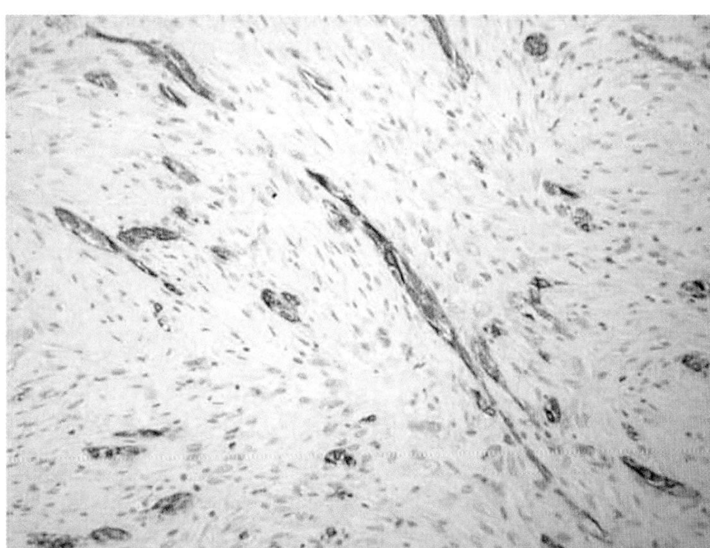

■ **FIGURE 24-25** Scattered spindle cells are positive for keratin stain, supporting the diagnosis of spindle cell metaplastic carcinoma (cytokeratin stain, ×200).

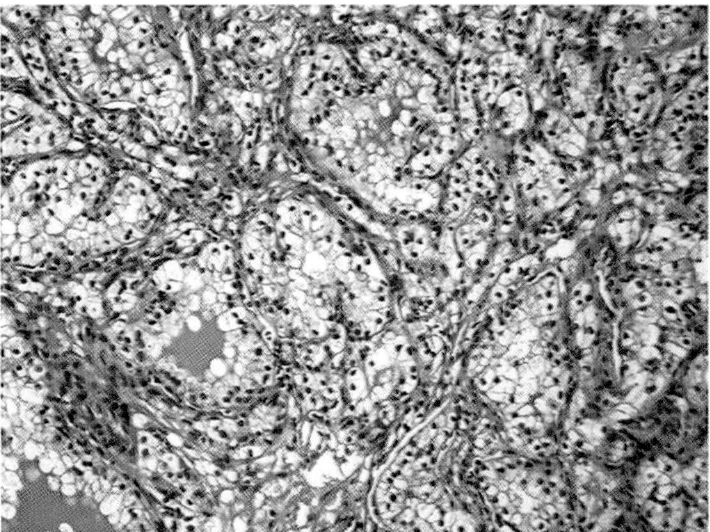

■ **FIGURE 24-26** Metastatic renal cell carcinoma to breast. Note the clear cells forming nests resembling clear cell type ductal carcinoma in situ (H&E, ×200).

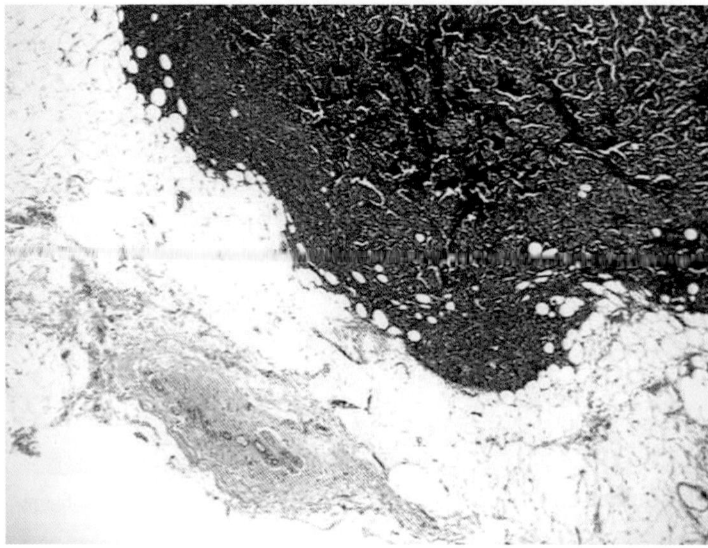

■ **FIGURE 24-27** Metastatic neuroendocrine carcinoma from colon to breast. Note the sharply demarcated tumor. No in situ carcinoma is seen from the breast tissue (H&E, ×40).

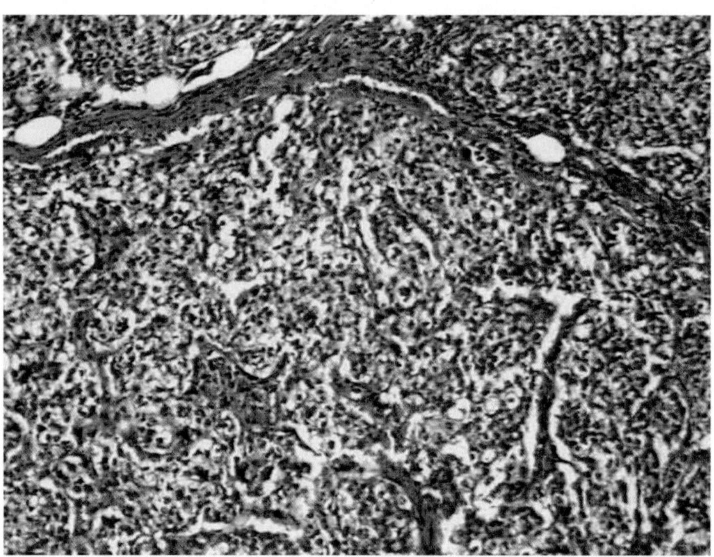

■ **FIGURE 24-28** Metastatic neuroendocrine carcinoma in same patient as in Figure 24-20 in high-power showing an organoid pattern (H&E, ×400).

usually show numerous psammomatous calcifications. Micropapillary carcinomas of the breast show clefts mimicking lymphovascular invasion with inverted epithelial membrane antigen (EMA) staining pattern by immunohistochemistry (Figs 24-29 to 24-31). Metastatic ovarian carcinoma to breast includes endometrioid and mucinous carcinomas.

Signet ring cell carcinoma from stomach and medullary carcinoma of thyroid resemble signet ring cell invasive lobular carcinoma and invasive lobular carcinoma trabecular/alveolar type, respectively (Figs 24-32 and 24-33). The presence of LCIS is helpful when looking to exclude possible metastatic diseases. Rare cases of metastatic choriocarcinoma of the breast in young female patients who had a history of molar pregnancy have been reported (Fig. 24-34).[22] The distinction between primary mammary tumors and metastasis in the breast is critical in clinical management and treatment because mastectomy and axillary lymph node dissection are not appropriate treatment of metastatic tumor. Systemic chemotherapy may be more appropriate depending on the specific primary neoplasm. The prognosis of patients with metastatic tumors depends on the nature of the primary tumor and the extent of disease.

Synopsis of Treatment Options

The distinction between primary breast and metastatic breast malignancy is critical for treatment. For primary breast tumors, the treatment options involve total mastectomy followed by irradiation and/or chemotherapy, depending on the nature of the tumor. For metastatic breast tumors, sampling of breast tissue either by fine-needle aspiration, core needle biopsy, or excision is required to

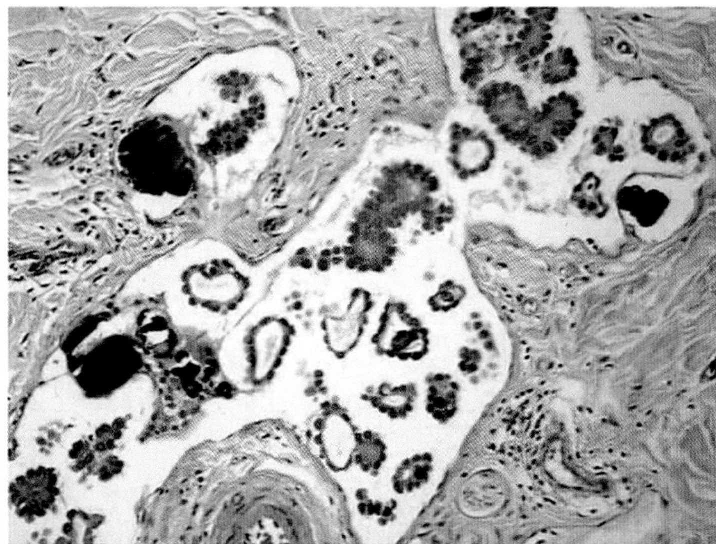

■ **FIGURE 24-29** Metastatic serous papillary carcinoma from the ovary filling the lymph-vascular spaces in the breast. Note the papillary pattern of tumor cells and psammomatous calcifications (H&E, ×200).

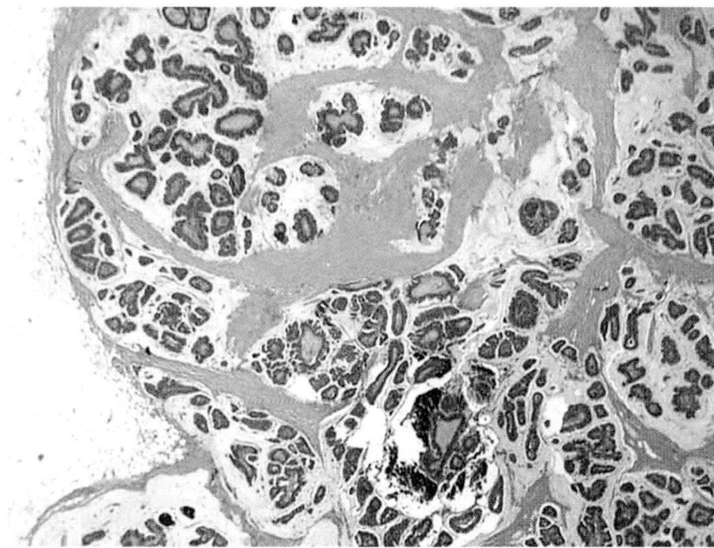

■ **FIGURE 24-30** Micropapillary carcinoma of the breast. Some clusters of tumor cells show papillary tufting but majority of tumor cells show clefts (H&E, ×100).

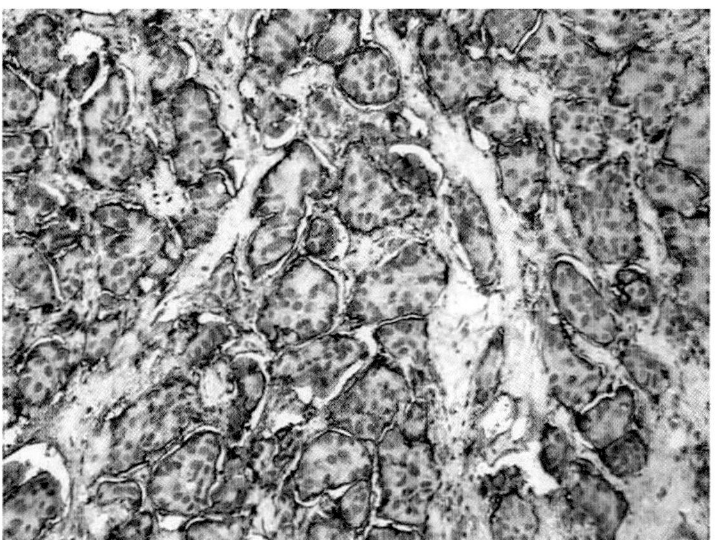

■ **FIGURE 24-31** Epithelial membrane antigen (EMA) stain shows "inside out" pattern (×200).

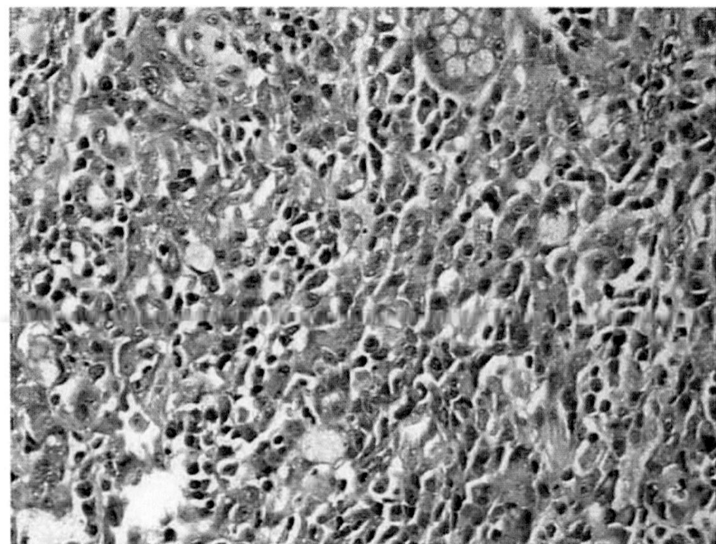

■ **FIGURE 24-32** Gastrointestinal signet ring cell carcinoma resembling invasive lobular carcinoma of signet ring cell type (H&E, ×200).

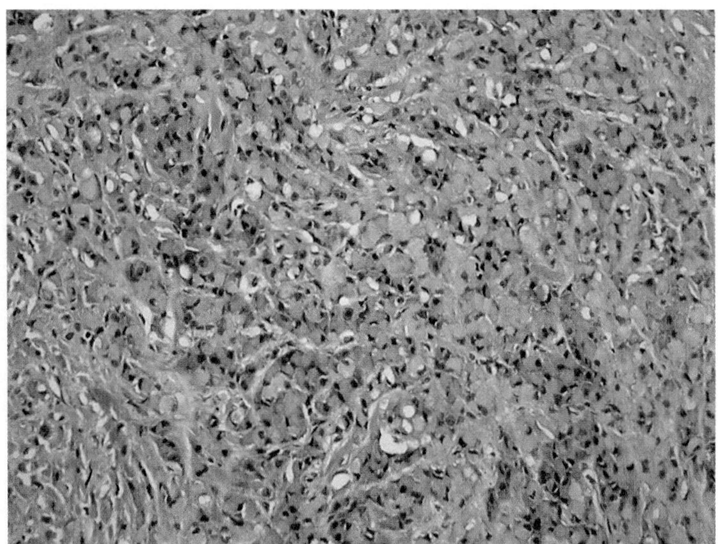

■ **FIGURE 24-33** Invasive lobular carcinoma signet ring cell type (H&E, ×200).

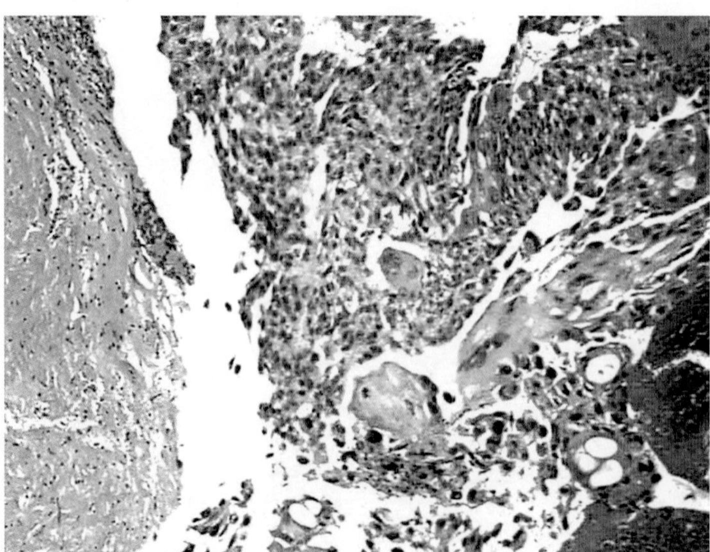

■ **FIGURE 24-34** Choriocarcinoma metastasized to breast in a young woman who had a recent history of pregnancy. Syncytiotrophoblastic (giant) cells and cytotrophoblastic cells are seen in the pools of blood (H&E, ×200).

establish the diagnosis. When an occult extramammary tumor presents as breast metastasis, clinical workup and additional body imaging studies are necessary. Mastectomy is usually not indicated for metastatic tumor to the breast, but it may be performed as a palliative therapy in the case of skin ulceration or local control of a bulky tumor. Chemotherapy is generally the first-line treatment option for metastatic breast malignancy.

KEY POINTS

- Primary lymphomas in the breast are extremely rare and non-Hodgkin lymphomas, specifically B-cell lymphomas, are the most common primary hematopoietic tumors of the breast.
- The diagnosis of primary breast lymphoma should be limited to patients without any evidence of other systemic hematopoietic malignancy.
- Malignant phyllodes tumors are biphasic tumors with both malignant stroma and benign intervening glands.
- The subclassification of phyllodes tumors is divided into three categories: benign, low-grade (borderline), and malignant.
- Pure primary sarcomas of the breast are exceedingly rare. Many primary sarcomas of the breast likely represent either matrix-producing stromal overgrowth of metaplastic carcinoma or malignant phyllodes tumors with heterologous differentiation in which the epithelial components have been undersampled and missed.
- Metastatic diseases to the breast from extramammary primary lesions are unusual. Metastatic lesions found in the breast from nonmammary malignant neoplasm are defined by tumor cells that originated from the other body sites and have no primary tumor within the breast parenchyma.
- The distinction between primary breast and metastatic breast malignancy is critical for treatment.

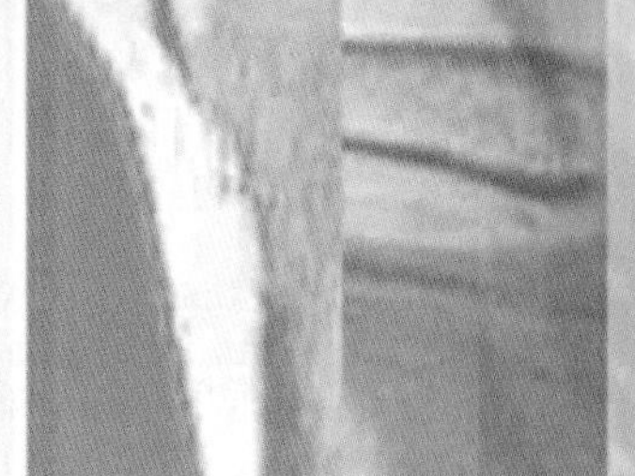

CASE STUDY

Chapter 24 Other Malignant Breast Diseases

HISTORY

A 64-year-old woman presented with a suspicious left breast mass at the upper inner position. Her family history is significant for breast cancer in a maternal aunt.

Physical examination of the left breast showed a palpable, mobile mass at the 10-o'clock position. No other masses are found in either axilla. No skin changes are seen.

FINDINGS

Mammogram showed a focal asymmetry at a posterior depth (Fig. 24-35). Directed ultrasonography of the left 10-o'clock position was performed and showed a hypoechoic area consistent with a solid mass measuring 30 mm × 12 mm × 5 mm (Fig. 24-36). Computed tomography of the chest, abdomen, and pelvis with and without contrast showed no other significant findings.

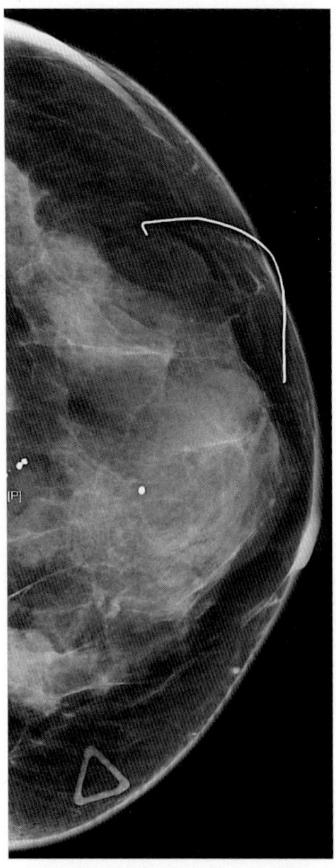

■ **FIGURE 24-35** Craniocaudal mammography view of the left breast demonstrates an asymmetry at a posterior depth.

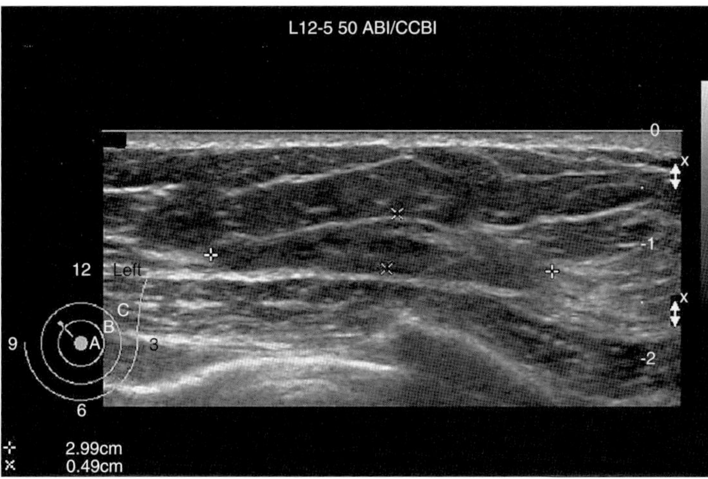

■ **FIGURE 24-36** Ultrasound image demonstrates a hypoechoic area consistent with a solid mass measuring 30 mm × 12 mm × 5 mm.

Fine-needle aspiration findings: Smears show cellular material of predominantly single, dyshesive cells with scant cytoplasm. The cells are uniform without variation of small, intermediate, and large size. Occasional prominent nucleoli are seen. The background shows numerous lymphoglandular bodies that are fragmented cytoplasm of lymphocytic cells (Fig. 24-37).

Excisional biopsy: The tumor shows well-demarcated borders from the adjacent fatty tissue of the breast. No definite evidence of lymph node structures in the intracapsular area, sinus, or medullary area is noted. A diffuse infiltrate of atypical lymphocytes is seen. There are sheets of large lymphoid cells, many with irregular nuclear outlines. The lymphoma infiltrates into breast tissue and the surrounding fat (Fig. 24-38). High-power view shows large nuclei with prominent central nucleoli and numerous mitotic figures (Fig. 24-39).

IHC stains are performed and the results are listed as follows:

- Pankeratin: Negative
- CD20: Positive
- CD3: Negative (positive in a few small lymphocytes)
- CD30: Negative
- CD45: Positive
- Bcl-6: Positive weak
- Bcl-2: Positive strong

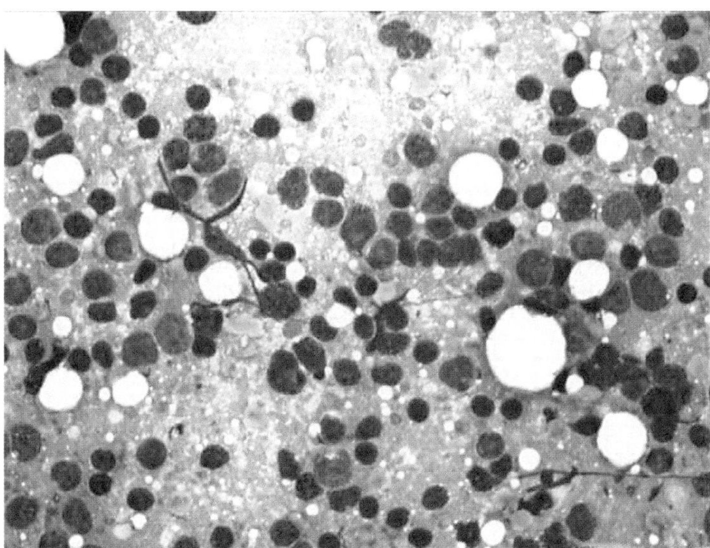

■ **FIGURE 24-37** Singly dispersed cells without cytoplasm and large nuclei with occasional prominent nucleoli (fine-needle aspiration May-Gruenwald Giemsa [MGG] stain, ×400).

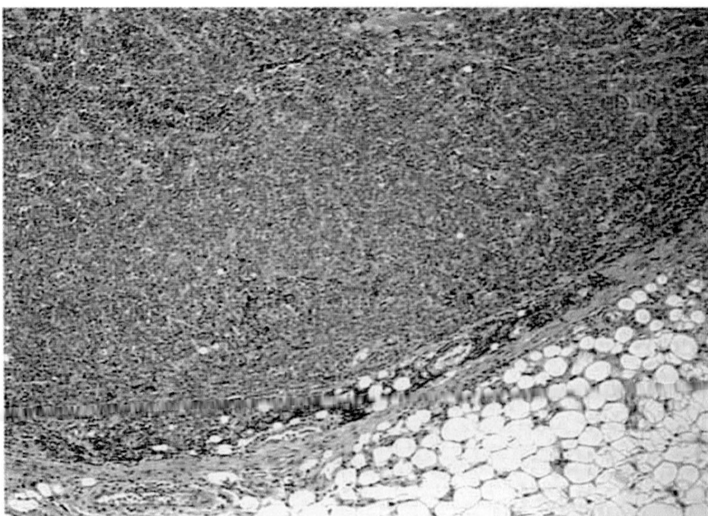

■ **FIGURE 24-38** Excisional biopsy from the same patient as in Figure 24-37 shows a fairly well circumscribed mass with diffuse infiltrate of lymphoid cells resembling lymph node (H&E, ×40).

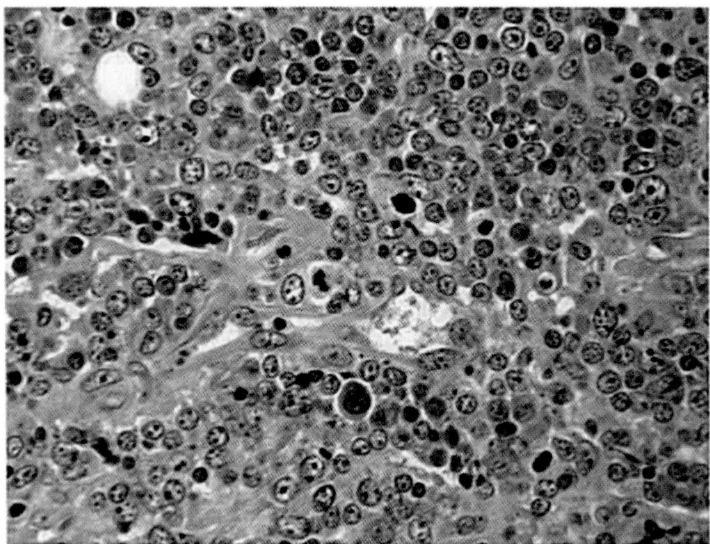

■ **FIGURE 24-39** Diffuse B-cell lymphoma. Same patient as in Figure 24-36 (H&E, ×400).

- Bcl-1: Negative
- Kappa: Positive
- Lambda: Negative
- Ki-67: Positive (60% of cells)

IHC stains are positive for CD20, Bcl-6, and Bcl-2 with kappa light chain restriction, supportive of large B-cell lymphoma. All other clinical findings are negative for hematopoietic malignancy.

DIFFERENTIAL DIAGNOSIS

The differential diagnosis includes:

- Invasive ductal carcinoma, poorly differentiated (Fig. 24-40)
- Intramammary lymph node
- Lymphoma
- Metastatic hematopoietic malignancy

DIAGNOSIS

Malignant lymphoma, diffuse large B-cell type, breast primary.

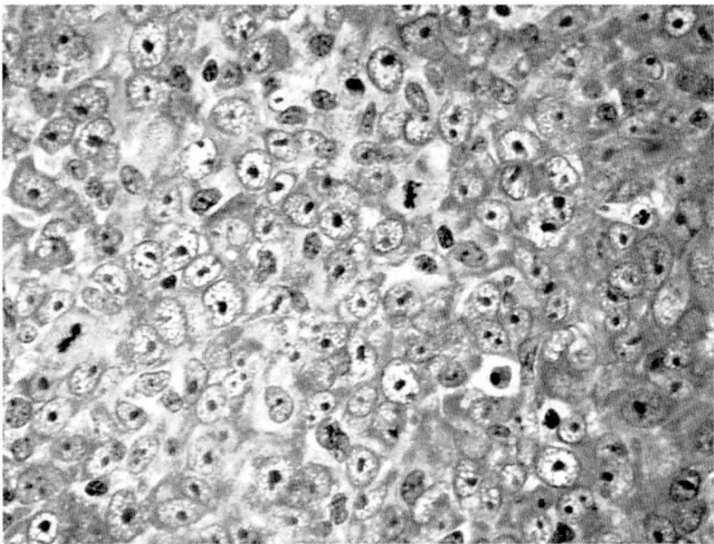

■ **FIGURE 24-40** Invasive ductal carcinoma (IDC), which is in the differential diagnosis of diffuse B-cell lymphoma. Cluster of neoplastic cells have large nuclei with prominent nucleoli and many mitotic figures (H&E stain, ×600).

COMMENTARY

The patient was treated with three cycles of CHOP chemotherapy (cyclophosphamide, doxorubicin, vincristine [Oncovin], prednisone) plus four doses of rituximab (Rituxan), followed by involved field radiotherapy.

SUGGESTED READINGS

Sebenik M, Ricci A Jr, DiPasquale B, Mody K, Pytel P, Jee KJ, et al. Undifferentiated intimal sarcoma of large systemic blood vessels: report of 14 cases with immunohistochemical profile and review of the literature. *Am J Surg Pathol* 2005;**29**:1184-9.

REFERENCES

1. Topalovski M, Crisan D, Mattson JC. Lymphoma of the breast. *Arch Pathol Lab Med* 1999,**123**:1208-18.
2. Donegan WL, Spratt JS, editors. *Cancer of the breast*. 4th ed. Philadelphia: WB Saunders; 1995.
3. Liberman L, Giess CS, Dershaw DD, Louie DC, Deutch BM. Non-Hodgkin's lymphoma of the breast: imaging characteristics and correlation with histopathologic findings. *Radiology* 1994;**192**:157-60.
4. Aguiler NS, Tavassoli FA, Chu WS, Abbondanzo SL. T-cell lymphoma presenting in the breast: a histologic, immunophenotypic and molecular genetic study of four cases. *Mod Pathol* 2000;**13**:599-605.
5. Lun AN, Lam TR, Khoo US. Subcutaneous panniculitislike T-cell lymphoma appearing as a breast mass: a difficult and challenging case appearing at an unusual site. *J Ultrasound Med* 2005;**24**:1453-60.
6. Grabowski J, Salzstein S, Sadler, Georgia, et al. Malignant phyllodes tumor, review of 752 cases. *Am Surg* 2007;967-9.
7. Reinfuss M, Mitus J, Duda K, Stelmach A, Rys J, Smolak K. The treatment and prognosis of patients with phyllodes tumor of the breast: an analysis of 170 cases. *Cancer* 1996;**77**:910-6.
8. Bernstein L, Deapen D, Koss RK. The descriptive epidemiology of malignant cystosarcoma phyllodes tumors of the breast. *Cancer* 1993;**71**:3020-4.
9. Noguchi S, Yokouchi H, Aihora T, Motomura K, Inaji H, Imaoka S, et al. Progression of fibroadenoma to phyllodes tumor demonstrated by clonal analysis. *Cancer* 1995;**76**:1779-85.
10. Asoglu O, Ugurlu M, Blanchard K, et al. Risk factors for recurrence and death after primary surgical treatment of malignancy phyllodes tumors. *Ann Surg Oncol* 2004;1011-7.
11. McGregor J. Liposarcoma of the breast. Case report and review of literature. *Can Med Assoc J* 1960;**82**:781-3.
12. Sabate J, Gomez A, Torrubia S, Flotats A. Osteosarcoma of the breast. *AJR Am J Roentgenol* 2002;**179**:277-8.
13. Glazebrook K, Magut M, Reynolds C. Angiosarcoma of the breast. *AJR Am J Roentgenol* 2008;**190**:533-8.
14. Yang WT, Hennessy BT, Dryden MJ, Valero V, Hunt KK, Krishnamurthy S. Mammary angiosarcomas: imaging findings in 24 patients. *Radiology* 2007;**242**:725-34.
15. Cancellieri A, Eusebi V, Mambelli V, Ricotti G, Gardini G, Pasquinelli G. Well differentiated angiosarcoma of the skin following radiotherapy. Report of two cases. *Pathol Res Pract* 1991;**187**:301-6.
16. Bohman L, Bassett L, Gold R, Voet R. Breast metastases from extra-mammary malignancies. *Radiology* 1982;**144**:309-12.
17. Wong K, Lee P, Chan Y. Case Report. Paraffinoma in the anterior abdominal wall mimicking liposarcoma. *Br J Radiol* 2003;**76**:264-7.
18. Abrams H, Spiro R, Goldstein N. Metastases in carcinoma: analysis of 1000 autopsied cases. *Cancer* 1950;**3**:74-85.
19. Sandison A. Metastatic tumors in the breast. *Br J Surg* 1959;**47**:54-8.
20. Hadju S, Urban J. Cancers metastatic to the breast. *Cancer* 1972;**29**:1691-1696.
21. Bartella L, Kaye J, Perry NM. Metastases to the breast revisited: radiological-histopathological correlation. *Clin Radiol* 2003;**58**:524-31.
22. Kalra N, Ojili V, Gulati M, Prasad GR, Vaiphei K, Suri S. Metastatic choriocarcinoma to the breast. Appearance on mammography and Doppler sonography. *AJR Am J Roentgenol* 2005;**184**:S53-5.

CHAPTER 25

The Effect of Neoadjuvant Chemotherapy and Radiation Therapy on Breast Tissue

Sophia Kim Apple, Erum W. Sethi, and Lawrence W. Bassett

NEOADJUVANT CHEMOTHERAPY

Since the early 1980s, neoadjuvant chemotherapy (NACT) has been part of the treatment approach to inoperable stage IV breast cancers. NACT is becoming more commonly used in the treatment of locally advanced breast cancer, and it is generally used in large, bulky primary tumors, often with involvement of the overlying skin or fixed ipsilateral underlying chest wall (inflammatory breast cancer), the presence of matted axillary lymph nodes or supraclavicular/subclavicular lymphadenopathy or a combination of those conditions. The expectation is that it can reduce the size of tumor enough to permit a surgical procedure with a reasonable degree of long term survival and a low incidence of local recurrence. Before the introduction of NACT these patients were treated almost exclusively with palliative therapy. One of the most apparent advantages of NACT is the clinically rapid reduction of tumor volume in the primary tumor site and enlarged lymph nodes, presumably due to metastatic disease. Tumor downstaging with NACT can convert inoperable disease to operable disease and can allow breast-conserving surgery in patients for whom mastectomy is the only option for local or regional control of disease. NACT also enables oncologists to determine tumor chemosensitivity in vivo. Another benefit of NACT is the downstaging of lymph node metastases. The National Surgical Adjuvant Breast and Bowel Project (NSABP) B-18 study[1] showed 36% of NACT patients who initially had clinically apparent positive lymph nodes were found to be node negative. This was compared with 14% of patients who received only postoperative chemotherapy. Both Rouzier and colleagues[2] and Kuerer and colleagues[3] demonstrated that NACT results in a complete axillary response for 23% of patients with cytology-proven lymph node metastases at the time of diagnosis.

There are several studies suggesting clinical or biological parameters that may predict response to NACT. Some studies have shown that high nuclear and histologic grade of the primary tumor is significantly associated with pathologic response to NACT, whereas others studies have not.[4] An association has been reported between negative estrogen receptor (ER)/progesterone receptor (PR) expression and improved pathologic response to NACT, which supports the results of several previous studies.[5,6] Furthermore, many groups have reported an association between increased Ki-67 expression and improved pathologic response.[5-7]

Human epidermal growth factor receptor 2 (HER-2)/neu amplified breast carcinoma tested by fluorescent in situ hybridization (FISH) has been associated with improved pathologic response with some chemotherapy regimens[8] but not with others.[9] Histologic subtype was significant in predicting pathologic response after NACT. Lobular carcinomas are less likely to show a complete pathologic response when compared with ductal carcinomas.[10,11] There is no single clinical or biological parameter identified as a reliable predictor of response, or of overall survival or disease-free survival, in breast cancer patients treated with NACT. Although the data are inconsistent, NACT may be more effective in killing tumor cells when tumor cells exhibit higher grade, higher Ki-67 rate, ER- and PR-negative, and HER-2/neu-negative (triple-negative) tumors.

Histologic changes in breast carcinoma after chemotherapy have been reported, including the presence of foam cells, confluent foci of fibrosis in lymph nodes, and bizarre cytologic changes in residual tumor cells.[12,13] Some other findings include cytoplasmic vacuolization, increased eosinophilia of cytoplasm probably due to anoxic changes, multinucleation of tumor cells, hyperchromasia and smudge appearance of nuclei, decreased nuclear-to-cytoplasmic ratio, decrease in mitotic figures, increased fibrosis, increased elastosis and hyalinization, and increase in inflammatory cells, including histiocytic collections and multinucleated giant cells around the tumor bed with chronic inflammation. Some of the chemotherapy effect on the normal breast tissue includes lobular atrophy, increased collagen deposition around the terminal ductal lobular unit (TDLU), lobular basement membrane thickness, and diffuse parenchymal fibrosis (Figs. 25-1 to 25-8). A similar finding occurs in carcinoma in situ, especially high-grade ductal carcinoma in situ (DCIS). Lobular carcinoma in situ (LCIS) often shows no significant changes as in invasive lobular carcinoma. The reason for this may be that most invasive lobular carcinomas are low grade with a low proliferation index and are ER- and PR-positive but HER-2/neu-negative tumors (Figs. 25-9 and 25-10).[11] With NACT, lymph nodes show diffusely hyalinized fibrotic stroma effacing the usual architecture of the lymph node. Within the extensive fibrosis are pockets of viable and degenerative tumor cells. One of the unexpected findings in our experience is lymphovascular invasion showing more viable tumor cells within vascular plugs. Rare cases show similar degenerative changes within lymphovascular invasion as is seen in the breast parenchymal tumor. Because most of the chemotherapeutic agents are delivered intravascularly, one may assume that lymphovascular invasion would the first to receive most of the effect of chemotherapy. Interestingly, we found that is not the case. Tumor cell viability was intact within lymphovascular invasion, even in a case of a complete pathologic response from the breast and lymph nodes.

Studies reporting the association of histologic effect after NACT with pathologic response and outcome have been conflicting. Some have reported these changes to be associated with better response and survival[14,15] whereas others have not.[16] The NSABP B-18 study[17] demonstrated that histologic signs of cell death are compatible with partial pathologic response but not overall and disease-free survival.

Classification of post-NACT primary tumors into the categories of partial and no pathologic response depends on an accurate measurement of residual tumor size. However, this is complicated by variable changes within the tumor bed and loss of viable tumor cells. From our institutional experience, clinical and radiologic studies after NACT

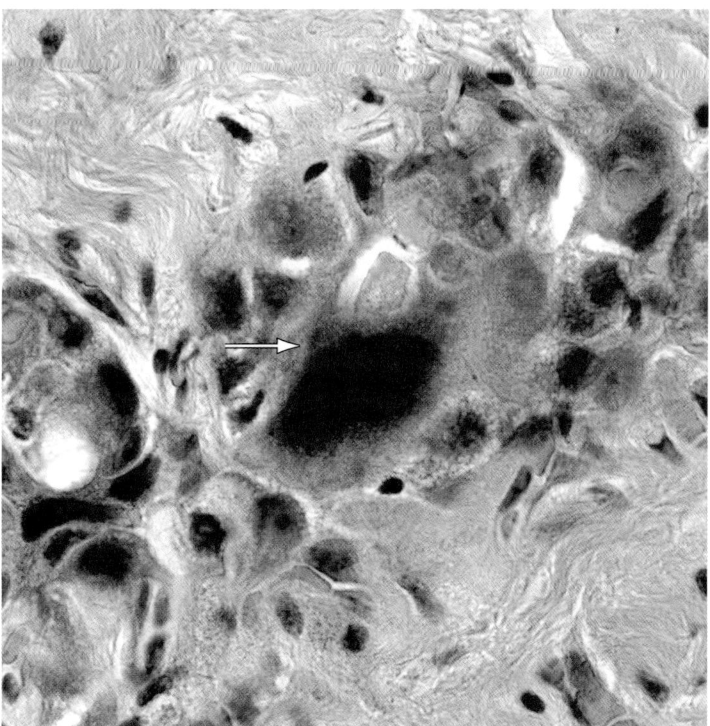

■ **FIGURE 25-1** Degenerated tumor cells after neoadjuvant chemotherapy (NACT). Large, bizarre nuclei with hyperchromatic and smudged appearance (*arrow*) in post-NACT carcinoma (H&E, × oil magnification). *(Courtesy of Peggy S. Sullivan, MD, Pathology & Lab Medicine Women's Health Fellow, University of California, Los Angeles.)*

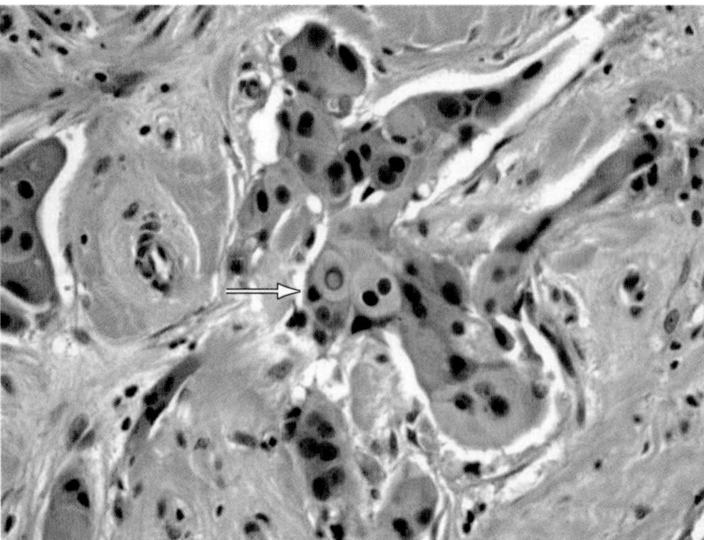

■ **FIGURE 25-2** Cytoplasmic ballooning after neoadjuvant chemotherapy (NACT). An increased amount of eosinophilic cytoplasm with well defined cytoplasmic border is present on invasive ductal carcinoma (*arrow*) (H&E, ×100). *(Courtesy of Peggy S. Sullivan, MD, Pathology & Lab Medicine Women's Health Fellow, University of California, Los Angeles.)*

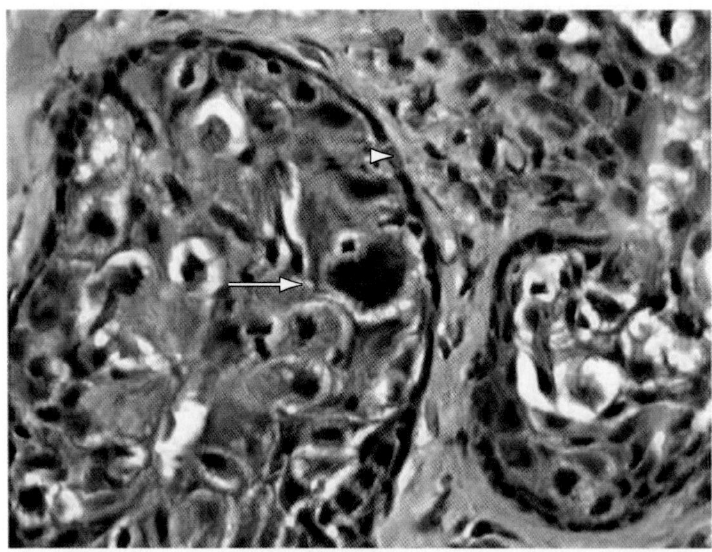

■ **FIGURE 25-3** Ductal carcinoma in situ (DCIS) after neoadjuvant chemotherapy (NACT). Note the similar degenerative changes within the DCIS cells (*arrow*) and accentuation of the myoepithelial cells (*arrowhead*) (H&E, ×400).

often overestimate the response rate: the size of the tumor after NACT is often smaller clinically and radiologically than the final pathologic size when tissue is thoroughly examined.[18] One reason is residual smaller pockets and viable tumor cells occupying the entire original volume of the tumor bed. One may assume that the tumor shrinks from the periphery and forms a central nidus. However, the pathologic size of the tumor spans the entire initial tumor size but the volume of the tumor within that span is smaller.

In reporting breast carcinoma cases after NACT, the pathologic report should provide detailed information, such as the extent of residual viable tumor, percent estimated necrosis induced by NACT, percent apoptosis, and any significant histologic changes, such as nuclear and cytoplasmic degenerative changes. Some authors recommend that the modified Scarff-Bloom-Richardson (SBR) grade should be determined after NACT.[19] This task is difficult with complete or near-complete pathologic response because many of the previously mentioned histologic changes after NACT preclude evaluation by modified SBR grade criteria. When the tumor shows no pathologic response after NACT, then modified SBR grade scoring is easily applicable and should be done. When the tumor shows a complete pathologic response, there is no need to document the results using the modified SBR grade scores. When the tumor shows a

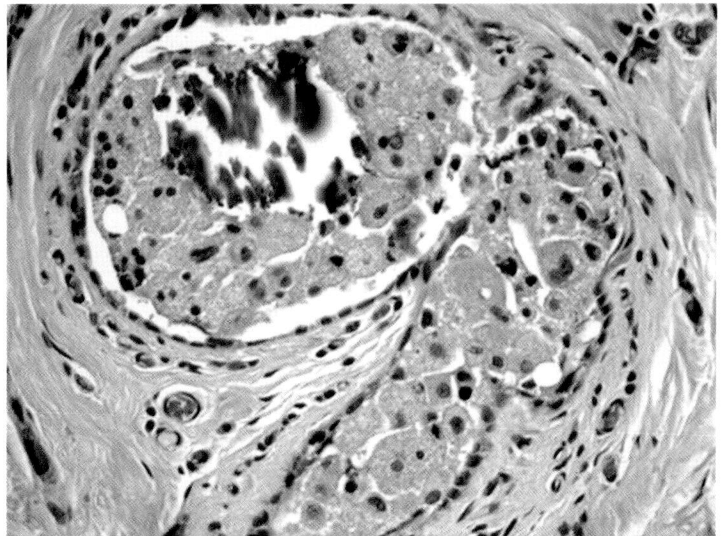

■ FIGURE 25-4 Ductal carcinoma in situ (DCIS) after neoadjuvant chemotherapy (NACT). Comedo necrosis type DCIS was present in the pre-NACT biopsy. The resection specimen shows an expanded terminal duct lobular unit (TDLU) replaced with necrosis (H&E, ×400).

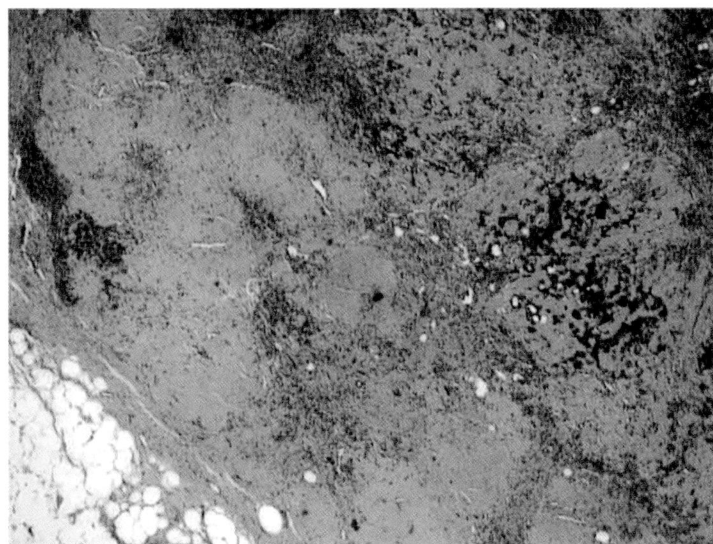

■ FIGURE 25-5 Lymph node after neoadjuvant chemotherapy (NACT). Metastatic tumor is replaced with fibrosis, foam cells, and occasional residual tumor cells with marked degenerative changes (H&E, ×40).

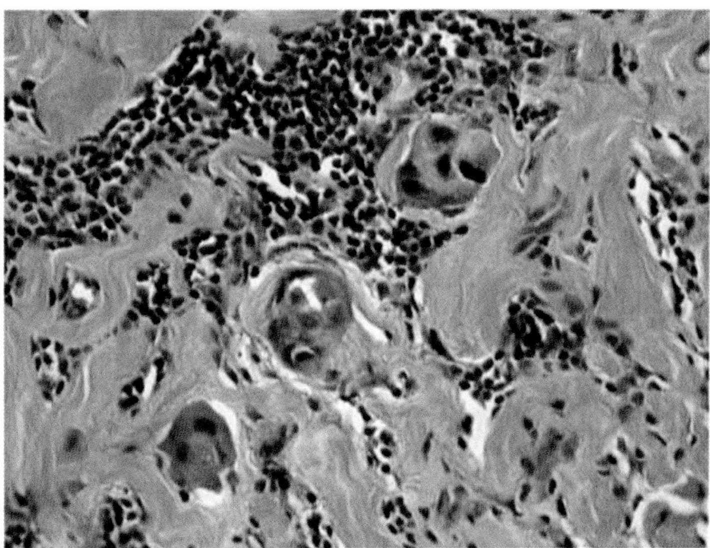

■ FIGURE 25-6 Lymph node showing a few aggregates of viable metastatic carcinoma embedded within the fibrosis (H&E, ×400).

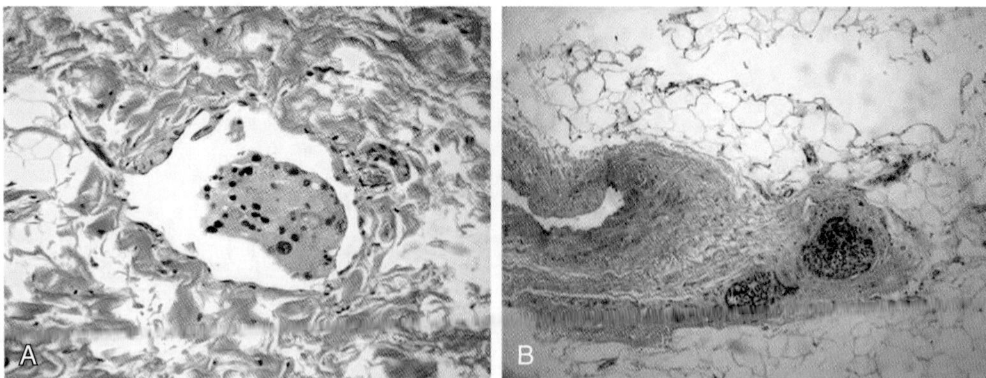

■ **FIGURE 25-7** Lymph-vascular invasion. Tumor cells are plugging the lymphatic spaces. **A,** No neoadjuvant chemotherapy (NACT) effect. **B,** NACT effect with dark, pyknotic nuclei with fragmentation and shrunken, abundant eosinophilic cytoplasm (H&E).

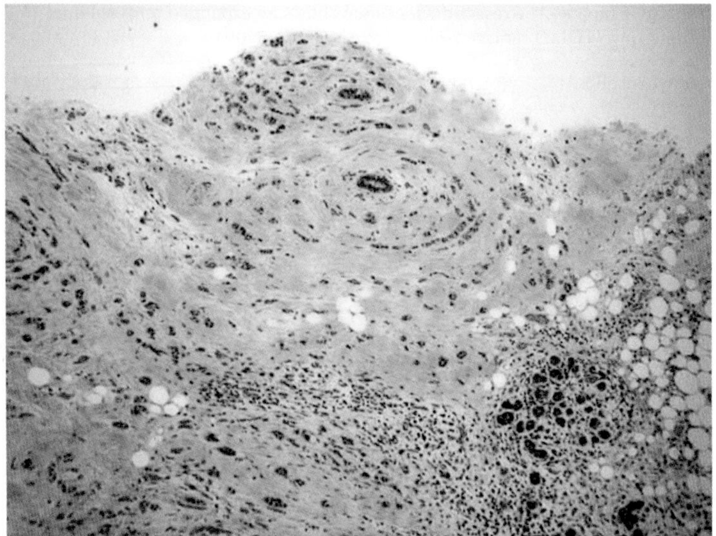

■ **FIGURE 25-8** Preneoadjuvant chemotherapy invasive lobular carcinoma. Tumor cells are in a targetoid and linear pattern (H&E, ×100).

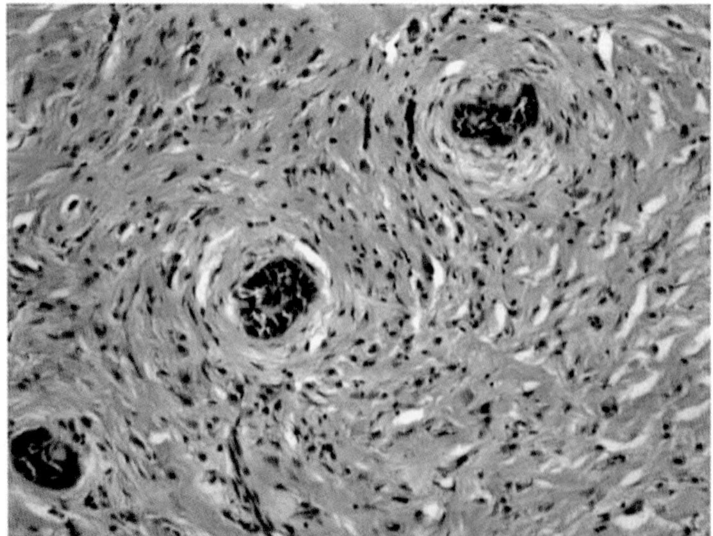

■ **FIGURE 25-9** Postneoadjuvant chemotherapy invasive lobular carcinoma. Same patient as in Figure 25-8. Essentially no chemotherapy effect is seen. The tumor cells are viable and maintaining a linear and targetoid pattern (H&E, ×100).

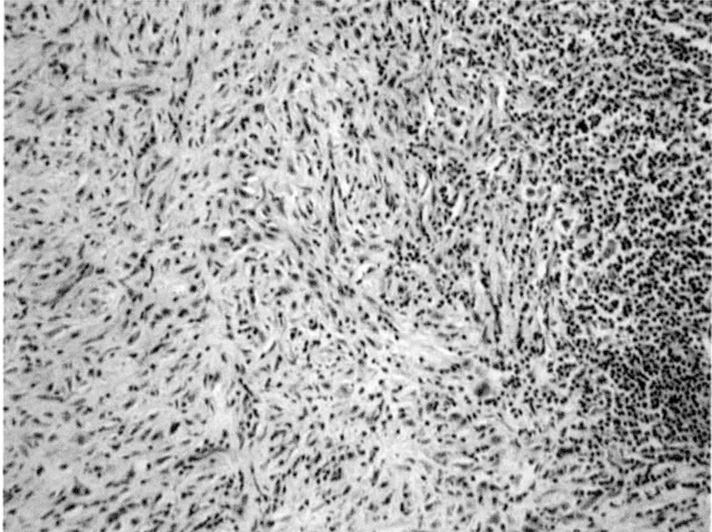

■ **FIGURE 25-10** Postneoadjuvant chemotherapy effect on lymph node with metastatic lobular carcinoma. Essentially no chemotherapy effect is seen. Tumor cells are viable, effacing the entire lymph node (H&E, ×200).

partial pathologic response, modified SBR grade scores cannot be done: nuclear pleomorphism is severe due to degenerative changes of tumor cells and mitotic rate is low after NACT.

The significance of the histologic changes in NACT-treated tissue is unclear. However, as chemotherapy becomes an important tool in the treatment of locally advanced breast cancer or even early breast cancer, pathologists will be required to recognize the histologic changes in the NACT-treated breast.

On mammography and ultrasonography, the most common response to NACT is reduction in tumor size and also a density difference of the mass on mammography[20] (Figs. 25-11 and 25-12). After NACT, magnetic resonance imaging (MRI) has also been increasingly used to depict residual disease (Fig. 25-13). To avoid harm and costs due to

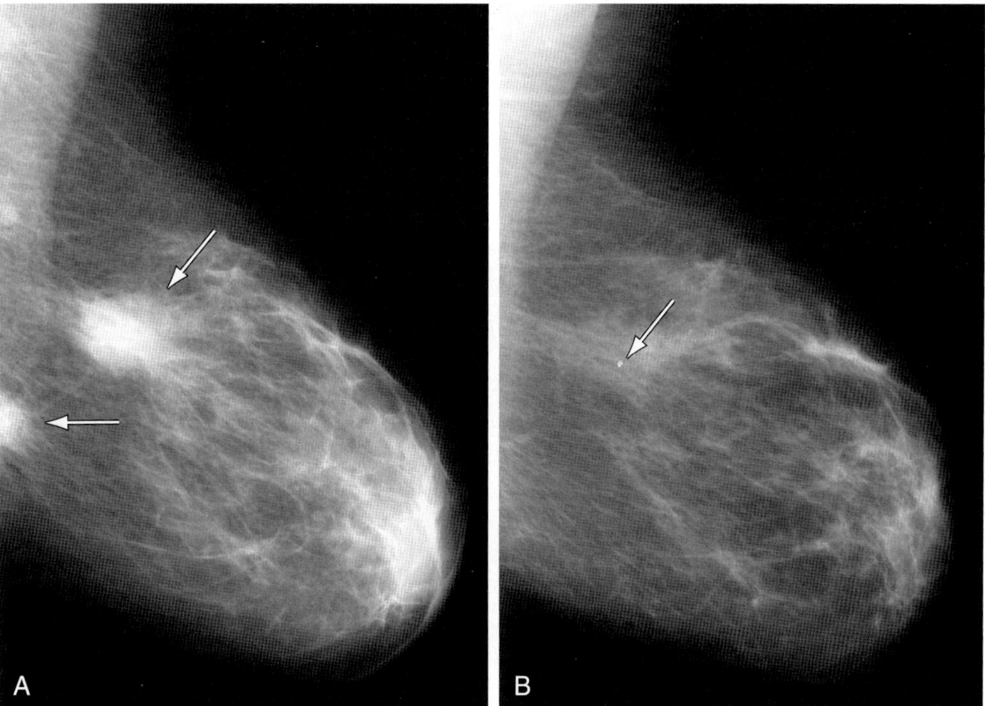

■ **FIGURE 25-11** Neoadjuvant chemotherapy (NACT) effect shown on mammography. **A,** Left mediolateral oblique mammogram in a woman with known invasive breast carcinoma demonstrates two irregular, dense spiculated masses (*arrows*) within the posterior breast. **B,** There is a significant reduction in the size and density of both masses status post-NACT. A microclip (*arrow*) denotes where the larger mass had been.

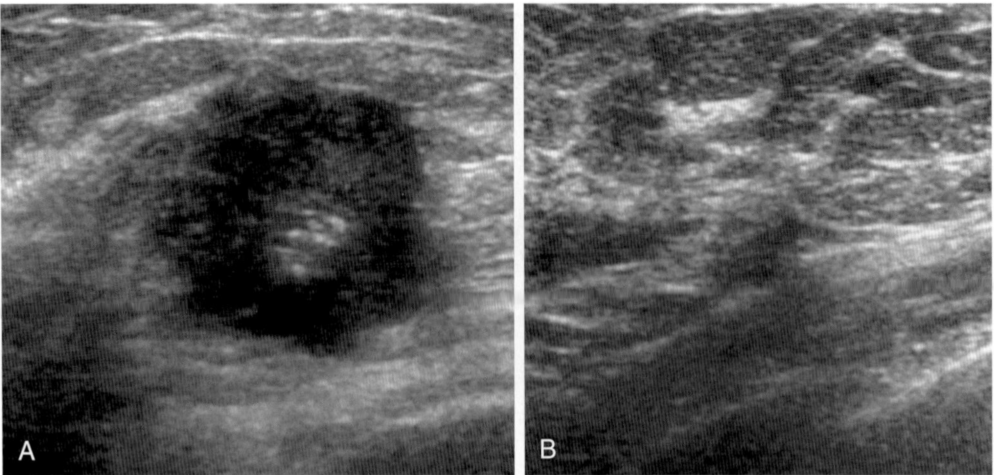

■ **FIGURE 25-12** Neoadjuvant chemotherapy (NACT) effect shown on ultrasonography. **A,** Directed ultrasound imaging of the larger irregular, microlobulated hypoechoic mass in the patient in Figure 25-11 with known invasive breast carcinoma. **B,** Directed ultrasound imaging in the same area status post-NACT demonstrates no definite mass.

inefficient treatment, it is beneficial to predict response to NACT as early as possible, ideally immediately after the first cycle. Several studies have investigated the confidence with which residual disease is demonstrated with different imaging modalities, and the results of these studies indicate that breast MRI is superior to conventional imaging and clinical breast assessment. MRI findings correlate significantly better with pathologic response. However, the correlation is not a perfect and even if an MRI study is negative, residual tumor may be identified in up to 30% of patients.[21]

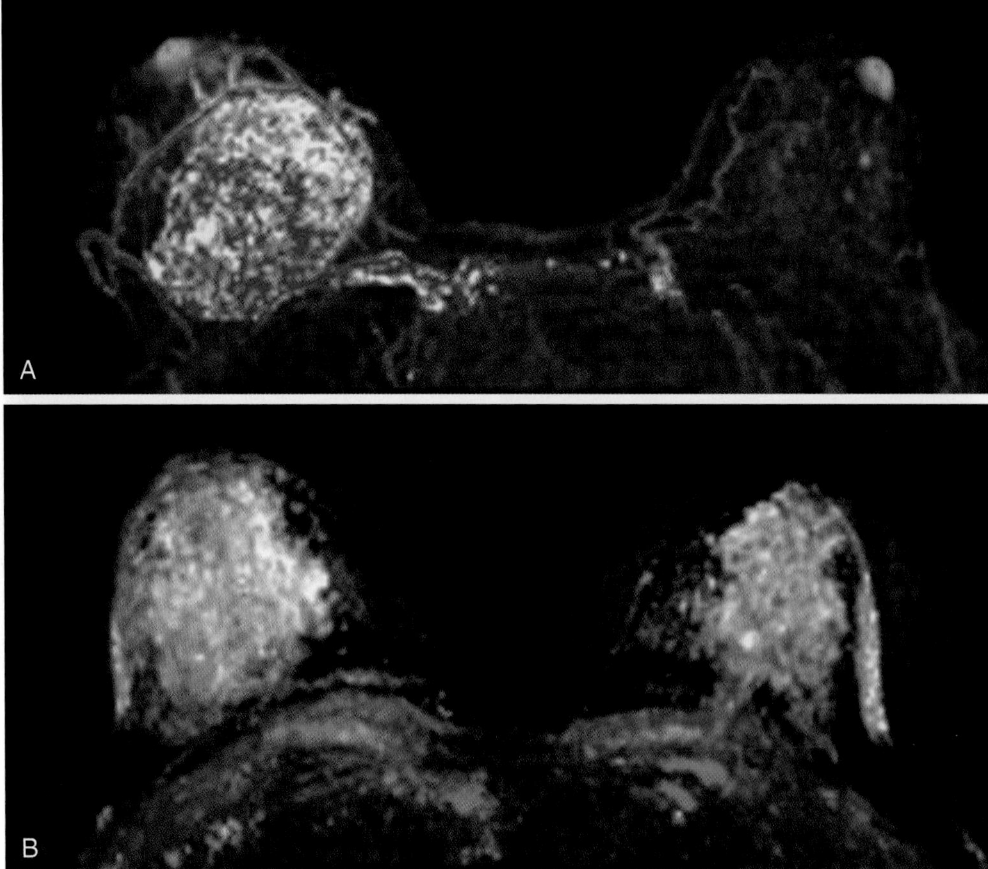

■ **FIGURE 25-13** Neoadjuvant chemotherapy (NACT) effect shown on magnetic resonance imaging (MRI). **A,** Maximum intensity projection (MIP) image with color-coded map overlay demonstrates a large oval enhancing mass within the right breast in a woman with known breast carcinoma. **B,** The mass shows marked reduction in tumor volume and enhancement status post-NACT, with no definite residual mass visualized.

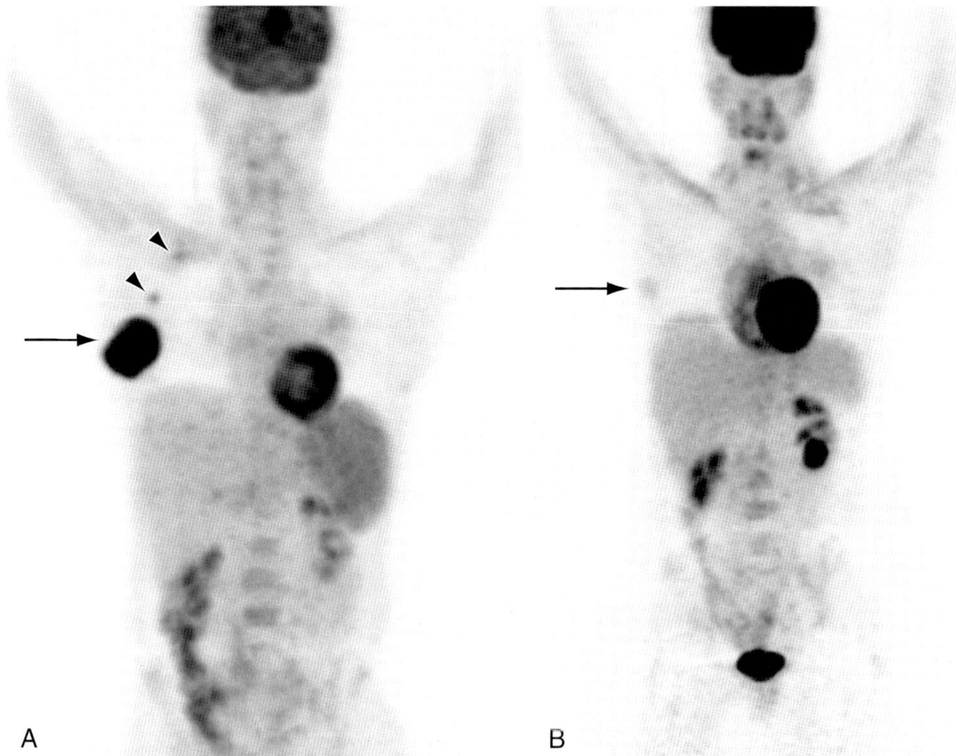

■ **FIGURE 25-14** Neoadjuvant chemotherapy (NACT) effect shown by positron emission tomography (PET). **A,** Maximum intensity projection (MIP) PET scan demonstrates a large focus of intense metabolic activity in the right breast that corresponds to patient's known breast cancer (*arrow*). There are smaller foci of uptake within the right axilla that correlate to axillary metastases (*arrowheads*). Smaller, less intense foci of mediastinal uptake are probably secondary to the patient's history of sarcoidosis. **B,** There is significant decrease in previously seen area of tumor uptake within the right breast status post-NACT with a small focus of residual uptake remaining (*arrow*). The foci within the right axilla are no longer visualized.

Serial fluorodeoxyglucose (FDG)-labeled positron emission tomography (FDG-PET) and combined FDG-PET with computed tomography (PET/CT) are also being used to assess response to NACT (Fig. 25-14). The majority of studies that evaluate FDG-PET to assess response to NACT have measured change in FDG uptake at mid-therapy compared with baseline as a measure of response.[22] A decline in primary tumor FDG uptake by about 50% or more is predictive of a good response to NACT, whereas a lesser decline is more characteristic of a nonresponder.[23] Early FDG-PET results are suggested to be predictive of final response.[22,24,25] FDG-PET that is performed after completion of therapy allows confirmation of gross residual disease but does not allow exclusion of residual microscopic malignancy.[26]

RADIATION THERAPY

Radiation therapy (RT) is used with increasing frequency as part of the breast-conserving treatment option. Histomorphologic alterations induced by RT are critical for a correct diagnosis, especially in the setting of questionable recurrence. Some women who have had breast conservation and RT may develop subsequent mammographic or clinically palpable lesions and will require either core needle biopsy or small excisional biopsy to rule out recurrence. It is critical to recognize morphologic alterations induced by RT to prevent misinterpretation of radiation atypia as malignant cells. RT is often not given twice to women, and thus the only option for recurrent breast malignancy is mastectomy. The morphologic changes of RT effect can be seen in as short as 1 month to several years (>6 years). The effect occurs in breast skin, endothelial cells, and epithelial cells (TDLU) within the breast parenchyma. The skin changes induced by RT include stromal fibrosis, endothelial cell hyperplasia with fibrinoid necrosis, and fat necrosis. Fat necrosis can present as a clinically palpable mass resembling recurrent breast cancer. Epithelial alterations induced by RT include enlargement of nuclei, marked hyperchromasia, smudging appearance, and cytoplasmic vacuolization. Nuclear-to-cytoplasmic ratio is low, unlike malignant cells (Fig. 25-15). Also, nucleoli and mitotic figures are inconspicuous. In addition, lobular atrophy and stromal hyalinization and fibrosis (involutional changes) are common morphologic features of RT (Fig. 25-16). Similar morphologic changes can also occur in adjuvant or neoadjuvant chemotherapy, or both. The most challenging differential diagnosis is distinguishing between radiation atypia and cancerization of lobules, which is the result of DCIS cells in the lobules (Fig. 25-17). This is particularly challenging in a case of recurrent DCIS and cancerization of lobules in the background of radiation atypia. However, in the absence of hyperplasia or pro-

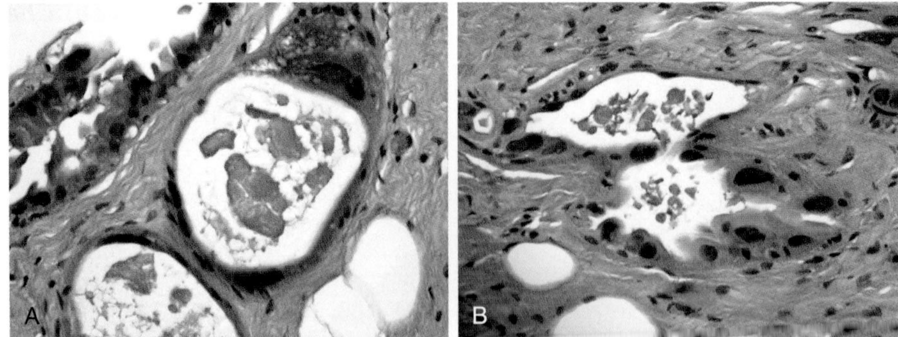

■ **FIGURE 25-15** A and B, Radiation-induced atypia of small ductules showing low nuclear-to-cytoplasmic ratio, marked nuclear hyperchromasia, smudged appearance of nuclei, and cytoplasmic vacuoles (H&E, ×400).

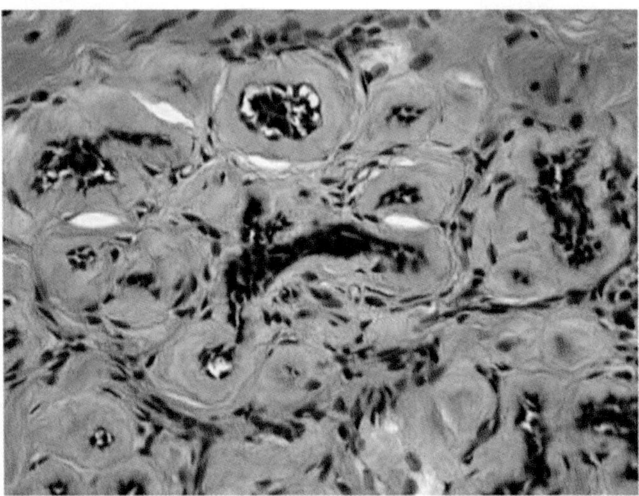

■ **FIGURE 25-16** Radiation-induced changes in normal breast parenchyma. Note marked fibrosis and atrophy of the terminal duct lobular unit (TDLU) (H&E, ×400).

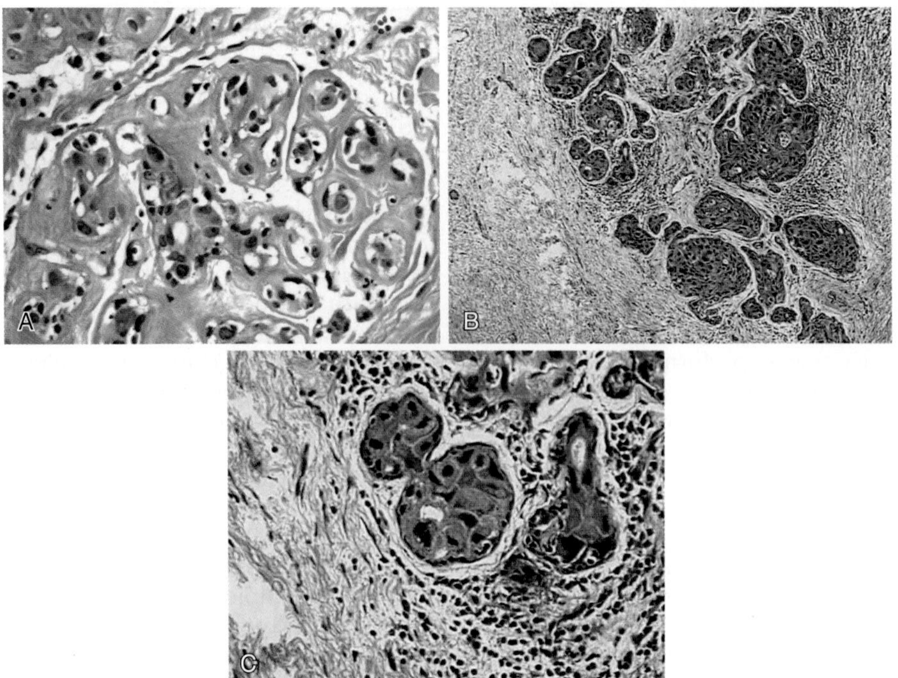

■ **FIGURE 25-17** Radiation-induced atypia in terminal duct lobular unit (TDLU). **A,** Small lobules mimic cancerization of lobules. Nuclei are mildly atypical, and the epithelial cells are surrounded by thickened fibrosis (H&E, x400). **B,** Cancerization of lobules recurred after radiation therapy many years previously. There are distended TDLUs with atypical epithelial proliferations (H&E, × 100). **C,** Higher magnification of cancerization of lobules (COL) recurrence after radiation therapy. Proliferation of TDLU is required to make the distinction between COL. (H&E, ×400).

liferation of epithelial cells, the diagnosis of recurrent malignancy such as DCIS or cancerization of lobules is unlikely.

Postirradiation changes include skin thickening, edema, trabecular thickening, increased focal and diffuse increased density of the breast parenchyma, and fat necrosis, as well as coarse pleomorphic and dystrophic calcifications. These changes can be easily demonstrated on mammography and ultrasonography (Figs. 25-18 and 25-19).

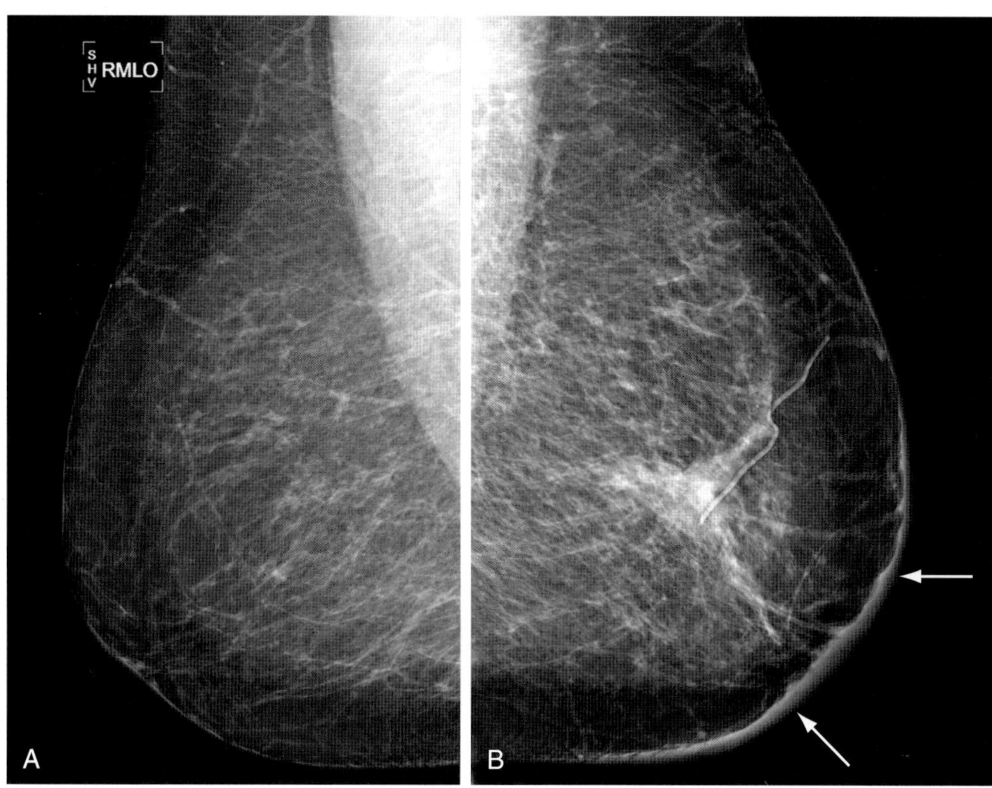

■ **FIGURE 25-18** Postirradiation changes. Right (**A**) and left (**B**) mediolateral oblique mammogram in a patient status post left lumpectomy and radiation therapy. There is skin thickening (*arrows*) and increased trabecular markings secondary to radiation changes within the left breast.

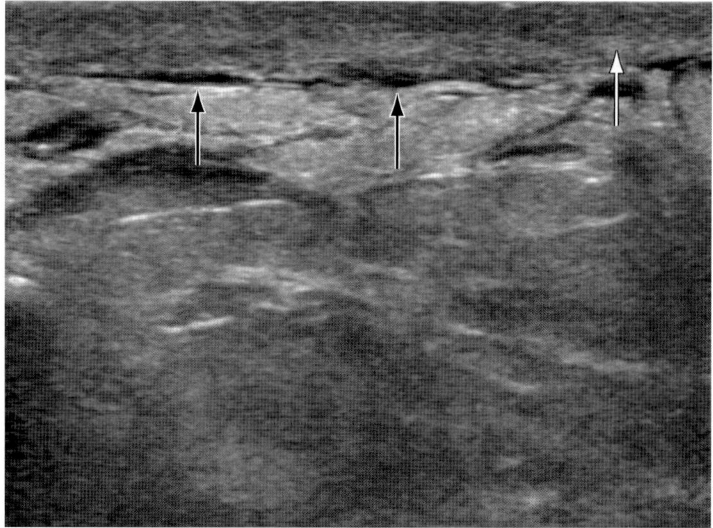

■ **FIGURE 25-19** Post-radiation changes. Ultrasound image of the breast in a patient status post lumpectomy and radiation demonstrates postirradiation skin thickening (*white arrow*) and edema (*black arrows*).

KEY POINTS

- Neoadjuvant chemotherapy (NACT) is becoming more commonly used in locally advanced breast cancer with the expectation that NACT can reduce the size of tumor enough to permit a surgical procedure with a reasonable degree of long term survival and a low incidence of local recurrence.
- No difference in survival benefit has been found between total mastectomy and breast-conserving surgery coupled with whole-breast irradiation.
- Radiation therapy cannot be given twice to women, and thus the only option for recurrent breast malignancy is mastectomy.
- Postirradiation changes include skin thickening, edema, trabecular thickening, increased focal and diffuse density of the breast parenchyma, and calcifications, including fat necrosis, which can be seen on mammography and ultrasonography.

SUGGESTED READINGS

Rosen EL, Eubank WB, Mankoff DA. FDG PET, PET/CT, and breast cancer imaging. *Radiographics* 2007;**27**(Suppl. 1):S215-29.

REFERENCES

1. Fisher B, Brown A, Mamounas E, Wieand S, Robidoux A, Margolese RG, et al. Effect of preoperative chemotherapy on local-regional disease in women with operable breast cancer: findings from National Surgical Adjuvant Breast and Bowel Project B-18. *J Clin Oncol* 1997;**15**:2483-93.
2. Rouzier R, Extra JM, Klijanienko J, Falcou MC, Asselain B, Vincent-Salomon A, et al. Incidence and prognostic significance of complete axillary downstaging after primary chemotherapy in breast cancer patients with T1 to T3 tumors and cytologically proven axillary metastatic lymph nodes. *J Clin Oncol* 2002;**20**:1304-10.
3. Kuerer HM, Sahin AA, Hunt KK, Newman LA, Breslin TM, Ames FC, et al. Incidence and impact of documented eradication of breast cancer axillary lymph node metastases before surgery in patients treated with neoadjuvant chemotherapy. *Ann Surg* 1999;**230**:72-8.
4. Pu RT, Schott AF, Sturtz DE, Griffith KA, Kleer CG. Pathologic features of breast cancer associated with complete response to neoadjuvant chemotherapy: importance of tumor necrosis. *Am J Surg Pathol* 2005;**29**:354-8.
5. Petit T, Wilt M, Velten M, Millon R, Rodier JF, Borel C, et al. Comparative value of tumour grade, hormonal receptors, Ki-67, HER-2 and topoisomerase II alpha status as predictive markers in breast cancer patients treated with neoadjuvant anthracycline-based chemotherapy. *Eur J Cancer* 2004;**40**:205-11.
6. MacGrogan G, Mauriac L, Durand M, Bonichon F, Trojani M, de Mascarel I, et al. Primary chemotherapy in breast invasive carcinoma: predictive value of the immunohistochemical detection of hormonal receptors, p53, c-erbB-2, MiB1, pS2 and GST pi. *Br J Cancer* 1996;**74**:1458-65.
7. Wang J, Buchholz TA, Middleton LP, Allred DC, Tucker SL, Kuerer HM, et al. Assessment of histologic features and expression of biomarkers in predicting pathologic response to anthracycline-based neoadjuvant chemotherapy in patients with breast carcinoma. *Cancer* 2002;**94**:3107-14.
8. Penault-Llorca F, Cayre A, Bouchet Mishellany F, Amat S, Feillel V, Le Bouedec G, et al. Induction chemotherapy for breast carcinoma: predictive markers and relation with outcome. *Int J Oncol* 2003;**22**:1319-25.
9. Tulbah AM, Ibrahim EM, Ezzat AA, Ajarim DS, Rahal MM, El Weshi AN, et al. HER-2/Neu overexpression does not predict response to neoadjuvant chemotherapy or prognosticate survival in patients with locally advanced breast cancer. *Med Oncol* 2002;**19**:15-23.
10. Cocquyt VF, Blondeel PN, Depypere HT, Praet MM, Schelfhout VR, Silva OE, et al. Different responses to preoperative chemotherapy for invasive lobular and invasive ductal breast carcinoma. *Eur J Surg Oncol* 2003;**29**:361-7.
11. Mathieu MC, Rouzier R, Llombart-Cussac A, Sideris L, Koscielny S, Travagli JP, et al. The poor responsiveness of infiltrating lobular breast carcinomas to neoadjuvant chemotherapy can be explained by their biological profile. *Eur J Cancer* 2004;**40**:342-51.
12. Aktepe F, Kapucuoglu N, Pak I. The effects of chemotherapy on breast cancer tissue in locally advanced breast cancer. *Histopathology* 1996;**29**:63-7.
13. Honkoop AH, Pinedo HM, De Jong JS, Verheul HM, Linn SC, Hoekman K, et al. Effects of chemotherapy on pathologic and biologic characteristics of locally advanced breast cancer. *Am J Clin Pathol* 1997;**107**:211-8.
14. Tomczykowski J, Szubstarski F, Kurylcio L, Stanislawek A, Barycki J, Baranowski W. Does the degree of cell lesion in breast cancer after inductive chemotherapy have any prognostic value? *Acta Oncol* 1999;**38**:949-53.
15. Ogston KN, Miller ID, Payne S, Hutcheon AW, Sarkar TK, Smith I, et al. A new histological grading system to assess response of breast cancers to primary chemotherapy: prognostic significance and survival. *Breast* 2003;**12**:320-7.
16. Gajdos C, Tartter PI, Estabrook A, Gistrak MA, Jaffer S, Bleiweiss IJ. Relationship of clinical and pathologic response to neoadjuvant chemotherapy and outcome of locally advanced breast cancer. *J Surg Oncol* 2002;**80**:4-11.
17. Fisher ER, Wang J, Bryant J, Fisher B, Mamounas E, Wolmark N. Pathobiology of preoperative chemotherapy: findings from the National Surgical Adjuvant Breast and Bowel (NSABP) protocol B-18. *Cancer* 2002;**95**:681-95.
18. Apple SK, Suthar F. How do we measure a residual tumor size in histopathology (the gold standard) after neoadjuvant chemotherapy? *Breast* 2006;**15**:370-6.
19. Amat S, Penault-Llorca F, Cure H, Le Bouedec G, Achard JL, Van Praagh I, et al. Scarff-Bloom-Richardson (SBR) grading: a pleiotropic marker of chemosensitivity in invasive ductal breast carcinomas treated by neoadjuvant chemotherapy. *Int J Oncol* 2002;**20**:791-6.
20. Vinnicombe SJ, MacVicar AD, Guy RL, Sloane JP, Powles TJ, Knee G, et al. Primary breast cancer: mammographic changes after neoadjuvant chemotherapy, with pathologic correlation. *Radiology* 1996;**198**:333-40.
21. Kuhl CK. Current status of breast MR imaging. Part 2. Clinical Applications. *Radiology* 2007;**244**:672-91.
22. Wahl RL, Zasadny K, Helvie M, Hutchins GD, Weber B, Cody R. Metabolic monitoring of breast cancer chemohormonotherapy using positron emission tomography: initial evaluation. *J Clin Oncol* 1993;**11**:2101-11.

23. Mankoff DA, Dunnwald LK. Changes in glucose metabolism and blood flow following chemotherapy for breast cancer. *PET Clin* 2006; 1:71-81.
24. Schelling M, Avril N, Nährig J, Kuhn W, Römer W, Sattler D, et al. Positron emission tomography using [(18)F]Fluorodeoxyglucose for monitoring primary chemotherapy in breast cancer. *J Clin Oncol* 2000;**18**:1689-95.
25. Smith IC, Welch AE, Hutcheon AW, Miller ID, Payne S, Chilcott F, et al. Positron emission tomography using [(18)F]-fluorodeoxy-D-glucose to predict the pathologic response of breast cancer to primary chemotherapy. *J Clin Oncol* 2000;**18**:1676-88.
26. Dershaw DD, Shank B, Reisinger S. Mammographic findings after breast cancer treatment with local excision and definitive irradiation. *Radiology* 1987;**164**:455-61.

SECTION

SIX

Appropriateness Criteria for Breast Imaging Workup

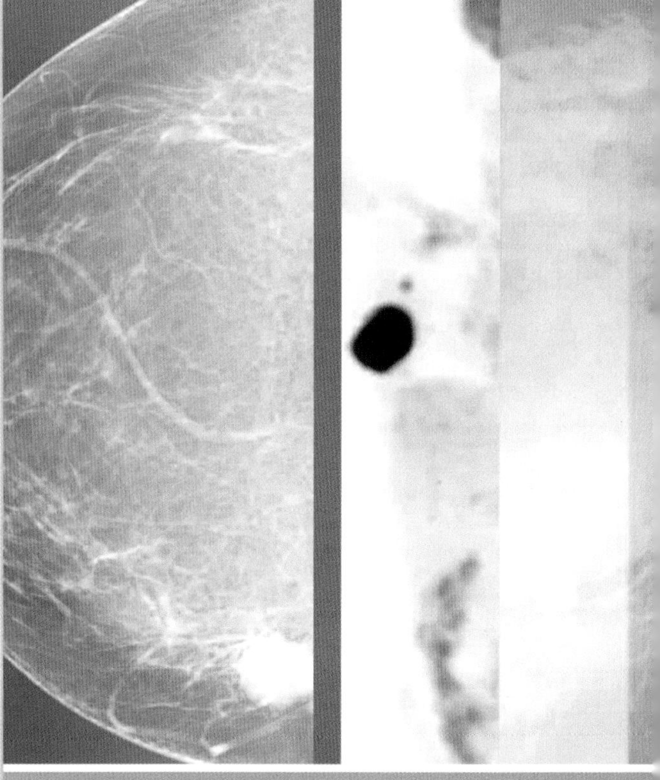

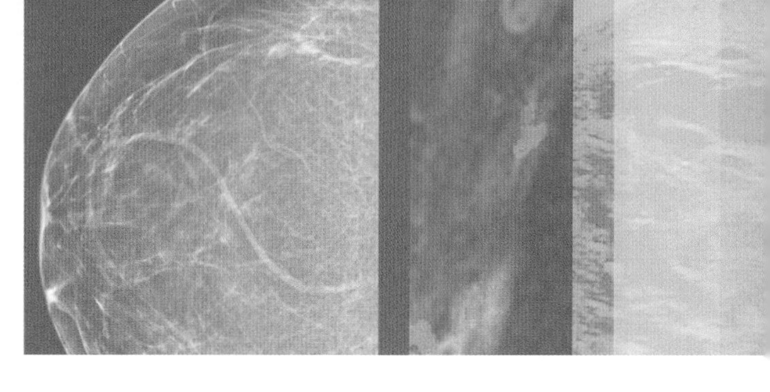

CHAPTER 26

American College of Radiology Appropriateness Criteria

Lawrence W. Bassett

Traditionally, guidelines for the appropriate performance of medicine were based on expert opinion, wherein the experts provided guidance based on their own experience and judgment. The limitation of this traditional approach is that individual experts might have biased and subjective opinions based on the nature of their own practices. Today, expert opinion has largely been supplanted in medicine by the use of evidence-based approaches to determine the criteria for optimal care.[1-3]

The American College of Radiology (ACR) Appropriateness Criteria (AC) are evidence-based guidelines designed to assist referring physicians and other providers in making the most appropriate imaging or treatment decisions.[4] The purpose of these guidelines is to help providers enhance quality of care and make the most efficacious use of radiology resources. This chapter will review the following: (1) The background leading to the development of the appropriateness criteria; (2) the methodology for developing the AC and the committee structure; (3) a discussion of the current need for the ACR AC, and controversies about the AC; and (4) the breast AC, and the future of the breast AC.

BACKGROUND

The ACR began the development of the AC in the early 1990s.This was largely in response to the changing health care environment, including the Clinton Administration's focus on the health care system, which included an emphasis on the efficient use of health care resources.[5] Additionally, there had been numerous requests from radiologists, hospitals and the payers for information on the most appropriate use of imaging examinations. It was clear that if our specialty did not take the leading role in establishing the appropriateness utilization of imaging studies, other entities would take on this role.

The crisis in health care costs has continued to spiral.[6] Total health care spending in 2008 reached $2.3 trillion, or $7,681 per person.[7] Total health care spending represented 17% of the gross domestic product (GDP), and U.S. health care spending is expected to increase at similar levels for the next decade, reaching $4.3 trillion in 2017, or 20% of the GDP.

Radiology services have been highlighted due to their growing percentage of total health care costs.

In creating the ACR AC, the original task force incorporated attributers for developing medical practice guidelines used by the Agency for Healthcare Research and Quality (AHRQ). These guidelines were designed by the Institute of Medicine (IOM),[8] which serves as an official advisor to our nation on improvement in healthcare. The IOM required attributers include:

1. *Validity:* Guidelines are valid if they lead to better outcomes. Validity assessment should be based on the quality of the scientific evidence and the method of evidence evaluation.
2. *Reliability/Reproducibility:* Another set of experts should be able to produce similar guidelines when using the same methodology to evaluate the same scientific evidence.
3. *Clinical applicability:* Guidelines should include an explicit description of the applicable patient population.
4. *Clinical flexibility:* Guidelines must specify known or expected exceptions.
5. *Clarity:* Guidelines must be unambiguous with clearly defined terms.

6. *Multidisciplinary process:* Affected provider groups should have representation in the guidelines development process.
7. *Scheduled review:* All guidelines should undergo scheduled review to determine whether revision is indicated based on current scientific evidence.
8. *Documentation:* The development procedure, the participants, the evidence, and the methods of analysis should be documented.

The AHRQ guidelines emphasize that scientific evidence should be used as much as possible, but acknowledges that expert group consensus will be necessary in the development of medical guidelines when adequate scientific evidence is lacking. The AHRQ provides a public resource for evidence-based clinical practice guidelines on the National Guidelines Clearinghouse (NGC) Web site.[9] Many of the ACR AC topics are included on this Web site.

To date, the ACR has established 17 expert panels to develop Appropriateness Criteria for diagnostic radiology and therapeutic radiology (radiation oncology). The diagnostic panels include cardiovascular, gastrointestinal, urologic, musculoskeletal, thoracic, neurological, pediatric, women's imaging, and women's imaging-breast.

METHODOLOGY

The ACR AC development process is designed to produce evidence-based information and recommendations.[10] The steps in the process are listed here:

1. The process starts with a formal review of the literature conducted by the lead author assigned by the chairperson of the expert panel. ACR staff provides a collection of scientific articles on the topics from sources such as the Library of Medicine.
2. The lead author reviews all relevant articles, selects the ones that are deserving of inclusion in the topic, and then reviews and rates these on the basis of the study design (e.g., prospective randomized control study, observational study, clinical reports, review articles). The lead author also evaluates the strength of the evidence and validity of the conclusions, and then writes a narrative based on these studies.
3. The relevant articles are included in an evidence table provided to committee members that includes the list of selected articles, and ratings based on the type of study (e.g., randomized, prospective, retrospective) and the validity of results (e.g., numbers of patients and if there are statistically significant results).
4. The lead author's narrative, evidence table, and suggested AC tables are forwarded to the panel members for review.
5. Panel members then individually vote on the appropriateness of a given imaging modality for the evaluation of a specific clinical problem (e.g., "palpable breast mass") listed in the AC table on a scale of 1 ("least appropriate") to 9 ("most appropriate"). In this first vote, the committee members do not have access to the votes from other committee members.
6. If consensus if not reached on any individual items, there is a revote of committee members (with voting and comments from other panel members available). If necessary, a second revote is conducted. Then, if necessary, a conference call is conducted to establish a final consensus among panel members.

DISCUSSION

The establishment of widely accepted AC developed by members of the radiology community has become more important than ever in the current healthcare environment. One of many challenges we face is the proposal for radiology benefits managers (RBMs) in a new health care system.[11] Using RBMs, payers would contract with third parties to act as gatekeepers for imaging coverage. RBMs would review a physician's imaging study orders, for prior authorization before allowing coverage. The federal government is being pressured to use this methodology for Medicare reimbursement. A major problem is that RBMs take decisions out of the hands of physicians and patients, and could potentially cause delays in treatment and potentially form barriers to necessary imaging care for patients.

It is important that radiologists provide the evidence-based guidelines for determining whether an imaging examination is warranted. However, there have been criticisms that the ACR AC need to be improved in terms of the nature of the literature review, clarity of recommendations, and training of expert panel members in the principles of the evidence-based approach.[12]

The ACR is continually working on improvements in the AC process.[10]

Another problem is underutilization of the ACR AC among our referring physicians. A survey of referring physicians in 2009 showed a surprisingly low utilization of the ACR AC (2.4%), which was attributed primarily to lack of awareness of the guidelines.[13] However, it should also be noted that 64% of those surveyed did actually consult a radiologist as one of their top three resources for guidance prior to ordering imaging studies. Other studies have shown that when the ACR AC are used by general practitioners there is better utilization of imaging technologies, such as magnetic resonance imaging (MRI).[14] Therefore, it is important to find better ways to reach this audience.

CURRENT BREAST APPROPRIATENESS CRITERIA TOPICS

The current ACR AC addresses "Workup of Palpable Breast Masses," "Workup of Nonpalpable Breast Masses," "Workup of Breast Calcifications," and "Stage I Breast Carcinoma." The most current AC guidelines are available online.[4]

KEY POINTS

- The appropriate utilization of imaging procedures should be evidence-based whenever possible.
- Appropriateness criteria may require expert opinion when there is insufficient scientific evidence (published scientific research studies).

SUGGESTED READINGS

Bettman MA. The appropriateness criteria: view from the committee chair. *J Am Coll Radiol* 2006;**3**:510–2.

Blackmore CC, Medina S. Evidence-based radiology and the ACR Appropriateness Criteria. *J Am Coll Radiol* 2006;**3**:505–9.

Sackett DL, Rosenberg WM, Gray JA, Haynes RB, Richardson WS. Evidence-based medicine: what it is and what it isn't. *BMJ* 1996;**312**:71–2.

REFERENCES

1. Sackett DL, Rosenberg WM, Gray JA, Haynes RB,Richardson WS. Evidence-based medicine: what it is and what it isn't. *BMJ* 1996;**312**:71–2.
2. Evidence-Based Working Group. Evidence-based medicine. A new approach to teaching the practice of medicine. *JAMA* 1992;**268**:2420–5.
3. Evidence-Based Radiology Working Group. Evidence-based radiology: a new approach to the practice of radiology. *Radiology* 2001;**220**:566–75.
4. American College of Radiology. *ACR Appropriateness Criteria*. 2008. Available at: www.acr.org/SecondaryMainMenuCategories/quality_safety/app_criteria.aspx.
5. Ginsberg PG. Controlling health care costs. *N Engl J Med* 2004;**351**:1591–3.
6. The Henry J. Kaiser Family Foundation. *Employee health benefits: 2008 annual survey*. September 2008. Available at http://ehbs.kff.org/images/abstract/7791.pdf.
7. http://www.chcf.org/publications/1010/04/health-care-costs-101.
8. Institute of Medicine. Guidelines for clinical practice: from development to use. Washington DC: National Academic Press, 1992.
9. National Guidelines Clearing House. Available at www.guideline.gov.
10. Bettman MA.The appropriateness criteria: view from the committee chair. *J Am Coll Radiol* 2006;**3**:510–2.
11. Insurers using radiology benefit managers to cut down on unnecessary, costly imaging procedures. 2008. Available at www.medicalnewstoday.com/articles/116595.php.
12. Blackmore CC, Medina S. Evidence-based radiology and the ACR Appropriateness Criteria. *J Am Coll Radiol* 2006;**3**:505–9.
13. Bautista AB, Burgos A, Nickel BJ, Yoon JJ, Tilara AA, Amorosa JK. Do clinicians use the American College of Radiology Appropriateness Criteria in the management of their patients? *AJR Am J Roentgenol* 2009;**192**:1581–5.
14. Levy G, Blachar A, Goldstein L, Paz I, Olsha S, Atar E, et al. Nonradiologist utilization of ACR appropriateness criteria in a preauthorization center for MRI requests: applicability and effects. *AJR Am J Roentgenol* 2006;**187**:855–8.

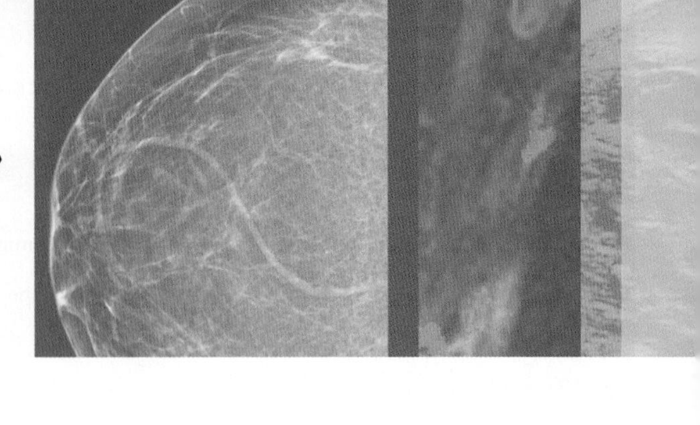

CHAPTER 27

Appropriate Management of Masses

Jennifer A. Harvey

Breast masses are a common finding on mammography. With the increasing use of screening mammography, the size of screening-detected carcinomas has decreased. A patient with a small invasive breast cancer may present with a developing focal asymmetry or mass on screening mammography. Additional imaging of a focal asymmetry may reveal a small mass. Developing focal asymmetries may require percutaneous biopsy even without evidence of a mass on additional imaging, because they represent a change over time. Benign masses, such as cysts and fibroadenomas, are common. As such, the positive predictive value of biopsy of breast masses is 10% to 30%.

WORKUP OF A POSSIBLE MASS ON SCREENING MAMMOGRAPHY

When a focal asymmetry or mass is identified on screening mammography, the area should be marked, described in the report, and recalled for additional diagnostic imaging (American College of Radiology Breast Imaging Reporting and Data System [BI-RADS] 0). Spot compression views of the possible mass with or without magnification apply focused compression to the area (Fig. 27-1). True masses typically become denser and more apparent with spot compression imaging (Fig. 27-2). Pseudomasses caused by overlapping breast tissue usually become less apparent or nonpersistent on spot compression views. Spot compression views can also be helpful to assess the margins of a mass.[1] Magnification with spot compression can also evaluate the area for associated microcalcifications. Other views that might be helpful include rolled craniocaudal (CC) views, true lateral views (either mediolateral or lateromedial), exaggerated CC views, and stepped oblique views. These views may determine if a mass is definitely or likely to be present, and define the location of the lesion.

Ultrasonography is often helpful in the evaluation of a mass or possible mass (see Fig. 27-2).[1] If a mass detected on screening mammography is likely to represent a cyst because it is round or oval with circumscribed margins, ultrasonography can be performed for evaluation as the primary step in additional imaging, because spot compression views are not likely to add useful information. Otherwise, ultrasonography usually follows spot compression and other special mammographic views. When a focal asymmetry is new or enlarging on screening mammography and the spot compression views are noncontributory, ultrasonography can sometimes demonstrate an underlying mass.

Magnetic resonance imaging (MRI) is not typically used in the workup of masses detected on screening mammography.[1] Occasionally, MRI may be helpful when the level of suspicion for an underlying lesion on mammography is high but the lesion cannot be localized for biopsy (Fig. 27-3). MRI should not replace diagnostic imaging, nor should it be used as an alternative to biopsy if a lesion is suspicious on mammography or ultrasonography.

Other imaging modalities, including scintigraphy, computed tomography (CT), and positron emission tomography (PET) are rarely indicated in the workup of a mammographically detected mass or focal asymmetry.[1]

Workup of a Palpable Mass

Patients with palpable breast masses should be evaluated with diagnostic imaging under direct supervision of a radiologist.[2] Ultrasonography is often the

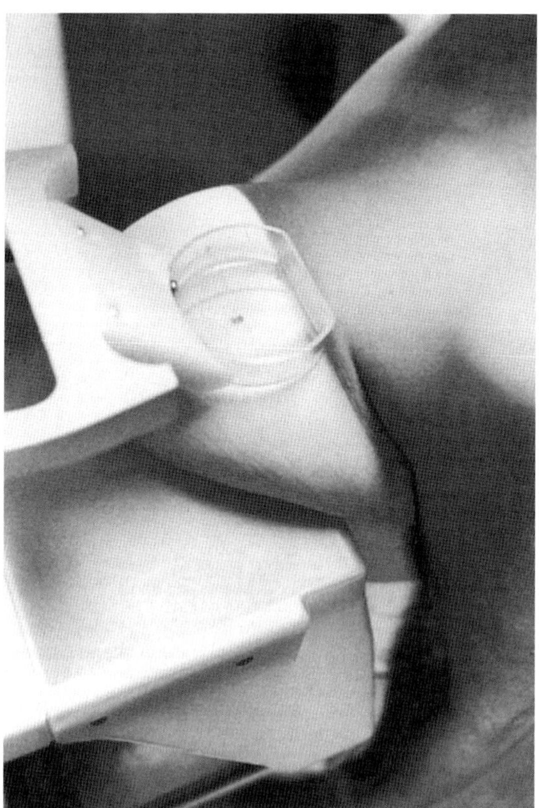

■ **FIGURE 27-1** Spot compression view of the right breast in the craniocaudal projection. During spot compression, only a portion of the breast is compressed with a clear plastic paddle. *(From Hendrick RE, et al. Mammography Quality Control Manual. Reston, Va.: American College of Radiology; 1999.)*

first diagnostic imaging for women younger than age 30 years, whereas mammography is usually performed first for women who are aged 30 years or older. The palpable lump should be marked with a radiopaque marker by the technologist before mammography. A bilateral study is usually performed unless a bilateral mammogram has been performed within the last 6 to 9 months. Spot compression views of the palpable lump, with or without magnification, improve sensitivity by about 9% and should be performed in both CC and mediolateral oblique (MLO) projections (Fig. 27-4).[3] Focused ultrasonography of the palpable area also improves sensitivity by another 6% and should be performed unless a specific benign lesion, such as a lipoma, is identified as the cause of the palpable mass on mammography.[4]

MRI typically is not indicated in the evaluation of a palpable breast mass.[2] However, MRI may occasionally prove useful in the setting of a concerning palpable breast mass with negative mammogram and ultrasound study. MRI should not replace appropriate diagnostic imaging. Other imaging modalities, including CT, PET, and scintigraphy are not typically indicated in the evaluation of a palpable mass.[2]

Benign Masses

Certain masses in the breast are clearly benign and do not typically require additional evaluation. On mammography, these include the circumscribed, fat-containing masses (Box 27-1) as well as circumscribed masses that contain coarse popcorn-like calcifications, indicating that they represent degenerating fibroadenomas. On ultrasonography, simple cysts are clearly benign.

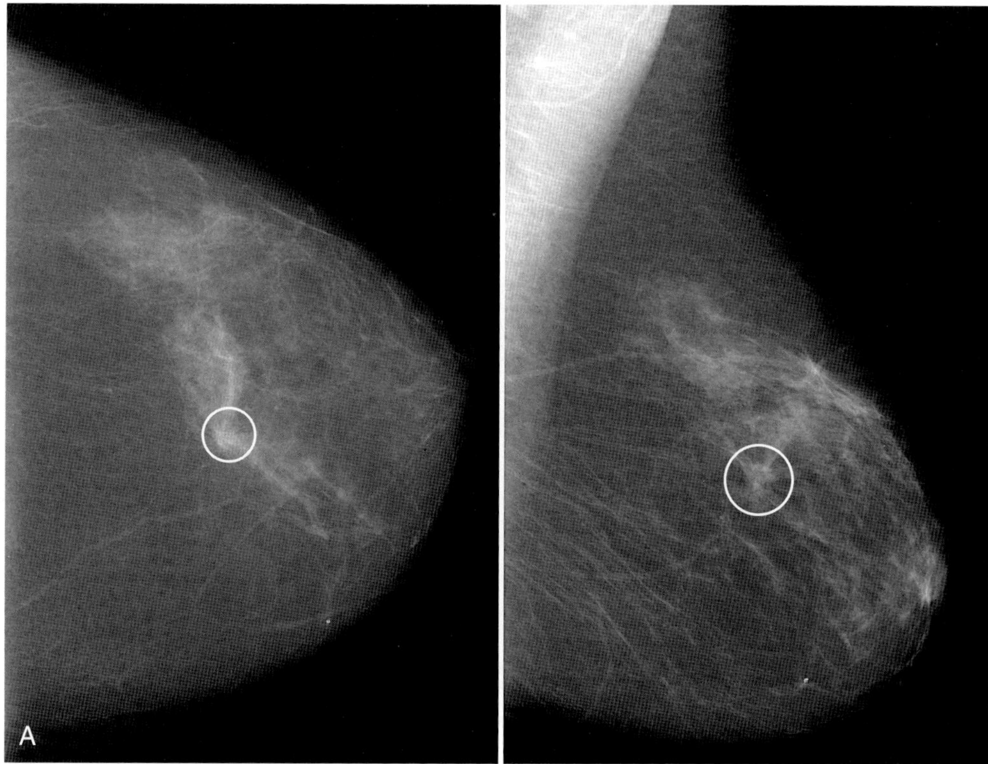

■ **FIGURE 27-2** Abnormal screening mammogram. **A,** Left craniocaudal and mediolateral oblique views from a screening mammogram show an irregular mass in the left breast at the 11-o'clock position, middle third (*circles*). Mammogram assessed as BI-RADS 0—Needs additional imaging.

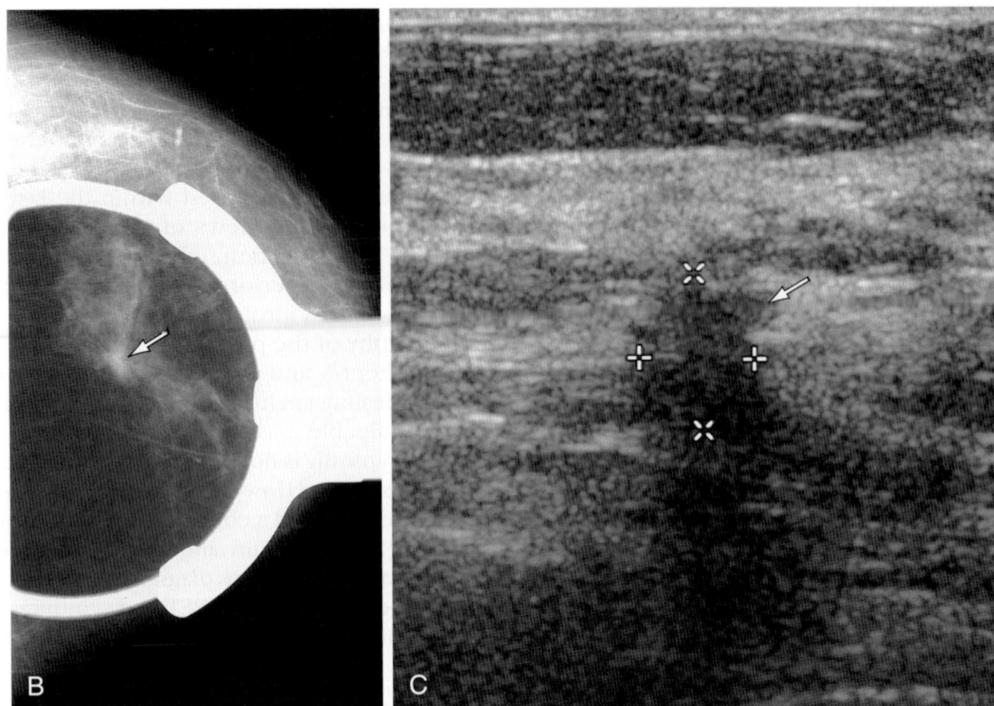

■ **FIGURE 27-2—cont'd** **B,** Spot compression view in the CC projection from the diagnostic mammogram shows a small irregular, high-density mass with spiculated margins (*arrow*). The diagnostic mammogram also included a spot compression view in the MLO projection and a mediolateral view (not shown). **C,** Ultrasound image shows a corresponding hypoechoic irregular solid mass (*arrow*) with microlobulated margin and posterior acoustic shadowing. Mammogram assessed as BI-RADS 4—Suspicious. Ultrasound-guided core needle biopsy showed invasive ductal carcinoma.

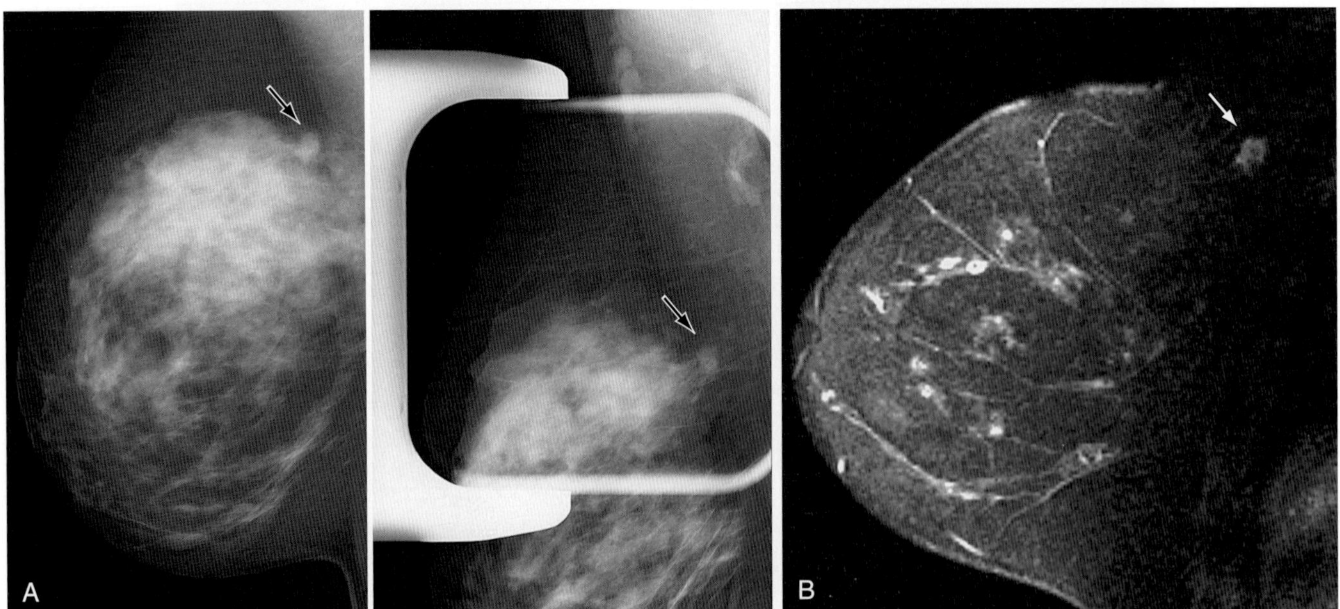

■ **FIGURE 27-3** Utility of magnetic resonance imaging (MRI) with an inconclusive mammogram. A 52-year-old woman presented with an abnormal screening mammogram. **A,** Diagnostic mammogram including mediolateral and spot compression views show a small oval, partially obscured mass in the posterior superior aspect of the right breast (*arrows*). Despite multiple views and the use of ultrasonography, the lesion could not be further localized in the breast. The lesion is too posterior to perform stereotactic biopsy. **B,** Sagittal T1-weighted contrast-enhanced MR image shows that the lesion on mammography represents an 8-mm irregular rim enhancing mass (*arrow*). The lesion was then successfully localized using targeted ultrasonography. Ultrasound-guided core needle biopsy showed invasive ductal carcinoma.

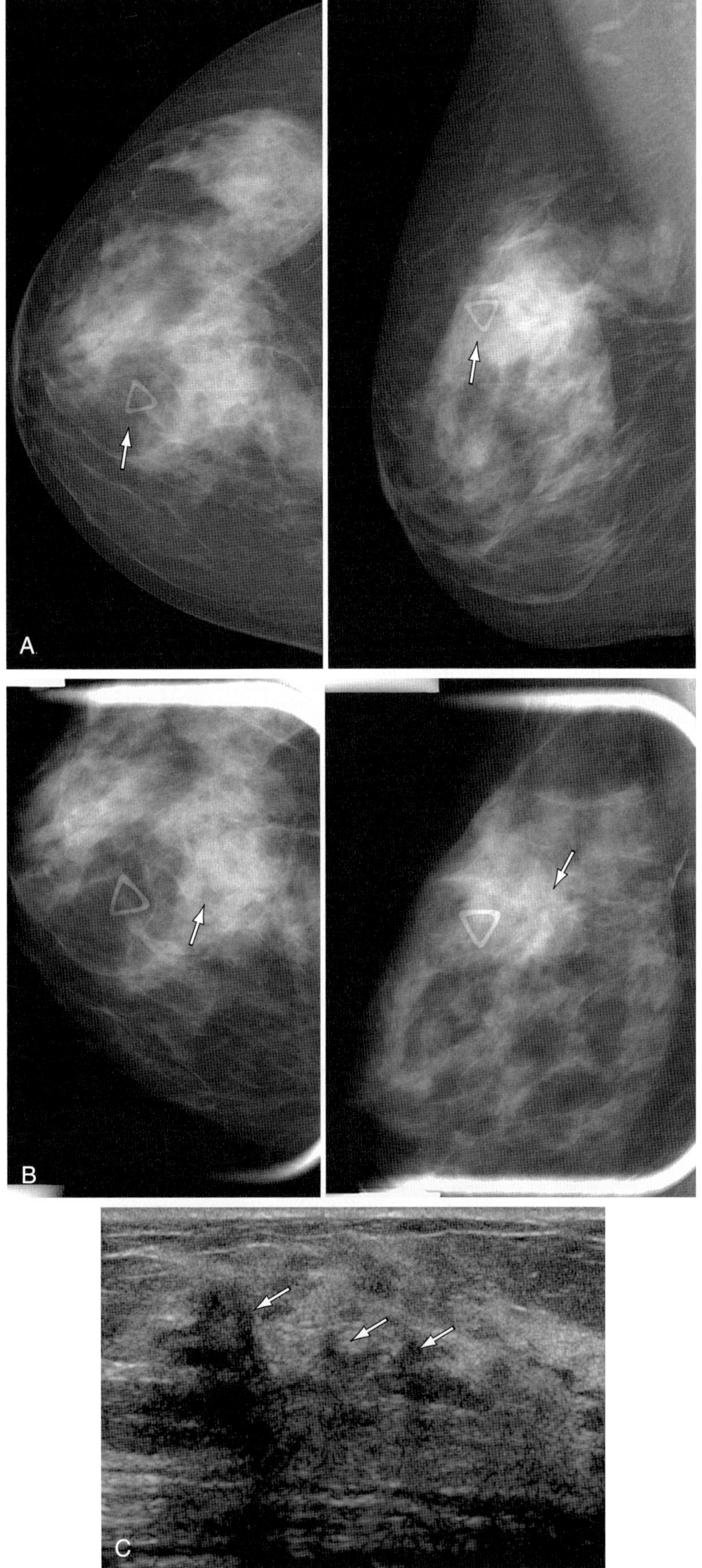

■ **FIGURE 27-4** Evaluation of a 48-year-old woman with a palpable lump in the right breast. **A,** Right diagnostic mammogram with the palpable lump marked by a radiopaque triangle (*arrow*) shows no obvious abnormality. **B,** Spot compression views of the palpable area show a possible partially obscured mass (*arrows*). **C,** Ultrasonography shows an irregular, microlobulated mass with posterior shadowing and mixed echogenicity in the area of the palpable finding (*arrows*). Ultrasound-guided core needle biopsy showed invasive lobular carcinoma.

BOX 27-1

CIRCUMSCRIBED, FAT-CONTAINING BREAST MASSES

Galactocele
Hamartoma
Lipoma
Lymph node
Oil cyst

Masses that clearly represent an oil cyst, hamartoma, lipoma, or degenerating fibroadenoma on screening mammography do not require recall for additional imaging evaluation. Galactoceles often present as palpable masses in women who are lactating and thus are more commonly seen in the diagnostic setting.

A Special Note Regarding Lymph Nodes

Lymph nodes with normal morphology identified on mammography or ultrasonography are typically benign and no further evaluation is usually indicated. Patients may palpate normal axillary or intramammary lymph nodes, particularly when the patient is thin.

Lymph nodes may be abnormal if there is thickening of the cortex greater than a few millimeters (Fig. 27-5),[5] loss of the fatty hilum, or an increase in size and density of the lymph nodes(s) compared with findings on prior mammograms. Further evaluation may be indicated in these cases.

Bilateral axillary adenopathy is often due to reactive hyperplasia. If mild and unchanged from prior mammograms, no further evaluation may be needed. However, if lymph nodes are enlarging compared with findings of prior mammograms, adenopathy could be due to known or undiagnosed lymphoma or leukemia or to metastatic disease from a nonbreast primary malignancy. Clinical evaluation of the patient by the referring health care provider may be useful in identifying a cause for bilateral adenopathy. If no cause for adenopathy is identified, biopsy may be indicated. Ultrasound-guided core needle biopsy can be performed of one of the concerning lymph nodes. Histologic diagnosis of lymphoma may be facilitated with core needle biopsy rather than with fine-needle aspiration biopsy. If the diagnosis of lymphoma is considered, a nonfixed sample may be evaluated with flow cytometry to assess for a monomorphic cell population, which is present in lymphoma.

Unilateral axillary adenopathy is of more concern for ipsilateral invasive breast carcinoma, especially in the presence of an abnormal mammogram (see Fig. 27-5). When the mammogram is otherwise normal, adenopathy may be due to a benign cause, such as a rash on the ipsilateral trunk or recent cellulitis of the ipsilateral arm. However, if a benign etiology is not identified, then unilateral adenopathy is of more concern for metastatic disease, and biopsy of a lymph node should be considered. This can be performed percutaneously using ultrasound guidance. Metastatic disease is most commonly due to an ipsilateral breast primary invasive carcinoma but may be due to other malignancies, particularly in women with history of other cancers, such as melanoma.

Focal Asymmetries

Small cancers may present initially as a focal asymmetry. The BI-RADS lexicon[6] defines a focal asymmetry as "...a finding that does not fit criteria of a mass...visible as a confined asymmetry with a similar shape on two views but completely lacking borders and the conspicuity of a true mass." Most focal asymmetries are benign, owing to overlapping normal breast tissue, and are a common source of screening false-positive results. However, the detection of small invasive cancers on screening mammography necessitates the recall of focal asymmetries that are somewhat mass-like or developing compared with prior mammographic findings.

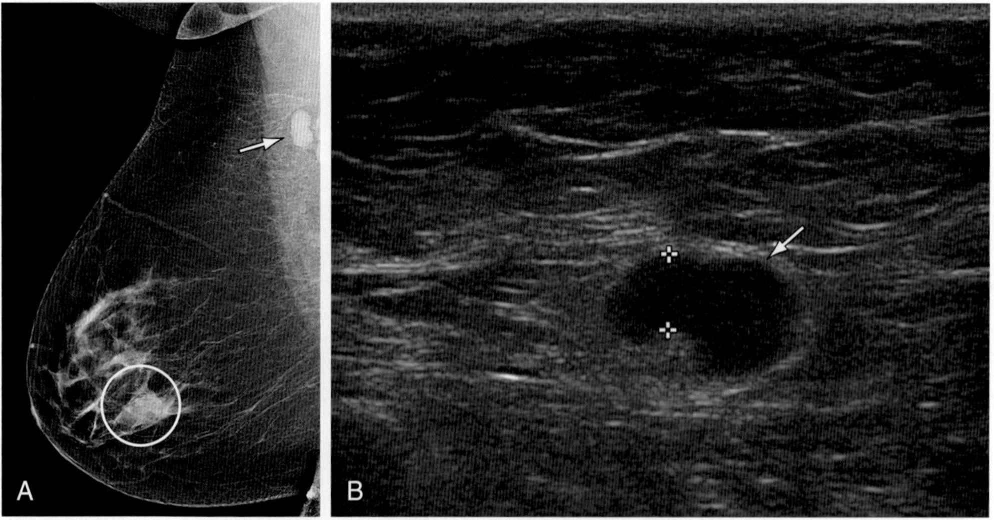

■ **FIGURE 27-5** Left mediolateral oblique view from a screening mammogram of a 54-year-old woman. An axillary lymph node appears dense with loss of the cortex (*arrow*). There is a subtle focal asymmetry in the inferior breast (*circle*). **B,** Ultrasound image of the left axilla shows a lymph node with diffuse cortical thickening (*arrow*). Additional images of the inferior left breast showed a solid suspicious mass. Fine-needle aspiration biopsy of the lymph node showed metastatic adenocarcinoma, consistent with a breast primary tumor. Core needle biopsy of the left breast mass showed invasive ductal carcinoma, grade III.

Diagnostic mammography, including spot compression views with or without magnification and a true lateral view, should be performed. The true lateral view is typically a mediolateral view if the lesion is lateral and a lateromedial view if the lesion is medial. This approach will result in the lesion being closer to the receptor, thus increasing sharpness of the image. Rolled CC views may help demonstrate whether the focal asymmetry represents overlapping tissue or a persistent focal asymmetry and may also help localize lesions seen only on the CC view. If a focal asymmetry identified on a baseline mammogram does not appear mass-like on spot compression and other additional views, the patient may return to her usual screening protocol.

When a focal asymmetry on a baseline mammogram persists on spot compression views (appears mass-like) or represents a developing asymmetry compared with older studies, ultrasonography is typically performed and may reveal an underlying mass. Ultrasound-guided biopsy with placement of a marking clip is useful to confirm that the ultrasonographic finding that underwent biopsy corresponded to the mammographic finding (Fig. 27-6). If the ultrasound image shows no underlying abnormality for patients with a persistent focal asymmetry on a baseline mammogram, short-term follow-up mammography in 6 months may be useful to confirm a benign cause. In the case of a focal asymmetry that is developing compared with older studies and is persistent on spot compression views, percutaneous sampling under stereotactic guidance or wire-localized surgical biopsy may be required even when additional mammographic views and ultrasonography are negative.

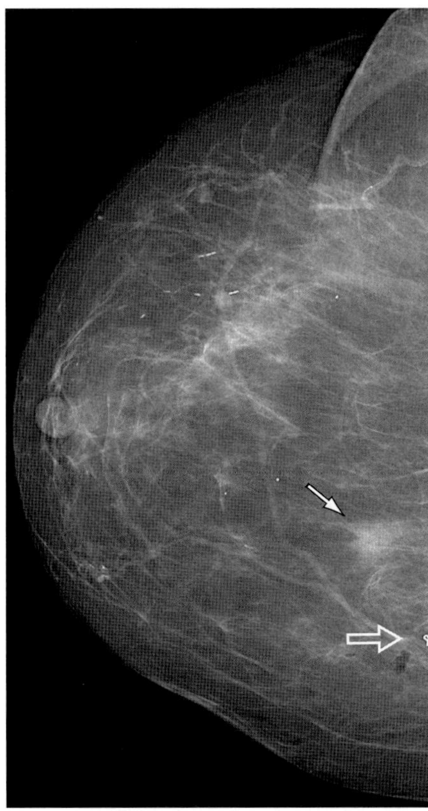

■ **FIGURE 27-6** An 80-year-old woman presented with developing focal asymmetry of the medial left breast (*arrow*) compared with older mammograms (not shown). The lesion was sampled using ultrasound guidance with clip placement (*open arrow*). The clip is not within the focal asymmetry. Biopsy histology showed only normal breast tissue and was considered discordant. Subsequent stereotactic biopsy showed invasive ductal carcinoma, grade II.

Masses with Benign Features

Mammography

Masses that are round, oval, or lobular that are of low or equal density to breast tissue with circumscribed margins on mammography are often benign, most commonly representing fibroadenomas or cysts. However, cancers may present as a mass with benign features. Therefore, management depends on whether the mass is single or one of multiple similar masses and is stable when compared with results of prior mammograms.

Multiple bilateral round or oval, circumscribed masses are benign findings (BI-RADS 2) (Fig. 27-7), and no further evaluation is needed. These masses typically represent multiple cysts or fibroadenomas. Leung and coworkers have shown that the risk of malignancy for these patients is similar to that of the overall screening population,[7] supporting the use of BI-RADS 2 and routine follow-up for these women.

When the patient has no prior mammograms and a dominant or single mass with benign features is identified on a screening mammogram, the patient should be recalled for diagnostic mammography that includes spot compression views to ensure that the margins are circumscribed.

Ultrasonography is often helpful to characterize the lesion. If the mass corresponds to a simple cyst, then no further evaluation is needed and routine follow-up can be recommended. If no lesion is identified on ultrasonography or if there is a complicated cyst or solid mass with no malignant features, then the mass can be considered probably benign (BI-RADS 3) (Fig. 27-8). Short-term follow-up can be performed with an ipsilateral mammogram in 6 months and bilateral mammograms at 12 and 24 months after the initial evaluation. The risk of malignancy in these cases is less than 2%. If the mass enlarges at any of the follow-up studies and is not identified as a simple cyst, then biopsy is indicated. When present, cancer is most frequently diagnosed at the first 6-month examination and is still typically stage I.

If prior mammograms are present, then comparison will influence management (Fig. 27-9). Therefore, an attempt should be made to obtain older studies for comparison, even if located at another institution. If the mass is new or enlarging, biopsy will usually be indicated unless it represents a simple cyst on ultrasonography. If the mass is unchanged in size, then a BI-RADS 2 is assigned and routine follow-up is usually all that is needed. Occasionally, old studies are less than helpful and stability cannot be assessed owing to considerable interval involution or far posterior location of the mass. Short-term follow-up may be reasonable in these cases.

Some patients are very anxious about waiting for 6 months to reassess the mass. Biopsy can be performed as an alternative to short-term follow-up if desired, although the vast majority of patients undergo short-term imaging.

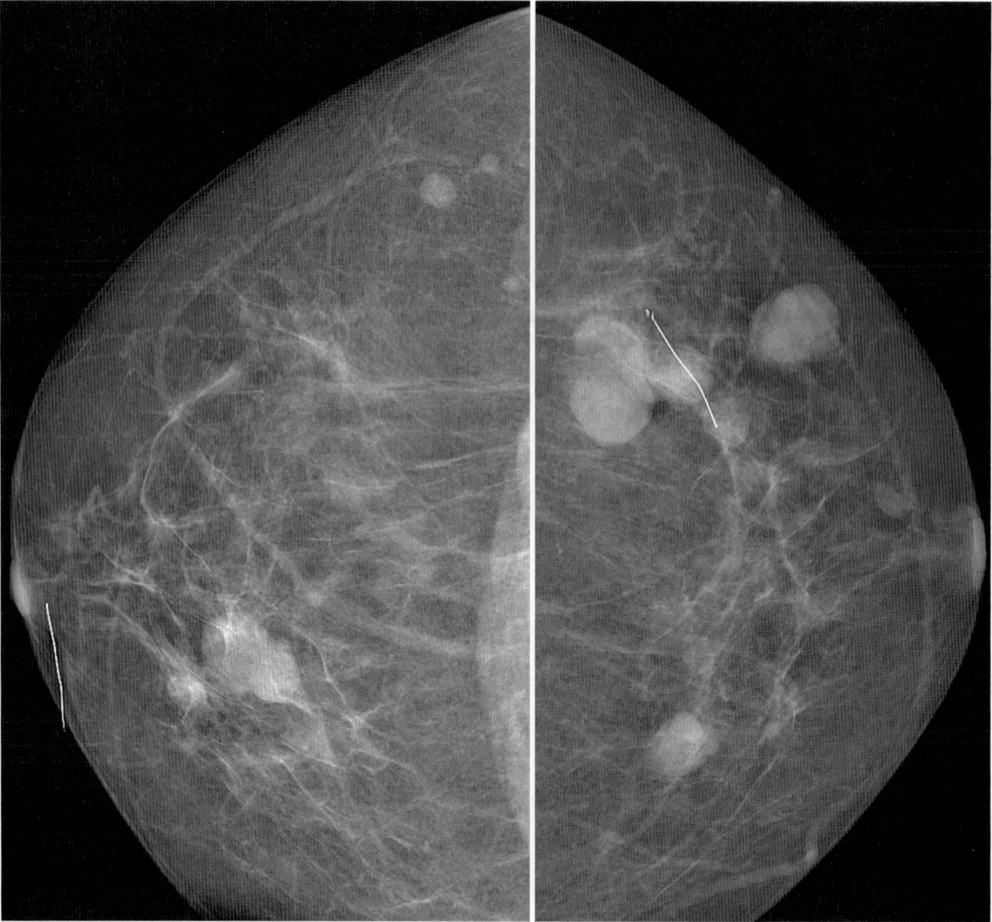

■ **FIGURE 27-7** Baseline screening mammogram (craniocaudal views shown) of a 43-year-old woman showing multiple bilateral circumscribed, round and oval masses, which is a BI-RADS 2—Benign finding.

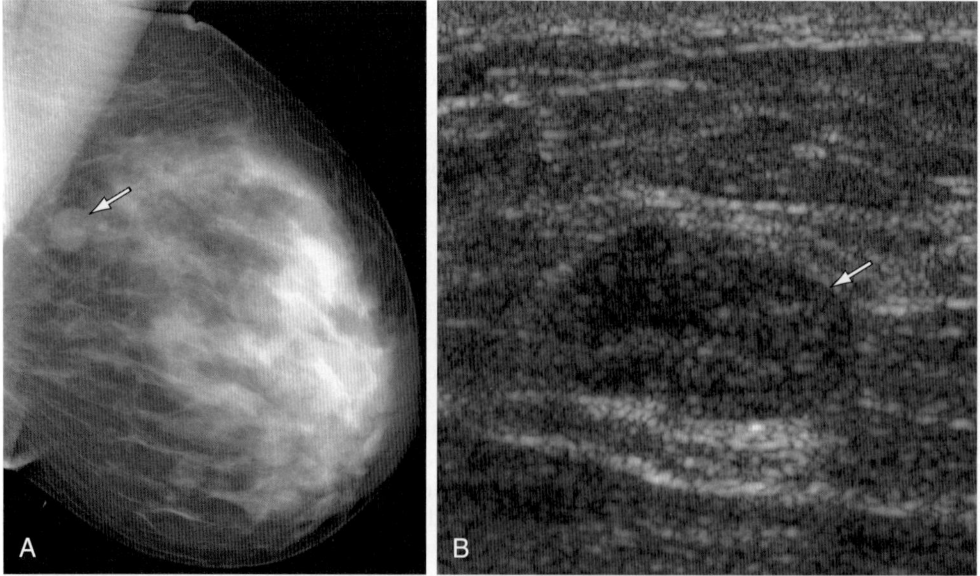

■ **FIGURE 27-8** Baseline mammogram of a 38-year-old woman. **A,** Right mediolateral oblique view demonstrates a round, circumscribed, equal density mass (*arrow*) at the 12-o'clock position, in the posterior third of the breast. **B,** Ultrasound image shows an oval, circumscribed, hypoechoic, solid mass (*arrow*). Because both the mammographic and ultrasonographic features suggest a benign etiology, BI-RADS 3—Short-interval follow-up recommended is appropriate for this case. The mass has been stable for more than 2 years at follow-up.

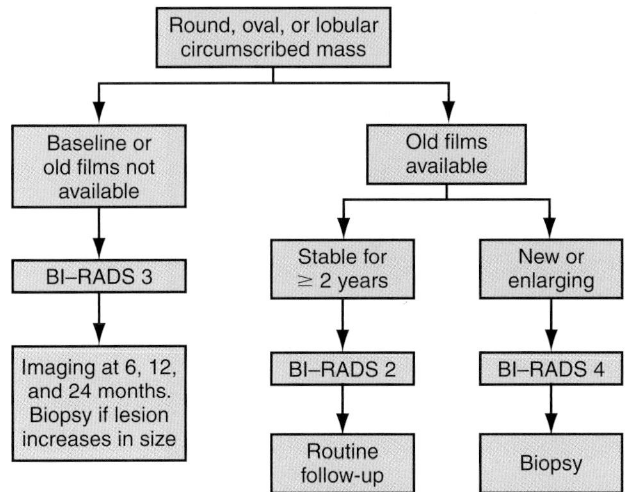

■ **FIGURE 27-9** Management of solid masses with benign features on mammography.

Immediate biopsy can also be considered if the patient may not or is not likely to comply with the short-term interval imaging due to travel or migrant behavior. For women with recently diagnosed cancer, biopsy of a probably benign lesion may influence surgical management. Biopsy can be helpful to ensure that breast conservation is an option if the lesion is in the ipsilateral breast. If the patient is considering autologous breast reconstruction, biopsy of a contralateral lesion may be helpful to ensure that bilateral reconstruction should not be considered.

If the oval, round, or lobular mass with circumscribed margins on mammography corresponds to a complex mass on ultrasonography (i.e., contains both cystic and solid components), then biopsy is indicated. Aspiration of the fluid with cytology is a low sensitivity test, such that ultrasound-guided core biopsy of the solid portion of the lesion or wire-localized excisional biopsy of the entire lesion is preferred. The risk of malignancy is 20% to 30%.

Ultrasonography

Round or oval circumscribed homogeneously hypoechoic masses with well-defined margins and orientation parallel to the chest wall on ultrasonography are usually benign. When the mass corresponds to a mammographic finding that is new or enlarging, biopsy should be considered despite benign ultrasonographic features. When the mass corresponds to a mammographic finding that is stable for 2 years or more on mammography, then no further evaluation is usually necessary. When there is no corresponding mammographic finding (e.g., an incidental finding on ultrasonography), then short-term follow-up may be reasonable, although there is less literature supporting this management than for mammographic findings.

Palpable Masses

There are an increasing number of studies that indicate that when a mass has benign features on mammography and ultrasonography and is palpable, it is also likely to be benign, and short-interval follow-up may be a reasonable alternative to biopsy.[8] However, the reports supporting this approach are ongoing.

Suspicious and Malignant Masses

Masses identified on mammography that are irregular in shape or have ill-defined, microlobulated, indistinct, or spiculated margins, or are of high density compared with breast parenchyma are of more concern for malignancy, and biopsy should be considered. Likewise, masses identified on ultrasonography that are of irregular shape, without well-defined margins, have an echogenic halo and posterior acoustic shadowing, and do not have an orientation that is parallel to the chest wall are suggestive of malignancy. Of note, correlation between modalities should be performed because some lesions that may be suspicious on ultrasonography, such as a degenerating fibroadenoma (Fig. 27-10), oil cyst, and scar, may be clearly benign on mammography. Assessment of stability by comparing with prior mammograms is much less important for suspicious masses because a lack of change over 1 or 2 years will not likely dissuade one from recommending biopsy.

When a lesion is identified on screening mammography, the patient should be recalled for diagnostic evaluation (BI-RADS 0). Evaluation with spot compression views with or without magnification is useful to define margins of the mass. A true lateral view, mediolateral for masses in the lateral breast or lateromedial for masses in the medial breast, are helpful for definitive localization in two views before ultrasonography and for biopsy planning. If the mammographic appearance suggests that the finding is related to prior surgery, repeat views with a wire on the skin to mark the scar may be helpful to confirm. If the lesion is likely due to prior surgery or trauma, short-term follow-up may be helpful to confirm the benign cause.

Ultrasonography can be used to characterize a mass identified on mammography. Identification of a benign simple cyst in the region of a suspicious mass identified on mammography should not circumvent the need for biopsy unless additional mammographic views confirm that the mass actually has circumscribed margins and is oval, round, or lobular. Ultrasound characterization may increase the level of suspicion to BI-RADS 4C or 5.

Choice of BI-RADS category depends on the level of suspicion. Masses that have benign features but that have increased in size might be assigned a BI-RADS 4A category, whereas an irregular mass that is not an obvious malignancy may be placed in the BI-RADS 4C category. Masses with multiple malignant features are usually assigned a BI-RADS 5 category.

When masses are very suspicious (BI-RADS 4C) or malignant (BI-RADS 5), additional evaluation of the patient for multifocal disease or metastatic ipsilateral adenopathy may be helpful. This may include ultrasound of the quadrant or ipsilateral breast of the suspicious lesion and ipsilateral axilla.

The majority of breast masses that are suspicious or malignant on mammography, ultrasonography, or MRI can undergo percutaneous core needle biopsy rather than open

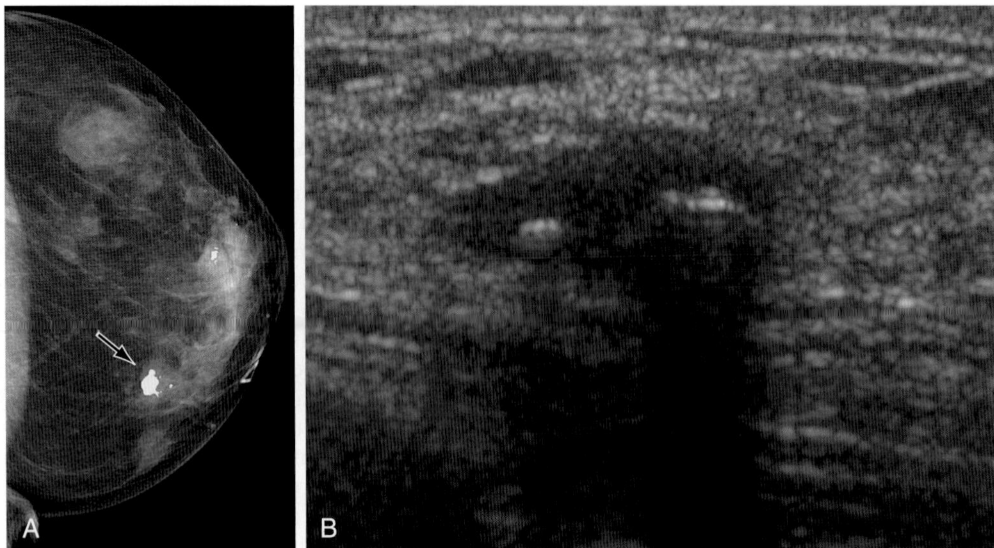

■ **FIGURE 27-10** A 45-year-old woman presented with a palpable lump in the medial right breast. **A,** *Triangle* marks the location of palpable lump that corresponds to a lobular, equal density mass with obscured margins and associated dystrophic calcifications (*arrow*). The mass is consistent with a degenerating fibroadenoma and was stable for at least 3 years on mammography. **B,** On an ultrasound image, the palpable finding corresponds to a hypoechoic, solid oval mass with circumscribed margins and associated shadowing calcifications. By ultrasonographic criteria, the mass is highly suspicious. However, correlation with the mammogram demonstrates that the ultrasound finding corresponds to the stable degenerating fibroadenoma and no further evaluation is needed.

surgical biopsy. Core needle biopsy is less invasive and more cost-effective than surgical biopsy. In some cases, the lesion may not be amenable to core needle biopsy owing to difficulty identifying a low density mass on stereotactic images or ultrasonography, small compressed breast thickness, and so on.

Once a breast lesion has been identified as malignant, MRI can be useful to evaluate the extent of disease in the ipsilateral breast. In addition, MRI can identify mammographically occult breast carcinoma in the contralateral breast in 3% of women with recently diagnosed breast cancer.[9] The use of MRI in evaluation of masses before sampling has not been shown to be as helpful.

SUMMARY

Masses and focal asymmetries that are new or enlarging or that have suspicious or malignant features on screening mammography should be recalled for further evaluation with diagnostic mammography and/or ultrasound (BI-RADS 0). Diagnostic mammography and ultrasonography are useful to characterize a mass, dismiss a focal asymmetry that may represent overlapping benign breast tissue, aid with biopsy planning, and evaluate for the extent of disease when a highly suspicious or malignant lesion is identified. Biopsy should be considered for focal asymmetries that appear mass-like on spot compression or other views or are new compared with findings of prior mammograms. Most masses and focal asymmetries identified on mammography are amenable to percutaneous sampling using either stereotactic or ultrasound guidance.

KEY POINTS

- A patient with a focal asymmetry or mass that is suggestive of malignancy on screening mammography should be recalled for diagnostic evaluation with mammography and/or ultrasonography.
- Spot compression views (with or without magnification) and targeted ultrasound evaluation of a palpable finding improve sensitivity for cancer detection.
- Certain masses, such as degenerating fibroadenoma or hamartoma on mammography and a simple cyst on ultrasonography, are typically benign, and routine follow-up is indicated.
- Lymph nodes identified in the breast or axilla on mammography or ultrasonography are usually benign, but loss of the fatty hilum or thickening of the cortex may indicate a pathologic process, especially in the setting of an ipsilateral breast carcinoma.
- A focal asymmetry that is clearly new or developing may require a tissue diagnosis, even when additional mammographic views and ultrasonography are negative.
- Masses with benign features on a baseline mammogram can undergo short-term follow-up (BI-RADS 3) rather than biopsy. If new or enlarging, then biopsy is often indicated.

REFERENCES

1. Nonpalpable breast masses. American College of Radiology. ACR Appropriateness Criteria. 2005. Available at: www.acr.org/SecondaryMainMenuCategories/quality_safety/app_criteria.aspx.
2. Palpable breast masses. American College of Radiology. ACR Appropriateness Criteria. 2006. Available at: www.acr.org/SecondaryMainMenuCategories/quality_safety/app_criteria.aspx.
3. Faulk RM, Sickles EA. Efficacy of spot compression-magnification and tangential views in mammographic evaluation of palpable breast masses. *Radiology* 1992;**185**:87-90.
4. Zonderland HM, Coerkamp EG, Hermans J, van de Vijver MJ, van Voorthuisen AE. Diagnosis of breast cancer: contribution of US as an adjunct to mammography. *Radiology* 1999;**213**:413-22.
5. Deurloo EE, Tanis PJ, Gilhuijs KG, Muller SH, Kröger R, Peterse JL, et al. Reduction in the number of sentinel lymph node procedures by preoperative ultrasonography of the axilla in breast cancer. *Eur J Cancer* 2003;**39**:1068-73.
6. D'Orsi CJ, Bassett LW, Berg WA, et al. *Illustrated breast imaging reporting and data system (BI-RADS)*. 4th ed. Reston, Va: American College of Radiology; 2003.
7. Leung JWT, Sickles EA. Multiple bilateral masses detected on screening mammography: assessment of need for recall imaging. *Am J Roentgenol* 2000;**175**:23-9.
8. Raza S, Chikarmane SA, Neilsen SS, Zorn LM, Birdwell RL. BI-RADS 3, 4, and 5 lesions: value of US in management-follow-up and outcome. *Radiology* 2008;**248**:773-81.
9. Lehman CD, Gatsonis C, Kuhl CK, Hendrick RE, Pisano ED, Hanna L, et al. MRI evaluation of the contralateral breast in women with recently diagnosed breast cancer. *N Eng J Med* 2007;**356**:1295-303.

CHAPTER 28

Appropriate Management of Calcifications

Jennifer A. Harvey

Some calcifications are frequently present on mammograms. Common typically benign calcifications are dermal, stromal, or vascular. The vast majority of breast calcifications are benign. However, calcifications related to the breast ductal system or lobules can be due to malignancy. The positive predictive value for calcifications that are biopsied, a desirable goal, varies from 19% to 22%.[1,2] When calcifications without a mass do turn out to be malignant they are due to ductal carcinoma in situ (DCIS) without an invasive carcinoma component in 65% to 70% of patients.[3,4] DCIS is the earliest form of breast carcinoma. When invasive carcinoma is present in a biopsy for suspicious calcifications, it often consists of a small focus of microinvasion.

Morphology, distribution, and change over time should be considered in the evaluation of mammographically-detected calcifications (Table 28-1). Fine, linear, branching, and fine pleomorphic morphology calcifications with a linear or segmental distribution have the highest probability of malignancy (see Table 28-1).[2,5] The term *linear* may refer to morphology or distribution of calcifications,[6] either of which is of concern for malignancy. The American College of Radiology (ACR) Breast Imaging Reporting and Data System (BI-RADS) lexicon divides calcification morphology types into three categories: typically benign, of intermediate concern, and higher probability of malignancy.[6]

Comparison with previous mammograms is helpful to determine whether calcifications are new or increasing in number. However, biopsy may be considered for calcifications that are of concern regarding morphologic appearance despite apparent stability. In one study of 105 women with malignant microcalcifications, 26 (25%) had microcalcifications that were stable for 8 to 63 months.[4] A more recent study, however, found no malignancy in 23 cases of stable microcalcifications that were sampled.[2] In general, calcifications that are unchanged for two or more years are considered benign. However, the morphology and distribution of the calcifications should be taken into account when deciding whether to biopsy.

EVALUATION OF CALCIFICATIONS

Calcifications that are of concern on screening mammography should be evaluated using magnification views. Digital zoom is not a substitute for magnification for full field digital mammography (Fig. 28-1).

Several techniques may improve the quality of magnification views. Spot compression applied with magnification reduces the breast thickness, which lowers exposure, reduces scatter, improves contrast, and minimizes motion-related blur. Collimating or coning the x-ray beam to the area of interest on the magnification view reduces scatter, resulting in improved image sharpness. A larger field of view may be useful, however, when evaluating the extent of calcifications. When a large field of view is desired, magnification views are performed using a larger spot compression paddle without coning of the x-ray beam.

Magnification views should be obtained in the craniocaudal (CC) and true lateral (90-degree) projections (either mediolateral or lateromedial). Milk of calcium, a benign process, may be difficult to discern from amorphous calcifications if magnification views are obtained with an oblique projection rather than a true lateral view.

A full breast lateral view, either a mediolateral or lateromedial view, is often helpful for stereotactic localization if biopsy is indicated. A lateromedial view may provide better clarity than a mediolateral view if the calcifications are in the medial breast because the calcifications will be closer to the image receptor, resulting in less scatter.

TABLE 28-1. Frequency of Carcinoma as a Function of Calcification Distribution and Morphology

	Morphology					
Distribution	**Linear**	**Fine, Pleomorphic**	**Coarse Pleomorphic**	**Amorphous**	**Punctate or Round**	**Total**
Linear	75-86%	67%	–	0%	0%	**67-68%**
Segmental	100%	67%	–	0-20%	–	**38-74%**
Clustered	36-75%	22%	7%	13-24%	0-11%	**16-36%**
Regional	0%	0%	–	67%	0%	**0-46%**
Diffuse	0%	–	–	–	–	**0%**
Total	**53-81%**	**29%**	**7%**	**13-26%**	**0-9%**	

Burnside ES, Ochsner JE, Fowler KJ, et al. Use of microcalcification descriptors in BI-RADS 4th edition to stratify risk of malignancy. *Radiology* 2007; 242:388-95; Liberman L, Abramson AF, Squires FB, Glassman JR, Morris EA, Dershaw DD. The breast imaging reporting and data system: positive predictive value of mammographic features and final assessment categories. *AJR Am J Roentgenol* 1998; 171:35-40.

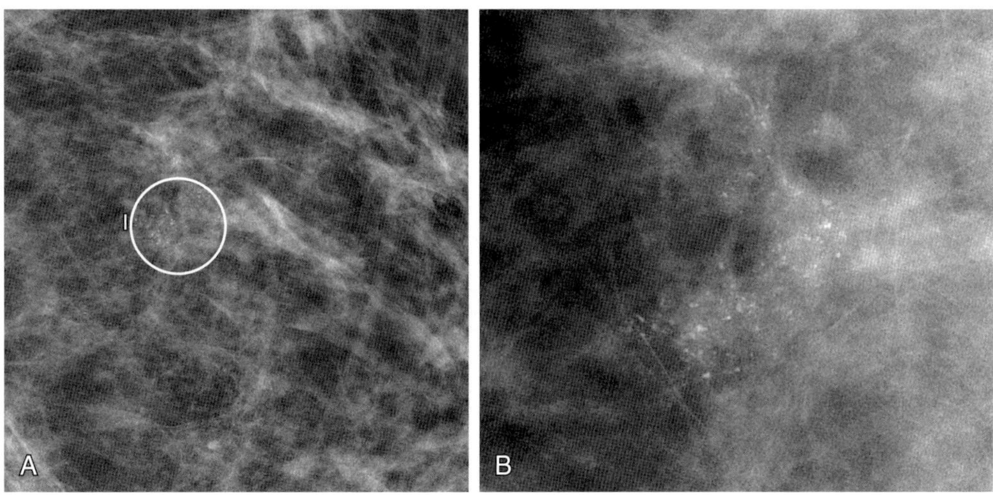

■ **FIGURE 28-1** True magnification views versus digital zoom. **A,** Zoomed cranio-caudal image from screening mammogram shows a cluster of calcifications with round and punctate morphology. **B,** True magnification cranio-caudal image shows fine pleomorphic and fine, linear branching and amorphous calcifications in a segmental distribution. The magnification views shift the BI-RADS final assessment from Category 4 (Suspicious) to Category 5 (Highly Suggestive of Malignancy).

Typically Benign Calcifications

The majority of calcifications identified on mammography are typically benign (Box 28-1, Fig. 28-2). Many calcifications, such as skin and suture calcifications, will be clearly benign on screening views, and diagnostic imaging usually will not be needed. Occasionally, the benign etiology of the calcifications may not be clear on a screening mammogram and diagnostic mammography including magnification or lateral views, or both, may be necessary. A tangential view may be useful to prove the dermal location of skin calcifications. An apparent change in morphology between the CC and 90-degree lateral magnification views from amorphous or round to linear suggests that the calcifications are benign and due to milk of calcium (Fig. 28-3).

BOX 28-1

TYPICALLY BENIGN BREAST CALCIFICATIONS

Coarse, popcorn-like
Dystrophic
Eggshell or rim
Large rod-like
Lucent-centered
Milk of calcium
Round, punctate
Skin (dermal)
Suture
Vascular

Round and Punctate Calcifications

Round and punctate calcifications are usually benign. However, patients with DCIS can occasionally present with round or punctate calcifications (Fig. 28-4). The distribution of round and punctate calcifications is helpful in deciding if recall for additional imaging is indicated. If the distribution is bilateral and scattered or regional, the etiology is usually benign and no further evaluation may be needed. Round or punctate calcifications that are in a segmental distribution are of more concern for DCIS, and biopsy may be indicated.

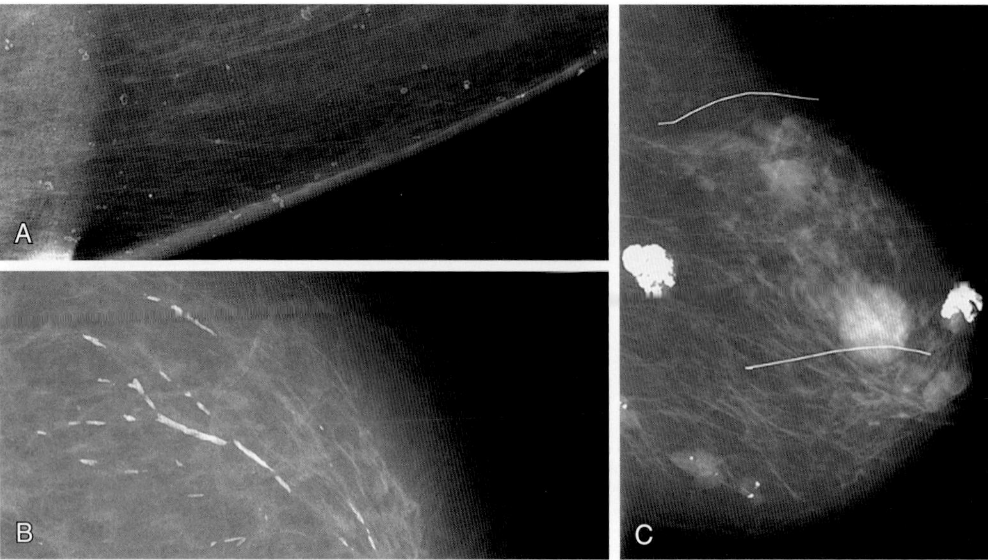

■ **FIGURE 28-2** Examples of typically benign breast calcifications on mammograms. **A,** Skin calcifications. Many can be seen located within the dermis. **B,** Large, rod-like calcifications. **C,** Coarse, popcorn-like calcifications in degenerating fibroadenomas. Note smaller developing coarse, heterogeneous calcifications in the lower breast that are earlier forms of coarse, popcorn-like calcifications within degenerating fibroadenomas.

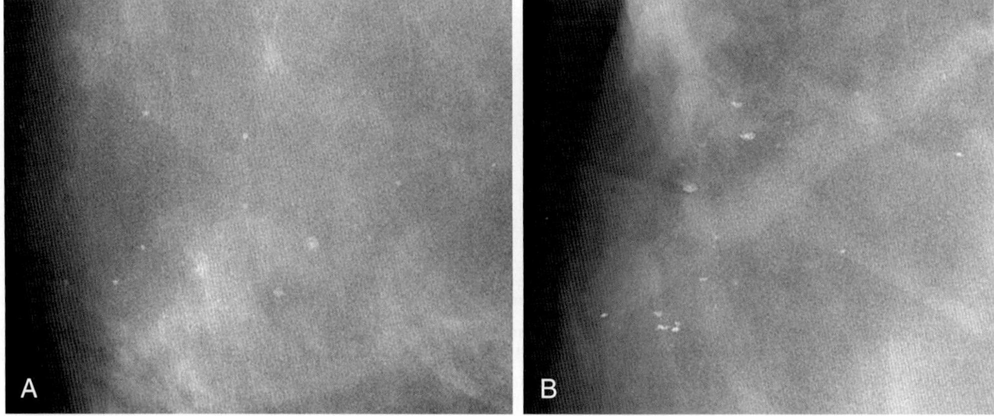

■ **FIGURE 28-3** Milk of calcium. **A,** Calcifications may appear amorphous and may be difficult to identify on the craniocaudal view. **B,** Calcifications form a meniscus or may appear linear on a true lateral magnification view.

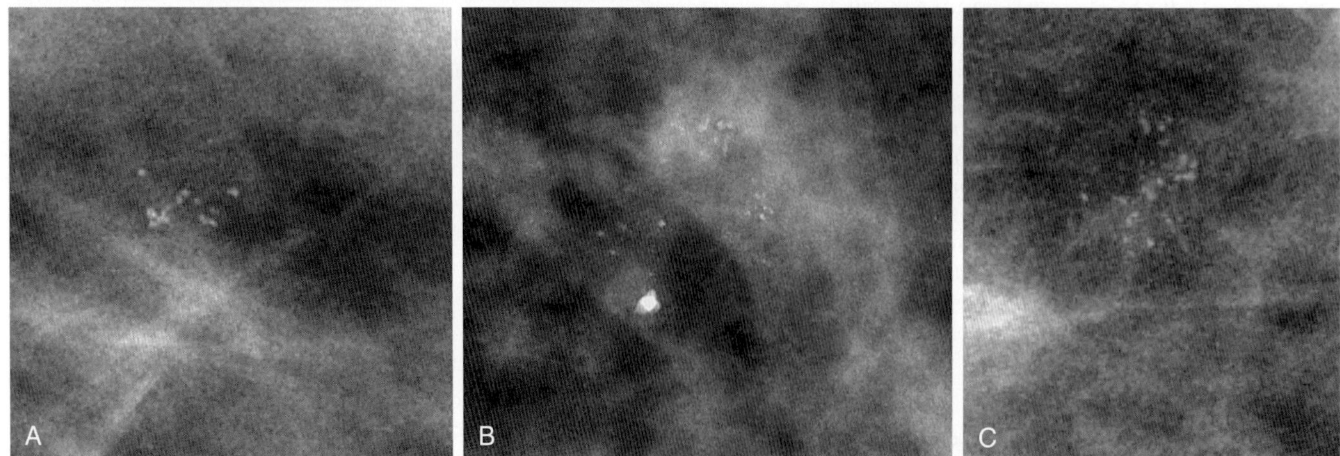

■ **FIGURE 28-4** Round calcifications. **A,** Grouped, round calcifications on a baseline mammogram that are well-defined and not associated with a soft tissue density or mass can undergo short-term follow-up (BI-RADS 3). Grouped, round calcifications that are new or increasing in number are suspicious (BI-RADS 4) and may represent ductal carcinoma in situ (DCIS) (**B**), or a benign etiology such as fibrocystic change (**C**).

When round or punctate calcifications are grouped or clustered, a benign cause is still most likely. Management is the same as for masses with benign features. If there is a group of round or punctate calcifications on a baseline mammogram, recall for magnification views should be performed. Short-interval follow-up at 6, 12, and 24 months after the initial assessment can be performed, usually with magnification views, to assess whether the findings have changed or remained stable.

If the patient has had previous mammograms, attempts should be made to obtain them for comparison. If the calcifications are new or increasing, then biopsy may be indicated. If the round, punctate calcifications are unchanged for at least 2 years, then a benign assessment is reasonable (BI-RADS 2).

Intermediate Risk Calcifications

Amorphous, Indistinct Calcifications

Amorphous, indistinct calcifications are often benign and due to columnar cell change or columnar cell hyperplasia, fibrocystic change, or sclerosing adenosis (Fig. 28-5). Berg and colleagues evaluated histology results for calcifications classified as amorphous that were sampled.[7] They found an 18% rate of malignancy for amorphous calcifications. When present, DCIS was usually low grade (60%),[7] such that comparison with previous studies is probably less helpful for amorphous calcifications than those of other morphologic appearances.

Distribution is helpful in the evaluation of amorphous calcifications. When the calcifications are bilateral and diffuse, no further workup is typically indicated. Amorphous calcifications are of more concern when grouped or clustered or when in a linear or segmental distribution. When multiple clusters of amorphous calcifications are present in a region of the breast, sampling of the most suspicious area is usually indicated.

Diagnostic mammography including magnification views in both CC and mediolateral projections is very important in the evaluation of amorphous calcifications. Milk of calcium calcifications may appear amorphous and indistinct on screening views, but the morphology usually becomes apparent as characteristically benign milk of calcium on a 90-degree lateral magnification view.

Coarse, Heterogeneous Calcifications

Coarse, heterogeneous calcifications are of intermediate risk for breast cancer (Fig. 28-6). Common benign causes of coarse heterogeneous calcifications include degenerating fibroadenoma, papilloma, fibrosis, and fibrocystic change. These calcifications are typically grouped and smaller than dystrophic calcifications. When the calcifications are not due to a benign etiology, the cause is usually DCIS (more commonly high grade than low grade). Comparison with previous mammograms is helpful in the evaluation of coarse heterogeneous calcifications, because benign causes typically result in slow change over time

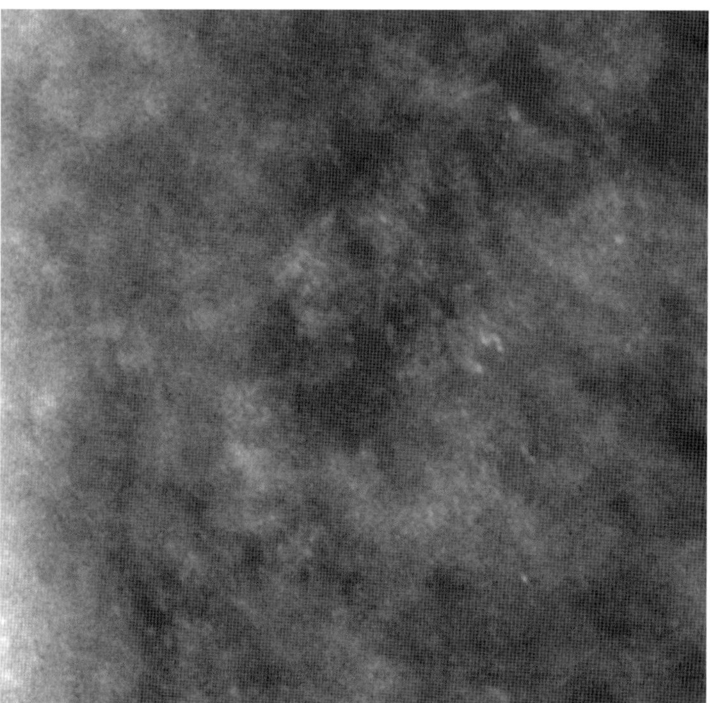

■ **FIGURE 28-5** Mammogram showing amorphous calcifications. Note the area of grouped, amorphous calcifications that are too numerous to count. They are difficult to see because of their indistinct morphology. Stereotactic-guided vacuum-assisted core needle biopsy of these calcifications showed sclerosing adenosis and fibrocystic change.

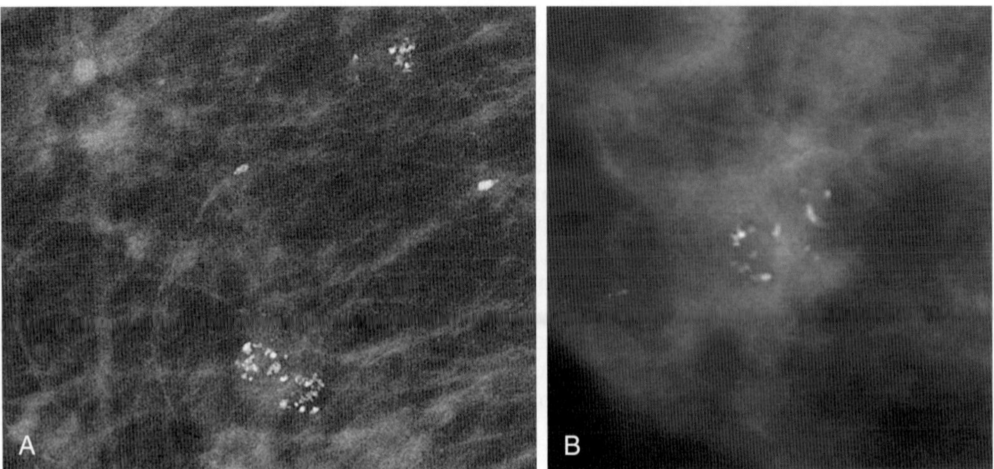

FIGURE 28-6 Mammograms shows coarse, heterogeneous calcifications. **A,** Two areas of grouped, coarse, heterogeneous calcifications stable for three years. **B,** New grouped, coarse heterogeneous calcifications. Stereotactic-guided core needle biopsy revealed high-grade ductal carcinoma in situ (DCIS).

in comparison with DCIS with this presentation. Coarse heterogeneous calcifications that are stable for 2 or more years can be usually be considered benign. When new or increasing in number, biopsy is often needed. Likewise, a linear or segmental distribution increases the likelihood of malignancy and biopsy is often indicated.

Suspicious and Malignant Calcifications

Fine, Pleomorphic Calcifications

Fine, pleomorphic calcifications are more conspicuous than amorphous calcifications and smaller than coarse heterogeneous calcifications (see Fig. 28-1).[6] They usually present in a grouped or segmental distribution. A regional or diffuse distribution is very uncommon. Fine pleomorphic calcifications cause concern. The likelihood of carcinoma is higher than for amorphous or coarse heterogeneous calcifications but not as high as for fine, linear branching calcifications (see Table 28-1).[2] Comparison with prior mammograms will not typically change recommendations for biopsy because these are of high suspicion based on morphology alone.

Fine, Linear Branching Calcifications

Calcifications that are fine in morphology and linear or branching in distribution are highly suspicious for DCIS (see Fig. 28-1) and often of high nuclear grade. Biopsy will nearly always be indicated. There are few benign causes of fine, linear branching calcifications, although early vascular calcifications may mimic these. Magnification views can help to differentiate vascular calcifications from early fine, linear branching calcifications. Occasionally, biopsy may be performed that shows atherosclerotic calcification as the only source of calcification in the sample.

Assessment of stability of the lesions by comparing them with previous mammograms is not typically useful. Assessment of distribution will not likely influence the need for biopsy, although a segmental distribution may result in a BI-RADS 5 assessment owing to the high likelihood of malignancy (see Table 28-1).

APPROACH FOR BIOPSY

Stereotactic-guided percutaneous biopsy is usually preferred to surgical biopsy owing to cost-effectiveness and absence of scarring. Diagnosis of cancer by stereotactic-guided biopsy helps surgical planning, including decisions regarding whether a sentinel node biopsy should be performed at the time of surgery. Stereotactic biopsy of additional areas of calcification in the ipsilateral breast may be helpful in evaluating the extent of DCIS, which may aid in decision-making regarding the likely success of breast conservation. In addition, suspicious calcifications of differing morphology should each undergo sampling because they will likely have differing causes (Fig. 28-7). Either area of differing calcifications may be malignant or benign and as such must be evaluated separately.

If suspicious calcifications are not amenable to stereotactic biopsy, pre-surgical needle localization is appropriate.

USE OF ULTRASONOGRAPHY AND MAGNETIC RESONANCE IMAGING (MRI) IN THE EVALUATION OF BREAST CALCIFICATIONS

For calcifications that have a benign morphology, no further imaging with ultrasonography or MRI is indicated. Likewise, the literature regarding the use of ultrasonography or MRI for suspicious calcifications of intermediate to higher risk is evolving.

When calcifications are present that suggest a high likelihood of malignancy, the presence of an associated mass is of concern for invasive carcinoma. Ultrasound evaluation of the area of high suspicion calcifications may be useful to identify an associated mass when the breast tissue is dense (Fig. 28-8).[8]

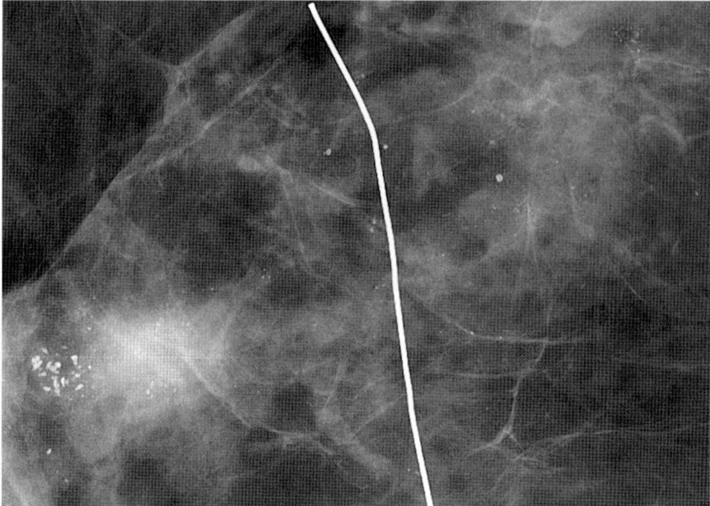

■ **FIGURE 28-7** Management of calcifications with differing morphologic appearances. Magnification view of the right breast in a 65-year-old woman. Mammogram shows grouped, coarse heterogeneous calcifications adjacent to subtle fine pleomorphic and amorphous calcifications in a segmental distribution. Stereotactic-guided core needle biopsy performed of both areas showed high-grade DCIS at the site of the coarse heterogeneous calcifications and fibrocystic changes at the site of the fine pleomorphic calcifications.

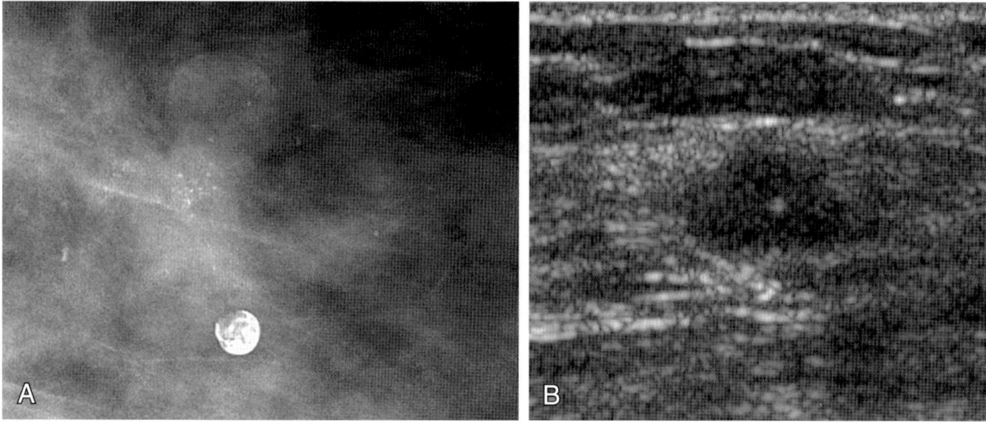

■ **FIGURE 28-8** A 74-year-old woman presented with new suspicious calcifications in the left breast. **A,** Mammography magnification view shows grouped fine pleomorphic calcifications in the left breast. The adjacent round, circumscribed mass was stable and represented a simple cyst on ultrasound evaluation. **B,** Ultrasound image of the area of microcalcifications in the left breast shows a corresponding oval, indistinet, hypoechoic, solid mass with ill-defined margins containing calcium. Ultrasound-guided core-needle biopsy showed DCIS and invasive ductal carcinoma.

Once a breast cancer is diagnosed by core needle biopsy, MRI is useful to evaluate the extent of the biopsy-proven breast carcinoma (Fig. 28-9), to identify other areas of cancer in the same breast, and to identify cancer in the contralateral breast.[8,9] There are little data on the usefulness of breast MRI in the evaluation of calcifications before biopsy. Because MRI is less sensitive for DCIS than invasive carcinoma,[10] a negative MRI should not be used to influence the decision to sample calcifications that are suspicious based on mammographic views.

SUMMARY

Microcalcifications are common in the breast and often have a typical benign appearance. Calcifications that are round or punctate are typically benign, such that short-term follow-up can be performed if they are grouped and appear on a baseline mammogram. Intervention may be indicated, however, if round or punctate calcifications are new or increasing compared with prior studies or have a worrisome distribution. Intermediate-risk calcifications, such as those that are amorphous or coarse and heterogeneous may require sampling,

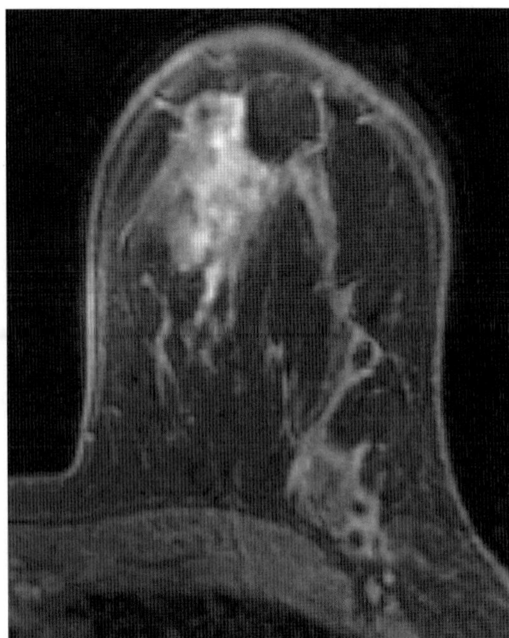

■ **FIGURE 28-9** A 45-year-old woman presented with biopsy-proven DCIS in the left breast and positive margins at lumpectomy. The postoperative mammogram (not shown) was normal, with no residual calcifications. T1-weighted axial MR image of the left breast with fat suppression after intravenous administration of gadolinium shows clumped, linear non-mass enhancement in a segmental distribution in the medial left breast.

unless they are reasonably stable or in a benign distribution. More suspicious calcifications, such as fine, pleomorphic, or fine, linear branching, will nearly always require tissue sampling. In general, calcifications should be judged on their worst features. Most suspicious calcifications can be sampled using stereotactic-guided vacuum-assisted core needle biopsy.

The ACR Breast Imaging Practice and Intervention Guidelines are a useful, up-to-date source of information to practicing radiologists.[11] Specific topics include the evaluation and management of breast calcifications, and these guidelines can be consulted for additional information and advice.

KEY POINTS

- Typically benign calcifications, such as suture, rim or lucent-centered, and skin, do not require additional imaging evaluation in most cases.
- Calcifications should be evaluated based on their morphology, distribution, and stability (if prior mammograms are available).
- Workup includes magnification views in the CC and 90-degree lateral (mediolateral or lateromedial) projections.
- Round or punctate calcifications, although typically benign, may require histologic diagnosis if grouped and new or increasing, or if linear or segmental in distribution. Grouped round and/or punctate calcification on a baseline mammogram may require short-term follow-up to establish stability.
- Amorphous or indistinct calcifications are of intermediate concern and often require sampling unless the distribution is bilateral and symmetric. Stability is a less helpful feature because low-grade DCIS is a common result at biopsy and may not manifest changes in annual mammograms.
- Coarse heterogeneous calcifications are now considered of intermediate concern. Comparison with prior mammograms and evaluation of their distribution can be helpful in determining whether they warrant a biopsy.
- Fine, pleomorphic calcifications usually require tissue sampling owing to the current higher level of concern for malignancy.
- Fine, linear branching calcifications are suspicious and should be biopsied after appropriate workup to rule out other etiologies (i.e., early vascular calcifications).
- Most suspicious calcifications in the breast are amenable to stereotactic vacuum-assisted core needle biopsy to establish a diagnosis.

SUGGESTED READINGS

D'Orsi CJ, Bassett LW, Berg WA, et al. *Breast Imaging Reporting and Data System: ACR BI-RADS-Mammography.* 4th ed. Breast calcification section, Reston, Va: American College of Radiology, 2003. Available at: www.acr.org/.

Monsees BS. Evaluation of breast microcalcifications. *Radiol Clin North Am* 1995;**33**:1109–21.

REFERENCES

1. Venkatesan A, Chu P, Kerlikowske K, Sickles EA, Smith-Bindman R. Positive predictive value of specific mammographic findings according to reader and patient variables. *Radiology* 2009;**250**:648–57.
2. Burnside ES, Ochsner JE, Fowler KJ, Fine JP, Salkowski LR, Rubin DL, et al. Use of microcalcification descriptors in BI-RADS 4th edition to stratify risk of malignancy. *Radiology* 2007;**242**:388–95.
3. Stomper PC, Geradts J, Edge SB, Levine EG. mammographic predictors of the presence and size of invasive carcinomas associated with malignant microcalcification lesions without a mass. *AJR Am J Roentgenol* 2003;**181**:1679–84.
4. Lev-Toaff AS, Feig SA, Saitas VL, Finkel GC, Schwartz GF. Stability of malignant breast microcalcifications. *Radiology* 1994;**192**:153–6.
5. Liberman L, Abramson AF, Squires FB, Glassman JR, Morris EA, Dershaw DD. The breast imaging reporting and data system: positive predictive value of mammographic features and final assessment categories. *Am J Roentgenol* 1998;**171**:35–40.
6. D'Orsi CJ, Bassett LW, Berg WA, et al. *Breast Imaging Reporting and Data System: ACR BI-RADS-Mammography*. 4th ed. Reston, Va: American College of Radiology; 2003. Available at: www.acr.org/.
7. Berg WA, Arnoldus CL, Teferra E, Bhargavan M. Biopsy of amorphous breast calcifications: pathologic outcome and yield at stereotactic biopsy. *Radiology* 2001;**221**:495–503.
8. Berg WA, Gutierrez L, NessAiver MS, Carter WB, Bhargavan M, Lewis RS, et al. Diagnostic accuracy of mammography, clinical examination,

US, and MR imaging in preoperative assessment of breast cancer. *Radiology* 2004;**233**:830–49.
9. Lehman CD, Gatsonis C, Kuhl CK, Hendrick RE, Pisano ED, Hanna L, et al. MRI evaluation of the contralateral breast in women with recently diagnosed breast cancer. *N Engl J Med* 2007;**356**:1295–303.
10. Neubauer H, Li M, Kuehne-Heid R, Schneider A, Kaiser WA. High grade and non-high grade ductal carcinoma in situ on dynamic MR mammography: characteristic findings for signal increase and morphological pattern of enhancement. *Br J Radiol* 2003;**76**:3–12.
11. ACR Breast Imaging and Intervention Practice Guidelines. 2008, Available at: www.acr.org/SecondaryMainMenuCategories/quality_safety/guidelines/breast.aspx.

SECTION

SEVEN

Interventional Approaches

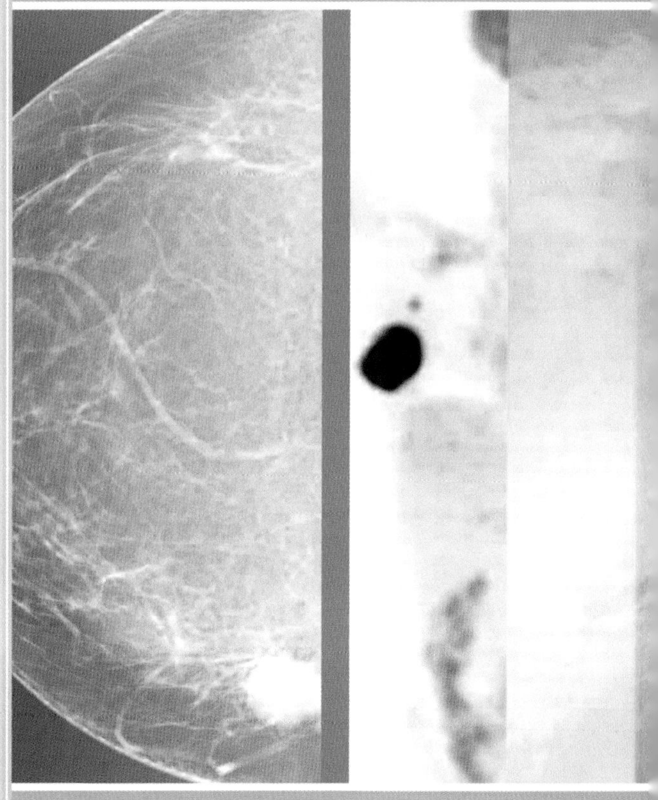

CHAPTER 29

Image-Guided Percutaneous Biopsy

Mary S. Newell and Mary Catherine Mahoney

Imaging-guided percutaneous tissue sampling of the breast has favorably altered the management of breast lesions, both benign and malignant, since its inception in the 1980s and subsequent acceptance in the 1990s.[1-3] Its safety, accuracy, and cost-effectiveness have been validated in several studies.[1-3] However, this set of procedures serves the patient best when performed by an operator with full appreciation of patient's salient imaging findings, a knowledge of the benefits and limitations of the chosen sampling method, and a thorough understanding of what constitutes an adequate and concordant pathologic specimen.

This chapter outlines a general approach to imaging-guided percutaneous breast biopsy, and discusses the specifics of the various available imaging modalities currently available for guidance.

VALIDATION OF IMAGING-GUIDED PERCUTANEOUS BIOPSY

About 1.6 million individuals in the United States will require biopsy for definitive diagnosis of a breast problem, either imaging-detected or clinically identified, each year. On an individual and population basis, any biopsy technique that minimizes patient discomfort, time away from routine duties, post-biopsy scarring and deformity, and cost would be the preferred method of tissue retrieval. This assumes, of course, that the technique has a comparable record of accuracy and safety when stacked up against other biopsy methods (i.e., surgical excision). Imaging-guided percutaneous tissue sampling provides such a technique.

Of the anticipated breast biopsies performed each year, the majority (approximately 80%) of results will be benign. Confidence in a benign, concordant imaging-guided needle biopsy allows avoidance of unnecessary surgery. Parker and coworkers showed an overall 1.5% false negative rate for percutaneous biopsy,[1] indicating that confidence in a negative biopsy result is warranted. Several authors have also confirmed the accuracy of a malignant biopsy result, with excellent histologic agreement between core needle biopsy results and subsequent examination of the excised specimen. Histologic underestimates with core biopsy do occur; however, if careful review of pathology results is performed, with recommendation for excision of lesions known to be subject to upgrade (e.g., atypical ductal hyperplasia), equality with surgical excision results can be achieved. In point of fact, core needle biopsy (CNB) has been shown to have a smaller "missed lesion" rate compared with surgical excision of nonpalpable lesions (1.1% for CNB vs. 2.6% for surgery).[2,3]

The safety of imaging-guided breast biopsies has been demonstrated, as well. Parker and coworkers showed a 0.2% rate of clinically significant complications (defined as ones that necessitated medical or surgical intervention) in a large multi-institutional cohort of patients (3765 cases) with both stereotaxis and ultrasound used for guidance of large core needles.[1]

The cost-effectiveness of percutaneous breast biopsy provides an additional impetus for its use. This occurs in large part due to the ability to defer surgery if benign, concordant results are returned, resulting in large savings, and which can safely occur in an estimated 71% to 85% of cases.[4] However, cost savings are also realized when core biopsy shows malignant results. A patient whose cancer is diagnosed via percutaneous biopsy can expect to undergo fewer surgeries compared with those whose cancer is diagnosed with surgical open biopsy (average of

1.25 surgeries vs. 2.01).[5] Due to its confirmed safety, accuracy and cost-effectiveness, CNB is widely accepted as the appropriate first-line tool for histologic confirmation of a breast abnormality.

ULTRASOUND-GUIDED PERCUTANEOUS TISSUE SAMPLING

Ultrasound-guided core needle biopsy (US-guided CNB) offers many advantages over the other available methods of imaging guided tissue retrieval (stereotactic and magnetic resonance imaging [MRI]-guidance). For the patient, it allows comfortable positioning compared with the other techniques. Real-time verification of sampling accuracy is possible. It is relatively quick in terms of room-time and physician requirement.[6] No ionizing radiation is used (as opposed to stereotactic procedures). There are no modality-based contraindications (as compared with MRI and, occasionally, stereotactic guidance) and its accuracy has been supported in the literature.[7,8] In general, when a suspicious lesion for which biopsy is warranted can be confidently visualized at ultrasound, and its location is reconciled with other imaging techniques, sonographic-guidance should be chosen.

Description, Equipment and Technique

High quality scanning technique and image recording is an obvious requisite for accurate US-guided CNB. As addressed in the American College of Radiology (ACR) Practice Guidelines, a high-resolution (center frequency at least 10 MHz) transducer, preferably linear-array, should be used during performance of imaging and biopsy.[9] Once a target for biopsy is identified, notation should be made on the images and in the written report in regard to the size (maximal dimension in at least 2 orthogonal planes), location (outlined as specifically as possible with regard to side, and position in the breast, using the "o'clock" method as well as number of centimeters that the target lies from the nipple), and transducer orientation ("transverse/longitudinal" or "radial/anti-radial"). This information is vital because it is quite possible that the biopsy procedure may be performed on a day different from the workup and/or by a different examiner. Using specific detail about the location of the lesion will allow even subtle findings to be re-identified accurately.

Equipment

A private single-patient procedure room should be used for biopsy. In this way, informed consent may be obtained and the patient's history discussed without fear of a privacy breach. Additionally, any complications can be dealt with without alarming other patients. The room should be large enough to accommodate the physician, the ultrasound technologist, a patient gurney (with room to maneuver it for optimal positioning), and, if possible, a few additional people (e.g., students or residents, the cytopathologist if needed, and as indicated, a family member). Temperature should be controlled such that patient is comfortable but not too warm. A sink should be available for handwashing. Lockable drawers and cabinets that allow for the securing of supplies and all medications should be in place. The patient gurney should be height-adjustable, on wheels, lockable and, if possible, able to be placed in Trendelenburg position in case of a vasovagal patient reaction during the procedure. A mobile procedure tray that can be placed near the physician allows the biopsy to proceed efficiently.

Each center or each physician may construct a sterile procedure tray to individual specifications. However, when there are multiple practitioners within a single center, standardization of set-up and supplies promotes quick patient turnaround and cost savings, as the technologist can more efficiently prepare the trays and fewer supplies need to be stocked. A typical sterile set-up (Fig. 29-1) may

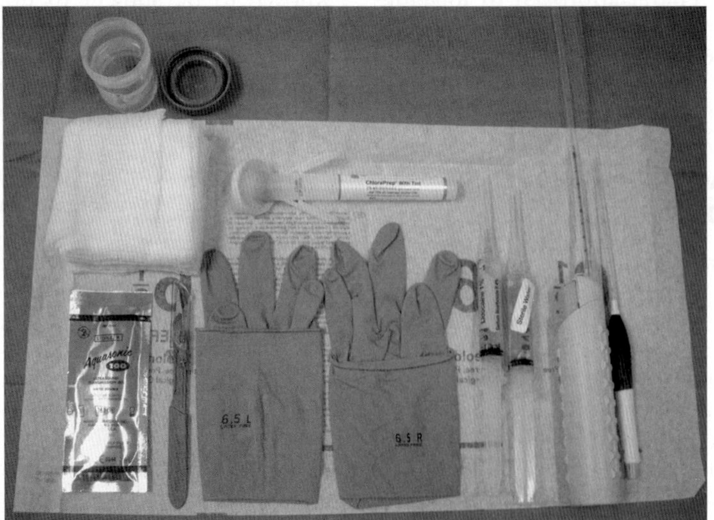

■ **FIGURE 29-1** Typical sterile biopsy tray set-up, which may include sterile gloves, gauze, local anesthetic with syringe clearly labeled, as well as additional items specific to the modality being used. Here, gel for acoustical coupling and saline in a syringe to aid in the transfer of tissue specimen from biopsy needle into formalin indicate that an ultrasound-guided core biopsy is being performed.

include sterile gloves, antiseptic, sterile gauze, sterile saline in a syringe to flush tissue sample from needle, sterile gel to allow transducer-skin acoustic coupling, and pre-drawn local anesthetic agent (clearly labeled as to exact content). Pre-constructed trays can be purchased from many vendors, and the client can determine the specific contents. While these promote efficiency, they may prove more costly than simply making up the trays on-site. Once the standard set-up is prepared by the technologist or aide, the needle selected for biopsy may be individualized to physician or specific lesion type, and opened at the time of actual biopsy.

The variety of available needles has increased significantly since Parker described the efficacy of the 14-gauge automated biopsy gun in 1993.[7] However, that needle remains a very reliable workhorse. Models are now available from many different vendors. The needle works via a springloaded device that is cocked in preparation for use. Upon firing, a solid needle having a recessed notch along its side rapidly traverses the targeted tissue. It is beveled at its tip, causing it to deflect as it travels. This is important, because once it reaches full throw, it re-straightens, forcefully impressing tissue into the notch. A hollow cutting cannula then slides over the needle, cleanly shearing the entrapped tissue (Fig. 29-2). This two-step action occurs in rapid sequence, nearly instantaneously, and is triggered by single button push. The needle is removed from the patient, partially re-cocked to expose the core sample, and then fully re-cocked in preparation for another pass.

Automated biopsy needles come in a variety of gauges, sampling notch lengths, and overall needle lengths. Most commonly used is a 14 gauge needle with a 22 mm throw. Literature supports the use of a 14 gauge or larger needle, a longer throw (22 vs. 11 mm) and an automated device over a nonautomated cutting needle.[10,11] Knowledge of the *throw* or length of automated tip-travel of the selected device is vital in order to prevent inadvertent penetration of adjacent tissue (e.g., blood vessel in the axilla). Although use of a *short throw* device (11 mm vs. 22 mm) is tempting in close anatomic quarters, the volume of tissue obtained is greatly diminished, usually by more than 50% (due to the lesser degree of needle deflection and tissue entrapment). If needle approach is planned carefully, the safe deployment of a long-throw device can almost always be ensured. Although somewhat controversial, likely a minimum of four samples should be obtained. Fragmented cores or those that float rather than sink in preservative should be viewed as potentially nondiagnostic.[12]

More recently, the use of vacuum-assisted devices, long the needle of choice for stereotactic core biopsies, have become accepted for use with ultrasound, with hand-held versions available. These systems may require the use of an external vacuum or can be self-contained. The external-vacuum systems have been used most extensively. Each system varies in its mechanism of action, but in general, the needle or probe is placed along the deep margin of the lesion in the closed position. It is then activated such that the inner cutting cannula is retracted, rendering the sampling notch sonographically visible relative to the biopsy target; any required adjustments to needle position can be made. Upon sampling, the vacuum pulls tissue into the notch and the inner cannula transects the tissue (Fig. 29-3). This core is then delivered retrograde for retrieval, either by an assistant using forceps or into a closed chamber for later collection, depending on the device. The systems that require each sample to be collected individually by an assistant result in a slightly longer procedure time and greater risk of exposure to blood products. However, they provide the advantage of confirming that an adequate core was obtained during each pass. As opposed to spring-loaded devices, these vacuum-assisted devices allow multiple contiguous samples to be taken during a single needle insertion, because the tissue is delivered externally while the needle remains poised for added cores. This biopsy method results in larger core samples.

Other devices are available that represent variants or hybrids of the above. Some have self-contained rather than external vacuums. These do not offer the benefit of contiguous biopsy and retrograde tissue delivery but do result in large core samples and negate the need for the space-occupying vacuum. Another advantage is that they can be "fired" into the lesion, as an automated device is, or can be "pre-fired" outside the patient in cases where

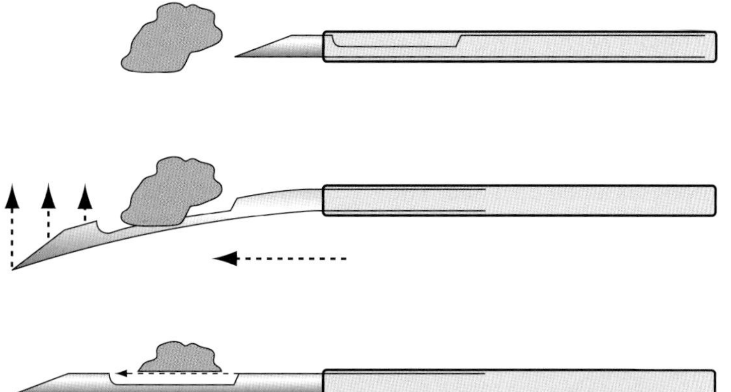

■ **FIGURE 29-2** Graphic depiction of automated core needle biopsy throw mechanism. The needle deploys as a multi-stage process. The portion of the needle containing the sampling notch has a beveled leading tip, causing it to arc as it deploys. Upon reaching full throw, it re-straightens, impressing the tissue firmly into the notch. A cutting cannula extends over the notch, shearing off a cylinder of tissue, the specimen.

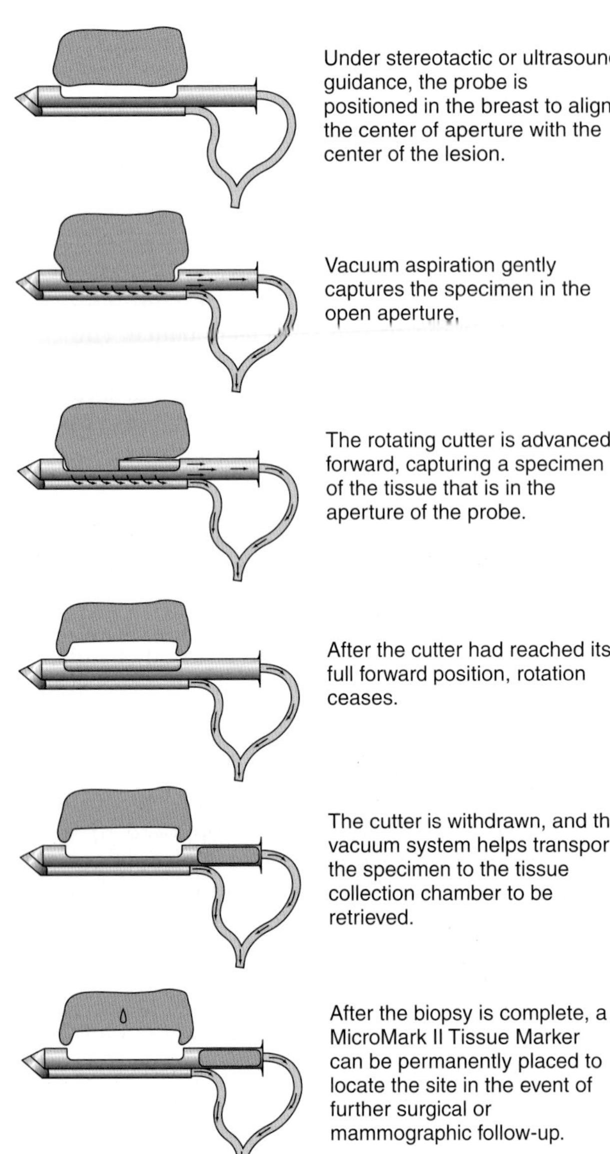

Under stereotactic or ultrasound guidance, the probe is positioned in the breast to align the center of aperture with the center of the lesion.
Vacuum aspiration gently captures the specimen in the open aperture.
The rotating cutter is advanced forward, capturing a specimen of the tissue that is in the aperture of the probe.
After the cutter had reached its full forward position, rotation ceases.
The cutter is withdrawn, and the vacuum system helps transport the specimen to the tissue collection chamber to be retrieved.
After the biopsy is complete, a MicroMark II Tissue Marker can be permanently placed to locate the site in the event of further surgical or mammographic follow-up.

■ **FIGURE 29-3** Cutting mechanism of a vacuum-assisted biopsy device. (*Courtesy of Ethicon Endo-surgery Inc.*)

forceful throw of the needle is not desired. Another unique system uses a 19-gauge forked needle at the lead of the device to traverse, immobilize and freeze (using CO_2 contained in the unit) that segment of the lesion, followed by tissue transaction via a cutting cannula that automatically extends over the 19-gauge lead needle.

The choice of needles or probes is a personal one. The automated biopsy needles are relatively cheap, light and easy to maneuver, require no significant capital expenditure for associated equipment (external vacuum), and are time-tested.[7] The vacuum-assisted devices allow tissue retrieval quickly and contiguously, and deliver larger samples, perhaps requiring fewer cores. While the advantage of larger samples has been confirmed when using stereotactic guidance, it remains controversial whether larger cores are as important with the lesions that are selected to undergo ultrasound-guided biopsy: largely masses with or without associated calcium. Some authors have demonstrated no significant difference between the two mechanisms of biopsy in terms of missed cancers, insufficiency, or histologic underestimation.[13] However, other authors have shown a smaller rate of histologic underestimation with vacuum-assisted devices, at least for atypical ductal hyperplasia.[14] Vacuum-assisted biopsies are more highly reimbursed than the other technique, but therefore also result in significantly higher procedure cost to the patient. Perhaps a lesion-specific choice of biopsy technique is appropriate, with an automated needle chosen for highly suspicious ACR's Breast Image Reporting and Data System (BI-RADS) 5 lesions or BI-RADS 4A lesions (e.g., probable fibroadenomas or equivocal intramammary lymph nodes), all of which are unlikely to be subject to histologic upgrade, and for which near complete lesion removal is not required for confident diagnosis.

Technique

Pre-Procedural Considerations

Written informed consent is an obligate requisite to the procedure. Each center will likely have an organization-composed and approved consent form. Some sites use a general form for all types of procedures and surgeries performed at that institution that outlines all potential risks, up to and including death; others use procedure-specific consent forms that are tailored to the appropriate set of risks and complications. If the former is required by the institution, this should be explained to the patient, telling her that some of the potential risks and complications mentioned are not considered applicable to her situation. However, all consents should make mention of bleeding, infection, pneumothorax, allergic reaction to administered medications and, if appropriate, implant rupture as potential complications of the procedure. Additionally, the patient should be fully informed about the benefits of the biopsy (e.g., deferral of surgery in the face of benign specific results; pre-operative verification of malignancy, allowing definitive surgical therapy in one setting) as well as the potential drawbacks (possible need for rebiopsy or excision in the face of nonspecific, insufficient or discordant pathology results). She should be told about the use of a marking clip. In the optimal setting, this material, as well as a general description of what she can expect during the procedure and its aftermath, will have been discussed with the patient ahead of time by a physician, technologist, nurse or physician-extender possibly at the time of her diagnostic workup or upon scheduling. However, the written informed consent should be obtained by the practitioner performing the biopsy, with a witness in attendance. For The Joint Commission (TJC)-accredited facilities, compliance with Universal Protocol (to prevent wrong site, wrong procedure, wrong person mishaps) is mandated. This requires marking of the side of biopsy (right/left), and completion of a time-out just prior to the start of the procedure to verify the identity of the patient, the site of the biopsy and the procedure to be performed, in the presence of the entire procedural team and the patient, all of whom must participate and be in agreement (See TJC policy for more detail at www.jointcommission.org). This process must be carried out by the physician or physician-extender who is performing the procedure, and not a surrogate (resident, nurse, technologist, other physician), and formally documented. Even if a facility is not subject to TJC accreditation, the process when used in some form can help prevent procedural errors. The patient should be queried directly by the physician about any allergies (including latex) as well as her medication history in regards to anticoagulation and bleeding diathesis status. While biopsy can be pursued even in the face of anticoagulation (see discussion under "Contraindications"), knowledge of her coagulation status may alter post-procedure care (e.g., longer compression time, etc.).

The patient is next placed in optimal position. For lesions in the outer, upper and lower breast, this will likely be in the oblique supine position, turned slightly to the opposite side so that the breast falls gently toward medial, with ipsilateral arm raised overhead (Fig. 29-4A). This decreases the tissue depth of the breast and firms up the skin surface, allowing easier needle penetration. For medial lesions, the patient can either lie supine or be placed slightly oblique toward the side the lesion is on, with the physician on her opposite side. In some small-breasted woman, or in males, adjustment may be needed to bolster the breast thickness to allow safe biopsy. For example, with lateral lesions in a small breast, the patient's arm may be left at her side and used to mound up tissue, or she may be placed laterally oblique rather than medially. For medial lesions, a similar bolstering technique can be used with the arm, or the patient may be rolled medially so that more tissue falls toward the biopsy quadrant (Fig. 29-4B).

Once the patient has given consent, the time-out has occurred, and she is positioned, pre-scanning should be performed in order to re-identify the target and plan a needle approach. The technologist will stand on the same side of the gurney as the ultrasound machine. The physician will stand on the other side. The patient can be positioned either with her head near the ultrasound unit or rotated 180 degrees such that her feet are near the unit, depending on the side and location of the lesion. For lesions in the lateral left breast or medial right breast, having the physician on the left side of the patient may be optimal; this can be reversed for lesions in the medial left breast or lateral right breast. In general the shortest route to the lesion that allows safe ingress of the needle (as well as adequate tissue beyond the lesion and a parallel-to-chest-wall orientation if a springloaded device with a throw is being used) is chosen. Pre-scanning can also help identify an optimal specific needle route. Fat is far easier to traverse with a needle than fibrous or parenchyma tissue. Adjustment of the transducer radially over the lesion may allow for identification of a *window* of fat between anticipated skin entry site and the lesion (Fig. 29-5).

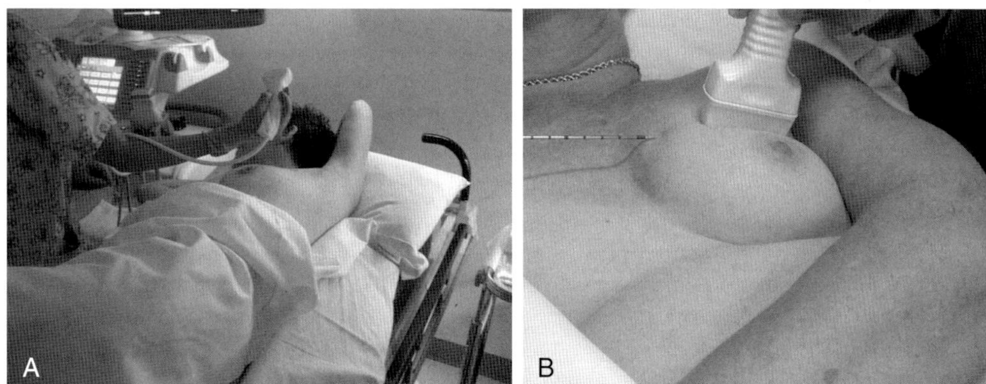

■ **FIGURE 29-4** Positioning for ultrasound-guided core biopsy. Typical position for most lesions in lateral, superior or inferior breast, with patient placed slightly oblique in the contralateral direction and arm raised over head (**A**). For small-breasted women or males, arm placement at the side may allow buttressing of tissue for greater breast thickness for either lateral lesion or medial lesions (**B**).

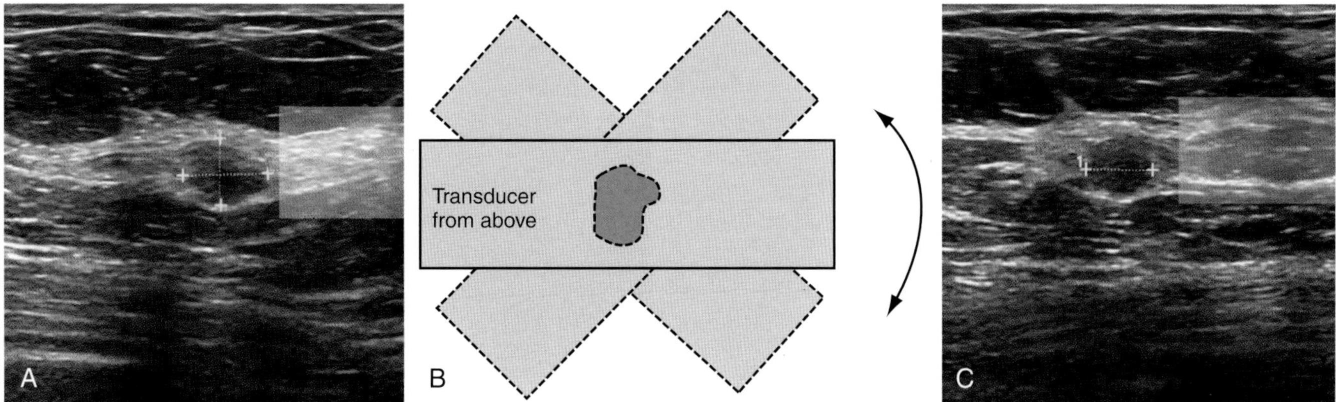

■ **FIGURE 29-5** If dense tissue plane is encountered along expected needle path (shaded area, [**A**]) during ultrasound-guided core needle biopsy, the transducer can be rotated over the lesion prior to puncture (**B**) in an attempt to identify a fat plane that may allow easier needle egress (shaded area [**C**]).

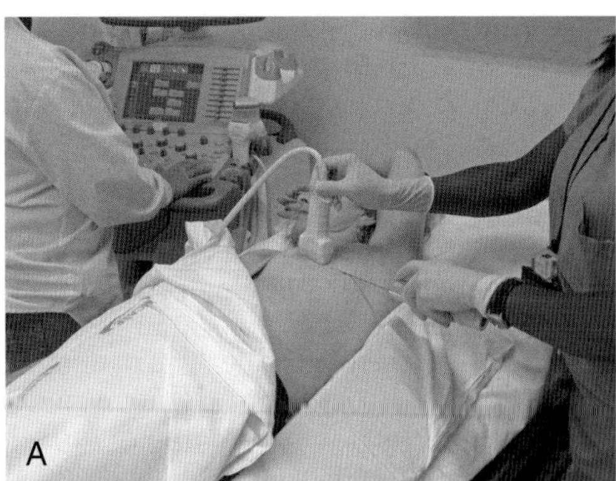

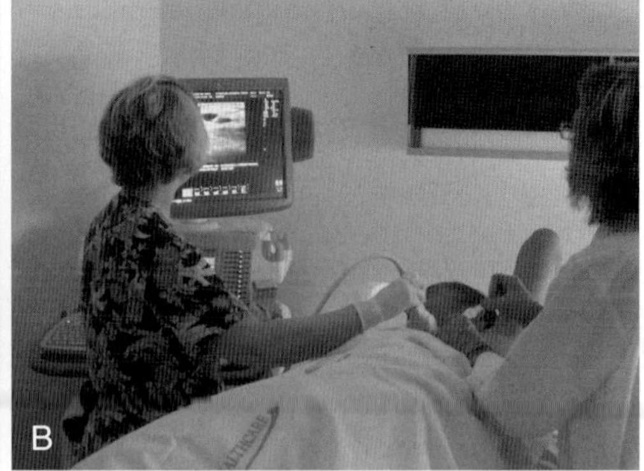

■ **FIGURE 29-6** Ultrasound-guided procedures may be performed, depending on personal preference, with the physician holding both the transducer and needle (**A**), or with the technologist scanning as the physician guides the needle (**B**).

The procedure may be either a one-person or two-person process (Fig. 29-6). Both work well, and it appears to be a matter of personal physician opinion, usually a strongly held one. Some practitioners prefer to hold the biopsy device and the transducer themselves. In this way extremely subtle adjustments to needle and transducer position can be made quickly and without discussion. However, the needle must be steered and deployed with one hand, and the transducer handed off between passes. Alternately, some physicians prefer to have a technologist or other person scan while they manipulate the needle. It seems as though this system would be unwieldy; however, many teams find that after just a few procedures performed in concert, the physician and assistant are able to anticipate needed adjustments and maintain excellent needle visualization during the procedure. This gives the physician two hands to steer and deploy the needle, and retrieve the tissue. Both choices require practice at keeping the transducer pointing at the skin entry site, such that the long axis of the transducer face is aligned with the needle trajectory, to ensure the continued ability to visualize the entire shaft of the needle during biopsy (Fig. 29-7).

Sterile Portion of the Procedure

Once the lesion is identified and the expected needle route is defined, the sterile portion of the procedure can commence. The transducer is covered with a sterile probe cover. The physician can "glove-up" and cleanse the biopsy site with antiseptic solution. Several solutions and preparations are available but there is evidence to suggest that chlorhexidine-based solutions provide better antisepsis than iodine-based solutions.[15]

For the vast majority of percutaneous breast biopsies, local anesthesia will suffice. Care should be taken to review the patient's allergy history prior to administration. This should be specifically done by the physician performing the procedure, even if a nurse or technologist has obtained such history as well. Many effective agents are available; the practitioner can acquaint himself or herself with dosage, side effects and contraindications of one or two of these drugs, one for routine use and another agent to use if an alternate is needed because of patient allergy. Preferably one routine drug can be chosen from the amide family (e.g., lidocaine, mepivacaine, prilocaine, bupivacaine) and one from the ester family (e.g., procaine, tetracaine), because cross-allergies only rarely occur between these groups. Lidocaine 1% is a common choice. For this agent, the maximum dose to be used in one setting is 4 mg/kg up to a maximum of 280 mg (28 mL). If epinephrine is added, maximum allowable dose is increased to 7 mg/kg (50 mL); this amount is rarely required. True allergy to the amide family of local anesthetics is rare and is usually reflects an allergy to the preservative or antimicrobial used in the

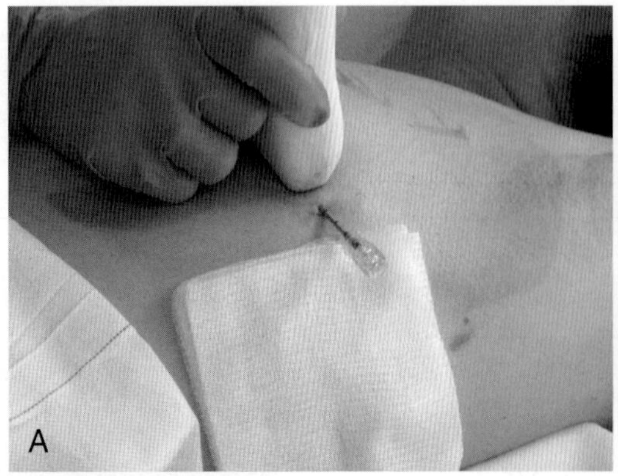

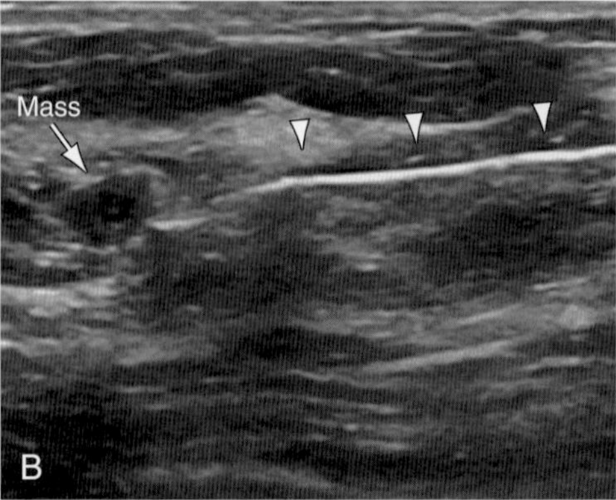

■ **FIGURE 29-7** When performing ultrasound-guided procedures, the biopsy needle or probe should be oriented along the long axis of the transducer (**A**), so that the needle (*arrowheads*) can be visualized in its entirety at all times, thereby ensuring that its tip position is always verified (**B**).

drug rather than the drug itself. The patient can be carefully questioned about the nature and symptoms of any prior "allergic" experience. Often, what she reports is "a racing heart" or palpitations related to the co-usage of epinephrine. If this is the case, the patient can be reassured about the cause of such a reaction, and epinephrine can be avoided. If a real allergy is confirmed, use of an agent in the alternate family (amide vs. ester) can be safely selected.

In selected cases, a topical anesthetic (e.g., EMLA Cream, AstraZeneca LP, Wilmington, Del) may be applied to the skin prior to administration of injectable local anesthesia to diminish pain at the injection site. However, as this requires pre-identification of the specific needle entry site and placement of the topical agent up to 1 hour prior to biopsy, this process results in significant lengthening of the procedure time, and should be reserved for patients who otherwise refuse the procedure or have a debilitating aversion to pain. Other methods are available to minimize the pain that accompanies injection of local anesthetic. A 25 gauge needle or smaller should be used for injection. The agent should be kept at room temperature. The skin may be cooled with ice or a quick spray of liquid nitrogen just before injection. Sodium bicarbonate (8.4%), when admixed with lidocaine in a dose of 1:9 parts bicarbonate-to-lidocaine, is very effective in correcting for the acidic nature of the agent, and thus minimizing the sting of the injection.

The local anesthetic agent can be applied along the entire expected route of the needle. It should be used most liberally at the needle entry site and around the accessible margin of the biopsy target, as these represent the sites of greatest pain, especially if the target is truly a cancer. Optimal skin numbing is provided when the anesthetic is instilled intradermally and, less importantly, subcutaneously. The raising of a generous skin wheal ensures good anesthesia over a large enough area to allow for a generous dermatotomy, as needed. Care should be taken to *backdraw* (apply negative pressure to) the syringe plunger prior to injection to minimize the possibility of intravascular administration.

Some physicians favor the addition of epinephrine 1:100,000 to 1:200,000 to the local anesthetic agent to prolong the duration of numbing and to aid in peri-lesion hemostasis, related to its vasoconstrictive properties. If used, a waiting period of about 5 minutes after injection will maximize its effectiveness. The patient may experience a sense of anxiety or the onset of temporary palpitations with its use, however, and should be warned ahead of time about this possibility. This solution can be purchased as a pre-mixed preparation.

The exact injection site will occur along an imaginary line paralleling the long axis of the transducer, at a variable distance from transducer, depending on the angle of approach to be taken. If a relatively steep angle of approach is expected, or for superficial targets, the site will be close to the transducer. As a more parallel-to-chest-wall approach is sought, the chosen entry site will migrate from the transducer (Fig. 29-8). The anesthetic needle is placed and the dermis and epidermis are numbed, creating a skin wheal. As deeper anesthetic is injected, the anesthetic needle position and course can be imaged in real time, allowing confirmation that an appropriate approach has been selected, a kind of test run. If not, either the entry site can be modified or compensatory techniques can be anticipated once the biopsy needle is placed. If the small gauge numbing needle does not reach the lesion, a spinal needle can be placed, for deeper anesthetic application.

After local anesthesia is achieved, the biopsy needle/device can be placed. Depending on the device being used, a dermatotomy can be performed with a scalpel. In general, these small (3-5 mm) skin nicks heal completely and are helpful in allowing unimpeded needle motion. They may prevent the need for an initial thrust to gain skin entry, preventing uncontrolled and unintended needle motion.

The choice of whether or not to use a coaxial system depends in part on personal choice and the needle system selected. Introducers allow easier reintroduction of the needle when using a device that requires needle removal for core retrieval. The introducer remains pointed at the biopsy site and the needle can quickly be replaced without need for significant retargeting. However, with each pass, a small amount of air is introduced with the needle, sometimes resulting in significant ring-down artifact, obscuring or partially obscuring the needle (Fig. 29-9). Slight parallel shifting of needle position can usually correct this.

Continuous real-time scanning should be performed during needle/introducer placement. Attempts should be made to identify the needle as soon as possible once it enters the breast. If the physician has chosen a long route to the lesion by necessity, the needle may not initially be in the field of the transducer. If there is a question as to whether an appropriate course or angle is being used, the transducer can be slid from the lesion toward the entry

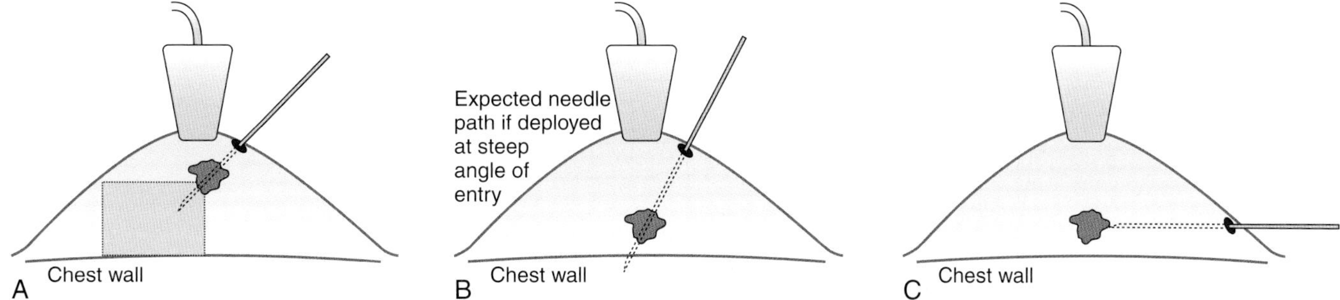

■ **FIGURE 29-8** A, For relatively superficial lesions, a steep needle approach allows needle entry adjacent to transducer. Care should be taken to examine the tissue beyond the lesion along the expected post-fire needle excursion to ensure that chest wall is not within reach (shaded area). **B**, If too steep an approach is taken with deep lesions, the risk of chest wall penetration occurs. **C**, When deep lesions are encountered, adjusting the skin entry site away from the transducer allows a parallel-to-chest-wall approach.

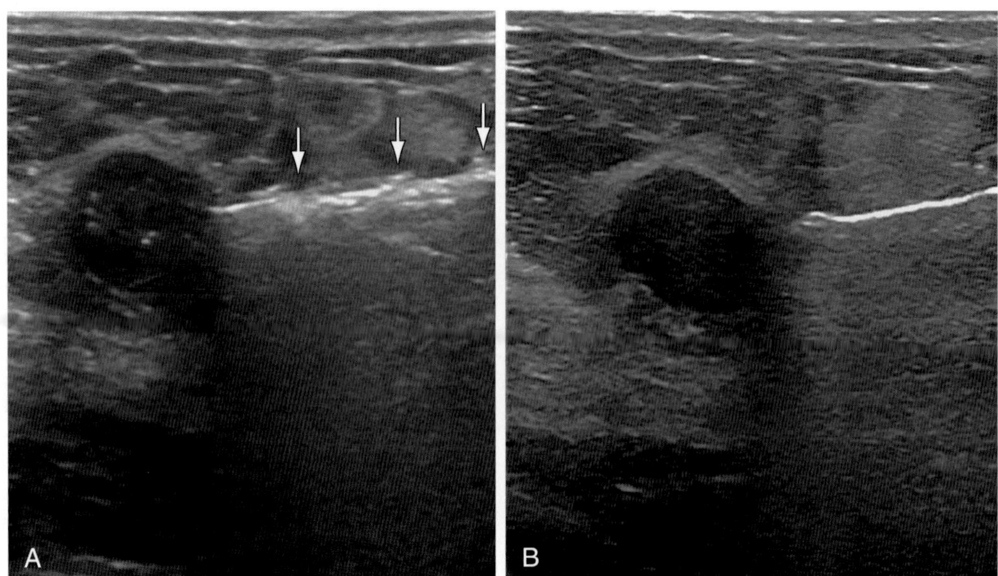

■ **FIGURE 29-9** Ultrasound images show how use of coaxial technique can result in the introduction of a small amount of air along the needle tract, causing obscuration of segments of the introducer (*arrows*) (**A**). This usually can be remedied by parallel shifting the coaxial device a few millimeters either way (**B**).

site along the expected course of the needle to intercept it. As needle progress is made, the transducer can be returned toward the lesion location, paired with the needle. It is imperative to know where the tip of the needle is at all times, thereby precluding the possibility of inadvertent puncture of an unintended structure (i.e., the chest wall). This can be guaranteed by consistently visualizing the uninterrupted embedded needle. If only segments of the shaft are seen, one cannot be sure what portion of the needle is being outlined and where the needle tip actually is. If the transducer and the needle maintain the same longitudinal axis, complete needle visualization is ensured. The first requirement is that the short end of the transducer remain "pointed at" the skin entry site. If change in transducer position is needed, it can be rotated like the hands on a clock, where the center of the clock is represented by the needle puncture site (Fig. 29-10). With a springloaded device, the needle/introducer is advanced until it reaches the edge of biopsy target. The operator should be sure that there is adequate tissue beyond the lesion along the needle trajectory to ensure safe firing, especially if the needle path is angled to posterior. An image should be obtained at this point to document accurate pre-fire placement (Fig. 29-11A). If an introducer is being used, the stylet is removed, and the needle is advanced until it reaches the end of the introducer. In either case, once the needle is pointed at the lesion, and is visualized in its entirety, the needle can be fired into the target for the first pass. An image should be taken of the needle traversing the lesion on this and all subsequent passes (Fig 29-11B). Annotation should be made on the image, numbering the individual passes for documentation. If a vacuum-assisted device is used, the probe should be positioned along the posterior/deep margin of the lesion in most cases. Once the sampling notch is exposed, care should be taken to ensure that the lesion in question lies within the confines of the notch; when it does, sampling may commence. The goal of the procedure is obviously to obtain enough tissue to verify a pathologic diagnosis but cause as little discomfort and chance of complication as possible; in short, to get just the right amount

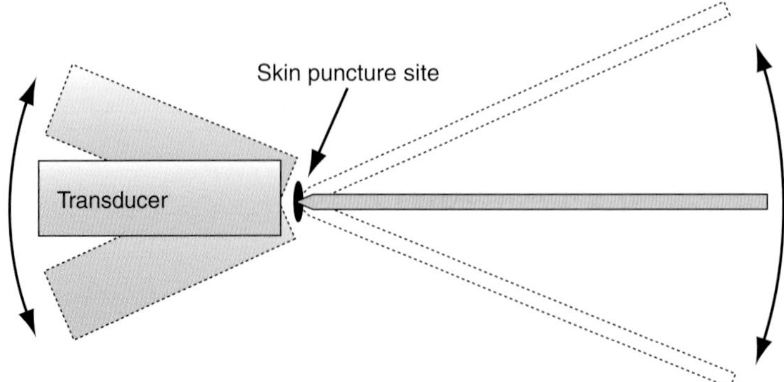

■ **FIGURE 29-10** If readjustment of transducer or needle position is required during ultrasound-guided biopsy, the transducer should be rotated radially around the skin entry site to ensure that the needle or probe can continue to be imaged along its entire long axis.

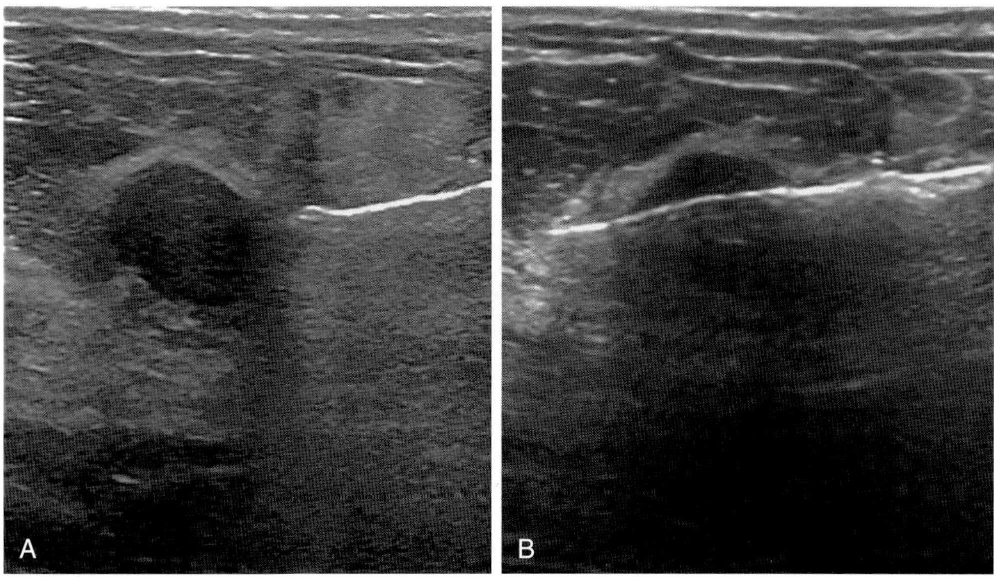

■ **FIGURE 29-11** Optimal needle positioning for ultrasound-guided core biopsy using an automated needle. The tip of the needle and/or introducer should be placed proximal to lesion (**A**), directed as parallel to chest wall as possible, with needle visualized along its entire long axis. Real-time imaging during and after sampling verifies that needle fires into the lesion (**B**), and should be documented with a post-fire image.

of tissue. Toward this end, attention should be paid to the quality of cores being obtained and the appearance of the lesion. If a springloaded or hybrid device is being used (where specimens are visualized between passes): Are the cores sinking rather than floating in preservative? Are they intact and firm rather than fragmented? Can air tracts be seen within the lesion between passes, confirming needle entry? (Fig. 29-12.) For vacuum-assisted devices, if the target lies in the notch at the start of sampling, high quality samples can be safely assumed. However, observing the lesion getting smaller as sampling progresses provides added confidence (Fig. 29-13).

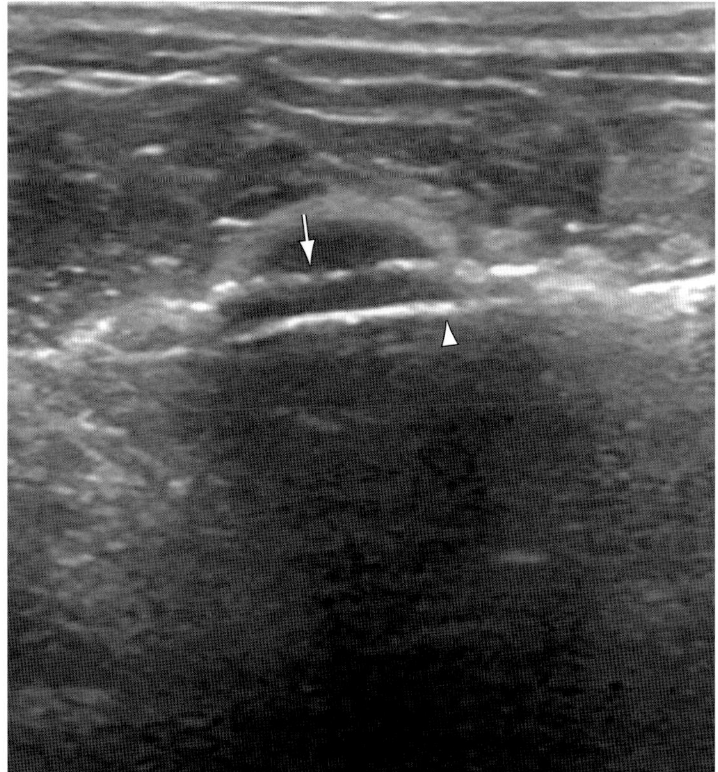

■ **FIGURE 29-12** Ultrasound image shows hyperechoic linear air tract (*arrow*) within mass, left by automated needle on prior pass, confirming accurate sampling. The needle can be seen penetrating the mass on the current pass (*arrowhead*), just posterior to the air tract.

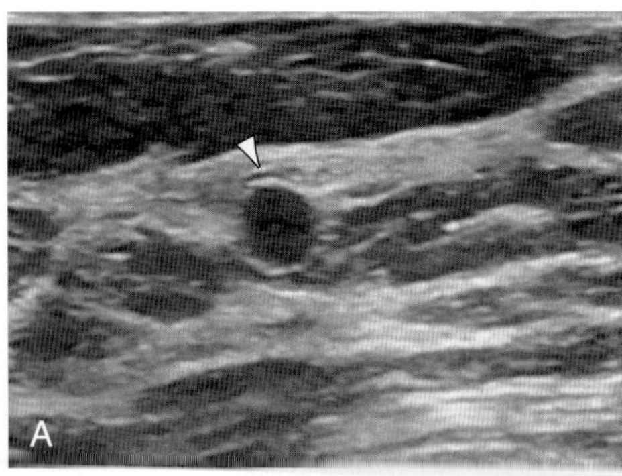

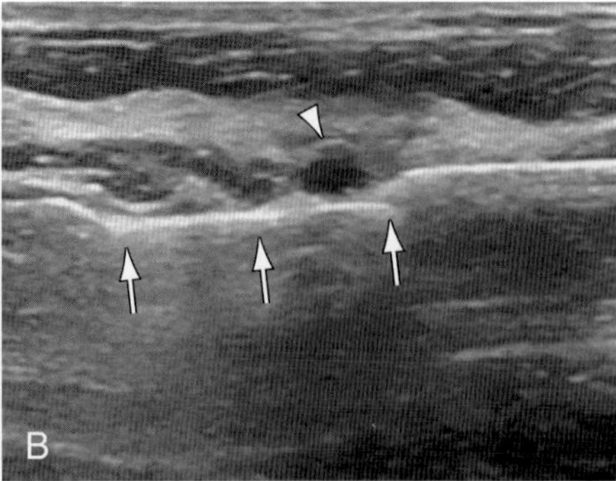

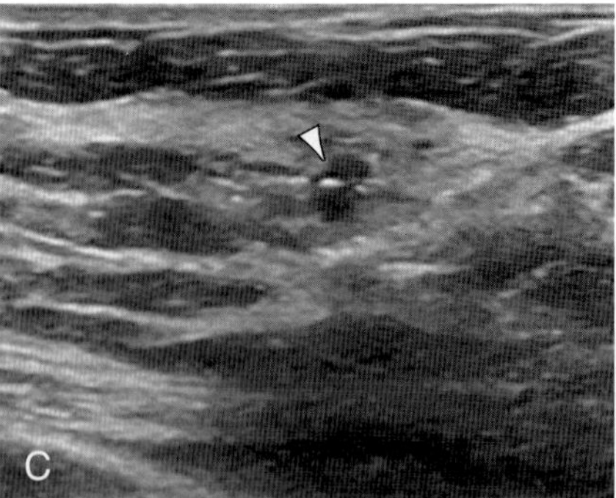

■ **FIGURE 29-13** Ultrasound image shows confirmation of sampling adequacy when using vacuum-assisted device. **A,** Solid mass (*arrowhead*) targeted for percutaneous biopsy. **B,** Mass (*arrowhead*) clearly seen in sampling notch of biopsy probe (*arrows*). **C,** Mass (*arrowhead*) is noted to be smaller post-procedure, suggesting sampling adequacy.

Once the operator is confident that adequate tissue has been retrieved, a marking clip should be placed directly in the lesion. If the clip is placed adjacent to (but on the same horizontal plane with the patient lying supine) rather than in the lesion, it will likely remain in relative close contiguity to the actual lesion. However, if the clip is inadvertently placed anterior or posterior to the site, it will likely end up lying quite far remote, as breast tissue "un-accordions" when the patient sits up. Marking devices come in many shapes and varieties, some consisting of simply a small titanium clip, which may be hard to detect at ultrasound. Others consist of a clip encased in other material (e.g., a collagen plug) that is subsequently absorbed and allows greater sonographic visibility. All clips are radiopaque on mammography and cause a small signal void on breast MRI. A post-procedure mammogram performed in orthogonal (craniocaudal and either mediolateral or lateromedial) projections confirms clip deployment and its accurate position. Some practitioners question whether a clip needs to be placed in all cases. Clip placement allows confirmation that the lesion that underwent biopsy was, indeed, the intended target, assuming it was initially detected on mammogram. It ensures that the lesion can be localized if surgical excision is mandated. Many patients with breast cancer now undergo neoadjuvant chemotherapy prior to surgical treatment; the presence of a clip ensures that a target for excision remains visible, even if the patient has a complete imaging response to therapy. Even in the case of a benign core biopsy result, the presence of a clip can assure future imagers that that particular site has been previously subjected to biopsy and may negate the need for additional intervention. In short, there are many compelling reasons to place a clip at the time of percutaneous biopsy. Practitioners who virtually always place a clip usually do not regret having done it. However, it adds cost to the procedure. Some patients are uncomfortable with the concept of having a clip in their breast; once educated about the nature and purpose of the clip, they usually can be persuaded to allow it. The intention to leave a clip should be included in the informed consent process. On occasion clip migration occurs, either due to inaccurate initial deployment or related to hematoma formation, and may cause confusion about the actual lesion location. Post-procedure mammograms should be closely correlated to pre-biopsy films, if the target was seen mammographically. Re-scanning the patient may allow confirmation of clip location relative to the lesion. If the clip lies a remote distance from its target, another should be placed accurately, preferably using a different clip type or shape.

Some lesions require a special approach. Deep lesions may be difficult to reach, especially if they lie near the chest wall. A remote skin entry site can be used to allow a horizontal needle or introducer path, but this requires traversing a large distance of tissue, and may be limited by device length. Another approach is to use a standard entry site, initially aim the needle at a steep angle toward the lesion and then, as the needle nears the target, torque the needle or introducer angle such that it approaches horizontal (Fig. 29-14). Targets that lie directly on pectoralis muscle or on an implant may be elevated away from those structures by instilling a volume of local anesthetic or sterile saline under them, thereby creating a safety zone. This technique can be used with very superficial lesions as well, especially when a vacuum-assisted device is being used and there is concern for inadvertent skin sampling (Fig. 29-15). Fluid is instilled between lesion and overlying skin. Additionally in such a case, the vacuum-assisted device can be placed anterior or superficial to the target and inverted, such that the notch is pointed deep, thereby precluding sampling of skin. When the location of the lesion requires a steep approach angle, the needle may be difficult to outline sonographically, given the angle of incidence of the acoustical beam. This can be corrected by either altering the needle angle or by angling the transducer face so that the perpendicular orientation of the acoustic beam and the needle shaft is re-established to as great a degree as possible (Fig. 29-16).

On occasion, the degree of breast density makes needle and/or introducer advancement very difficult. In these cases, instillation of local anesthetic through this tissue with a spinal needle may loosen it up enough to allow the biopsy needle or probe to be placed. Another technique is to use a springloaded device and an introducer. The introducer is advanced as far as possible. The automated gun is placed via the introducer and fired into the dense tissue, and the introducer then advanced over it, similar to a Seldinger technique. The introducer will thus have been advanced the length of the needle throw. This process can be repeated until the introducer has reached the actual biopsy target.

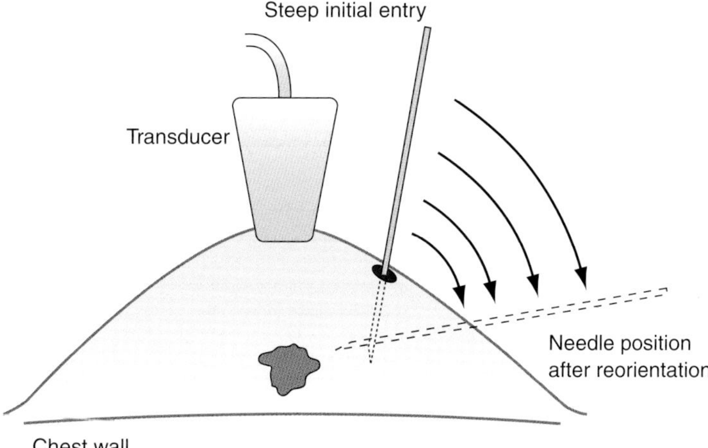

■ **FIGURE 29-14** Needle reorientation to maintain a horizontal needle course. In order to allow a parallel-to-chest wall needle throw, the needle may be placed via a steep initial approach, with entry site near transducer, then re-angled toward horizontal.

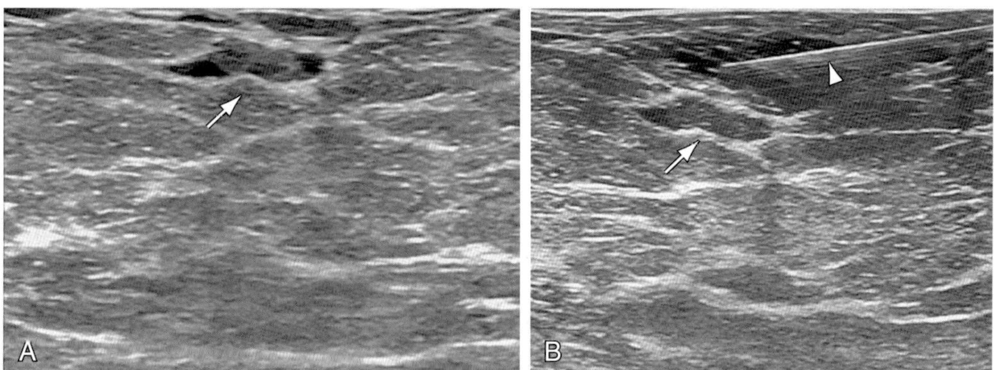

■ **FIGURE 29-15** Ultrasound images illustrate creating a safe zone when lesion is near skin. If target of biopsy lies too close to the skin to allow biopsy, especially when a vacuum-assisted device is being employed, the distance from lesion to skin can be increased by instillation of local anesthetic or saline between the two structures. **A,** Intraductal mass (*arrow*) lies within a few millimeters of skin. **B,** 25-Gauge needle (*arrowhead*) is used to inject lidocaine between the mass and overlying skin. This method can be used to increase distance between a deep lesion and chest wall, as well.

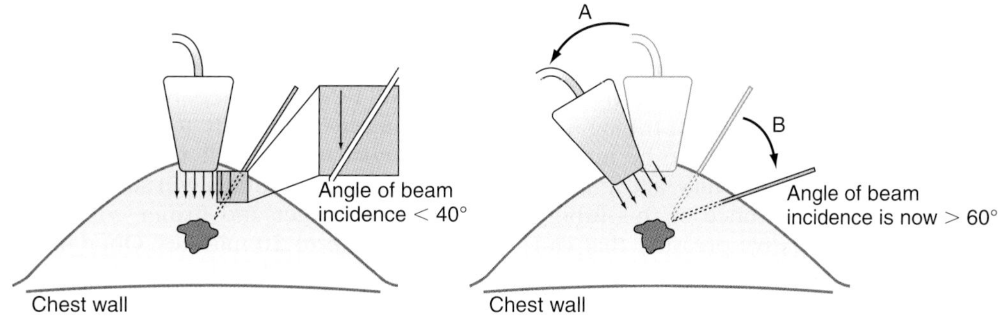

■ **FIGURE 29-16** Difficulty in sonographic needle visualization with steep needle entry. When steep needle entry is used, the acute angle of incidence of the ultrasound beam can result in poor visualization of the needle shaft (**A**). Alteration of the transducer or the needle orientation results in an increase in the beam angle of incidence toward 90 degrees, optimizing visualization (**B**).

When biopsying small targets with an automated system, it should be remembered that only a portion of the thrown needle represents the sampling notch and that it is possible that if the needle tip has been placed directly at the edge of the lesion in pre-fire position, the notch may actually lie beyond the lesion when fired. In these cases, some passes should be made with the needle positioned proximal to the lesion so that it can confidently be expected to lie in the notch when the needle is deployed (Fig. 29-17). With large lesions, it is a good idea to vary

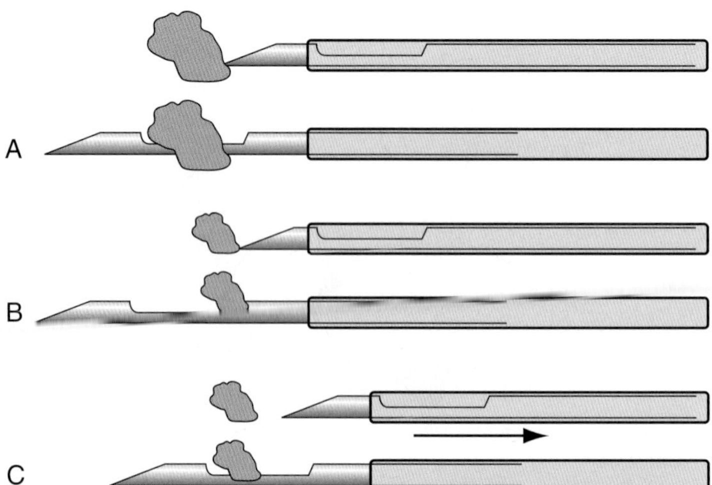

■ **FIGURE 29-17** Optimal needle placement. For moderate to large masses, the automated device may be placed at lesion edge (**A**). However, for small masses, placement directly at the lesion edge may cause the inadequate sampling, due to throw of the sampling notch beyond the mass (**B**). In such cases, the needle may be placed short of the lesion, such that upon firing, the mass is centered within the notch (**C**).

needle position during the biopsy to ensure that the various components of the lesion have been sampled. If a mass appears necrotic, cores from the periphery of the lesion must be obtained to ensure that viable tissue is included in the submitted material.

Cyst Aspiration

In general, simple cysts can be safely dismissed as BI-RADS 2—benign lesions that do not require intervention. However, occasionally aspiration is indicated, possibly only for symptomatic relief and not for the purpose of obtaining a tissue diagnosis. As a result, core biopsy is not needed and a standard hypodermic needle (18-25 gauge) is perfectly appropriate. Because this needle will be placed in and not beyond the cyst, the shortest possible route to the cyst can be taken without concern for angle of approach. As described earlier, if a steep angle is used, however, needle visualization may be impeded, and either alteration of the needle or transducer angle may be required. Once the cyst is entered, its contents can be aspirated, either via a syringe attached directly to the needle or with intervening extension tubing. The inclusion of this tubing allows the needle to be maneuvered separately from the syringe and may allow more delicate steering. However, the presence of this tubing does decrease the amount of negative pressure that can be delivered to the needle, sometimes important when a cyst with inspissated contents is encountered. When such a cyst cannot be completely evacuated, a larger needle may be required, or even subsequent core biopsy to ensure that a complex mass rather than a complicated cyst is not the target of biopsy.

If the cyst is completely collapsed upon aspiration, and yields non-hemorrhagic fluid, the fluid can be discarded, the patient reassured that the finding was a benign cyst and returned to routine follow-up. If suspicious fluid (bloody or mucinous) is aspirated, or if the cyst is not able to be fully emptied, the fluid should be sent for cytologic evaluation. In these cases, it is imperative that a marking clip be placed at the site so that it can be found again if needed. The operator does not want to experience aspirating a cyst to completion, sending the fluid for evaluation and have it return as atypical or malignant only to realize that the target may be difficult or impossible to confidently relocate.

If the aspiration has been performed to ensure that a patient or physician-identified palpable mass correlates to a sonographically-identified cyst and not an imaging-occult malignancy, the patient and/or referring physician should re-examine area of clinical concern as soon after aspiration as possible, so that the absence or persistence of the physical finding can be confirmed. If the aspiration has been performed to ensure concordance between a mammographic mass and the cyst in question, a post-procedure mammogram should be obtained to prove that the mammographic mass is gone.

Post-Procedure Considerations

After the biopsy device has been removed, pressure can be applied manually to the breast by the physician, technologist or assistant for several minutes. For most patients, 5 to 10 minutes will suffice; if the patient is anticoagulated, longer and firmer compression is required, sometimes up to 20 minutes. Once hemostasis has been achieved, a sterile dressing can be applied to the wound. The patient is instructed in post-procedure wound care, informed about what events are normal post-biopsy sequelae (minor pain and bruising) and what constitute cause for concern (signs of infection, an expanding hematoma, shortness of breath). She should be told what to do in case of a problem, and given contact numbers. All these instructions should be given to her in written form, as well. In addition, the patient should be informed about how she will receive her biopsy results, and when. At this point, a post-procedure mammogram can be obtained if needed.

The obtained core samples should be placed in preservative. If a specimen radiograph is to be obtained (to confirm the presence of suspected calcifications), the samples may be placed on a Petri dish or other appropriate vessel, radiographed, and then placed in preservative. While a technologist or assistant may aid in packaging the specimen for transport and delivery to pathology, it is ultimately the responsibility of the practitioner to ensure that the specimen container is accurately labeled, and that a pathology requisition form is filled out with appropriate history and the specifics of the specimen's source. If the patient has had biopsy from more than one site, the specimens should be very specifically labeled as to the location of the respective biopsy sites (e.g., "Specimen #1: left breast, 2:00, 3 cm/nipple; Specimen #2: left breast 4:00, 5 cm/nipple"). When calcifications are expected or known to be a component of the lesion, the pathologist should be cued to search for them, with specific instructions on the pathology request. If the patient has prior radiation therapy to the affected breast, that information should be noted on the requisition, because post-radiation atypia may prove difficult to differentiate from ductal carcinoma in situ (DCIS) or other atypia,[16] but obviously has markedly different management implications. Similarly, if the patient has been undergoing neoadjuvant chemotherapy, this should be noted on the pathology request.

A written permanent procedure report should be constructed that outlines the nature, side, and location of each biopsy target, the type of device used for core biopsy, the number of samples obtained, whether a marking clip was placed, the location of the clip relative to the target, if a post-procedure mammogram was obtained, and any complications that were encountered during the procedure. This report should subsequently be amended when the pathology results are returned, with concordance or discordance noted, and further appropriate management or follow-up recommendations outlined. When the pathology results are returned, the case should be reviewed in its entirety, including perusal of all recent imaging performed. Concordance between initial imaging and the final pathology results can be assessed. If discordant results are returned, arrangements should be made for additional tissue sampling, either by repeat CNB or by excision. Additionally, the physician can make sure that additional areas do not now require further intervention, based on the newly available pathologic information. For example, if malignancy is confirmed, consideration may be now given to pursuing biopsy of another area previously deemed a BI-RADS 3 lesion. A well-defined policy should be in place outlining how the patient will be informed of her results. The policy must ensure that no patient will remain unapprised of her diagnosis, and this is likely best achieved when the biopsying physician (or delegate) takes responsibility for the task. In this way, it will never be simply assumed that the referring physician has conveyed the results. The patient may be informed of the results in person (via an additional office visit) or by telephone. If malignancy has been found, arrangements can be made for referral to other members of the breast cancer treatment team (surgical oncology, medical oncology) as indicated. If benign results are returned, the recommended follow-up can be outlined to the patient. If an atypical or discordant diagnosis has been rendered, discussion can be made with the patient about the need for further intervention. The conveyance of results and recommendations should be documented, preferably as an addendum to the formal biopsy report.

Indications

Due to patient comfort, cost, lack of ionizing radiation, and speed of procedure, ultrasound should be the guidance modality of choice for any lesion confidently seen sonographically. This would include any BI-RADS 4—suspicious or 5—highly suspicious lesion for which biopsy has been recommended. Although BI-RADS 3—probably benign findings are suitable for short-term follow up rather than biopsy, in some cases, core of the lesions may be preferred instead. Some examples would include patients who have a highly suspicious lesion elsewhere in either breast, those with a known synchronous breast cancer where management may be altered by the presence another cancer, patients who are undergoing fertility treatment or anticipate getting pregnant in the near future, those with a strong family history, and those for whom the anxiety of short-term follow-up outweighs the benefit of avoiding biopsy.

If multiple suspicious findings are present, biopsy of as many targets as needed to outline the full extent of malignant disease and direct appropriate future management should be carried out. For example, if five small suspicious masses are present in one breast, core of at least two of these should be performed, preferably those lying at the greatest distance from each other, to fully establish extent of disease and help determine the need for mastectomy versus breast conserving surgery. However, biopsy of all five masses is probably not needed.

If suspicious axillary, supra- or infraclavicular, or internal mammary chain lymph nodes have been identified during diagnostic workup in a patient with a suspicious breast finding, these, too, can be targeted for biopsy, with the understanding that a positive result confirms nodal spread but that a negative result by no means excludes nodal metastases. This can be performed using CNB technique, or if there is concern for adjacent structures, with fine-needle aspiration cytology (FNAC). Most sonographic targets consist of masses or areas of reproducible shadowing. Suspicious calcifications are usually biopsied with stereotactic guidance. However, with the high-frequency transducers used today, calcifications can often be confidently identified sonographically, and targeted for core biopsy. This is especially true if there is an associated mass, in which case biopsy with sonographic rather than stereotactic guidance may actually help allow core of the highest-stage portion of the lesion (e.g., invasive tumor rather than just DCIS). Specimen radiography should be obtained in cases where calcifications are expected to be part of the lesion.

If ultrasound guidance is being used to biopsy a lesion discovered by another modality (mammography, MRI, or positron emission tomography [PET]), great care must be taken to ensure that the sonographic lesion indeed represents the finding seen on the other imaging technique. This requires a good working knowledge of the other modality, the ability to translate expected lesion position from one modality to another, meticulous radiologic-pathologic correlation when the results are returned, and the knowledge to obtain imaging follow-up either immediately post-biopsy or in a delayed manner, or even rebiopsy, as needed. Identifying surrogate sonographic targets for findings seen with other modalities, especially MRI, can be especially challenging. If there is any question as to whether an accurate correlate has been chosen, biopsy should probably proceed guided by the modality that originally found the lesion. Image-guided biopsies, in general, are best performed by a physician with the above-described knowledge and skill set who, in most cases, is a radiologist.

Contraindications

Few contraindications to US-guided CNB exist. Biopsy should not be performed on a patient who has no intention of seeking treatment if a cancer is diagnosed, due to co-morbid conditions or other reasons. Anticoagulation has traditionally been considered a relative contraindication for core biopsy, with the patient asked to cease therapy prior to biopsy if possible. However, recent literature suggests no significant difference in hematoma rate between anticoagulated and nonanticoagulated patients (on either warfarin or nonsteroidal anti-inflammatory products).[17] In implant patients, if rupture appears unavoidable, core biopsy should be avoided; however, with careful planning, this should be a rare situation. The potential for implant rupture should be clearly delineated to the patient during the consenting process.

Potential Complications of Ultrasound-Guided Core Biopsy

Complications during US-guided CNB are relatively rare but potentially include: hematoma formation, infection, pneumothorax, allergic reaction to local anesthetic, and vagal reaction. A small amount of bleeding is not unusual during core biopsy but occasionally, needle transection of a vessel can result in more profuse bleeding. This is most certainly not a life-threatening event but can result in hematoma formation. The ultimate size of the hematoma can be minimized by firm compression over the area at the end of the procedure, to include the segment of breast from needle entry site to lesion. If a springloaded needle is being used, transducer pressure can be applied between passes to staunch potential bleeding. If it occurs early in the procedure or is arterial in origin, the bleeding can result in target obscuration. When it is apparent that this is occurring as real-time scanning proceeds, the transducer should be maintained in vigilant position over the target and a clip placed as quickly and accurately as possible so the lesion can be identified for re-biopsy or excision, if needed.

If sterile technique is respected, infection should be rare. Using some needle set-ups (e.g., reusable needle holders), the procedure at some point becomes *clean* rather than *sterile*; however, if sterility of the needle and skin is maintained, the expectation of a germ-free environment can be achieved. If infection is reported by the patient, she should be asked to come in so that the radiologist can inspect the wound, ensure that abscess is not a possibility, and assess whether the infection is not simply a reaction to tape or bandage material. If infection is confirmed, the physician can choose to prescribe antibiotics as appropriate, and arrange to see the patient in follow-up.

Vagal reactions (bradycardia with hypotension) are not uncommon during breast procedures, but occur relatively less often during US-guided CNB, in part owing to the patient's supine positioning for the procedure. The vast majority of vagal reactions respond immediately to simple conservative treatment: elevation of patient's feet/placement in Trendelenburg position, squeezing of calf muscles to restore blood return to head, application of a cool cloth to neck or forehead, and calm reassurance. Oxygen may be administered but is rarely required. As she recovers, the patient should be warned that she will soon experience the onset of shaking, as release of epinephrine by her system occurs. If the patient does not respond to these conservative measures, an IV may started and consideration given to pharmacologic support (atropine). Allergic or anaphylactoid reactions must be recognized and treated promptly. In the rare case of suspected pneumothorax, a chest x-ray film can be obtained and further treatment as needed pursued. With these latter types of more complicated or severe events, the biopsying physician has the ultimate responsibility for patient outcome. As a result, it is the obligation of any physician taking on the privilege of performing such procedures to also assume the responsibility of knowing how to manage minor complications, including a working knowledge of the medications and interventions involved. However, ultimately the best interest of the patient is paramount, and if the biopsying physician needs assistance in an acute situation, help should be sought promptly, up to and including sending the patient to the emergency room or calling a "code."

Epithelial displacement of tumor cells along the percutaneous needle tract has been discussed as a potential risk of core biopsy. Seeding of the tract does appear to occur, in an estimated 22% of cases. However, a systematic review of the available literature by Liebens and associates did not show evidence of increased local recurrence rate in patients undergoing pre-operative diagnosis via percutaneous biopsy who subsequently underwent conservative therapy and radiation, or increased morbidity in patients who had core biopsy of malignant lesions.[18]

STEREOTACTIC-GUIDED PERCUTANEOUS BREAST BIOPSY

The accuracy and cost-effectiveness of stereotactic-guided vacuum-assisted core biopsy have been well validated in the literature. A multicenter study of 2874 patients showed only 1 false negative result (negative predictive value of 99.50%) in the study population.[19] Other authors confirmed a high degree of accuracy, especially after an initial learning curve, with a 0.6% false negative biopsy rate achieved after performing more than 15 cases.[20] In addition, cost-effectiveness of the technique has been demonstrated, allowing deferral of surgical intervention in 76% of cases and decreasing the cost/diagnosis by 20% versus surgical biopsy.[21]

Description, Equipment and Technique

Stereotactic assistance for needle placement allows for localization of a target in *three* dimensions, while using only *two* dimensional images for guidance, exploiting the geometry of parallax shift. For example, when performing a traditional needle localization procedure, the lesion can be easily targeted in the x and y planes by simply obtaining a mammographic image with an alpha-numeric grid superimposed on the region of breast in question: a needle can be inserted perpendicular to the skin surface with every expectation that the lesion will be "skewered." However, the depth of the lesion relative to the needle tip remains unknown, and an orthogonal image is required to determine their relative positions. While this is acceptable for a localization procedure, it is not feasible to accurately place a needle for percutaneous biopsy in such a manner. Stereotactic technique allows that third plane, the exact depth of the lesion, or its z axis position, to be determined without obtaining the disruptive orthogonal view. This is achieved by obtaining a standard scout image (x-ray beam direction perpendicular to the detector) and 2 subsequent *swing views*, in which the beam is angled plus and minus 15 degrees off perpendicular. On these two images, the target lesion will appear to shift away from its original position on the scout view, along the same axis in which the x-ray arm is swung (the x axis). The target will shift in an amount that is proportional to its distance from the detector (parallax shift). Lesions that lie in the portion of the compressed breast close to the detector will "shift" in position less than those lying more distant from the detector and closer to the x-ray source (Fig. 29-18). Many of variables required to locate a point in space are known (the beam angulation, the distance from source to detector, the amount of apparent lesion shift on the swing views), and can be conveyed to a computer by placing a cursor on the lesion in both angled views. The z position, or depth, of the target can be easily computed and its location in all three dimensions of space accurately determined.

Equipment

Two broad categories of stereotactic units are available: the dedicated prone unit and the nondedicated add-on unit, with which the patient may be positioned sitting upright or in the lateral decubitus position. Originally, some units used screen-film images, requiring significant delays during the procedure while awaiting film development. Now, digital image acquisition is the rule. Most centers use a dedicated prone table, where the patient is positioned prone and the breast undergoing biopsy is placed dependently through an opening in the table. The table is raised, allowing the physician access to the breast while comfortably seated. This approach has many advantages, including a relatively unencumbered workspace for the physician and a virtual barrier of sorts between the patient and the biopsy site, such that she does not see the procedure as it unfolds (Fig. 29-19). Because she lies horizontal in position, vagal episodes are unusual. However, this prone unit requires significant capital outlay and dedication of a procedure room for the single use of stereotactic core biopsy. Prone positioning may be difficult for some patients, especially those with kyphosis. Some far-posteriorly situated lesions may prove inaccessible with the prone tables. If the breast is too small in compressed thickness, the biopsy may not be possible.

Add-on units are used less commonly and at first glance may seem "user-unfriendly" but offer some advantages. These units may serve as regular mammogram machines and can be up-fitted with the add-on stereotactic device when needed to perform a biopsy. They can be configured

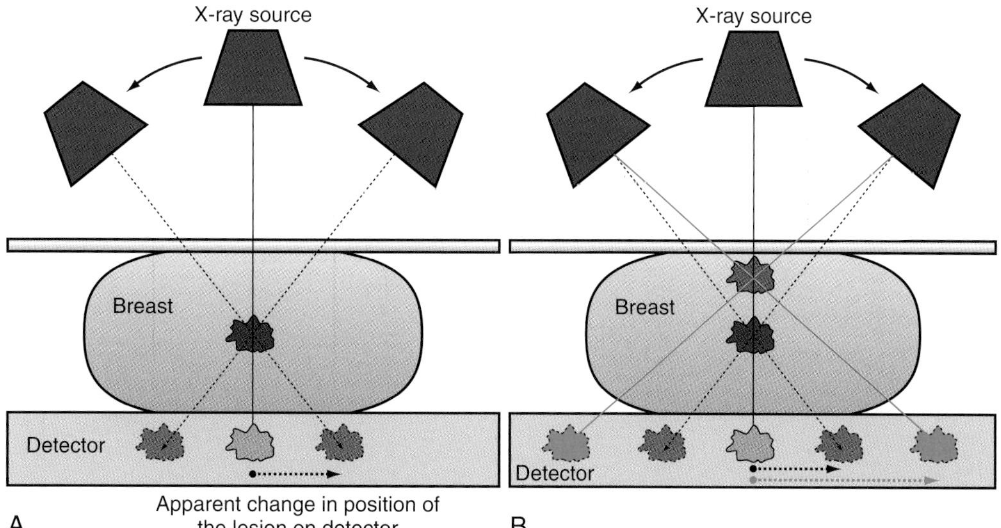

■ **FIGURE 29-18** Schematic representation of the concept of stereotaxis. Whereas a lesion will project on the detector directly under its location in the breast on images obtained with the beam perpendicular to the plate, its position will appear to migrate when imaged with angled views (**A**). The degree of "migration" (or parallax shift) will depend on how close or far the lesion lies from the detector (**B**). When its apparent location on each angled view is conveyed to the computer by cursor placement at the workstation, the z-axis position of the biopsy target can be calculated.

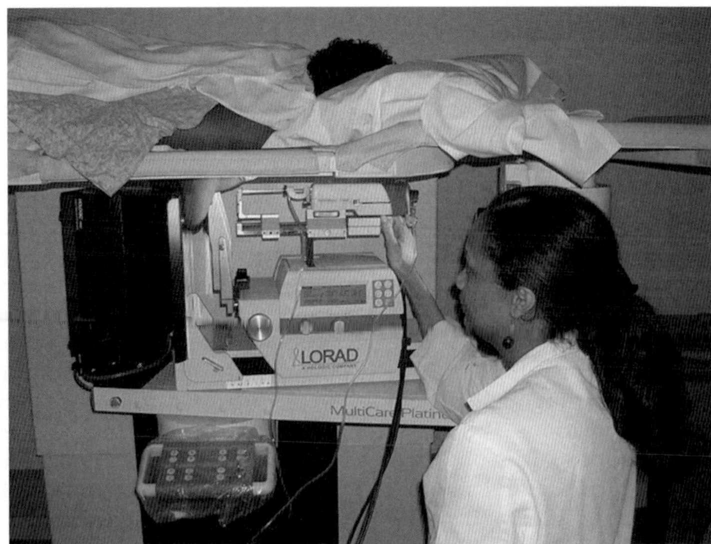

■ **FIGURE 29-19** Prone stereotactic breast table. The dedicated prone table allows the physician unfettered access to the breast, while providing a barrier between the patient and the biopsy procedure in progress.

in several ways. The needle may be positioned in the same manner as with prone technique (i.e., oriented parallel to the direction of the x-ray beam and perpendicular to compression paddle/detector) or via a sidearm needle holder, such that the needle is oriented parallel to the compression device (Fig. 29-20). Additionally, the patient may sit upright or may be positioned in the lateral decubitus position (Fig. 29-21). These add-on units are cheaper, can be used for routine mammographic imaging, and do not require a dedicated room. However, the process of converting the machine to its biopsy mode and performing required quality assurance testing may, in practice, be time-consuming enough to discourage use of the unit and room for routine mammography. Posterior lesions are commonly more accessible with the add-on unit compared with the prone table. Patients with most body habitus can be accommodated with the add-on unit, especially with decubitus positioning. The upright patient is more at risk for vagal reaction, especially as the procedure is carried out in her plain sight, as opposed to the prone table. The effective work area for the physician is diminished with the add-on unit compared with the prone table. All in all, either unit can be effective in obtaining high quality tissue samples. The pluses and minuses of each unit can be weighed in the context of any individual practice and a satisfactory decision achieved. Once the purchase is made, each practitioner will discover how to address any minor limitations the unit might present.

Although early stereotactic biopsies were carried out using automated biopsy needles, and even FNAC, vacuum-assisted directional biopsy devices, generally 11-gauge or larger, have become the standard choice. This is in part because of lack of real-time sampling verification, as occurs during US-guided CNB. In addition, as calcifications represent the most common target for stereotactic guidance, retrieving a large volume of tissue minimizes insufficiency rates and histologic upgrades. Because the needle is relatively fixed in position by a needle holder during the stereotactic sampling process as opposed to a US-guided CNB, where free-hand technique allows needle manipulation, the rotational/directional aspect of the vacuum-assisted device is vital in ensuring broad tissue sampling.

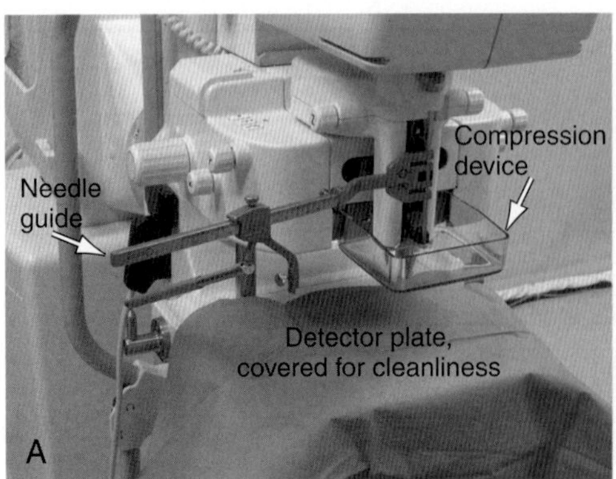

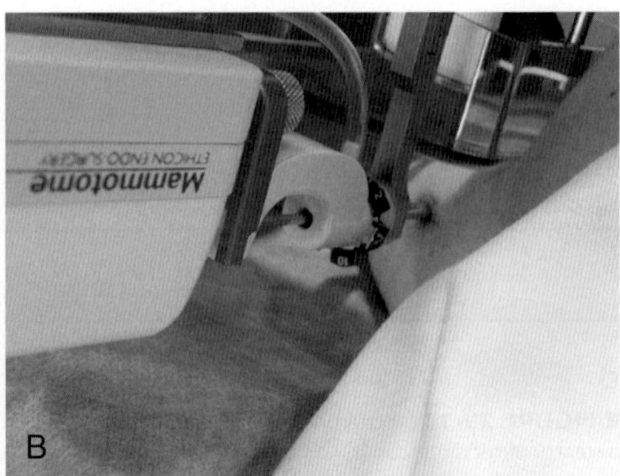

■ **FIGURE 29-20** Add-on stereotactic unit set-up with side arm needle guide (**A**). The needle guide holds the vacuum-assisted probe such that the needle enters the breast parallel to the detector and the plane of compression (**B**), rather than perpendicular, as occurs with a prone table.

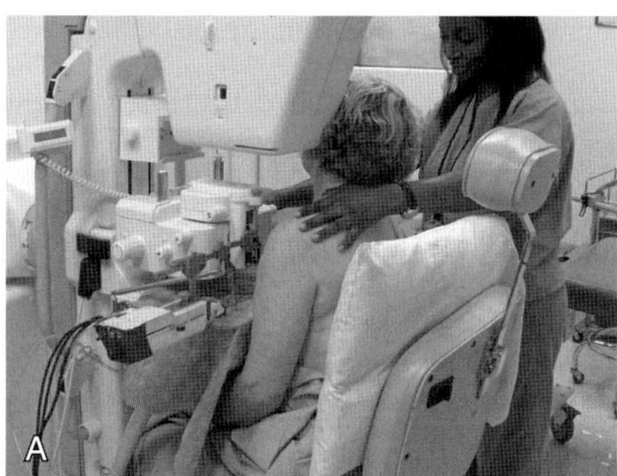
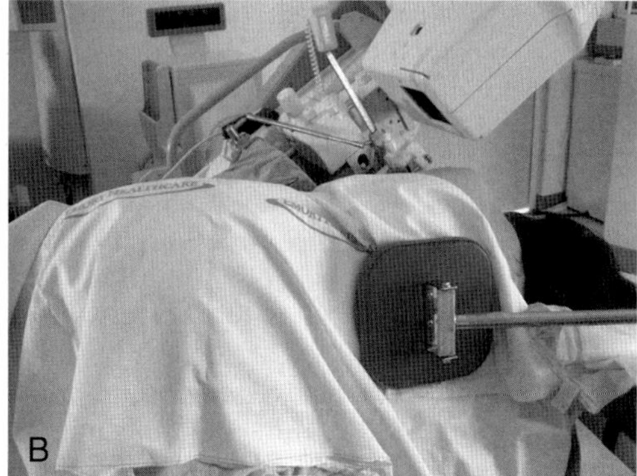

■ **FIGURE 29-21** Add-on stereotactic unit. The patient may sit upright (**A**) or lie in the lateral decubitus position (**B**). In both cases shown here, the left breast is being biopsied from a lateral approach, compressed in the craniocaudal position, relative to the patient (see Fig. 29-20B).

The device is placed using the coordinates calculated during the targeting portion of the procedure. Once accurate needle placement is confirmed by additional paired stereotactic images, with the target seen to lie adjacent to the needle, sampling can proceed. The vacuum pulls tissue into the recessed sampling notch, which lies on the side of the needle, and an inner cannula transects the tissue (see Fig. 29-3). This core is then delivered retrograde for retrieval, either by an assistant using forceps or into a closed chamber for later collection, depending on the device. The systems that require each sample to be collected individually by an assistant result in a slightly longer procedure time and greater risk of exposure to blood products. However, they provide the advantage of confirming that an adequate core was obtained during each pass. The vacuum-assisted biopsy process allows multiple contiguous samples to be taken during a single needle insertion, because the tissue is delivered externally while the needle remains poised for added cores.

As with US-guided percutaneous tissue sampling, stereotactic-guided core needle biopsies (SCNBs) must be performed in a private single-patient procedure room. In this way, informed consent may be obtained and the patient's history discussed without fear of a privacy breach. Additionally, any complications can be dealt with without alarming other patients. The room should be large enough to accommodate the physician, the technologist, the stereotactic unit, and, if possible, a few additional people (e.g., students or residents, and in rare cases, a family member). Temperature should be controlled such that patient is comfortable but not too warm. A sink should be available for hand-washing and other uses. Lockable drawers and cabinets that allow for the securing of supplies and all medications should be in place. A mobile procedure table that can be placed near the physician allows the biopsy to proceed efficiently.

Each center or each physician may construct a sterile procedure tray to individual specifications. However, when there are multiple practitioners within a single center, standardization of set-up and supplies promotes quick patient turnaround and cost savings, as the technologist can more efficiently prepare the trays and fewer supplies need to be stocked. A typical sterile set-up may include sterile gloves, antiseptic, sterile gauze, pre-drawn local anesthetic agent (clearly labeled as to exact content). Sterile forceps or "pick-ups" should be available to the technologist to retrieve the core samples from the device, if they are not transmitted automatically to a collection chamber. Pre-constructed trays can be purchased from many vendors, and the client can determine the specific contents. While these promote efficiency, they may prove more costly than simply making up the tray on-site. Once the standard set-up is prepared by the technologist or aide, the needle selected for biopsy may be individualized to physician or specific lesion type, and opened at the time of actual biopsy.

Technique

Pre-Procedural Considerations

Written informed consent is an obligate requisite to the procedure. Each center will likely have an organization-composed and approved consent form. Some sites use a general form for all types of procedures and surgeries performed at that institution that outlines all potential risks, up to and including death; others use procedure-specific consent forms that are tailored to the appropriate set of risks and complications. If the former is required by the institution, this should be explained to the patient, telling her that some of the potential risks and complications mentioned are not considered applicable to her situation. However, all consents should make mention of bleeding, infection, pneumothorax, allergic reaction to administered medications and, if appropriate, implant rupture as potential complications of the procedure. Additionally, the patient should be fully informed about the benefits of the biopsy (e.g., deferral of surgery in the face of benign specific results; pre-operative verification of malignancy, allowing definitive surgical therapy in one setting) as well as the potential drawbacks (possible need for re-biopsy or excision in the face of nonspecific, insufficient or discordant pathology results). She should be told about the use of a marking clip. In the optimal setting, this material, as well as a general description of what she can expect during the procedure and its aftermath, will have been discussed with the patient ahead of time by a physician, technologist, nurse or physician-extender, possibly at the time of her diagnostic workup or upon scheduling. However, the written informed consent should by obtained by the practitioner performing the biopsy, with a witness in attendance. For TJC-accredited facilities, compliance with Universal Protocol (to prevent wrong site, wrong procedure, wrong person mishaps) is mandated. This requires marking of the side of biopsy (right/left), and completion of a time-out just prior to beginning the procedure to verify identity of the patient, the site of the biopsy and the procedure to be performed. This takes place in the presence of the entire procedural team and the patient, all of whom must participate and be in agreement (see TJC policy for more detail at www.jointcommission.org). This process must be carried out by the physician or physician extender who is performing the procedure, not a surrogate (resident, nurse, technologist, other physician) and must be formally documented. Even if a facility is not subject to TJC accreditation, the process, when used in some form, can help prevent procedural errors. The patient should be queried directly by the physician about any allergies (including latex) as well as her medication history in regard to anticoagulation status. While biopsy can be pursued even in the face of anticoagulation (see discussion under "Contraindications"), knowledge of her coagulation status may alter post-procedure care (e.g., longer compression time, etc.).

The patient is positioned as comfortably as possible, since lack of motion is vital once the breast is compressed and the scout images are obtained. Any subsequent patient movement may result in inaccurate needle placement, as the calcifications will have moved. The biopsy needle approach is determined by reviewing the mammograms leading to the biopsy, and determining which projection provides the best visualization of the lesion and the shortest distance from the skin to the lesion. The breast is placed and compressed such that the target is expected to lie in the field of view of the scout image. With prone tables, the direction of compression (mediolateral versus lateromedial; craniocaudal versus caudocranial) is usually chosen based on the shortest distance from skin to target. Once the target is visualized on the scout image, the angled paired stereotactic views are obtained. Cursors are placed on the target in each of the paired images. If calcifications are the subject of biopsy, the same single piece of calcium should be targeted in each view; if discordant individual targets are chosen on the two different views, the computer may be "fooled" into choosing a random point in space that does not correspond to either of the two targets chosen. Once a target is chosen on each swing view, the scout view should be re-examined to ensure that the chosen targets refer back to a specific calcification (automatically highlighted by a cursor) that appears similar in morphology to what was elected on the swing views (Fig. 29-22). If it does not, either the patient moved between the scout and the swing views,

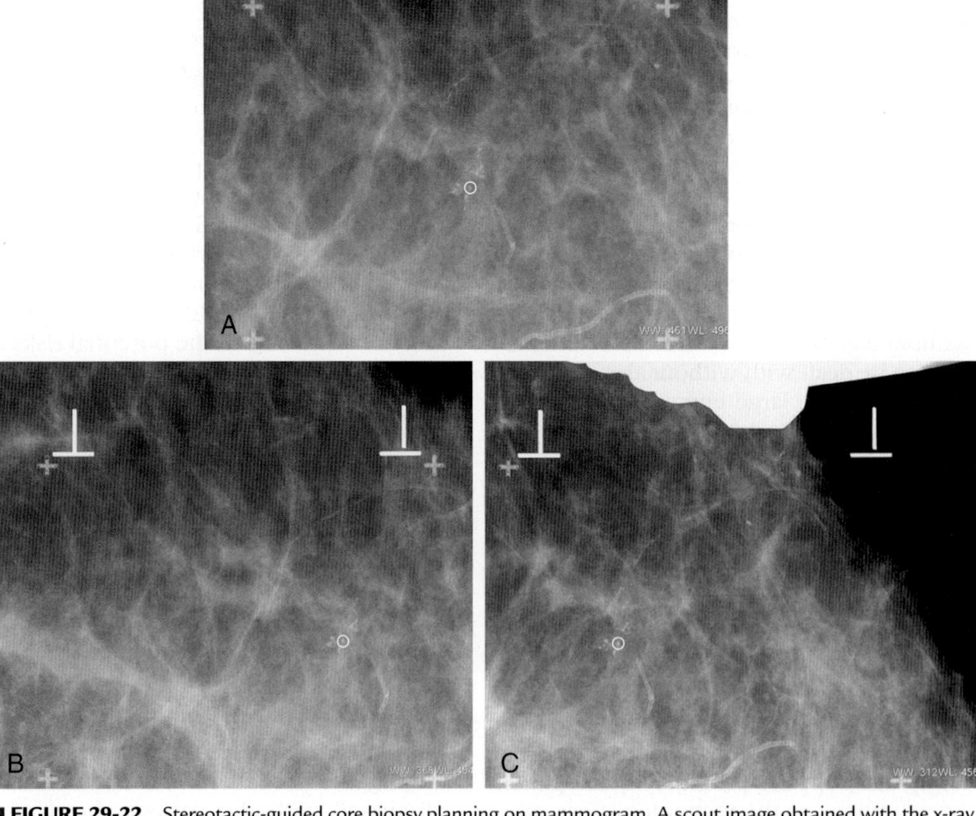

■ **FIGURE 29-22** Stereotactic-guided core biopsy planning on mammogram. A scout image obtained with the x-ray beam oriented perpendicular to the detector shows the target (pleomorphic calcifications) to lie centrally in the field of view (**A**). Swing views are obtained with the beam angled plus and minus 15 degrees off perpendicular, resulting in apparent movement in the x axis (parallax shift) of the calcifications. A discrete piece of calcium is marked by cursor placement (*white circle*) on each of these views (**B**). Note that the cursor refers to the same discrete piece of calcium on the scout (*white circle in A*), confirming that the same calcification was correctly targeted on each swing view. If no unique form can be identified on both swing views, the cursor may be placed in the center of the cluster (**C**).

or the targets chosen on the swing views are not a concordant individual piece of calcium. If the calcifications in the lesion are too similar to each other or too amorphous to allow identification of a unique form, or if the target is a mass, asymmetry or architectural distortion, the center of lesion may be chosen, and checked on the scout view for verification. This information is sent to the biopsy platform to be used for subsequent needle positioning.

Sterile Portion of the Procedure

Once the lesion has been targeted and the coordinates conveyed to the unit, the biopsy probe can be directed toward the lesion while still external to the patient by "zeroing out" all but the z (depth) coordinate. The z coordinate may be dialed in just to the point where the needle approaches the skin surface, thereby divulging the correct skin entry site. At this point, the sterile portion of the procedure can commence. The skin surface may be cleansed with antiseptic solution. Several solutions and preparations are available but there is evidence to suggest that chlorhexidine-based solutions provide better antisepsis than iodine-based solutions.[15]

For the vast majority of percutaneous breast biopsies, local anesthesia will suffice. Care should be taken to review the patient's allergy history prior to administration. This should be specifically done by the physician performing the procedure, even if a nurse or technologist has obtained such history as well. Many effective agents are available; the practitioner can acquaint himself or herself with dosage, side effects and contraindications of one or two of these drugs, one for routine use and another agent to use if an alternate is needed because of patient allergy. Preferably one routine drug can be chosen from the amide family (e.g., lidocaine, mepivacaine, prilocaine, bupivacaine) and one from the ester family (e.g., procaine, tetracaine), because cross-allergies only rarely occur between these groups. Lidocaine 1% is a common choice. For this agent, the maximum dose to be used in one setting is 4 mg/kg up to a maximum of 280 mg (28 mL). If epinephrine is added, maximum allowable dose is increased to 7 mg/kg (50 mL), although this amount is rarely required. True allergy to the amide family of local anesthetics is rare and usually reflects an allergy to the preservative or antimicrobial used in the drug rather than the drug itself. The patient can be carefully questioned about the nature and symptoms of any prior "allergic" experience. Often, what she reports is "a racing heart" or palpitations related to the co-usage of epinephrine. If this is the case, the patient can be reassured about the cause of such a reaction, and epinephrine can be avoided. If a real allergy is confirmed, use of an agent in the alternate family (amide vs. ester) can be safely selected.

In selected cases, a topical anesthetic (e.g., EMLA Cream, AstraZeneca LP, Wilmington, Del) may be applied to the skin prior to administration of injectable local anesthesia to diminish pain at the injection site. However, as this requires pre-identification of the specific needle entry site and placement of the topical agent up to 1 hour prior to biopsy, this process results in significant lengthening of the procedure time, and should be reserved for patients who otherwise refuse the procedure or have a debilitating aversion to pain. Other methods are available to minimize the pain that accompanies injection of local anesthetic. A 25 gauge needle or smaller should be used for injection. The anesthetic agent should be kept at room temperature. The skin may be cooled with ice or a quick spray of liquid nitrogen just before injection. Sodium bicarbonate (8.4%), when admixed with lidocaine in a dose of 1:9 parts bicarbonate to lidocaine, is very effective in correcting for the acidic nature of the agent, and thus minimizing the sting of the injection.

The local anesthetic agent can be applied along the entire expected route of the needle. It should be used most liberally at the needle entry site and in the biopsy bed, as these represent the sites of greatest pain, especially if the target is truly a cancer. Optimal skin numbing is provided when the anesthetic is instilled intradermally and, less importantly, subcutaneously. The raising of a generous skin wheal ensures good anesthesia over a large enough area to allow for a generous dermatotomy, as needed. Care should be taken to *backdraw* (apply negative pressure to) the syringe plunger prior to injection to minimize the possibility of intravascular administration.

Some physicians favor the addition of epinephrine 1:100,000 to 1:200,000 to the local anesthetic agent to prolong the duration of numbing and to aid in peri-lesion hemostasis, related to its vasoconstrictive properties. If so, a waiting period of about 5 minutes after injection will maximize its effectiveness. The patient may experience a sense of anxiety or the onset of temporary palpitations with its use, however, and should be warned ahead of time about this possibility. This solution can be purchased as a pre-mixed preparation.

The exact injection tract will occur along an imaginary line outlining the long axis of the needle, estimated by viewing the needle orientation. The anesthetic needle is placed and the dermis and epidermis are numbed, creating a skin wheal. Deeper administration can be obtained using a spinal needle. One trick to ensuring accurate instillation of anesthetic directly to the biopsy bed is to place the spinal needle along the expected needle course and lesion depth, take either of the two swing views, and confirm that the tip of the spinal needle is in the region of the target. If needed, additional agent can be instilled once the biopsy probe is placed, via the probe itself. If the target of biopsy is noncalcified, it is important to remember that instillation of lidocaine directly at the bed may obscure the lesion, as both are of soft tissue density.

After local anesthesia is achieved, some practitioners favor retargeting the lesion with scout and swing views, believing that the volume of the injected anesthetic may result in target displacement. When the probe is ready to be placed, a dermatotomy can be performed with a scalpel, as needed. In general, these small skin incisions heal completely and are helpful in allowing unimpeded needle motion. They may prevent the need for an initial thrust to gain skin entry, preventing uncontrolled and unintended needle motion.

Once the needle has been placed, paired swing views should be obtained with the needle in pre-fire position to confirm accurate placement. When using the prone table or the upright unit with standard needle holder, these paired images will display the needle somewhat foreshortened in appearance (because the needle is oriented along the same general axis, angled at 15 degrees), directed at, but just short of, the target in both views, if accurately positioned (Fig. 29-23). If needle position varies from this optimal position, careful review of both images allows determination of which axis or axes are errant (Fig. 29-24) and corrections may be made as needed.

A number of potential problems specific to the prone biopsy table (or upright unit using a standard needle holder) may be encountered during stereotactic biopsy. These include a negative or inadequate stroke margin and difficult-to-reach lesions. A patient with thin or small breasts may not have an adequate tissue depth after compression to permit the biopsy needle to be positioned for targeting without passing entirely through the breast to strike the image receptor distally. The same problem arises in the patient whose lesion lies close to the distal skin surface. There are a number of approaches to remedy a negative stroke margin. First, the planned approach for the needle can be changed. With the breast compressed in the orthogonal position, the location of a lesion may change sufficiently to allow safe insertion of the needle. Second, injecting an additional amount of anesthetic into the tissues may add sufficient depth for a stroke margin that is only slightly negative. Third, the needle may be positioned slightly proximal to the targeted location. Although this places the lesion in the distal aspect of the sampling notch, rather than centered within the sampling notch, adequate tissue samples of the lesion can still be obtained. Fourth, manufacturing adaptations include use of a lateral arm to perform the biopsy from an orthogonal approach to the compressed breast (Siemens AG, Munich, Germany), or 180-degree rotation of the biopsy device (Hologic Inc, Bedford, Mass). Lastly, the air gap technique may be used, in which a second compression plate is placed between the undersurface of the breast and the image receptor, with the open biopsy window of both compression plates in line with the lesion. Once inserted, if the needle passes through the breast and exits the skin on the opposite side, it will enter an air space, rather than striking the image receptor. Lesions close to the chest wall or high in the axillary tail of the breast may be difficult to sample using

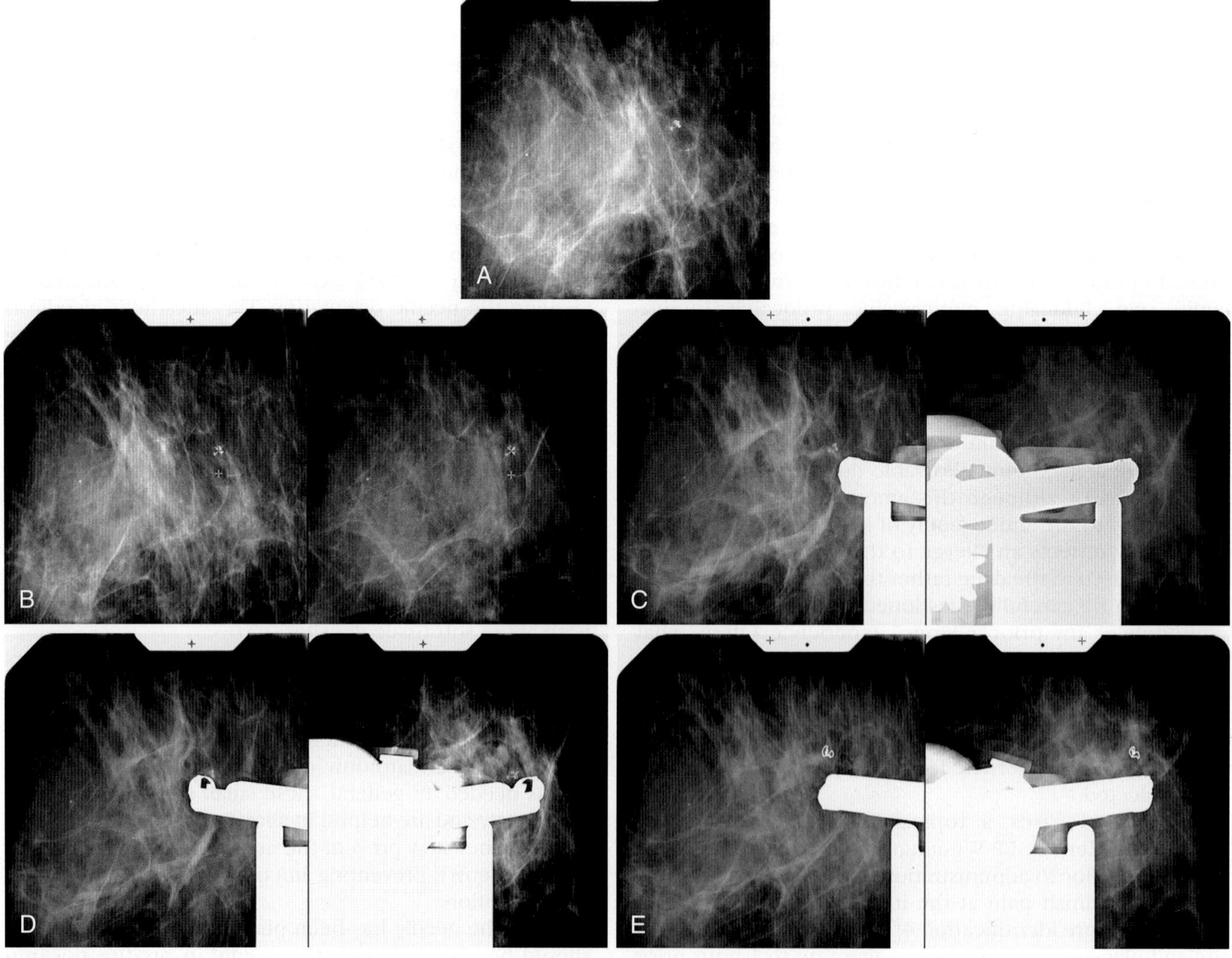

■ **FIGURE 29-23** **A,** The scout mammogram view from a stereotactic biopsy demonstrates the targeted cluster of coarse, heterogeneous microcalcifications. **B,** The stereo pair images demonstrate the targeted calcifications. **C,** Pre-fire images from both stereo images demonstrate the needle tip at the cluster of calcifications. **D,** The post-fire stereo pair images demonstrate the clustered calcifications to be within the sample notch region of the needle. **E,** Post-biopsy images demonstrate removal of the targeted calcifications and a tissue marker in the biopsy site.

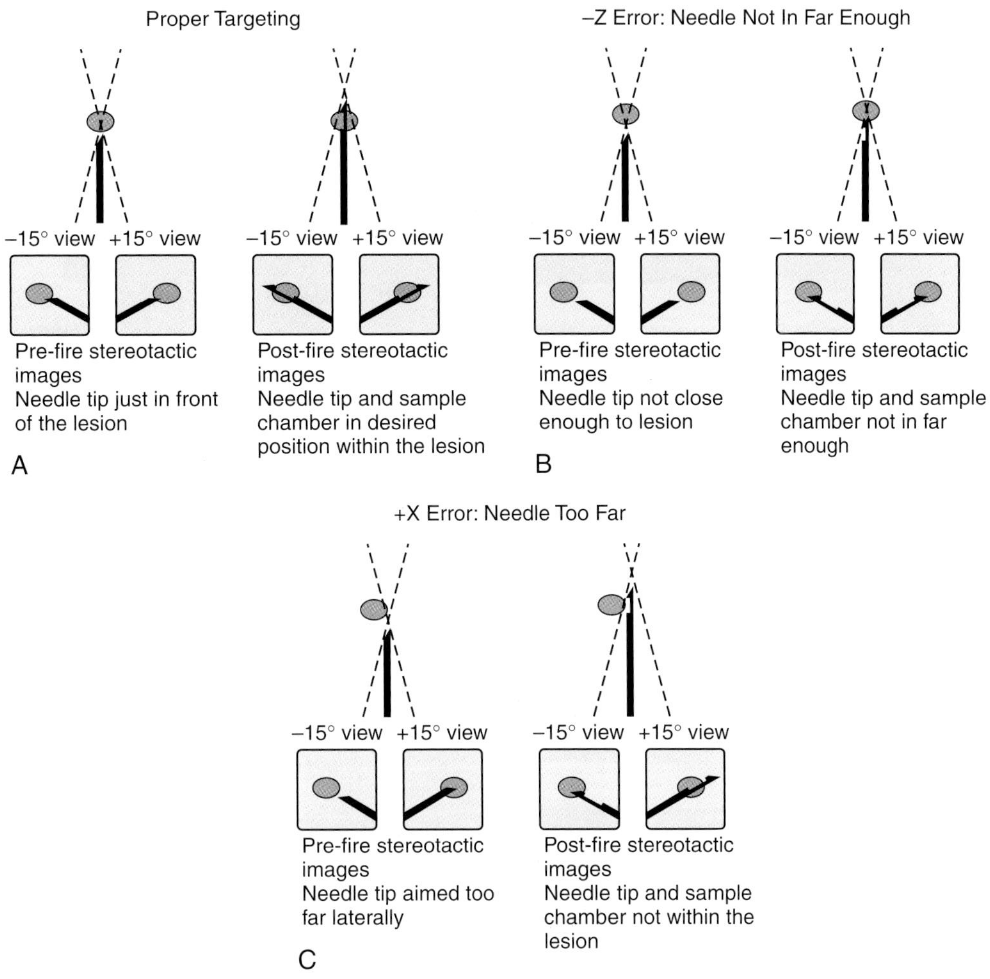

■ **FIGURE 29-24** **A,** Example of proper stereotactic targeting when using a prone table. **B,** Example of minus-Z error: Needle is not advanced deep enough into the breast. **C,** Example of plus-X error: Needle is positioned too far laterally with respect to the lesion.

the prone stereotactic technique. By rolling the patient toward the table aperture and passing the arm and shoulder through the opening, more of the posterior and axillary tissues can be brought into the biopsy window.

Confirmation of targeting accuracy with the side-arm needle holder presents a different set of images, as well as considerations, compared with the prone table or (upright unit using a standard needle holder). As the needle is traveling perpendicular to the direction of the x-ray beam (and parallel to the detector), the needle will be pointed in the same direction on both swing views. Pre-fire images should show the probe pointing directly at, but lying just short of, the lesion. The post-fire, pre-sampling images should show the lesion lying in close contiguity to the sampling notch, which is seen in profile. The target may lie somewhat anterior, superimposed or posterior to the notch (the vacuum will allow target retrieval), but must overlap, at least in part, the notch along the long axis of the needle (Fig. 29-25). If the sampling notch is not located in contiguity with the lesion, retargeting may be needed. However, in most cases, adjustment can be made by altering the needle holder position coordinates, either with the needle still in place, or by removing the needle, making changes in needle coordinates, and replacing the needle. It is obvious from consulting the post-fire images when changes are required in the x axis (parallel to chest wall along the axis of the needle) or the y axis (anterior or posterior change). However, because of the needle orientation, the relationship of the target to the needle in the z axis is not easily discernable. However, as the breast is compressed in that plane as well, it is rare that the z axis alignment is incorrect.

Once sampling notch position is deemed correct, sampling proceeds. A minimum of 12 specimens should be obtained. In general, these are retrieved by rotating the probe around its 360-degree radius. However, in some cases, the target is noted to lie in a more focal location relative to the probe; when this is the case, the directional nature of the probe can be exploited to aim the sampling aperture at the target and obtain samples from a more limited area. When adequate tissue is believed to have been retrieved, and calcifications were the original target, a specimen radiograph, using either a dedicated specimen radiography device, or magnification specimen radiography using a standard mammographic unit, should be obtained (Fig. 29-26). Some centers prefer to separate and mark the tissue cores containing calcifications prior to submitting the tissue to pathology. Even if a noncalcified lesion was targeted, a specimen radiograph may help confirm specimen adequacy, showing some margin detail or an interface between fat and the suspected lesion. If the

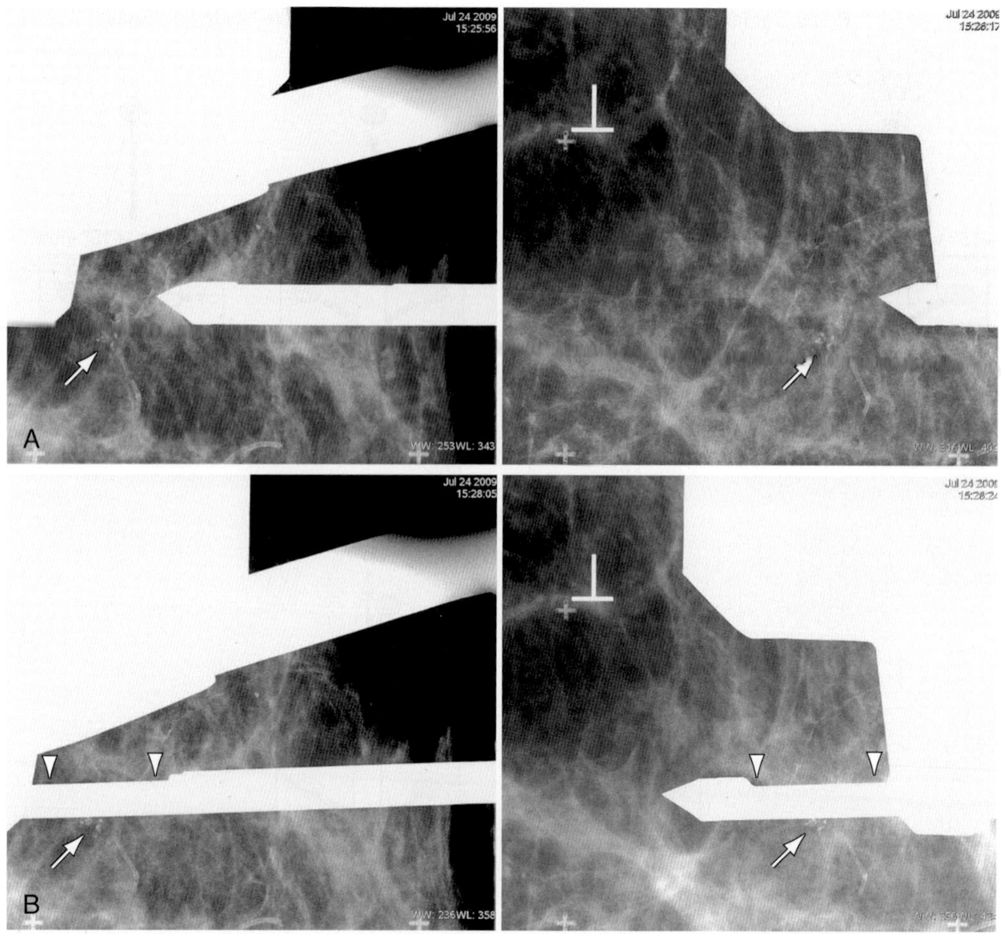

■ **FIGURE 29-25** Mammographic verification of accurate stereotactic-guided probe placement with "add-on" unit. Paired pre-fire swing images show the probe short of but directed at the linearly distributed punctate and amorphous targeted calcifications (*arrow*) in both views (**A**). Post-fire swing views (**B**) confirm that the calcifications will lie in the confines of the sampling notch (*arrowhead, currently directed anteriorly*), once it is directed posteriorly, utilizing the directional function of the probe.

specimen radiograph confirms lesion inclusion, a titanium marking clip can be placed at that point. A variety of marking clips are available from different vendors. While some practitioners do not place a clip if residual calcifications are suspected, others leave a clip in all cases. The only way to know if residual calcifications remain with certainty is to re-expose the breast with an added view. Even if residual target remains, the presence of a clip can ensure that the target remains visible if hematoma forms and helps ensure that what was actually biopsied does, indeed, represent the intended biopsy target, especially if multiple relatively similar findings are present. Some patients are uncomfortable with the concept of having a clip in their breast; once educated about the nature and purpose of the clip, they can usually be persuaded to allow it. The intention to leave a clip should be included in the informed consent process. Once the clip has been deployed, the probe is rotated 180 degrees (so that the smooth side of the probe abuts the clip) and closed (so that the sampling notch is covered, preventing "hooking" the clip as the needle is removed). A single swing view may be obtained at this point, prior to probe removal, to ensure successful clip deployment. Upon probe removal, the breast is compressed, either manually or by using the unit compression paddle. The former allows the patient to lie supine during compression, and also lets the technologist have a face-to-face discussion with the patient about post-procedure wound care. For most patients, 5 to 10 minutes will suffice; if the patient is anticoagulated or has a bleeding diathesis, longer and firmer compression is required, sometimes up to 20 minutes. Once hemostasis is achieved, the entry site can be temporarily dressed with a Steri-strip. A post-procedure two-view mammogram (craniocaudal and 90° lateral views) should be obtained at this point, to ensure that the correct target underwent biopsy and to assess for clip migration, either due to inaccurate initial deployment, accordion effect upon removal of breast compression, or related to hematoma formation. The post-procedure mammograms should be closely correlated to pre-biopsy films. The biopsy bed/location of original target, if remote from the clip, should be outlined on the films and note made in the report about the exact position of the clip relative to the target.

If microcalcifications cannot be found histologically, the paraffin blocks should be radiographed to direct additional sections for the pathologist, and a polarized lens may be used to identify unstained calcium oxylate crystals. If calcifications still are not identified, the patient should undergo follow-up mammographic images to confirm that the proper site was sampled.

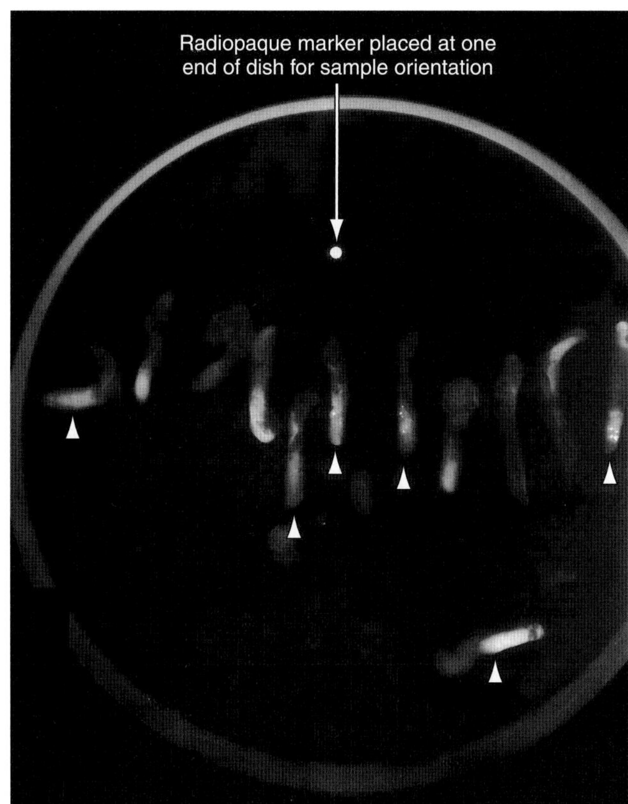

■ **FIGURE 29-26** Specimen radiograph of core biopsy samples containing calcifications (*arrowheads*).

Post-Procedure Considerations

Once hemostasis has been achieved and the post-procedure mammogram has been obtained, a final sterile dressing can be applied to the wound. The patient is instructed in post-procedure wound care, informed about what events are normal post-biopsy sequelae (minor pain and bruising) and what constitute cause for concern (signs of infection, an expanding hematoma, shortness of breath). She should be told what to do in case of a problem, and given contact numbers. All these instructions should be given to her in written form, as well. Additionally, the patient should be informed about how she will receive her biopsy results, and when.

The obtained core samples should be placed in preservative. While a technologist or assistant may aid in packaging the specimen for transport and delivery to pathology, it is ultimately the responsibility of the practitioner to ensure that the specimen container is accurately labeled, and that a pathology requisition form is filled out with appropriate history and the specifics of the specimen source. If the patient has had biopsy from more than one site, the specimens should be very specifically labeled as to the location of the respective biopsy sites (e.g. "Specimen #1: left breast, upper outer quadrant, posterior depth; Specimen #2: left breast subareolar region, middle depth"). When calcifications are expected or known to be a component of the lesion, the pathologist should be cued to search for them via specific instructions on the pathology request. If the patient has prior radiation therapy to the affected breast, that information should be noted on the requisition, as postradiation atypia may prove difficult to differentiate from DCIS or other atypia, but obviously has markedly different management implications. Similarly, if the patient has been undergoing neoadjuvant chemotherapy, this should be noted on the pathology request.

A written permanent procedure report should be constructed that outlines the nature, side, and location of each biopsy target, the type of device used for core biopsy, the number of samples obtained, the confirmed presence of calcifications in the cores as demonstrated on specimen radiograph, whether a marking clip was placed, the location of the clip relative to the target, if a post-procedure mammogram was obtained, and any complications that were encountered during the procedure. This report should subsequently be amended when the pathology results are returned, with concordance or discordance noted, and further appropriate management or follow-up recommendations outlined. When the pathology results are returned, the case should be reviewed in its entirety, including perusal of all recent imaging performed. Concordance between initial imaging and the final pathology results must be assessed. If discordant results are returned, arrangements should be made for additional tissue sampling, either by repeat percutaneous biopsy or by excision. In addition, the physician can make sure that additional areas do not now require further intervention, based on the newly available pathologic information. For example, if malignancy is confirmed, consideration may be now given to pursuing biopsy of another area previously deemed a BI-RADS 3 lesion. A well-defined policy should be in place outlining how the patient will be informed of her results. The policy must ensure that no patient will remain unapprised of her diagnosis, and this is likely best achieved when the biopsying physician (or his delegate) takes responsibility for the task. In this way, it will never be simply assumed that the referring physician has conveyed the results. The patient may be informed of the results in person (via an additional office visit) or by telephone. If malignancy has been found, arrangements can be made for referral to other members of the breast cancer treatment team (surgical oncology, medical oncology) as indicated. If benign results were returned, the recommended follow-up can be outlined to the patient. If an atypical or discordant diagnosis has been rendered, discussion can be made with the patient about the need for further intervention. The conveyance of results and recommendations should be documented, preferably as an addendum to the formal biopsy report.

Indications

Stereotactic technique should be used to guide biopsy of any BI-RADS 4—suspicious or 5—highly suspicious lesion seen only, or most conspicuously, on mammogram. This would include most cases of suspicious calcifications, but might also include masses, asymmetries or architectural distortions not indentified by ultrasound. Although BI-RADS 3—probably benign findings are by definition suitable for short-term follow up rather than biopsy, in some cases, core of the lesions may be preferred instead. Some examples would include patients who have a highly suspicious lesion elsewhere in either breast, those with a known synchronous breast cancer where management may be altered by the presence another cancer, patients who are undergoing fertility treatment or anticipate getting pregnant in the near future, those with a strong family history, and those for whom the anxiety of short-term follow-up outweighs the benefit of avoiding biopsy.

If multiple suspicious findings are present, biopsy of as many targets as needed to outline the full extent of malignant disease and direct appropriate future management should be carried out. For example, if multiple clusters of suspicious calcifications are present in one breast, core of at least two of these can be performed, preferably those lying farthest apart, to fully establish extent of disease and help determine the need for mastectomy versus breast conserving surgery. However, biopsy of all clusters is probably not needed. The fewest number of biopsies that will firmly establish surgical management is optimal.

If stereotactic guidance is being used to biopsy a lesion discovered by another modality (MRI, or PET), great care must be taken to ensure that the mammographic target is concordant with the image that originally detected the target. This requires a good working knowledge of the other modality, the ability to translate expected lesion position from one modality to another, meticulous radiologic-pathologic correlation when the results are returned, and the knowledge to obtain imaging follow-up either immediately post biopsy or in a delayed manner, or even rebiopsy, as needed. If there is any question as to whether an accurate correlate has been picked, biopsy should probably proceed, guided by the modality that originally found it. Another corollary here is that imaging guided biopsies, in general, are best performed by a physician with the above-described knowledge and skill set, and that physician, in most cases, is a radiologist.

Contraindications

Few contraindications to stereotactic-guided core biopsy exist. Biopsy should not be performed on a patient who has no intention of seeking treatment if a cancer is diagnosed, due to co-morbid conditions or other reasons. However, this type of patient is also not a candidate for screening or diagnostic evaluation. Any patient who has reservations about signing the consent or undergoing biopsy should not be coerced into it, even if it is likely in her best interest. To do so may constitute battery. The procedure should be cancelled and rescheduled as indicated, and the referring physician alerted. Additional discussion about the risks and benefits of the procedure and why it is indicated can be carried out on a different day. The events and subsequent communications with the patient should be documented. Anticoagulation has traditionally been considered a relative contraindication for core biopsy, with the patient asked to cease therapy prior to biopsy if possible. However, recent literature suggests no significant difference in hematoma rate between anticoagulated patients (on either warfarin or nonsteroidal anti-inflammatory products) and other patients undergoing core biopsy.[17] In implant patients, if rupture appears likely, core biopsy should be avoided; however, with careful planning, use of implant-displacement with compression of the breast, and exploitation of the ability to rotate the sampling notch so that the vacuum is directed away from the implant, this should be a rare situation. The potential for implant rupture should be clearly delineated to the patient during the consenting process.

Potential Complications of Stereotactic-guided Core Biopsy

As with US-guided core biopsy, complications during stereotactic-guided core biopsy are relatively rare but potentially include: hematoma formation (not uncommon), infection, pneumothorax (rare), allergic reaction to local anesthetic, and vagal reaction. A small amount of bleeding is not unusual during core biopsy but occasionally, needle transection of a vessel can result in more rapid bleeding. This is most certainly not a life-threatening event but can result in significant hematoma formation. The ultimate size of the hematoma can be minimized by firm compression over the area at the end of the procedure, to include the segment of breast from needle entry site to lesion. If it occurs early in the procedure or is arterial in origin, the bleeding can result in target obscuration or displacement. If this is recognized (large amount of blood being returned via or around needle), a clip may be placed as quickly as possible so the lesion can be re-identified for re-biopsy or excision (especially with non-calcified targets) in case the procedure needs to be prematurely aborted.

If sterile technique is respected, infection should be rare. At some point in the biopsy process, the procedure becomes *clean* rather than *sterile*; however, if sterility of the needle and skin is maintained, the expectation of a germ-free environment can be achieved. If infection subsequently is reported by the patient, she should be asked to come in so the physician can inspect the wound, ensure that abscess is not a possibility, and assess whether the infection is not simply a reaction to tape or bandage material. If infection is confirmed, the physician can choose to prescribe antibiotics as appropriate, and arrange to see the patient in follow-up.

Vagal reactions (bradycardia with hypotension) are not uncommon during breast procedures, but occur relatively less often during most stereotactic biopsies, in part owing to the patient's prone or decubitus positioning for the procedure. However, when upright positioning is used with some add-on units, it is not uncommon. The vast majority of vagal reactions respond immediately to simple conservative treatment: placing the patient in a horizontal position, elevation of patient's feet/placement in Trendelenburg with squeezing of calf muscles to restore blood return to the head; application of a cool cloth to the neck or forehead; calm reassurance. Oxygen may be administered but is rarely required. As she recovers, the patient should be warned that she will soon feel the onset of shaking, as release of epinephrine by her system occurs. If the patient does not respond to these conservative measures, an IV may started and consideration given to pharmacologic support (atropine). Allergic or anaphylactoid reactions must be recognized and treated promptly. In the rare case of suspected pneumothorax, a chest radiograph can be obtained and further treatment pursued as needed. With these latter types of more complicated or severe events, the biopsying physician has the ultimate responsibility for patient outcome. As a result, it is the obligation of any physician taking on the privilege of performing such procedures to also assume the responsibility of knowing how to manage minor complications, including knowledge of the medications and interventions involved. However, ultimately the best interest of the patient is paramount, and if the biopsying physician needs assistance in an acute situation, help should be sought promptly, up to and including sending the patient to the Emergency Room or calling a "code."

Epithelial displacement of tumor cells along the percutaneous needle tract has been discussed as a potential risk of core biopsy. Seeding of the tract does appear to occur, in an estimated 22% of cases. However, a systematic review of the available literature by Liebens and associates did not show evidence of increased local recurrence rate in patients undergoing pre-operative diagnosis via percutaneous biopsy who subsequently underwent conservative therapy and radiation or increased morbidity in patients who had core biopsy of malignant lesions.[18]

MRI-GUIDED PERCUTANEOUS TISSUE SAMPLING

Breast MRI has gained acceptance as a highly sensitive technology for the detection of breast cancer, not uncommonly finding lesions occult on mammogram and ultrasound. Because of this, it becomes quickly apparent to practitioners of breast MRI that the ability to biopsy these lesions with MRI-guidance is an absolute must. While some of the lesions can be identified retrospectively with other modalities (usually via "second-look" ultrasound), others cannot, mandating the use of MRI-guidance for accurate sampling. Centers performing breast MRI should therefore expect to develop an MRI breast biopsy program. If this is not feasible for some extenuating reason, a close working relationship with another site that does perform MRI-guided biopsies should be established. That site should be privy to the original center's reports, all of the patient's salient imaging (including mammograms and ultrasound images) and should have a way to view the original breast MRI exam in a way that allows the target lesion to be definitively identified.

The efficacy and safety of MRI-guided percutaneous biopsy has been validated in multiple studies. Liberman and colleagues demonstrated a 97% technical success rate, median biopsy time of 33 minutes, minimal complication rate (1 of 98 patients experienced a vagal episode), and a positive predictive value (PPV) of 25% (within the range of PPVs of other percutaneous biopsy methods). Seventy-eight percent of cases were spared diagnostic surgical biopsy because MRI-guided biopsy was performed.[22] Mahoney reported similar results in 55 lesions with 31% of patients demonstrating malignancy or atypia.[23]

Equipment and Technique

Equipment

As with the other forms of imaging-guided biopsy, high-quality image acquisition is a requisite for success. Variability among centers occurs in regards to specific scanning parameters. However, images should be obtained on a unit of adequate field strength to ensure an optimal signal-to-noise ratio. In most cases, this will likely be 1.5 Tesla or higher. However, some 1.0 Tesla units have been shown to offer high quality images. Use of a dedicated breast coil is required. As with stereotactic-guided procedures, a vacuum-assisted 11-gauge (or larger) biopsy device is standard, with use of springloaded devices discouraged.[24] This maximizes the volume of tissue retrieved and diminishes the chance of insufficiency, especially important with MRI-guided biopsies, because real-time monitoring of sampling accuracy is not possible (as occurs with ultrasound), lesions are often smaller than those detected with other modalities, and there is no confirmatory method such as specimen radiography to ensure sample adequacy. Because the needle is relatively fixed in position by a needle holder during the sampling process (as opposed to an ultrasound-guided CNB, where free-hand technique allows needle manipulation), the rotational/directional aspect of the vacuum-assisted device is vital in ensuring accurate tissue sampling. Obviously, this equipment must be MRI-compatible. Most of these devices use an external vacuum, which is placed outside the MRI suite. The probe is placed, guided by coordinates calculated during pre-procedure scanning. Once accurate needle placement is confirmed by additional MR images, sampling can proceed. The vacuum pulls tissue into the recessed sampling notch, which lies on the side of the probe and an inner cannula transects the tissue (see Fig. 29-3). This core is then delivered retrograde for retrieval, either by an assistant using forceps or into a closed chamber for later collection, depending on the device. The systems that require each sample to be collected individually by an assistant result in a slightly longer procedure time and greater risk of exposure to blood products. However, they provide the advantage of confirming that an adequate core was obtained during each acquisition. The vacuum-assisted biopsy process allows multiple contiguous samples to be taken during a single needle insertion, as the tissue is delivered externally while the needle remains poised for added cores. Hand-held self-contained devices are available, as well, and their efficacy is supported in the literature.[25]

Since the procedure room in this case actually constitutes the MRI suite, provisions should be made to ensure patient privacy during positioning as well as during the procedure. As personnel will be entering and leaving the room multiple times during the procedure, a screen may be used to shield the patient from others passing the doorway. A separate private room should be available to consult with and obtain consent from the patient prior to the procedure.

Each center or physician may construct a sterile procedure tray to individual specifications. However, when there are multiple practitioners within a single center, standardization of set-up and supplies promotes quick patient turnaround and cost savings, as the technologist can more efficiently prepare the trays and fewer supplies need to be stocked. A typical sterile set-up may include sterile gloves, antiseptic, sterile gauze, forceps for specimen retrieval (depending on the biopsy device being used), pre-drawn local anesthetic agent (clearly labeled as to exact content). Pre-constructed trays can be purchased from many vendors, and the client can determine the specific contents. While these promote efficiency, they may prove more costly than simply making up the trays on-site. Once the standard set-up is prepared by the technologist or aide, the device selected for biopsy may be individualized to physician or specific lesion type, and opened at the time of actual biopsy.

Technique

Pre-Procedural Considerations

Written informed consent is an obligate requisite to the procedure. Each center will likely have an organization-composed and approved consent form. Some sites use a general form for all types of procedures and surgeries performed at that institution that outlines all potential risks, up to and including death; other use procedure-specific consent forms that are tailored to the appropriate set of risks and complications. If the former is required by the institution, this should be explained to the patient, telling her that some of the potential risks and complications mentioned are not considered applicable to her situation. However, all consents should make mention of bleeding, infection, pneumothorax, allergic reaction to administered medications and contrast and, if appropriate, implant rupture as potential complications of the procedure. Additionally, the patient should be fully informed about the benefits of the biopsy (e.g., deferral of surgery in the face of benign specific results; pre-operative verification of malignancy, allowing definitive surgical therapy in one setting) as well as the potential drawbacks (possible need for re-biopsy or excision in the face of non-specific, insufficient or discordant pathology results). She should be told about the use of a marking clip. In the optimal setting, this material, as well as a general description of what she can expect during the procedure and its aftermath, will have been discussed with the patient ahead of time by a physician, technologist, nurse or physician-extender, possibly at the time of her diagnostic workup or upon scheduling. However, the written informed consent should by obtained by the practitioner performing the biopsy, with a witness in attendance. For TJC-accredited facilities, compliance with Universal Protocol (to prevent wrong site, wrong procedure, wrong person mishaps) is mandated. This requires marking of the side of biopsy (right/left), and completion out a time-out just prior to beginning the procedure to verify identity of the patient, the site of the biopsy and the procedure to be performed in the presence of the entire procedural team and the patient, all of whom must be in agreement (See TJC policy for more detail at www.jointcommission.org). This process must be carried out by the physician or physician-extender who is performing the procedure, and not a surrogate (resident, nurse, technologist, other physician) and formally documented. Even if a facility is not subject to TJC accreditation, the process when used in some form can help prevent procedural errors. The patient should be queried directly by the physician about any allergies (including latex) as well as her medication history in regards to anticoagulation status. While biopsy can be pursued even in the face of anticoagulation (see discussion under "Contraindications"), knowledge of her coagulation status may alter post-procedure care (e.g., longer compression time, etc.). In addition, if the patient is new to the facility, she should be thoroughly screened for any contraindications to MRI, unlikely as she has presumably already safely undergone a preliminary breast MRI.

The patient is then placed prone on the MRI table with the breast/breasts (if she is undergoing bilateral biopsies) positioned within the confines of the dedicated surface breast coil system. The physician, having reviewed the original study, should be involved in positioning, thereby maximizing the likelihood that the lesion can be accessed. The breast will be lightly to moderately compressed between the plates of a dedicated biopsy compression device (which allows access to the lateral or medial skin surface of the breast, or both); the degree of compression should be tight enough to discourage patient motion and to minimize breast deformity during needle placement, but light enough to allow full vascular perfusion, thereby insuring optimal lesion enhancement (Fig. 29-27). Most commonly, the lesion is approached laterally. Some guidance systems allow a medial approach

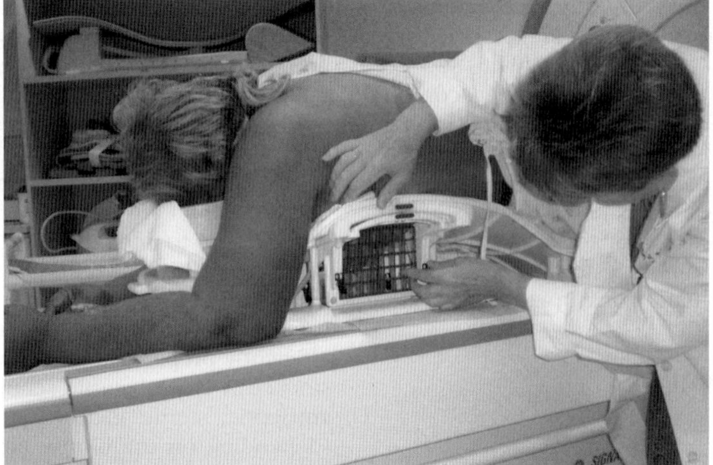

■ **FIGURE 29-27** Positioning for magnetic resonance imaging (MRI)-guided breast biopsy. Patient is positioned for left breast biopsy, using lateral approach. Participation in positioning by the physician, after review of the case, can help ensure lesion accessibility.

to the breast. In general, this is more cumbersome, as the physician is working under the table from the contralateral side. Generally, less posterior tissue is accessible via a medial approach. However, for a lesion that is quite medial (and not too far posterior), a medial approach may be desired and a biopsy system that offers this approach is preferred. Once proper positioning has been achieved, the patient should be instructed to lie still, and not raise her head when the staff re-renters the room. Lack of patient movement may be confirmed by placing an ink mark on the skin at the edge of the open grid. A vitamin E capsule should be placed on one of the horizontal grid slats near the expected lesion location, to be used either for primary targeting reference or as a backup reference, if a computer-aided detection (CAD) guidance system is being used (Fig. 29-28). The patient is placed in the gantry and pre-scanning commences.

Pre-contrast images are optional; however, they are often extremely helpful. The visibility of the system's intrinsic fiducial markers (or the vitamin E tablet) can be established before contrast injection. The expected location of the lesion (based on consultation of landmarks on the original study) can be confirmed to lie within the confines of available grid openings. Adjustments can then be made to either of these variables prior to giving contrast. In that way, the pre-contrast images may be repeated after any needed change in positioning, and accurate subtraction images subsequently generated, which may be useful in targeting subtle lesions. In general, meticulous technique similar to that used for the site's diagnostic breast MRIs should be employed, to best replicate the lesion. In about 12% of cases, nonvisualization of the original target may occur upon scanning the day of biopsy.[26] This most commonly occurs with lesions detected in pre-menopausal women undergoing high-risk screening.[26] If the lesion is not demonstrated, even after delayed images are performed, the procedure should be cancelled. However, short-term follow-up is recommended in these cases; Hefler and colleagues showed a 7% (2 of 29 lesions) malignancy rate in lesions that were not visualized the day of biopsy but were demonstrated on follow-up performed 4 to 24 hours after the cancelled procedure.[27] Alternatively, Liberman and colleagues found no cancers among 13 cases that underwent follow-up (median follow-up interval equals 5 months) due to non-visualization.[28] While follow-up of such nonvisualized lesions seems prudent, there is no clearly defined optimal follow-up interval at this time, with a 0- to 12-month range described in the literature; common sense would suggest that the interval chosen should take into consideration the degree of initial suspicion for malignancy.

Once the lesion is confidently identified on post-contrast images, it can be accurately targeted by various methods. Most simply, a cursor can be placed on the lesion, and the series scrolled back to the image on which the grid device with Vitamin E capsule is visible. The capsule is used as a reference: by knowing its grid location, the correct grid opening for needle placement can be surmised (e.g., the cursor overlies a grid two units in the caudal direction relative to the capsule). One can then determine what specific portion of that grid needs to be accessed by noting where the cursor lies within it on the review station (Fig. 29-29). Needle depth can be calculated by multiplying the number of slices one scrolled through from the target to the grid times the individual slice thickness. Using a CAD system may allow a somewhat more elegant approach to planning. Instead of a vitamin E capsule serving as reference, system-specific fiducial markers are used. These may consist of drops of gadolinium placed in designated areas of the grid frame or a block containing paramagnetic material that is placed in

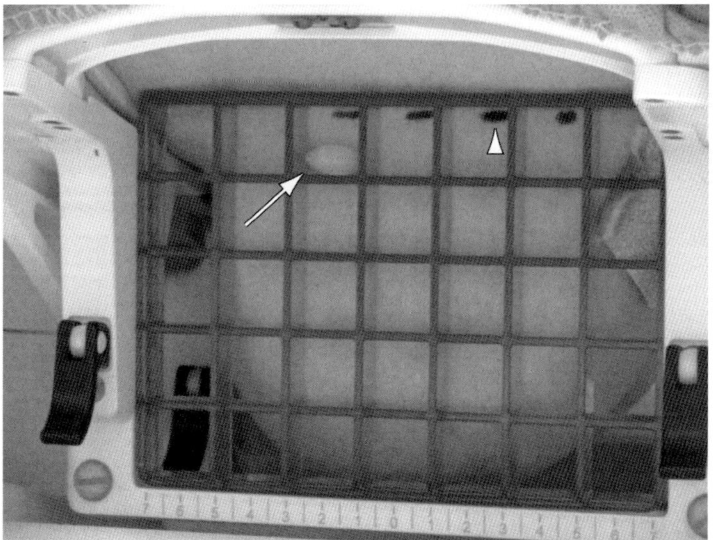

■ **FIGURE 29-28** Preparation for magnetic resonance imaging (MRI)-guided biopsy. The breast is immobilized using the biopsy grid, compressed tightly enough to discourage motion but lightly enough to allow adequate breast vascular perfusion. The skin may be marked at grid edge (*arrowhead*) to confirm lack of patient motion. A vitamin E tablet, which will be visible upon scanning, is placed in one of the grid squares (*arrow*), and can be used to guide subsequent needle placement.

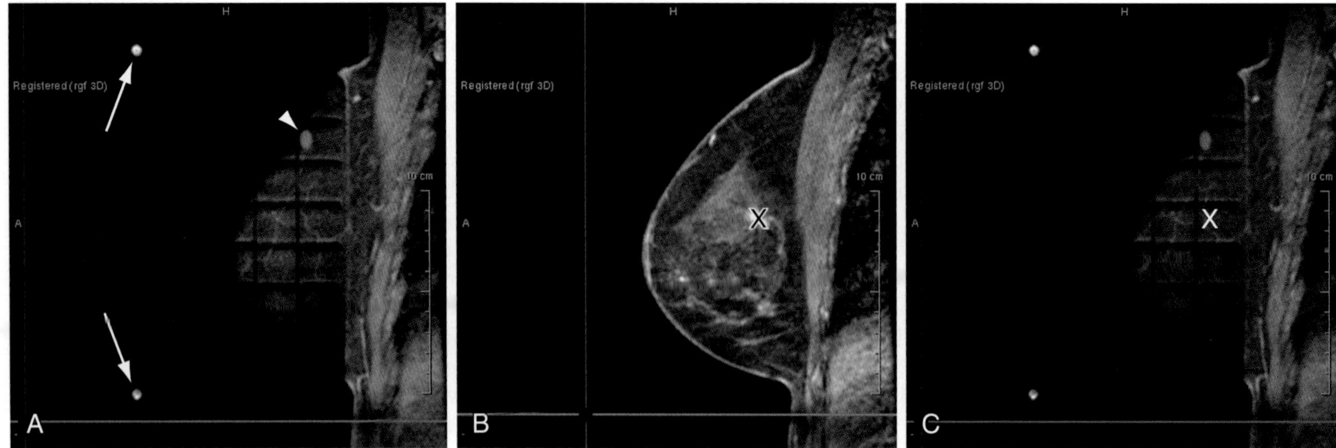

■ **FIGURE 29-29** Magnetic resonance imaging (MRI)-guided breast biopsy: pre-biopsy planning. **A**, Slice showing the unit's intrinsic fiducials (*arrows*), used to plan a biopsy with CAD-assistance, and a vitamin E tablet (*arrowhead*) that has been placed on the biopsy grid and is faintly visible after scanning. The vitamin E tablet may be used to determine in which grid square the needle guide will be placed by referencing its position relative to cursor placed on biopsy target (**B**), and then scrolling out to the grid image (**C**). In this case, the correct grid square, outlined by prior cursor placement on lesion, lies two units toward the patient's feet from the vitamin E tablet.

one of the grid openings and used for reference. The CAD device can detect these fiducials automatically. Once the lesion is identified and targeted by cursor placement, the CAD device calculates and pictorially displays the correct grid opening, specific aperture in the needle guide and the lesion depth (Fig. 29-30).

Posteriorly-situated lesions may be difficult to access. Removing the pad on the table allows greater tissue inclusion. Angling the patient by raising her contralateral side slightly may help include more posterior tissue, especially with lateral lesions. Some of the biopsy compression devices may be slid upward (i.e., toward posterior on the patient) to gain more posterior access. Some systems now offer a needle holder that can be angled anteriorly or posteriorly as needed, in addition to the fixed grid system. One potential drawback of these *pillar and post* systems is that there is more needle dead space outside the patient, resulting in significantly less depth accessibility. Additionally, care must be taken when posterior needle angulation is used, to avoid chest wall penetration, which does not occur with the fixed system unless there is a targeting error.

Sterile Portion of the Procedure

Once the lesion is identified and the biopsy route determined, the sterile portion of the procedure can commence. The physician may now "glove-up" and cleanse the skin surface with antiseptic solution. Several solutions and preparations are available but there is evidence to suggest that chlorhexidine-based solutions provide better antisepsis than iodine-based solutions.[15]

For the vast majority of percutaneous breast biopsies, local anesthesia will suffice, although an oral benzodiazepine agent may be a useful adjunct in selected patients, especially those with claustrophobia. Care should be taken to review the patient's allergy history prior to administration. This should be specifically done

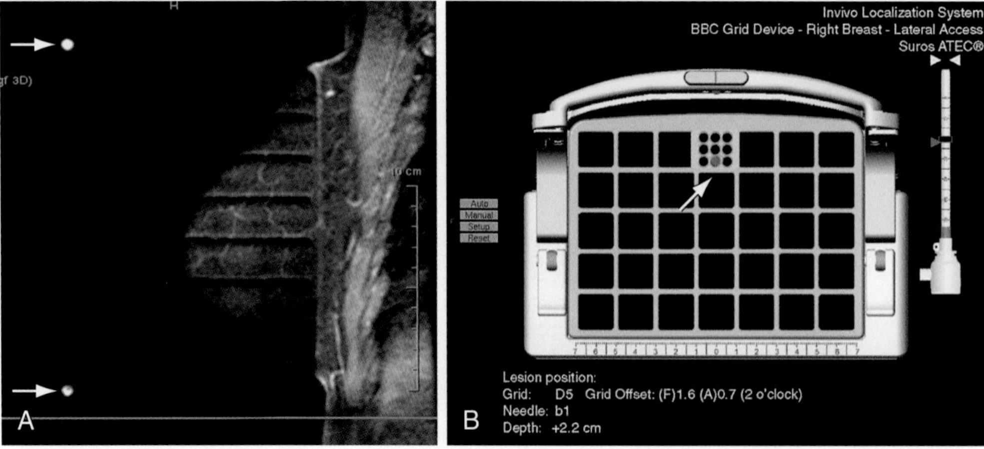

■ **FIGURE 29-30** Magnetic resonance imaging (MRI)-guided biopsy using CAD planning technique. The system can detect intrinsic fiducials, which are unique to each system. **A**, This system uses drops of gadolinium placed in two wells in the biopsy grid frame, seen as hyperintense dots on the scout images (*arrows*), and are automatically detected by the system. Once detected, a cursor may simply be placed over the biopsy target on the appropriate slice and (**B**) the unit will pictorially and graphically (*lower left corner*) outline the correct grid square (*arrow*), specific needle hole (*shaded circle*) and lesion depth.

by the physician performing the procedure, even if a nurse or technologist has obtained such history as well. Many effective local anesthetic agents are available; the practitioner can acquaint himself or herself with dosage, side effects and contraindications of one or two of these drugs, one for routine use and another agent to use if an alternate is needed because of patient allergy. Preferably one routine drug can be chosen from the amide family (e.g., lidocaine, mepivacaine, prilocaine, bupivacaine) and one from the ester family (e.g., procaine, tetracaine), because cross-allergies only rarely occur between these groups. Lidocaine 1% is a common choice. For this agent, the maximum dose to be used in one setting is 4 mg/kg up to a maximum of 280 mg (up to 28 mL). If epinephrine is added, maximum allowable dose is increased to 7 mg/kg (up to 50 mL). This amount is rarely required. True allergy to the amide family of local anesthetics is rare and usually reflects an allergy to the preservative or antimicrobial used in the drug rather than the drug itself. The patient can be carefully questioned about the nature and symptoms of any prior "allergic" experience. Often, what she reports is "a racing heart" or palpitations related to the co-usage of epinephrine. If this is the case, the patient can be reassured about the cause of such a reaction, or epinephrine can be avoided, or both. If a real allergy is confirmed, use of an agent in the alternate family (amide vs. ester) can be safely selected.

Methods are available to minimize the pain that accompanies injection of local anesthetic. A 25 gauge needle or smaller should be used for injection; 30 gauge needles are available and work well. The agent should be kept at room temperature. The skin may be cooled with ice or a quick spray of liquid nitrogen just before injection. Sodium bicarbonate (8.4%), when admixed with lidocaine in a dose of 1:9 parts bicarbonate-to-lidocaine, is very effective in correcting for the acidic nature of the agent, and thus minimizing the sting of the injection.

The local anesthetic agent can be applied along the entire expected route of the needle. It should be used most liberally at the needle entry site and at the biopsy bed (location can be estimated), as these represent the sites of greatest pain, especially if the target is truly a cancer. Optimal skin numbing is provided when the anesthetic is instilled intradermally and, less importantly, subcutaneously. The raising of a generous skin wheal ensures good anesthesia over a large enough area to allow for a generous dermatotomy, as needed. Care should be taken to *backdraw* (apply negative pressure to) the syringe plunger prior to injection to minimize the possibility of intravascular administration.

Some physicians favor the addition of epinephrine 1:100,000 to 1:200,000 to the local anesthetic agent to prolong the duration of numbing and to aid in peri-lesion hemostasis, related to its vasoconstrictive properties. If so, a waiting period of about 5 minutes after injection will maximize its effectiveness. The patient may experience a sense of anxiety or the onset of temporary palpitations with its use, however, and should be warned ahead of time about this possibility. This solution can be purchased as a pre-mixed preparation.

The exact injection site can be identified when the needle guide is placed. The anesthetic needle is placed and the dermis and epidermis are numbed, creating a skin wheal. If the small gauge numbing needle does not reach the anticipated lesion depth, a spinal needle can be placed, for deeper anesthetic application.

After local anesthesia is achieved, the biopsy trocar/introducer can be placed to its predetermined depth. Depending on the device being used, a dermatotomy may be indicated. In general, these small skin nicks heal completely and are helpful in allowing unimpeded needle motion. The introducer apparatus also varies depending on the device being used. Some consist of a sharp metal stylet covered by a plastic introducer sheath (Fig. 29-31); once the stylet and sheath are placed in the breast, the stylet is removed and replaced by a localizing obturator, whose tip location represents the center of the needle's sampling notch and which should lie at the lesion when subsequently imaged on pre-biopsy scanning. Sagittal images will show the obturator in cross-section, as a small circle (either as a signal void or a hyperintense circle, depending on the system being used). Axial confirmatory scans will show the obturator in profile, along its full length (Fig. 29-32). Another system uses a sharp ceramic introducer whose distal side contains a recessed notch that couples with the sampling notch of the biopsy device once it is placed. The lesion should be seen adjacent to this introducer's notch upon confirmatory pre-sampling imaging in the axial projection. If pre-sampling imaging demonstrates lesion migration or inaccurate introducer placement, adjustments should be made at that time, with rescanning post manipulation. If the error is simply one of

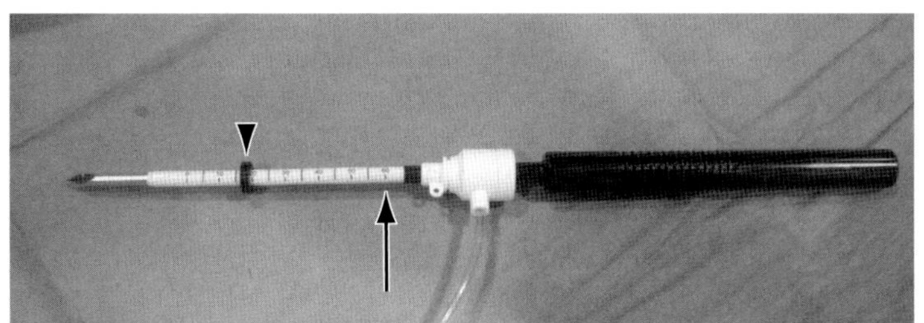

■ **FIGURE 29-31** Magnetic resonance imaging (MRI)-guided biopsy introducer apparatus. One type of biopsy device uses an MR-compatible metallic stylet, covered by a plastic sheath (*arrow*), to access the breast tissue. The black rubber ring (*arrowhead*) is set to the proper position on the sheath, as determined during the planning stage of the procedure. This introducer apparatus is then advanced to that depth as it is placed in the breast. The stylet is replaced by a rod-like obturator, and the breast is scanned to confirm accurate positioning.

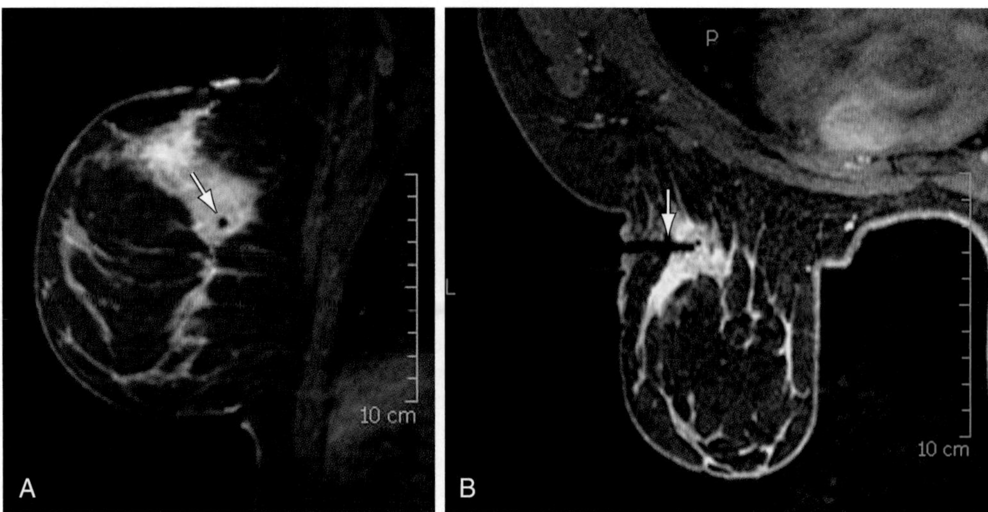

■ **FIGURE 29-32** Obturator placement during magnetic resonance imaging (MRI)-guided biopsy. Obturator appears as an area of black or signal void, seen in cross-section (*arrow*) during sagittal scanning (**A**), and en face (*arrow*) when imaged axially (**B**). Note that the obturator tip lies at the target, an area of regional enhancement. The position of the obturator tip corresponds to the center of the probe sampling notch, once the probe is placed. Hence, accurate sampling can be expected in this case.

depth, the introducer can be manipulated along its long axis to the proper depth. However, if the error is along the x or y axis, and the lesion is anticipated to lie more than about 5 mm from the needle, complete repositioning of the device may be required. Once accurate obturator/introducer placement is confirmed, the vacuum-assisted biopsy device can be placed and samples obtained. Many physicians prefer to target directly adjacent to the lesion rather than at the center of the lesion, itself, in order to minimize the possibility of lesion migration/displacement when the needle is placed. If this is the case, the directional nature of these devices can be exploited to sample maximally in the appropriate radian. The optimal number of specimens has not been firmly established in the literature. Liberman and coworkers retrieved a minimum of six and a median of eight samples using a 9-gauge vacuum-assisted breast biopsy device when describing their initial experience with MRI-guided biopsies.[28] However, the 2006 European consensus meeting on MR-guided vacuum-assisted breast biopsy recommended, on average, that at least 24 samples (using an 11-gauge probe) be obtained.[24] Lee et al showed no significant difference in the likelihood of DCIS underestimation as a function of the number of samples (=10 vs. >10 specimens) retrieved,[29] nor a difference in the rate of imaging-histologic discordance (=8 vs. >8) depending on specimen count.[30] The general range of 8 to 12 specimens as an initial acquisition set appears to be most commonly described. Once adequate samples are retrieved, the patient should be re-imaged to confirm lesion removal or partial removal. If it is unclear that the lesion has been sampled (i.e., it is seen to lie remote from the biopsy bed or it has not changed significantly in size, or both), re-biopsy, either at that time if possible, or in a delayed manner with repeat needle biopsy or MRI-guided localization, is indicated. If the biopsy appears to have been accurate, a marking clip should be placed at that time, important for several reasons. The patient may be undergoing neoadjuvant chemotherapy and the clip may represent the only remnant of the target. Subsequent localization may be required post-biopsy; a clip ensures that this may be mammographically or sonographically guided, rather than necessitating MRI guidance. The lesion may well be completely removed at biopsy. If follow-up is needed to monitor a benign biopsy site, the presence of a clip allows delineation of the exact site. In short, while the placement of a clip may be redundant with some highly conspicuous lesions, its presence rarely confuses matters, and placement infrequently is regretted, whereas lack of clip placement can confound management, especially in complex cases. For these reasons, we recommend that a clip be placed at the time of virtually every biopsy.

Post-Procedure Considerations

After the biopsy apparatus has been removed, firm pressure can be applied manually to the breast (from skin entry site to biopsy bed) by the physician, technologist or assistant for several minutes. For most patients, 5 to 10 minutes will suffice; if the patient is anticoagulated, longer and firmer compression is required, sometimes up to 20 minutes. This can be performed with the patient still prone, using the far grid plate for counter pressure, or with the patient supine. Once hemostasis has been achieved, a sterile dressing can be applied to the wound. The patient is instructed in post-procedure wound care, informed about what things are normal post-biopsy sequelae (minor pain and bruising) and what constitutes cause for concern (signs of infection, an expanding hematoma, shortness of breath). She should be told what to do in case of a problem, and given contact numbers. All these instructions should be given to her in written form, as well. In addition, the patient should be informed about how she will receive her biopsy results, and when. At this point, a post-procedure two view (craniocaudal and ML/LM views) mammogram can be obtained.

The obtained core samples should be placed in preservative. While a technologist or assistant may aid in packaging the specimen for transport and delivery to pathology, it is ultimately the responsibility of the practitioner to ensure that the specimen container is accurately labeled, and that a pathology requisition form is filled out with appropriate history and the specifics of the specimen's source. If the patient has had biopsy from more than one site, the specimens should be very specifically labeled as to the location of the respective biopsy sites (e.g.,"Specimen #1: left breast, upper outer quadrant; Specimen #2: left breast lower outer quadrant"). When calcifications are expected to be a component of the lesion, the pathologist should be cued to search for them, with specific instructions on the pathology request. If the patient has prior radiation therapy to the affected breast, that information should be noted on the requisition, because post-radiation atypia may prove difficult to differentiate histologically from DCIS or other atypia,[16] but obviously has markedly different management implications. Similarly, if the patient has been undergoing neoadjuvant chemotherapy, this should be noted on the pathology request.

A written permanent procedure report should be constructed that outlines the nature, side, and location of each biopsy target, the type of device used for core biopsy, the number of samples obtained, what adjustments to probe position were made during the procedure, whether a marking clip was placed, if a post-procedure mammogram was obtained, and any complications that were encountered during the procedure. An accurate assessment as to whether the lesion appeared partially or completely removed, or may not have been sampled, should be noted. This report should subsequently be amended when the pathology results are returned, with concordance or discordance noted, and further appropriate management or follow-up recommendations outlined. When the pathology results are returned, the case should be reviewed in its entirety, including perusal of all recent imaging performed. Concordance between initial imaging and the final pathology results must be assessed. If discordant results are returned, arrangements should be made for additional tissue sampling, either by repeat CNB or by excision. Additionally, the physician can make sure that additional areas do not now require further intervention, based on the newly available pathologic information. For example, if malignancy is confirmed, consideration may be now given to pursuing biopsy of another area previously deemed a BI-RADS 3 lesion. A well-defined policy should be in place outlining how the patient will be informed of her results. The policy must ensure that no patient will remain unapprised of her diagnosis, and this is likely best achieved when the biopsying physician (or delegate) takes responsibility for the task. In this way, it will never be simply assumed that the referring physician has conveyed the results. The patient may be informed of the results in person (via an additional office visit) or by telephone. If malignancy has been found, arrangements can be made for referral to other members of the breast cancer treatment team (surgical oncology, medical oncology) as indicated. If benign results are returned, the recommended follow-up can be outlined to the patient. If an atypical or discordant diagnosis has been rendered, discussion can be made with the patient about the need for further intervention. The conveyance of results and recommendations should be documented, preferably as an addendum to the formal biopsy report.

Indications

MRI guidance should be used to biopsy any suspicious lesion detected only or most definitively on breast MRI. This would include any BI-RADS 4—suspicious or 5—highly suspicious lesion for which biopsy has been recommended. Although BI-RADS 3—probably benign findings are by definition suitable for short-term follow up rather than biopsy, in some cases, immediate biopsy of the lesions may be preferred instead. Some examples would include patients who have a highly suspicious lesion elsewhere in either breast, those with a known synchronous breast cancer where management may be altered by the presence another cancer, patients who are undergoing fertility treatment or anticipate getting pregnant in the near future, those with a strong family history, and those for whom the anxiety of short-term follow-up outweighs the benefit of avoiding biopsy.

If multiple suspicious findings are present, biopsy of as many targets as needed to outline the full extent of malignant disease and direct appropriate future management should be carried out. For example, if multiple enhancing suspicious masses are seen in one breast, biopsy of at least two of these can be performed, preferably those lying farthest apart, to fully establish extent of disease and help determine the need for mastectomy versus breast conserving surgery. However, biopsy of all masses is likely not needed. The fewest number biopsies that will firmly establish surgical management is optimal.

Because of the relative cost and ease of percutaneous biopsy using ultrasound guidance versus MRI guidance, attempts are often made to identify the suspicious MRI lesion sonographically and biopsy with that modality. This requires a good working knowledge of both modalities, the ability to translate expected lesion position from one modality to another, meticulous radiologic-pathologic correlation when the results are returned, and the knowledge to obtain imaging follow-up either immediately post-biopsy or in a delayed manner, or even rebiopsy, as needed. If there is any question as to whether an accurate correlate has been picked, biopsy should likely proceed guided by MRI. If there is low likelihood that a sonographic target will be found, especially in small or non-masslike enhancements, so-called *second-look* ultrasound may be deferred in favor of promptly proceeding with MRI-guided biopsy. A corollary to this discussion is that imaging guided biopsies, in general, are best performed by a physician with the above-described knowledge and skill set, and that physician, in most cases, is a radiologist.

Contraindications

A few contraindications to MRI-guided core biopsy exist. It is obviously contraindicated in those patients who cannot undergo MRI, due to implanted metallic or electromagnetic devices or allergy to MRI contrast material. Biopsy should not be performed on a patient who has no intention of seeking treatment if a cancer is diagnosed, due to co-morbid conditions or other reasons. Anticoagulation has traditionally been considered a relative contraindication for core biopsy, with the patient asked to cease therapy prior to biopsy if possible. However, recent literature suggests no significant difference in hematoma rate between anticoagulated patients (on either warfarin or nonsteroidal anti-inflammatory products) and other patients undergoing core biopsy.[17] In implant patients, if implant rupture appears likely, core biopsy should be avoided; however, with careful planning, use of implant-displacement upon compression of the breast, and exploitation of the ability to rotate the sampling notch so that the vacuum is directed away from the implant, this should be a rare situation. The potential for implant rupture should be clearly delineated to the patient during the consenting process. Claustrophobia represents a relative contraindication and can often be mitigated by oral administration of an anti-anxiety agent from the benzodiazapam family of medications prior to the procedure (and after written consent has been obtained).

Potential Complications of Magnetic Resonance Imaging-Guided Vacuum-Assisted Breast Biopsy

Complications during MRI-guided vacuum-assisted breast biopsy are relatively rare but potentially include: hematoma formation (not uncommon), infection, pneumothorax (rare), allergic reaction to local anesthetic or MRI contrast material, and vagal reaction. A small amount of bleeding is not unusual during vacuum-assisted breast biopsy but occasionally, needle transection of a vessel can result in more rapid bleeding. This is most certainly not a life-threatening event but can result in significant hematoma formation. The ultimate size of the hematoma can be minimized by firm compression over the area at the end of the procedure, to include the segment of breast from needle entry site to lesion. If it occurs early in the procedure or is arterial in origin, the bleeding can result in target obscuration or displacement. If is apparent that this is occurring as biopsy proceeds (large amount of blood being returned via or around needle), a clip may be placed as quickly as possible so that the area can be re-identified for re-biopsy or excision, if the procedure needs to be prematurely ended.

If sterile technique is respected, infection should be rare. At some point in the biopsy process, the procedure becomes *clean* rather than *sterile*; however, if sterility of the probe/needle and skin is maintained, a germ-free environment can be achieved. If infection subsequently is reported by the patient, she should be asked to come in so that the physician can inspect the wound, ensure that abscess is not a possibility, and assess whether the infection is not simply a reaction to tape or bandage material. If infection is confirmed, the physician can choose to prescribe antibiotics as appropriate, and arrange to see the patient in follow-up.

Vagal reactions (bradycardia with hypotension) are not uncommon during breast procedures, but occur relatively less often during most MRI-guided vacuum-assisted breast biopsy, in part owing to the patient's prone positioning for the procedure. The vast majority of vagal reactions respond immediately to simple conservative treatment: placing the patient in a horizontal position, elevation of patient's feet/placement in Trendelenburg with squeezing of calf muscles to restore blood return to head; application of a cool cloth to neck or forehead; calm reassurance. Oxygen may be administered but is rarely required. As she recovers, the patient should be warned that she will soon experience the onset of shaking, as release of epinephrine by her system occurs. If the patient does not respond to these conservative measures, an IV may started and consideration given to pharmacologic support (atropine). Allergic or anaphylactoid reactions must be recognized and treated promptly. In the rare case of suspected pneumothorax, a chest radiograph can be obtained and further treatment as needed pursued. With these latter types of more complicated or severe events, the biopsying physician has the ultimate responsibility for patient outcome. As a result, it is the obligation of any physician taking on the privilege of performing such procedures to also assume the responsibility of knowing how to manage minor complications, including a working knowledge of the medications and interventions involved. However, ultimately the best interest of the patient is paramount, and if the biopsying physician needs assistance in an acute situation, help should be sought promptly, up to and including sending the patient to the Emergency Room or calling a "code."

FINE-NEEDLE ASPIRATION CYTOLOGY

The above discussions have centered on use of large core biopsy devices to retrieve tissue via imaging guidance. Another method of obtaining material involves use of FNAC technique to obtain cytologic (rather than histologic) material. While still used extensively at some centers, its use has in general waned as core and vacuum-assisted devices have been introduced. Duijm and colleagues report that over the course of their observation from 1995 to 2005, the percentage of malignant cases diagnosed pre-operatively by way of FNAC decreased from 91.3% to 14.5%, while those diagnosed by core biopsy (either using ultrasound or stereotactic guidance) increased from 8.7% to 86.5%.[31] One reason for this includes the relatively high rate of insufficiency noted with FNAC technique. The results of a multicenter trial assessing the diagnostic accuracy of imaging-guided FNAC directed at non-palpable breast lesions, conducted by the Radiologic Diagnostic Oncology Group V, demonstrated a 35.4% insufficiency rate. In addition, a 12% false negative rate for FNAC would have occurred if it had been relied upon as proof of diagnosis.[32] In fact, during an interim analysis of the data, the rate of FNAC insufficiency was considered to be so high that the FNA arm of the study was closed.[33] Accurate FNAC is achieved at some centers, but requires practiced technique in obtaining and handling the cytologic material and availability of dedicated cytopathologists. Not all of the centers involved in the multicenter trial had these prerequisites; however, the group felt that the cross-section of centers involved accurately reflected the pattern of care most frequently encountered across the country, and as a result, opined that FNAC was impractical for diagnosis of nonpalpable breast lesions. Other potential shortcomings involve the inability to differentiate between invasive and noninvasive cancers, and lack of sufficient tissue to define tumor biomarker status. Proponents of FNAC point out that an immediate diagnosis can be rendered, thereby lessening time-to-diagnosis and patient anxiety. However, this is only helpful if the diagnosis rendered is accurate. If immediacy is desired, Jones and colleagues report that using imprint cytology technique (dragging an ultrasound-guided core sample across a dry slide to yield cytologic material, with subsequent immediate evaluation) on US-guided CNB specimens can provide same-day answer similar in accuracy to that achieved with FNAC, but still allowing more definitive evaluation of the larger core samples.[34] However, in reality, the complete evaluation of a potential breast cancer is rarely achieved with immediacy. The retrieval of cancer cells is only one part of the process. Thorough and sometime extensive imaging, as well as physical exam, is required to assess for extent of disease. Involvement of the breast imager, surgeon, medical and radiation oncologist add time to the evaluation, but are vital. As a result, corners should not be cut in the desire for immediate diagnosis, if more accurate information can be obtained by waiting a few days for definitive histologic information. The patient can usually accept this if educated about its importance.

CONCLUSION

Imaging-guided percutaneous biopsy, using either core or vacuum-assisted technique combined with a variety of guidance modalities, proves to be a safe, accurate, cost-effective method of establishing the tissue diagnosis of imaging-detected breast abnormalities, thereby either mitigating the need for surgical biopsy when benign pathology is demonstrated or allowing definitive single-stage surgical therapy in most cases, if malignant results are returned. Careful attention to technique and radiologic-pathologic concordance is required, best ensured when performed by an operator well versed in multi-modality image interpretation.

KEY POINTS

- Imaging guided percutaneous breast biopsy has been validated as a safe, cost-effective, accurate method of tissue sampling. It is now widely accepted as the first-line technique for establishing the benign or malignant nature of an imaging-detected breast abnormality, supplanting surgical biopsy in most cases.
- Ultrasound-guidance, mammographic stereotactic-guidance, and MRI-guidance are all effective methods of performing percutaneous breast biopsy.
- Of these methods, ultrasound guidance is preferred, when possible, because of patient comfort, cost and real-time imaging capabilities.
- Fine-needle aspiration cytology is less accurate than core biopsy, and should be used in limited circumstances.
- A successful percutaneous breast biopsy program demands disciplined radiologic-pathologic correlation and is best performed by a practitioner well-versed in multi-modality imaging interpretation.

SUGGESTED READINGS

Heywang-Kobrunner SH, Sinnatamby R, Lebeau A, Lebrecht A, Britton PD, Schreer I. Interdisciplinary consensus on the uses and technique of MR-guided vacuum-assisted breast biopsy (VAB): results of a European consensus meeting. *Eur J Radiol* 2009;**72**:289-94.

Liberman L. Percutaneous imaging-guided core breast biopsy: state of the art at the millennium. *AJR Am J Roentgenol* 2000;**174**:1191-9.

Parker SH, Jobe WE, Dennis MA, Stavros AT, Johnson KK, Yakes WF, et al. US-guided automated large-core breast biopsy. *Radiology* 1993;**187**:507-11.

Parker SH, Klaus AJ. Performing a breast biopsy with a directional, vacuum-assisted biopsy instrument. *RadioGraphics* 1997;**17**:1233-52.

Reynolds H. Core needle biopsy of challenging benign breast conditions: a comprehensive literature review. *AJR Am J Roentgenol* 2000;**174**:1245-50.

Youk JH, Kim EK, Kim MJ, Lee JY, Oh KK. Missed cancers at US-guided core needle biopsy: how to reduce them. *RadioGraphics* 2007;**27**:79-94.

REFERENCES

1. Parker SH, Burbank F, Jackman RJ, Aucreman CJ, Cardenosa G, Cink TM, et al. Percutaneous large core breast biopsy: a multi-institutional study. *Radiology* 1994;**193**:359-64.
2. White RR, Halperin TJ, Olson Jr JA, Soo MS, Bentley RC, Seigler HF. Impact of core needle biopsy on the surgical management of mammographic abnormalities. *Ann Surg* 2001;**233**:769-77.
3. Jackman RJ, Marzoni Jr FA. Needle-localized breast biopsy: why do we fail? *Radiology* 1997;**204**:677-84.
4. Gruber R, Bernt R, Helbich TH. [Cost-effectiveness of percutaneous core needle breast biopsy (CNBB) versus open surgical biopsy (OSB) of nonpalpable breast lesions: metaanalysis and cost evaluation for German-speaking countries.]. *Rofo* 2008;**180**:134-42.
5. Smith DN, Christian R, Meyer JE. Large core needle biopsy of nonpalpable breast cancers. The impact on subsequent surgical excisions. *Arch Surg* 1997;**132**:256-9.
6. Mainiero MB, Gareen IF, Bird CE, Smith W, Cobb C, Schepps B. Preferential use of sonographically guided biopsy to minimize patient discomfort and procedure time in a percutaneous image-guided breast biopsy program. *J Ultrasound Med* 2002;**21**:1221-6.
7. Parker SH, Jobe WE, Dennis MA, Stavros AT, Johnson KK, Yakes WF, et al. US-guided automated large-core breast biopsy. *Radiology* 1993;**187**:507-11.
8. Schueller G, Jaromi S, Ponhold L, Fuchsjaeger M, Memarsadeghi M, Rudas M, et al. US-guided 14-gauge core needle breast biopsy: results of a validation study in 1352 cases. *Radiology* 2008;**248**:406-13.
9. American College of Radiology. *American College of Radiology Practice Guidelines and Technical Standards-2008*. p. 572.
10. Helbich TH, Rudas M, Haitel A, Kohlberger PD, Thurnher M, Gnant M, et al. Evaluation of needle size for breast biopsy: comparison of 14-, 16-, and 18-gauge biopsy needles. *AJR Am J Roentgenol* 1998;**171**:59-63.
11. Nath ME, Robinson TM, Tobon H, Chough DM, Sumkin JH. Automated large-core needle biopsy of surgically removed breast lesions: comparison of samples obtained with 14-, 16- and 18-gauge needles. *Radiology* 1995;**197**:739-42.
12. Fishman JE, Milikowski C, Ramsinghani R, Velasquez MV, Aviram G. US-guided core needle biopsy of the breast: how many specimens are necessary? *Radiology* 2003;**226**:779-82.
13. Philpotts LE, Hooley JR, Lee CH. Comparison of automated versus vacuum-assisted biopsy methods for sonographically guided core biopsy of the breast. *AJR Am J Roentgenol* 2003;**180**:347-51.
14. Jang M, Cho N, Moon WK, Park JS, Seong MH, Park IA. Underestimation of atypical ductal hyperplasia at sonographically guided core biopsy of the breast. *AJR Am J Roentgenol* 2008;**191**:1347-51.

15. Mimoz O, Villeminey S, Ragot S, Dahyot-Fizelier C, Laksiri L, Petitpas F, et al. Chlorhexidine-based antiseptic solution vs alcohol-based povidone-iodine for central venous catheter care. *Arch Intern Med* 2007;**167**:2066–72.
16. Ellis IO, Humphreys S, Mitchell M, Pinder SE, Wells CA, Zakhour HD, for the UK National Coordinating Committee for Breast Screening Pathology; European Commission Working Group on Breast Screening Pathology. Best practice No 179: guidelines for breast needle biopsy handling and reporting in breast screening assessment. *J Clin Pathol* 2004;**57**:897–902.
17. Somerville P, Seifert PJ, Destounis SV, Murphy PF, Young W. Anticoagulation and bleeding risk after core needle biopsy. *AJR Am J Roentgenol* 2008;**191**:1194–7.
18. Liebens F, Carly B, Cusumano P, Van Beveren M, Beier B, Fastrez M, et al. Breast cancer seeding associated with core needle biopsies: a systematic review. *Maturitas* 2009;**62**:113–23.
19. Kettritz U, Rotter K, Scheer I, Murauer M, Schulz-Wendtland R, Peter D, et al. Stereotactic vacuum-assisted breast biopsy in 2874 patients: a multicenter study. *Cancer* 2004;**100**:245–51.
20. Pfarl G, Helbich TH, Riedl CC, Wagner T, Gnant M, Rudas M, et al. Stereotactic 11-gauge vacuum-assisted breast biopsy: a validation study. *AJR Am J Roentgenol* 2002;**179**:1503–7.
21. Liberman L, Sama MP. Cost-effectiveness of stereotactic 11-gauge directional vacuum-assisted breast biopsy. *AJR Am J Roentgenol* 2000;**175**:53–8.
22. Liberman L, Bracero N, Morris E, Thornton C, Dershaw DD. MRI-guided 9-gauge vacuum-assisted breast biopsy: initial clinical experience. *AJR Am J Roentgenol* 2005;**185**:183–93.
23. Mahoney MC. Initial clinical experience with a new MRI vacuum-assisted breast biopsy device. *J Magn Reson Imaging* 2008;**28**:900–5.
24. Heywang-Kobrunner SH, Sinnatamby R, Lebeau A, Lebrecht A, Britton PD, Schreer I. Consensus Group: Interdisciplinary consensus on the uses and technique of MR-guided vacuum-assisted breast biopsy (VAB): results of a European consensus meeting. *Eur J Radiol* 2009;**72**:289–94.
25. Ghate S, Rosen E, Soo MS, Baker JA. MRI-guided vacuum-assisted breast biopsy with a handheld portable biopsy system. *AJR Am J Roentgenol* 2006;**186**:1733–6.
26. Perlet C, Heywang-Kobrunner S, Heinig A, Sittek H, Casselman J, Anderson I, et al. Magnetic resonance-guided, vacuum-assisted breast biopsy: results from a European multicenter study of 538 lesions. *Cancer* 2006;**106**:982–90.
27. Hefler L, Casselman J, Amaya B, Heinig A, Alberich T, Koelbl H, et al. Follow-up of breast lesions detected by MRI not biopsied due to absent enhancement of contrast medium. *Eur Radiol* 2003;**13**:344–6.
28. Liberman L, Morris E, Dershaw DD, Thornton CM, Van Zee KJ, Tan LK. Fast MRI-guided vacuum-assisted breast biopsy: initial experience. *AJR Am J Roentgenol* 2003;**181**:1283–93.
29. Lee J, Kaplan J, Murray MP, Mazur-Grbec M, Tadic T, Stimac D, et al. Underestimation of DCIS at MRI-guided vacuum-assisted breast biopsy. *AJR Am J Roentgenol* 2007;**189**:468–74.
30. Lee J, Kaplan J, Murray MP, Bartella L, Morris EA, Joo S, et al. Imaging-histologic discordance at MRI-guided 9-gauge vacuum-assisted breast biopsy. *AJR Am J Roentgenol* 2007;**189**:852–9.
31. Duijm L, Groenewoud J, Roumen RM, de Koning HJ, Plaisier ML, Fracheboud J. A decade of breast cancer screening in The Netherlands: trends in the preoperative diagnosis of breast cancer. *Breast Cancer Res Treat* 2007;**106**:113–9.
32. Pisano E, Fajardo L, Caudry DJ, Sneige N, Frable WJ, Berg WA, et al. Fine-needle aspiration biopsy of nonpalpable breast lesions in a multicenter clinical trial: results from the Radiologic Diagnostic Oncology Group V. *Radiology* 2001;**219**:785–92.
33. Pisano E, Fajardo L, Tsimikas J, Sneige N, Frable WJ, Gatsonis CA, et al. Rate of insufficient samples for fine-needle aspiration for nonpalpable breast lesions in a multicenter trial: the Radiologic Diagnostic Group 5 study. *Cancer* 1998;**82**:679–88.
34. Jones L, Lott MF, Calder CJ, Kutt E. Imprint cytology from ultrasound-guided core biopsies: accurate and immediate diagnosis in a one-stop breast clinic. *Clin Radiol* 2004;**59**:903–8.

CHAPTER 30

Galactography

Mary Catherine Mahoney, Valerie P. Jackson, and Lawrence W. Bassett

Galactography (ductography) is a mammographic study involving the injection of water-soluble contrast material into a breast duct. It is indicated for evaluation of spontaneous, unilateral, bloody, serous, or clear nipple discharge that originates from one or two ducts. Many women will experience discharge that is elicited when the breast and nipple are vigorously compressed or manipulated.[1] Therefore, galactography is performed only in cases of spontaneous discharge. A hemoglobin reagent stick can be used to test the discharge for blood. Other types of discharge (e.g., yellow, green, or milky) are usually physiologic and not associated with breast tumors.[1,2] The incidence of abnormal discharge caused by carcinoma has ranged widely in the literature. A review of the literature by Tabar and colleagues in 1983 demonstrated a 10% frequency of carcinoma in women undergoing surgery for nipple discharge. The frequency was higher for bloody discharge (13%), compared with serous discharge (7%).[3] Cytologic analysis of nipple discharge has a high false-negative rate and is therefore unreliable for evaluation of nipple discharge.[1-3] Although less frequent, false-positive cytology results for nipple discharge have also been reported.[1-3]

PROCEDURE

A woman presenting with bloody or serous nipple discharge should undergo diagnostic mammographic evaluation as the primary imaging modality. If no mammographic abnormalities are found to account for the discharge, galactography can then be performed. Ultrasonography also may be helpful in the evaluation of nipple discharge to search for a dilated duct, an intraductal mass, or ductal irregularity.

Discharge must be present on the day of the ductogram so that the discharging duct can be identified. The woman is asked to check for discharge on the day of her appointment to ensure that the discharge is present. It is important for the patient to elicit only a small amount of discharge so that fluid will be available at the time of the procedure to guide cannulation of the appropriate duct.

At the time of the procedure, a small amount of discharge is elicited by the physician to determine the appropriate duct for cannulation. It is unusual for there to be a palpable mass associated with nipple discharge. However, there is often a *trigger point*. This is a point at which pressure will elicit the discharge, and it is often easily identified by the patient.

The equipment needed for galactography includes a 30-gauge, angled, blunt needle-catheter with attached tubing (Ranfac Corporation, Avon, Mass). This is filled with a water-soluble contrast agent such as iothalamate meglumine (Conray-60, Mallinckrodt Inc, St. Louis) and connected to a 1-mL syringe. The system must be completely filled with contrast medium and free of air bubbles, which would appear as filling defects if injected into the ductal system. Although nonionic contrast material can be used (because of the possibility of contrast extravasation from duct perforation), this precaution is unnecessary, as there are no reports in the literature regarding adverse effects from extravasation of ionic contrast material into the breast tissue.[4] A high-intensity lamp provides additional light for better visualization, and its warmth often assists in dilatation of the ductal orifice. Magnifying glasses are needed for optimal visualization of the duct orifice as well.

The patient is usually in a supine or semi-reclining position. The breast is cleansed with an antiseptic solution to remove dried secretions. The radiologist then gently expresses a small amount of discharge onto the nipple surface to identify the correct ductal orifice. Once the appropriate ductal orifice is identified, the cannula is easily inserted into the orifice. The nipple should be stabilized between the thumb and forefinger of one hand. The cannula is held in the opposite hand, and the radiologist carefully probes the area of discharge to guide the catheter into the appropriate ductal orifice. No pressure should be applied. In some cases, it may be helpful to elongate the nipple to firmly seat the catheter into the ductal orifice. If cannulation is unsuccessful, warm compresses applied to the nipple areolar complex may help dilate the opening and ease cannulation. However, if cannulation is still unsuccessful, it is often helpful for a different radiologist to make another attempt. In the rare event that catheter placement is still not possible, the patient should be rescheduled for another attempt 1 to 2 weeks later.

When ductal cannulation is achieved, the needle should not be forced because perforation may occur. The contrast injection rate will be slow because of both the small needle size and the high viscosity of the contrast agent. Approximately 0.4 mL of contrast medium is administered. Injection should be continued until the patient feels fullness or when the contrast agent refluxes onto the nipple surface. Injection should be stopped if the patient experiences pain or a burning sensation, because this usually indicates extravasation. In most cases, less than 1 mL of contrast agent is used.

Magnification craniocaudal (CC) and 90-degree lateral mammograms are obtained with mild to moderate compression. Additional mammographic views are performed as needed if there is superimposition of the opacified ducts. Although the needle may be taped to the nipple during mammographic imaging, it is preferable to remove the needle to prevent dislodging or contamination during positioning. It is usually easy to recannulate the duct if a second injection is necessary for further duct filling or clarification of a potential abnormality. Contrast material may leak out during positioning and mammographic imaging, but this is usually minimal.

The patient is given gauze pads to place in her brassiere after the procedure. She is advised to expect increased discharge for 1 or 2 days after the procedure and even new bloody discharge during this time. Patients are instructed to call the breast imaging center for any symptoms of mastitis, including redness, swelling, and increased warmth of the breast.

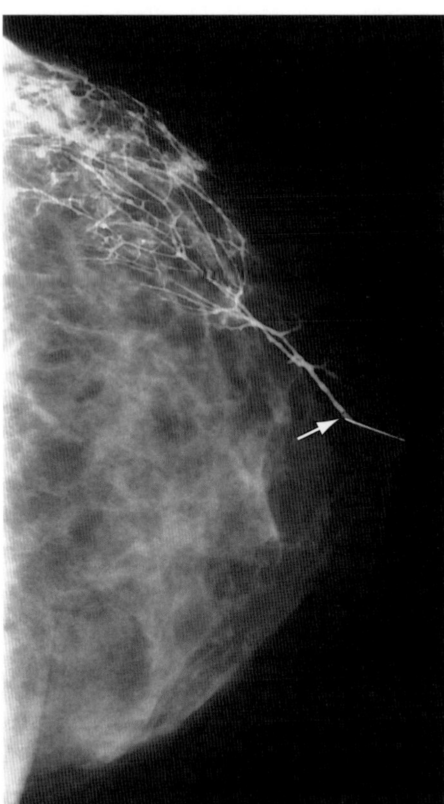

■ **FIGURE 30-1** Normal galactogram (left craniocaudal projection). There is normal arborization of the ductal system, with lobular filling. A small air bubble can be seen near the catheter tip (*white arrow*).

INTERPRETATION

A normal study demonstrates filling of the lactiferous sinus, the arborizing ductal system, and even the lobules (Fig. 30-1). The lactiferous sinus is a fusiform dilated ductal segment immediately posterior to the nipple. There may be intercommunication between ducts, and the ducts may extend in unexpected directions from the nipple.[4,5]

Generalized ductal ectasia may occur in secretory disease (Fig. 30-2), and filling of small cysts may be seen with fibrocystic changes of the breast (Fig. 30-3).[6] The normal duct caliber is variable, and there are no well-established normal limits.[5,6] The lobular "blush" is due to contrast agent filling the lobular portion of the terminal ductal lobular unit (TDLU) (Fig. 30-4).[4]

Papillomas are the most common cause of spontaneous bloody nipple discharge.[2,4] These lesions are usually mammographically occult but may present as a small circumscribed mass or as clustered microcalcifications.[6-8] At galactography, papillomas cause a round (Fig. 30-5) or lobulated (Figs 30-6 and 30-7) filling defect within the duct.[6-8] They may also

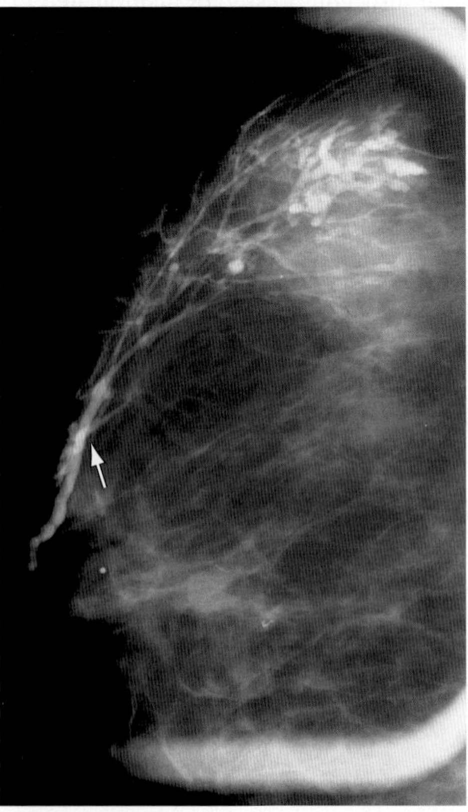

■ **FIGURE 30-2** Duct ectasia. This magnification left mediolateral galactogram demonstrates diffuse mild dilation of the duct (*arrow*). There were no filling defects.

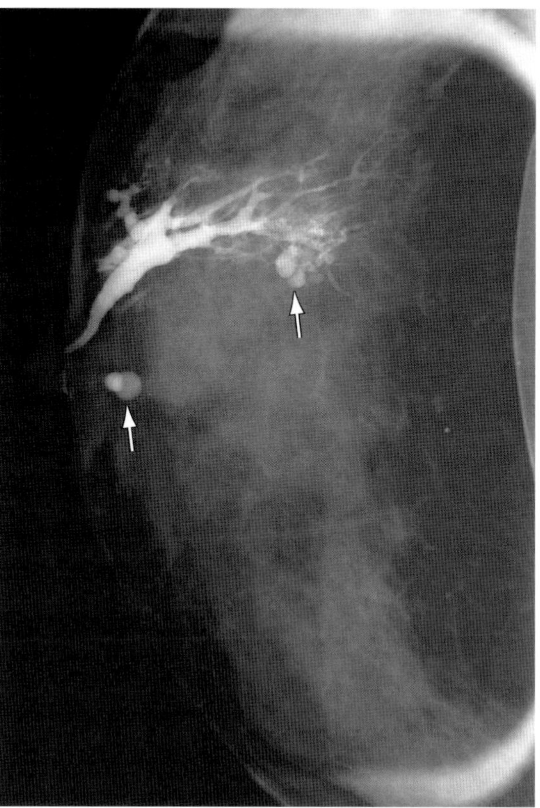

■ **FIGURE 30-3** Cysts on galactography. Contrast agent fills the arborizing duct system on this magnification right craniocaudal galactogram. Several small cysts are filled with contrast agent (*white arrows*).

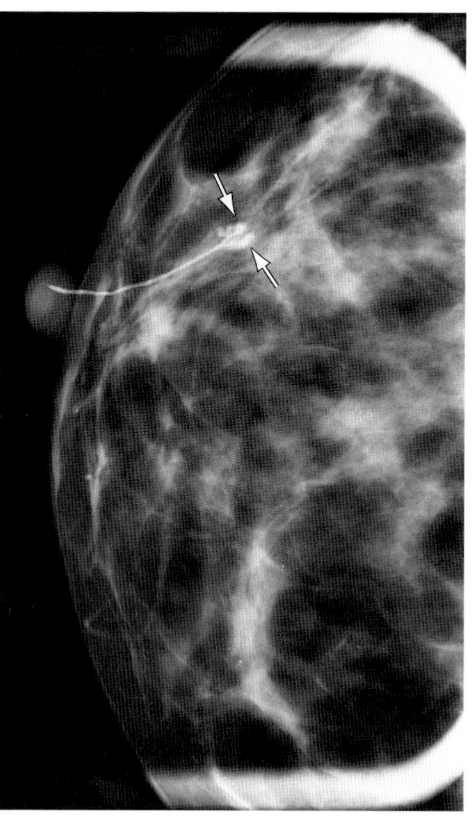

■ **FIGURE 30-4** Normal galactogram with lobular filling (*arrows*).

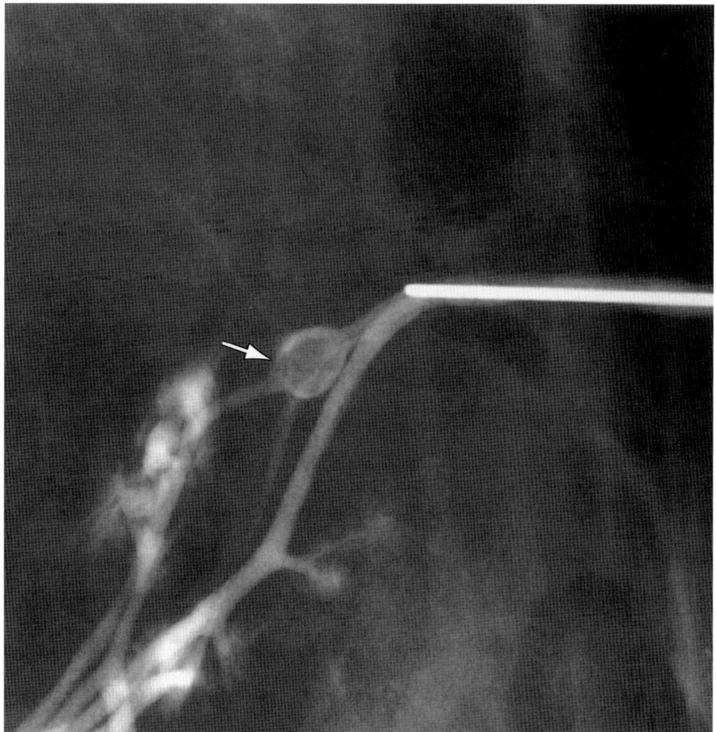

■ **FIGURE 30-5** Solitary papilloma. A 49-year-old woman presented with spontaneous nipple discharge. The 5-mm round circumscribed filling defect seen on galactogram (*arrow*) was identified as a papilloma at excisional biopsy.

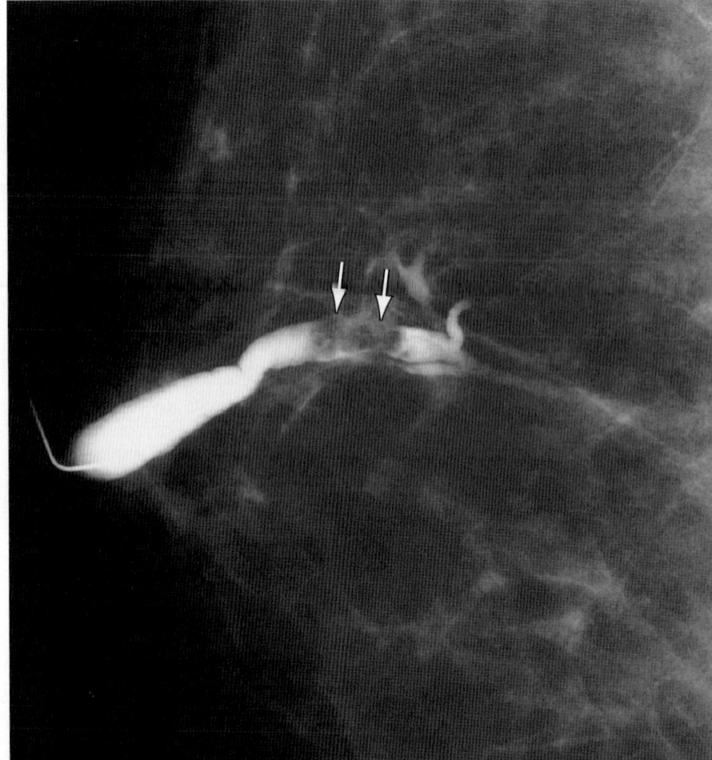

■ **FIGURE 30-6** Solitary papilloma. The patient is a 72-year-old woman with bloody nipple discharge produced by a 9-mm lobulated filling defect (*arrows*). At surgical biopsy this was determined to be a benign solitary papilloma.

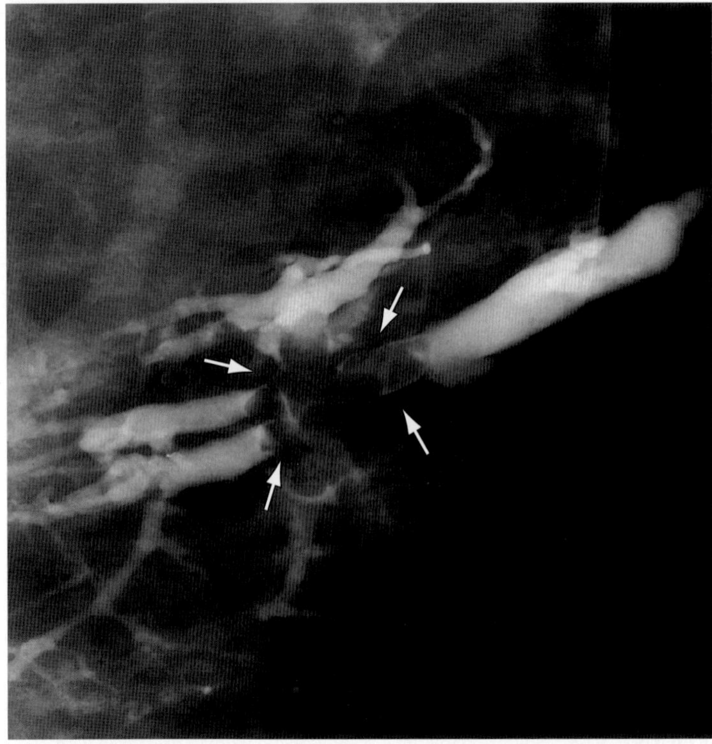

■ **FIGURE 30-7** Solitary papilloma. Bloody nipple discharge occurred in a 65-year-old woman due to a 1.5-cm lobulated papilloma (*arrows*).

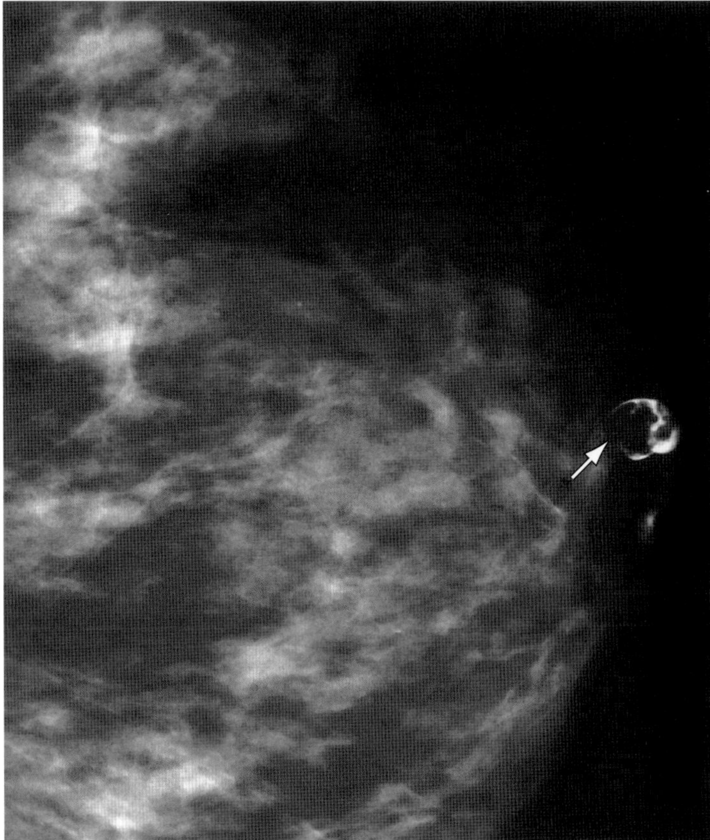

■ **FIGURE 30-8** Solitary papilloma. Magnification left craniocaudal galactogram demonstrating a lobulated filling defect (*arrow*) that completely obstructs the passage of contrast agent.

cause ductal dilation due to the copious secretions produced by the tumor.[4,6,7] Occasionally, a large papilloma may completely obstruct the duct, preventing passage of contrast material beyond the lesion (Fig. 30-8).[6,7]

Intraductal carcinoma may produce filling defects that are indistinguishable from papillomas on galactography.[4,6] Intraductal carcinoma may also cause wall irregularity, abrupt caliber changes, and blunt cutoff of the duct on galactography (Figs. 30-9 and 30-10).[6] These are suspicious changes but not reliable in the differentiation of carcinoma and papilloma.[5,6]

Perforation of the duct causes extravasation of contrast medium. An irregular extraluminal collection of contrast agent obscures the ductal anatomy and prevents completion and interpretation of the galactogram (Figs. 30-11 and 30-12).

OTHER MODALITIES

Ultrasonography can also be used for evaluation of the ducts. High-frequency ultrasound transducers (10-15 MHz) allow visualization of ductal structures and intraductal abnormalities (Fig. 30-13). However, it may be difficult to confirm that the sonographically visualized ductal structures are the cause of the patient's discharge. Ultrasound-guided percutaneous galactography has been described in patients for whom conventional ductal cannulation is unsuccessful.[9] Contrast-enhanced magnetic resonance imaging (MRI) has also been used to evaluate breast ducts.[10] The sensitivity of MRI is high and may be better than galactography in the detection of cancer.[10] However, enhancement patterns are variable and the specificity for distinguishing papillomas, ductal hyperplasia, and intraductal carcinoma is not well studied. Nonetheless, contrast-enhanced MRI is an option for women with nipple discharge that is of concern and for whom ductal cannulation and successful galactography cannot be achieved (Fig. 30-14).

CONTRAINDICATIONS AND COMPLICATIONS

Galactography is not indicated for evaluation of discharge that is not bloody, serous, or clear, because other types of discharge are usually physiologic.[2,4,8] Similarly, it is not indicated for women with any type of discharge that is multiductal and bilateral or in pregnant or lactating women.[8] Benign bloody discharge may occur in the second and third trimesters of pregnancy and may persist in the postpartum period.[11]

A relative contraindication to galactography is the presence of mastitis.[6] The procedure is not performed because of the risk of spreading the infection and increasing the inflammation. Galactography is usually not performed in women with known hypersensitivity to radiographic

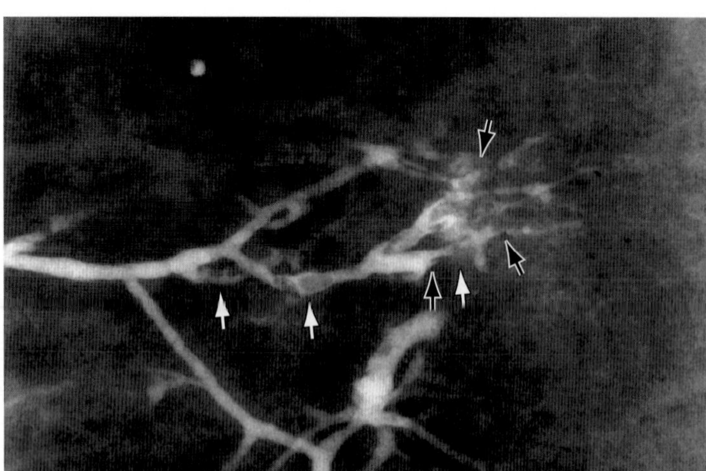

■ **FIGURE 30-9** Ductal carcinoma in a 50-year-old woman with spontaneous bloody nipple discharge. The magnification right craniocaudal galactogram shows multiple small filling defects (*white arrows*), wall irregularity (*black arrows*), and abrupt cutoff of the column of contrast agent.

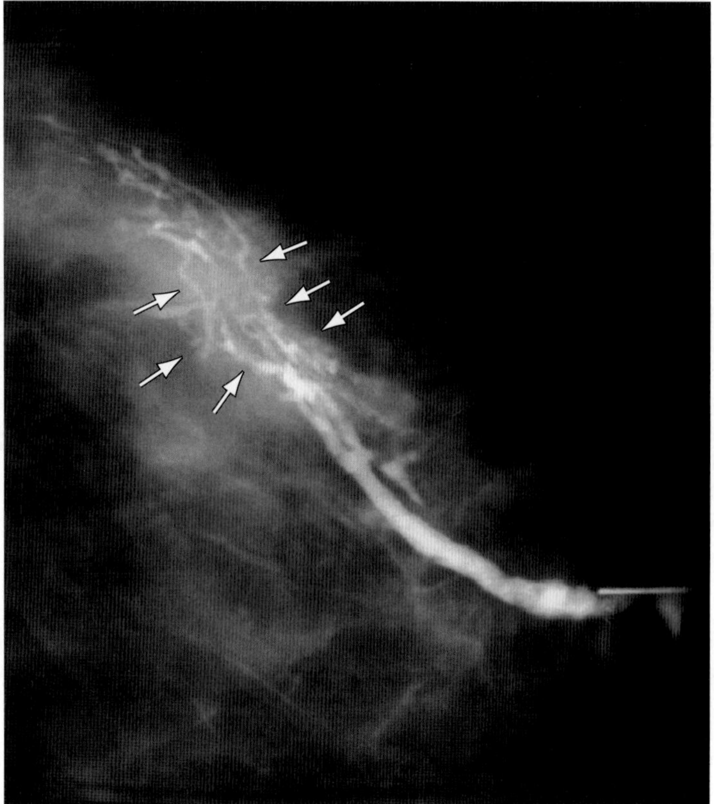

■ **FIGURE 30-10** Ductal carcinoma in situ in a 60-year-old woman with bloody nipple discharge. The left craniocaudal galactogram shows wall irregularity and minimal narrowing (*arrows*).

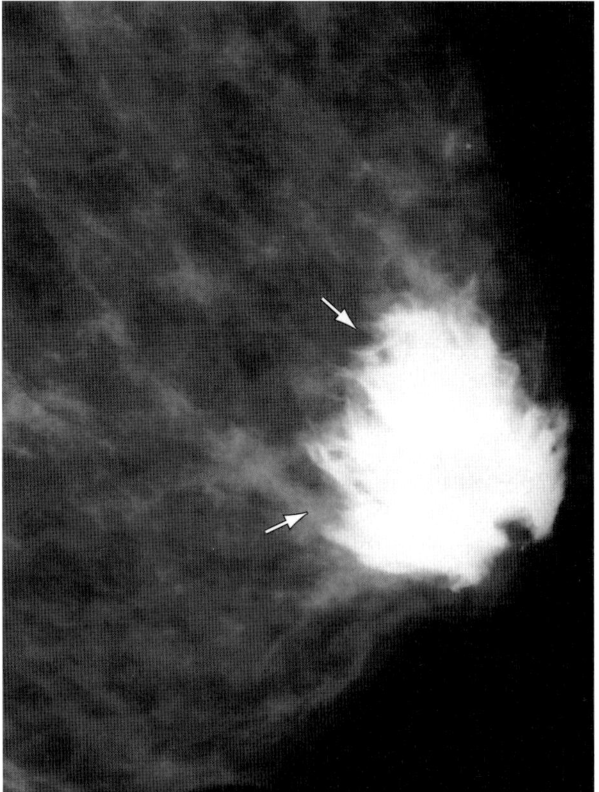

■ **FIGURE 30-11** Contrast extravasation (*arrows*) from perforation of the duct in the immediate subareolar region.

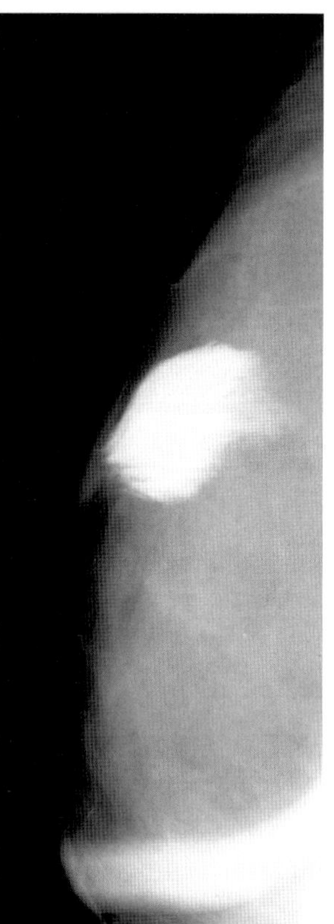

■ **FIGURE 30-12** Contrast extravasation from perforation of the duct in the subareolar region.

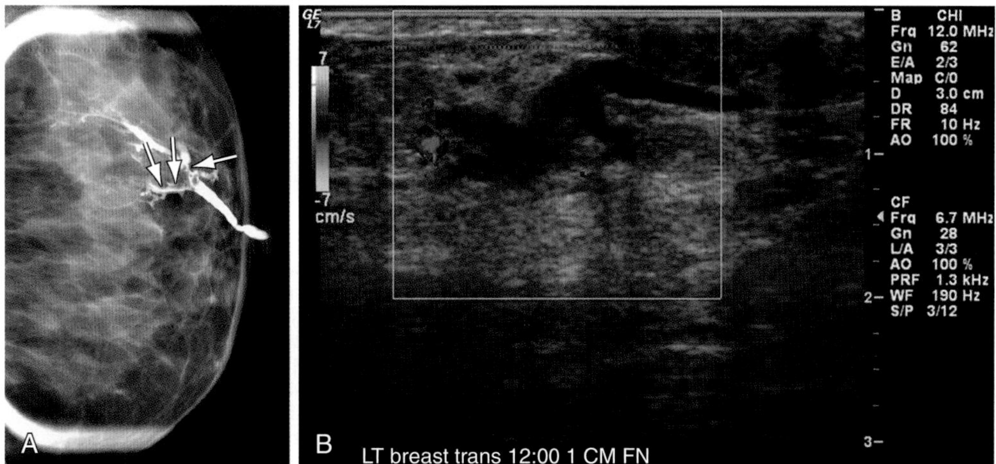

■ **FIGURE 30-13** Ductal carcinoma in a 69-year-old woman. **A,** Galactogram demonstrates multiple irregular filling defects and wall irregularity. **B,** Ultrasound image shows a dilated ductal segment containing a branching, irregular solid mass.

contrast media. Although there are no reports of reactions to contrast agents after galactography, the potential for contrast medium to enter the vascular system exists.[4] In these cases, ultrasound evaluation is usually performed. Additional contraindications to galactography include severe nipple retraction or previous nipple surgery with cannulation of the ducts.[4]

There are two potential complications of galactography. The first is perforation of the duct with extravasation of contrast medium into the breast tissue. The procedure cannot be completed, and no diagnostic information is obtained. This necessitates a repeat attempt, usually 1 to 2 weeks later. The extravasation itself is of no clinical consequence, owing to the very small amount of the contrast agent used.[4]

The second potential complication of galactography is mastitis. Strict attention to sterile technique is important. The patient should be instructed regarding the signs and symptoms of mastitis so that she can seek medical attention immediately if an infection develops.

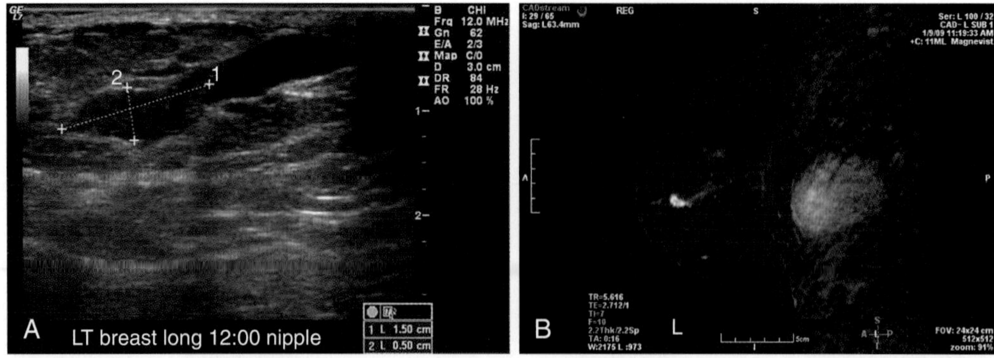

■ **FIGURE 30-14** Intraductal papilloma in a 50-year-old woman with bloody nipple discharge. A, Ultrasound image demonstrates a 1.5-cm solid intraductal mass. **B,** Contrast enhanced subtraction magnetic resonance (MR) image demonstrates a corresponding enhancing mass.

Vasovagal reactions can occur during any interventional procedure. Although it is rare for a vasovagal reaction to occur during galactography, the patient should be supervised throughout the procedure.

MANAGEMENT

When a lesion is identified on galactography, surgical excision is recommended because of the possibility of malignancy.[1,2] Although some surgeons prefer to dissect the discharging duct without preoperative galactography, many surgeons use a galactographic "road map" to guide them to the site of the tumor.[5,10] The procedure is repeated on the day of surgery with a 1:1 ratio of radiographic contrast medium and methylene blue.[4,5,12] This allows the surgeon to visually identify the abnormal ductal system. Placement of a drop or two of collodion on the nipple orifice will prevent leakage before surgery. Alternatively, needle localization can be performed prior to surgery. Repeat galactography can be performed, and localization can be directed toward the visualized filling defect.[13]

Percutaneous image-guided biopsy is an alternative to surgery for histologic sampling of lesions identified on galactography. The galactogram is repeated at the time of biopsy, and targeting is directed toward the filling defect identified within the duct. Guidance with ultrasound, stereotactic, and MRI systems has been used to direct biopsy devices for sampling of intraductal lesions.[14-16]

Galactography is not a perfect test, and its usefulness is controversial. Both false-positive and false-negative rates of 20% have been reported.[1,17,18] The management of women with abnormal discharge, but normal galactographic findings remains controversial. In some published series, if the fluid cytology findings are normal, clinical follow-up rather than biopsy is performed.[1] However, most authors advocate surgical duct excision for bloody nipple discharge despite normal results of galactography.[1]

REFERENCES

1. Funderburk WW, Syphax B. Evaluation of nipple discharge in benign and malignant diseases. *Cancer* 1969;**24**:1290-6.
2. Winchester DP. Nipple discharge. In: Harris JR, Lippman ME, Morrow M, Hellman S, editors. *Diseases of the breast*. Philadelphia: Lippincott-Raven; 1996. p. 106-10.
3. Tabar L, Dean PB, Pentek Z. Galactography: the diagnostic procedure of choice for nipple discharge. *Radiology* 1983;**149**:31-8.
4. Slawson SH, Johnson BA. Ductography: how to and what if? *Radiographics* 2001;**21**:133-50.
5. Fajardo LL, Jackson VP, Hunter TB. Interventional procedures in diseases of the breast: needle biopsy, pneumocystography, and galactography. *AJR Am J Roentgenol* 1992;**158**:1231-8.
6. Cardenosa G, Doudna C, Eklund GW. Ductography of the breast: technique and findings. *AJR Am J Roentgenol* 1994;**162**:1081-7.
7. Woods ER, Helvie MA, Ikeda DM, Mandell SH, Chapel KL, Adler DD. Solitary breast papilloma: comparison of mammographic, galactographic, and pathologic findings. *AJR Am J Roentgenol* 1992; **159**:487-91.
8. Piccoli CW, Feig SA, Vala MA. Breast imaging case of the day. *Radiographics* 1998;**18**:783-6.
9. Rissanen T, Typpo T, Tikkakoski T, Turunen J, Myllymäki T, Suramo I. Ultrasound-guided percutaneous galactography. *J Clin Ultrasound* 1993;**21**:497-502.
10. Orel SG, Dougherty CS, Reynolds C, Czerniecki BJ, Siegelman ES, Schnall MD. MR imaging in patients with nipple discharge: initial experience. *Radiology* 2000;**216**:248-54.
11. Lafreniere R. Bloody nipple discharge during pregnancy: a rationale for conservative treatment. *J Surg Oncol* 2006;**43**:228-30.
12. Hou MF, Huang TJ, Huang YS, Hsieh JS. A simple method of duct cannulation and localization for galactography before excision in patients with nipple discharge. *Radiology* 1995;**195**:568-9.
13. Koskela A, Berg M, Pietilainen T, Mustonen P, Vanninen R. Breast lesions causing nipple discharge: preoperative galactography-aided stereotactic wire localization. *AJR Am J Roentgenol* 2005;**184**:1795-8.
14. Guenin MA. Benign intraductal papilloma: diagnosis and removal at stereotactic vacuum-assisted directional biopsy guided by galactography. *Radiology* 2001;**218**:576-9.
15. Dennis MA, Parker S, Kaske TI, Stavros AT, Camp J. Incidental treatment of nipple discharge caused by benign intraductal papilloma through diagnostic Mammotome biopsy. *AJR Am J Roentgenol* 2000;**174**:1263-8.
16. Sardanelli F, Imperiale A, Zandrino F, Calabrese M, Bonifacio A, Canavese G, et al. Breast intraductal masses: US-guided fine-needle aspiration after galactography. *Radiology* 1997;**204**:143-8.
17. Dawes LG, Bowen C, Venta LA, Morrow M. Ductography for nipple discharge: no replacement for ductal excision. *Surgery* 1998;**124**: 685-91.
18. Baker KS, Davey DD, Stelling CB. Ductal abnormalities detected with galactography: frequency of adequate excisional biopsy. *AJR Am J Roentgenol* 1994;**162**:821-4.

CHAPTER 31

Presurgical Needle Localization

Mary Catherine Mahoney and Valerie P. Jackson

The increased use of mammographic screening has generated an increasing number of nonpalpable breast lesions requiring histologic evaluation.[1,2] Most of these lesions undergo percutaneous biopsy as the primary method of diagnosis. The many advantages of percutaneous biopsy compared with surgical excisional biopsy are well recognized.[3,4] However, once a malignancy or high-risk lesion is identified, surgical excision becomes necessary. A preoperative localization procedure is performed to identify nonpalpable breast lesions for successful surgical excision.[1,5,6]

PROCEDURE

Preoperative localization can be performed with mammographic imaging, ultrasonography, computed tomography (CT), and magnetic resonance imaging (MRI). Although the guidance method may differ, the procedure remains based on that originally developed for mammographically guided needle localizations.

Before any localization procedure, the radiologist must review the imaging studies to be sure that the lesion has been appropriately evaluated. A complete imaging workup is essential to ensure that the lesion is a true finding and that the biopsy is appropriate. The radiologist must know the exact location of the lesion, so as to plan a suitable approach. Although suspicious lesions are occasionally identified in only one mammographic projection, this is an unusual occurrence when appropriate imaging evaluation has been performed.[7]

The needle or hook wire system used for presurgical localization depends on the specific preference of the radiologist and surgeon. Some surgeons prefer to have a rigid needle left in place, allowing incision in the periareolar region or another location distant from the localization entry site. In these cases, the needle serves as a palpable localizer for the surgeon.[5] However, other surgeons prefer to have only the wire left in place and usually make the incision at the entry site of the localizing wire.[1,5] Although blue dye has been used as a localizing marker in the past and continues to be used with sentinel lymph node mapping and biopsy, it is seldom used for presurgical localization procedures today.[8,9] A newer technique involves the placement of a radioactive seed at the site of the breast abnormality. This allows the localization procedure to be performed one or more days before surgery, reducing scheduling pressures on the date of the surgical excisional biopsy.[10]

Informed consent is obtained from the patient before all needle localization procedures. It is important that the patient not be premedicated before localization to allow for appropriate informed consent and to allow the patient to cooperate with positioning for the localization procedure.[11]

The technique for mammographic localization with a fenestrated mammography compression plate is simple and accurate. The original mammograms are reviewed to determine the appropriate needle length and the skin surface closest to the lesion (Fig. 31-1A through 31-1C). Although the approach is usually from the superior, inferior, lateral, or medial aspect of the breast, any degree of angulation is possible. In some situations, the patient's body habitus may preclude an inferior approach. In these cases, the breast can be rolled to allow an oblique approach or the procedure can be performed with patient in the recumbent position. In all cases, the needle should be positioned parallel to the chest wall.[12,13]

The procedure is usually performed with the patient sitting. The breast is positioned with the opening of the fenestrated paddle against the proposed skin entry surface. A scout film is obtained, and the breast is left in compression while the image is evaluated. Digital imaging has greatly speeded the process of needle localization procedures, with one study demonstrating a 50% reduction in the time needed for a localization procedure compared

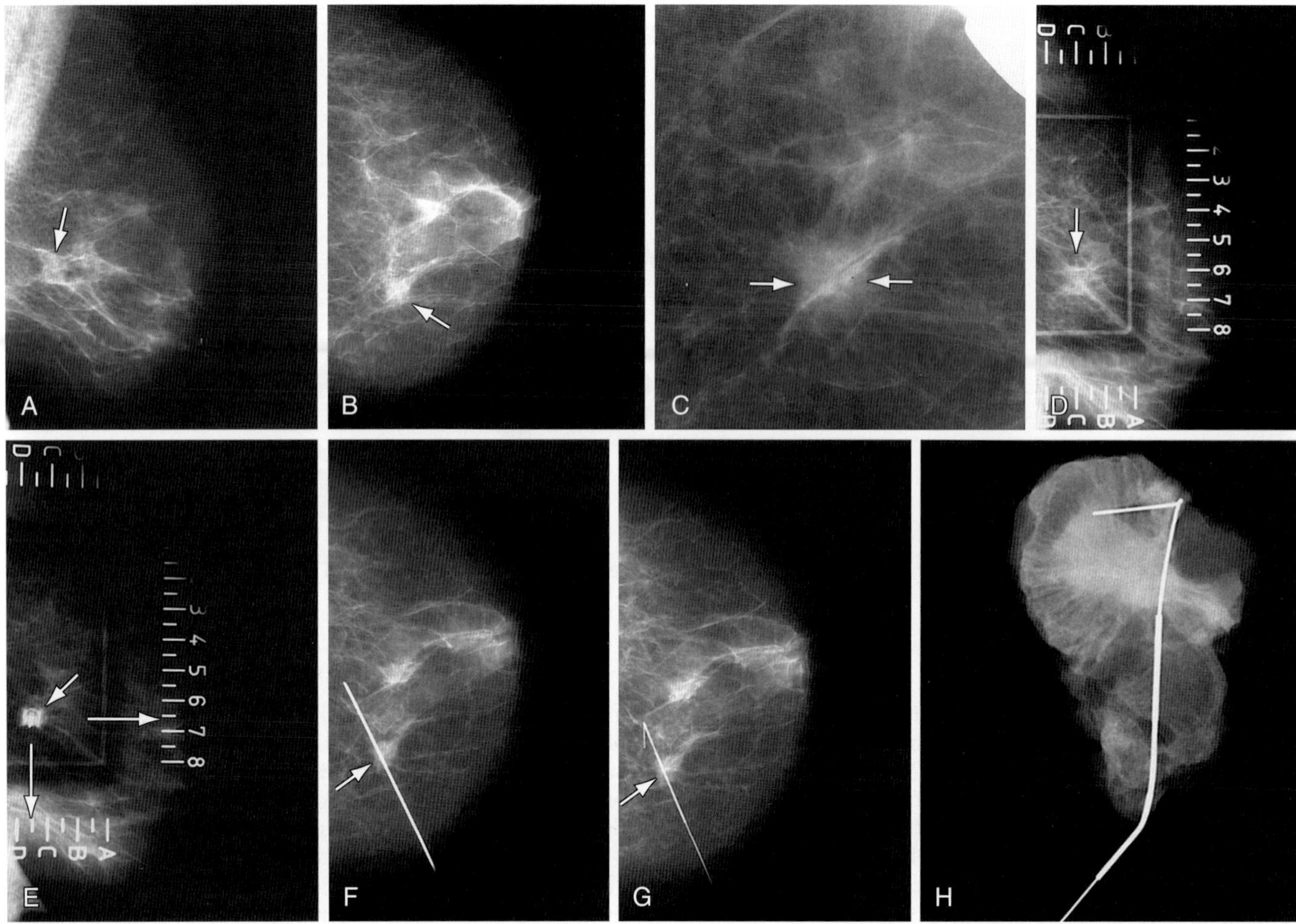

■ **FIGURE 31-1** A 60-year-old woman presented with a 1.2-cm spiculated mass in the left breast seen on mammogram (*arrows*). The lateromedial (**A**), craniocaudal (**B**), and spot compression magnification craniocaudal (**C**) views show the irregular, spiculated and indistinct mass located at the 9-o'clock region of the medial aspect of the breast. **D,** The fenestrated compression paddle has been placed against the medial aspect of the breast, which is the skin surface closest to the lesion (*arrow*). The breast remains compressed until image processing is completed and the exam reviewed. **E,** The needle (*short arrow*) has been inserted into the mass at the coordinates shown by the *long arrows.* **F,** Craniocaudal view shows the needle entering the medial aspect of the breast and coursing through the mass (*arrow*). The distance from the mass to the end of the needle was measured, and the needle was pulled back 2 cm, to the level of the far edge of the mass. If there is any doubt as to the position of the needle, another image should be obtained before the wire is afterloaded. **G,** Craniocaudal view demonstrating the mass (*arrow*) at the thick part of the wire. The hook is approximately 1 cm beyond the mass. **H,** Specimen radiograph showing the hook wire and spiculated mass.

with the screen-film technique.[14] If the lesion is not identified within the open window of the compression paddle, the breast is repositioned until the lesion is accessible. A cursor is placed over the lesion and the coordinates of the lesion are then identified using the markings along the open window of the compression paddle (Fig. 31-1D) The skin is cleansed with an aseptic solution. Although local anesthesia is considered optional, it is routinely used at our institution.[8,11,15] Usually, 1 mL of buffered 1% lidocaine is administered into the skin and subcutaneous tissue, with an additional 3 to 4 mL placed into deeper tissues when necessary. In addition, compression leads to some degree of numbness of the breast.

There are numerous needle and hook wire devices available. Regardless of the specific device used, the procedure is similar. The needle is positioned using the localizing light of the mammography unit. The needle is placed into the breast as straight as possible, with the shadow of the needle hub superimposed on the skin entry site (Fig. 31-1E).[2,11] No attempt should be made to gauge the distance from the skin to the lesion in this position. Instead, the needle should be passed as far as possible into the breast. An image is obtained in this first projection to verify that the needle is superimposed on the lesion. While the radiologist has control of the needle to maintain its depth within the tissue, the compression paddle is carefully removed and the patient's breast is repositioned in the orthogonal projection. This second view is usually performed with a small spot compression device overlying the expected location of the distal needle shaft and tip (Fig. 31-1F). If the proper needle length has been chosen, the needle will have traveled beyond the lesion and is then slightly pulled back before deploying the wire. If the needle tip is proximal (short) of the lesion, the needle should be removed and the procedure repeated with a longer needle. Advancement of a needle that is short of the lesion is inaccurate. The needle may deviate away from the lesion, and its exact location can no longer be confirmed.[2]

Once appropriate positioning of the needle is confirmed, the hook wire is deployed. Ideally, the hook of the wire should be positioned approximately 1 cm beyond the lesion (Fig. 31-1G). If it is the preference of the surgeon, the needle can be removed at this time. A final mammographic image is obtained, demonstrating the final position of the needle or wire. Most needles are marked at 1-cm intervals, allowing the distance from the skin to needle tip to be determined.

The needle or wire is secured and bandaged with gauze. The initial mammographic films, demonstrating the lesion, and the localization films, demonstrating the needle or wire, accompany the patient to the surgical suite for the surgeon's review. The entire localization procedure is usually completed in 15 to 20 minutes using digital mammography equipment.

Challenges

The localization of faint microcalcifications or vague masses can be challenging. The relative lack of compression in the open window of the compression paddle leads to poor tissue contrast. Additional tissue contrast can be achieved by stretching a sterile adhesive, such as Tegaderm, across the compression paddle window. The taut plastic adhesive provides a small amount of compression and may allow successful localization through better visualization of the lesion. The patient's skin must be cleansed before placement of the sterile adhesive over the compression paddle window, because the adhesive dressing will adhere to the breast surface. Once the lesion is visualized, the anesthetic and localization needles are placed into the breast through the adhesive.

In some cases it may be necessary to use a magnification technique to adequately visualize faint microcalcifications with screen-film technique.[16] The use of digital mammography allows electronic magnification of the image, obviating the need for true magnification in most cases.

When multiple suspicious abnormalities are present, multiple localization devices may be placed to mark each lesion individually. When a large abnormality, such as an extensive area of microcalcifications, is to be localized, multiple devices are used to bracket the boundaries of the lesion (Fig. 31-2). This helps the surgeon remove the entire area at the initial excision.[17]

Complications

All localization procedures carry the potential risks of bleeding, infection, and vasovagal reaction. Bleeding is rarely, if ever, a problem for needle localization procedures because of the small-gauge needle that is routinely used. Sterile techniques should be used to minimize the chance of an infection. A vasovagal reaction is the most dramatic and severe complication of presurgical needle localization procedures.[11,18] After the needle has been placed, the patient should never be left alone. A crash cart and basic resuscitation equipment should be nearby at all times. The patient must be alert and able to cooperate with the procedure. Therefore, no preoperative sedative medication should be given before the localization procedure.[11]

The free-hand localization method, with an anterior approach, carries the additional risk of pneumothorax.[1,2,11] Therefore, the free-hand method of localization is used only with ultrasound guidance, in which there is direct visualization of the needle at all times. Placement of the needle parallel to the chest wall is still routinely performed with ultrasound localization to avoid pneumothorax. Pneumothorax is usually not a problem with the open compression paddle technique, which also routinely utilizes a parallel approach to the chest wall.[1]

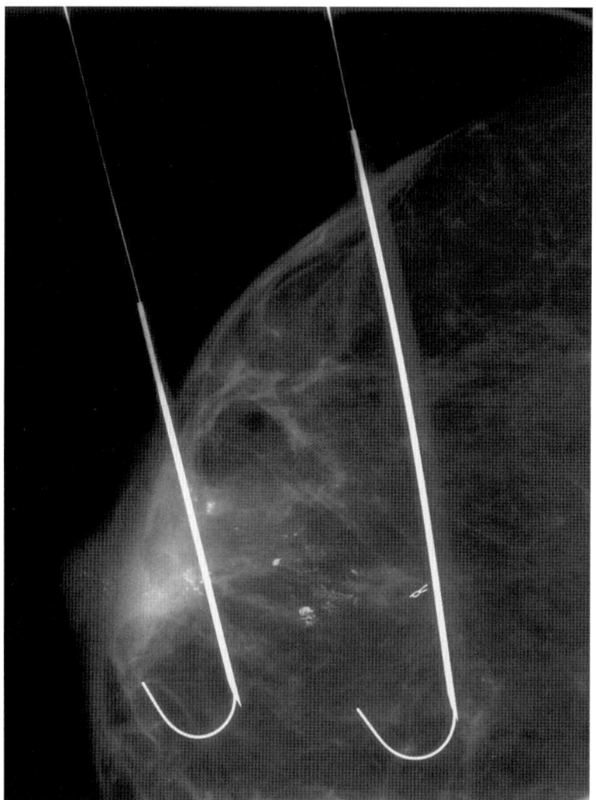

■ **FIGURE 31-2** Localization radiograph with bracketing needles and wires used to mark the boundaries of widespread microcalcifications and tissue marker from previous stereotactic biopsy yielding ductal carcinoma in situ (DCIS).

Specimen Radiography

Obtaining a specimen radiograph is an important part of the localization and surgical biopsy procedure for all types of nonpalpable breast lesions. It allows documentation that both the lesion and localizing device have been removed and demonstrates the location of the abnormality within the tissue for the pathologist (Fig. 31-3).[2,19,20] A specimen radiograph should be performed for all lesions (including calcified and noncalcified lesions) to ensure that the lesion and the localizing device have been removed. Magnification and compression are usually used for specimen radiographs.[2] There has been speculation that the use of compression in specimen radiography may lead to inaccurate assessment of the histologic margin.[21] Nonetheless, most radiologists do require compression with specimen radiography to identify the presence of the lesion.[2]

Specimen radiography can be performed on a standard mammographic unit or with a dedicated specimen x-ray machine. Low kilovolts peak (kVp) technique (20-23 kVp) can be used.[2] The specimen radiographs

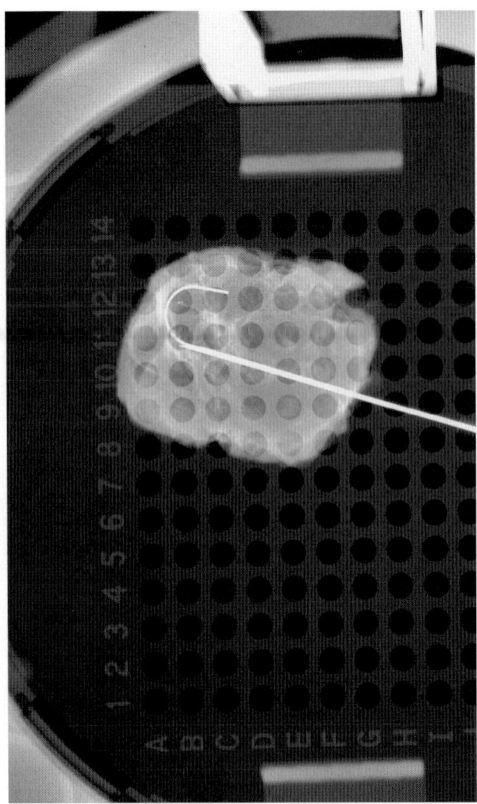

■ **FIGURE 31-3** **A,** Specimen radiograph demonstrates localizing needle and wire with spiculated mass. **B,** Specimen radiograph demonstrates localizing wire and tissue marker from previous magnetic resonance imaging (MRI)-guided percutaneous biopsy.

should be reviewed while the patient is still in the operating room. The radiologist who performed the localization should evaluate the specimen radiograph. If the lesion is not seen within the specimen, the surgeon should be notified so that additional tissue can be resected.[19] The radiologist should also evaluate the specimen radiograph to determine that the entire localizing device has been removed. The surgeon should be notified of these findings as well.

For vague noncalcified masses, the specimen radiograph may be equivocal. Turning the specimen 90 degrees and taking another specimen radiograph may allow visualization of the lesion.[2,22] Although specimen radiography is poor for predicting the margin status of a resected carcinoma, it remains an important part of the procedure to document removal of at least a portion of the lesion.[21,23] The specimen is oriented by the surgeon with clips or sutures, or both, to assist in evaluation of the margins. If both the specimen radiograph and pathology findings are equivocal, repeat mammography should be performed within 2 to 3 months of surgery to determine if the lesion has been removed.

The specimen radiograph should be marked with the location of the lesion to assist the pathologist in evaluating the correct area histologically.[2] This marking is easily accomplished in that most specimen handling systems have an alphanumeric coordinate system imbedded within the immobilization device with coordinates visible on the specimen radiograph (Fig. 31-4). It is occasionally necessary to image the specimen blocks to precisely localize the lesion, particularly microcalcifications, within the tissue

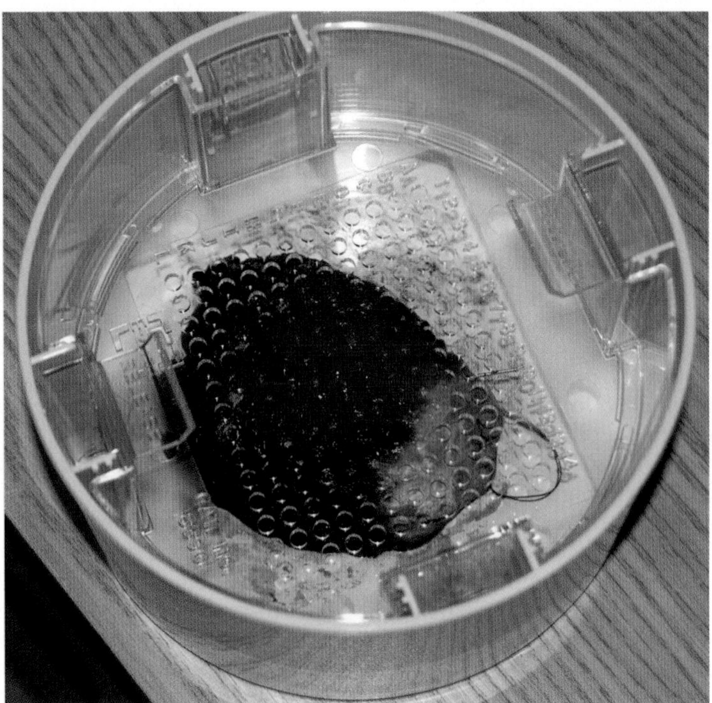

■ **FIGURE 31-4** Gross surgical specimen in container for transport and specimen radiography. The alphanumeric coordinate system built into the container is visible on the specimen radiograph and can assist the pathologist in identifying the targeted lesion within the specimen.

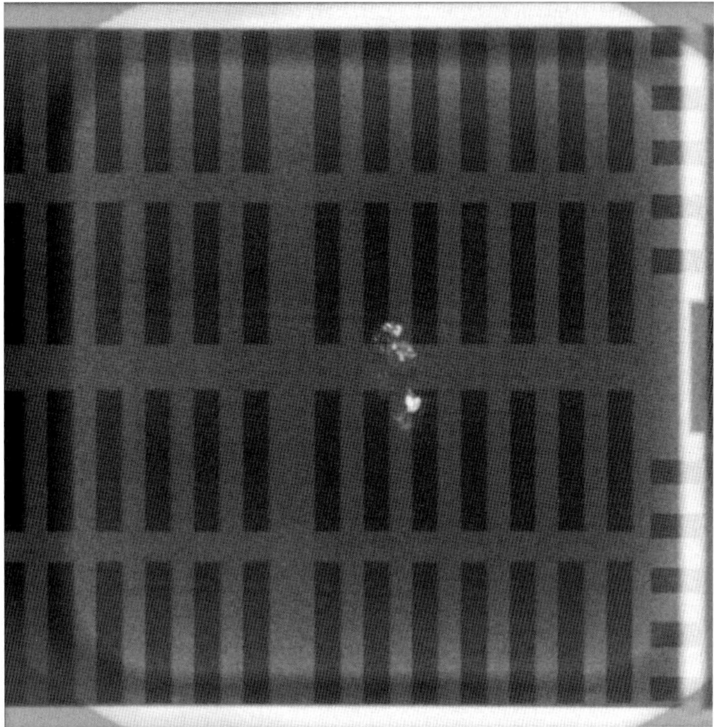

■ **FIGURE 31-5** Specimen radiograph of the pathology tissue block identifies coarses, heterogeneous microcalcifications.

for the pathologist (Fig. 31-5).[2,11] In the event that localization is performed ultrasonographically for a nonpalpable, nonmammographically detected lesion, specimen evaluation should be performed with ultrasonography. However, in some cases these lesions may be visible on x-ray specimen radiography.[2] Unfortunately, there is no optimal method for specimen radiography to evaluate lesions that are visible only with MRI.[2] Therefore, postsurgical breast MRI may be necessary to document removal of the lesion.

KEY POINTS

- A preoperative localization procedure is performed to identify nonpalpable breast lesions for successful surgical excision.
- Localization using mammographic imaging and an open window compression plate is simple and accurate.
- The needle tip and hook wire should be positioned approximately 1 cm beyond the lesion.
- A large abnormality, such as extensive microcalcifications, requires multiple wires to bracket the boundaries of the lesion.
- Specimen radiography documents removal of the targeted lesion and localization device.

SUGGESTED READINGS

D'Orsi CJ. Management of the breast specimen. *Radiology* 1995; **194**:297-302.

Kopans DB, Swann CA. Preoperative imaging-guided needle placement and localization of clinically occult breast lesions. *AJR Am J Roentgenol* 1989;**152**:1-9.

REFERENCES

1. Kopans DB, Lindfors K, McCarthy KA, Meyer JE. Spring hookwire breast lesion localizer: use with rigid-compression mammographic systems. *Radiology* 1985;**157**:537-8.
2. D'Orsi CJ. Management of the breast specimen. *Radiology* 1995;**194**:297-302.
3. Liberman L, LaTrenta LR, Dershaw DD, Abramson AF, Morris EA, Cohen MA, et al. Impact of core biopsy on the surgical management of impalpable breast cancer. *AJR Am J Roentgenol* 1997;**168**: 495-9.

4. Meyer JE, Christian RL, Lester SC, Frenna TH, Denison CM, DiPiro PJ, et al. Evaluation of nonpalpable solid breast masses with stereotaxic large-needle core biopsy using a dedicated unit. *AJR Am J Roentgenol* 1996;**167**:179-82.
5. Homer MJ. Localization of nonpalpable breast lesions with the curved-end, retractable wire: leaving the needle in vivo. *AJR Am J Roentgenol* 1988;**151**:919-20.
6. Homer MJ, Pile-Spellman ER. Needle localization of occult breast lesions with a curved-end retractable wire: technique and pitfalls. *Radiology* 1986;**161**:547-8.
7. Kopans DB, Waitzkin ED, Linetsky L, Swann CA, McCarthy KA, Hall DA, et al. Localization of breast lesions identified on only one mammographic view. *AJR Am J Roentgenol* 1987;**149**:39-41.
8. Reynolds HE, Jackson VP, Musick BS. A survey of interventional mammography practices. *Radiology* 1993;**187**:71-3.
9. Czarnecki DJ, Feider HK, Splittgerber GF. Toluidine blue dye as a breast localization marker. *AJR Am J Roentgenol* 1989;**153**:261-3.
10. Gray RJ, Salud C, Nguyen K, Dauway E, Friedland J, Berman C, et al. Randomized prospective evaluation of a novel technique for biopsy or lumpectomy of nonpalpable breast lesions: radioactive seed versus wire localization. *Ann Surg Oncol* 2001;**8**:711-5.
11. Kopans DB, Swann CA. Preoperative imaging-guided needle placement and localization of clinically occult breast lesions. *AJR Am J Roentgenol* 1989;**152**:1-9.
12. Pisano ED, Hall FM. Preoperative localization of inferior breast lesions. *AJR Am J Roentgenol* 1989;**153**:272.
13. Homer MJ. Preoperative needle localization of lesions in the lower half of the breast: needle entry from below. *AJR Am J Roentgenol* 1987;**149**:43-5.
14. Dershaw DD, Fleischman RC, Liberman L, Deutch B, Abramson AF, Hann L. Use of digital mammography in needle localization procedures. *AJR Am J Roentgenol* 1993;**161**:559-62.
15. Reynold HE, Jackson VP, Musick B. Preoperative needle localization in the breast: utility of local anesthesia. *Radiology* 1993;**187**:503-5.
16. Berkowitz JE, Horan PM. Preoperative needle localization of subtle breast calcifications: magnification technique. *Radiology* 1992; **185**:277.
17. Liberman L, Kaplan J, Vanzee KJ. Bracketing wires for preoperative breast needle localization. *AJR Am J Roentgenol* 2001; **177**:565-72.
18. Helvie MA, Ikeda DM, Adler DD. Localization and needle aspiration of breast lesions: complications in 370 cases. *AJR Am J Roentgenol* 1991;**157**:711-4.
19. Homer MJ, Berlin L. Radiography of the surgical breast biopsy specimen. *AJR Am J Roentgenol* 1998;**171**:1197-9.
20. Stomper PC, Davis SP, Sonnenfeld MR, Meyer JE, Greenes RA, Eberlein TJ. Efficiency of specimen radiography of clinically occult noncalcified breast lesions. *AJR Am J Roentgenol* 1988;**151**:43-7.
21. Graham RA, Homer MJ, Katz J, Rothschild J, Safaii H, Supran S. The pancake phenomenon contributes to the inaccuracy of margin assessment in patients with breast cancer. *Am J Surg* 2002;**184**:89-93.
22. Rebner M, Pennes DR, Baker DE, Adler DD, Boyd P. Two-view specimen radiography in surgical biopsy of nonpalpable breast masses. *AJR Am J Roentgenol* 1987;**149**:283-5.
23. Graham RA, Homer MJ, Sigler CJ, Safaii H, Schmid CH, Marchant DJ, et al. The efficacy of specimen radiography in evaluating the surgical margins of impalpable breast carcinoma. *AJR Am J Roentgenol* 1994;**162**:33-6.

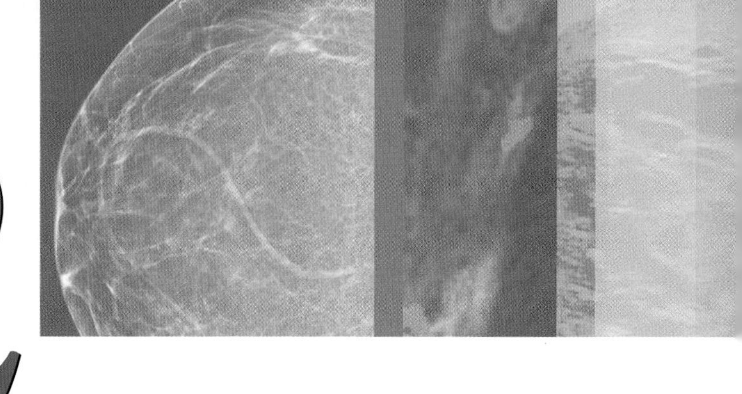

CHAPTER 32

Specimen Processing in Pathology

Sophia Kim Apple

Pathology departments receive many different types of breast specimens. Some of the different types of breast specimens include plastic surgical specimens for cosmetic purposes, diagnostic breast tissue such as excision and mastectomy with or without axillary lymph node dissection, core needle biopsy and fine-needle aspiration. The primary function of the pathologist includes providing an accurate diagnosis, and providing prognostic and predictive analysis of breast diseases. In this chapter, the proper handling of different types of breast specimens to achieve accurate diagnosis and to optimize further clinical management of breast cancer patients will be described. And when appropriate, each variable technique with advantages and disadvantages will be presented.

FINE-NEEDLE ASPIRATION (FNA) OF BREAST LESIONS

In 1847, the earliest report on usage of FNA was by Kun of Strasbourg. Later in London, descriptions were made of the use of a grooved needle and microscopy for diagnosis, especially for diseases of the breast. In the early 1900s, military doctors aspirated lymph nodes to diagnose trypanosomes. Actual aspiration using an 18-guage needle with a 20 mL syringe was not common until 1926. For many years, cytology was dormant in the United States, but European countries were accepting and evolving the practice. Over the past 25 years, FNA became more accepted and used in the United States. The principle preoperative diagnosis of FNA usage gained acceptance in breast, salivary glands, thyroid and lymph nodes. It was in the 1930s that FNA of breast lesions was introduced and now has become widely accepted as a first-line diagnostic procedure[1]. Currently there is a national trend away from FNA of breast lesions and increased use of core needle biopsy (CNB) as the first line diagnostic method in many settings. Use of FNA of breast lesions has also decreased in the United Kingdom and Canada.[2] Some of the advantages of using breast FNA as a first line diagnostic procedure are minimal invasiveness, cost-effectiveness, rapid turn-around time, less discomfort for patients, and accurate diagnosis with a high positive predictive value. Some of the disadvantages of using FNA of breast lesions are inability to distinguish an in situ lesion from the invasive carcinoma, a higher rate of non-diagnostic or insufficient materials when compared with core needle biopsy, lack of experienced cytopathologists at individual institutions leading to more diagnostic errors, and some limitations in performing breast biomarkers studies such as HER-2/neu. The first limitation (inability to diagnose in situ versus invasive carcinoma from FNA) is an important issue since most surgeons prefer to procure sentinel lymph node(s) if the lesion is deemed invasive carcinoma at the time of the first therapeutic surgery. More recently, neoadjuvant chemotherapy is offered to the patient who has advanced breast cancer and for this, an accurate HER-2/*neu* analysis is needed to design appropriate chemotherapy agents. HER-2/*neu* testing is done by either an immunohistochemical (IHC) test or a fluorescent in situ hybridization (FISH) test, both which are approved by the U.S. Food and Drug Administration (FDA). Most of the FNA smears are alcohol fixed or air-dried, which are not ideal solutions for FDA approved HER-2/*neu* tests unless FNA materials are washed in the 10% formalin as a cell block directly. The FNA procedure is highly dependent on the operator who is performing and interpreting the findings. Non-diagnostic or insufficient amount of material to accurately evaluate FNA sample of breast lesions ranges from 0% to 50%[3-7].

The non-diagnostic rate of CNB is less than FNA, and has been reported to range from 3% to 7%.[8,9] Diagnostic accuracy, however, is the same or slightly better for FNA when compared with CNB. Recently published sensitivity and specificity ranges are from 75.8% to 98.7% for sensitivity, and 60% to 100% for specificity of breast FNAs. [5,7,10,11] The accuracy of CNB in diagnosing breast cancer depends on the size of the needle and number of samples taken. Based on a meta-analysis, Dillon and colleagues reported false negative rate ranges from 0% to 13% for palpation guided CNB, 0% to 12% for ultrasound guided CNB and 0.2% to 8.9% for stereotactic CNB.[12] Some comparisons of sensitivity and specificity rates between FNA and CNB studies report that FNA had a higher accuracy rate in diagnosing breast cancers. Ballo and coworkers[13] reported sensitivity and specificity of 97.5% and 100% respectively in FNA, when compared to 90% and 100% respectively in CNB. Antley and colleagues[14] also reported sensitivity and specificity of 99% and 99.5% respectively in FNA when compared to 85% and 100% respectively in CNB. The number of samples obtained directly correlates to a higher diagnostic accuracy in both FNA and CNB. Brenner and colleagues recommended collecting between 5 and 15 cores (up to 22 cores) on nonpalpable breast lesions such as mass, microcalcifications and architectural distortions, depending on the type of lesion seen on imaging.[15] There is also a trend toward using larger bore needles (typically 14-7 gauge) to increase sensitivity of diagnostic accuracy.[16,17]

Patients tolerate FNA procedures better because they are less painful. Typical fine-needle bore size is 25 gauge, and sometimes 27 gauge, often attached to a 10 cc vacuum syringe. The larger bore needle, such as 23 or 18 gauge, tends to induce more bleeding and obscure the cells obtained from the FNA procedure, which hinders the interpretation. FNA is typically performed with 3 to 5 passes into different areas and directions depending on the size and the location of the targeted mass. The aspirated materials are expressed on glass slides. Some of the samples are fixed immediately into 95% alcohol solution and these alcohol fixed slides are stained with Papanicolaou (PAP) which is green to blue color. It is critical to fix the slides into alcohol immediately after making smears to prevent air-drying artifact. Some of the samples from the aspirated materials are air-dried and these can be used to stain with May-Grunewald Giemsa (MGG) stains. PAP and MGG stains are commonly used in conventional FNA settings. Cell block sections can be made by rinsing the needles with 10% buffer formalin solution, which can be spun with a centrifuge. The supernatant is discarded and the pellet is used to make a paraffin block section similar to CNB sample. The cell block material, then, can be used to study any IHC stains for future studies if necessary. FNA is useful if there are mass lesions; however, it is not a recommended procedure if the breast lesion is an architectural distortion or microcalcifications. It is essential that *triple test* correlation is used on every patient when dealing with breast lesions. Triple test is defined as clinical impression, radiological findings, and pathology findings with either FNA or CNB results. All three parameters have to be concordant. If any of these parameters is discordant, an open biopsy or further workup is necessary to resolve discordant findings. Some of the classic FNA diagnostic materials are shown in Figures 32-1 to 32-3.

CORE NEEDLE BIOPSY OF BREAST LESIONS

CNBs of breast lesions are often performed by radiologists using necessary image guidance such as mammogram, ultrasound, or magnetic resonance imaging (MRI). An advantage of the CNB is less morbidity compared with surgery, and it is also less expensive than an excisional biopsy. A successful imaging-guided core needle biopsy program requires a strong working relationship between the radiologist(s) and the pathologist(s). An experienced breast pathologist who is aware of sampling limitations

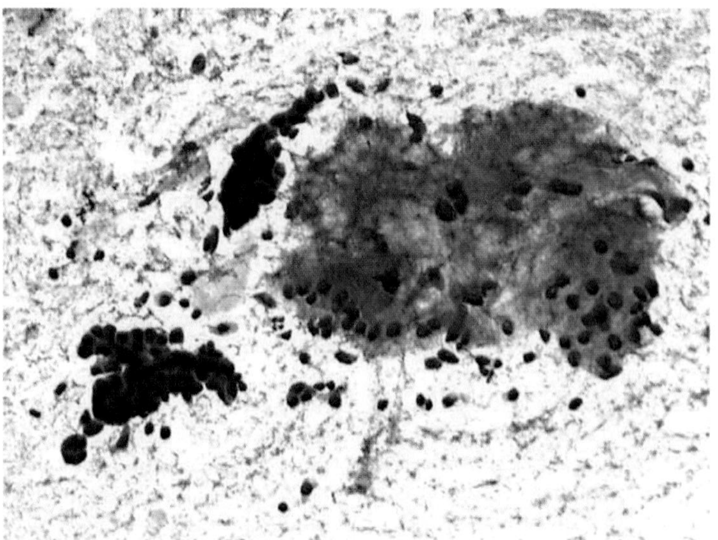

■ **FIGURE 32-1** Fine-needle aspiration specimen stained with May-Grunewald Giemsa (MGG) of fibroadenoma showing tightly cohesive groups of epithelial cells admixed with spindle cells (myoepithelial cells). The background shows naked nuclei, which are bare myoepithelial nuclei and stromal component. The stroma shows bland-appearing spindle cells without increased cellularity with myxoid changes ×200.

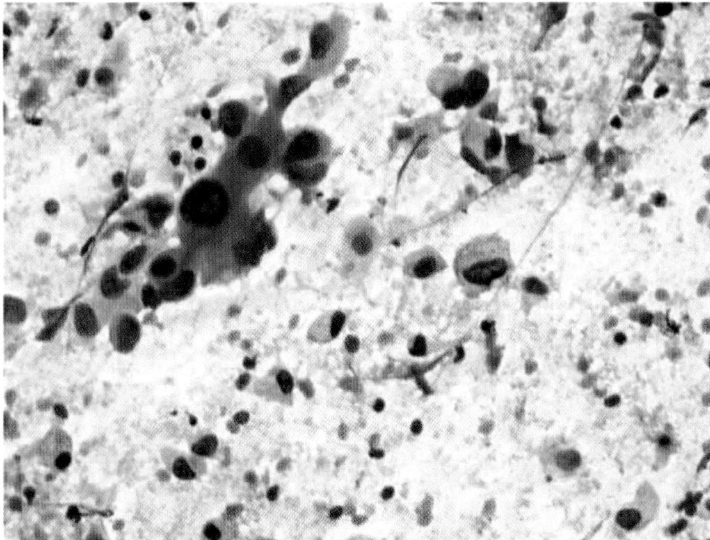

■ **FIGURE 32-2** In invasive ductal carcinoma stained with Papanicolaou (PAP), the smears are highly cellular with loosely cohesive and single malignant cells with high nuclear to cytoplasmic (N/C) ratio, irregular nuclear chromatin, variable sizes and shapes of nuclear shapes and contours. Single cells with retained cytoplasm are characteristic of malignant breast cancer in fine-needle aspiration (FNA) samples. The background shows necrosis.

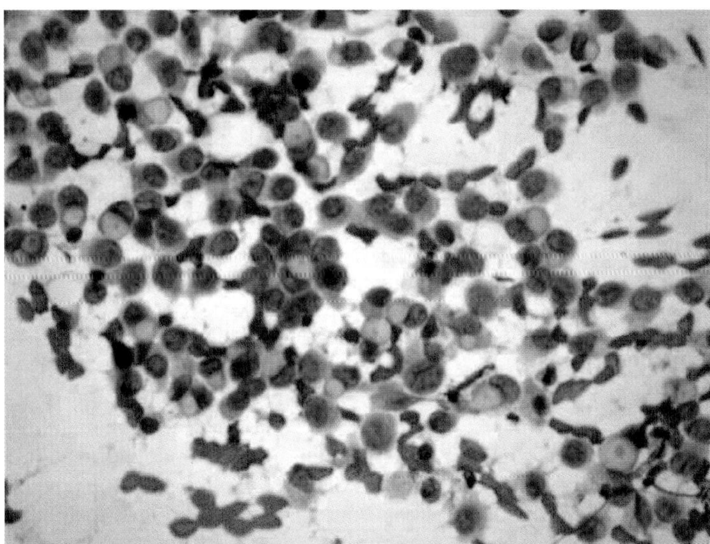

■ **FIGURE 32-3** In invasive lobular carcinoma stained with Papanicolaou (PAP), the smears are loosely cohesive cells with a single-file or small aggregates of tumor cells with intracytoplasmic vacuoles and bland to only mildly irregular nuclei ×400.

and problem lesions at CNB is an essential component of accurate diagnosis with breast CNB.Therefore, it is important that the pathologist has adequate clinical information and knowledge of radiological findings when evaluating CNB specimens.The information needed from the radiologist includes location of the lesion (crucial if more than one biopsy site), most relevant imaging findings (e.g., mass, calcifications, architectural distortion) and the radiologist's degree of concern regarding the likelihood of malignancy by using American College of Radiology (ACR) Breast Imaging Reporting and Data System (BI-RADS). After CNB samples are done, careful removal of the fresh tissue from the core needle is essential to not further disrupt and fragment the specimens.The fresh tissue should be laid on slightly moist paper with saline solution to be flattened and straightened. For stereotactic-guided biopsy for calcifications, radiographs of the specimens and the pathology report should document the presence of calcifications. If x-ray of the specimens shows no microcalcifications from the targeted lesion, it is extremely helpful that this finding is reported in the pathology requisition form, so that the pathologist avoids looking for microcalcifications on the slides and performing additional steps to search for microcalcifications.The tissue with calcifications should be picked up gently with forceps and transferred into either the cassette provided by the pathology department, or into a tea-bag.The entire specimen should then be placed in a 10% formalin bottle with patient identification.When the pathologist receives this type of specimen, the designated calcification cores are submitted into a different cassette (Cassette A) and the remaining non-designated cores are submitted into another cassette. (Cassette B). There are mainly two types of calcifications. Most breast microcalcifications are calcium phosphate, showing dark blue-purple concretion readily visible by light microscope. (Fig. 32-4). The other type of microcalcification is calcium oxalate crystals, which are not visible under light microscope but are visible under a polarizing lens (Figs. 32-5 and 32-6). All CNB specimens are routinely evaluated at multiple levels to ensure inclusion of representative areas for histological study. Intervening levels of unstained tissue slides can be stored for possible use of IHC stains. Each slide is 4 to 5 microns thick and each of the levels is 50 microns thick. If there is no evidence of microcalcifications seen from the initial three levels, pathologists will examine polarizable microcalcifications such as calcium oxalate using a polarizing lens. If there are no polarizable microcalcifications, then the designated cassette with microcalcifications documented by x-ray is further sectioned into 10 to 20 slides until no tissue remains on the block. Many times, additional slides from these intervening slides will show the presence of microcalcifications. If a biopsy is performed on more than one lesion, the specimens should be properly labeled and submitted separately (e.g., specimen #1 is right at 12:00 o'clock and specimen #2 is right at 4:30 o'clock).

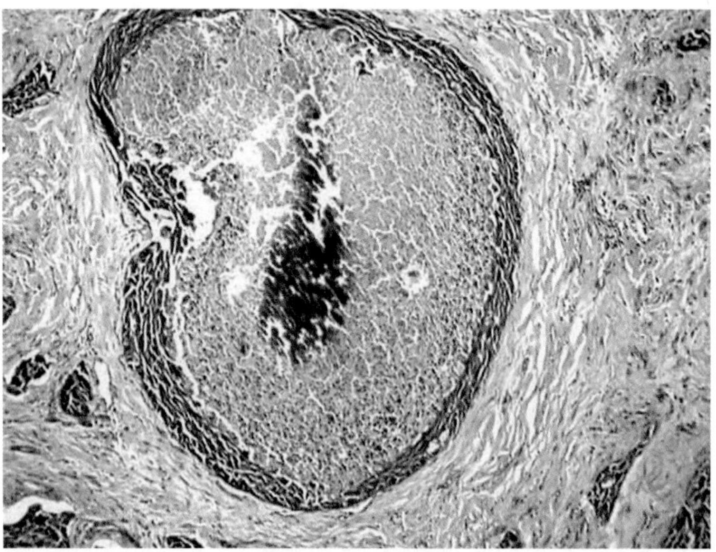

■ FIGURE 32-4 Hematoxylin and eosin stain of calcium phosphate showing dark purple color concretion within the lumen of breast ducts. Calcium phosphate calcifications are seen with all types of breast lesions such as benign, ductal carcinoma in situ (DCIS), and invasive cancers ×100.

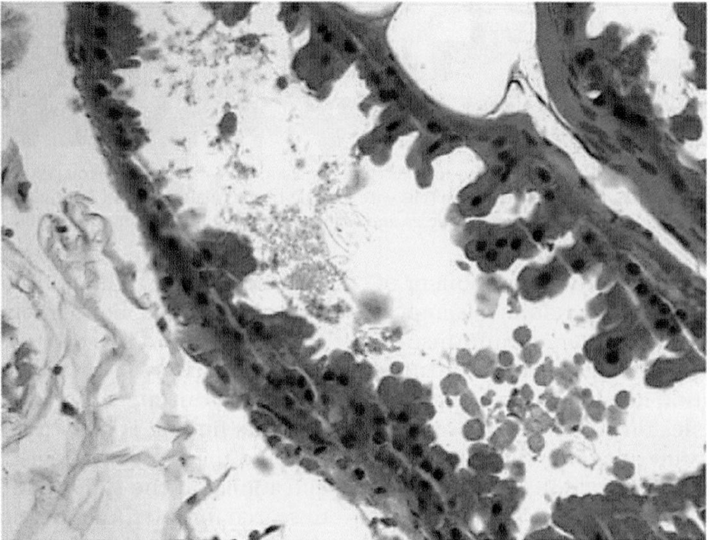

■ FIGURE 32-5 Hematoxylin and eosin stain ×400 of calcium oxalate showing refractile clear crystals that are difficult to visualize by light microscope but can be seen with polarizing lens. Of note, calcium oxalate calcifications are often seen in association with apocrine microcysts and are usually an indication of benign process.

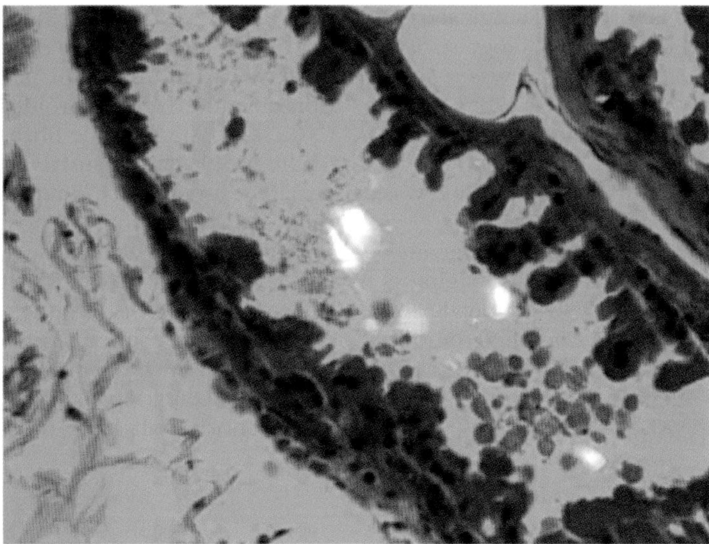

■ **FIGURE 32-6** Polarized lens ×400 showing visible calcium oxalate crystals.

The assessment for concordance of imaging and pathology findings is based on the *triple test*, first developed for breast FNA biopsy and standardized under the auspices of the National Cancer Institute in 1996.[18] Based on the triple test, if there is any discordance between clinical, imaging and pathology findings, an open (excisional) biopsy should be performed. The assessment for concordance can be performed in a number of ways:

1. A case-by-case or scheduled meeting with the pathologist(s) and radiologist(s).
2. Reviewing the imaging findings alongside the written pathology report by radiologist(s).
3. Comparing the written imaging and pathology reports for concordance by clinician(s).

Once the imaging-pathology assessment for concordance has been completed, a management plan is devised. Concordant malignant cases are referred to surgeons for a definitive treatment. Concordant benign cases are placed in follow-up imaging because there is a 2% reported false negative rate for CNB[19]. An alternative for definite benign results (imaging likely fibroadenoma and pathology diagnosis of fibroadenoma) is routine follow-up with annual mammogram. Discordant cases and those with possible underestimation of disease require an open biopsy and this recommendation should be directly communicated to the referring health care provider. The discordant rates range from 1.7% to 4.8 %.[20] Among the reported discordant cases, as much as 47% to 50% had carcinoma on re-biopsy or excisional biopsy.[21]

Limitations of Core Needle Biopsy

The most important limitation of CNB is sampling error. In addition, several uncommon benign and high-risk CNB pathology diagnoses have been linked to a potential underestimation of disease. For example, some benign histologic findings have been shown to frequently coexist with carcinoma, and a cancer could have been missed due to sampling error. If there is imaging-pathology discordance or possible underestimation of disease, an open biopsy should be performed.

In general, the larger core needles size provide better sensitivity and specificity for diagnosis. With a 14 gauge needle, the sensitivity and specificity is reported to be nearly 100% and 100% respectively. With a 16 gauge needle, the sensitivity and specificity is reported as 92% and 100% respectively. With an 18 gauge needle, the sensitivity and specificity is reported as 65% and 100%.[22]

Underestimation of Disease

Although the subsequent management of patients who had CNB diagnosis of invasive cancer, ductal carcinoma in situ (DCIS), and most benign lesions is straightforward, there are certain nonmalignant lesions that pose dilemmas with regard to the most appropriate clinical management. The need for excisional biopsy for these CNB histologic diagnoses has been controversial. These include atypical ductal hyperplasia (ADH), lobular neoplasia (atypical lobular hyperplasia and lobular carcinoma in situ[LCIS]), papillary lesions, radial scars, fibroepithelial lesions, mucocele-like lesions, and columnar cell lesions.[23] Detailed discussion on each section is covered on the specific entity from the chapters 17 through 19.

False Positive Core Needle Biopsy

A false positive CNB is defined as a pathology interpretation of malignancy with subsequent determination that the findings were benign on excision. If a false positive CNB is suspected because surgical excision did not identify malignancy, several courses of action should be undertaken:

1. The entire breast specimen should be processed for the histological examination by the pathologist.
2. The pathologist needs to find a prior biopsy site with changes such as fat necrosis, hemorrhage and/or a surgical clip within the breast specimen.

3. The original CNB specimens that led to surgical excision should be re-reviewed. If the pathology review only shows a benign lesion, the CNB was a false positive.
4. If the CNB review confirms malignancy, repeat imaging (postsurgical excision image study) should be performed to verify that the imaging finding was removed at the time of the surgical excision.
5. If the pathologic review confirmed a malignancy in the CNB specimens and postsurgical imaging is negative, it is likely that the small suspicious lesion was entirely removed by the CNB. Complete removal of lesion is more likely to occur with the more efficient sampling devices such as the 8- and 11-gauge vacuum-assisted device (VAD).

Sclerosing adenosis is one of the most common potential false positive CNB results that can be diagnosed as invasive carcinoma by the pathologist. It is a benign condition characterized by proliferation of lobules and fibrous tissue. Occasionally the fibrosis is so severe that the acini of the lobules are distorted enough to mimic well differentiated ductal carcinoma or invasive tubular carcinoma. (Fig. 32-7) Sclerosing adenosis can be seen with DCIS or LCIS, which may also cause it to be misdiagnosed as invasive carcinoma (Fig. 32-8). Histologically, on high power, sclerosing adenosis has a two cell layer epithelium, identified by the presence of myoepithelial cells; but invasive carcinoma will have only a one cell layer epithelial lining with no myoepithelial cells. On low power, sclerosing adenosis will have lobular configurations, whereas

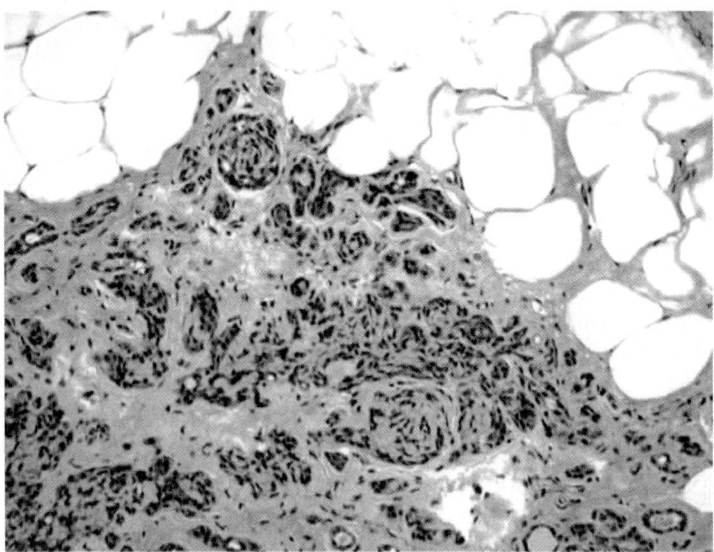

■ **FIGURE 32-7** Sclerosing adenosis with H&E stain ×200 small ductal proliferation within sclerotic background. This lesion mimics invasive carcinoma due to haphazard arrangement of terminal ductal-lobular units.

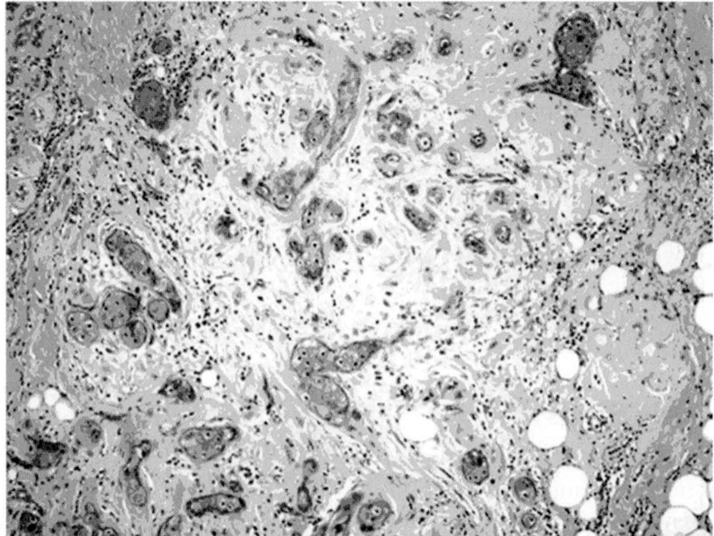

■ **FIGURE 32-8** Ductal carcinoma in situ (DCIS) involving sclerosing adenosis H&E stain ×200. DCIS cells are seen within lobules; cancerization of lobules involving sclerosing adenosis H&E stain: in low power, this area mimics invasive carcinoma.

carcinoma will have haphazard patterns. If there is any doubt, Immunohistochemical (IHC) stains for myoepithelial cells can aid in the correct diagnosis. The most sensitive and specific myoepithelial cell markers are smooth muscle myosin heavy chain (SMMHC) and p63 stains.[24,25] The presence of myoepithelial cells support sclerosing adenosis, but the absence of staining is supportive of invasive carcinoma (Figs. 32-9 and 32-10).

Potential False Negatives and Follow-up for Benign Core Needle Biopsy

A false negative CNB is defined as one diagnosed as benign on pathology but cancer is detected at the biopsy site within two years in the same quadrant of the breast. A false negative CNB does not include cases with discordance or underestimation of disease when excisional biopsy was performed identifying a cancer without significant delay in diagnosis. The false negative rate for CNB is approximately 2%.[19] Imaging follow-up is recommended to avoid delay in diagnosis of a possible false negative CNB. For most benign concordant biopsy results, a 6-month follow-up is recommended. One study suggests that a 1-year follow-up is adequate for definite benign cases, such as a typical fibroadenoma at imaging with a concordant pathology diagnosis of fibroadenoma.[19] The follow-up imaging modality should be the one which best demonstrated the original lesion; that is, if the mass was initially detected by ultrasound, the follow-up image should be ultrasound. It is important to be aware that compliance with follow-up recommendations presents another problem, so documentation regarding a noncompliant patient is important. One study reported that only 74% of patients complied with recommendations for excisional biopsy and only 54% complied with recommended short-term follow-up imaging studies.[26]

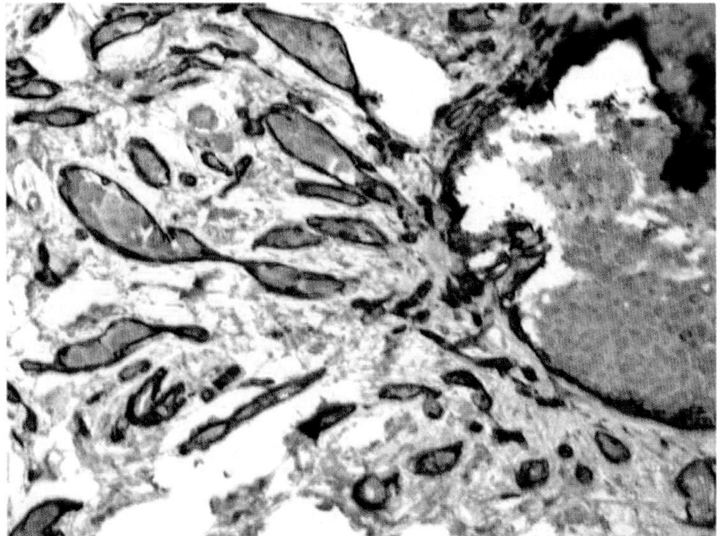

■ **FIGURE 32-9** Smooth muscle myosin heavy chain (SMMHC) IHC positive stain around the cytoplasm of myoepithelial cells.

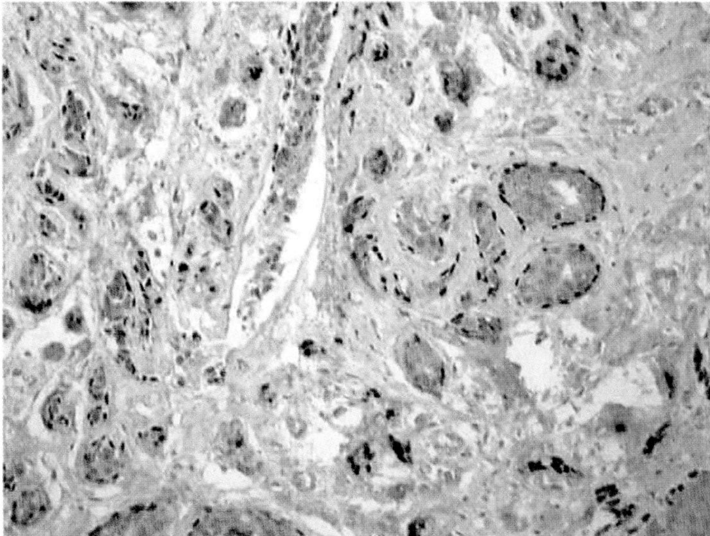

■ **FIGURE 32-10** p63 IHC positive stain in the nuclei of myoepithelial cells.

Communicating Results after Core Needle Biopsy

Most patients have considerable anxiety related to their biopsy findings and hence the results should be obtained in a reasonable time period and quickly communicated to them. Usually this can be accomplished in two to three business days without compromising accuracy. When there is a delay, it is usually because of additional time necessary to perform IHC stains. The most common situations for using IHC stains are to verify the presence of myoepithelial cells for microinvasive carcinoma or sclerotic lesions that mimic invasive carcinoma, delineating ductal or lobular neoplasia, ruling out possible metastatic tumors to breast, and classifying hematopoietic malignancy for primary breast lymphoma. It is important to avoid communicating "preliminary" pathology readings because changing a diagnosis from a benign to a malignant final interpretation or vice versa can be devastating for patients. In our practice, the pathologist communicates the final result to both the referring health care provider and to the radiologist. The final pathology report also will show documentation that communication to the referring physician was performed, with a specific date and time. Also in our practice, a regular meeting between pathologists and radiologists is done on a case-by-case basis. Once a management plan is devised (e.g., 6 month follow-up or surgical excision), the result is communicated to the referring clinician and the patient by the radiologist. The radiologist conveys the recommendations to the health care provider in two ways. First, a phone call is made to the referring physician with the results and management recommendations. In addition, an addendum to the original CNB report is made.

INCISIONAL BIOPSY OF BREAST LESION

Incisional biopsy is often performed by the surgical oncologist when inflammatory breast cancer and/or advanced breast cancers are suspected and a cancer diagnosis and breast biomarkers are needed to plan for neoadjuvant chemotherapy. A skin sample can be included to rule-in dermal lymphatic invasion and Paget disease. An incisional biopsy is usually a fragment or multiple fragments of breast tissue containing tumor measuring approximately 1 cm. No suture orientations are given since margin assessment is not needed.

EXCISIONAL BIOPSY OF BREAST LESION

Excisional biopsy is done for both benign and malignant breast lesions. An excisional specimen should be submitted as one intact tissue with suture orientations by oncologic surgeons. Multiple fragments of breast tissue are not ideal since the surgical margins will be compromised. In our institution, lumpectomy and mastectomy specimens are almost always designated with a short suture for superior and a long suture for lateral (SS and LL). For benign breast lesions such as fibroadenoma, representative sections of the specimen will be sufficient, provided that the cut surface at the time of gross pathology is homogenous. At times, a J-wire is placed in the area of mammographic abnormality. Ideally, a copy of the radiographic finding localized by J-wire should be given to the pathologist. This will better enable the pathologist to sample thoroughly the abnormal area for histological examination. If the excisional biopsy is done for malignant lesions, clinical information regarding prior FNA or CNB should be given to the pathologist, especially if the initial workup was done from an outside institution. FNA induces tissue hemorrhage, infarct, hemosiderin deposit, granulation tissue, inflammatory reaction and epithelial cell displacement of in situ lesion mimicking invasive carcinoma on the excisional biopsy sample.[27] Epithelial displacement is more commonly seen after CNB than FNA. Displaced epithelium can also be seen in the vascular lymphatic space [27-29] (Fig. 32-11).

If the excisional biopsy was done for a malignant lesion, two important features should be evaluated by the

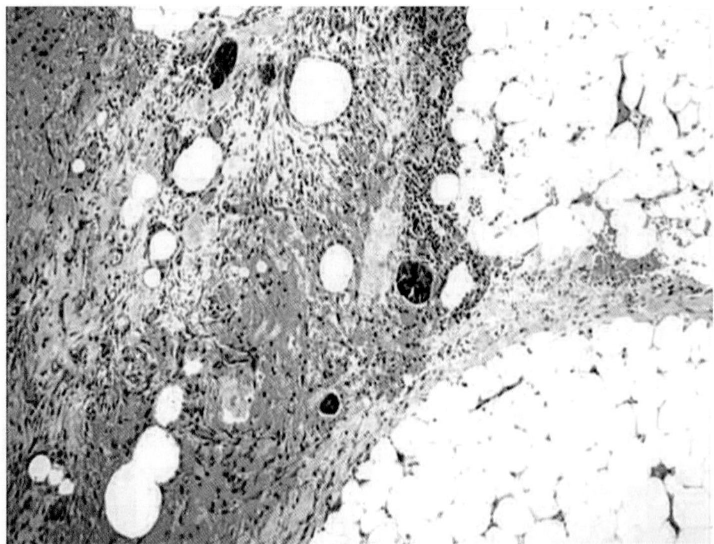

■ **FIGURE 32-11** Hematoxylin and eosin stain ×200 needle track after core needle biopsy of ductal carcinoma in situ (DCIS). Aggregates of tumor cells from DCIS are dislodged and sitting on hemorrhagic needle track of a prior biopsy site, resembling invasive carcinoma.

pathologist: tumor size and margin status. These two factors are dependent on how the gross examinations are done. The most important prognostic factor is the lymph node metastasis. The tumor size is the second most important prognostic factor in determining disease-free survival in invasive breast cancer. This fact is particularly true in cases of node-negative invasive breast cancers where the stage becomes almost completely dependent on the tumor size. Even in node-positive breast cancer, the tumor size is an essential element in the TNM staging system (**t**umor size, lymph **n**odes affected, **m**etastases) and the one measurable variable of utmost consequence.[30] The type and extent of subsequent surgical and oncological management is heavily dependent on the tumor size. The guidelines of American Joint Committee on Cancer (AJCC) for breast tumors classifies them pathologically into four groups for staging purposes: T0 refers to tumors that are not grossly visible, T1 for those measuring less than or equal to 2 cm, T2 for those greater than 2 cm but not more than 5 cm, and T3 for tumors greater than 5 cm in the greatest dimension.[31] Therefore, accurate measurement of an invasive breast cancer is crucial for appropriate patient management. There are various methods for determining tumor size including palpation on physical examination, breast-imaging studies including mammography, ultrasound, and more recently MRI. Pathology, however, is considered to be the gold standard method for measurement of tumor size. However, neither AJCC nor International Union Against Cancer (IUCC) staging manuals specify how breast tumors are to be measured by gross or microscopic methods.[32,33] The College of American Pathologists (CAP), however, recommends that the microscopic measurement of tumor should be used as the actual tumor size for staging.[33-35] The gross assessment of tumor size is not accurate and yet many pathology laboratories stage the tumor size by gross examination.[36,37]

In this age of cost containment, it is necessary to consider the extent of sampling for histologic evaluation. Many different institutions have their own policy on how to perform a gross examination and how much tissue is to be sampled from the excisional biopsy specimens. For large invasive ductal carcinomas proven by CNB, representative sections of the tumor and extensive sampling of the margin may be fairly accurate. However, for the smaller tumor detected only by imaging without clinical palpation, DCIS and many invasive lobular carcinoma cases, a sequential and careful grossing technique is essential to be able to reconstruct the 3-dimensional view by microscopic examination to determine an accurate tumor size.[38]

GROSS TUMOR SIZE MEASUREMENT METHOD

All specimens are received with orientation and are grossly examined in the fresh state, or after being fixed in 10% buffer formalin overnight (Fig. 32-12). It is absolutely essential to fix the breast tissue more than 6 hours and not longer than 48 hours to have reliable breast biomarker results by IHC stains, particularly for HER-2/*neu*.[39] Gross examination consists of describing the specimen and placing all or parts of it into a small plastic cassette that holds the tissue

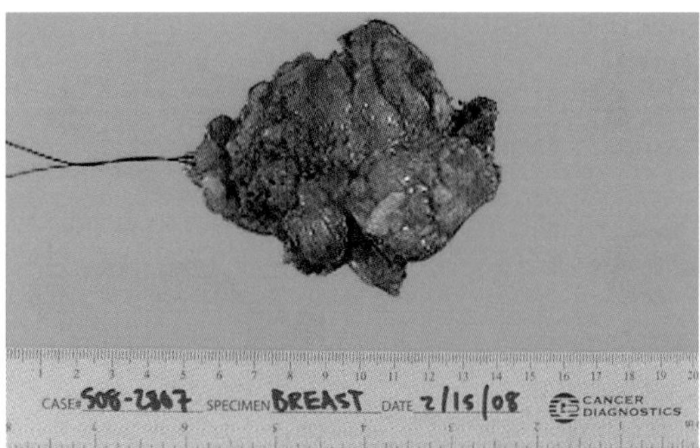

■ **FIGURE 32-12** An intact specimen is received with sutures designation by surgeon.

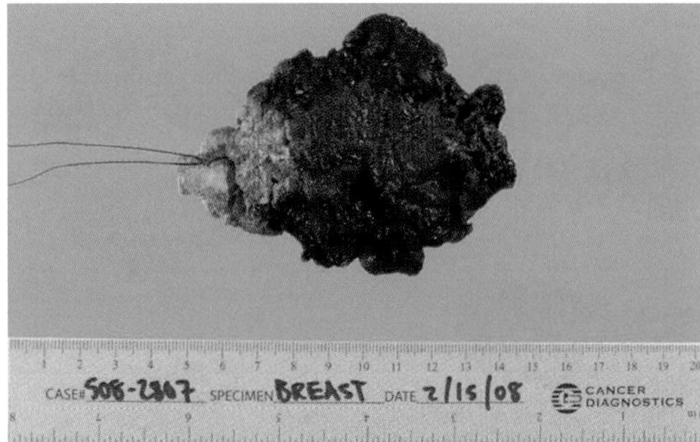

■ **FIGURE 32-13** Specimen is inked with different colors.

while it is being processed to a paraffin block. Initially, the cassettes are placed into a fixative. Initially, all margins are painted with different colored inks (Fig. 32-13). In our institution, six colors are applied as follows for all excisional biopsy specimens: superior—blue, inferior—green, lateral—yellow, medial—violet, superficial—red, and deep—black. It is important to air-dry the specimen painted with ink before cutting into it. This will minimize ink seeping into the breast tissue and compromising accurate surgical margin assessment. This can be done in several ways, such as a using a low voltage, cool hair dryer or a brief application of Bouin solution to coagulate the ink. Specimens are then cut bread-loaf style into 0.3 to 0.5 cm thick levels from the longest axis, usually medial to lateral. All slices are laid consecutively for inspection and palpation (Fig. 32-14). Most invasive tumors are grossly visible with the naked eye and firm to palpation (Fig. 32-15). Most carcinoma in situ lesions are not visible and palpable unless DCIS is comedo type in which case it may show small areas of punctuated (comedo) necrosis. The grossly identifiable tumors are measured in three dimensions at the time of gross examination. The gross size is recorded as "no mass identified" when the dissector is unable to identify a definite tumor within the fibroadipose tissue. When the mass is seen by gross examination, the distance between the mass and each margin also is recorded at the time of grossing the specimen. In addition, mass characteristics such as borders (e.g., well circumscribed, irregular, or infiltrative), consistency (e.g., soft, rubbery, or firm), and other features (e.g., cystic, necrotic or hemorrhagic) should be documented. The edges of the specimen, most medial and most lateral margins are each further cut perpendicularly along the longest axis and placed in separate cassettes.

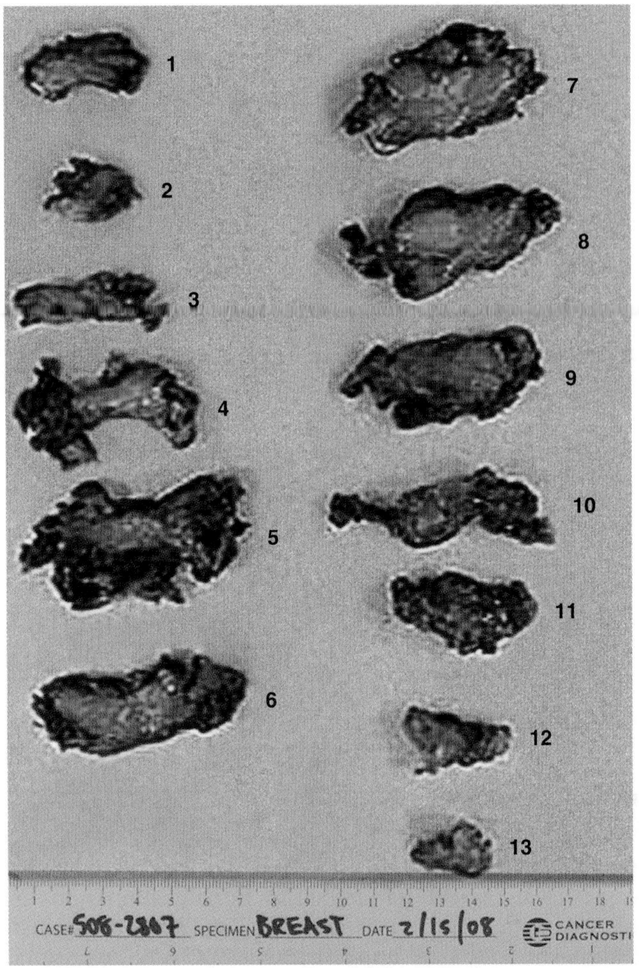

■ **FIGURE 32-14** Specimen is serially cut into slices.

The remainder of the levels is entirely submitted from medial to lateral for microscopic examination. All cassettes are sequentially numbered for each case. If the lumpectomy is larger in size (in our institution, greater than 5 cm), each level is sampled in its entirety; however, trimmed tissue is not submitted. For instance, each level is cut at 0.5 cm intervals, and each level is further sliced into 0.25 cm sections to fit into the cassette. The trimmed tissue thickness of 0.25 cm is not submitted. It is important not to stuff the cassette with tissue because the processing solution during the tissue processing has to be able to penetrate the tissue (Fig. 32-16).

MICROSCOPIC TUMOR SIZE MEASUREMENT METHOD

The exact tumor size is determined by first measuring in centimeters the microscopic extensions of the invasive carcinoma in six directions, that is, medial, lateral, superior, inferior, anterior, and posterior. The measurements are then compiled by multiplying the number of levels showing the invasive cancer by the thickness of each level. In cases where the maximum dimension of the tumor is only on one slide, the linear dimension of the invasive cancer on that slide is measured and recorded as the maximum tumor size. In-situ carcinoma sizes can be measured by using the same method as invasive carcinoma cases (Fig. 32-17).

RE-EXCISIONAL BIOPSY AFTER LUMPECTOMY

The widespread use of breast-conserving therapy in the treatment of breast cancer has resulted in increasing numbers of re-excision specimens. Re-excisional biopsy is

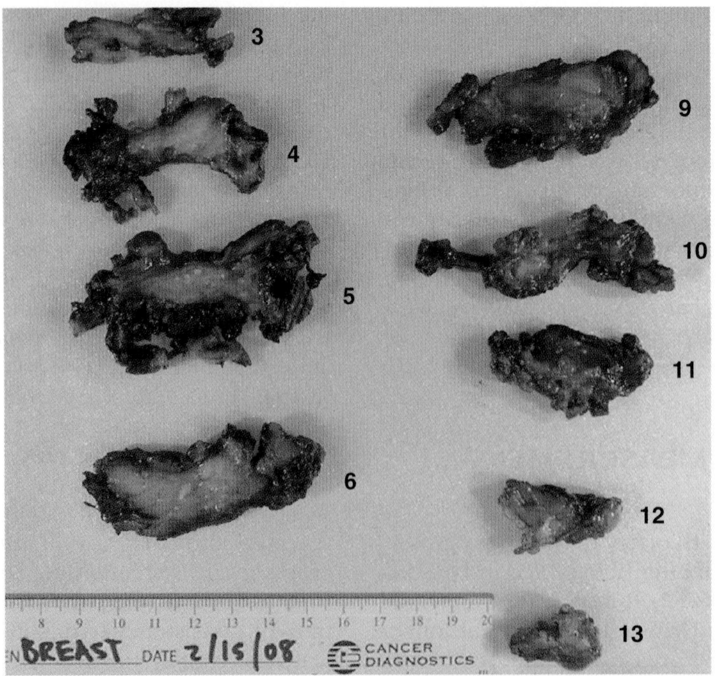

■ **FIGURE 32-15** On levels 5 and 6, the tumor is visible. The tumor is seen in the central portion of the specimen, punctuated white to tan in color, and closely approaching to multiple margins.

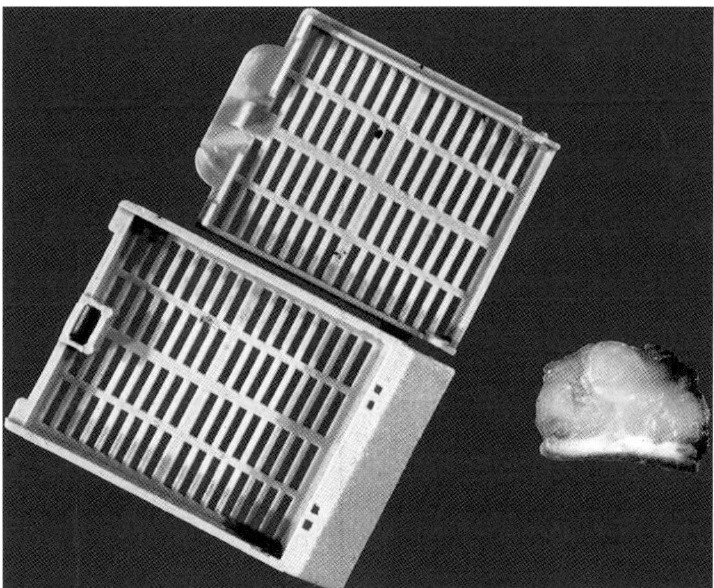

■ **FIGURE 32-16** A standard cassette size is 3.5 cm in length and 2.5 cm in width. Tissue should not fill the entire area within the cassette for proper penetration of different solutions during processing. The ideal size and the thickness of each tissue is shown.

usually done due to tumor present at or near the initial excisional margin. Re-excisional specimens usually contain a large biopsy cavity with a seroma in the center. Many re-excisions are performed for only microscopically positive or close margins, and therefore specimens often appear grossly negative. Suture orientations by surgeons are necessary for evaluation of the re-excisional biopsy. The gross examination of a re-excision specimen is similar to the initial lumpectomy specimen. The presence or absence of residual tumor and the margin assessment are most important components to be determined by the pathologist. Adequate sampling is essential for microscopic analysis. Abraham and coworkers studied the extent of sampling for histological samples in 97 consecutive re-excision specimens for in situ and invasive carcinoma. The authors reported that with a 52% reduction in number of paraffin blocks they would have missed 47 positive specimens, 30 of which resulted in a major change in patient management (recommendation for additional surgery), 10 of which resulted in minor changes (alteration in radiation dose or adjuvant chemotherapy regimen), and 7 of which did not alter management. In contrast, two blocks per centimeter would have missed an average of less than one case each of diagnoses resulting in major and minor therapy changes (0.9 and 0.8 cases, respectively), with a 17% reduction in number of tissue blocks.[40] It is critical to examine the specimen thoroughly and when possible, all surgical margins should be examined by histological evaluation and two blocks per 1 cm biopsy cavity area are recommended.

MASTECTOMY

It is not possible to submit all tissue from a mastectomy for microscopic examination. Hence, careful inspection and dissection of mastectomy specimens is an essential part of gross examination. If gross examination is poorly done without detecting a mass or masses, margin assessment and searching for all lymph nodes, microscopic examination is meaningless. The quality assurance rendered by surgical pathology services is rarely measured by accuracy in the grossing technique of the mastectomy specimen. There are only a handful studies on quality assurance on this topic.[41] The first necessary action for the pathologist is to read the imaging findings and clinical findings, such as the location of the mass or masses, and the expected size of the mass or masses. Additional critical information such as previous CNB or lumpectomy is necessary to know prior to handling a mastectomy specimen. A small tumor with prior history of CNB can be difficult to find within a mastectomy specimen. DCIS is usually not palpable or visible during gross examination and hence it is important to know how extensive are the microcalcifications found by imaging studies, and which quadrant or quadrants are involved. The imaging and clinical findings of each case will determine the quantity of sample sections to be taken for mastectomy.

All mastectomies without axillary dissection (simple mastectomy) should be oriented by the surgeon with sutures. The gross description includes the specimen's size dimensions, weight, presence of skin and nipple, location of tumor or tumors in terms of quadrant and the relationship to the margins. Special attention should be paid to the deep margin and should note whether skeletal muscle is present or not. The presence of fascia is not grossly visible. Previous biopsy site observations such as skin scar should be documented. The specimen is sectioned into 1 cm intervals (bread loaf) from medial to lateral. The protocol for re-excision biopsy applies to the mastectomy specimen. Shaved representative margins of grossly negative margin by tumor and perpendicular margin of grossly close margin by tumor samples, as well as representative sections of each slice (or at least from each quadrant) is recommended. At a minimum, the representative sections from a mastectomy specimen

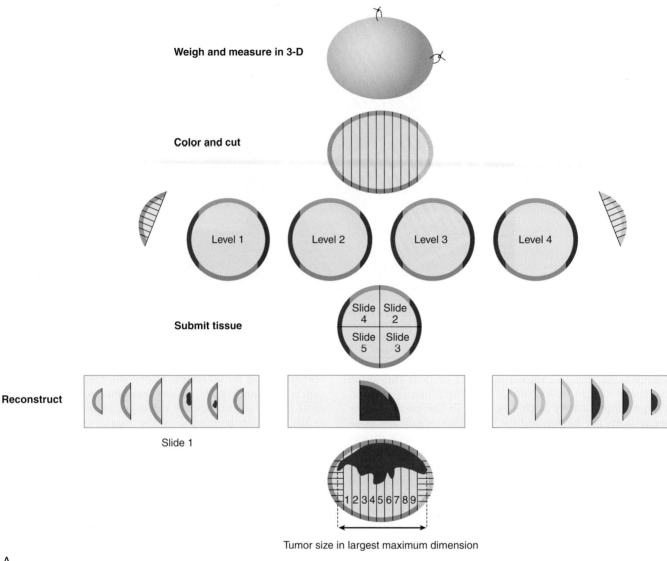

Weigh and measure in 3-D

Color and cut

Level 1 Level 2 Level 3 Level 4

Submit tissue

Slide 4 Slide 2 Slide 5 Slide 3

Reconstruct

Slide 1

1 2 3 4 5 6 7 8 9

Tumor size in largest maximum dimension

A

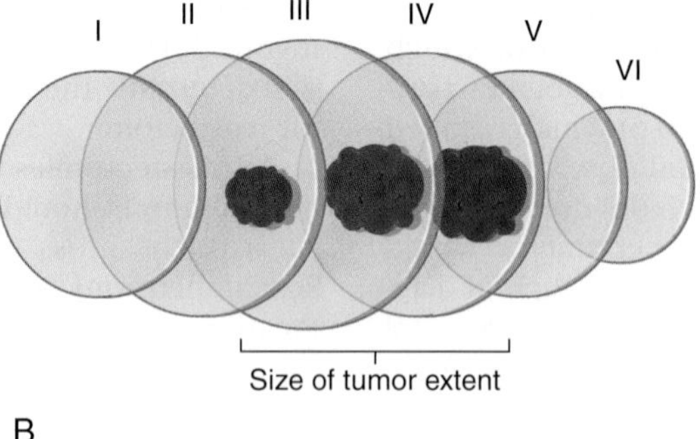

B

■ **FIGURE 32-17** The specimen is received oriented with two sutures and inked with six different colors (anteriorly, posteriorly, superiorly, inferiorly, medially, and laterally). The medial and lateral margins are cut followed by serial sectioning of the remainder of the specimen. Each level is completely submitted in cassettes and examined microscopically for the presence of invasive carcinoma or ductal carcinoma in situ (DCIS). (Purple striped area is invasive cancer which was reconstructed after reviewing all slides.) The tumor configuration and size can be reconstructed.

include nipple, areolar area, skin with scar area, any skin lesion, tumor section (at least 1 block per 1 cm), prior CNB biopsy site, biopsy cavity (2 blocks/1.0 cm), one or more sections of margins, normal breast tissue from each quadrant and all lymph nodes. If a lymph node is grossly positive for metastatic carcinoma and is large, one representative section of the longest axis including adjacent fatty tissue can be submitted. If lymph node is grossly negative, the entire lymph node is submitted by cutting it serially into 0.2 to 0.3 cm thicknesses.

MICROSCOPIC EVALUATION OF SURGICAL MARGINS

When a tumor is removed, some adjacent normal breast tissue is also removed. Margins refer to the distance between a tumor and the edge of the surrounding normal tissue that is removed along with it. The outer edges of normal-appearing breast tissue are inked by the pathologist as described earlier. The outer edges often show cautery artifact since many surgeons use Bovie (electrocautery) to decrease the amount of bleeding during the operation. This artifact often helps pathologists define a true margin that can often be seen with thick ink applied during gross examination of the specimen. Bovie-induced cautery artifact and ink are clearly visible under a light microscope. Bovie artifact also hinders the accurate evaluation of ductal structures due to the burned appearance of tissue. Depending upon what the pathologist sees, the margins of a tumor are described as:

- Positive margins: Cancer cells are present at the ink.
- Negative margins: No cancer cells are found at the ink.
- Close margins: Any situation that falls between positive and negative is considered *close*. Close margin should have specifications as to the distance between the tumor cells to the edge of the margin where the ink is, such as 1 mm, 2 mm, and so on. In our institution, we report margins within 10 mm distance from the tumor to the specific margin. (If more than 10 mm, we consider negative margin)

The definition of *negative margins* varies from one institution to another. Knowing the accurate margin status from the conservative surgical tissue is critical in making additional surgical treatment decisions. If the margins are positive, more surgery is needed. If the margins are close, surgery may or may not be necessary. If the margins are negative, no additional surgery is needed.

There are basically two ways to evaluate resection margins; by creating shaved or perpendicular margins.

Shaved margins are obtained as an "orange peel" where the inked edges are peeled 2 to 3 mm thick, from the main tissue (Fig. 32-18). The shaved surface is submitted for histological evaluation. One of the benefits of this technique is that a larger area can be examined versus perpendicular sections. However, one disadvantage is that if a shaved margin is positive by tumor cells, the assessment of tumor at the margin is unclear as to whether the tumor is actually close or positive at the margin. Shaved margins are either positive or negative.

Perpendicular margins are created by cross sectioning the breast tissue. Margin is considered positive when tumor cells extend to the inked surface. This technique allows an accurate assessment on either positive or close relationship to the tumor, and the distance is measured directly on the slide. The disadvantage of the perpendicular margin assessment is that it requires more sections and blocks to evaluate the entire excisional biopsy specimen surface. In our institution, perpendicular margins are taken for excision and re-excision (any type of breast conservative surgery) and shaved margins are taken for mastectomy.

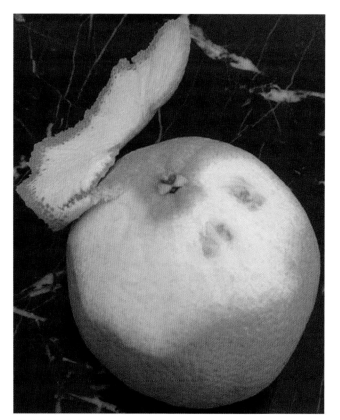

■ **FIGURE 32-18** Orange peel (shaved margin): lumpectomy specimen margin is cut by peeling.

Even for mastectomy, if the tumor is closely approximating the margin by gross examination, a perpendicular margin should be taken.

Problems can occur during the evaluation of surgical margins. Firstly, if a surgeon submits multiple fragments of breast tissue without orientation, accurate assessment of the resection margin will be compromised. Secondly, extensive Bovie or cautery artifacts distort the cellular architecture and cytologic findings that are critical to the pathologist (Fig. 32-19). Thirdly, ink sometimes flows from the surface to underlying tissue through defects and crevices. This is particularly true in cystic lesions, papillary lesions, biopsy cavity sites and necrotic tumor areas. Hence, the presence of tumor cells at the ink alone may not necessarily indicate a positive margin.

SENTINEL LYMPH NODE SAMPLE

Axillary sentinel lymph node biopsy is becoming a popular method for assessing lymph node status to avoid the morbidities caused by full axillary lymph node dissection. Sentinel lymph node sampling for breast cancer is presumed to be the first lymph node drainage from the primary site of breast cancer. This lymph node is identified by the surgeon after injection of isosulfan blue dye or a radioactive substance (usually injection of technetium Tc 99 sulfur colloid), or both, at the primary breast cancer site. Sentinel lymph nodes are harvested as those lymph nodes that have an elevated gamma count and by the presence of visible blue dye. Sentinel lymph node can be one or multiple. Standard practice is to forgo a more extensive

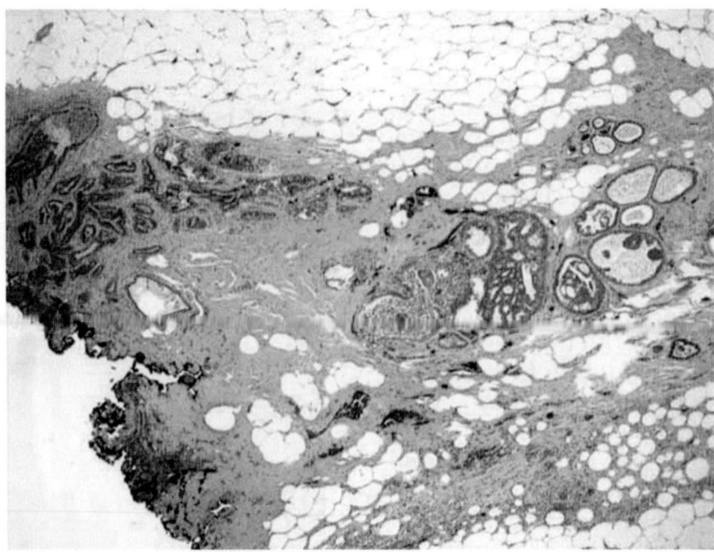

■ **FIGURE 32-19** H&E stain ×100 showing cauterized and inked edge. Ductal structures show burned artifact and nuclear detail is lost.

axillary lymph node dissection if sentinel lymph node is found to be negative for metastatic carcinoma. There is still no unanimity of opinion regarding the sentinel lymph node sampling procedure as the standard of care in all invasive breast cancer and DCIS.[42] There is also no unanimity of opinion regarding how to optimize and handle sentinel lymph node samples in pathology. How many levels of hematoxylin and eosin (H&E) stains should be obtained for each sentinel lymph node? Should cytokeratin IHC stain studies routinely be performed on all sentinel lymph nodes, and if so, how many different kinds of cytokeratin stains and how many levels should be undertaken on each node? Is there any clinically significant prognostic value on immunohistochemically detected cells in the sentinel lymph node or any node for that matter? How many sentinel lymph nodes are enough? What is the next step when micrometastatic carcinoma or isolated tumor cells are found in the sentinel lymph node? Should isolated tumor cells or micrometastatic carcinoma to sentinel lymph node be treated with chemotherapy? All these questions still remain to be conclusively answered.

Although there are many controversial issues around the sentinel lymph node protocol, most pathology laboratories perform a focused study on the sentinel lymph node that includes multiple sections of H&E stained tissue levels, and by IHC stains. In our institution, each sentinel lymph node is cut 2 mm thick, in the longest axis. Each 2 mm thick section is then further cut into 100 to 150 micron thickness onto glass slides. The entire lymph node is submitted and embedded. First, third and fifth slides are stained with H&E stains and second and fourth slides are stained with cytokeratin IHC stains. (Fig. 32-20) Macrometastatic disease is present when more than 2 mm of metastatic tumor cells are identified in the sentinel lymph node. In this situation, a full axillary lymph node dissection is recommended. The literature indicates that approximately 50% of patients may end up having additional positive metastatic disease in axillary lymph nodes.[43-46] Micrometastatic disease is present when from greater than 0.2 mm to less than 2 mm of metastatic tumor cells are seen within the sentinel lymph node. In this situation, a full axillary lymph node dissection is usually recommended (Fig. 32-21). The literature indicates that approximately 7% to 40% of patients may have additional positive metastatic disease in axillary lymph nodes.[45,47-52] Isolated tumor cells (ITC) is reported when less than 0.2 mm of metastatic tumor cells are seen within the sentinel lymph node (Fig. 32-22). The tumor cells are either single cells or a few clusters located within the subcapsular sinus of lymph node. These can be identified by either H&E stains or IHC

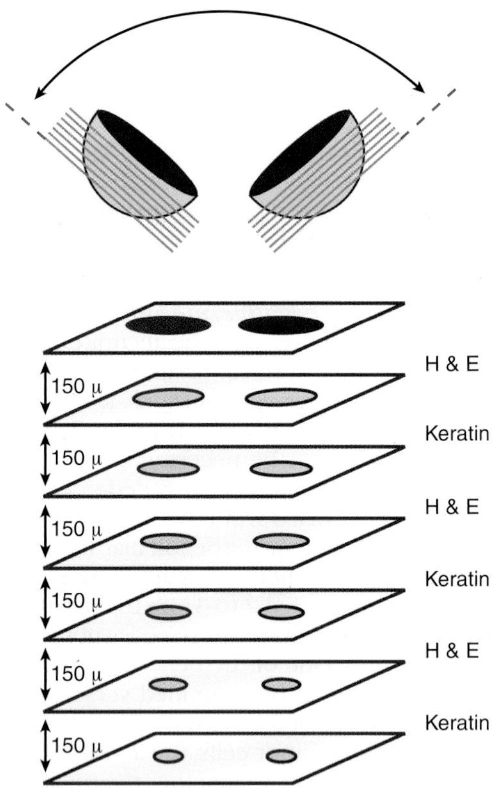

■ **FIGURE 32-20** Sentinel lymph node protocol: Lymph nodes are cut into 2mm thickness in a longest axis. Three H&E stains and two IHC cytokeratin stains are performed for each lymph node.

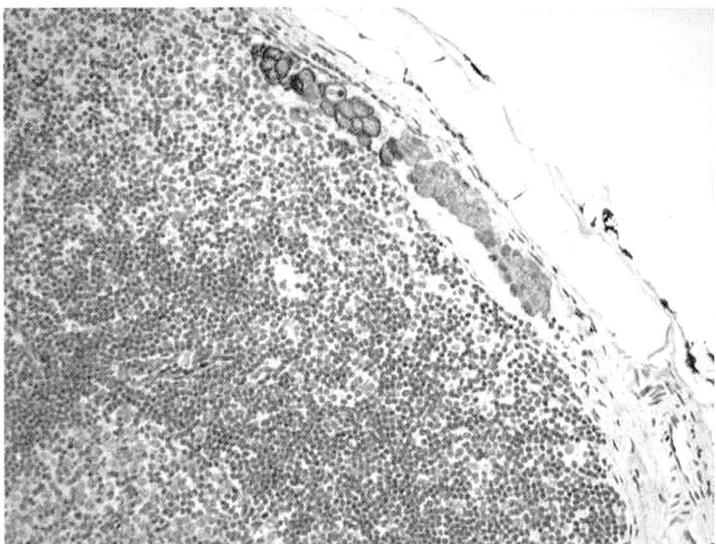

■ **FIGURE 32-21** pN1mi: micrometastasis (>0.2 mm, not > 2.0 mm). The immunohistochemical (IHC) stain for keratin shows 0.4 mm linear pattern of metastatic carcinoma located at subcapsular area of the lymph node.

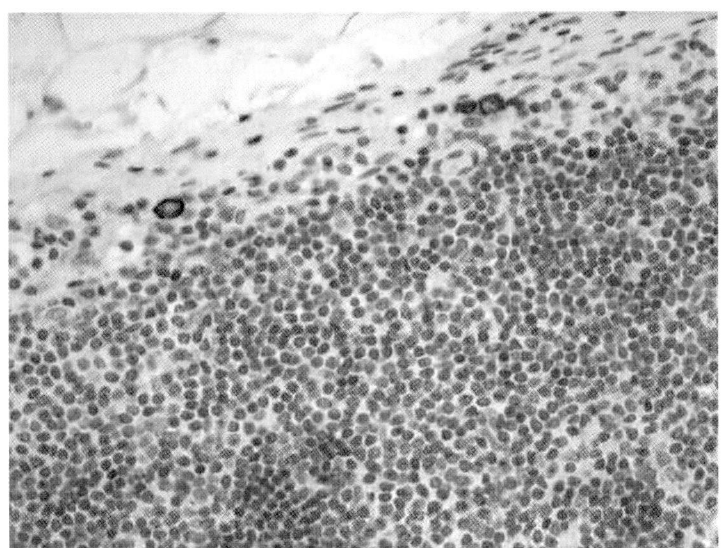

■ **FIGURE 32-22** pN0 (i+): metastatic focus <0.2 mm detected by hematoxylin and eosin or cytokeratin immunohistochemical (IHC) stain (isolated tumor cells). In this case, IHC-detected single cell to two cells in aggregate is seen.

stains. In this situation, it is still controversial whether or not a full axillary lymph node dissection is needed. A paucity of literature is devoted to this situation. A balanced discussion between the surgeon and patient is needed to consider what the best treatment options are. Considerations include larger primary tumor size, lymph vascular invasion, or both. Approximately 6% to 9% of patients may have additional positive metastatic disease in axillary lymph nodes after isolated tumor cells are seen in the sentinel lymph node.[48,51]

The role of radiation therapy after positive sentinel lymph node has not been well studied. AMAROS, a clinical trial from the European Organization for Research and Treatment of Cancer, is designed to address this issue. When the study is completed, we may have better insight into whether radiation therapy can substitute for surgical axillary lymph node dissection. Although both therapies can cause complications, surgical axillary dissection is associated with significant morbidity including pain, lymphedema, nerve injury, shoulder dysfunction, axillary web syndrome, compromised functionality and quality of life, and complex wound care.

INTRAOPERATIVE CONSULTATION/ FROZEN SECTION

At times during the performance of surgical procedures, surgeons may deem it necessary to get a rapid diagnosis from the pathologist. The surgeon may want to know sentinel lymph node status, margin status of malignant neoplasm before closing, or an unexpected disease process may be found requiring rapid diagnosis to decide what to do next. Another indication for using a frozen section is to determine if the appropriate tissue has been removed for further workup of a disease process. This is accomplished through use of a frozen section by snap freezing small pieces of tissue in a cold liquid or cold environment (-20° C to -70° C). Freezing with an instrument known as the cryostat makes the tissue solid enough to section with a microtome. The cryostat is simply a refrigerated box containing a microtome. The temperature inside the cryostat is -20° C to -30° C. The frozen tissue sections are cut, picked up on a glass slide and stained with H&E stain. The entire process can be done within 5 to 10 minutes. However, artifacts caused by freezing and poor preservation of cellular details often preclude an accurate diagnosis in breast tissue because of the high content of fatty tissue. Margin assessment, small tumor (size ≤1 cm) and initial diagnostic evaluation of breast lesions are cases in which preparation of frozen sections is not recommended due to the high percentage of discrepancies between frozen sections and permanent section diagnoses.[53,54]

BREAST BIOMARKERS

There are exciting advancements in breast cancer treatments, with intensive efforts to provide and identify new biological and molecular indicators of clinical outcome and response to therapy. A prognostic indicator is a factor capable of providing information on clinical outcome at the time of diagnosis, such as axillary lymph node status. A predictive indicator is a factor capable of providing information on likelihood of response to a given therapeutic modality such as estrogen receptor (ER), progesterone receptor (PR) studies and HER-2/*neu* status. Predictive and prognostic indicators are not mutually exclusive. For instances, ER status is mostly a predictive indicator to tamoxifen therapy, but it is also a weak prognostic indicator in that most ER-positive tumors have better prognosis than ER-negative tumors. Most institutions require breast biomarker studies to be done on all breast cancers, which include ER, PR, and HER-2/*neu*, and Ki-67 biomarker studies. All breast biomarkers are currently being done by IHC stains using formalin fixed paraffin blocks. HER-2/*neu* can be done with both IHC staining and FISH. Approximately 55% to 70% of primary breast carcinomas are ER positive and 45% to 60% are PR positive. Breast tumors co-expressing both ER and PR are more likely to respond to endocrine therapy.[55,56] Women whose breast cancer is ER positive have a 60% overall response rate, a 30% higher 5-year disease-free survival rate, and an average of 20% to 30% lower recurrence rate with adjuvant endocrine therapy.[57] ER positive status but loss of PR by tumor cells is associated with a worse prognosis.[58] The 5-year disease-free survival rate is 20% higher if the tumor is both ER and PR positive, than ER positive and PR negative tumors, confirming PR status as a useful predictor for endocrine therapy response.[57] Currently, ER and PR are tested via IHC assay, which has replaced the earlier ligand-binding biochemical assay. The IHC assay is beneficial because of use of paraffin-embedded blocks for the tumor, rather than requiring fresh frozen tissue as in ligand-binding biochemical assays. Most of the clinical outcome studies are done with ligand-binding biochemical assays. Hence, it is most ideal if the IHC assay is calibrated by a ligand-binding biochemical assay. The ligand-binding biochemical assay evaluates both ERα and ERβ. The IHC assay, however, only tests for ERα (Fig. 32-23). There may be a merit to studying ERβ because one study showed that ERβ has been detected in 47% of ERα negative tumors. Women with ERβ positive tumors receiving adjuvant endocrine therapy with tamoxifen were found to have better survival rates among both node positive and node negative tumors when compared with ERβ negative tumors.[59]

The cut-off value as to what is positive and negative on ER and PR in terms of quantification and qualification of IHC stain interpretation has not been standardized. Some authors consider 5% of tumor cells displaying easily discernible nuclear staining as positive.[60] Other authors require nuclear immunoreactivity in more than 10% of the tumor cells.[61] The Allred Score is a microscopic method conveying the estimated proportion and intensity of positive tumor cells (range from 0-8) (Fig. 32-24). This scoring system was developed more than a decade ago and has been used and validated for several markers, including

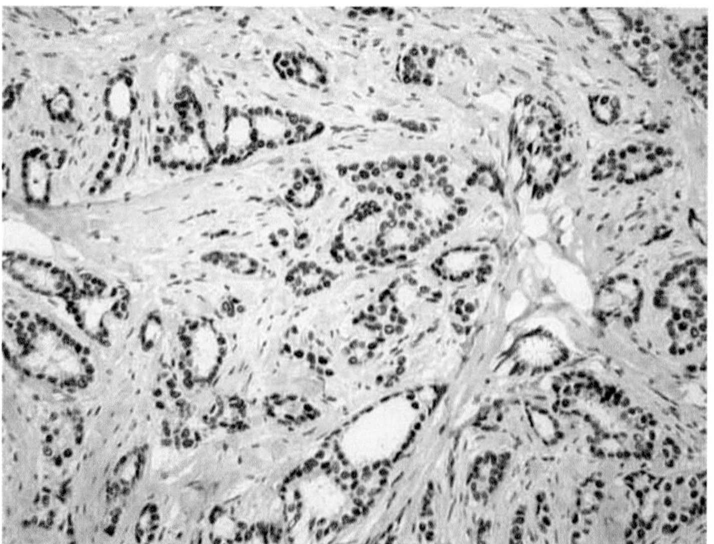

■ **FIGURE 32-23** Invasive ductal carcinoma with estrogen receptor (ER) (Antibody 6F11) immunohistochemical (IHC) stain: all nuclei of tumor cells are positive with +3 intensity.

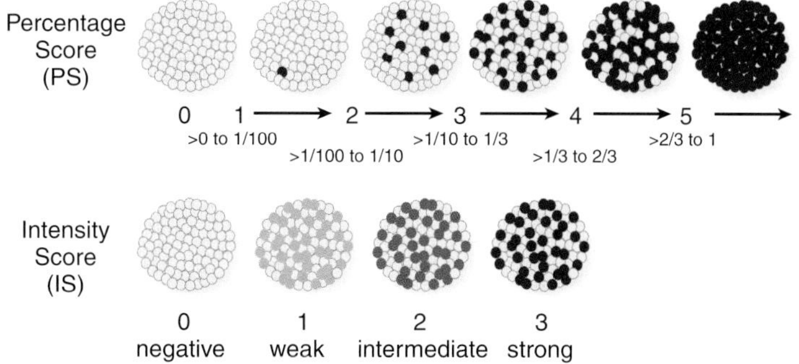

■ FIGURE 32-24 Allred Score, which is a microscopic method conveying the estimated proportion (range from 0-5) and intensity (range from 0-3) of positive tumor cells.

ER, PR, HER-2/*neu*, and p53. Based on several large clinical studies using this scoring system and an assay based on an antibody for ER, it has been determined that 3 (corresponding to 1%-10% positive cells) is the optimum score for defining ER-positive breast cancer.[62-64]

HER-2/*neu* is an oncogene located on chromosome 17q12-21.32 that encodes a 185-kilo-dalton transmembrane protein. (Fig. 32-25) It codes for a receptor for a particular growth factor that causes cells to grow. Normal epithelial cells contain two copies of the HER-2/*neu* gene and produce low levels of the Her-2 protein on the surface of their cells. The HER-2/*neu* gene is amplified, which means far too many copies are produced and its protein is over-expressed resulting in an abnormally large amount of the protein being produced. Most of the time, the HER-2/*neu* gene is both amplified and overexpressed. In about 20% to 30% of invasive breast cancers HER-2/*neu* is overexpressed and amplified. HER-2/*neu* is not unique to breast cancer but overexpressed and amplified in many other cancers such as ovarian and bladder cancers. HER-2/*neu* overexpressed tumors tend to grow more aggressively and resist hormonal therapy and some chemotherapy such as cyclophosphamide, methotrexate, and 5-flourouracil. Patients generally have a poorer prognosis. HER-2/*neu* positive tumors are more sensitive to doxorubicin (adriamycine) therapy. HER-2/*neu*-positive tumors are susceptible to trastuzumab (Herceptin), a drug therapy that was targeted for the HER-2/*neu* protein. Herceptin is an FDA-approved drug that is given to node-positive breast cancer patients. Herceptin may be used alone or with other chemotherapy agents but is only useful in those who have HER-2/*neu* amplification and protein overexpression. HER-2/*neu* positive tumors are reported to have reduced tumor progression in 28% in women treated with Herceptin and chemotherapy compared with 14% of women treated with chemotherapy alone.[65] The development of this specialized therapy has increased the use of HER-2/*neu* testing. There are two main methods to test HER-2/*neu* status: IHC (Figs. 32-26 through 32-29) and FISH (Fig. 32-30). Both methods are approved by the FDA. IHC measures the amount of HER-2/*neu* protein present. FISH looks at the genetic level for actual gene amplification — the number of copies of the gene present. IHC is currently the most widely used testing method and many institutions use this test. The HercepTest is an FDA-approved IHC test that uses a polyclonal antibody manufactured by DakoCytomation. The IHC stains are scored by the intensity and quantity of membrane staining around the invasive tumor cells. Several studies have reported that FISH is a more sensitive and specific method to evaluate HER-2/*neu*, because of variability in testing using different methodologies, reporting and scoring of the HER-2/*neu* IHC test. During the ASCO 2000 meeting, it was reported that the HER-2/*neu* IHC results were discrepant when the IHC test was done at reference center. A prospective randomized trial of 2700 patients with HER-2/*neu* positive breast cancer was conducted by a large cooperative group (NSABP B-31 study). One of the aims of this study was to assess the concordance between local and central HER-2/*neu* testing. A central review of the first 104 cases entered on the trial based on IHC results was conducted. It showed that only 84 of 104 were found to be HER-2/*neu* positive by HercepTest (IHC) and 82 of 104 were found to be HER-2/*neu* positive by PathVysion (FISH). There was less discrepancy between results when a high-volume lab performed the assay: 18 of 75 cases

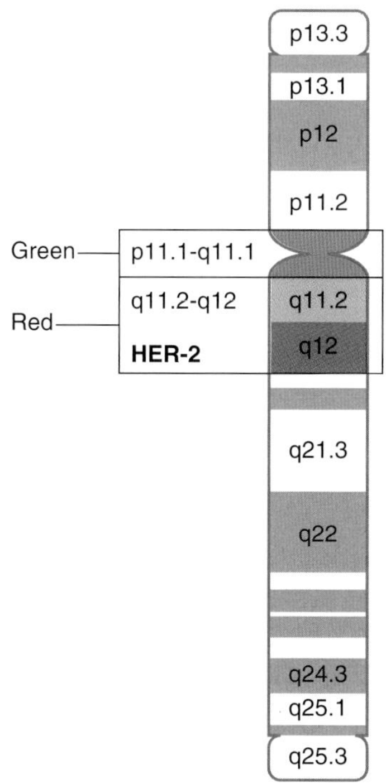

■ FIGURE 32-25 Diagram of HER-2/*neu* is located on chromosome 17q12-21.32.

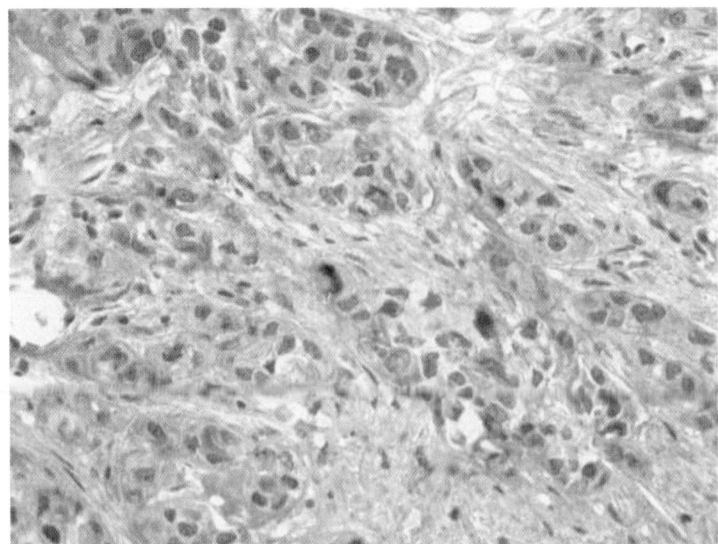

■ **FIGURE 32-26** HercepTest (Dako) ×200. Immunohistochemical (IHC) is scored on a 0 to 3+ scale based on staining intensity and completeness of membrane staining. No membrane staining is observed in tumor cells. Score is 0.

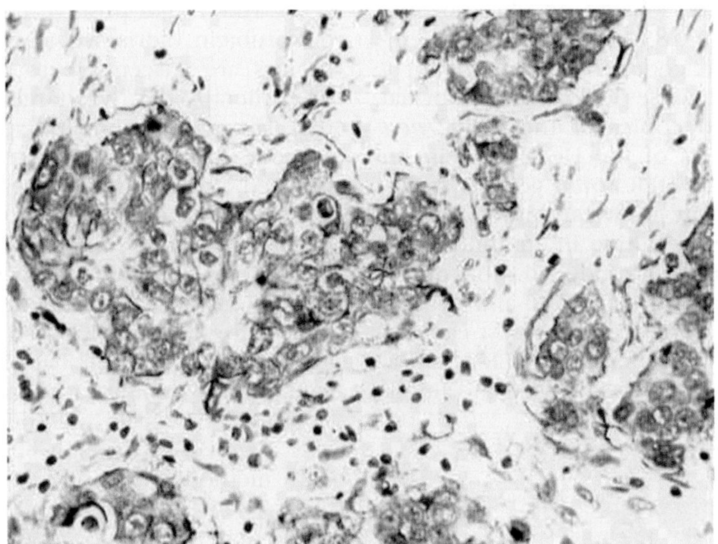

■ **FIGURE 32-27** HercepTest (Dako) ×200. Weak and incomplete membrane staining is observed in tumor cells. Score is +1.

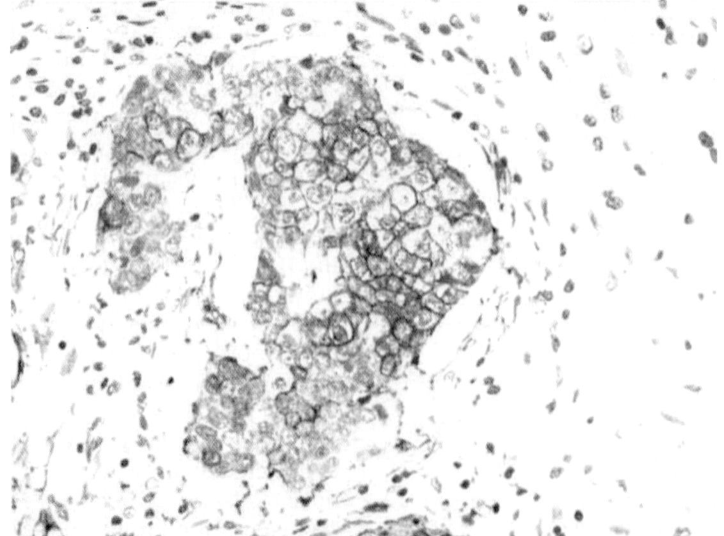

■ **FIGURE 32-28** HercepTest (Dako) ×200. Partial to complete membrane staining is observed in some tumor cells. Score is +2.

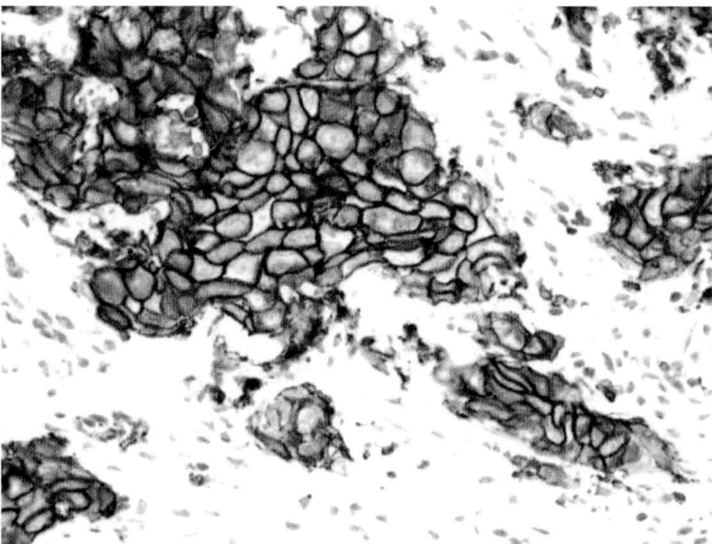

■ **FIGURE 32-29** HercepTest (Dako) ×200. Complete membrane staining is observed in all tumor cells. Score is +3.

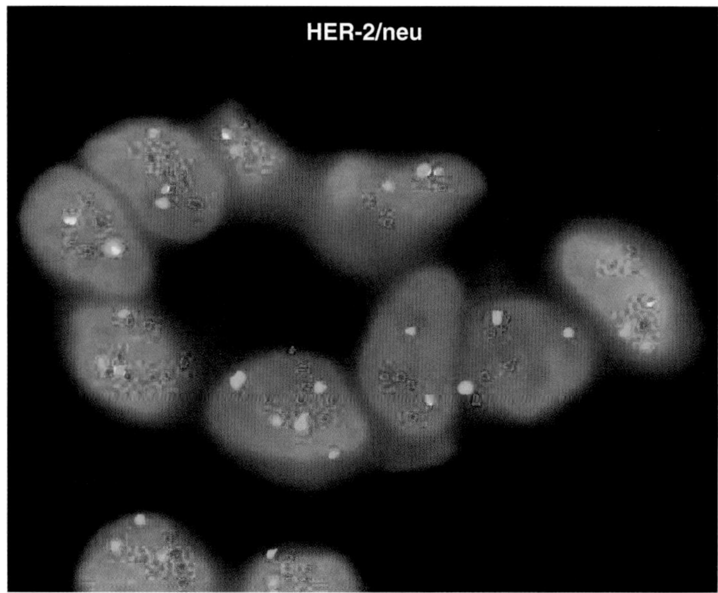

■ **FIGURE 32-30** HER-2/*neu* fluorescent in situ hybridization (FISH): Red and green signals within each nuclei are counted. In this case, there are six red signals and three green signals with ratio of red/green of 2.0.

from low-volume labs were false positives and 1 of 29 cases from high-volume labs was a false positive. High-volume labs were defined as those performing more than 100 cases per month. Recently, guidelines have been established to regulate and improve the HER-2/*neu* IHC test.[39] Concordance between IHC and FISH HER-2/*neu* test results was as high as 88%.[66] There is strong correlation between IHC and FISH in negative (immunoreactivity of 0 to +1) overexpressed and strongly overexpressed (immunoreactivity of +3) tumor cases. Immunoreactivity of +2 is weak overexpression of HER-2/*neu* and in this situation, it is not correlated well with FISH amplification. Ridolfi and coworkers reported that only 36% of tumors with +2 immunoreactivity were amplified by FISH.[67] For this reason +2 immunoreactivity is considered indeterminate, and the FISH method is often performed as a follow-up test. There are rare cases where HER-2/*neu* IHC test is overexpressed with +3 and FISH test is not amplified. Chromosome 17 polysomy is a major factor in strong Her-2 protein overexpression in 3+ nonamplified cases.[68] There are also rare cases where HER-2/*neu* is not overexpressed with 0 to +1 score in IHC assay and FISH is amplified. The etiology of such cases is not well understood or well described in current literature. More studies are necessary, especially studies that address Herceptin treatment and overall survival benefit.

REPORT FOR BREAST CANCER SPECIMENS

The CAP distributed guidelines for reporting cancer specimens in 1998. Accu-rate pathology reporting is important for treatment of breast cancer. Table 32-1 lists breast biomarkers and Table 32-2 lists pathology reporting guidelines for breast cancer.

TABLE 32-1. Report Breast Biomarkers

Result: Estrogen and Progesterone Receptors		
	Estrogen Receptors	**Progesterone Receptors**
Antibody	Clone 6F11	Clone 636
%Tumor Staining		
Intensity (1+ to 3+)		

Result: HER-2/*neu* (using FDA-approved Dako HercepTest):

Test Score		
0	Absent membrane staining	No overexpression
1+	Weak, or partial membrane staining	No overexpression or low expression
2+	Weak-to-moderate membrane staining of entire membrane	Indeterminate
3+	Strong, uniform membrane staining in >30% of tumor	Overexpression

Score 0: No staining is observed in invasive tumor cells. (No overexpression)

Score 1: Weak, incomplete membrane staining in any proportion of invasive tumor cells, or weak, complete membrane staining in less than 10% of cells. (No overexpression)

Score 2: Complete membrane staining that is non-uniform or weak but with obvious circumferential distribution in at least 10% of cells, or intense complete membrane staining in 30% or less of tumor cells (Indeterminate)

Score 3: Uniform intense membrane staining of more than 30% of invasive tumor cells. (Overexpression)

HER-2/*neu*: Overexpression, Indeterminate, No overexpression

HER-2 gene amplification by FISH: amplified/not amplified

Ki-67: in __ %

TABLE 32-2. Checklist for Reporting Breast Cancer Specimen:

1. Type of tumor:	
Infiltrating ductal carcinoma, not otherwise specified	
Infiltrating lobular carcinoma	
Infiltrating mammary carcinoma, specialized type	
Modified Scarff-Bloom-Richardson grading system :	
Tubule formation:	
>75% of the tumor	1
10-75%	2
<10 %	3
Nuclear pleomorphism:	
Small regular, uniform cells	1
Moderate increase in size and shape variability	2
Marked variation in size and shape	3
Mitotic counts of tumor: field diameter 0.59 mm/0.274 mm^2	
0-9/10 high power field (HPF)	1
10-20	2
>20	3
Mitotic counts of tumor: field diameter 0.44 mm/0.152 mm^2	
0-5/10HPF	1
6-10	2
>11	3
Grade 1: well differentiated ductal carcinoma	3-5
Grade 2 : moderately differentiated ductal carcinoma	6-7
Grade 3: poorly differentiated ductal carcinoma	>8-9
2. Preinvasive tumor:	
Ductal carcinoma in situ (DCIS)	
Types (i.e., comedo, solid, cribriform, micropapillary, clinging, apocrine, mucinous, endocrine etc)	
Nuclear grade, 1 of 3, 2 of 3, 3 of 3.	
With or without central necrosis.	
Cancerization of lobules (DCIS in lobules)	Present/absent
Atypical ductal hyperplasia	Present/absent
Lobular carcinoma in situ (LCIS)	Present/absent
Atypical lobular hyperplasia (ALH)	Present/absent.
3. Size of the invasive tumor, cm:	
4. Surgical margins:	
Positive for tumor (report both invasive and in situ components)	
Close margins: specify within 1 cm	
Negative for tumor: specify clear greater than 1 cm	
5. Extensive intraductal components (>20%)	Present/absent.
6. Microcalcifications	Absent/ present associated with invasive tumor/DCIS/ benign breast tissue.
7. Lymphovascular invasion	Absent/present
8. Benign breast tissue: status post biopsy site	Present/absent
9. Lymph nodes	
Report number of lymph nodes examined	
Report how many lymph nodes are positive/ negative for metastatic carcinoma and what levels (level I, level II or level III).	
If lymph node is positive, report:	
Maximum dimension of metastatic carcinoma size (macrometastasis, micrometastasis, isolated tumor cells)	
Extracapsular invasion	Absent/present
10. Skin: dermal lymphatic invasion	Present/absent.
11. Skeletal muscle	Not applicable/ tumor invasion is present/ absent.
12. Nipple	
Dermal lymphatic invasion	Present/absent
Paget disease	Present/absent.
13. Tumor stage:	TNM (AJCC 2003)[69]

Tissue Processing and Permanent Sections

Tissues from the breast are processed in the histology laboratory to produce microscopic slides that are viewed under the microscope by pathologists.The individuals who do the tissue processing and make the glass microscopic slides are histotechnologists. The purpose of fixation is to preserve tissues permanently. Fixation should be carried out as soon as possible after removal of the tissues.A variety of fixatives are available for use, depending on the type of tissue present and features to be demonstrated. The most frequently used and recommended fixative for breast tissue is 10% buffered formalin in neutral pH. The technique for getting fixed tissue into paraffin is called tissue processing. The main steps in this process are dehydration and clearing. The above processes are almost always automated for the large volumes of routine tissues processed. Automation consists of an instrument that moves the tissues around through the various agents on a preset time scale. Due to the fatty content of breast tissue, the entire time takes longer, usually 8 to 12 hours. Tissues that come off the tissue processor are still in the cassettes and must be manually put into the blocks by a histotechnician who must pick the tissues out of the cassette and pour molten paraffin over them. This embedding process is very important, because the tissues must be aligned, or oriented properly in the block of paraffin. Once the tissues have been embedded, they must be cut into sections that can be placed on a slide. This is done with a microtome; a knife with a mechanism for advancing a paraffin block across standard distances. Tissues can be sectioned at anywhere from 3 to 10 microns, usually 4 to 6 microns. Once the ribbons or tissue slides are made from the microtome sections, the tissue sections are dipped into a water bath. The water bath releases wrinkles and allows the tissue to be uniformly spread out. The histotechnician then picks up one of the sections by using a glass slide. The glass slides with tissue on top are then stained with H&E. Hematoxylin, a basic dye, has an affinity for the nucleic acids of the cell nucleus. Eosin, an acidic dye, has an affinity for the cytoplasmic components of the cell. The stained section on the slide must be covered with a thin piece of plastic or glass to protect the tissue from being scratched, to provide better optical quality for viewing under the microscope, and to preserve the tissue section for years to come. This process is called *coverslipping*. In order to adhere the coverslip, a small amount of glue is applied between the glass slide and coverslip (Figs. 32-31 through 32-35).

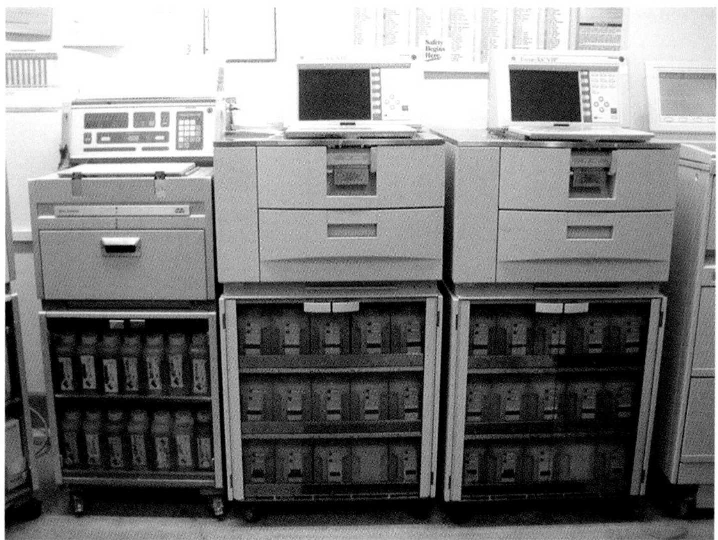

■ FIGURE 32-31 Processing machine in pathology. All cassettes are placed inside the machine and many different solutions fix and process the tissue within the cassettes overnight ×400.

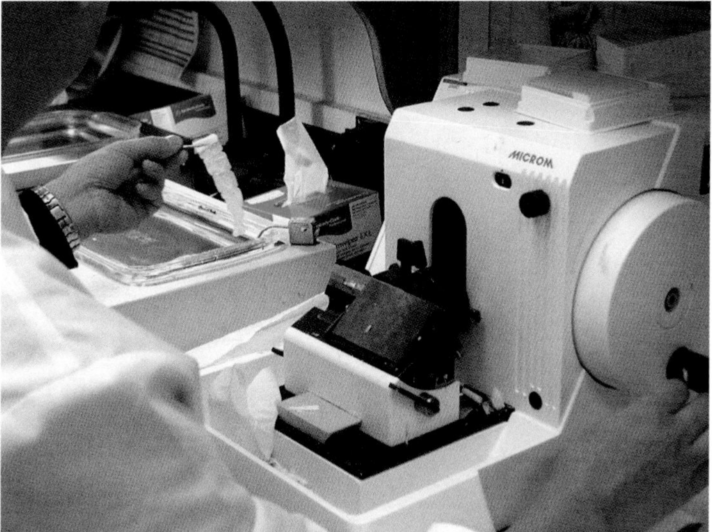

■ FIGURE 32-32 Paraffin block is made from each cassette and tissue is cut 4 to 5 microns thick by a histology technician ×400.

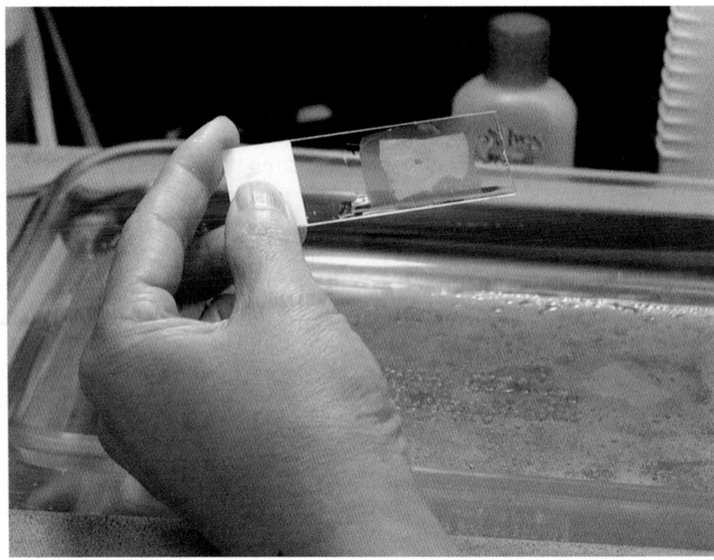

■ **FIGURE 32-33** After paraffin section is cut, it is placed in a water bath and picked up by glass slide ×100.

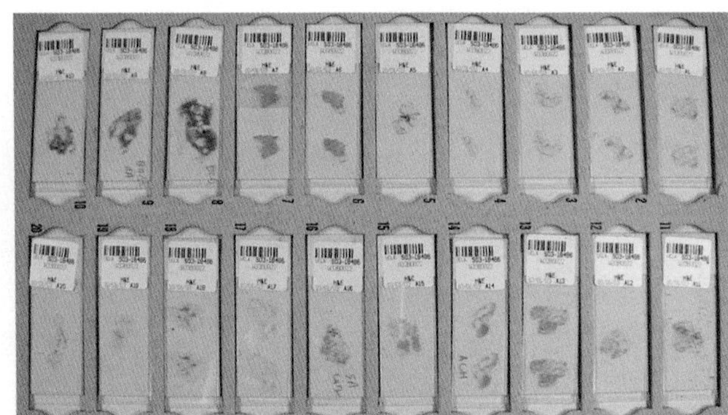

■ **FIGURE 32-34** Each glass slide is stained with hematoxylin and eosin for color contrast. Each slide is then labeled with a unique surgical number in sequential manner.

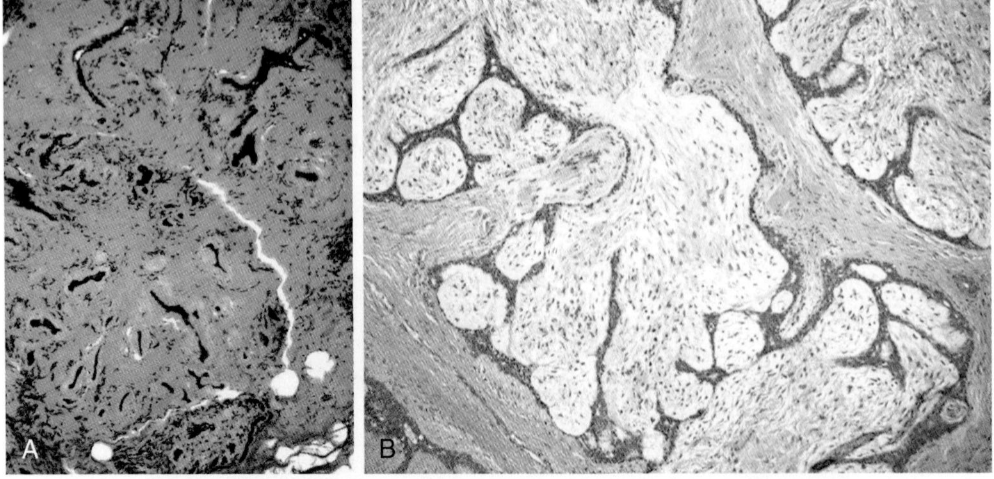

■ **FIGURE 32-35** Hematoxylin and eosin stain ×100. Unfixed tissue (**A**) versus well-fixed tissue histology section (**B**). Both are fibroadenoma.

SUMMARY

In this chapter, the proper handling of different breast specimens, reporting pathologic findings and specimen tissue processing are described to achieve a high accuracy in diagnosis and to optimize clinical management of breast cancer patients.

KEY POINTS

- It is essential that triple test correlation is used on every patient when dealing with breast lesions. *Triple test* is defined as clinical impression, radiological findings, and pathology findings with either FNA or CNB results.
- There are various methods to determine tumor size including palpation on physical examination, breast-imaging studies including mammography, ultrasound, and more recently MRI. Pathology, however, is considered to be the gold standard method for measurement of tumor size.

SUGGESTED READINGS

Jacobs TW, Connolly JL, Schnitt SJ. Nonmalignant lesions in breast core needle biopsies: to excise or not to excise? *Am J Surg Pathol* 2002;**26**:1095-110.

Singletary SE, Greene FL, Sobin LH. Classification of isolated tumor cells: clarification of the 6th edition of the American Joint Committee on Cancer Staging Manual. *Cancer* 2003;**98**:2740-1.

Reynolds HE. Core needle biopsy of challenging benign breast conditions: a comprehensive literature review. *Am J Roentgenol* 2000;**174**:1245-50.

REFERENCES

1. Ellis EB, Martin HE. Aspiration biopsy. *Surg Gynecol Obstet* 1934;**59**:578-89.
2. Cobb CJ, Raza AS. Alas poor FNA of breast-we know thee well. *Diagn Cytopathol* 2005;**32**:1-4.
3. O'Neil S, Castelli M, Gattuso P, Kluskens L, Madsen K, Aranha G. Fine-needle aspiration of 697 palpable breast lesions with histopathologic correlation. *Surgery* 1997;**122**(4):824-8.
4. Wells CA, Castelli M, Gattuso P, Kluskens L, Madsen K, Aranha G. Fine needle aspiration cytology in the UK breast screening program. *Breast* 1999;**8**:261-6.
5. Ariga R, Bloom K, Reddy VB, Kluskens L, Francescatti D, Dowlat K, et al. Fine-needle aspiration of clinically suspicious palpable breast masses with histopathologic correlation. *Am J Surg* 2002;**184**:410-3.
6. Chaiwun B, Settakorn J, Ya-In C, Wisedmongkol W, Rangdaeng S, Thorner P. Effectiveness of fine-needle aspiration cytology of breast: analysis of 2,375 cases from northern Thailand. *Diagn Cytol* 2002;**26**:201-5.
7. Ljung BM, Drejet A, Chiampi N, Jeffrey J, Goodson WH 3rd, Chew K, et al. Diagnostic accuracy of fine-needle aspiration biopsy is determined by physician training in sampling technique. *Cancer* 2001;**93**:263-8.
8. Dronkers DJ. Stereotactic core biopsy of breast lesion. *Radiology* 1992;**183**:631-4.
9. Liberman L, Dershaw DD, Rosen PP, Abramson AF, Deutch BM, Hann LE. Stereotactic 14-gauge breast biopsy: how many core biopsy specimens are needed? *Radiology* 1994;**192**:793-5.
10. Chaiwun B, Thorner P. Fine needle aspiration for evaluation of breast masses. *Curr Opin Obstet Gynecol* 2007;**19**:48-55.
11. Pisano ED, Fajardo LL, Caudry DJ, Sneige N, Frable WJ, Berg WA, et al. Fine-needle aspiration biopsy on nonpalpable breast lesions in a multicenter clinical trial: results form the Radiology Diagnostic Oncology Group V. *Radiology* 2001;**219**:785-92.
12. Dillon M, Hill ADK, Quinn CM, O'Doherty, McDermott EW, et al. The accuracy of ultrasound, stereotactic, and clinical core biopsies in the diagnosis of breast cancer, with an analysis of false negative cases. *Ann Surg* 2005;**242**:701-7.
13. Ballo MS, Sneige N. Can core needle biopsy replace fine needle aspiration cytology in the diagnosis of palpable breast carcinoma? *Cancer* 1996;**78**:773-7.
14. Antley CM, Eoghan E, Mooney MB, Layfield LJ. A comparison of accuracy rates between open biopsy, cutting needle biopsy and fine needle aspiration biopsy of the breast: a 3 year experience. *The Breast Journal* 1998;**4**(1):3-7.
15. Brenner JR, Fajardo L, Fisher PR, Dershaw DD, Evans PW, Bassett L, et al. Percutaneous core biopsy of the breast: effect of operator experience and number of samples on diagnostic accuracy. *AJR Am J Roentgenol* 1996;**166**:341-6.
16. Silverstein MJ, Lagios MD, Recht A, Allred DC, Harmes SE, Holland R, et al. Image detected breast cancer: state of the art diagnosis and treatment. Special report: International Consensus Conference II. *J Am Coll Surg* 2005;**201**:586-97.
17. Russin LD, Jackson VP, Gin FM, Madden CM, Hawes DR. Large-gauge core needle biopsy of the breast. *Breast J* 1996;**2**:370-3.
18. The Uniform approach to breast fine needle aspiration biopsy: a synopsis. Developed and approved at the National Cancer Institute Sponsored Conference, Bethesda, Md, September 9-10, 1996. *Breast J* 1996;**2**:357-63.
19. Lee CH, Philpotts LE, Horvath LJ, Tocino I. Follow-up of breast lesions diagnosed as benign with stereotactic core needle biopsy: frequency of mammographic change and false-negative rate. *Radiology* 1999;**212**:189-94.
20. Liberman L, Drotman M, Morris EA, LaTrenta LR, Abramson AF, Zakowski MF, et al. Imaging-histologic discordance at percutaneous breast biopsy. *Cancer* 2000;**98**:2538-46.
21. Stolier AJ. Stereotactic breast biopsy: A surgical series. *J Am Coll Surg* 1997;**185**:224-8.
22. Reynolds HE. Core needle biopsy of challenging benign breast conditions: a comprehensive literature review. *Am J Roentgenol* 2000;**174**:1245-50.
23. Jacobs TW, Connolly JL, Schnitt SJ. Nonmalignant lesions in breast core needle biopsies: to excise or not to excise? *Am J Surg Pathol* 2002;**26**:1095-110.
24. Kalof AN, Tam D, Beatty B, Cooper K. Immunostaining patterns of myoepithelial cells in breast lesions: a comparison of CD10 and smooth muscle myosin heavy chain. *J Clin Pathol* 2004;**57**:625-9.
25. Barbareschi M, Pecciarini L, Cangi MG, Macrì E, Rizzo A, Viale G, et al. p63, a p53 homologue, is a selective nuclear marker of myoepithelial cells of the human breast. *Am J Surg Pathol* 2001;**25**:1054-60.
26. Goodman KA, Birdwell RL, Ikeda DM. Compliance with recommended follow-up after percutaneous breast core biopsy. *AJR Am J Roentgenol* 1998;**170**:89-92.
27. Connolly JL, Schnitt SJ. Evaluation of breast biopsy specimens in patients considered for treatment by conservative surgery and radiation therapy for early breast cancer. *Pathol Annals* 1988;**23**(Pt 1):1-23.

28. Phelan S, O'Doherty A, Hill A, Quinn CM. Epithelial displacement during breast needle core biopsy causes diagnostic difficulties in subsequent surgical excision specimens. *J Clin Pathol* 2007;**60**:373–6.
29. Youngston BJ, Cranor M, Rosen PP. Epithelial displacement in surgical breast specimens following needling procedures. *Am J Surg Pathol* 1994;**18**:896–903.
30. Lagios MD. Pathologic practice standards for breast carcinoma: tumor size, reliable data, or miscues? *J Am Coll Surg* 2003;**196**:91–2.
31. Greene FL, Page DL, Fleming ID, Firtz AG, Balch CM, Haller DG, et al., editors. *American Joint Committee on Cancer (AJCC) Cancer Staging Manual*. 6th ed New York: Springer; 2002. p. 221–40.
32. Sobin LH, Wittekind CH. *TNM Classification of Malignant Tumors*. 6th ed. New York: Wiley; 2002.
33. Fitzgibbons PL, Page DL, Weaver D, Thor AD, Allred DC, Clark GM, et al. Prognostic factors in breast cancer: College of American Pathologists consensus statement 1999. *Arch Pathol Lab Med* 2000;**124**:966–78.
34. Campton CC, Hensen DE, Hammond EH, Schramm JB. *Reporting on cancer specimens: protocols and case summaries*. Northfield, Il: College of American Pathologists; 1998.
35. Fitzgibbons PL, Connolly JL, Page DL. Updated protocol for the examination of specimens from patients with carcinoma of the breast. A basis of checklists. *Arch Pathol Lab Med* 2000;**124**:1026–33.
36. Lagios MFD. Problems in the assessment of tumor size: an elusive grail in current practice. *Semin Breast Dis* 2005;**8**:24–30.
37. Shin SJ, Osborne MP, Moore A, Hayes MK, Hoda SA. Determination of size of invasive breast carcinoma. *Am J Clin Pathol* 2000;**113**(Suppl. 1):S19–29.
38. Moatamed NA, Apple SK. Extensive sampling changes t-staging of infiltrating lobular carcinoma of breast: a comparative study of gross versus microscopic tumor sizes. *Breast J* 2006;**6**:511–7.
39. Wolff AC, Hammond ME, Schwartz JN, Hagerty KL, Allred DC, Cote RJ, et al. American Society of Clinical Oncology/College of American Pathologists guideline recommendations for human epidermal growth factor receptor 2 testing in breast cancer. *J Clin Oncol* 2007;**25**:118–45.
40. Abraham SC, Fox K, Fraker D, Solin L, Reynolds C. Sampling of grossly benign breast reexcisions: a multidisciplinary approach to assessing adequacy. *Am J Surg Pathol* 1999;**23**:316–22.
41. Wiley E, Keh P. Diagnostic discrepancies in breast specimens subjected to gross examination. *Am J Surg Pathol* 1999;**23**:876–81.
42. Moffat FL. Sentinel node biopsy is not an alternative to axillary dissection in breast cancer. *J Surg Oncol* 2001;**77**:153–6.
43. Kim T, Giuliano AE, Lyman GH. Lymphatic mapping and sentinel lymph node biopsy in early-stage breast carcinoma. A metaanalysis. *Cancer* 2006;**106**:4–16.
44. Chu KU, Turner RR, Hansen NM, Brennan MB, Bilchik A, Giuliano AE. Do all patients with sentinel lymph node metastasis from breast carcinoma need complete axillary node dissection? *Ann Surg* 1999;**229**:536–41.
45. Rahusen FD, Torrenga H, van Diest PJ, Pijpers R, van der Wall E, Licht J, et al. Predictive factors for metastatic involvement of nonsentinel nodes in patients with breast cancer. *Arch Surg* 2001;**136**:1059–63.
46. Reynolds C, Mick R, Donohue JH, Grant CS, Farley DR, Callans LS, et al. Sentinel lymph node biopsy with metastasis: can axillary dissection be avoided in some patients with breast cancer? *J Clin Oncol* 1999;**17**:1720–6.
47. Veronesi U, Paganelli G, Viale G, Luini A, Zurrida S, Galimberti V, et al. A randomized comparison of sentinel-node biopsy with routine axillary dissection in breast cancer. *N Engl J Med* 2003;**349**:546–53.
48. Katz A, Niemierko A, Gage I, Evans S, Shaffer M, Fleury T, et al. Can axillary dissection be avoided in patients with sentinel lymph node metastasis? *J Surg Oncol* 2006;**93**:550–8.
49. Cserni G, Gregori D, Merletti F, Sapino A, Mano MP, Ponti A, et al. Meta-analysis of non-sentinel node metastases associated with micrometastatic sentinel nodes in breast cancer. *Br J Surg* 2004;**91**:1245–52.
50. Turner RR, Chu KU, Qi K, Botnick LE, Hansen NM, Glass EC, et al. Pathologic features associated with non-sentinel lymph node metastases in patients with metastatic breast carcinoma in a sentinel lymph node. *Cancer* 2000;**89**:574–81.
51. Schrenk P, Konstantiniuk P, Wölfl S, Bogner S, Haid A, Nemes C, et al. Prediction of non-sentinel lymph node status in breast cancer with a micrometastatic sentinel node. *Br J Surg* 2005;**92**:707–13.
52. Dabbs DJ, Fung M, Landsittel D, McManus K, Johnson R. Sentinel lymph node micrometastasis as a predictor of axillary tumor burden. *Breast J* 2004;**10**:101–5.
53. Association of Directors of Anatomical and Surgical Pathology. Immediate management of mammographically detected breast lesions. *Am J Pathol* 1993;**17**:850–1.
54. Zarbo RJ, Hoffman GG, Howanitz PJ. Interinstitutional comparison of frozen section consultation. A College of American pathologists Q-probe Survey of 79,647 consultations in 297 North American Institutions. *Arch Pathol Lab Med* 1991;**115**:1187–94.
55. Stanford JL, Szklo M, Brinton LA. Estrogen receptor and breast cancer. *Epidemiol Rev* 1986;**8**:42–56.
56. Elledge RM, Allred DC. Clinical aspects of estrogen and progesterone receptors. In: Harris JR, Lippman ME, Morrow M, Osborne CK, editors. Diseases of the breast. Philadelphia: Lippincott Williams & Wilkins; 2004. p. 603–17.
57. Allred DC, Harvey JM, Berardo M, Clark GM. Prognostic and predictive factors in breast cancer by immunohistochemical analysis. *Mod Pathol* 1998;**11**:155–68.
58. McGuire WL, Clark GM. The role of progesterone receptors in breast cancer. *Semin Oncol* 1985;**12**(Suppl.):12–6.
59. Mann S, Laucirica R, Carlson N, Younes PS, Ali N, Younes A, et al. Estrogen receptor beta expression in invasive breast cancer. *Hum Pathol* 2001;**32**:113–8.
60. Battifora H, Mehta P, Ahn C, et al. Estrogen receptor immunohistochemical assay in paraffin-embedded tissue. A better gold standard? *Appl Immunohistochem* 1993;**1**:39–45.
61. De Mascarel I, Soubeyran I, MacGrogan G, et al. Immunohistochemical analysis of estrogen receptors in 938 breast carcinomas. Concordance with biochemical assay and prognostic significance. *Appl Immunohistochem* 1995;**3**:222–31.
62. Harvey JM, Clark GM, Osborne CK, Allred DC. Estrogen receptor status by immunohistochemistry is superior to the ligand-binding assay for predicting response to adjuvant endocrine therapy in breast cancer. *J Clin Oncol* 1999;**17**:1474–81.
63. Elledge RM, Green S, Pugh R, Allred DC, Clark GM, Hill J, et al. Estrogen receptor (ER) and progesterone receptor (PgR), by ligand-binding assay compared with ER, PgR and pS2, by immuno-histochemistry in predicting response to tamoxifen in metastatic breast cancer: a Southwest Oncology Group Study. *Int J Cancer* 2000;**89**:111–7.
64. Love RR, Duc NB, Allred DC, Binh NC, Dinh NV, Kha NN, et al. Oophorectomy and tamoxifen adjuvant therapy in premenopausal Vietnamese and Chinese women with operable breast cancer. *J Clin Oncol* 2002;**20**:2559–66.
65. Slamon D, Leyland-Jones B, Shak, et al. Addition of Herceptin (humanized anti-Her-2 overexpressing metastatic breast cancer (Her-2+?MBC) markedly increases anticancer activity: A randomized multinational controlled phase III trial. abstract *Proc ASCO* 1998;**17**:98a.
66. Kakar S, Puangsuvan N, Stevens JM, Serenas R, Mangan G, Sahai S, et al. HER-2/neu assessment in breast cancer by immunohistochemistry and fluorescence in situ hybridization: comparison of results and correlation with survival. *Mol Diagn* 2000;**5**:191–2.
67. Ridolfi R, Jamehdor MR, Arber JM. Her-2/neu testing in breast carcinoma: a combined immunohistochemical and fluorescence in situ hybridization approach. *Mod Pathol* 2000;**12**:866–73.
68. Varshney D, Zhou YY, Stephen Geller SA, Alsabeh R. Determination of HER-2 status and chromosome 17 polysomy in breast carcinomas comparing HercepTest and PathVysion FISH Assay. *Am J Clin Pathol* 2004;**121**:70–7.
69. Singletary SE, Greene FL, Sobin LH. Classification of isolated tumor cells: clarification of the 6th edition of the American Joint Committee on Cancer Staging Manual. *Cancer* 2003;**98**:2740–1.

CHAPTER 33

Post-Biopsy Management

Anne C. Hoyt and Lawrence W. Basset

Over the past decade, image-guided breast core needle biopsy (CNB) has become the most common biopsy performed at our facility for nonpalpable and many palpable breast lesions. It is now a widely used and widely accepted, cost-effective alternative to open surgical biopsy.[1,2] The use of needle biopsy to obtain a histologic diagnosis of breast lesions requires that the physician performing the procedure have a good understanding of postprocedural responsibilities and management. After the biopsy, the physician must evaluate the results for concordance between imaging and pathology findings, carry out appropriate patient follow-up, develop a management plan, and communicate results to the referring health care provider, the patient, or both.

Once the technical component of the examination is completed, important patient management and follow-up issues must be addressed. In our experience, patients rarely have significant physical problems after the procedure, other than temporary discomfort and bruising at the site of the biopsy. However, they do experience considerable anxiety about the biopsy findings, so results should be obtained in a reasonable time and communicated to them. Usually this goal can be accomplished in 2 to 3 days without compromising accuracy. We avoid asking for and communicating "wet" or "stat" readings from the pathologist, because changing a diagnosis from a benign (negative) wet reading to a malignant (positive) final reading can be devastating for the patient.

ASSESSING FOR CONCORDANCE

The process of assessing concordance involves comparison of the imaging findings that led to the biopsy with the pathology results. Success of an image-guided needle biopsy program requires a good working relationship between radiologist and pathologist. To optimize the process, the pathologist must have adequate clinical information.

To assist the pathologist with this process, we have devised a modified imaging/pathology requisition form for needle biopsy cases (Fig. 33-1). The form includes the following information:

- Location of the lesion
- The most relevant imaging findings (e.g., mass versus calcifications)
- The probability of malignancy; we use a modified American College of Radiology Breast Imaging Reporting and Data System (BI-RADS) numbering system, wherein the *suspicious* category is subdivided into 4A (mild suspicion), 4B (moderate suspicion), and 4C (high suspicion).

When a high likelihood of malignancy is communicated in the pathology requisition (e.g., 4C or 5), the pathologist frequently telephones us if he or she does not find a cancer. When calcifications are present in the biopsy specimen, the specimens that contain the calcifications are placed in a separate bag (called a *tea bag*) within the specimen jar. The pathologist re-cuts the specimen if imaging demonstrated calcifications but none were identified in the initial histologic slides.

After the biopsy is performed and interpreted, the next step is to assess the pathology results for concordance with the imaging findings that led to the biopsy and with any relevant clinical findings. The concept of concordance has origins in the fine-needle aspiration biopsy triple test protocol, which compares clinical findings, imaging findings, and pathology results.[3] If the results are *benign triplets* (clinical, imaging, and pathology findings are benign), the patient is followed clinically or with further imaging in 6 months. If the results are *malignant triplets* (all three types of findings indicate malignancy), definitive surgery can be planned. When pathology findings are malignant, definitive surgery would follow pathologic confirmation (permanent or frozen section). *Mixed triplets* or *inconclusive triplets* mandate an open biopsy. These basic principles for

BIOPSY DATA ENTRY FORMS

[Place ID Sticker here or Print below]

1. **UCLA ID Number** ______	**Accession #** ______
2. **Last Name** ______	**Referring MD.** ______ **Pager:** ______ **Contacted: Yes / No**
First Name ______ **Age** ___	**Ph. Number:** ______

4. **Referred for: (Circle appropriate box)** | Screening | Diagnostic | US | O |

5. **Final Interpretation** based on: | Screening | Diagnostic | US | Outside films |

6. **Mammography findings:** | Calcs / Mass / a Rch / Evolving Density / Negative / Other / O |

7. **US** findings: | B/9 mass | Malig Mass | Negative | O |

8. R L

Faculty	9. BI-RADS						
LB	2	3	4A	4B	4C	5	6
ND	2	3	4A	4B	4C	5	6
AH	2	3	4A	4B	4C	5	6
CP	2	3	4A	4B	4C	5	6
CW	2	3	4A	4B	4C	5	6
	2	3	4A	4B	4C	5	6

10. Procedure: | Stereo | US-Guided | Core | Wire Loc | FNAC | Palpable |

11. **Core Biopsy date:**____/____/____ **Radiologist:** ______

Calcifications in x-ray specimens: **Yes / No / O ; In histology specimens: Yes / No**

12. **CNB** path results (abbreviations from other side): ______ **Malig / High Risk / B9**

Reviewed at Rad Path on ____/____/____ | **Concordant** | **Discordant** |

13. **Interpretation Outcome** (Rad Path Conference)

	Malig	Benign
Positive	**TP**	**FP**
Negative	**FN**	**TN**

14. **Final CNB Outcome**

	Malig	Benign
4, 5	**TP**	**FP**
1, 2, 3	**FN**	**TN**

15. **Management recommendation(s):** | Surgery | 6 Mo f/u | Other |

FNAC date ____/____/____ : Benign / Malignant / Atypical / Insufficient

Concordant / Discordant

16. **Surgery** date: ____/____/____ 17. **Where done:** UCLA / Other ______

18. **Surgery/Loc results: (using abbreviations)** ______ Malig / High Risk / Benign

19. **Final Outcome from Surgery or Long Term Follow-up: Cancer / No cancer**

	Malignant	Benign
4, 5	**TP**	**FP**
1, 2, 3	**FN**	**TN**

■ **FIGURE 33-1** Imaging/pathology form for breast core needle biopsy.

correlating clinical, imaging, and pathology findings can be applied to CNB.

The assessment for concordance can be done in a number of ways:

- A case-by-case or regularly scheduled meeting with the pathologist (Fig. 33-2).
- Viewbox review of mammographic images alongside the written pathology reports.
- Comparison of written imaging reports and pathology reports for concordance.

The correlation process involves determining whether pathology results adequately explain imaging findings. The imaging documentation of the procedure is reviewed to verify that the lesion was accurately targeted (e.g., in ultrasonography-guided biopsies, the needle traversed the lesion) and that post-biopsy images confirm that the lesion was sampled. For stereotactically guided biopsies of calcifications, the specimen radiograph is reviewed to verify that the specimens contained adequate numbers of calcifications. *Concordance* means that the imaging findings of concern are adequately explained by the pathology results. *Discordance* indicates that the imaging findings are not consistent with or are not adequately explained by the pathology results.

Once concordance or discordance between imaging and pathology findings has been established, a post-CNB management plan is devised. In our practice, patients with discordant findings and patients in whom accurate targeting or limited sampling is a concern are referred for open surgical biopsy. Patients with positive results, in which cancer is diagnosed, are referred to a surgeon for definitive treatment.

For most patients with benign concordant imaging-biopsy findings, a 6-month follow-up is recommended to identify any false-negative results as soon as possible. The modality used for follow-up imaging (mammography or ultrasonography) should be the modality that better demonstrates the lesion. Some investigators believe that a 1-year follow-up is adequate for definite benign cases, such as a typical fibroadenoma identified at imaging with a CNB diagnosis of fibroadenoma in a 25-year-old woman (Fig. 33-3). We review each case individually and assign annual follow-up for definite benign cases and 6-month follow-up for concordant benign cases. Our 6-month follow-up protocol reflects our experience with two phyllodes tumors that were diagnosed as fibroadenomas on CNB.

A *false-negative CNB result* is defined as a benign CNB finding in a patient in whom cancer is detected at the biopsy site within 2 years after the biopsy (Fig. 33-4). Reports in the literature indicate that the false-negative rate for breast CNB is approximately 2%.[4] However, this rate may be lower when the physician performing the biopsy is experienced.[5]

Understanding the limitations of CNB is important. Several uncommon "benign" and "high-risk" pathology diagnoses have been linked to underestimation of disease, because adjacent carcinoma was missed as a result of sampling error. When there is the possibility of underestimation of disease, open biopsy should be performed. There is universal agreement that after a CNB diagnosis of atypical ductal hyperplasia (ADH), open biopsy should be performed to rule out underestimation of disease. The need for open biopsy is controversial for the following conditions: radial scar, papillary lesions, lobular carcinoma in situ (LCIS), atypical lobular hyperplasia (ALH), and columnar cell lesions. In addition, approximately 10% of cases with CNB diagnosis of ductal carcinoma in situ (DCIS) show evidence of invasive carcinoma at surgical excision, another example of underestimation of disease.

ATYPICAL DUCTAL HYPERPLASIA

ADH is the classic high-risk lesion in terms of possible underestimation of disease. Surgical excision after a CNB diagnosis of ADH can yield in situ or invasive carcinoma in a significant number of cases. For this lesion, underestimation is defined as a diagnosis of ADH on CNB with identification of DCIS or invasive ductal carcinoma in the

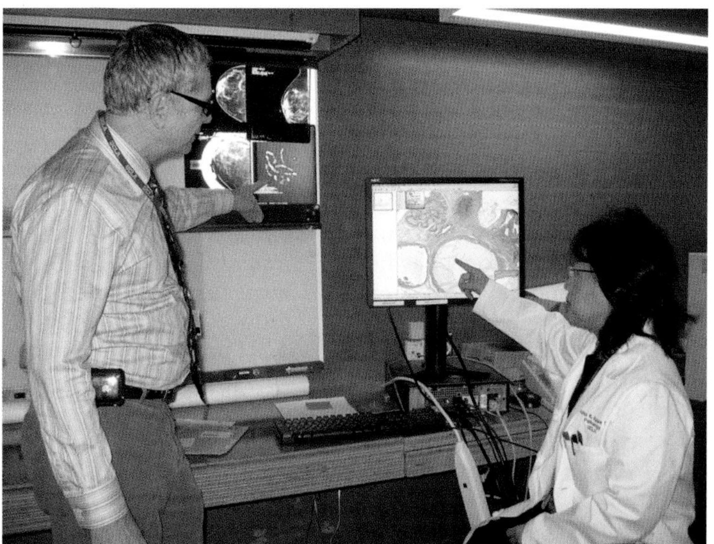

■ **FIGURE 33-2** Radiology/pathology correlation conference. The radiologist presents the history and imaging findings. The pathologist shows the histologic findings. Concordance or discordance is determined, and a management plan is developed.

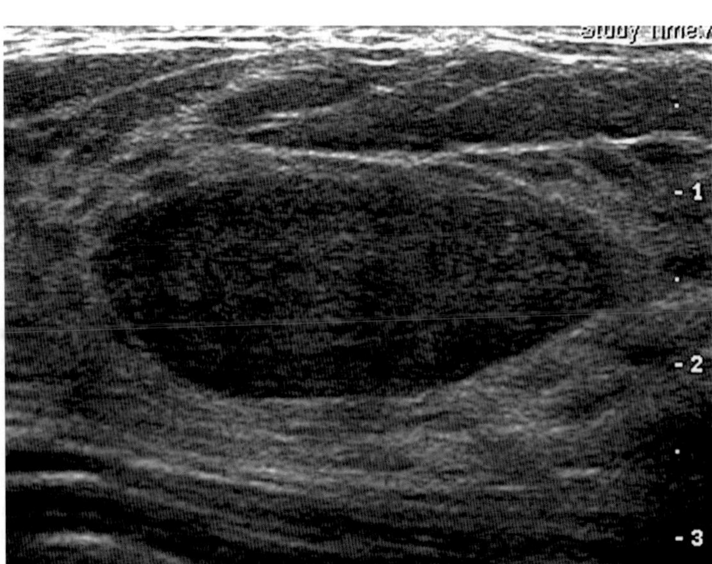

■ **FIGURE 33-3** Definite benign. A 25-year-old woman presented with a palpable breast mass. Ultrasonography shows an oval solid mass oriented parallel to the skin surface (wider than tall), with circumscribed margins and a thin echogenic rim, considered typical of fibroadenoma.

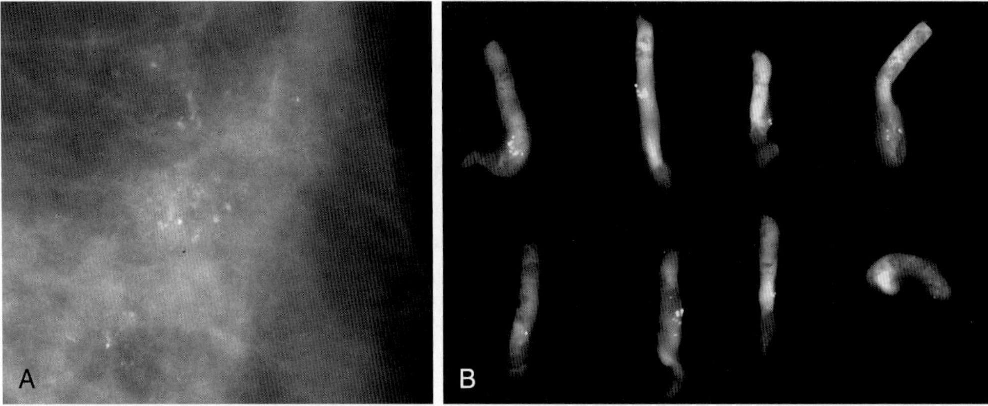

■ **FIGURE 33-4** False-negative result of core needle biopsy (CNB) in a 47-year-old woman. **A,** Magnification mammography shows numerous amorphous and punctate calcifications in a segmental distribution. **B,** Breast core needle biopsy (CNB) specimen radiograph confirms inclusion of numerous targeted calcifications in most of the specimens. Subsequent, routine screening and diagnostic mammography showed a questionable increase in the number of calcifications. Excisional biopsy was recommended and revealed a mucocele-like tumor with 3 cm of low-grade ductal carcinoma in situ (DCIS).

subsequent surgically excised specimen. Underestimation rates for ADH vary with the type of biopsy device used. Underestimation of in situ or invasive carcinoma has been reported in 20% to 25% of CNB diagnoses of ADH, even with the use of an 11-gauge vacuum-assisted device.[6,7] Use of 14-gauge automated (spring-loaded) biopsy devices has underestimation rates of up to 58%.[8-11]

The post-biopsy management of this entity is universally agreed upon. When ADH is identified after CNB, surgical excision is indicated. Even complete removal of the mammographic lesion during CNB does not ensure benign findings at subsequent surgical excision.[12-14] Both histologic and mammographic factors make accurate diagnosis difficult. Some cases of ADH have a similar histologic appearance to that of DCIS, making differentiation difficult. Individual pathologists may disagree on whether borderline cases are ADH or DCIS. Furthermore, the two entities frequently coexist and may manifest as mammographically identical microcalcifications (Fig. 33-5). Increasing the number of CNB specimens obtained can reduce the frequency of ADH diagnoses and the rates of ADH underestimation.[10]

RADIAL SCAR

Management of radial scars is controversial. For the patient in whom mammographic findings suggest radial scar, many investigators suggest that open biopsy rather than CNB should be performed.[15-17] Typically, radial scars manifest as an area of architectural distortion with a lucent center (Fig. 33-6). However, confident imaging diagnosis of radial scar is difficult because the

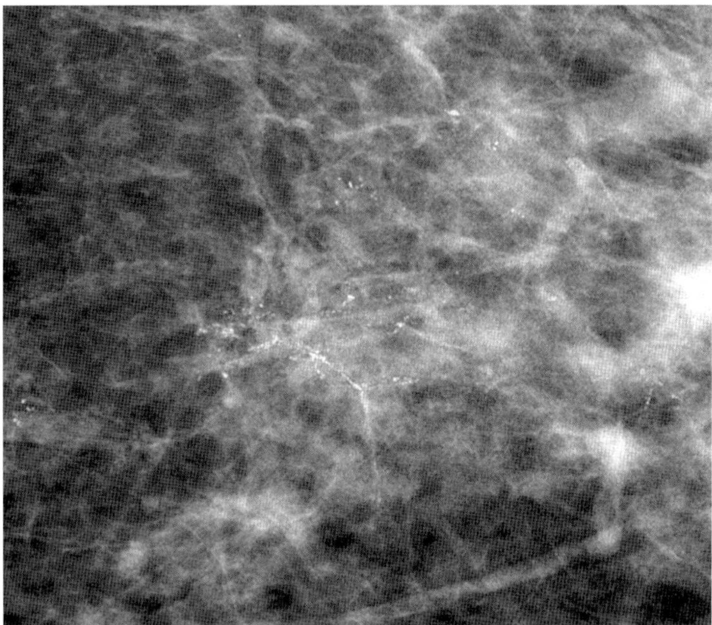

■ **FIGURE 33-5** Atypical ductal hyperplasia (ADH) versus ductal carcinoma in situ (DCIS). In a 61-year-old woman, the mammogram shows fine linear, branching punctate amorphous calcifications in a segmental distribution that are considered suggestive of DCIS. Breast core needle biopsy (CNB) revealed ADH approaching DCIS. Excisional biopsy was recommended based on the presence of ADH and concern for sampling error. The surgical specimen yielded both ADH and DCIS.

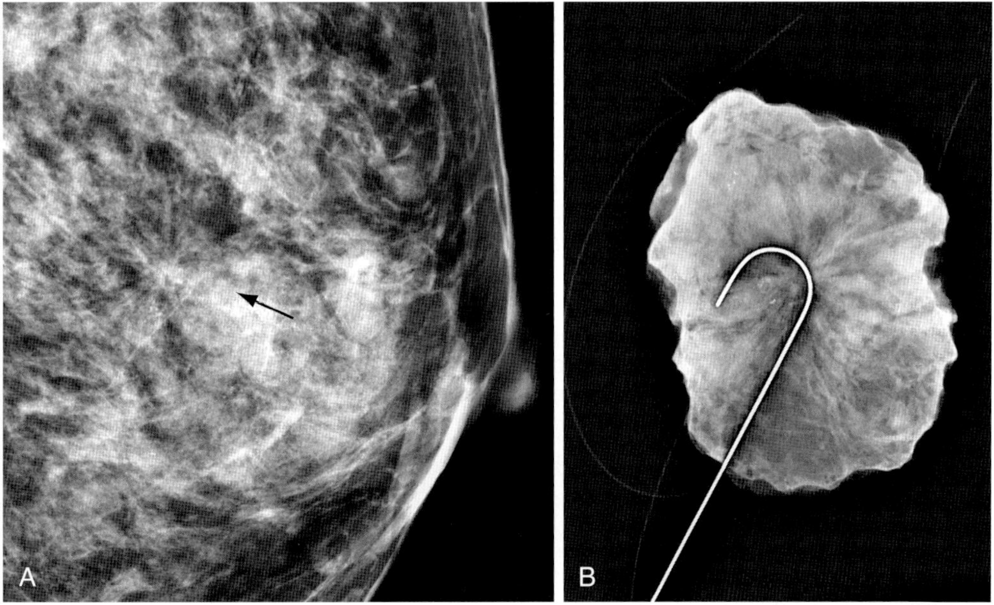

■ **FIGURE 33-6** Radial scar in a postmenopausal woman with an abnormal mammogram. **A,** Mediolateral spot compression mammogram shows an architectural distortion (spicules with no central mass) deep to the nipple (*arrow*). Differential diagnosis was radial scar versus carcinoma. Excisional biopsy was performed. **B,** The surgical specimen radiograph shows the classic architectural distortion and lucent center to better advantage. Histologic diagnosis was radial scar and ductal carcinoma in situ (DCIS).

architectural distortion may look identical to invasive carcinoma. Furthermore, an unexpected histologic diagnosis of radial scar is not uncommon, because lesions can manifest as a mass or calcifications. Other radial scars are small, microscopically visible lesions, incidentally identified in a pathologic specimen.

Experts no longer believe that radial scar itself is a high-risk lesion or precursor of tubular carcinoma, but it may coexist with DCIS or invasive carcinoma.[18] Histologically, radial scars harbor an array of proliferative elements. The ducts within a radial scar are often distorted by a central fibroelastic core but maintain both epithelial and myoepithelial cell layers with a surrounding basement membrane. This two-cell layer and basement membrane differentiates radial scar from tubular carcinoma, which has only a single cell layer and no basement membrane.

Reported rates of carcinoma found at excision of radial scars vary from 0% to 40%; however, the total number of cases is small.[2,9,19] A large multi-institutional study of 157 cases of radial scar diagnosed at CNB found carcinoma in 8% at surgical excision.[20] The risk was 28% if the radial scar was associated with atypia (ADH, ALH, LCIS) but was 4% if no atypia was present. Furthermore, the cancer miss rate was 0 in cases in which 12 or more CNB specimens were obtained. Our current policy is to recommend excisional biopsy for imaging-expected radial scars, for CNB-diagnosed radial scars associated with atypia, and for imaging/pathology discordance.

PAPILLARY LESIONS

Papillomas are a diverse group of lesions ranging from a typically solitary, large central duct papilloma to multiple peripheral papillomas. A papilloma is composed of arborescent fronds of fibrovascular stroma with a stalk that arises from the duct lumen. The fronds are usually covered with a benign two-cell epithelial layer; however, this lining may undergo hyperplasia and evolve into ADH, DCIS, or invasive papillary carcinoma. As with ADH, there is variability among pathologists in differentiating borderline benign from malignant lesions. The appearance of this epithelial lining determines whether the papilloma is benign, high-risk, or malignant or not commonly an admixture of one or more epithelial cell types resulting in lesion heterogeneity. Epithelial heterogeneity within a single papilloma increases the risk of CNB sampling errors.

Mammographically, a papilloma may appear as a circumscribed mass with or without microcalcifications or a cluster of microcalcifications (Fig. 33-7). Clinical features of central large duct papillomas include bloody or clear nipple discharge, whereas peripheral papillomas are more likely to be asymptomatic. It used to be thought that multiple peripheral papillomas raised a woman's risk of breast cancer but central solitary papillomas did not. However, a study by Page and colleagues[21] documented that increased risk from papilloma was related to the presence or absence of ADH in a papilloma rather than the papilloma's location.

A CNB-diagnosed papilloma warrants open biopsy if ADH is found in its epithelium. However, routine performance of open biopsy after a CNB diagnosis of papilloma without atypia remains controversial. Many investigators believe that 11-gauge vacuum-assisted devices adequately sample papillomas and that open biopsy is not necessary unless atypia is identified or there is imaging-pathology discordance.[19,22,23] A large study of 46 papillary lesions subjected to biopsy with either 14-gauge, automated, large core, or 11- or 14-gauge vacuum-assisted devices further support the latter recommendation.[24] However, review of the recent literature reveals variable upgrade rates of CNB-diagnosed, otherwise benign papillomas (i.e., no associated atypia, imaging-pathology discordance or suspicious imaging) that when excised were found to be malignant.[25-32] If the total number of otherwise benign, surgically excised papillomas is extracted from these data sets, the upgrade rates average approximately 6% (range: 0-29%). Based on these high upgrade rates, some authors recommend excision of all otherwise benign papillary lesions diagnosed on CNB.[25,29,31] At our facility, we recommend excision for all CNB-diagnosed papillomas unless the papilloma is small and appears to have been completely excised by the CNB.

LOBULAR NEOPLASIA

Lobular neoplasia (LN) comprises a spectrum of lesions, from LCIS to ALH to ductal involvement with cells of ALH. ALH confers a 3-fold to 5-fold increase in the risk of developing breast cancer while LCIS confers a 7-fold to 10-fold increase. LCIS is divided into four subtypes: classic, signet ring, apocrine, and pleomorphic. Histologically, LCIS is characterized by a lobule distended by small, uniform cells. When the same small uniform cells proliferate but do not distend the lobule, ALH is diagnosed. Cancerization of the lobules occurs when DCIS grows retrograde into the lobules from the involved ducts, and this condition can mimic LCIS. Because cancerization

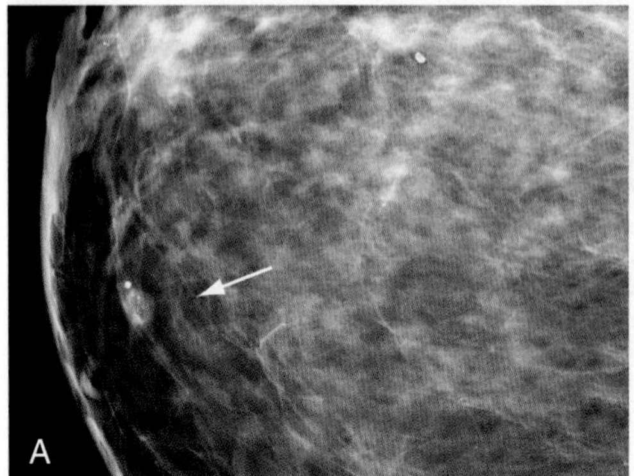

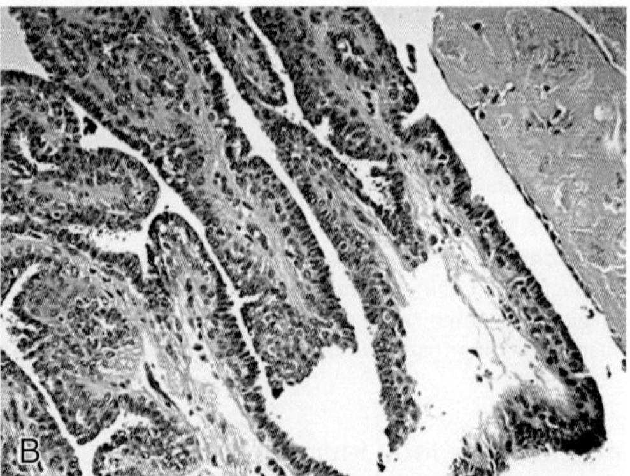

■ **FIGURE 33-7** Papilloma. **A,** In a 59-year-old woman, craniocaudal spot compression mammogram shows a 4 mm periareolar round mass (*arrow*) with partially circumscribed and partially indistinct margins with a few associated microcalcifications. The patient elected surgical excisional biopsy over CNB. Pathologic examination revealed an intraductal papilloma. **B,** Intraductal mass arising from the duct lumen composed of arborescent fronds of fibrovascular stroma covered with a benign two-cell epithelial layer (H&E, ×100).

of the lobules requires lumpectomy and radiation treatment, the pathologist must be able to differentiate these two conditions.

LN does not have any clinical or mammographic features although it is commonly identified on biopsies performed for microcalcifications; identification of lobular neoplasia after biopsy of a mass is less common.

Our understanding of LN is evolving and current concepts reflect these changes. It used to be believed that LN was not a precursor to malignancy but, rather, a marker that identified an increased risk of development of invasive breast cancer in either breast due to its multicentric nature. Page and associates[33] found that the relative risk of development of breast cancer after a benign biopsy showing ALH was 3.1. Furthermore, subsequent breast cancers were approximately three times more likely to develop in the ipsilateral breast than in the contralateral breast of women with such biopsy findings. These investigators therefore suggest that ALH may be a lesion intermediate between a local precursor and a generalized bilateral risk factor for breast cancer. In contrast, subsequent breast cancers in women with a prior biopsy showing LCIS appear to develop nearly equally in either breast.

The necessity for open biopsy after a CNB diagnosis of LN (LCIS, ALH) remains controversial. This is in part because these lesions are relatively uncommon, with an incidence of less than 2% in most CNB studies.[19,34,35] A paper by Liberman and associates suggests some potential guidelines.[35] In this paper, excisional biopsy was recommended only when there was overlap of the histologic features of LCIS and DCIS, when imaging-histologic discordance was identified, or when the LCIS coexisted with a high-risk lesion (radial scar, ADH). The current literature remains divided on the appropriate management of patients with LN diagnosed after CNB.[36-44] In these studies upgrade rates range from 1% to 37%. Investigators with upgrade rates of 8% to 37% suggest excision in all patients whereas those with upgrade rates of less than about 8% do not believe that surgical excision is warranted in all cases. Furthermore, the subtype of LCIS may influence the risk of an associated malignancy, with the pleomorphic subtype carrying a worse prognosis and a higher risk of underestimation of malignancy. Accordingly, different experienced radiologists use different approaches to manage LN when diagnosed at CNB. More investigation is necessary before there is a clear answer to this question.

COLUMNAR CELL LESIONS

Breast biopsy for microcalcifications may reveal a columnar cell lesion (CCL). The microcalcifications associated with CCLs tend to be very faint clusters, with morphologies ranging from punctate to round to amorphous to pleomorphic.[45] State-of-the-art digital imaging and its associated high image contrast have increased the detection of these faint clusters of calcium. This may explain the recent increase in CNB diagnoses of this entity.

Columnar cell lesions include a wide variety of pathologic lesions distinguished by columnar epithelial cells lining dilated acini within the terminal duct lobular unit (TDLU).[46-48] Benign and atypical columnar changes of the TDLU acini were previously described by a wide variety of terms such as *blunt duct adenosis, columnar alteration of the lobules, metaplasie cylindrique*, and *columnar alteration with prominent apical snouts and secretions* (CAPSS).[49,50] The varied terminology and pathologic descriptors were standardized by Schnitt and Vincent-Salomon in 2003 by establishing a practical classification system for CCLs.[51] This classification system divides lesions into columnar cell change (CCC), columnar cell hyperplasia (CCH), and flat epithelial atypia (FEA). Like many breast lesions, CCLs may show no atypia, associated atypia, or atypia bordering on DCIS.

CCC is characterized by variably dilated acini lined by one to two layers of columnar epithelial cells with uniform bland, ovoid nuclei, possible apical snouts, and no cytologic atypia. CCC may be associated with luminal secretions with or without microcalcifications. CCH is similar to CCC except that the acini are lined by more than two layers of stratified columnar cells; apical snouts and luminal secretions with microcalcification are usually present. FEA encompasses both CCC and CCH lesions with cuboid to columnar epithelial cells showing cytologic atypia[47] (Fig. 33-8). CCC and CCH are considered benign lesions whereas FEA may be a precursor to low-grade ductal carcinoma with a very low risk of progression to invasive carcinoma.[48,52]

Management of CCLs diagnosed by CNB remains somewhat unclear. However, there is agreement that CCC and CCH lesions are considered benign and do not require surgical excision. Short interval follow-up imaging is performed in some practices. Because FEA may be associated with ADH, DCIS, invasive tubular carcinoma, or lobular neoplasia, surgical excision is currently warranted.[45,53-55] Identification of FEA in a CNB specimen should prompt the pathologist to search for a more significant lesion in deeper sections and in any subsequent surgical specimen.[52,56] However, large studies clearly elucidating the upgrade rate to carcinoma are lacking. The literature contains only a small number of studies addressing this issue, many of which were performed on small study populations or are only in abstract form. Three published studies[57-59] show upgrade rates of 12% to 21%. Larger studies are needed to complete our understanding and validate CNB management of this complex entity.

SCLEROSING ADENOSIS

Sclerosing adenosis is a benign proliferative condition characterized by proliferation of the lobules (adenosis) and fibrous tissue. Occasionally, the associated fibrosis is so severe that the lobules are distorted enough to mimic invasive carcinoma. Mammographically, sclerosing adenosis is characterized by a cluster of microcalcifications that can range from uniform and round to pleomorphic or linear. Less commonly, it may manifest as a mass. Sclerosing adenosis does not carry a significantly increased risk of future malignancy, but it can lead to a false-positive CNB diagnosis of malignancy. A *false-positive CNB diagnosis* occurs when the CNB result is interpreted as malignant but surgical excision reveals a benign condition and re-evaluation of the original CNB pathologic specimen indicates that the diagnosis

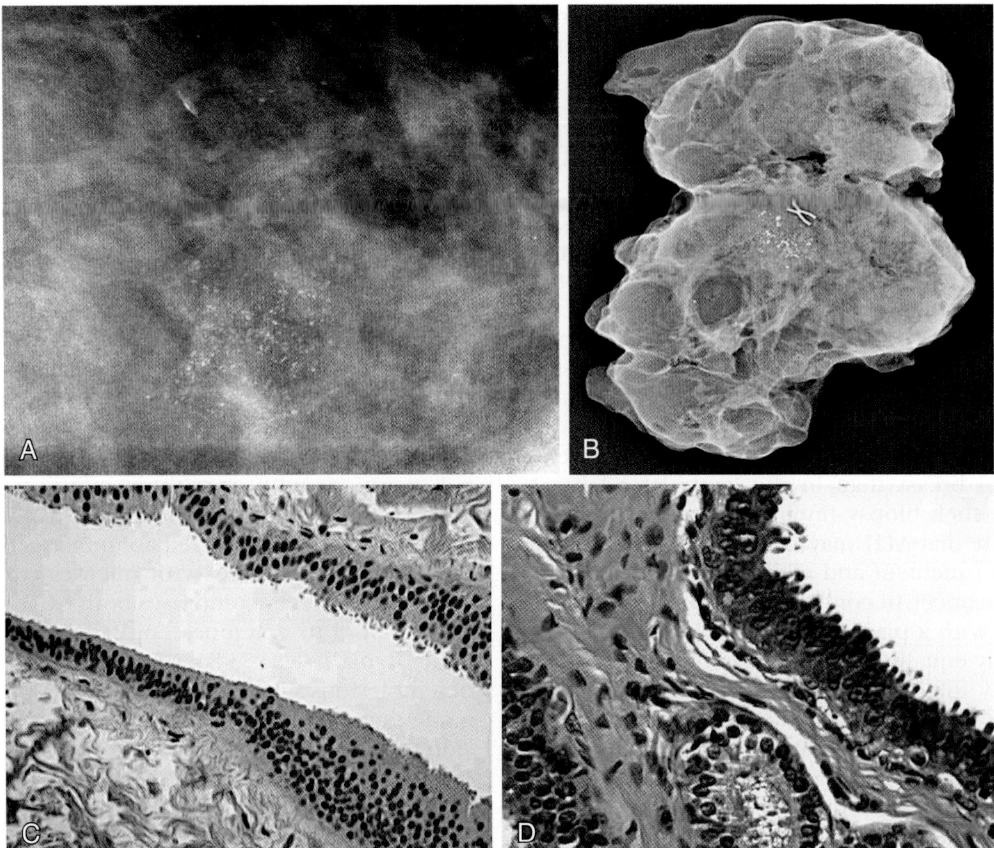

■ **FIGURE 33-8** Columnar cell lesions. **A,** Digital magnification mammography shows clustered amorphous, fine linear and punctuate microcalcifications. Core needle biopsy (CNB) was performed and revealed columnar cell hyperplasia (CCH), which is considered a benign lesion. **B,** A 44-year old woman presented with new clustered microcalcifications. The CNB showed flat epithelial atypia (FEA), and surgical excision was recommended. Surgical pathologic study revealed FEA and a 0.2 mm focus of invasive tubular carcinoma. The surgical specimen radiograph (**B**) illustrates this cluster of microcalcifications with amorphous and punctuate morphologies. **C,** Transition from columnar cell change (CCC; *left side of slide*) where one to two cell layers of columnar epithelial cells line a dilated acinus to CCH (*right side of slide*) where more than two cell layers of stratified columnar epithelium line the acinus, often with apical snouts, luminal secretions, and microcalcifications (not shown). Both are considered benign and have no cytologic atypia (H&E, ×200.) **D,** FEA with multiple stratified layers of cuboidal to columnar epithelial cells with cytologic atypia characterized by loss of polarity of nuclei with round, hyperchromatic, mildly enlarged nuclei with occasional prominent nucleoli (H&E, ×400).

should have been sclerosing adenosis rather than invasive cancer. We have encountered only two false-positive CNB results. In both cases, sclerosing adenosis mimicked an invasive carcinoma. Subsequent review by an expert in breast pathology found that the correct diagnosis was sclerosing adenosis, not carcinoma. If there is doubt, special stains can be used on the pathologic specimen to identify the presence of myoepithelial cells, which are seen in sclerosing adenosis but are not seen in carcinoma (Fig. 33-9).

FALSE-POSITIVE RESULTS

As already mentioned, a false-positive CNB result consists of an original pathologic interpretation of malignancy with subsequent decision that the original diagnosis should have been benign. If a false-positive CNB result is suspected because the surgical excision specimen does not demonstrate carcinoma, the original pathologic specimen should be reviewed. If the review finds a benign lesion, the CNB result was a false-positive finding. If the review confirms a malignancy, then further imaging is performed to verify that the mammographic abnormality was removed at the surgical excision. If the postoperative imaging finding is negative and pathologic review confirmed a malignancy in the CNB specimen, it is likely that the original lesion was removed entirely during the CNB. Complete removal of lesions is more likely to occur with the more efficient sampling devices, such as the 8- and 11-gauge, vacuum-assisted devices.

COMMUNICATION RESPONSIBILITIES

Communicating post-biopsy management recommendations to the referring health care provider is an important responsibility of the physician performing the CNB. In many practices, it is the radiologist who directly conveys the pathology results to the patient. A study from Stanford University found poor patient compliance with recommendations for CNB follow-up management; only 74% of patients acted on recommendations for open surgical biopsy, and only 54% returned for the recommended short-term follow-up imaging studies.[60]

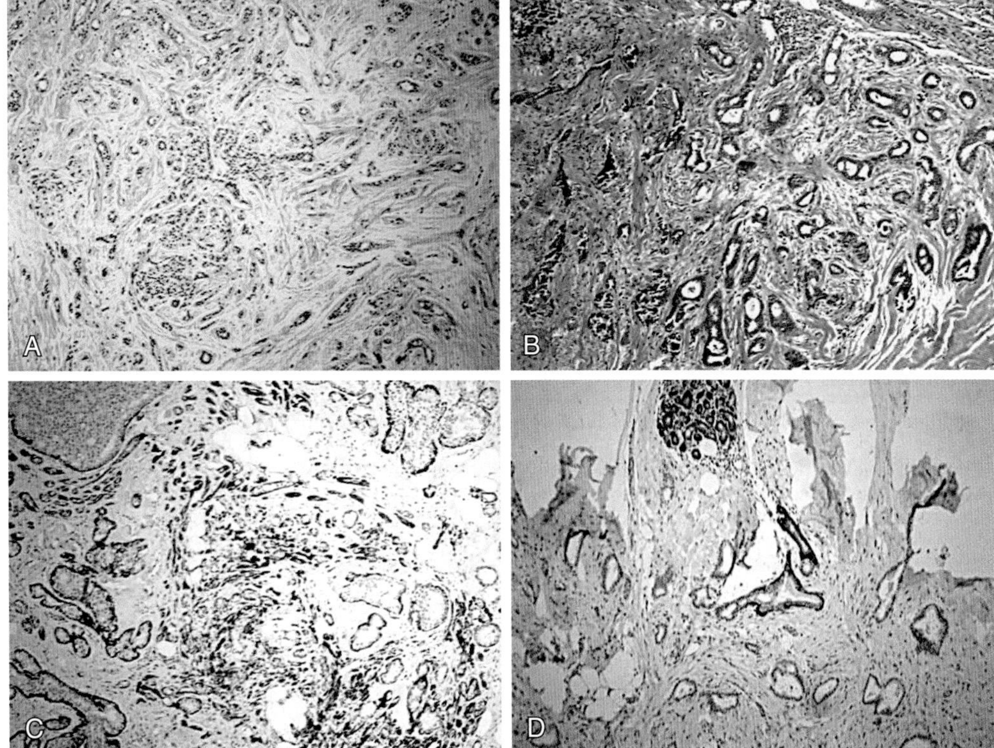

■ **FIGURE 33-9** A, Sclerosing adenosis. Ductal epithelial cells are proliferating in a lobulated pattern with sclerotic stroma. The differential diagnosis is invasive ductal carcinoma (H&E, ×200). **B,** Invasive ductal carcinoma, well differentiated. Atypical ductal epithelial cells are in haphazard pattern and the stroma shows desmoplasia (H&E, ×200). **C,** Anti-smooth muscle myosin heavy chain (SMMHC) for histologic section in **A** shows uptake of the stain by myoepithelial cells, indicating the diagnosis is sclerosing adenosis. **D,** Anti-SMMHC stain for histologic section in **B** shows no uptake of the stain, indicating absence of myoepithelial cells and a diagnosis of invasive tubular carcinoma at the bottom. Top portion shows a normal lobule and middle portion shows a normal duct: SMMHC stain is highlighting the presence of myoepithelial cells.

Once a management plan is devised (6-month follow-up or surgical excision), the results are communicated to the referring clinician and the patient. In our practice, the referring clinician usually conveys the results and recommendations to the patient; however, we assume this role whenever this task is not easily or quickly accomplished by the referring clinician. We convey our recommendations to the health care provider in two ways. First, a telephone call is made to the referring physician with the results and management recommendations. Second, an addendum to the original biopsy report is issued that summarizes the recommendations from the radiology/pathology correlation conference as well as our post-CNB management recommendations.

SUMMARY

Management of the patient undergoing breast CNB does not end with the performance of the biopsy. Follow-up management includes correlating pathology results and imaging findings for concordance, developing a patient management plan, communicating this plan to the referring health care provider and patient, and monitoring compliance with the recommendations.

KEY POINTS

- Understanding pathology is crucial to performing core needle biopsy.
- Assessment of imaging/pathology concordance is essential and can be performed in several ways.
- A false-negative result occurs when the biopsy specimen was benign but cancer was present.
- Undication of post-biopsy management recommendations is essential.erestimation of disease may occur after a diagnosis of a high-risk lesion.
- The management of some high-risk lesions continues to be controversial.
- Commun

SUGGESTED READINGS

Brandt SM, Young GQ, Hoda SA. The "Rosen Triad": tubular carcinoma, lobular carcinoma in situ and columnar cell lesions. *Adv Anat Pathol* 2008;**15**:140-6.

Collins LC, Schnitt SJ. Papillary lesions of the breast: selected diagnostic and management issues. *Histopathology* 2008;**52**:20-9.

Feeley L, Quinn CM. Columnar cell lesions of the breast. *Histopathology* 2008;**52**:11-9.

Pinder SE, Provenzano E, Reis-Filho JS. Lobular in situ neoplasia and columnar cell lesions: diagnosis in breast core biopsies and implications for management. *Pathology* 2007;**39**:208-16.

REFERENCES

1. Bassett L, Winchester DP, Caplan RB, Dershaw DD, Dowlatshahi K, Evans 3rd WP, et al. Stereotactic core-needle biopsy of the breast: a report of the Joint Task Force of the American College of Radiology, American College of Surgeons, and College of American Pathologists. *CA Cancer J Clin* 1997;**47**:171-90.
2. Lee CH, Egglin TK, Philpotts L, Mainiero MB, Tocino I. Cost-effectiveness of stereotactic core needle biopsy: analysis by means of mammographic findings. *Radiology* 1997;**202**:849-54.
3. The uniform approach to breast fine needle aspiration biopsy: a synopsis. developed and approved at the National Cancer Institute-Sponsored Conference, Bethesda, Md, September 10, 1996. *Breast J* 1996;**2**:357-63.
4. Lee CH, Philpotts LE, Horvath LJ, Tocino I. Follow-up of breast lesions diagnosed as benign with stereotactic core-needle biopsy: frequency of mammographic change and false- negative rate. *Radiology* 1999;**212**:189-94.
5. Pfarl G, Helbich TH, Riedl CC, Wagner T, Gnant M, Rudas M, et al. Stereotactic 11-gauge vacuum-assisted breast biopsy: a validation study. *AJR Am J Roentgenol* 2002;**179**:1503-7.
6. Brem RF, Behrndt VS, Sanow L, Gatewood OM. Atypical ductal hyperplasia: histologic underestimation of carcinoma in tissue harvested from impalpable breast lesions using 11-gauge stereotactically guided directional vacuum-assisted biopsy. *AJR Am J Roentgenol* 1999;**172**:1405-7.
7. Philpotts LE, Shaheen NA, Carter D, Lange RC, Lee CH. Comparison of rebiopsy rates after stereotactic core-needle biopsy of the breast with 11-gauge vacuum suction probe versus 14-gauge needle and automatic gun. *AJR Am J Roentgenol* 1999;**172**:683-7.
8. Brenner RJ, Bassett LW, Fajardo LL, Dershaw DD, Evans 3rd WP, Hunt R, et al. Percutaneous core breast biopsy: a multi-institutional prospective trial. *Radiology* 2001;**218**:866-72.
9. Jackman RJ, Nowels KW, Rodriquez-Soto J, Marzoni Jr FA, Finkelstein SI, Shepard MJ. Stereotactic, automated, large-core needle biopsy of nonpalpable breast lesions: false-negative rates and histologic underestimation rates after long-term follow-up. *Radiology* 1999; **210**:799-805.
10. Jackman RJ, Nowels KW, Shepard MJ, Finkelstein SI, Marzoni Jr FA. Stereotaxic large-core needle biopsy of 450 nonpalpable breast lesions with surgical correlation in lesions with cancer or atypical hyperplasia. *Radiology* 1994;**193**:91-5.
11. Liberman L, Cohen MA, Dershaw DD, Abramson AF, Hann LE, Rosen PP. Atypical ductal hyperplasia diagnosed at stereotaxic core biopsy of breast lesions: An indication for surgical biopsy. *AJR Am J Roentgenol* 1995;**164**:1111-3.
12. Jackman RJ, Birdwell RL, Ikeda DM. Atypical ductal hyperplasia: Can some lesions be defined as probably benign after stereotactic 11-gauge vacuum-assisted biopsy, eliminating the recommendation for surgical excision? *Radiology* 2002;**224**:548-54.
13. Liberman L, Dershaw DD, Rosen PP, Morris EA, Abramson AF, Borgen PI. Percutaneous removal of malignant mammographic lesions at vacuum-assisted biopsy. *Radiology* 1998;**206**:711-5.
14. Liberman L, Kaplan JB, Morris EA, Abramson AF, Menell JH, Dershaw DD. To excise or to sample the mammographic target: What is the goal of stereotactic 11-gauge vacuum-assisted breast biopsy? *AJR Am J Roentgenol* 2002;**179**:679-83.
15. Ciatto S, Morrone D, Catarzi S, Del Turco MR, Bianchi S, Ambrogetti D, et al. Radial scars of the breast: Review of 38 consecutive mammographic diagnoses. *Radiology* 1993;**187**:757-60.
16. Frouge C, Tristant H, Guinebretiere JM, Meunier M, Contesso G, Di Paola R, et al. Mammographic lesions suggestive of radial scars: Microscopic findings in 40 cases. *Radiology* 1995;**195**:623-5.
17. Kopans DB. Pathologic, mammographic, and sonographic correlation. In: *Breast Imaging*. 2nd ed. Philadelphia: Lippincott-Raven; 1998. p. 551-615.
18. Anderson JA, Gram JB. Radial scar in the female breast: a long term follow-up of 32 cases. *Cancer* 1984;**15**:2557-60.
19. Philpotts LE, Shaheen NA, Jain KS, et al. Uncommon high-risk lesions of the breast diagnosed at stereotactic core-needle biopsy: clinical importance. *Radiology* 2000;**216**:831-7.
20. Brenner RJ, Jackman RJ, Parker SJ, Evans 3rd WP, Philpotts L, Deutch BM, et al. Percutaneous core needle biopsy of radial scars of the breast: When is excision necessary? *AJR Am J Roentgenol* 2002;**179**:1179-84.
21. Page DL, Salhany KE, Jensen RA, Dupont WD. Subsequent breast carcinoma risk after biopsy with atypia in a breast papilloma. *Cancer* 1996;**78**:258-66.
22. Liberman L, Bracero N, Vuolo MA, Dershaw DD, Morris EA, Abramson AF, et al. Percutaneous large-core biopsy of papillary breast lesions. *AJR Am J Roentgenol* 1999;**172**:331-7.
23. Mercado CL, Hamele-Bena D, Singer C, Koenigsberg T, Pile-Spellman E, Higgins H, et al. Papillary lesions of the breast: evaluation with stereotactic directional vacuum-assisted biopsy. *Radiology* 2001;**221**:650-5.
24. Rosen EL, Bentley RC, Baker JA, Soo MS. Imaging-guided core needle biopsy of papillary lesions of the breast. *AJR Am J Roentgenol* 2002;**179**:1185-92.
25. Skandarajah AR, Field L, Yuen Larn Mou A, Buchanan M, Evans J, Hart S, et al. Benign papilloma on core biopsy requires surgical excision. *Ann Surg Oncol* 2008;**15**:2272-7.
26. Ko ES, Cho N, Cha JH, Park JS, Kim SM, Moon WK. Sonographically guided 14-gauge core needle biopsy of papillary lesions of the breast. *Korean J Radiol* 2007;**8**:206-11.
27. Rizzo M, Lund MJ, Oprea G, Schniederjan M, Wood WC, Mosunjac M. Surgical follow-up and clinical presentation of 142 breast papillary lesions diagnosed by ultrasound-guided core-needle biopsy. *Ann Surg Oncol* 2008;**15**:1040-7.
28. Kil WH, Cho EY, Kim JH, Nam SJ, Yang JH. Is surgical excision necessary in benign papillary lesions initially diagnosed at core biopsy? *Breast* 2008;**17**:258-62.
29. Tseng HS, Chen YL, Chen ST, Wu YC, Kuo SJ, Chen LS, et al. The management of papillary lesion of the breast by core needle biopsy. *Eur J Surg Oncol* 2009;**35**:21-4.
30. Sohn V, Keylock J, Arthurs Z, Wilson A, Herbert G, Perry J, et al. Breast papillomas in the era of percutaneous needle biopsy. *Ann Surg Oncol* 2007;**14**:2979-84.
31. Mercado CL, Hamele-Bena D, Oken SM, Singer CI, Cangiarella J. Papillary lesions of the breast at percutaneous core-needle biopsy. *Radiology* 2006;**238**:801-8.
32. Sydnor MK, Wilson JD, Hijaz TA, Massey HD, Shaw de Paredes ES. Underestimation of the presence of breast carcinoma in papillary lesions initially diagnosed at core-needle biopsy. *Radiology* 2007;**242**:58-62.
33. Page DL, Schuyler PA, Dupont WD, Jensen RA, Plummer Jr WD, Simpson JF. Atypical lobular hyperplasia as a unilateral predictor of breast cancer risk: A retrospective cohort study. *Lancet* 2003; **361**:125-9.
34. Berg WA, Mrose HE, Ioffe OB. Atypical lobular hyperplasia or lobular carcinoma in situ at core-needle breast biopsy. *Radiology* 2001;**218**:503-9.
35. Liberman L, Sama M, Susnik B, Rosen PP, LaTrenta LR, Morris EA, et al. Lobular carcinoma in situ at percutaneous breast biopsy: surgical biopsy findings. *AJR Am J Roentgenol* 1999;**173**:291-9.
36. Mahoney MC, Robinson-Smith TM, Shaughnessy EA. Lobular neoplasia at 11-gauge vacuum-assisted stereotactic biopsy: correlations with surgical excisional and mammographic follow-up. *AJR Am J Roentgenol* 2006;**187**:949-54.
37. Foster MD, Helvie MA, Gregory NE, Rebner M, Nees AV, Paramagul C. Lobular carcinoma in situ or atypical lobular hyperplasia at core-needle biopsy: is excisional biopsy necessary? *Radiology* 2004;**231**:813-9.
38. Cangiarella J, Guth A, Axelrod D, Darvishian F, Singh B, Simsir A, et al. Is surgical excision necessary for the management of atypical lobular hyperplasia and lobular carcinoma in situ diagnosed on core needle biopsy?: a report of 38 cases and a review of the literature. *Arch Pathol Lab Med* 2008;**132**:979-83.
39. Londero V, Zuiani C, Linda A, Vianello E, Furlan A, Bazzocchi M. Lobular neoplasia: core needle breast biopsy underestimation of malignancy in relation to radiologic and pathologic features. *Breast* 2008;**17**:623-30.
40. Brem RF, Lechner MC, Jackman RJ, Rapelyea JA, Evans WP, Philpotts LE, et al. Lobular neoplasia at percutaneous breast biopsy: variables associated with carcinoma at surgical excision. *AJR Am J Roentgenol* 2008;**190**:637-41.
41. Elsheikh TM, Silverman JF. Follow-up surgical excision is indicated when breast core needle biopsies show atypical lobular hyperplasia or lobular carcinoma in situ: a correlative study of 33 patients with review of the literature. *Am J Surg Pathol* 2005;**29**:534-43.

42. Nagi CS, O'Donnell JE, Tismemetsky M. Lobular neoplasia on core needle biopsy does not require excision. *Cancer* 2008;**112**:2152–8.
43. Hwang H, Barke LD, Mendelson EB, Susnik B. Atypical lobular hyperplasia and classic lobular carcinoma in situ in core biopsy specimens: routine excision is not necessary. *Mod Pathol* 2008;**21**:1208–16.
44. Sohn VY, Arthurs ZM, Kim FS, Brown TA. Lobular neoplasia: is surgical excision warranted? *Am Surg* 2008;**74**:172–7.
45. Pandey S, Kornstein MJ, Shank W, de Paredes E. Columnar cell lesions of the breast: mammographic findings with histopathologic correlation. *Radiographics* 2007;**27**:S79–89.
46. Jacobs TW, Connolly JL, Schnitt SJ. Nonmalignant lesions in breast core needle biopsies: to excise or not to excise? *Am J Surg Pathol* 2002;**26**:1095–110.
47. Feeley L, Quinn CM. Columnar cell lesions of the breast. *Histopathology* 2008;**52**:11–9.
48. Lerwill MF. Flat epithelial atypia of the breast. *Arch Pathol Lab Med* 2008;**132**:615–21.
49. Page DL, Anderson TJ. *Diagnostic Histopathology of the Breast*. Edinburgh: Churchill Livingstone; 1987.
50. Trojani M. *Atlas en couleurs d'histopathologie mammaire*. Paris: Maloine; 1988.
51. Schnitt SJ, Vincent-Salomon A. Columnar cell lesions of the breast. *Adv Anat Pathol* 2003;**10**:113–24.
52. Schnitt SJ, Collins LC. Columnar cell lesions and flat epithelial atypia of the breast. *Semin Breast Disease* 2005;**8**:100–11.
53. Brandt SM, Young GQ, Hoda SA. The "Rosen Triad": tubular carcinoma, lobular carcinoma in situ and columnar cell lesions. *Adv Anat Pathol* 2008;**15**:140–6.
54. Rosen PP. Columnar cell hyperplasia is associated with lobular carcinoma in situ and tubular carcinoma. *Am J Surg Pathol* 1999;**23**:1561.
55. Fraser JL, Raza S, Chorny K, Connolly JL, Schnitt SJ. Columnar alteration with prominent apical snouts and secretions: a spectrum of changes frequently present in breast biopsies performed for microcalcifications. *Am J Surg Pathol* 1998;**22**:1521–7.
56. Jara-Lazaro AR, Tse GM, Tan PH. Columnar cell lesions of the breast: an update and significance on core biopsy. *Pathology* 2009;**41**:18–27.
57. Kunju LP, Kleer CG. Significance of flat epithelial atypia on mammotome core needle biopsy: should it be excised? *Hum Pathol* 2007;**38**:35–41.
58. Guerra-Wallace MM, Christensen WN, White Jr RL. A retrospective study of columnar alteration with prominent apical snouts and secretions and the association with cancer. *Am J Surg* 2004;**188**:395–8.
59. Lim CN, Ho BC, Bay BH, Yip G, Tan PH. Nuclear morphometry in columnar cell lesions of the breast: is it useful? *J Clin Pathol* 2006;**59**:1283–6.
60. Goodman KA, Birdwell RL, Ikeda DM. Compliance with recommended follow-up after percutaneous breast biopsy. *AJR Am J Roentgenol* 1998;**170**:89–92.

SECTION

EIGHT

The Surgically Altered Breast

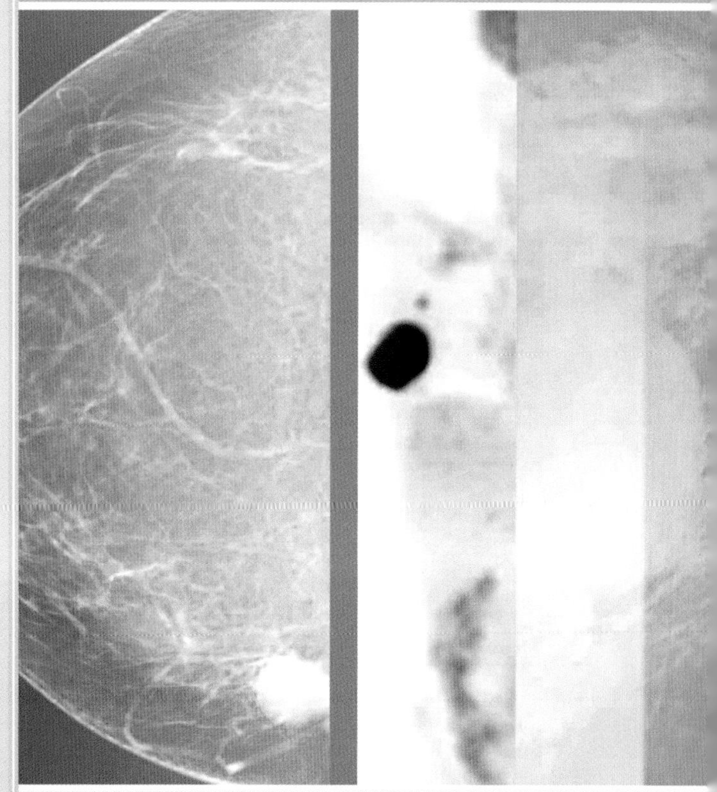

CHAPTER 34

The Conservatively Treated Breast

D. David Dershaw and Adam Bracha

Unlike mastectomy, in which the sole goal of treatment is to cure the patient of her disease, breast-conserving therapy has two goals: cure the disease and achieve an acceptable cosmetic result. Before a patient can be offered breast-conserving therapy, it must be possible to resect the cancer without causing unacceptable breast deformity. Because the radiologist is often able to determine the extent of tumor before surgery more accurately than the surgeon, the role of the radiologist is integral to the decision-making process about treatment options. Cancer can recur in the treated breast and early detection of recurrence can improve the likelihood of survival, so the radiologist also has a responsibility to monitor the breast after therapy to detect recurrences as early as possible and to provide information for patients and surgeons about the possibility of breast conservation.

CLINICAL TRIALS OF BREAST-CONSERVING THERAPY

Breast-conserving therapy has been tested in large numbers of controlled, prospective clinical trials, and its results have been reported in multiple retrospective single-institution studies. Of these investigations, seven randomized clinical trials are the most important.[1] In these trials, women with stage I or stage II breast cancers (invasive tumors no larger than 5 cm in greatest diameter) were treated. These women had no evidence of distant metastases and did not have fixed axillary lymph nodes. Presence of nonfixed but clinically involved axillary nodes at the time of enrollment into a study was not considered a reason for exclusion. In these randomized trials, women were treated either with mastectomy or with resection of the breast cancer and total breast irradiation of 45 to 50 Gy.

Survival rates for women treated with breast conservation versus mastectomy are comparable for overall disease-free survival. Women treated with breast conservation, however, have a risk for local treatment failure (recurrence of tumor in the treated breast), which cannot occur in the woman treated with mastectomy. Reports of the incidence of local failure have ranged from 3% to 19% at 8 years for women in high-risk groups; local recurrence rates of 20% to 40% have been reported.[2]

SELECTION OF WOMEN FOR BREAST-CONSERVING THERAPY

The appropriateness of this treatment depends on an assessment of the extent of tumor within the breast to ascertain whether the cancer can be resected without causing unacceptable breast deformity. The determination of the extent of local disease is made by the surgeon, pathologist, and radiologist, each using different modalities to identify the extent of tumor within the breast. Therefore, any of these physicians can recommend mastectomy as the appropriate therapy if the physical findings, histologic assessment of tumor margins, or size of tumor as determined on imaging studies indicate that it is too large to be resected without significant deformity of the breast (Figs 34-1 and 34-2).

Beyond those with extensive tumors, women for whom conservation is inappropriate include those in the first or second trimester of pregnancy or with a history of prior therapeutic irradiation to the breast. Women in early pregnancy must have the pregnancy terminated if they wish to undergo breast-conserving therapy. Women in late pregnancy may elect to delay therapy until after delivery. For women who have had prior therapeutic irradiation to the breast, additional irradiation is not possible because the total dose would not be tolerated. Therefore, women who have undergone previous breast-conserving therapy with irradiation and those who have been treated for Hodgkin disease with a mantle-type field of radiation are not eligible for breast-conserving therapy. In instances in which conservative treatment did not include radiation, such as

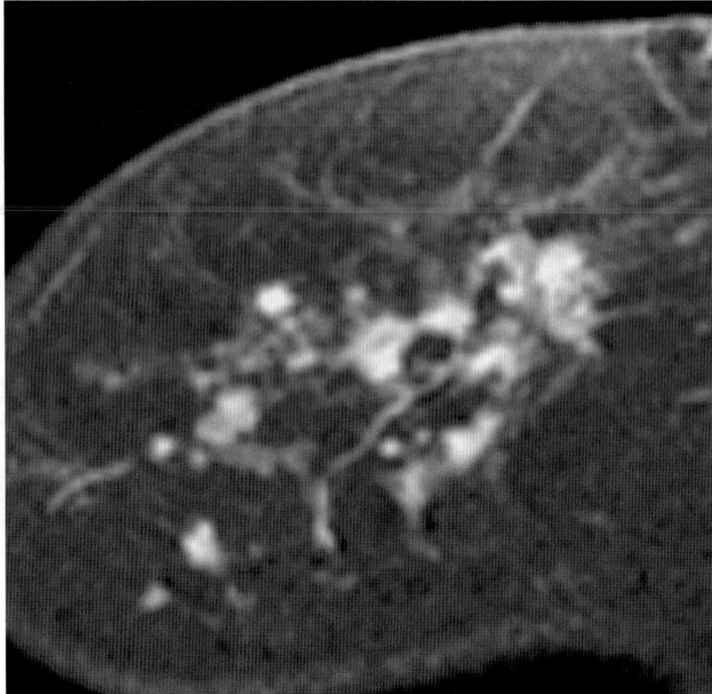

■ **FIGURE 34-1** Postcontrast magnetic (MR) image shows clumped, regional enhancement due to multicentric carcinoma. Breast conservation is not possible in this patient.

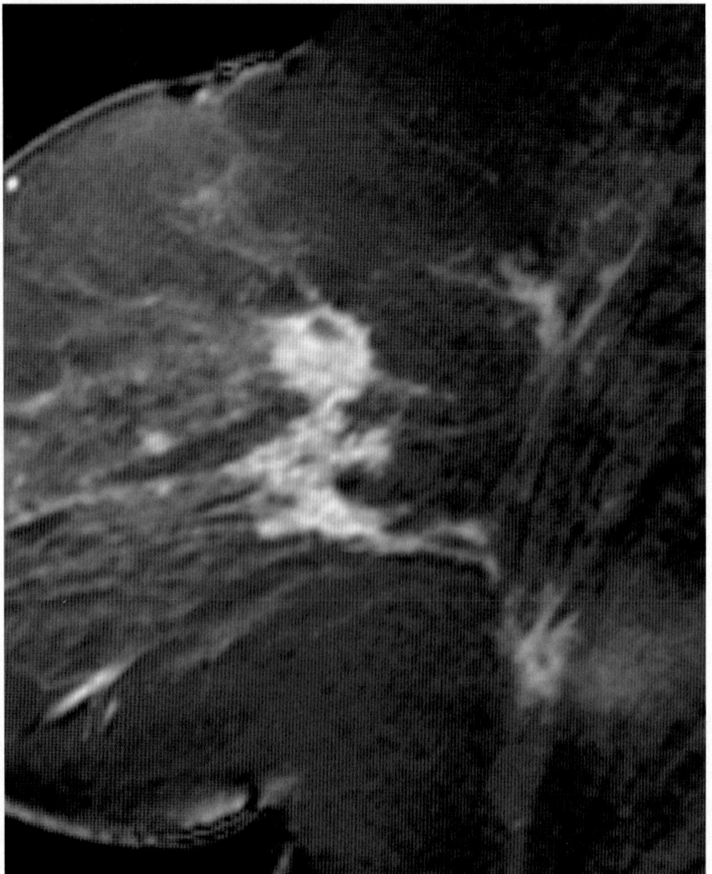

■ **FIGURE 34-2** Postcontrast magnetic resonance (MR) image shows an irregular, spiculated heterogeneously enhancing mass with areas of enhancement in the pectoralis. This finding indicates tumor involvement of the chest wall musculature and modifies the surgical approach to the carcinoma.

for small foci of ductal carcinoma in situ (DCIS), a second attempt at conservation is possible.

Women should be queried about a history of collagen vascular disease, which is a relative contraindication to breast-conserving therapy. If the disease is quiescent, the radiotherapist may determine that treatment may proceed. Active collagen vascular disease, however, often leads to significant complications after radiation therapy and may make the patient ineligible for such treatment.

The completion of radiation therapy usually takes 4 to 6 weeks. Women who have difficulty traveling to a radiation treatment center because of distance or because of infirmity that makes traveling a problem, as well as women who may not be sufficiently responsible to complete their course of therapy, may not be appropriate candidates for breast conservation.

Tumor size is an important determinant of whether a woman can undergo breast-conserving therapy, but absolute measurements of tumor size are not used. The determining factor is the ratio of the size of the tumor to the size of the breast. In a large breast, a large tumor can be resected with good cosmetic results. In a small breast, a large tumor may be impossible to excise without causing such severe deformity as to make breast-conserving therapy inappropriate. Although the large size of a tumor is not an absolute contraindication, randomized prospective studies included only tumors up to 5 cm in diameter, and data are not available on the appropriateness of therapy for larger cancers.

Imaging Indications and Algorithm

The goal of imaging in breast conservation is to assist in the selection of appropriate women for this treatment, evaluation of adequacy of surgical excision, and follow-up of the patient to detect recurrence at the earliest possible stage, if this occurs, and to obviate the need for surgical biopsy if benign but suspicious sequelae develop.

Mammography, often augmented by magnetic resonance imaging (MRI), is the imaging tool that is most important in evaluating these women. A suggested algorithm for mammography and MRI in this setting is shown in Tables 34-1 and 34-2.

Imaging Technique and Findings

Imaging evaluation of adequacy of treatment begins while the patient is undergoing surgery. Intraoperatively, specimen radiography is useful in assessing adequacy of tumor resection. Extension of tumor mass or calcifications to the margin of the lumpectomy specimen suggests that residual tumor may be present in the breast at that margin (Fig. 34-3). Further resection and specimen radiography of that margin is appropriate at the time the patient is in surgery.

Because the mammographic changes of surgical distortion and hematoma formation that occur at the surgical site obscure findings related to unresected uncalcified carcinoma, postoperative preradiation mammography need not be performed in these cases. However, the calcifications of carcinoma are not obscured by these immediate

TABLE 34-2. Uses for Magnetic Resonance Imaging in Breast Conservation

Preoperative	Assess extent of disease: particularly useful for invasive lobular, large DCIS, suspected chest wall involvement; identify unknown primary lesions; assess the opposite breast
Postoperative	Assess residual disease in close or positive margins; may be appropriate for any women undergoing additional surgery for re-excision
Suspected recurrence	After 18 months can be useful to differentiate recurrence from scar

TABLE 34-1. Memorial Sloan-Kettering Schedule for Mammography in Patients Treated with Breast-Conserving Therapy

Timing	Study	Technique	Comments
Preoperative	Bilateral mammogram	Routine views; use magnification and coned views as needed to assess full extent of tumor	Determine presence and extent of multiplicity of tumor to assess possibility of breast conservation; evaluate other breast
Intraoperative	Specimen radiography	May require at least two orthogonal views and magnification view; compression useful for masses	Determine whether lesion of interest has been sampled; if malignant, determine whether tumor extends to margins of resection, requiring further surgery
Before radiation therapy	Unilateral mammograms for women whose tumors contained calcifications	If no calcifications present at lumpectomy site, perform magnification view; if calcium present, perform magnification view to determine extent	Assess completeness of tumor excision by mammographic criteria; if re-excision performed, repeat this study
Post-therapy baseline	Unilateral mammogram	Do at 3-6 months after radiation therapy; if calcium was present in original cancer and magnification view was not previously performed do it now	Re-establish baseline mammographic pattern
Routine follow-up	Annual bilateral mammogram	Additional views as clinically indicated	To detect early recurrence
Area of clinical concern	Diagnostic mammogram	Two-view mammogram with additional views as needed	Evaluate new area of concern

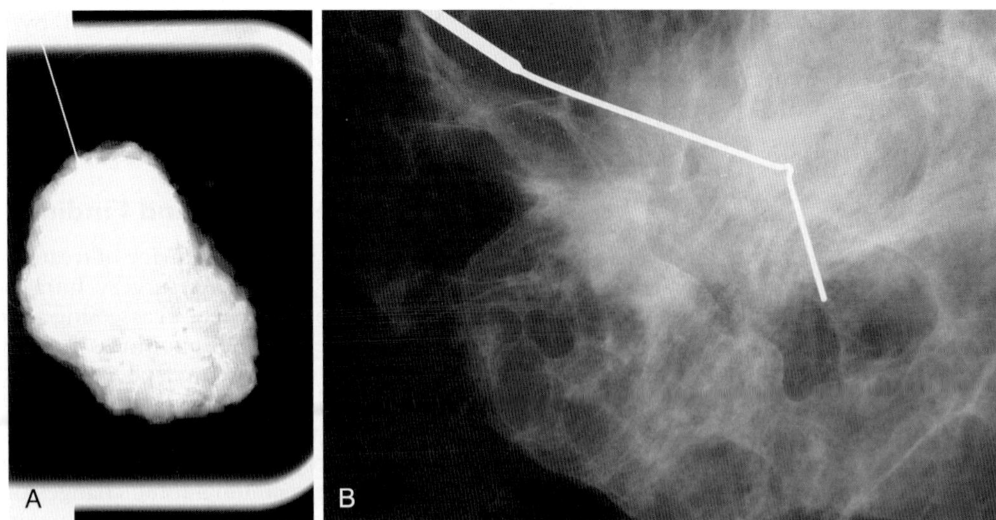

■ **FIGURE 34-3** **A,** Specimen radiography shows calcium at the margin of the excised specimen. Calcium was due to ductal carcinoma in situ (DCIS). Its presence at the margin of the specimen resulted in excision of more tissue to attempt to clear the breast of cancer. **B,** A spiculated carcinoma is seen in this specimen. Spicules and mass extend to the resected margin because of transection of tumor. Additional tissue was excised to clear the breast of cancer.

postoperative findings, and postoperative mammography is worthwhile to seek evidence of incomplete resection of a calcified tumor in the form of residual calcifications (Fig. 34-4). Because microscopic residual tumor will presumably be sterilized by postoperative radiotherapy,[3] evidence of minimal residual tumor may not require further surgery. However, large volumes of residual tumor will not be adequately treated by postoperative irradiation and will have to be excised.[4] In addition to determining whether a re-excision may be necessary, the postoperative preradiation mammogram is useful in establishing a new baseline image of the calcifications remaining in the breast. If the residual calcifications at the lumpectomy site are not re-excised, it is important to be able to determine on later mammograms whether the pattern of calcifications is stable or if they have increased in number or extent.

Magnification views are useful to determine more accurately the number and extent of residual calcifications. Occasionally, when routine views of the lumpectomy site do not show residual calcium, this finding might be evident on magnification imaging.[5] Therefore, the routine use of magnification in at least one view may be desirable in postoperative imaging. Punctate benign microcalcifications can be seen postoperatively at the lumpectomy site. Comparison with the preoperative mammogram should be made to be certain that calcium at this site is residual tumoral calcium and not postoperative benign calcification.

The precise number of residual microcalcifications that require a re-excision has not been determined. One or two calcifications suggest the presence of minimal residual tumor. Although this residual tumor may be sterilized with radiation, some routinely recommend re-excision of any residual microcalcifications.[6] A large number of residual calcifications indicates a large volume of tumor that must be surgically excised. The histologic assessment of the margins of the resected specimen should also be considered in the determination of the need for re-excision.

Postoperative mammography to exclude residual calcifications that may necessitate re-excision may be performed at any time before the start of radiotherapy. After a re-excision, another postoperative mammogram should be obtained to determine the adequacy of re-excision and

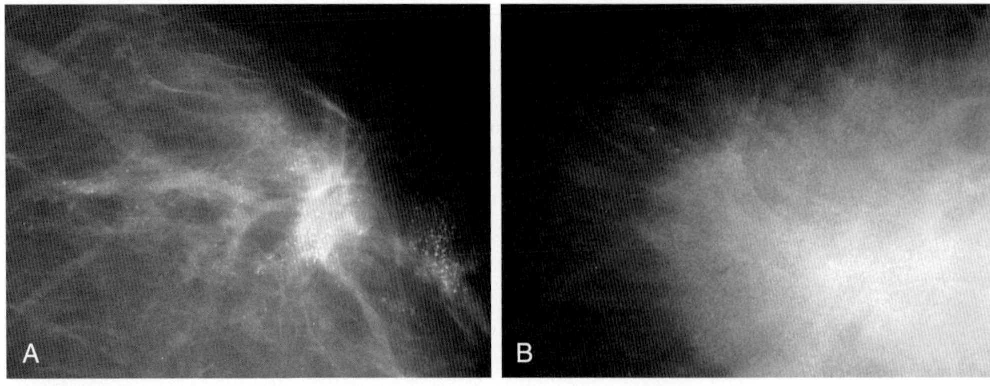

■ **FIGURE 34-4** **A,** Preoperative mammogram shows a cluster of fine, pleomorphic calcifications due to ductal carcinoma in situ (DCIS). **B,** A postoperative mammogram shows a spiculated scar. Residual tumoral calcifications are present because of incomplete excision of DCIS. Additional tissue was removed to clear the breast of tumor associated calcifications.

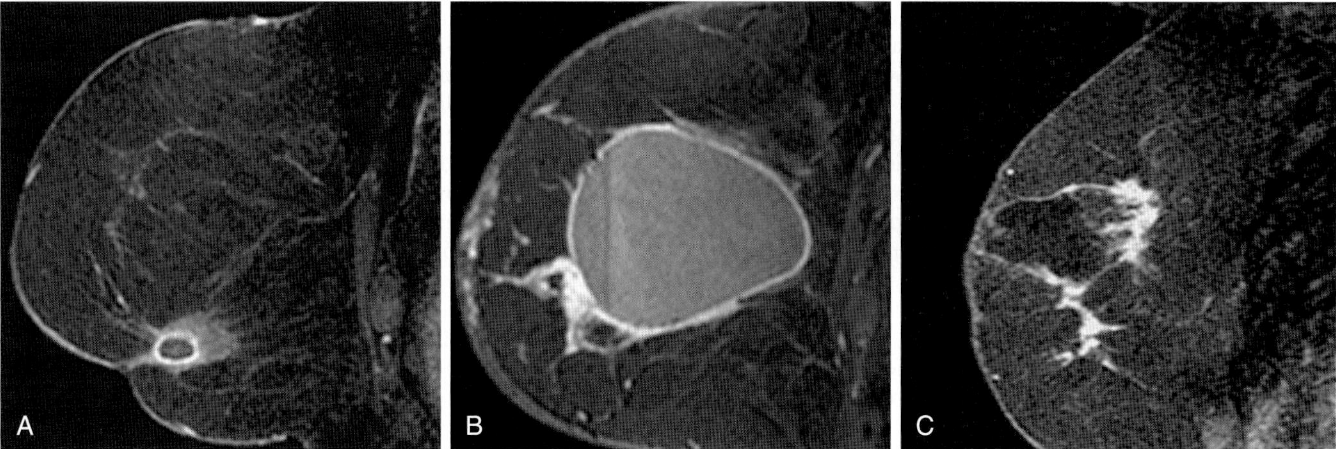

■ **FIGURE 34-5** **A,** Shortly after lumpectomy, a contrast-enhanced magnetic resonance (MR) image shows a rim enhancement in the wall of the seroma that has formed at the operative site. **B,** Clumped enhancement at the anterior seroma margin was due to residual tumor. The lumpectomy specimen showed tumor extension to the anterior margin of the removed tissue. **C,** The posterior and inferior margins of the seroma are contaminated by residual tumor depicted as focal clumped enhancement. Magnetic resonance imaging (MRI) is helpful in this case in mapping the extent of carcinoma left in the breast.

to establish a new baseline. Because the breast may be tender after re-excision, compression to immobilize the breast during the two standard radiographic exposures should be no greater than the patient can tolerate.

Residual microcalcifications at the lumpectomy site do not invariably imply the presence of residual tumor. In one study of 29 women who underwent re-excision of a focus of mammographically evident residual microcalcifications, 69% were found to have residual carcinoma.[7] The women who were found not to have residual cancer were usually those in whom small numbers of residual calcifications had been seen. Although the calcifications were pleomorphic, they were found to be associated with sclerosing adenosis, fat necrosis, and foreign-body reaction. In the same study, 64% of 14 women in whom tumor-associated calcifications had been completely excised had no residual tumor at re-excision. Because a carcinoma may not have calcifications throughout its entire extent, it is not surprising that the removal of all calcifications does not always result in complete excision of the tumor.[8,9] Thus, the removal of all tumor-associated calcifications does not ensure the total removal of the tumor.

In women with positive margins histologically, MRI has been found to be able to demonstrate the extent of residual carcinoma in the breast that might otherwise be unsuspected.[10,11] A pattern of smooth enhancement around the lumpectomy site due to granulation tissue is normal, but clumped or irregular enhancement can be found in women with residual carcinoma (Fig. 34-5). Accurate mapping of the extent of residual tumor can spare the patient multiple trips to surgery, for procedures that only "chip away" at the cancer, by demonstrating the extent of tumor requiring resection or treatment with mastectomy.

ROUTINE MAMMOGRAPHY AFTER RADIATION THERAPY

After the completion of radiation therapy, routine mammography is performed to detect recurrent tumor as early as possible, to characterize any palpable abnormality that develops in either breast, and to screen for cancer in the untreated breast. Mammography of the untreated breast should be performed annually. The treated breast requires a baseline mammogram after the completion of radiotherapy and routine follow-up thereafter. It has been the policy at my institution to perform the initial post-treatment mammogram of the irradiated breast 3 to 6 months after completion of therapy. If the breast becomes red, firm, and tender, the mammogram is done at 6 months, at which time the breast is usually less tender, allowing for more effective compression. For those women in whom only minimal radiation reaction is seen on physical examination, the mammogram is performed 3 months after the completion of radiation therapy.

Routine mediolateral oblique (MLO) and craniocaudal (CC) views are obtained. It is important that the tumorectomy site be imaged as completely as possible, because that is the area at greatest risk for recurrent cancer. Because a recurrence may be manifest merely as a subtle change in the scar, additional images of the lumpectomy site, including spot cone views, are often obtained to document the post-treatment size and configuration of the scar. Additional views that are needed at the time of this initial post-treatment mammogram to fully image the surgical bed are routinely included in follow-up mammograms to screen for tumor recurrence. If the original tumor contained microcalcifications, and magnification views were not obtained before radiation therapy, it is the policy at my institution to obtain these views as part of the postirradiation baseline study to allow any calcifications near the scar to be fully documented. If later in the course of follow-up a patient is seen at my institution for the first time and magnification views have not yet been obtained or are unavailable, and either the original tumor contained calcifications or its mammographic appearance is unknown, a magnification view of the lumpectomy site is obtained as part of the initial assessment of the patient.

The timing of further mammograms is a source of debate. Some authorities have suggested follow-up mammograms at 6-month intervals for the first 2 to 5 years.[12,13] However, no existing data suggest that routine follow-up at intervals shorter than 1 year result in a diagnosis of recurrence at an earlier stage. For women who do not undergo radiation therapy, the initial mammogram is performed within a few months of surgery to establish a new baseline, and thereafter mammography follows the same schedule as for patients who have undergone radiation therapy.

The changes seen in the mammogram after breast-conserving therapy include focal alterations at the lumpectomy site resulting from surgery and more diffuse changes caused by radiation therapy. All, some, or none of the following changes may be present in any individual case.

Seromas and Hematomas

In the initial postoperative period, a new round or oval mass at the lumpectomy site usually represents a seroma or hematoma (Fig. 34-6).[14] The seroma occasionally contains a fat-fluid or air-fluid level that is visible on a 90-degree lateral view. These masses are clinically unimportant, tend to resolve slowly (sometimes over a period of a year), and may be replaced by a scar in the form of a spiculated mass that should not be mistaken for recurrent cancer.[5]

Scars

Scars and areas of parenchymal distortion are often evident at the lumpectomy site. It is imperative that the radiologist know the location of this site to be certain that the spiculated mass is a scar. Surgical clips that are placed at the lumpectomy site to accurately target the boost dose of radiation are helpful in defining the lumpectomy bed for the radiologist (Fig. 34-7). The surgical site can also localized by reference to the preoperative mammogram (if it showed the cancer) or the postoperative mammogram. Although some radiologists have suggested the placement of radiopaque skin markers at the cutaneous scar to localize the area of resection, the skin incision is often far removed from the site of resection.

The scar may be associated with a contour deformity and focal skin thickening, which can also be useful in localizing the surgical site. In the early postoperative period, edema may obscure the scar, which then becomes increasingly apparent as the edema subsides. Careful attention to the earlier mammogram may show that an increasingly apparent spiculated mass is the scar that was "silhouetted" by the edema on earlier studies and does not represent a new lesion. The scar may also be characterized by a pattern that is more prominent on one orthogonal view than on the other. Although cancer occasionally may look similar, this pattern supports the diagnosis of a scar. Scars may contain a central focus of fat owing to the herniation of fat into the lumpectomy site and the occurrence of fibrosis around it. Finally, in some conservatively treated breasts, no scar may be evident in mammograms.

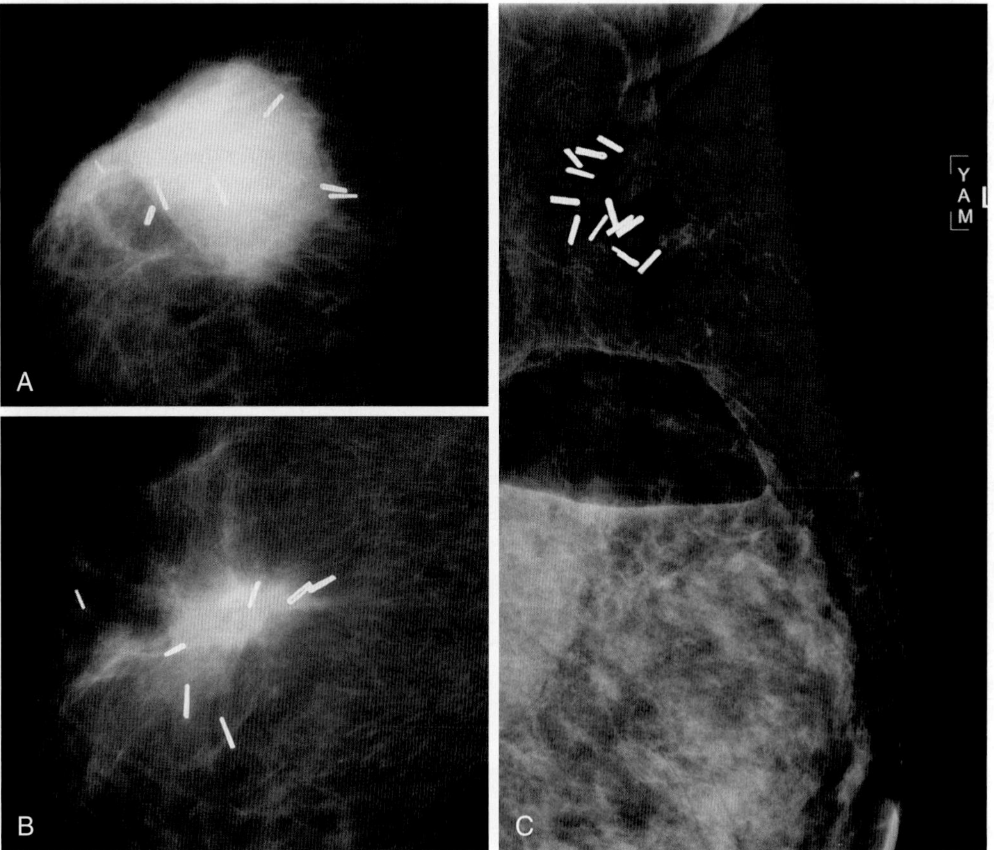

■ **FIGURE 34-6** **A,** On mammography, weeks after surgery, an oval partially circumscribed and partially indistinct, high density mass is present at the lumpectomy site. This is a postoperative seroma. Surgical clips have been placed at the margins of resection to facilitate accurate treatment planning for the boost dose of radiation to the lumpectomy bed. **B,** Six months later, the seroma has become smaller irregular in shape and more spiculated, a normal evolution of the mammographic changes at the operative site. **C,** In another patient, the mammogram performed 2 weeks after surgery shows an air-fluid level at the lumpectomy site on the mediolateral oblique (MLO) view. This finding, due to acute changes, is a normal pattern shortly after lumpectomy.

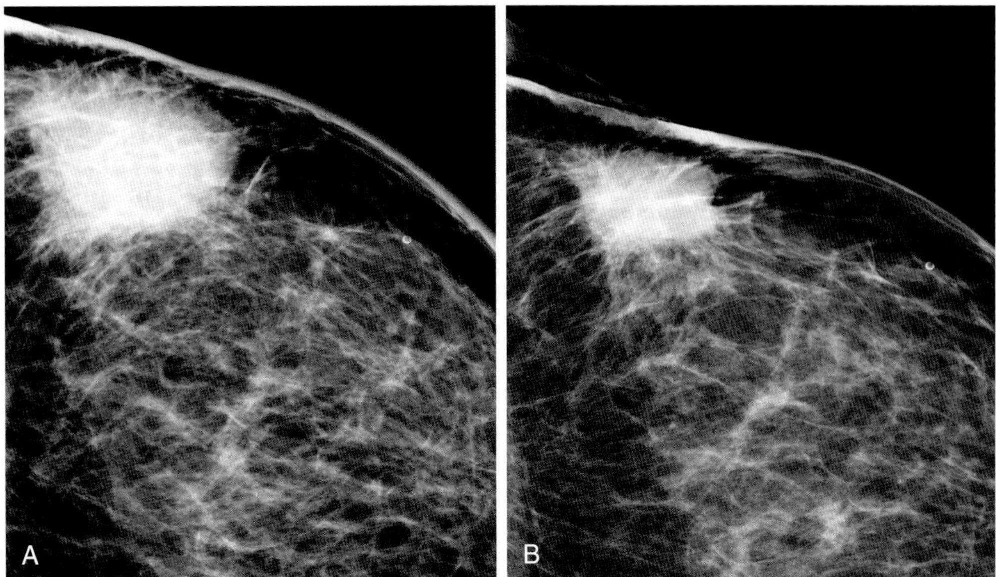

■ **FIGURE 34-7** **A,** Within the first few months after lumpectomy, the scar is as large as it should ever be. An oval indistinct and spiculated mass at the lumpectomy site on this mammogram is a small seroma. Note the tethered contour of the skin due to surgical deformity. **B,** One year later, the scar is smaller, and spiculation is slightly more prominent. This is a normal pattern of scar formation.

In one series, a scar was evident on the mammograms in only one fourth of the women who underwent breast-conserving therapy.[15]

On MRI the surgical site initially demonstrates smooth, rim enhancement. As the seroma involutes, this pattern can become more irregular. Enhancement at the surgical site can persist for several years. Clumped enhancement should not occur without residual or recurrent disease.[16]

Diffuse Mammographic Changes

Superimposed on the focal changes at the surgical site are diffuse alterations in the mammogram that are due to radiation. Histologically, the early changes resulting from radiation therapy result from edema, and the more chronic alterations are caused by fibrosis.[17] Mammographically, these changes are manifested as skin thickening, trabecular thickening, increase in the density of the parenchyma, and diffuse increase in the density of the breast (Fig. 34-8). These changes are identical to those that result from inflammatory breast cancer, mastitis, lymphoma, and obstructed lymphatic or venous drainage. A patient may have none, some, or all of these findings, and their occurrence is not related to radiation dose.[18] On serial examinations, these findings may remain unaltered, may decrease, or may completely resolve. After the initial baseline mammogram, any progression of findings is worrisome and should lead to an investigation of the cause.

Skin Changes

Thickening of the skin may be diffuse or localized to the surgical site or dependent portion of the breast.[15] Skin changes are more common in women who have also undergone axillary node dissection. Diffuse skin thickening may be apparent only on comparison of the mammogram of the treated breast with that of the breast before treatment or with the mammogram of the other breast. Skin thickening is the most common change on the mammogram after breast-conserving therapy, being reported in up to 90% of cases.[15] The radiologist should remember that this finding is more conspicuous on mammograms performed with full breast digital imaging than with screen-film technique. Thickened skin returns to normal by 2 to 3 years after therapy in 46% to 60% of cases.[15]

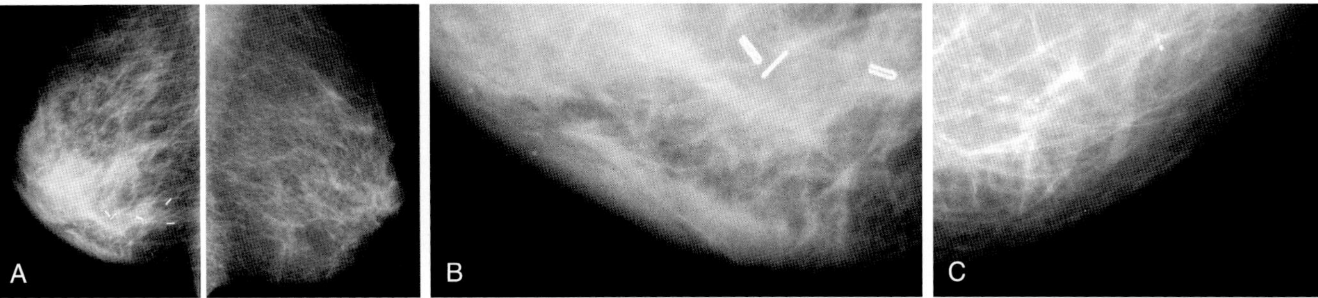

■ **FIGURE 34-8** **A,** Mediolateral oblique (MLO) mammographic views of treated *(left)* and untreated *(right)* breasts 1 year after radiation. Close-up views of the lower portions of the left (**B**) and right (**C**) breasts show skin thickening on the left. The treated left breast also shows diffuse increase in density and diffuse coarsening of the breast trabecula, due to inflammation, that have occurred in response to radiation.

Parenchymal Changes

Postirradiation changes of the parenchyma include coarsening of the fibrous supportive tissues of the breast (thickening of the trabeculae), an increase in the density and apparent volume of the ductal and glandular elements, and a diffuse increase in the density of the entire breast. In addition to the edema and fibrosis caused by radiation, increased flow through the lymphatic channels and small blood vessels causes them to become distended, contributing to this pattern. In the dense breast, trabecular thickening may be most apparent in the subdermal fat, especially when the mammogram is examined with bright light. Although these changes may be nonexistent or subtle in some women, they may be accentuated in women undergoing chemotherapy.[15]

Calcifications

Calcifications develop in one third to one half of women who have undergone breast radiation therapy, sometimes after a delay of up to 5 years.[15] Calcified suture material and coarse calcifications of fat necrosis are commonly apparent in the irradiated breast, particularly at the site of tumorectomy and the boost dose of radiotherapy (Fig. 34-9). The calcifications of fat necrosis tend to be round, may have radiolucent centers, and usually do not develop sooner than 2 years after treatment. They reflect the trauma of radiotherapy and surgery. Radiopaque surgical clips may also be present at the surgical site. Microcalcifications, if not fully excised at surgery, may increase, decrease, or remain stable in number. The calcifications that decrease in number are presumably associated with cancer that has responded to radiotherapy. An increase in number of microcalcifications raises the concern about an associated viable growing tumor, and biopsy is indicated. The radiologist should be aware that nonmalignant processes can also cause microcalcifications to develop; these are discussed later. Microcalcifications that remain stable may reflect viable tumor whose growth has been retarded by radiotherapy. Such stable calcifications followed for several years with mammograms to confirm that they remain unchanged do not signal the presence of viable tumor.

Magnetic Resonance Imaging Post-treatment Changes

In addition to changes at the seroma noted above, skin thickening and decreased size of the breast may be noted. Often, parenchymal enhancement and cyst formation are suppressed by radiation. This is most obvious by comparison with the contralateral breast, particularly in the premenopausal woman.

TUMOR RECURRENCE IN THE IRRADIATED BREAST

Mammographic follow-up after breast-conserving therapy is undertaken to detect recurrent tumor in the treated breast (local treatment failure) as early as possible. Local treatment failure is reported to occur at a rate of 5% at 5 years and of 10% to 15% at 10 years after completion of therapy.[19] Because the stage of tumor recurrence is related to the likelihood of survival, the early diagnosis of recurrence is of extreme importance.[20,21] The woman whose recurrent cancer is diagnosed while it is still intraductal or whose invasive cancer is less than 2 cm in diameter has the best prognosis. Survival rates decrease with increasing tumor size.

Although local treatment failure can occur in any woman who has undergone breast-conserving therapy, certain women are at a higher risk. Some risk factors remain controversial but include younger age at the time of treatment, an extensive intraductal component of the tumor, and vascular invasion by the tumor.[2] Also implicated in increasing the likelihood of recurrence are multiple cancers at the time of the original treatment, tumor involvement at the margin of resection, lymphatic invasion by tumor, high histologic grade,

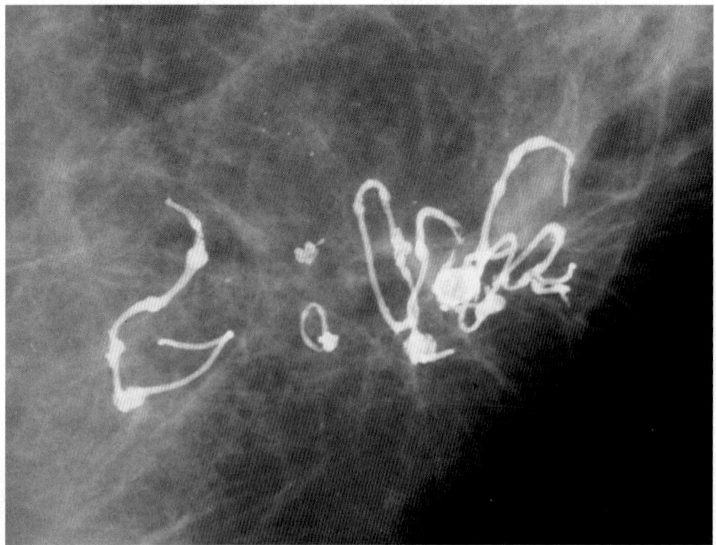

■ **FIGURE 34-9** Linear calcifications are due to calcified suture material at the lumpectomy site. Clumped, eggshell calcifications and punctate calcifications are foci of fat necrosis.

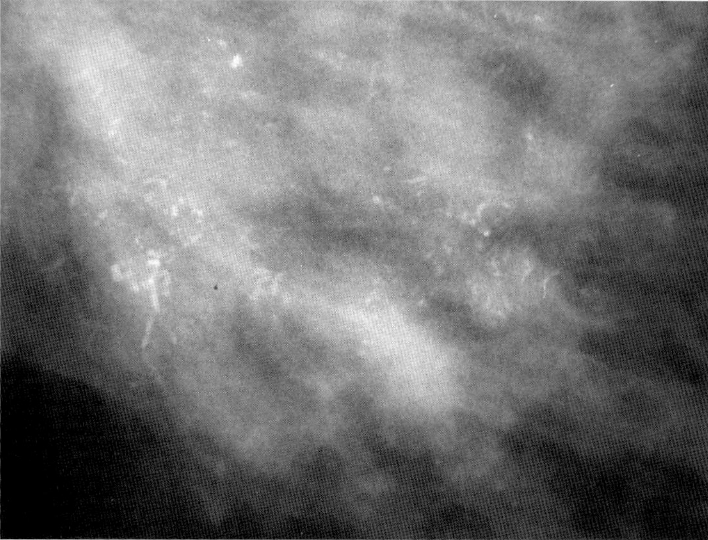

■ **FIGURE 34-10** Fine linear and fine pleomorphic, (microcalcifications in a regional distribution) developed at the lumpectomy site of this women owing to local recurrence of ductal carcinoma in situ (DCIS).

larger tumor size, nonductal histologic type, and monocellular reaction to the tumor.[22] Chemotherapy has been reported to lower the incidence of recurrence.[22]

The ability of mammography to identify recurrent cancer after breast-conserving therapy is compromised compared with its ability to detect cancer in the untreated breast. This is because of the surgical distortion and increased breast density that result from treatment. Mammography reportedly has been unable to detect 19% to 50% of local recurrences.[20,23,24] However, 29% to 42% of local recurrences have been reported to be detected only by mammography. Compared with local recurrences detected on physical examination, those found by mammography are more often DCIS, whereas those found on physical examination are more often invasive (Fig. 34-10).[23] Recurrences consisting of invasive lobular histology can be extremely difficult to detect mammographically.

To optimize the efficacy of mammography of the treated breast, it is extremely important that careful communication between the clinician and the radiologist occurs and that subtle mammographic signs of tumor recurrences be vigorously sought. The signs are those of breast cancer superimposed on the findings characteristic of an irradiated breast. They include the development of new, pleomorphic microcalcifications or a new mass (see Fig. 34-10). Enlargement of the scar may signal the recurrence of tumor (Fig. 34-11). Enlargement of axillary nodes can result from metastatic tumor, causing an axillary

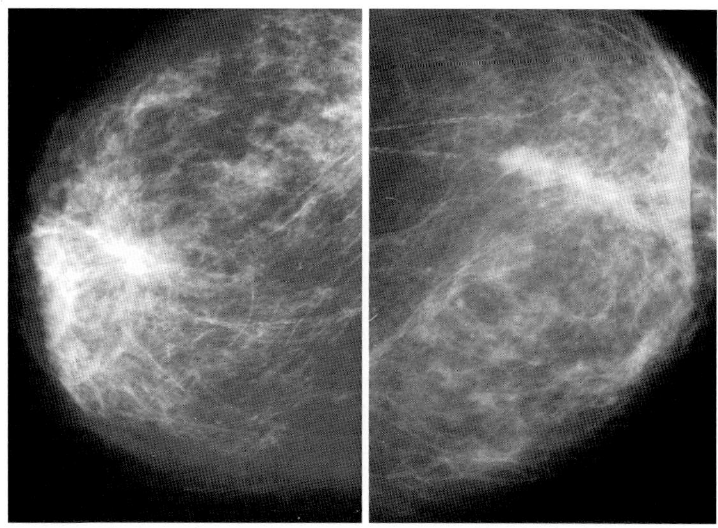

■ **FIGURE 34-11** *Left,* a mammogram performed 2 years after treatment shows an irregular spiculated mass. *Right,* A year later, the central scar has become elongated and lobulated. This change was due to recurrence of invasive ductal carcinoma.

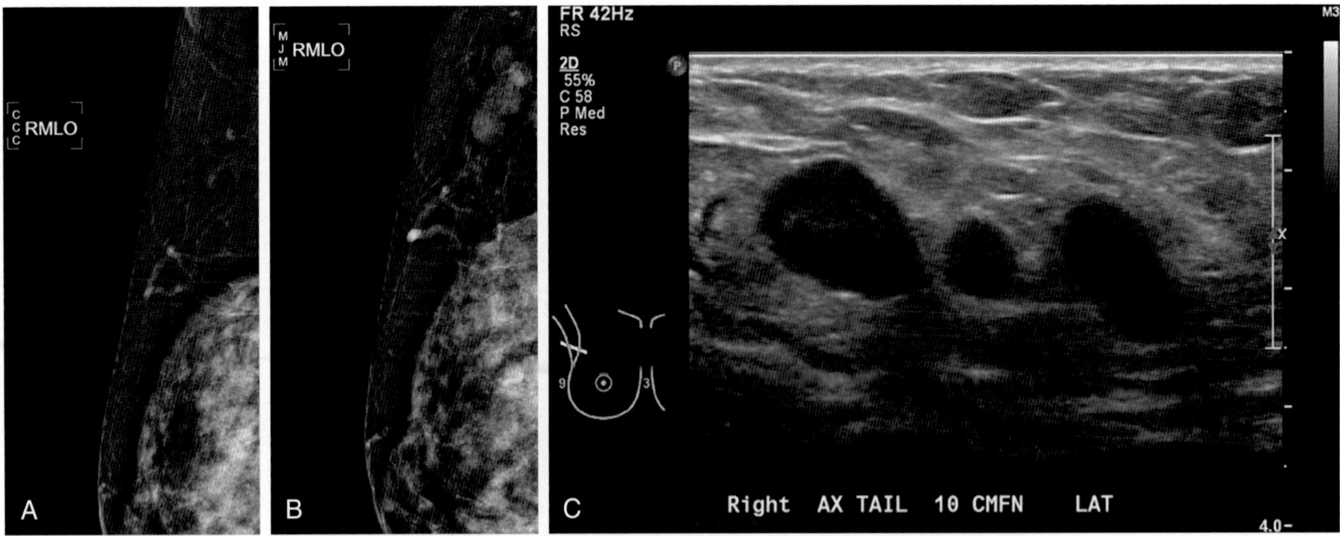

■ **FIGURE 34-12** **A,** A mammogram performed 1 year after treatment shows no abnormal axillary lymph nodes. **B,** A year later, numerous round, circumscribed masses compatible with nodes are present in the axilla due to an axillary recurrence. **C,** Ultrasonography of the adenopathy revealed numerous oval masses without the distinct echogenic center identified with normal nodes. Ultrasound-guided fine-needle aspiration confirmed the diagnosis of recurrent carcinoma.

recurrence (Fig. 34-12). As noted previously, an increase in breast density or in skin thickening should be viewed with suspicion, and the cause should be investigated. The other breast must also be monitored, because it is always at risk for cancer.

In the event of failure of local treatment, the site in the breast at which the new tumor occurs is related to the time from completion of treatment. A carcinoma that arises within 4 to 6 years after therapy is usually the result of failure to eradicate the original tumor. The tumor recurrence usually occurs at or near the site of the original cancer.[12,22,25] Recurrences rarely occur earlier than 18 months after adequate therapy. It is important during this follow-up period that the lumpectomy site be fully imaged. Treatment of the patient's original cancer usually sterilizes undetected sites of tumor within the breast. It usually takes at least 4 to 6 years for new cancers to grow in the breast and become detectable. Therefore, starting at 4 to 6 years after therapy, the breast is at risk for the development of a new cancer, usually arising in a different quadrant from that in which the original cancer developed.

The MRI findings of recurrent tumor are those seen in cancers in the nonirradiated breast superimposed on the pattern or the treated breast. It should be noted that rim enhancement at the lumpectomy site can persist for several years after treatment and should not be mistaken for tumor recurrence.

BENIGN SEQUELAE MIMICKING RECURRENCE

Although the development of a palpable mass or mammographic abnormality after breast-conserving therapy raises the specter of recurrent carcinoma, complications of treatment can mimic recurrent cancer and yet be clinically innocent. Fat necrosis and fibrosis can be caused by surgery or radiation, and radiation can produce a new mass and pleomorphic microcalcifications, findings identical to those of recurrent tumor (Figs 34-13 and 34-14). In one reported series of patients treated with breast-conserving therapy, 19 of 29 women who underwent breast biopsy for suspected recurrence had benign disease.[26]

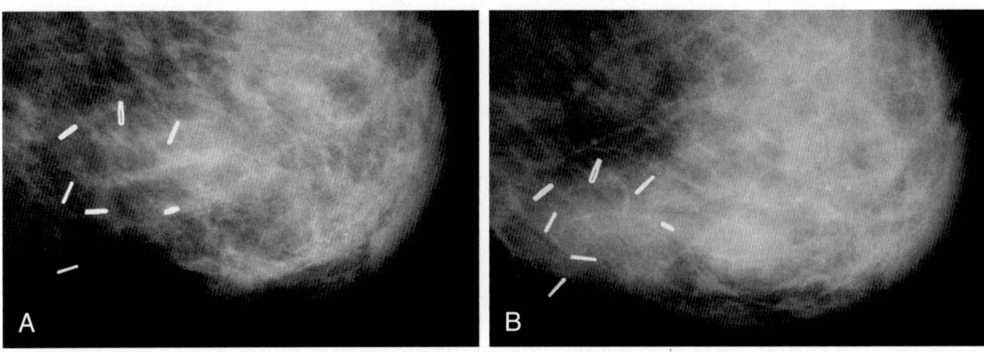

■ **FIGURE 34-13** **A,** One year after treatment, baseline changes are evident on a mammogram. **B,** A year later, a new asymmetry is surrounded by the surgical clips at the lumpectomy site. A palpable mass had also developed here. Biopsy revealed fat necrosis.

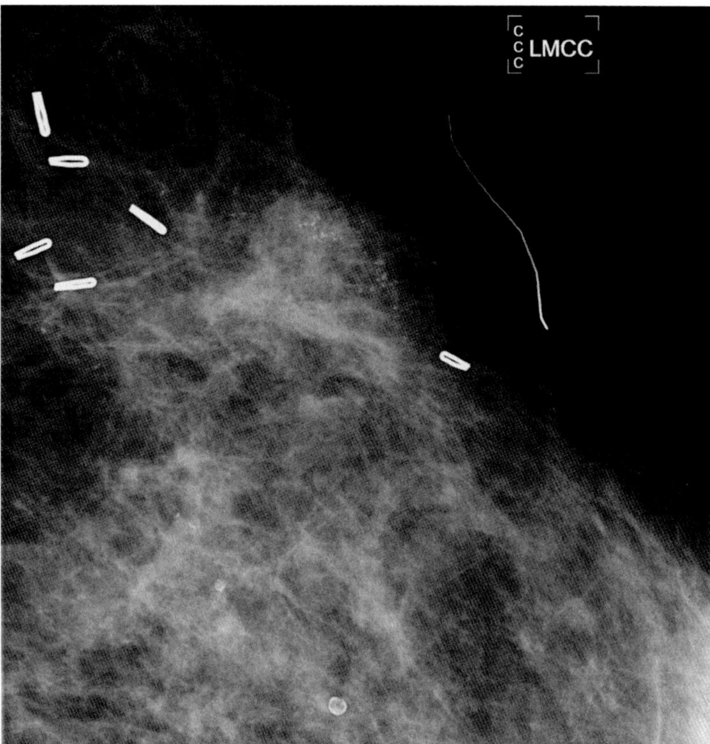

■ **FIGURE 34-14** A cluster of punctate and amorphous calcifications evident on the mammogram developed as a new finding at the lumpectomy site. Biopsy was done, and histologic examination showed only dystrophic calcifications.

It is important to attempt to differentiate fat necrosis and fibrosis from recurrent tumor. Surgical biopsy can compromise the cosmetic result of breast-conserving surgery, and scarring may be worsened.

It should be remembered that both benign and malignant processes can coexist in the treated breast. The presence of obvious fat necrosis does not negate the possibility of recurrent tumor (Fig. 34-15). Therefore, all findings should be adequately assessed to ensure that the breast is free of detectable tumor.

When it is not possible to determine whether the findings are due to carcinoma, fibrosis, or other benign processes, biopsy should be performed. Percutaneous needle biopsy may be useful in differentiating tumor from scar.[27]

MRI of the lumpectomy site has also been shown to be reliable in differentiating scar from tumor recurrence. Because breast cancers are vascular and scars are hypovascular or avascular, the enhancement of the cancers after the intravenous administration of gadolinium has enabled them to be distinguished from nonenhancing scars (Fig. 34-16).[28] However, during the first 18 months after therapy, both scars and cancers tend to enhance with administration of a contrast agent, and MRI patterns are not reliable during this period. Fortunately, recurrences are rare this

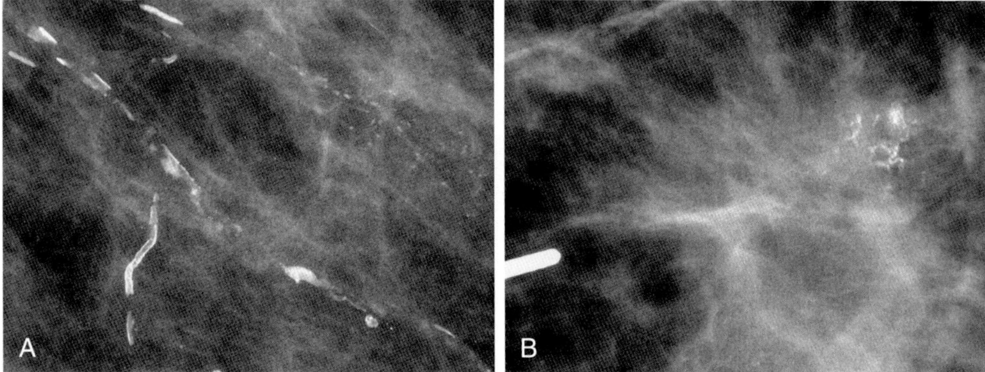

■ **FIGURE 34-15** **A,** Multiple patterns of calcifications are present at the lumpectomy site in this patient. There are vascular calcifications as well as an eggshell calcification due to fat necrosis. Additionally, pleomorphic microcalcifications have formed because of recurrent ductal carcinoma. **B,** Against a background pattern of architectural distortion from previous lumpectomy, a coarse dystrophic calcification is seen along with multiple, pleomorphic calcifications due to recurrent carcinoma.

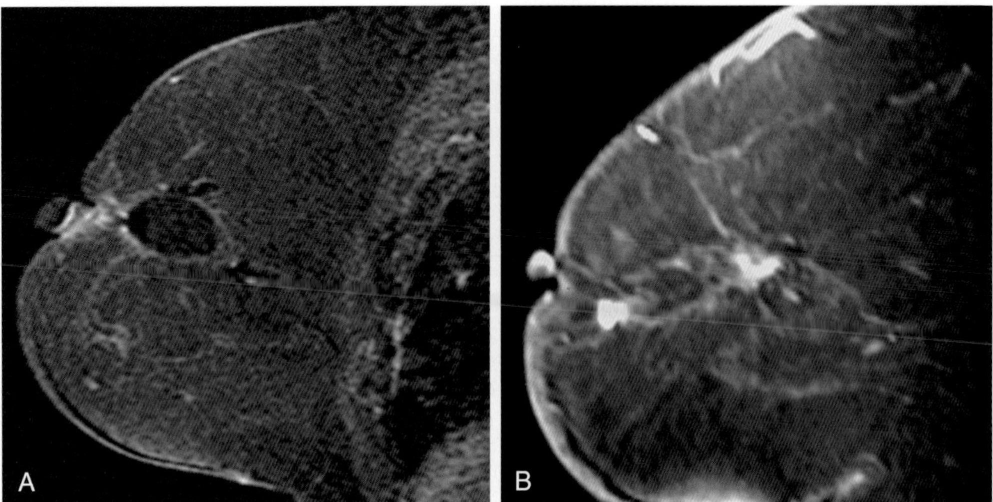

■ **FIGURE 34-16** **A,** Two years after surgery, there is no enhancement on contrast-enhanced magnetic resonance imaging (MRI) of a seroma. Note the artifact from clips next to the seroma and normal enhancement of the nipple. **B,** Three years after treatment, enlargement of the surgical scar was further evaluated with contrast MRI. Clumped enhancement is due to recurrent invasive carcinoma.

early. Also, enhancing scars have been reported more than 18 months after treatment, although they also seem to be unusual.[26]

Although a valuable tool in other situations in breast imaging, ultrasonography has limited usefulness in the irradiated, conserved breast. Changes of seroma formation and fibrosis at the surgical site are identical to those seen with carcinoma, and the differentiation of the two using ultrasonography is often impossible. Because the similarity of these findings is more likely to muddy the diagnosis, often pushing the patient to biopsy, it is often better to avoid sonography of the lumpectomy bed than to use it to clarify clinical issues.[29] Some have recommended that ultrasonography is valuable in the serial examination of the scar when the full mammographic imaging of the site is compromised owing to proximity to the chest wall. In this case, serial measurements are made to ensure that the scar is not enlarging.

KEY POINTS

- Imaging is an important tool in selecting women for breast conservation.
- Specimen radiography can suggest the presence of residual disease in the breast while the patient is undergoing surgery.
- A postsurgical mammogram is important to determine the presence or absence of calcifications in the breast. Without this mammogram, evaluation of breast calcifications after treatment may be impossible without biopsy.
- The extent of residual tumor in the breast may be best measured with MRI. Before re-excision for positive margins, MRI should be considered.
- Annual mammography should be used to assess the breast for possible recurrence of disease. Special views may be necessary to adequately image the lumpectomy site.
- Fat necrosis and fibrosis can mimic recurrent tumor. Biopsy may be necessary to differentiate the two, although MRI also is a valuable tool for this.
- Because of the similarity of ultrasonographic findings for scar and tumor, ultrasonography has a limited role to play in the management of these patients.

SUGGESTED READINGS

Chan HR, Bland KL. An overview of breast-conserving surgery in breast cancer treatment. *Breast J* 1995;**1**:91-5.

Dershaw DD. Breast Imaging and the conservative treatment of breast cancer. *Radiol Clin North Am* 2002;**40**:501-16.

Dershaw DD. Mammography in patients with breast cancer treated by breast conservation (lumpectomy with or without radiation). *Am J Roentgenol* 1995;**164**:309-16.

Kaplan J, Dershaw DD. Posttherapeutic magnetic resonance imaging. In: Morris EA, Liberman L, editors. *Breast MRI*. New York: Springer; 2005. p. 227-37.

Morrow M, Harris JR, editors. *Practice guideline for breast conservation therapy in the management of invasive breast carcinoma*. Reston, Va: Practice Guidelines and Technical Standards. American College of Radiology; 2006. p. 443-68.

Morrow M, Harris JR, editors. *Practice guideline for the management of ductal carcinoma in-situ of the breast (DCIS)*. Reston, Va: Practice Guidelines and Technical Standards. American College of Radiology; 2006. p. 469-93.

Recht A. Selecting patients for breast-conserving therapy. *Semin Breast Dis* 2001;**4**:198-206.

Schwartz GF, Veronesi U, Clough KB, Dixon JM, Fentiman IS, Heywang-Kobrunner SH, et al. Proceedings of the consensus conference on breast conservation, April 28 to May 1, 2005, Milan, Italy. *Cancer* 2006;107:242-50.

REFERENCES

1. Dershaw DD. Breast Imaging and the conservative treatment of breast cancer. *Radiol Clin North Am* 2002;**40**:501-16.
2. Borger J, Kemperman H, Hart A, Peterse H, van Dongen J, Bartelink H. Risk factors in breast-conservation therapy. *J Clin Oncol* 1994;**12**:653-60.
3. Hellman S, Harris JR. Breast Cancer: considerations in local and regional treatment. *Radiology* 1986;**164**:593-8.
4. Harris JR, Lippman ME, Veronesi U, Willett W. Medical progress: Breast Cancer (2). *N Engl J Med* 1992;**327**:390-8.
5. Dershaw DD. Mammography in patients with breast cancer treated by breast conservation (lumpectomy with or without radiation). *AJR Am J Roentgenol* 1995;**164**:309-16.
6. Morrow M, Strom EA, Bassett LW, Dershaw DD, Fowble B, Harris JR, et al. Standard for the management of ductal carcinoma in situ of breast. *CA Cancer J Clin* 2002;**52**:256-76.
7. Gluck BS, Dershaw DD, Liberman L, Deutch BM. Microcalcifications on postoperative mammograms as an indicator of adequacy of tumor excision. *Radiology* 1993;**188**:469-72.
8. Gefter WB, Friedman AK, Goodman RL. The role of mammography in evaluating patients with early carcinoma of the breast for tylectomy and radiation therapy. *Radiology* 1982;**142**:77-80.
9. Homer MJ, Schmidt-Ulrich R, Safaii H. Residual breast carcinoma after biopsy: role of mammography in evaluation. *Radiology* 1989;**170**:75-7.
10. Orel SG, Reynolds C, Schnall MD, Solin LJ, Fraker DL, Sullivan DC. Breast carcinoma: MR imaging before re-excisional biopsy. *Radiology* 1997;**205**:429-36.
11. Sonderson CE, Harms SE, Farrell Jr RS, Pruneda JM, Flamig DP. Detection with MR imaging of residual tumor in the breast soon after surgery. *AJR Am J Roentgenol* 1997;**168**:485-8.
12. Hassell PR, Olivotto IA, Mueller HA, Kingston GW, Basco VE. Early breast cancer: Detection of recurrence after conservative surgery and radiation therapy. *Radiology* 1990;**176**:731-5.
13. Rebner M, Pennes DR, Adler DD, Helvie MA, Lichter AS. Breast microcalcifications after lumpectomy and radiation therapy. *Radiology* 1989;**170**:691-3.
14. Harris KM, Costa-Greco MA, Baratz AB, Britton CA, Ilkhanipour ZS, Ganott MA. The mammographic features of the postlumpectomy, postirradiation breast. *Radiographics* 1989;**9**:253-68.
15. Dershaw DD, Shank B, Reisinger S. Mammographic findings after breast cancer treatment with local excision and definitive irradiation. *Radiology* 1987;**164**:455-61.
16. Heywane-Kobrunner SH, Schlegel A, Beck R, Wendt T, Kellner W, Lommatzsch B, et al. Contrast-enhanced MRI of the breast after limited surgery and radiation therapy. *J Comput Assist Tomogr* 1993;**17**:891-900.
17. Schnitt SJ, Connolly JL, Harris JR, Cohen RB. Radiation induced changes in the breast. *Hum Pathol* 1984;**15**:545-50.
18. Bloomer WD, Berenberg AL, Weissman BN. Mammography of the definitely irradiated breast. *Radiology* 1976;**118**:425-8.
19. Osborne MP, Borgen PL. Role of mastectomy in breast cancer. *Surg Clin North Am* 1990;**70**:1023-46.
20. Fowble B, Solin LJ, Schultz DJ, Rubenstein J, Goodman RL. Breast recurrence following conservative surgery and radiation: Patterns of failure, prognosis and pathologic findings from mastectomy specimens with implications for treatment. *Int J Radiat Oncol Biol Phys* 1990;**19**:833-42.
21. Kurtz JM, Almaric R, Brandone H, et al. Results of wide excision for local recurrence after breast-conserving therapy. *Cancer* 1988;**61**:1969-72.
22. Harris JR, Recht A. Conservative surgery and radiotherapy. In: Harris JR, Hellman S, Henderson IC, Kinne DW, editors. *Breast Diseases*. 2nd ed. Philadelphia: JB Lippincott; 1991. p. 388-419.
23. Dershaw DD, McCormick B, Osborne MP. Detection of local recurrence after conservative therapy for breast carcinoma. *Cancer* 1992;**70**:493-6.
24. Stomper PC, Recht A, Berenberg AL, Jochelson MS, Harris JR. Mammographic detection of recurrent cancer in the irradiated breast. *AJR Am J Roentgenol* 1987;**148**:39-43.
25. Kurtz JM, Amalric R, Brandone H, Ayme Y, Jacquemier J, Pietra JC, et al. Local recurrence after breast-conserving surgery and radiotherapy: frequency, time course and prognosis. *Cancer* 1989;**63**:1912-7.
26. Dershaw DD, McCormick B, Cox L, Osborne MP. Differentiation of benign and malignant local tumor recurrence after lumpectomy. *AJR Am J Roentgenol* 1990;**155**:35-8.
27. Liberman L, Dershaw DD, Durfee S, Abramson AF, Cohen MA, Hann LE, et al. Recurrent carcinoma after breast conservation: diagnosis with stereotaxic core biopsy. *Radiology* 1995;**197**:735-8.
28. Dao TH, Rahmouni A, Campana F, Laurent M, Asselain B, Fourquet A. Tumor recurrence versus fibrosis in the irradiated breast: differentiation with dynamic gadolinium-enhanced MR imaging. *Radiology* 1993;**187**:751-5.
29. Baker JA, Soo MS, Rosen E. Artifacts and pitfalls in sonographic imaging of the breast. *AJR Am J Roentgenol* 2001;**176**:1261-6.

CHAPTER 35

The Augmented Breast

Nanette D. DeBruhl, Dawn C. Nwamuo, and David P. Gorczyca

METHODS OF BREAST AUGMENTATION AND RECONSTRUCTION

During the last century, many different methods were used for augmentation and reconstruction of the breast. Unfortunately, the majority of the methods attempted were disappointing and were sometimes associated with adverse complications.[1-3] Methods for augmentation and reconstruction of the breast can be divided into the following three different groups: (1) autogenous tissue transplantation; (2) injectable materials; and (3) implanted prostheses. This chapter deals with the latter two types of augmentation.

Injectable Materials

Beginning in the late 1800s, a variety of different materials were injected into the breast for augmentation purposes. Paraffin was one of the earliest such materials, and demonstrated some success. Several other materials, including fat, mineral oil and Vaseline were also injected. All had unacceptable cosmetic outcomes and complications. The complications of injected materials ranged from granulomatous and inflammatory reactions, which presented clinically as breast lumps, skin necrosis, pulmonary embolism, and even death.[1]

The injection of liquid silicone into the breast was reportedly first attempted in Japan in the late 1940s.[2] By the 1960s this method was very popular in the United States, however, it too became associated with complications similar to the other injectables. The most notable complications included migration of silicone in fascial planes, thickening, breast lumps, and deformity.[3] Silicone injections into the breast over time resulted in palpable masses that mimicked carcinoma. The problem of differentiating these silicone granulomas from cancerous tumor was further complicated by the limited visualization of the parenchyma on mammograms of patients with silicone injections (Fig. 35-1). Other imaging modalities including ultrasound, computed tomography (CT) and magnetic resonance imaging (MRI) have all been tried as a alternative methods for evaluating the silicone granuloma. Each modality has its limitations. Ultrasound can distinguish silicone granuloma from mass if associated with an implant; however, it is essentially useless in a breast that has had a large amount of silicone injections. CT may identify implant rupture; however, silicone granulomas are difficult to distinguish on CT compared with the surrounding breast tissue. If intravenous contrast is given, CT can identify occult cancers as enhancing lesions relative to surrounding parenchymal tissue. MRI has been shown to be the most valuable in imaging implant rupture, silicone granulomas, and occult tumors and has the added benefit of no radiation.

Currently, dynamic contrast-enhanced (DCE) magnetic resonance imaging has been shown to be the best method for screening women for breast cancer in whom the other imaging modalities are not effective. For further discussion, see Chapter 12, MRI Indications and Interpretation.

Implantable Prostheses

The 1950s also saw the first use of synthetic implantable sponge prostheses. The first implantable prosthesis was composed of polyvinyl alcohol (Ivalon). The results of this new method of breast augmentation were initially promising. Unfortunately, the development of abundant reactive scar tissue caused these implants to have a hard consistency and to actually shrink over time.

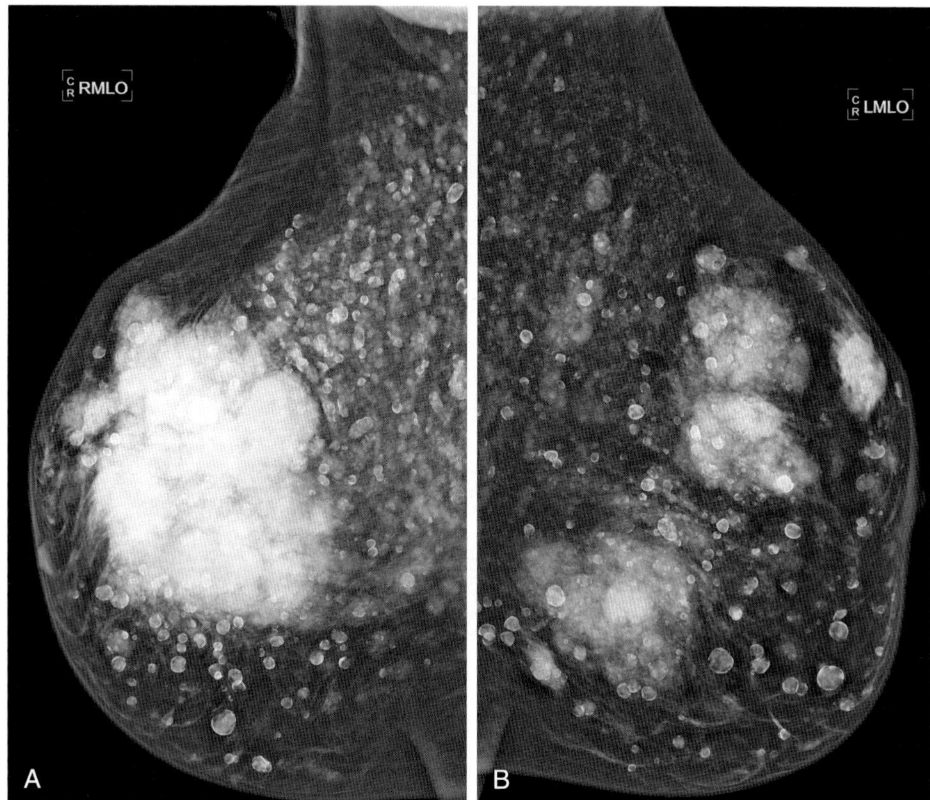

■ **FIGURE 35-1** Silicone injections. **A,B.** Bilateral digital mediolateral oblique (MLO) mammograms demonstrating silicone injections forming eggshell calcifications surrounding granulomas throughout the breast and axillae.

Undaunted, investigators tried other synthetic materials, such as etheron, polyether polyurethane, polypropylene, and even polytef (Teflon). All of these implants eventually had complications, including undesirable cosmetic effects.[1,3]

In 1963, Cronin and Gerow[4] described the first use of a silicone gel prosthesis. This method revolutionized plastic surgery of the breast. The majority of silicone implants are composed of an outer membrane made of silicone that surrounds and contains the silicone gel. The composition of the silicone membrane is an elastic polymer of silicone. It is the "liquid" silicone gel within the membrane that gives the implant its desirable feel and mobility. Manufacturers initially developed two basic types of breast implants: single chambered silicone gel and inflatable saline implants (Fig. 35-2). Saline implants could either be prefilled with sterile saline or filled at the time of surgery (Fig. 35-3). The variations of style, size, and texture with silicone or saline implants were quite extensive. Many were customized by the plastic surgeons, and new models were continuously introduced and discontinued by the manufacturers.[1,5] Each model type had its own set of problems that potentially could occur. One popular variation combined the two basic types and consisted of an inner silicone gel chamber surrounded by an outer saline chamber. This model is known as a dual chamber or double lumen implant (Fig. 35-4). Variations of this model type were also manufactured.

By 1993, it was estimated that more than 1. 5 million American women had had either breast augmentation or reconstruction with silicone and saline implants.[3]

According to recent data, American women are having increasing numbers of breast augmentation and reconstructive procedures. In 1997, there were reportedly about 100,000 breast augmentations performed and 27,000 reconstructive surgeries, compared with 2008 when there were more than 300,000 augmentations and more than 79,000 reconstruction procedures performed. Of those women who had augmentation in 2008, 53% of the implants were saline and 47% were silicone gel prosthesis. In the reconstructive group, American women had surgeries using autologous tissue (muscle flaps and fat), implants or both.[6]

For augmentation mammoplasty, implants are usually placed either anterior (subglandular) or posterior (subpectoral) to the pectoralis major muscle or in a dual plane position that is between the pectoralis major muscle and the pectoralis minor muscle. Insertion of a subglandular implant requires less complicated and less expensive surgery. The surgical insertion of sub-pectoral implants is technically more difficult, but sub-pectoral implants interfere less with visualization of the breast tissue at mammography, have a lower incidence of capsular contractures, and are associated with less obvious surgical scars.[1,3]

Imaging Indications and Algorithm

Silicone Breast Implants

As indicated previously, silicone breast prostheses have been manufactured for more than 40 years. There has been an evolution of breast implants from the first

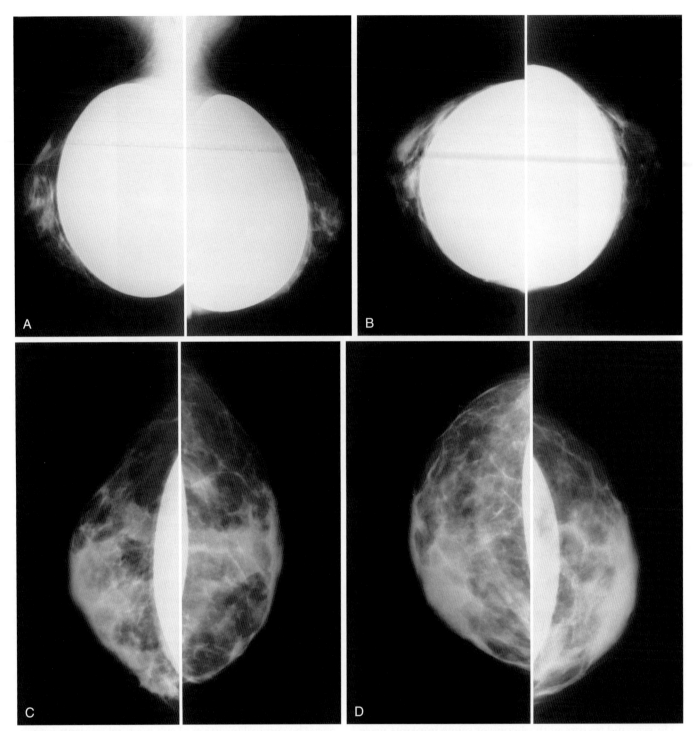

■ **FIGURE 35-2** Subglandular silicone implant. Implant-included mammograms, mediolateral oblique (MLO) (**A**) and subglandular saline implant (MLO) (**B**) mammographic views performed with moderate compression, required manual technique because the implants were over the photocell. Ninety-degree lateral medial (LM) (**C**) and craniocaudal (CC) implant-included (**D**) mammographic views allow for compression of tissue anterior to implants and can be done with automatic exposure control as long as the breast tissue covers the photocell completely.

generation type reported by Cronin that had thick gel and shell, to more viscous gel, with thinner shells to the latest fifth generation cohesive gel implant with a near solid gel and thicker layered shell.[7] During the early years as the various models were manufactured for augmentation and reconstruction, complications with silicone implants were frequent. These complications included rupture and leakage, migration of silicone through fascial planes, fibrous or calcific contracture of the tissue capsule that forms around the implant, localized pain, and paresthesias.[3,7]

As a result of reported complications, in 1992 the U.S. Food and Drug Administration (FDA) restricted the use of silicone gel implants.[1,8] Silicone gel-filled implants were allowed on the market only under controlled clinical adjunct studies for reconstruction after mastectomy,

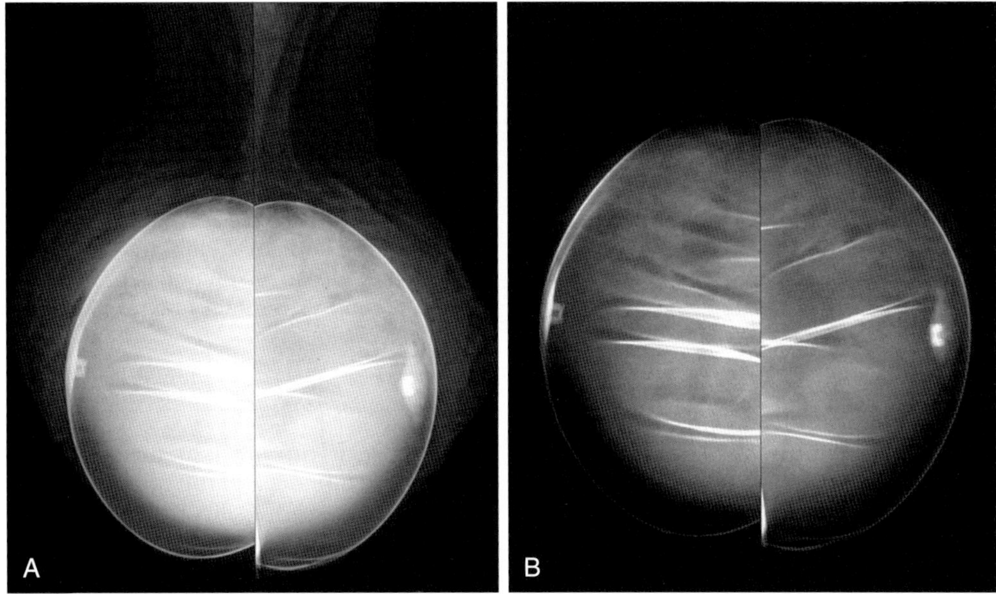

■ **FIGURE 35-3** Subpectoral implants. **A,** Digital mammographic mediolateral (MLO) images of saline implants in the implant-included view optimized for imaging soft tissues. **B,** Digital mammogram with windowing and leveling, which optimizes the image of the implant.

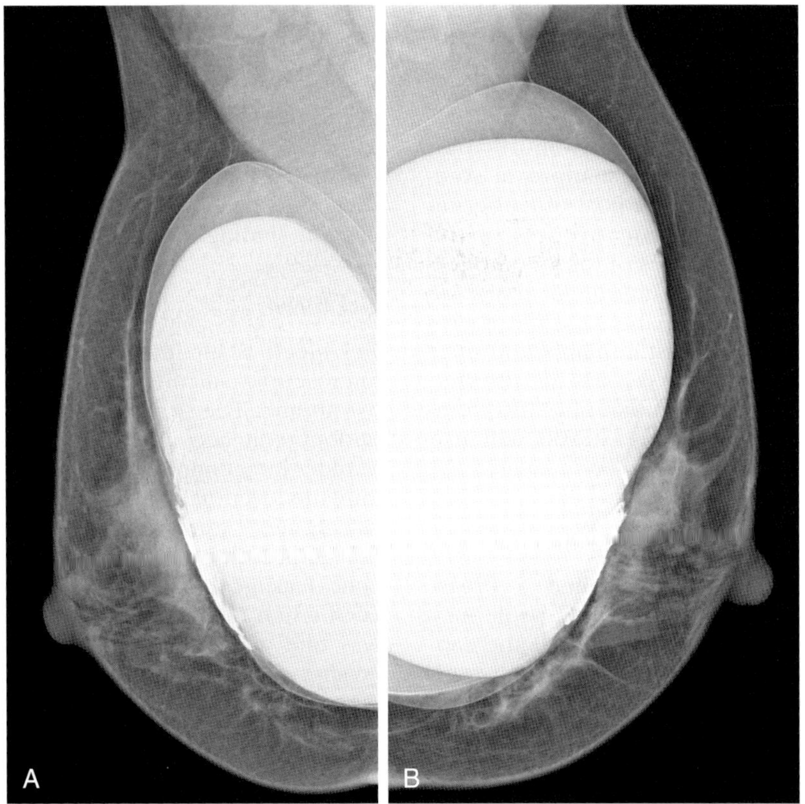

■ **FIGURE 35-4** Subpectoral dual chamber (double lumen) implants, **A**, **B**. Digital mammographic images of saline outer chamber and silicone inner chamber implants (mediolateral oblique views) with dense peri-implant calcifications in the anterior aspect at the level of the nipple.

correction of congenital deformities, or replacement of silicone gel-filled implants that were ruptured, for medical or surgical reasons. The use of implants for cosmetic enhancement or augmentation was postponed until the results of the adjunct studies were reported.

Silicone alternatives were also marketed during this time, but quickly fell out of favor because of increases in rupture rate and inflammatory reactions from the rupture contents of hydrogel products, hydroxypropyl cellulose, and those from guar gum, povidone, and soya bean.[7]

The much-publicized debate in the early 1990s over the association of connective tissue and autoimmune disorders including fibromyalgia with intact and ruptured silicone gel implants were not substantiated. Numerous studies could not find a direct cause and effect link to silicone implants to explain the affected women's symptoms.[9]

While the manufacturers were conducting the required studies, saline-filled breast implants remained on the market and were used for both reconstructive and augmentation procedures. By the year 2000, saline implants were given premarket approval by the FDA. This allowed the approved manufacturers to market these implants without informed consent of consumers.

In 1998, research conducted by individual manufacturers allowed a limited number of patients to participate in breast augmentation with silicone implants through investigational device exemption (IDE) studies. These studies required informed consent from women who would receive the implants through a protocol or plan that had been approved by a research site's review board, which was to be composed of scientists, health professionals, and community members.

In 2005, the FDA approved the silicone gel-filled breast implants for marketing with a number of conditions. The conditions included: continuation of its core study to complete a 10 year investigation by tracking each implant using MR imaging of the implants every other year; laboratory evaluation to characterize types of device failure; and dissemination of product-information updates to physicians and patients. Post-approval studies are expected to continue with the goal of gathering information about the safety and effectiveness of the implants. Evaluation will include rates of local complications, connective tissue disease, and neurological disease including all signs and symptoms; and possible reproductive effects in women with breast implants, and their children. Rates of cancer, suicide, reports of interference of breast implants with mammography, MRI compliance rates and rupture rates on breast MRI will also be tracked.[10]

Encapsulation of Silicone Gel Implants

A fibrous capsule invariably forms around a breast implant after it is placed in the breast. The capsule may be soft and impalpable or hard and resistant. If the capsule becomes hardened, the breast is likely to have an undesirable contour and feel.[11] Encapsulation of the implant with scar tissue has been the most common clinical problem associated with a silicone or saline implant that is often associated with breast pain and deformity. The reported causes were numerous: infection, hematomas, and foreign body reaction. Some suggested silicone gel migration through the implant shell was also a cause.[7] Closed capsulotomy, a procedure by which the surgeon uses vigorous manual compression to disrupt a hard fibrous capsule, was once used to restore the more natural feeling of the augmented breast. Closed capsulotomy is no longer performed because of its association with significant herniations and rupture of silicone breast implants.[11]

Rupture

Implant rupture can be divided into two major categories: intracapsular and extracapsular.[12]

Intracapsular Rupture

The most common type, intracapsular rupture is a rupture or tear of the implant membrane (elastomer envelope) that allows the release of silicone gel. The extruded silicone gel is contained by an intact fibrous capsule, surrounding the shell or envelope.

Extracapsular Rupture

Extracapsular rupture is defined as rupture of both the implant membrane and the fibrous capsule, which leads to extravasation of the silicone into the surrounding breast tissue.

Implant rupture has been postulated to be the result of several factors. Some suggest the tear in the silicone shell or envelope occurs at the time of surgery secondary to the technique used or an inadvertent puncture, or both. Another cause may be from prolonged focal folding that ultimately weakens the outer shell.[13] Common areas for this folding are along the medial or lateral chest wall. The third cause may be prosthetic fatigue and this occurs from a natural breakdown of the envelope. The imaging findings of rupture from any of these causes may not be evident for several years, as it may take time for the silicone shell to collapse from the weight of the free silicone between the shell and the fibrous capsule. Thus, there is spectrum of imaging findings depending on the age of the rupture.

Gel Bleed

Gel bleed is an interesting phenomenon. It represents microscopic silicone leakage through an intact implant membrane. This leakage across the silicone membrane undoubtedly accounted for the sticky feel on the surface of older intact implants. It was believed that most, if not all implants eventually have some gel bleed, but the bleed is usually not extensive enough to be detectable. Although not detectable, a patient was potentially exposed to silicone leakage into the breast and throughout the body even when her silicone implants were intact. This theory was one of the reasons the double lumen implant was developed. By placing a saline outer chamber over an inner silicone chamber, a barrier was created to reduce the diffusion of silicone gel to the surrounding tissues. The idea of silicone migration was supported by reports of free silicone with lymph nodes and other organs with intact and ruptured implants.[7,14] Whether gel bleed is ever great enough to be detectable by imaging methods was and still is controversial. Some investigators have reported visualization of silicone outside the membrane on MRI and ultrasound without evidence of a rupture of the silicone membrane and have attributed this finding to excessive gel bleed.[13] Other investigators believe that occult tears in the silicone membrane are present whenever this phenomenon occurs and that these tears can be found if the surgeon looks carefully enough.[15]

IMAGING TECHNIQUE AND FINDINGS

Imaging After Breast Implants

Mammography

Women with silicone breast implants are not at increased risk for development of breast cancer, so regular mammography screening is recommended at intervals appropriate for the woman's age. However, the presence of silicone implants usually limits the amount of tissue that can be visualized on mammograms. Clinical reports have suggested a possible delay in breast cancer diagnosis, but epidemiologic studies have not supported these claims.[16]

It is important to emphasize that the proper mammographic positioning of the breasts of women with silicone gel implants requires that radiologic technologists have special training and experience. In general, more tissue can be visualized in the mammograms of women with subpectoral implants than in the mammograms of women with subglandular implants. Special views called implant-displaced (ID) views have been developed to better visualize the breast tissue anterior to a silicone breast implant.[17]

Mammography of women with subglandular implants requires the use of the ID views, or "push-back" views, whenever possible (see Fig. 35-2). Implant-included views are performed first through the use of only moderate compression. ID views are done next. The posterior displacement of the implant during the ID maneuvers allows for greater compression of the tissue anterior to the implants and also provides an opportunity to visualize more breast tissue.[17] ID views cannot be performed if an implant is hard and fixed, a change due to exuberant formation of the fibrous capsule that prevents mobility of the implant.

Imaging implants with digital mammography has markedly reduced the number of additional exposures needed, because the modality enables the operator to "window" and level the post-acquisition images at the console and at the workstation.[18] The surrounding tissue and implants can be evaluated independently with the window and leveling technique, improving overall visualization (see Fig. 35-3).

There are a few case reports and incidents submitted to the FDA of implant rupture due to mammography compression.[19] Although new, non-implanted silicone gel implants can withstand considerable mammographic compression, it is suspected that over time, implanted silicone gel implants may be subject to fatigue and trauma, making them more vulnerable to mammographic compression. Therefore, radiologists should at least be aware of the potential for implant rupture during mammography and should have a protocol within their facilities to deal with any complications that may arise. Clinical signs of implant rupture include palpable silicone nodules, decreased breast size, asymmetry, tenderness, and a change in texture of the implant. Breakage of the fibrous capsule around the implant may occur with compression and may be accompanied by an audible "pop." Thus, mammographic compression can potentially convert an intracapsular rupture—one contained by the fibrous capsule—to an extracapsular rupture if the fibrous capsule is broken.

The American College of Radiology has not to date suggested the use of signed informed consent prior to imaging implants, but does encourage providing educational information to such women.[20]

Mammographic findings that may be encountered in women with implants are as follows: (1) a measurable peri-prosthetic dense band or rim of tissue that corresponds to the fibrous capsule around the implant; (2) peri-prosthetic calcification; (3) peri-implant fluid collections; (4) asymmetry of implant size or shape; (5) focal herniations of the implant; and (6) implant rupture with deflation of the envelope and extravasation of silicone beyond the membrane[21] (see Figs. 35-4 and 35-5). Free silicone in the breast may manifest as a dense mass, linear streaks, or lymph node opacification (see Fig. 35-5).

Mammography for the Evaluation of Implant Rupture

Rupture of a saline implant is clinically obvious, because the implant deflates rapidly. The body quickly absorbs the saline, so that by the time a woman undergoes imaging, only a collapsed outer membrane is visible on mammography (Fig. 35-6). Ultrasonography and MRI are not required for the diagnosis of a saline implant rupture.

Because clinical examination may fail to disclose an implant rupture and its extent, radiologists often are asked to evaluate the integrity of breast prostheses. In our experience, mammography has not been useful

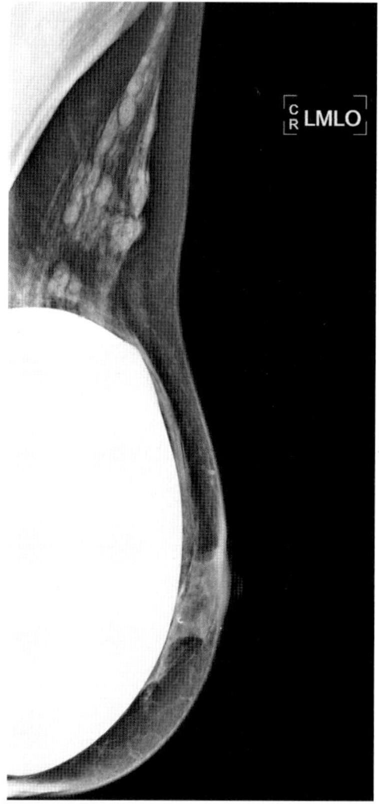

■ **FIGURE 35-5** Silicone adenopathy. Left mediolateral oblique (MLO) digital mammogram of subpectoral silicone implant associated with dense silicone laden lymph nodes.

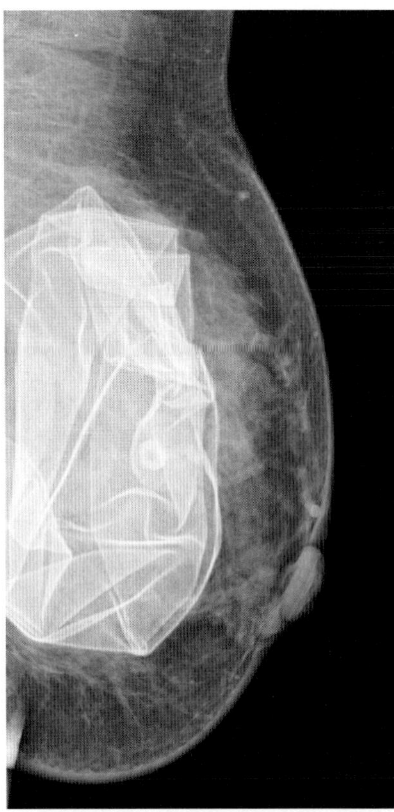

■ **FIGURE 35-6** Digital left mediolateral oblique (MLO) view of deflated saline implant.

in the detection of intracapsular implant rupture, the more common type of rupture. Although mammography can identify free silicone after an extracapsular silicone implant rupture, the silicone may be obscured by the overlying implant. After the removal of ruptured silicone implants, there may be residual silicone in the form of granulomas that appear as dense masses in the breast tissue (Fig. 35-7). These granulomas may be confused with breast lesions. Another source of confusion may occur if the implants were replaced and the granulomas not removed. If the prior films or history were not available at the time of imaging it would be difficult to prove the current implants were intact and not the source of free silicone.

Because of the limitations of clinical breast examination and mammography in the evaluation of breast implants, MRI and ultrasonography have been investigated as adjunctive methods for the evaluation of implants, especially for the identification of rupture.

Magnetic Resonance Imaging

MRI has proved to be the most accurate method for the detection of breast implant ruptures.[22,23] Familiarity with the MRI characteristics of silicone is helpful in understanding the MRI sequences that are used to distinguish silicone from surrounding breast parenchyma. The chemical composition of most medical-grade silicones is dimethylpolysiloxane with varying degrees of polymerization.[1,24] The MRI signal is derived from the protons of the methyl groups.

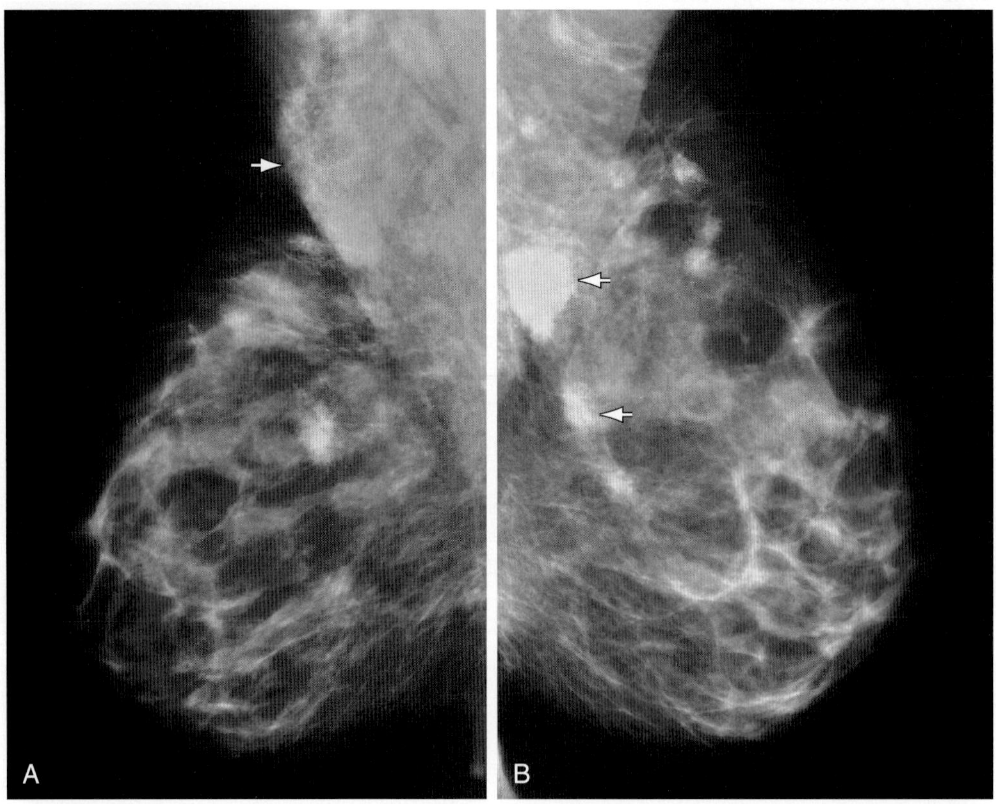

■ **FIGURE 35-7** Residual silicone after removal of ruptured implants. Right (**A**) and left (**B**) mediolateral oblique (MLO) mammograms obtained several years after explantation show multiple dense, irregular masses (*arrows,* **B**), which are silicone granulomas. Silicone can be seen to have extended into the axilla on the right (*arrow,* **A**).

The implant membrane is also composed of silicone but differs from the gel in chemical structure because of the many additional cross-linkages between the methyl groups, resulting in an elastic solid. Although the implant membrane is composed of silicone, only minimal MRI signal is produced from the membrane (envelope, shell) because of these additional methyl groups' cross-linkages.

Technical Factors

A variety of pulse sequences are available for imaging silicone implants. In general, the selection of MRI pulse sequences used to image breast implants is determined by the relative Larmor precession frequencies, as well as the T1 and T2 properties of the tissues (fat, water, and silicone). The relative resonance frequency of silicone is approximately 100 Hz lower than that of fat and 320 Hz lower than that of water at 1.5 Tesla (T) (Fig. 35-8). Because the resonance frequency of silicone is close to that of fat, the MRI signal from silicone behaves similarly to that of fat when chemical suppression techniques (chemical fat or water suppression) are applied. As a result, the silicone signal is high when chemical water suppression is used and low when chemical fat suppression is used. Table 35-1 presents a summary of the relative signal intensities of silicone, fat, and water with different pulse sequences.

One can use MRI sequences that selectively emphasize the signal from silicone by taking advantage of the different relative relaxation times of fat, silicone, and water. The relaxation time of fat is shorter than that of silicone. Therefore, one can use this difference to suppress the fat signal while maintaining a strong signal from silicone. It has been found that the use of an inversion recovery sequence with a short inversion time (short-tau inversion recovery [STIR]) suppresses the signal from fat while maintaining high signal from silicone.[14,25] The use of a chemical water-suppression pulse in conjunction with a STIR sequence results in a silicone-selective sequence.

Imaging Protocols

In our practice, the patient undergoing MRI lies prone with the breasts in a dedicated dual-breast coil. The 1.5 or 3.0 T superconducting magnet is used to acquire the images. There is one basic protocol for scanning implants and that is axial and sagittal imaging of both breasts using T2 weighted sequences with and without water suppression. The protocol is modified depending on the type of scanner used to acquire the images. Currently we use both General Electric (GE) and Siemens MRI units. An initial 30-second two-dimensional (2D) 3-plane scout image is taken to ensure the breasts have been properly positioned. The second sequence is a 2 to 3 minute axial fast inversion recovery (IR)(GE) or integrated parallel acquisition technique (iPAT) or Blade (3.0T)(Siemens) T2 weighted series without water saturation. The last sequence is an 8 to 10 minute sagittal fast IR (GE) or turbo inversion recovery (Siemens) of both breasts with water suppression. To achieve adequate water suppression for the sagittal images we pre-scan the breast automatically, and then perform a manual pre-scan for the evaluation of the water, fat and silicone peaks. If needed, the water peak will be suppressed using manual technique (see Fig. 35-8).

The parameters for the axial images on average use a 320 × 192 matrix or higher, 1 number of excitations (NEX) acquisition, with a slice thickness of 3 to 4 mm with a 1 mm skip to cover the entire implant. For sagittal imaging,

TABLE 35-1. Signal Intensities of Silicone, Fat, and Water with Different Magnetic Resonance Imaging (MRI) Pulse Sequences for Evaluation of Silicone Implants

	Signal Intensity		
MRI Sequence	**Silicone**	**Fat**	**Water**
Fast spin echo (FSE) T2-weighted (TR/TE >5000/200)	High	Medium	Very high
FSE with water suppression	High	Medium	Low
Inversion recovery FSE (IRFSE) (TR/TE >5000/90, TI = 150)	High	Low	Very high
IRFSE with water suppression	High	Low	Low

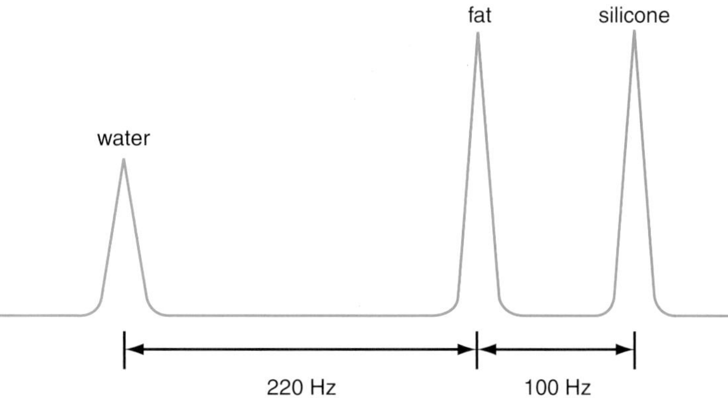

■ **FIGURE 35-8** Relative resonance frequencies of water, fat, and silicone at 1.5 Tesla (T). The resonance frequency of silicone is approximately 320 Hz lower than that of water and 100 Hz lower than that of fat.

a 256 × 192 matrix or higher, 2 NEX and a slice thickness of 4 to 5 mm with a 1-mm skip to cover the entire implant is used.

Frequency direction is anterior to posterior (AP) on axial images and right to left (RL) for sagittal images to reduce the artifact created by heart motion in the phase-encoding direction. We prefer scanning in axial and sagittal planes and using T2 weighted scans. However, some institutions and practices also use the coronal plane and T1 imaging. The IR sequence, designed to suppress signal from fat, increases the conspicuity of the silicone implant and the extravasation of silicone gel within the tissues. We do not add fat suppression as part of the silicone-specific sequences, as the suppression of the breast tissue with the IR imaging is more than adequate. Heavily T2-weighted fast spin echo (FSE) images can also be used; the echo time (TE) should be set at approximately 200 to decrease the signal from the breast adipose tissue while keeping the signal from the silicone fairly high.

This examination requires 20 to 30 minutes to complete, depending on the number of sequences performed and patient set-up time. We always give a contrast agent as part of the breast tissue evaluation, for occult cancers could be present. Imaging of the implants without contrast should only be performed if the patient is fully aware that the study is optimized for the evaluation of silicone and not breast parenchyma, thus potentially missing occult cancers. If silicone only imaging is to be performed, it may be best to have signed informed consent to ensure the patient understands the difference in imaging and the limitations of evaluating for cancer if contrast is not given.

Appearance of Normal Implants

On MRI, a normal single-lumen silicone implant contains homogeneous high-signal-intensity silicone (Fig. 35-9). A double-lumen silicone implant typically has an inner lumen of high-signal-intensity silicone surrounded by a smaller outer lumen that contains saline with different signal intensities, depending on the pulse sequence (see Table 32-1; Fig. 35-10). A variety of other types of implantable prostheses are occasionally encountered that alter the MRI appearance; they include expander implants, reverse double-lumen implants (saline in the inner lumen, silicone in the outer lumen), multicompartmental implants (silicone in silicone), foam implants, and single-lumen silicone implants into which saline was injected into a posterior compartment or directly into the silicone gel at the time of surgery.

Two or more implants placed in one breast, one on top of the other, are commonly known as *stacked implants*.[13] Some implants in the past had a coating of polyurethane covering the surface of the silicone envelope. A moderate to large amount of reactive fluid typically surrounded such an implant. This type of implant was discontinued in the United States in 1991 due to fragmentation of the coating. There have been recent reports this implant coating may be tried again.

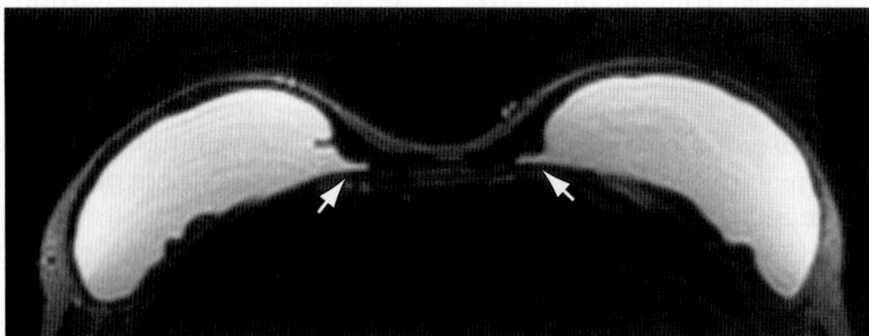

■ **FIGURE 35-9** Axial T2-weighted magnetic resonance (MR) images showing intact subpectoral single-lumen silicone implants. Finger-like projections are shown medially. This finding, which has been reported as the rat-tail sign (*arrows*), is not associated with implant rupture.

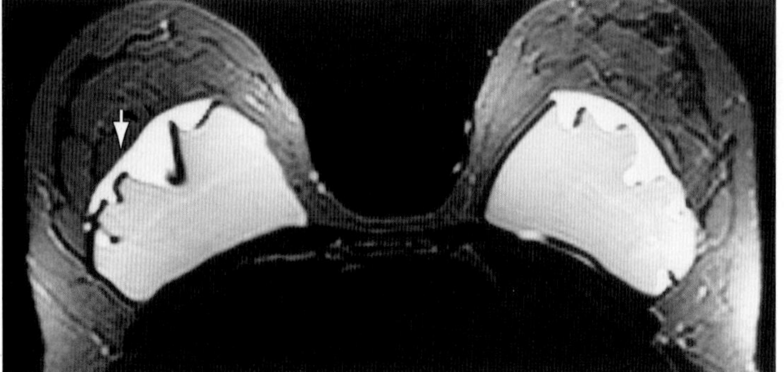

■ **FIGURE 35-10** Axial T2-weighted magnetic resonance (MR) image (without water suppression) of breasts, with bilateral intact double-lumen implants. The saline outer chambers (*arrow*) have higher signal intensity than the inner chambers containing silicone gel.

One of the most commonly encountered mammographic findings in normal implants is the presence of prominent radial folds that represent normal infolding of the Silastic elastomer membrane (Fig. 35-11). The folds may be prominent enough to suggest an appearance of implant rupture. However, even very prominent radial folds can be recognized as such because they extend to the periphery of the implant and are relatively few in number (see Fig. 35-11).

Signs of Intracapsular Rupture

Linguine Sign and Subcapsular Line Sign

The most reliable sign of intracapsular rupture on MRI is the presence of multiple, curvilinear low signal intensity lines within the high signal intensity silicone gel, the so-called linguine sign[22] (Fig. 35-12). These curvilinear lines represent the collapsed implant membrane that seems to be floating within the silicone gel.

In the very early stages, the curvilinear lines may be found close to the periphery of the implant rather than centrally located. This finding is known as the subcapsular line sign[26] (Fig. 35-13). Phase encoding artifacts caused by motion of the patient can be misinterpreted as the subcapsular sign if located in the anterior periphery of the implant. Changing the direction of the phase encoding direction on a repeat scan, or the same direction of the phase with less motion can confirm the finding or resolve the artifact. A type of multi-compartment implant (silicone in silicone) may also be misinterpreted as the subcapsular sign (Fig. 35-14).

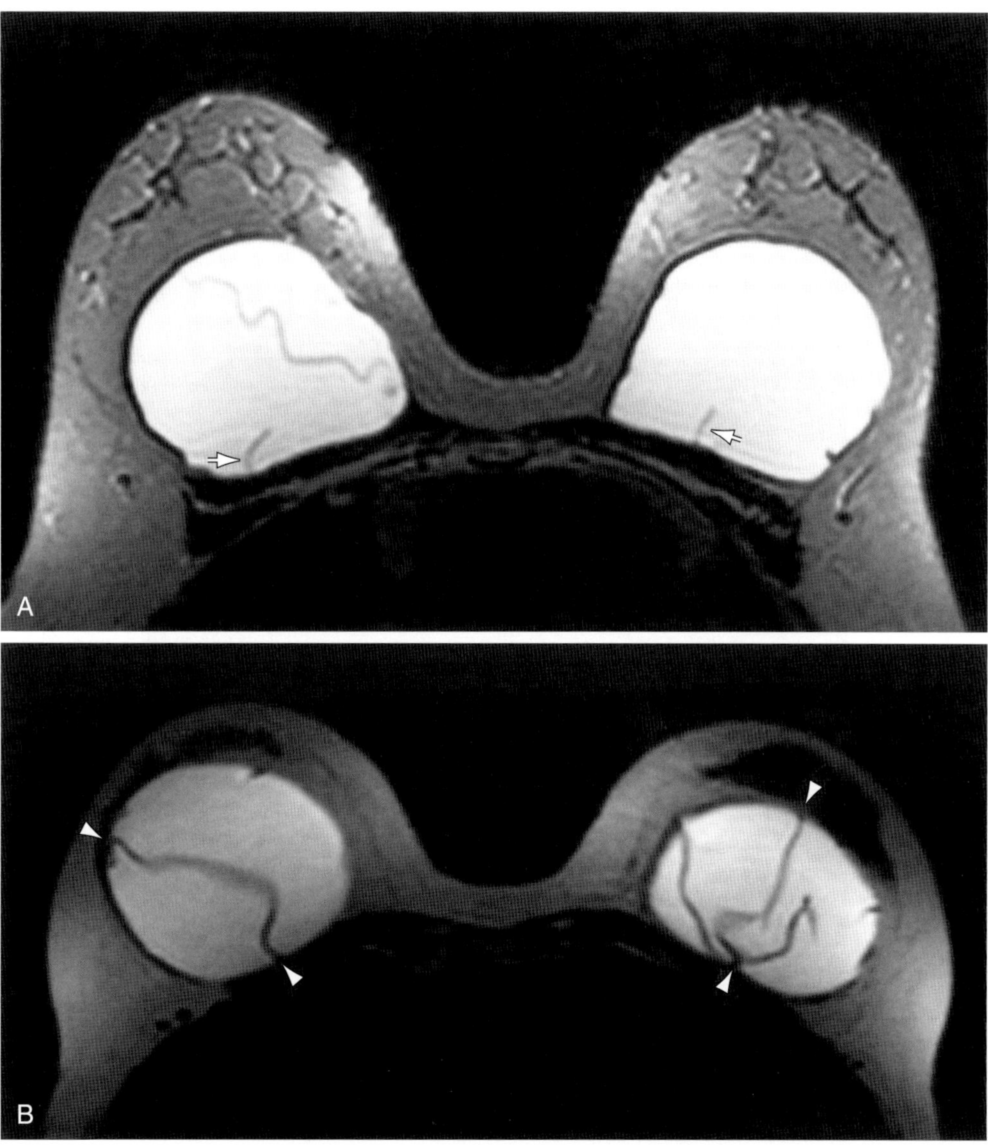

■ **FIGURE 35-11** Radial folds. **A**, Magnetic resonance (MR) axial T2-weighted fast spin echo (FSE) image with water suppression shows a normal implant with bilateral low signal intensity radial folds (*arrows*) that extend to the periphery of the implant. **B**, MR axial T2-weighted FSE image with water suppression shows prominent radial folds in a single-lumen implant. Radial folds can be distinguished from a collapsed implant shell because the folds extend to the periphery of the implant and are usually few in number (*arrowheads*).

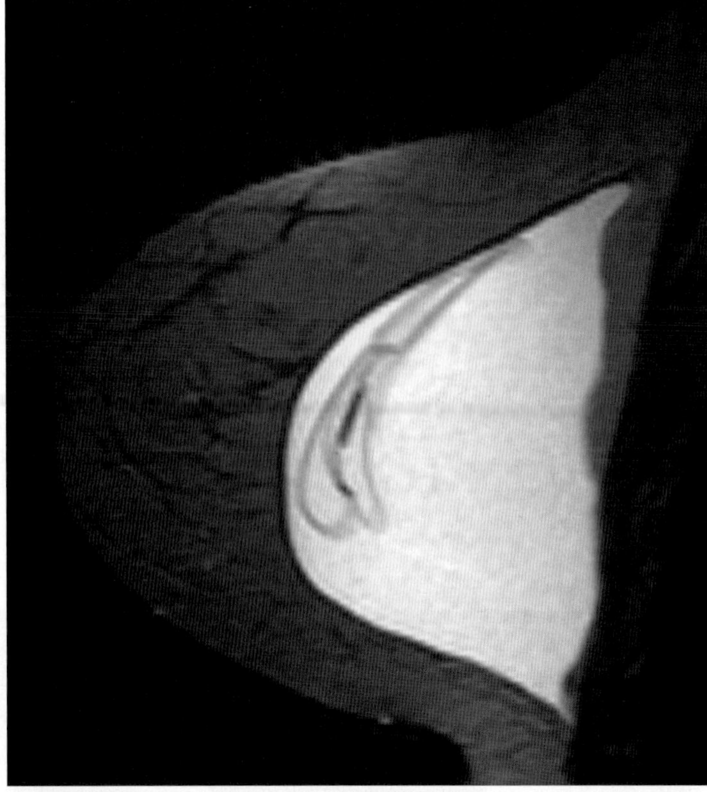

■ **FIGURE 35-12** Intracapsular rupture. Sagittal short-tau inversion recovery (STIR) T2-weighted magnetic resonance (MR) image shows multiple curvilinear low signal intensity lines within the left implant (linguine sign), representing a collapsed implant shell.

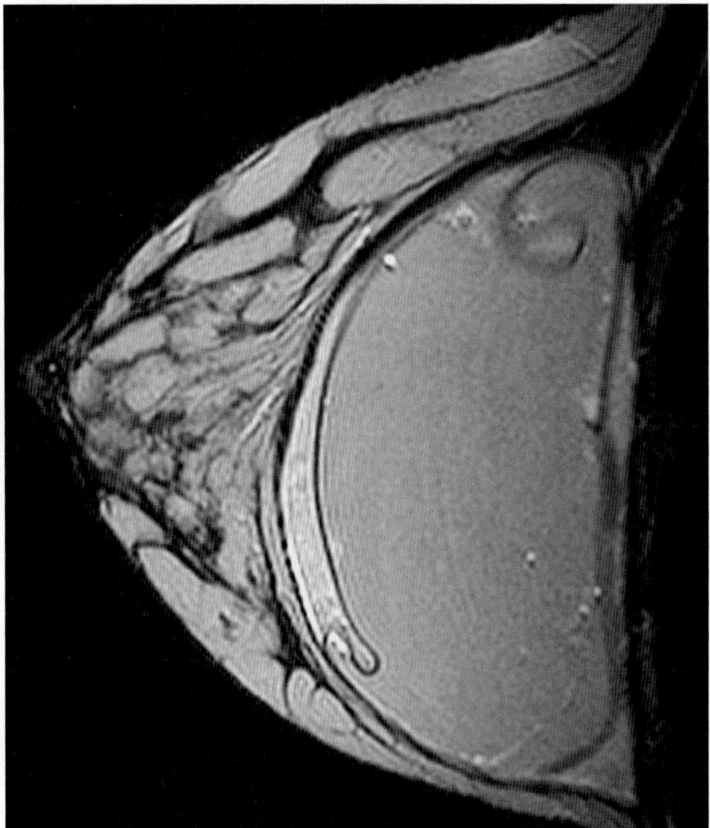

■ **FIGURE 35-13** Subcapsular line. Sagittal magnetic resonance (MR) image of subpectoral silicone implant with a linear low intensity line along the anterior aspect of the implant indicating early intracapsular rupture.

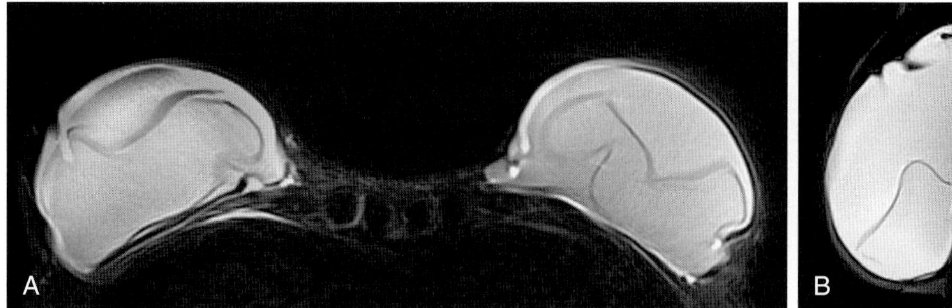

■ **FIGURE 35-14** Multi-compartment implant. **A,** Axial short-tau inversion recovery (STIR) magnetic resonance (MR) image of bilateral intact subpectoral silicone implants with silicone outer chamber and silicone inner chamber. Inner chamber may be mistaken for subcapsular line. **B,** Sagittal STIR MR image of right implant with a thick linear line delineating the inner silicone chamber.

Teardrop, Keyhole, or Noose Sign

The teardrop, keyhole, or noose sign is sometimes the only indication of implant rupture.[13,22,23,26] This sign represents silicone that has leaked out of the ruptured silicone implant and entered one of the radial folds on the exterior of the implant (Fig. 35-15). Whether this finding may exclusively result from a small tear or be associated with gel bleed from an intact implant has been controversial.

Inconclusive Signs of Intracapsular Rupture

Water Droplets

The appearance of multiple round hyper-intense foci within the implant lumen on T2-weighted images or multiple hypo-intense foci on water-suppression images within the gel of ruptured implants is known as the droplet sign[27] (Fig. 35-16). These water droplets can alone be an early sign of implant rupture or a result of inadvertent breach of the implant shell during injections of steroid, saline or povidone-iodine at the time of placement to reduce capsular contractures. Folding of the implant may also cause a weakening in the implant and the droplets can be focally located within the implant. If imaging is early, this may be the only finding. In our practice, we have seen numerous cases in which these small water droplets have been present in patients with intact implants. These finding have been noted to be more common in the older implants placed prior to 1995. If the findings for rupture are indeterminate, follow-up MRI can be performed in 6 to 12 month intervals to confirm progression or stability of findings.

Contour Deformities

Bulges and other contour deformities are not reliable signs of implant rupture and may be seen with intact implants. Finger-like medial projections along the chest wall—the rat-tail sign—can be mistaken for signs of implant rupture[23] (see Fig. 35-9).

Fluid on the Periphery of the Implant

Fluid may be seen around the periphery of intact implants and therefore is not considered a sign of rupture. This fluid may represent saline in the outer component of a double-lumen implant or, possibly, reactive fluid in surrounding tissue (Fig. 35-17).

Signs of Extracapsular Rupture

The presence of free silicone in the breast parenchyma is the definitive sign of an extracapsular rupture. On MRI, free silicone appears as focal areas of high signal

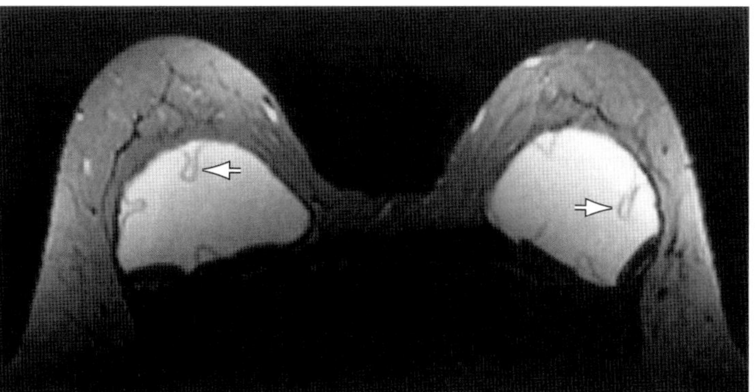

■ **FIGURE 35-15** Teardrop sign. Magnetic resonance (MR) axial T2-weighted image shows bilateral subpectoral implants with radial folds (*arrows*) containing silicone gel. At surgery, silicone gel was seen outside the implant shells. Careful inspection revealed a small tear in each implant shell.

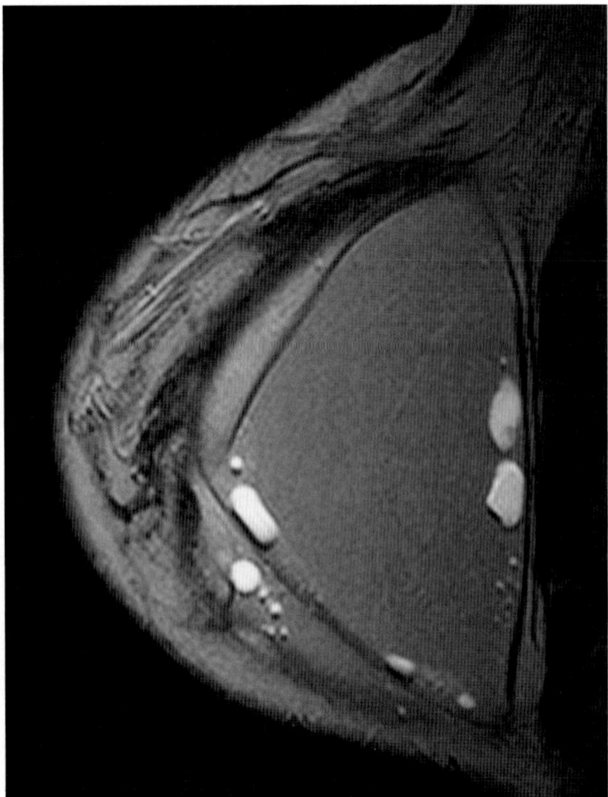

■ **FIGURE 35-16** Water droplet sign. Round fluid collections with high signal on magnetic resonance (MR) T2 imaging. Sagittal MR image of a breast implant with high signal intensity within the implant.

intensity outside the confines of the implant[14,23,27] (Fig. 35-18). Because of its multi-planar capabilities and its ability to identify even small foci of silicone, MRI can provide precise localization of free silicone deposits in the breast and surrounding structures. However, previous silicone injections or silicone remaining from a previous rupture of a silicone implant that has been removed can give rise to the same finding, so careful history-taking is essential before the diagnosis of extracapsular implant rupture is made.

Signs of intracapsular rupture are expected to be present in extracapsular rupture. For example, the linguine sign, the most reliable sign of intracapsular rupture, is almost always seen in extracapsular rupture

While the implant controversy and ultimate restrictions on silicone implants in the 1990s primarily affected the United States, many countries in Europe continued to use silicone implants for augmentation and reconstruction. A study reported in 2009 evaluated a cohesive gel implant that was developed and implanted from about 1995 to 2001 at several sites in different countries. This implant was restructured to make the gel less fluid-like and more cohesive, the implant contoured to the shape of the breast, and changes made to improve the shell, making it less permeable to gel bleed. The authors reported a decrease in capsular contractures, less folding and, thus, fewer ruptures. Free extracapsular silicone was not associated with the implant ruptures in this study.[28]

Gel Fracture

Although the cohesive gel implants have reportedly fewer intracapsular ruptures, there have been reports of what is known as gel fracture. [7] Gel fracture occurs when the filler is forcibly separated, and if intrinsic limits are exceeded, the shape is no longer maintained and the implant will require replacement. Fractures potentially occur during insertion, and to avoid this, longer incisions may be necessary to aid in the insertion of the anatomically shaped prostheses.[7] Fracture also may potentially occur if there are stresses on folded areas that, again, could weaken the gel. Rotation of the implant or severe folding should be avoided if possible. Gel fracture may present with similar signs of intracapsular implant rupture depending upon the timing of imaging relative to the age of the fracture.

Ultrasonography

Investigations into the usefulness of ultrasonography in detecting implant ruptures have reported conflicting results.[27,29] The variation in these results may reflect the technical factors employed. In our experience, the accuracy of ultrasonography is operator dependent, and the best results are achieved with on-site, real-time evaluation by an experienced radiologist.[29] We use an L12-5 MHz 38 mm transducer to evaluate the integrity of a silicone implant. High resolution is needed to identify subtle implant abnormalities; however, 5 MHz may be required to show the posterior aspects of the implant or adequately depict a subpectoral implant. The ultrasonography examination should be done systematically to ensure that all aspects of the implant are seen, including the surrounding breast and axilla. Clockwise scanning of the breast is used in our practice to ensure that the examination is complete. Selected hard-copy images can be obtained for documentation, or preferably images sent to a picture archiving and communication systems (PACS), and digital workstation.

Normal Sonographic Findings

The most reliable sign of an intact implant is an anechoic interior (Fig. 35-19). However, reverberation artifacts can be encountered in the anterior aspects of intact implants, and these echoes should not be considered abnormal (Fig. 35-20). As a general rule, the reverberation artifacts should be no thicker than the breast tissue anterior to the implant. The implant membrane, sometimes visualized as a thin echogenic line at the parenchymal tissue-implant interface, should be intact throughout.

On ultrasonography, radial folds are depicted as echogenic lines extending from the periphery of the implant to the interior (Fig. 35-21). Radial folds are normal infolding of the implant membrane into the silicone gel, but they may be more prominent in association with capsular contracture.

Ultrasonographic Signs of Implant Rupture

The reported ultrasonographic signs of implant rupture include hyperechoic or hypoechoic masses, dispersion of the ultrasonographic beam (*snowstorm*

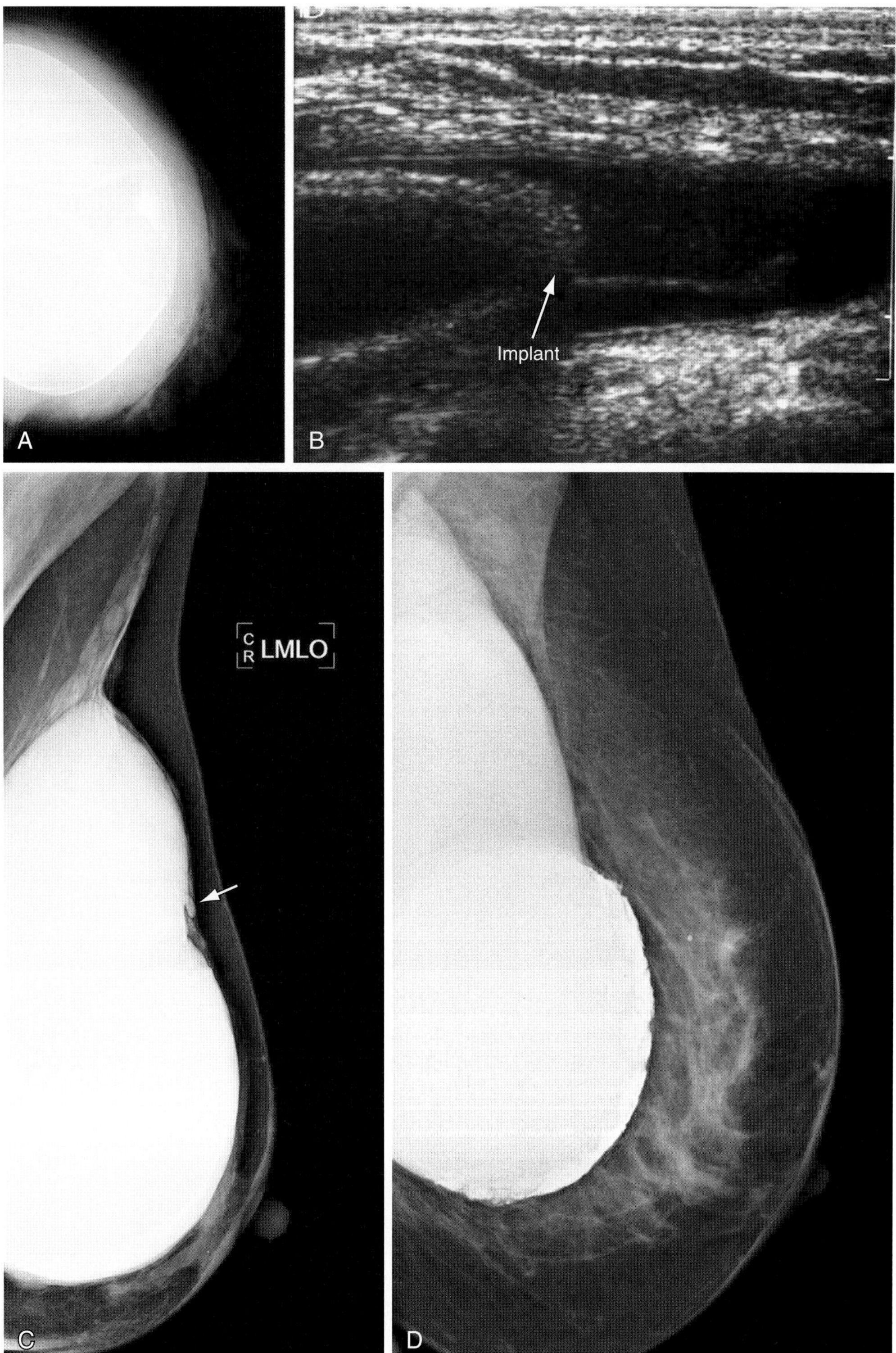

■ **FIGURE 35-17** A, Reactive fluid. Mediolateral oblique (MLO) mammogram of a single-lumen implant with peri-implant fluid collection of serous fluid due to inflammation. Fluid surrounding the implant expands the fibrous capsule. **B,** Ultrasound confirms that the fluid collection is external to the implant and adjacent to the implant edge. **C,** Ruptured subglandular implant. Elongation of the implant with free extracapsular silicone (granuloma; *arrow*) adherent to the outside of the fibrous capsule. **D,** Peri-implant calcifications and elongation of implant. Left MLO mammogram of a ruptured silicone implant shows dense calcifications circumferentially involving the surface of the implant. There is a sheet-like extension of the silicone superiorly associated with loss of anterior-posterior (AP) diameter.

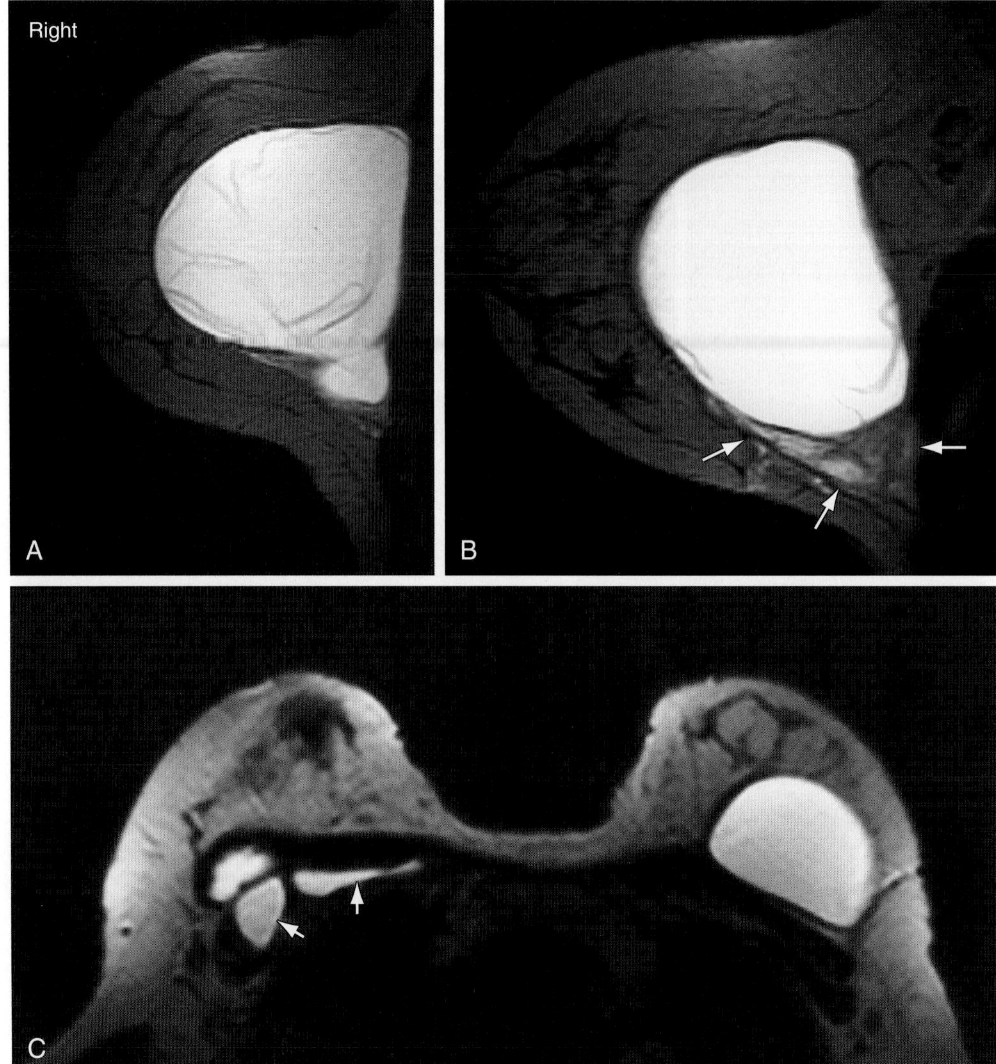

■ **FIGURE 35-18** Extracapsular rupture. **A,** Sagittal short tau inversion recovery (STIR) magnetic resonance (MR) image shows extravasated silicone migrating along the inferior aspect of the implant. The edges of the collapsed implant shell can be seen in the center and peripheral regions of the implant. **B,** Silicone granulomas (*arrows*) along the inferior aspect of the same implant with less intense signal than silicone within the implant. **C,** Axial T2-weighted MR image of a different patient demonstrates silicone granuloma formation (*arrows*) in the superior aspect of the right implant. The left implant is intact.

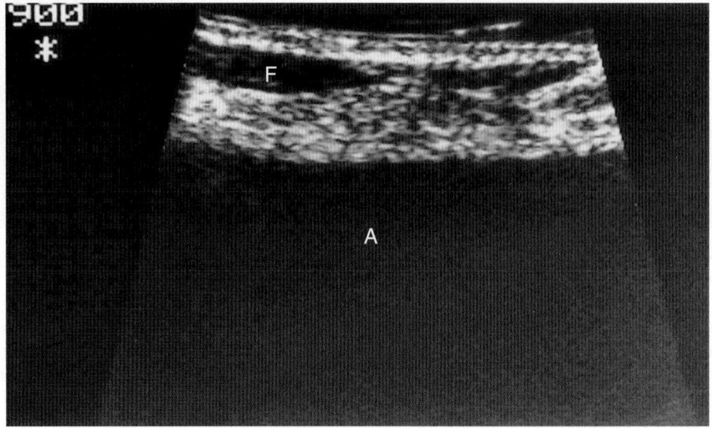

■ **FIGURE 35-19** Ultrasonography of intact subglandular implant. A, anechoic implant interior; F, subcutaneous fat.

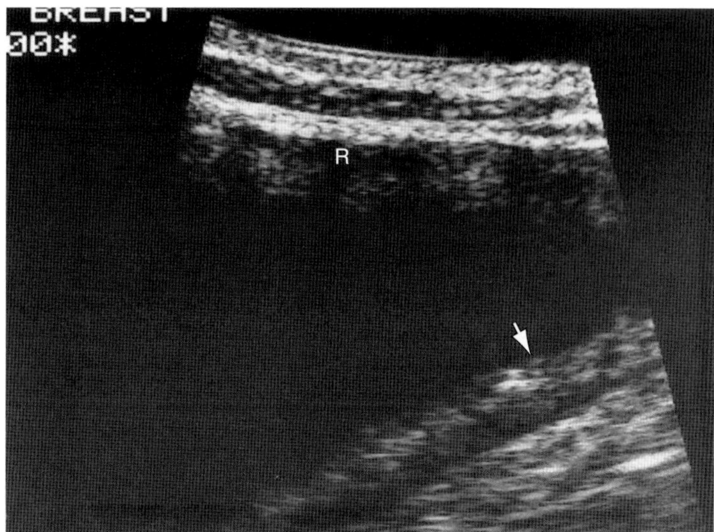

■ **FIGURE 35-20** Reverberation artifact (R), which is commonly seen at the anterior border of implants on ultrasonography, should not be mistaken for evidence of rupture. The implant is otherwise anechoic. *Arrow* indicates the posterior border of the implant.

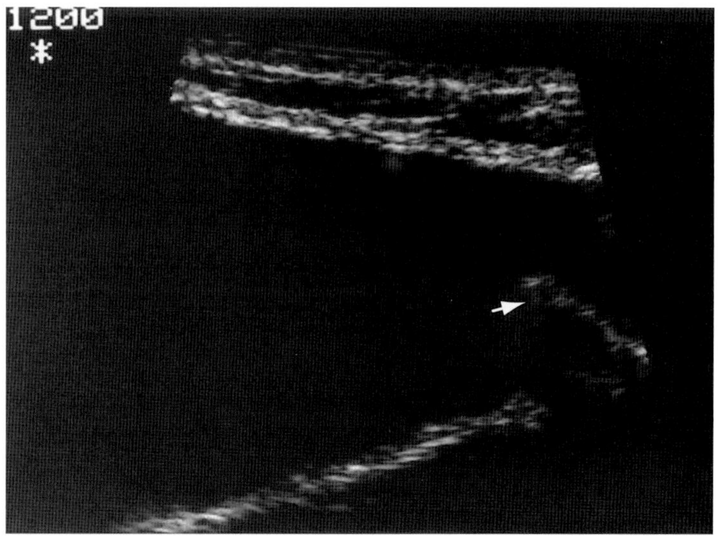

■ **FIGURE 35-21** Ultrasonography of an intact silicone implant with radial fold (*arrow*), manifested as a single echogenic line that extends to the periphery of the implant.

or *echogenic/echodense noise*), discontinuity of the implant membrane, multiple parallel echogenic lines within the implant interior (stepladder sign), and aggregates of medium- to low-level echoes in the interior of the implant.[27,29]

Intracapsular Ruptures

In our experience, the stepladder sign is the most reliable ultrasonographic evidence of an intracapsular rupture.[29] As previously mentioned, the stepladder sign consists of a series of horizontal echogenic straight or curvilinear lines, somewhat parallel, traversing the interior of the implant (Fig. 35-22). This sign represents the collapsed implant membrane floating within the silicone gel and is analogous to the linguine sign seen on MRI. The continuity of these echogenic lines is usually not obvious on ultrasonography, as it is on MRI, because of the narrow field of view of the ultrasonographic image. However, the continuity of the lines representing the floating membrane usually can be visualized with scanning along the lateral and medial aspects of the implant.

In our experience, the presence of aggregates of low- to medium-level echoes within the implant has not been a reliable sign of intracapsular rupture. The etiology of these aggregates of echoes is uncertain, but it has been hypothesized that chemical and physical changes of the silicone gel occur secondary to its exposure to tissue fluids.

Extracapsular Rupture

The most reliable sonographic sign of an extracapsular rupture is the presence of hyperechoic or hypoechoic nodules, often surrounded by a hyperechoic border

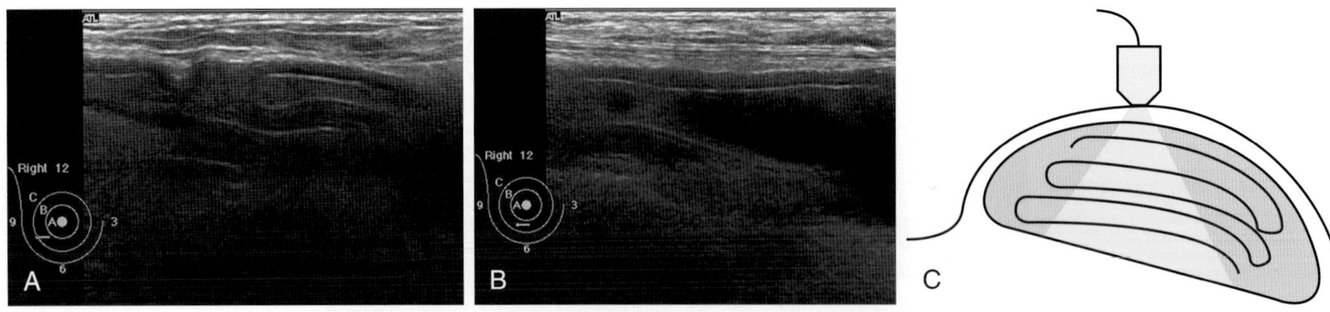

■ FIGURE 35-22 Ultrasonography of intracapsular rupture of a breast implant. **A**, The collapsed implant shell is signified by the stepladder sign, multiple horizontal echogenic lines (*arrows*) that are roughly parallel to one another. **B**, Peripheral curvilinear lines (subcapsular sign) consistent with the intracapsular rupture. **C**, The diagram shows how the stepladder sign of ultrasonography is related to the linguine sign seen on magnetic resonance imaging.

within the parenchyma (Figs. 35-23 and 35-24). The nodules represent silicone granulomas outside the confines of the fibrous capsule. The hyperechoic border around the nodules is believed to reflect the surrounding fibrous tissue reaction.[27,29] The granulomas have been associated with distal loss of ultrasonographic information, and dispersion of the ultrasound beam, a phenomenon termed echogenic/echodense noise. This noise can be present with or without any recognizable nodules. When a discrete silicone nodule is visualized and appears hypoechoic, an echogenic/echodense line can be seen along the posterior border of the granuloma[27] (see Fig. 35-23). This discrete finding of a thick linear echogenicity is usually not seen with breast tumors and maybe helpful in differentiating hypoechoic nodules of silicone from a lesion. The granulomas are best differentiated from breast tumors through the correlation of clinical, mammographic, ultrasonographic findings, and, when available, MR findings.

Occasionally, extracapsular rupture is associated with discontinuity of the breast-implant fibrous capsule interface along the anterior border of the implant (Fig. 35-25). This discontinuity may represent the extrusion of silicone through the ruptured fibrous capsule and into the anterior breast tissue. This apparent discontinuity could also occur when the fibrous capsule has calcified.

Ultrasonographic signs of intracapsular rupture, specifically the stepladder sign, can be expected to accompany extracapsular ruptures (see Fig. 35-25). When ultrasonographic signs of intracapsular rupture are present, a thorough search for extracapsular rupture should be performed, including careful scanning of the axilla to look for silicone granulomas.

Limitations of the Ultrasonographic Evaluation of Implants

We have identified some significant limitations to the ultrasonographic evaluation of silicone implants. Because of the marked attenuation of the ultrasound beam by silicone, ultrasonography is of limited use in the evaluation of the posterior wall of the implant as well as the tissue posterior to it. Another limitation is the prominent reverberation artifacts that are encountered

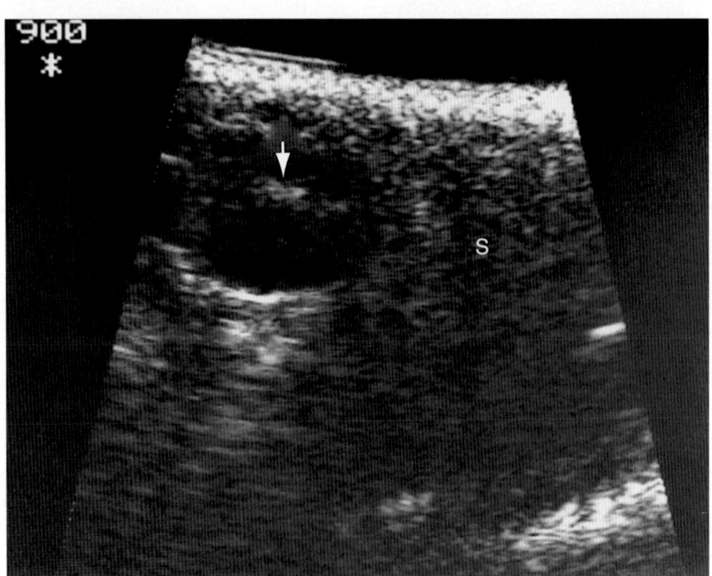

■ FIGURE 35-23 Ultrasonography of breast after silicone injections. Dispersion of the ultrasound beam is referred to as a *snowstorm* appearance (S). A hypoechoic silicone granuloma (*arrow*) is identified in the parenchyma. A hyperechoic interface (*asterisk*) is seen directly posterior to the granuloma.

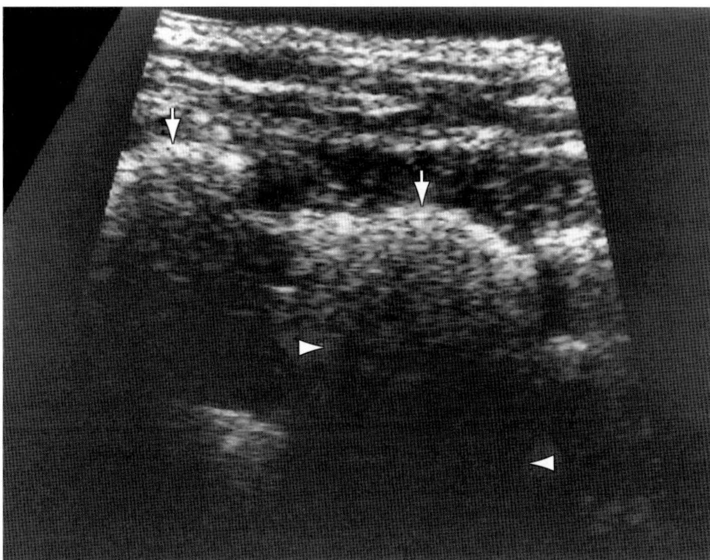

■ **FIGURE 35-24** Ultrasonography of silicone granulomas formed in the breast after extracapsular rupture. There are hyperechoic shadowing, masses of granuloma formation around extravasated silicone (*arrows*). Note the loss of ultrasonographic information posterior to the implants due to beam absorption by the silicone granuloma (*arrowheads*).

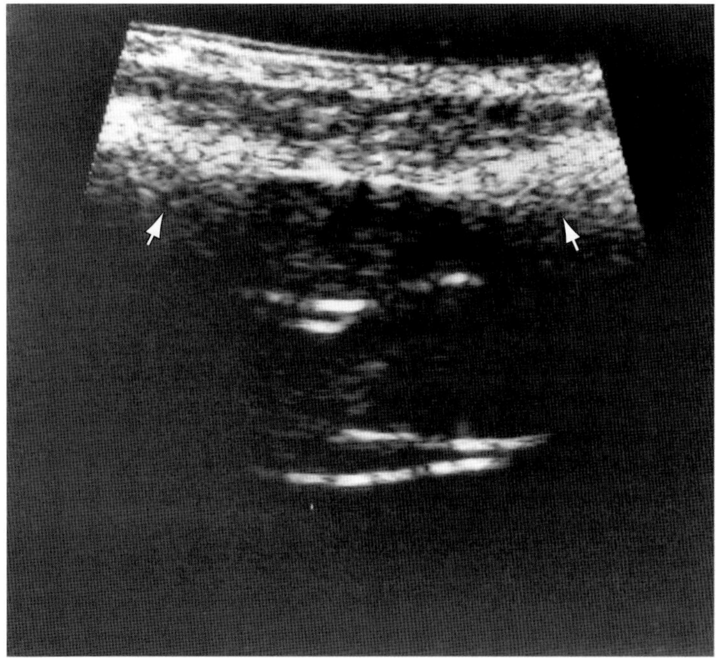

■ **FIGURE 35-25** Ultrasonographic findings of an implant with extracapsular rupture. Discontinuity of the echogenic breast-implant fibrous capsule interface along the anterior border of the implant (*arrows*) due to extracapsular implant rupture. Note the stepladder sign (multiple parallel echogenic lines) in the posterior aspect of the implant.

and can be confused with implant abnormalities. If a woman had silicone injections before undergoing placement of silicone implants, ruling out extracapsular rupture with ultrasonography may be impossible. Additionally, if the silicone injections are extensive, it can be extremely difficult to evaluate the interior of a subsequently placed silicone implant because of attenuation of the ultrasound beam by residual injected silicone and granuloma formation. In the same way, residual silicone granulomas from a previous extracapsular rupture of explanted silicone implants can compromise the evaluation of new implants. Peri-implant calcifications can create a dispersion of the beam similar to echodense noise and create a false positive for implant rupture. Sonographic findings should be correlated with mammographic findings.

COMPARISON OF DIFFERENT IMAGING MODALITIES

Mammography, ultrasonography, MRI, and CT have all been used to evaluate the integrity of silicone breast implants.[13,22,27,29,30] Overall, MRI appears to be the most accurate method for evaluating the integrity of breast implants, with a reported sensitivity of 94% and specificity of 97% when two orthogonal sequences are used to evaluate the implant.[22]

CT also is accurate in detecting intracapsular rupture and is capable of depicting the linguine sign originally described on MR images. The ability of CT to detect extracapsular rupture is less effective.[30] CT is not the modality of choice for imaging a young woman with implants because of the radiation exposure entailed. However, it is worthwhile for radiologists to become familiar with the CT findings of implant rupture, because silicone implants may be encountered during CT examinations of the chest and upper abdomen (Fig. 35-26).

As indicated earlier, mammography has only a limited ability to detect silicone rupture and leakage and is not appropriate for the evaluation of intracapsular rupture.[27] Ultrasonography is capable of detecting both intracapsular and extracapsular ruptures, with a reported sensitivity of 70% and specificity of 92%.[29] We have found, however, that the success of ultrasonography in this endeavor depends largely on the individual operator. A steep learning curve is needed for the development of proficiency in the ultrasonographic evaluation of silicone implants. Thus, the sensitivity of ultrasonography in the detection of implant rupture approaches that of MRI only when the examination is performed by an experienced operator who evaluates and records the findings at the time of the actual scanning.

SUMMARY

Despite the years of controversy surrounding breast augmentation with silicone implants, this procedure is extremely popular. If the newer generation implants prove to be more stable with fewer complications, then there is no doubt that the use of silicone implants will continue to increase and be considered safe for not only augmentation but breast reconstruction as well.

KEY POINTS

- Breast MR is the most effective method for detection of silicone implant rupture, symptomatic or asymptomatic.
- Ultrasound and mammography are most effective in symptomatic ruptures and can identify silicone within the breast tissue.
- Reliable signs of implant rupture seen on MR: linguine, subcapsular line, teardrop, keyhole or noose, droplet, fracture, and silicone granulomas.

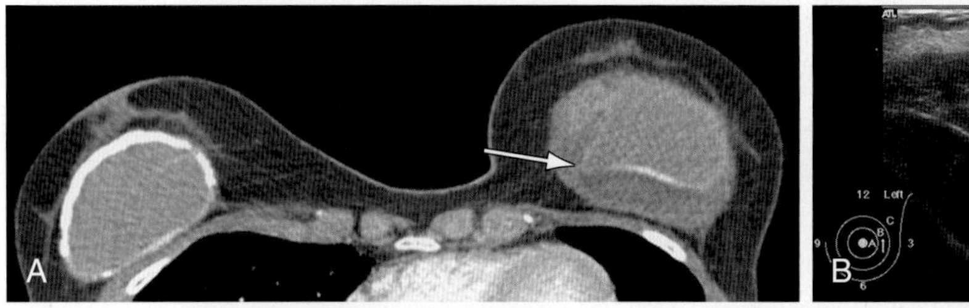

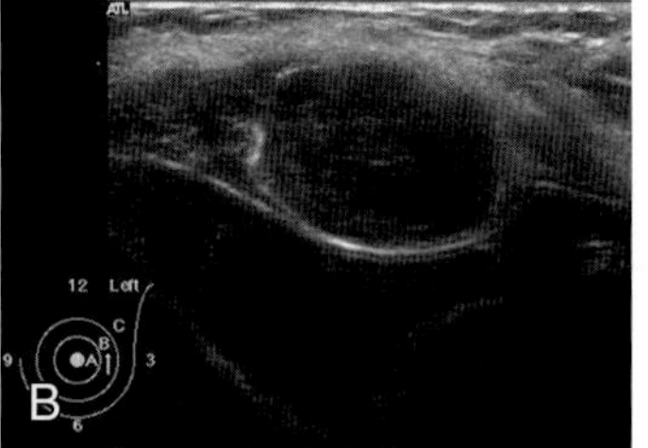

■ FIGURE 35-26 Computed tomography (CT) scan of implant rupture. Axial image of bilateral implants. Left implant has a dense curvilinear line within the central aspect of the implant. The right implant has dense calcification deposition and represents the bright signal surrounding the surface of the implant. **B**, Ultrasound of the left implant noting curvilinear lines, and echogenic material within the implant consistent with rupture.

SUGGESTED READINGS

Berg WA, Caskey CI, Hamper UM. Diagnosing breast implant rupture with MRI, US, and mammography. *Radiographics* 1993;**13**:1323-36.

Berry MG, Davie DM. Breast augmentation: Part I - A review of the silicone prosthesis. *J Plast Reconstr Aesthet Surg* 2010;**63**:793-800.

Everson LI, Parantainen H, Detlie T, Stillman AE, Olson PN, Landis G, et al. Diagnosis of breast implant rupture: imaging findings and relative efficacies of imaging techniques. *AJR Am J Roentgenol* 1994;**163**:57-60.

Ikeda DM, Borofsky HB, Herfkens RJ, Sawyer-Glover AM, Birdwell RL, Glover GH. Silicone breast implant rupture: pitfalls of magnetic resonance imaging and relative efficacies of magnetic resonance, mammography, and ultrasound. *Plast Reconstr Surg* 1999;**104**:2054-62.

Middleton MS, McNamara Jr MP. Breast implant classification with MR imaging correlation. *Radiographics* 2000;**20**:E1.

Mund DF, Farria DM, Gorczyca DP, DeBruhl ND, Ahn CY, Shaw WW, et al. MR imaging of the breast in patients with silicone-gel implants: spectrum of findings. *AJR Am J Roentgenol* 1993;**161**:773-8.

REFERENCES

1. Committee on the Safety of Silicone Implants. Institute of Medicine: Introduction. In: Bondurant S, Ernster V, Herdman R, editors. *Safety of silicone breast implants*. National Academy Press Washington, DC; 2000. pp. 20-3.
2. Ohtake N, Koganei Y, Itoh M, Shioya N. Postoperative sequelae of augmentation mammaplasty by injection method in Japan. *Aesthetic Plastic Surg* 1989;**13**:67-74.
3. Steinbach BG, Hardt NS, Abbitt PL. Mammography: breast implants-types, complications and adjacent breast pathology. *Curr Probl Diagn Radiol* 1993;**22**:43-86.
4. Cronin TD, Gerow F. Augmentation mammoplasty: a new "natural feel" prosthesis. In: *Transactions of the Third International Congress of Plastic Surgeons*. Amsterdam: ExcerptaMedica; 1964.
5. Middleton MS, McNamara Jr MP. Breast implant classification with MR imaging correlation. *Radiographics* 2000;**20**:E1.
6. American Society for Aesthetic Plastic Surgery. *ASAPS 12 year comparison of breast augmentation procedures*. Accessed website Sept 1; 2009.
7. Berry MG, Davies DM. Breast augmentation: Part I -A review of the silicone prosthesis. *J Plast Reconstr Aesthet Surg* (article in press) 2010;**63**:793-800.
8. Kessler DA. The basis of the FDA's decision on breast implants. *N Engl J Med* 1992;**326**:1713-5.
9. Holmich LR, Lipworth L, McLaughlin JK. Breast implant rupture and connective tissure disease: a review of the literature. *Plast Reconstr Surg* 2007;**120**:625-95.
10. U.S. Food and Drug Administration. *FDA approves silicone gel-filled breast implants after in-depth evaluation*. FDA News Release November17, available at www.fda.gov/newsevents/newsroom/pressannouncements/2006/ucm108790.htm; 2006.
11. Gruber RP, Jones HW. Review of closed capsulotomy complications. *Ann Plast Surg* 1981;**6**:271-5.
12. Ahn CY, Shaw WW, Narayanan K, Gorczyca DP, Sinha S, Debruhl ND, et al. Definitive diagnosis of breast implant rupture using magnetic resonance imaging. *Plast Reconstr Surg* 1993;**92**:681-91.
13. Mund DF, Farria DM, Gorczyca DP, DeBruhl ND, Ahn CY, Shaw WW, et al. MR imaging of the breast in patients with silicone-gel implants: spectrum of findings. *AJR Am J Roentgenol* 1993;**161**:773-8.
14. Flassbeck D, Pfleiderer B, Klemens P, Heumann KG, Eltze E, Hirner AV. Determination of siloxanes, silicon, and platinum in tissues of women with silicone gel-filled implants. *Anal Bioanal Chem* 2003;**375**:356-62.
15. Middleton MS. Does silicone gel really bleed? *Radiology* 1995; **197**:370-1.
16. Skinner KA, Silberman H, Dougherty W, Gamagami P, Waisman J, Sposto R, et al. Breast cancer after augmentation mammoplasty. *Ann Surg Oncol* 2001;**8**:138-44.
17. Eklund GW, Busby RC, Miller SH, Job JS. Improved imaging of the augmented breast. *AJR Am J Roentgenol* 1988;**151**:469-73.
18. Diekmann S, Diekmann F, Hauschild M, Hamm B. Digital full field mammography after breast augmentation. *Radiology* 2002;**42**:275-9.
19. Brown SL, Todd JF, Luu HM. Breast implant adverse events during mammography: reports to the Food and Drug Administration. *J Womens Health (Larchmt)* 2004;**13**:371-80.
20. Bassett LW, Brenner RJ. Considerations when imaging women with breast implants. *AJR Am J Roentgenol* 1992;**159**:979-81.
21. Destouet JM, Monsees BS, Oser RF, et al. Screening mammography in 350 women with breast implants: prevalence and findings of implant complications. *AJR Am J Roentgenol* 1992;**159**:973-8.
22. Gorczyca DP, Sinha S, Ahn C, DeBruhl ND, Hayes MK, Gausche VR, et al. Silicone breast implants in vivo: MR imaging. *Radiology* 1992;**185**:407-10.
23. Ikeda DM, Borofsky HB, Herfkens RJ, Sawyer-Glover AM, Birdwell RL, Glover GH. Silicone breast implant rupture: pitfalls of magnetic resonance imaging and relative efficacies of magnetic resonance, mammography, and ultrasound. *Plast Reconstr Surg* 1999;**104**:2054-62.
24. Habal MB. The biologic basis for the clinical application of the silicones. *Arch Surg* 1984;**119**:843-8.
25. Mukundan S, Dixon WT, Kruse BD, Monticciolo DL, Nelson RC. MR imaging of silicone gel-filled breast implants in vivo with a method that visualizes silicone selectively. *J Magn Reson Imaging* 1993;**3**:713-7.
26. Soo MS, Kornguth PJ, Walsh R, Elenberger CD, Georgiade GS. Complex radial folds versus subtle signs of intracapsular rupture of breast implants: MR findings with surgical correlation. *AJR Am J Roentgenol* 1996;**166**:1421-7.
27. Berg WA, Caskey CI, Hamper UM. Diagnosing breast implant rupture with MRI, US, and mammography. *Radiographics* 1993;**13**:1323-36.
28. Heden P, Bronz G, Elberg JJ, Deraemaecker R, Murphy DK, Slicton A, et al. Long-term safety and effectiveness of style 410 highly cohesive silicone breast implants. *Aesthetic Plast Surg* 2009;**33**:430-6.
29. DeBruhl ND, Gorczyca DP, Ahn CY, Shaw WW, Bassett LW. Silicone breast implants: US evaluation. *Radiology* 1993;**189**:95-8.
30. Everson LI, Parantainen H, Detlie T, Stillman AE, Olson PN, Landis G, et al. Diagnosis of breast implant rupture: imaging findings and relative efficacies of imaging techniques. *AJR Am J Roentgenol* 1994;**163**:57-60.

CHAPTER 36

Reduction Mammoplasty

Valerie P. Jackson and Katherine H. Walker

Reduction mammoplasty is a plastic surgical procedure done for the treatment of macromastia. Macromastia is a condition that can lead to a number of problems, including poor posture, kyphosis, back pain, deep grooves and skin ulceration in the shoulders from the pressure of brassiere straps, brachial plexus pressure symptoms, and chronic intertrigo under the breasts. Reduction mammoplasty is also used to achieve symmetry in women with congenital hypoplasia or aplasia of the contralateral breast. The procedure is also performed following contralateral mastectomy with reconstruction, large segmental resection for breast cancer, or severe trauma. Of women with breast carcinoma treated with mastectomy and reconstruction, 6% to 36% undergo reduction mammoplasty to achieve symmetric breast size.[1]

There are a number of surgical techniques for reduction mammoplasty.[2,3] Most involve removal of breast tissue and repositioning of the nipple-areolar complex (Figs 36-1 and 36-2). Nipple repositioning may be achieved by two types of procedures: pedicle flaps with nipple transposition, in which the nipple remains connected to the subareolar ducts; or pedicle flaps with full-thickness nipple-areolar grafts, in which the ducts are severed.[4] The most commonly used surgical techniques lead to a characteristic scar in the circumareolar region, extending down the inferior aspect of the breast and along the inframammary fold (Fig. 36-3). In recent years, circumareolar techniques and liposuction have also been used, but the imaging findings are not yet fully understood.

Imaging Indications and Algorithm

Most plastic surgeons recommend preoperative mammography for all women undergoing reduction mammoplasty, particularly if older than the age of 35 years.[3,5,6–12] The major value of the preoperative mammogram is to detect a lesion that requires further investigation or removal at the time of the reduction procedure. Ozmen and associates[13] recommended specimen radiography of the removed breast tissue to evaluate for abnormalities such as breast carcinoma, but this is rarely done and is probably unnecessary if preoperative mammography has been performed. Because major imaging changes occur after the surgical procedure, the preoperative mammogram is of little value after the reduction procedure. Many plastic surgeons advocate establishing a new baseline with mammography 3 to 12 months after the reduction procedure.[5,6–9,12] We have found this follow-up to be extremely useful in our own practice. It is often helpful to wait at least 6 months after surgery to minimize patient discomfort during the mammogram and allow the postoperative changes within the breasts to diminish.[8]

Early complications of reduction mammoplasty include seromas, hematomas, areolar necrosis, infection, and delayed skin healing. Most of these are handled clinically and do not require imaging.[14] However, imaging is indicated if a woman develops a new clinical abnormality beyond the initial postoperative period. Many benign breast masses occur as a result of the surgery, including hematomas, fat necrosis, and fibrous scars.[9] Mammography can definitively diagnose many of these lesions, which should not be assumed to be benign based on clinical breast examination.

There is evidence that women have a somewhat decreased risk of breast cancer after reduction mammoplasty.[15] The reason for the change in risk is unknown but may be related to the decreased amount of breast tissue. The prognosis and mortality rates for patients with breast cancer after breast reduction are the same as for women with breast cancer in the general population.[16] Nonetheless, it is important to remember that all women older than age 40 should have annual screening mammography. Women who have reduction mammoplasty to achieve symmetry after treatment for contralateral breast carcinoma are at increased risk for development of additional breast cancer and require annual imaging of the reduced breast regardless of their age.

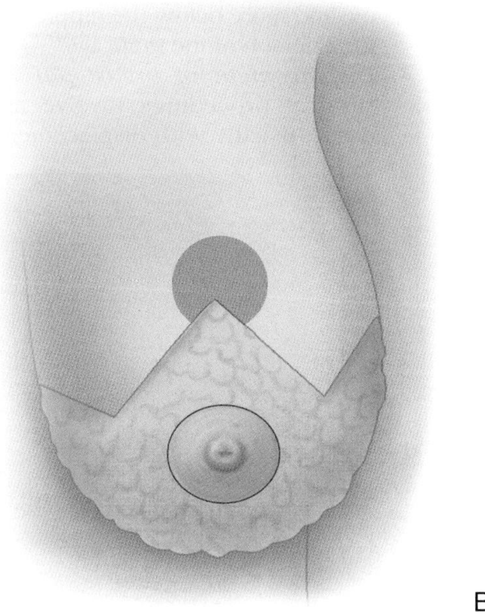

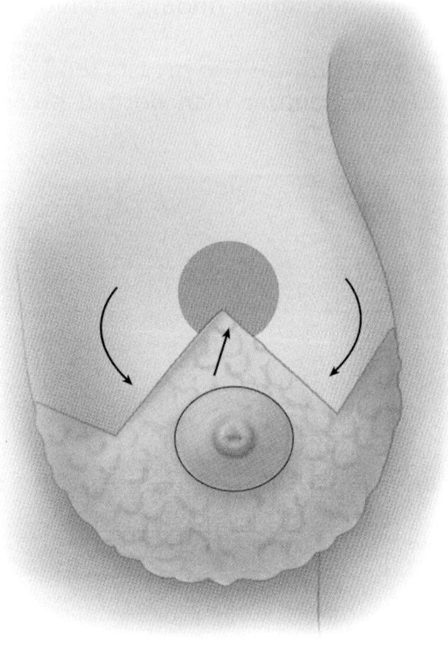

■ **FIGURE 36-1** Typical pattern of excision for reduction mammoplasty with nipple transplantation. **A,** The inferior, medial, and lateral breast tissue is resected with removal of the nipple. **B,** The upper aspects of the breasts are brought inferiorly (*curved arrows*) and the nipple-areolar complex is transplanted superiorly as a full-thickness graft (*straight arrow*).

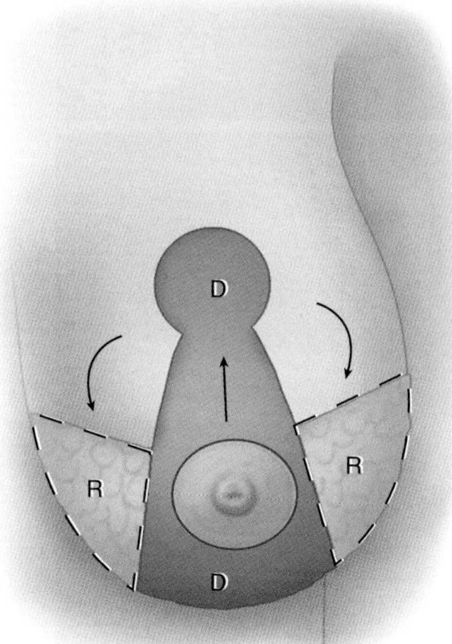

■ **FIGURE 36-2** Typical pattern of excision for reduction mammoplasty with nipple transposition. The skin and parenchymal tissue within the triangular areas (R) are resected. The nipple-areolar complex remains intact, but the surrounding region (D) is de-epithelialized. When the nipple is transposed superiorly into the "keyhole," it remains attached to the underlying ducts and vascular pedicle. The upper aspects of the breast are brought inferiorly as shown by the *curved arrows*.

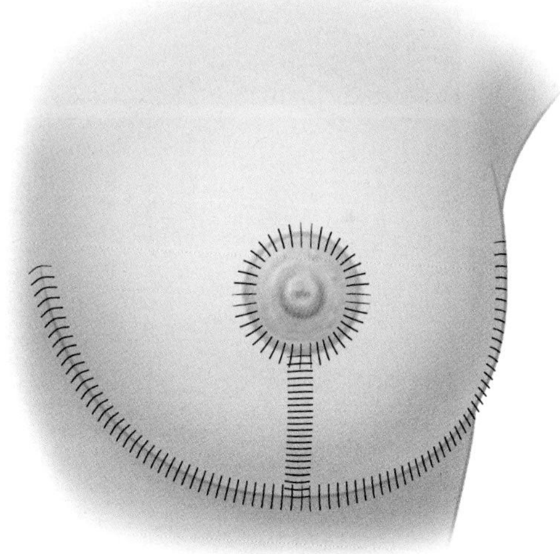

■ **FIGURE 36-3** Typical postoperative appearance after reduction mammoplasty. Surgical scars are found in the circumareolar region, inframammary fold, and at the 6-o'clock position (*cross-hatched lines*).

Imaging Technique and Findings

A number of characteristic mammographic changes have been reported after reduction mammoplasty (Box 36-1). Regardless of the exact type of reduction procedure performed, the changes reflect the removal and repositioning

BOX 36-1 Mammographic Changes After Reduction Mammoplasty

Alteration of breast contour
Architectural distortion
Displacement of breast parenchyma
Disruption of subareolar ducts
Elevation of the nipple
Fat necrosis
Retroareolar fibrotic band
Skin thickening

of breast tissue and the nipple-areolar complex. The commonly encountered mammographic findings include:

1. *Alteration of breast contour.* The breasts tend to be higher and flatter in contour than normal breasts[6] (Fig. 36-4).
2. *Elevation of the nipple.* There is less skin above the nipple and more below the nipple than in normal breasts for a person of the same age[6,7,17] (see Fig. 36-4).
3. *Displacement of breast parenchyma.* All of the surgical procedures involve movement of breast tissue, usually with displacement of tissue from the

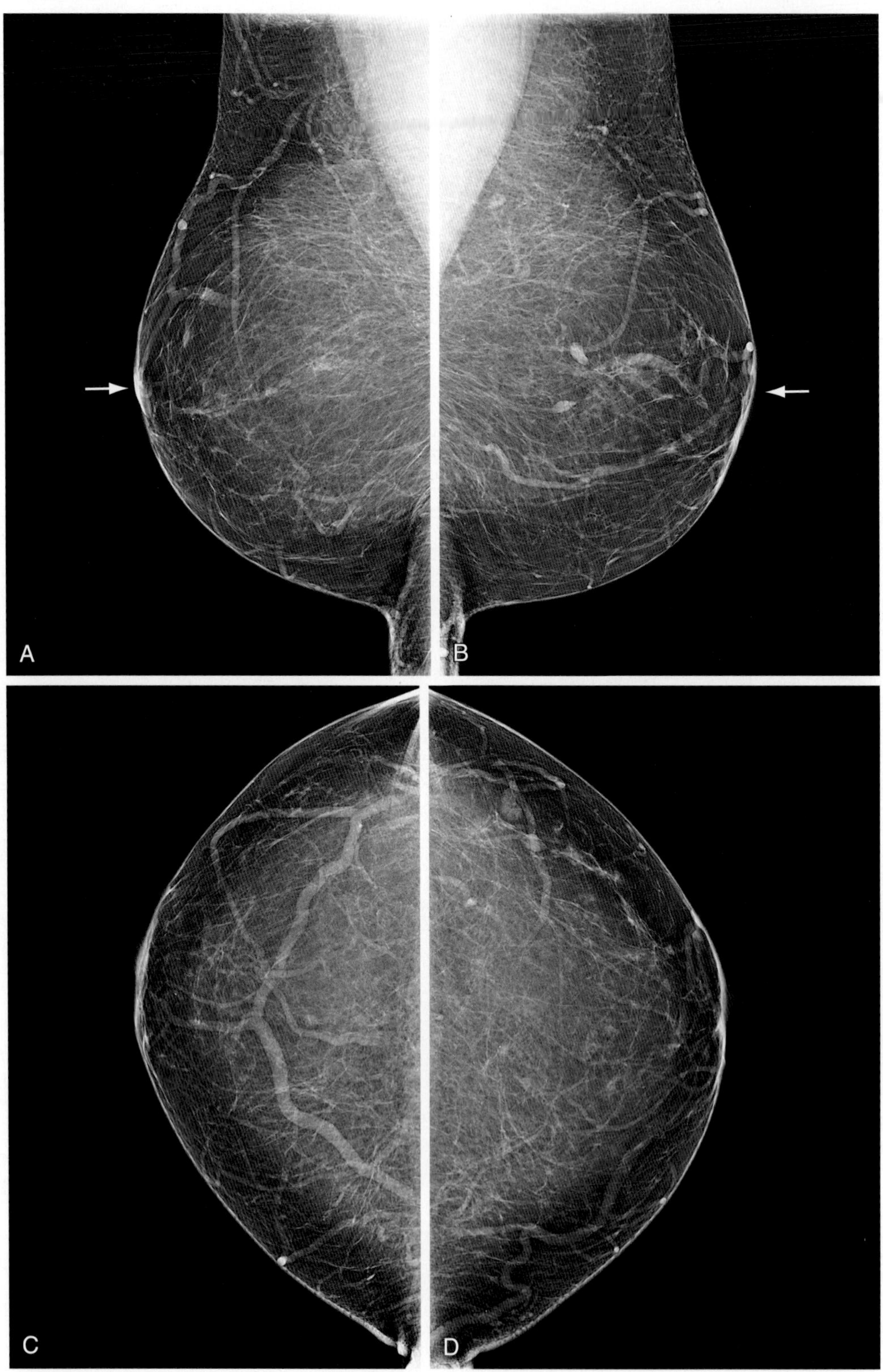

■ **FIGURE 36-4** Right and left mediolateral oblique (MLO) (**A** and **B**) and craniocaudal (CC) (**C** and **D**) mammograms 2 years after reduction mammoplasty in a 50-year-old woman. This patient was difficult to position for the MLO views, leading to suboptimal visualization of pectoralis muscles. The breasts are higher and flatter in contour than normal breasts, and the nipples (*arrows*) are elevated.

upper portions of the breast to the lower aspects of the breast. This leads to movement of fibroglandular tissue, which is normally most prominent in the upper outer quadrant, to the inferior aspect of the breast.[6,7,17,18] This is best seen on the mediolateral oblique (MLO) and lateral (mediolateral [ML] or lateromedial [LM]) views (Fig. 36-5). The pattern of fibroglandular density often becomes asymmetric[6] (see Fig. 36-5).

4. *Architectural distortion*. Postsurgical scarring and displacement of fibroglandular tissue usually leads to distortion of the normal breast architecture.[17,18] One of the most common findings is a "swirled" pattern of architectural distortion or lines seen inferiorly on the MLO or lateral (ML or LM) views[18] (Figs 36-5 and 36-6). This is more prominent in breasts with fibroglandular tissue than in breasts that are almost completely fatty. Areas of more focal asymmetry and architectural distortion are not uncommon (Fig. 36-7).
5. *Skin thickening*. This finding is most commonly seen in the areas of surgical anastomoses in the areolar region and the inferior aspect of the breast[6,7,18] (Fig. 36-8).
6. *Retroareolar fibrotic band*. This is a radiopaque band less than 0.5 cm thick that runs parallel to the skin line and is best seen on the craniocaudal (CC) view.[6,7,17] This is evident in nipple-areolar transposition procedures[17] (see Fig. 36-8).

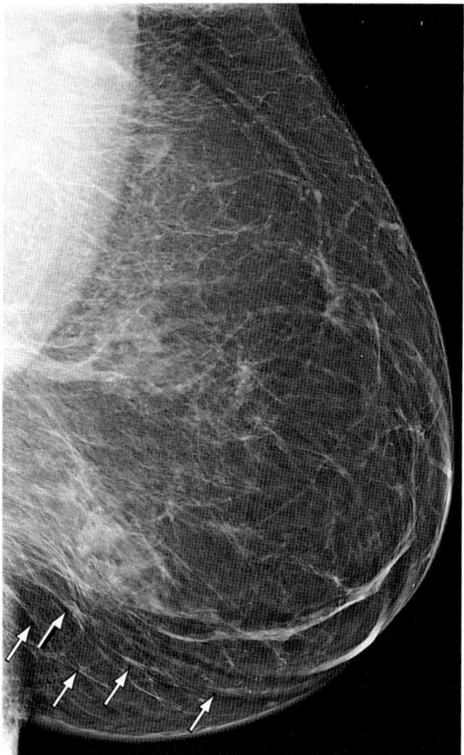

■ **FIGURE 36-6** Left mediolateral oblique (MLO) mammogram view demonstrates swirled lines of fibroglandular tissue (*arrows*) at the inferior aspect of the left breast 5 years after reduction mammoplasty.

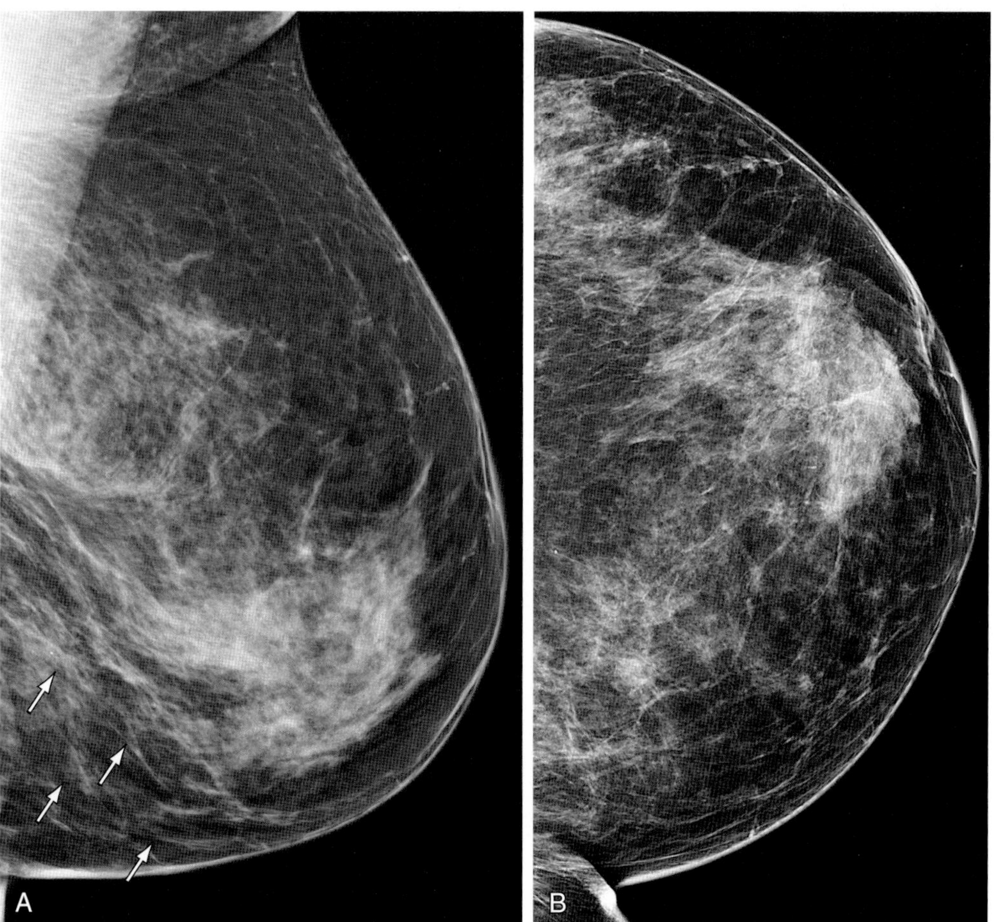

■ **FIGURE 36-5** Left mediolateral oblique (MLO) (**A**) and craniocaudal (CC) (**B**) mammograms, 4 years after reduction mammoplasty in a 45-year-old woman. Displacement and distortion of fibroglandular tissue is present. The swirled pattern of fibroglandular tissue is present in the posterior inferior aspect of the left breast (*arrows*).

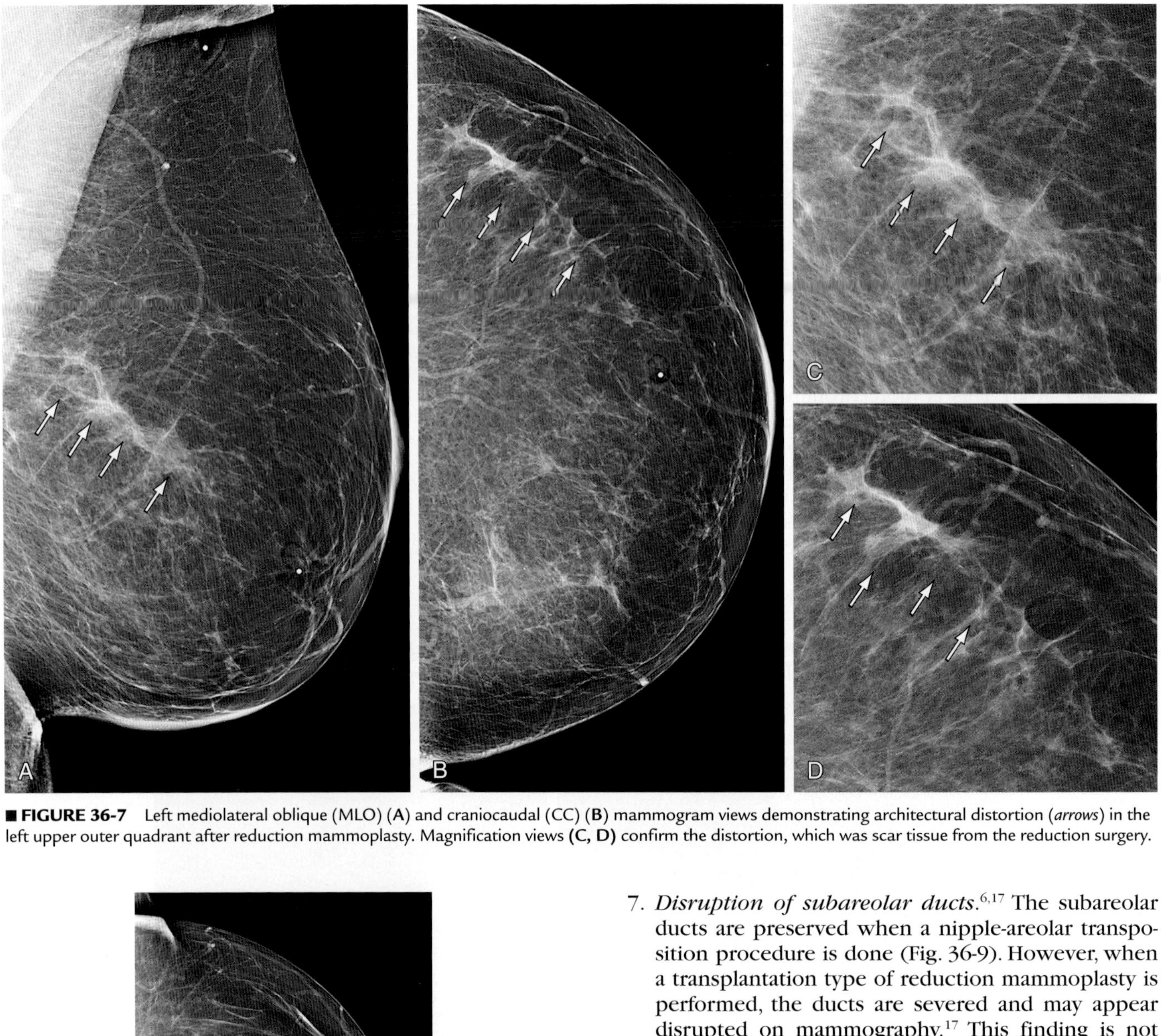

■ **FIGURE 36-7** Left mediolateral oblique (MLO) (**A**) and craniocaudal (CC) (**B**) mammogram views demonstrating architectural distortion (*arrows*) in the left upper outer quadrant after reduction mammoplasty. Magnification views (**C, D**) confirm the distortion, which was scar tissue from the reduction surgery.

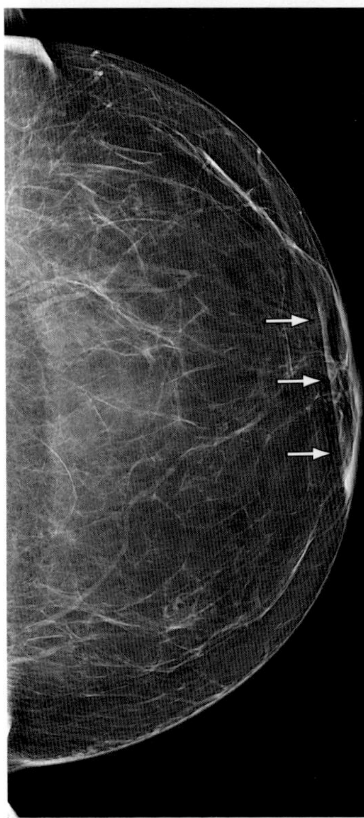

■ **FIGURE 36-8** Left craniocaudal (CC) mammogram demonstrating the retroareolar fibrotic band (*arrows*) in a woman 2 years after reduction mammoplasty with a nipple transposition procedure.

7. *Disruption of subareolar ducts.*[6,17] The subareolar ducts are preserved when a nipple-areolar transposition procedure is done (Fig. 36-9). However, when a transplantation type of reduction mammoplasty is performed, the ducts are severed and may appear disrupted on mammography.[17] This finding is not apparent in women with breasts that are nearly or completely fatty.[17]
8. *Fat necrosis.* Fat necrosis is a common consequence of extensive surgery, such as reduction mammoplasty. The most common findings are oil cysts, often with spherical lucent centered, eggshell, or dystrophic calcifications[4,6,7,18-20] (Fig. 36-10).

Unusual mammographic findings include spiculated scars,[18] epidermal inclusion cysts,[21] and suture calcifications.[18]

Brown and colleagues[6] followed women with serial mammography after reduction procedures and found that the architectural changes, such as periareolar and inferior breast alterations, were most prominent on the first postoperative mammogram and usually diminished over time. In none of their patients did these changes increase on subsequent mammograms. Asymmetric tissues were found in 50% of cases in the first year after surgery but in only 25% of cases after 2 years. In patients in whom the asymmetries persisted, they usually decreased in size and prominence and did not increase. Calcifications tended to develop later and therefore could represent more of a diagnostic problem. Only 3% of women had calcifications within the first year, 20% had

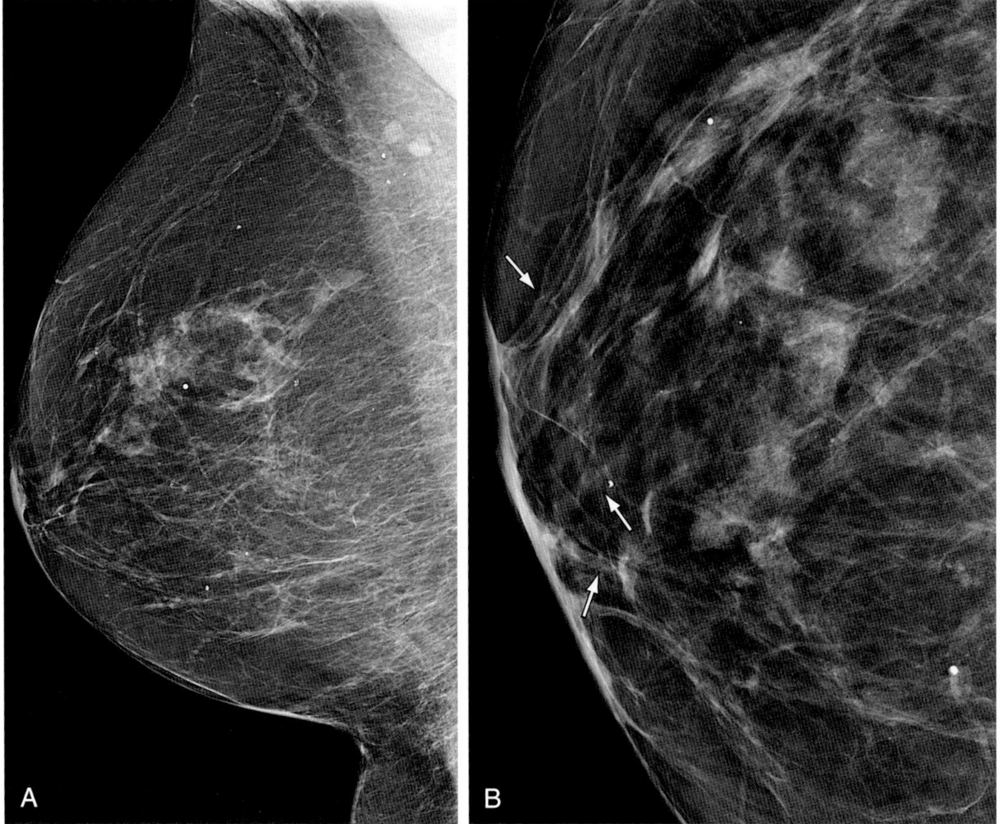

■ **FIGURE 36-9** **A,** Mammogram shows preservation of subareolar ducts in a woman with a nipple-areolar transposition type of reduction mammoplasty. **B,** Close-up shows the preserved ducts (*arrows*).

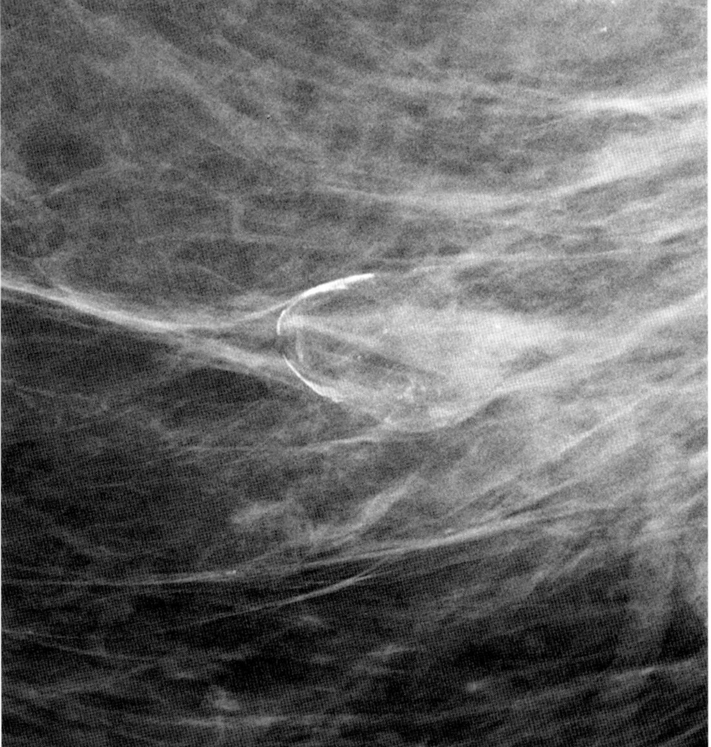

■ **FIGURE 36-10** Eggshell calcifications compatible with benign fat necrosis seen on mammography after reduction mammoplasty.

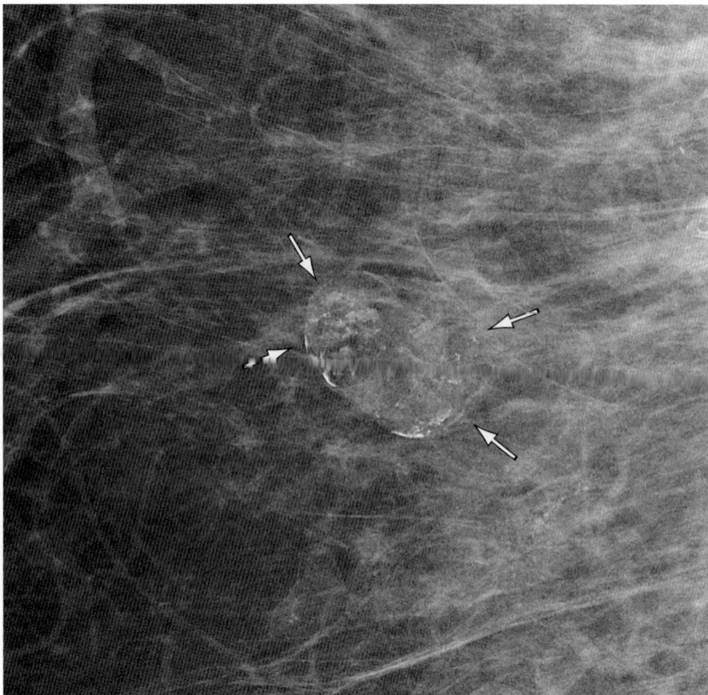

■ **FIGURE 36-11** Mammography shows early partial eggshell calcifications compatible with early benign fat necrosis calcifications (*arrows*) that could be confused with suspicious microcalcifications without the clinical history.

them by the second year, and more than 40% had developed calcifications after 2 years. While the number and extent of calcifications increased over time, the calcifications were usually typical postsurgical calcifications and obviously benign (see Fig. 36-10). However, early fat necrosis calcifications may rarely be fine and pleomorphic, mimicking malignant microcalcifications (Fig. 36-11).

Liposuction for breast reduction is gaining popularity. Unfortunately, the descriptions of postprocedure mammographic findings are limited and no long-term follow-up studies have yet been published. Reported follow-up periods range from 6 months to 2 years, and findings include smaller breasts, relative increase in fibroglandular tissue, and development of benign calcifications when compared with the preoperative mammograms.[22-24] However, it is highly likely that larger long-term studies will show the development of suspicious microcalcifications, spiculated masses, and architectural distortion from the fat necrosis and scarring.

Breast cancers in women with prior reduction mammoplasties have the same imaging features as in normal women. However, the changes from reduction mammoplasty may cause confusion, particularly if prior mammograms are not available for comparison. If one is aware of the typical changes of reduction and careful to compare with previous mammograms, it is possible to detect early breast carcinoma in these women.[25] In cases with indeterminate findings, image-guided automated large core or vacuum-assisted needle biopsies can be used to differentiate postsurgical changes from malignancy.

KEY POINTS

- Screening mammography should be performed before reduction mammoplasty, particularly for women older than age 40 years.
- It is helpful to have a mammogram performed 6 to 12 months after reduction surgery to re-establish baseline findings.
- The mammographic changes are the result of removal and movement of breast tissue and are usually obviously benign.

SUGGESTED READINGS

Brown FE, Sargent SK, Cohen SR, Morain WD. Mammographic changes following reduction mammaplasty. *Plast Reconstr Surg* 1987;**80**:691-8.

Danikas D, Theodorou SJ, Kokkalis G, Vasiou K, Kyriakopoulou K. Mammographic findings following reduction mammoplasty. *Aesthetic Plast Surg* 2001;**25**:283-5.

Leibman AJ, Kruse BD. Imaging of breast cancer after reduction mammoplasty. *Breast Dis* 1991;**4**:261-70.

Miller CL, Feig SA, Fox JW. Mammographic changes after reduction mammoplasty. *AJR Am J Roentgenl* 1987;**149**:35-8.

REFERENCES

1. Greco RJ, Dascombe WH, Williams SL, Johnson RR, Kelly JL. Two-staged breast reconstruction in patients with symptomatic macromastia requiring mastectomy. *Ann Plast Surg* 1994;**32**:572-9.
2. Hidalgo DA, Franklyn EL, Palumbo S, Casas L, Hammond D. Current trends in breast reduction. *Plast Reconstr Surg* 1999; **104**:806-15.
3. Strombeck JO. Reduction mammaplasty. In: Strombeck JO, Rosato FE, editors. *Surgery of the breast; diagnosis and treatment of breast diseases*. New York: Georg Thieme; 1986. p. 277-311.
4. Mendelson EB. Imaging the post-surgical breast. *Semin Ultrasound CT MR* 1989;**10**:154-70.
5. Beer GM, Kompatscher P, Hergan K. Diagnosis of breast tumors after breast reduction. *Aesthetic Plast Surg* 1996;**20**:391-7.
6. Brown FE, Sargent SK, Cohen SR, Morain WD. Mammographic changes following reduction mammaplasty. *Plast Reconstr Surg* 1987;**80**:691-8.
7. Danikas D, Theodorou SJ, Kokkalis G, Vasiou K, Kyriakopoulou K. Mammographic findings following reduction mammoplasty. *Aesthetic Plast Surg* 2001;**25**:283-5.
8. Howrigan PJ. Reduction and augmentation mammoplasty. *Obstet Gynecol Clin North Am* 1994;**21**:539-49.
9. Isaacs G, Rozner L, Tudball C. Breast lumps after reduction mammaplasty. *Ann Plast Surg* 1985;**15**:394-9.
10. Keleher AJ, Langstein HN, Ames FC, Ross MI, Chang DW, Reece GP, et al. Breast cancer in mammaplasty specimens: case reports and guidelines. *Breast J* 2003;**9**:120-5.
11. Perras C, Papillon J. The value of mammography in cosmetic surgery of the breasts. *Plast Reconstr Surg* 1973;**52**:132-7.
12. Spear SL, Antoine GA. Surgery for mammary hypertrophy. In: Nonne RB, editor. *Plastic and reconstructive surgery of the breast*. Philadelphia: BC Decker; 1991. p. 189-94.
13. Ozmen S, Yavuzer R, Latifoglu O, Ayhan S, Tuncer S, Yazici I, et al. Specimen radiography: an assessment method for reduction mammaplasty materials. *Aesthetic Plast Surg* 2001;**25**:432-5.
14. Lejour M. Vertical mammaplasty: early complications after 250 personal consecutive cases. *Plast Reconstr Surg* 1999;**104**:764-70.
15. Brown MH, Weinberg M, Chong N, Levine R, Holoway E. A cohort study of breast cancer risk in breast reduction patients. *Plast Reconstr Surg* 1999;**103**:1674-81.
16. Tang CL, Brown MH, Levine R, Sloan M, Chong N, Holoway E. A follow-up study of 105 women with breast cancer following reduction mammaplasty. *Plast Reconstr Surg* 1999;**103**:1687-90.
17. Miller CL, Feig SA, Fox JW. Mammographic changes after reduction mammoplasty. *AJR Am J Roentgenol* 1987;**149**:35-8.
18. Swann CA, Kopans DB, White G, et al. Observations on the postreduction mammoplasty mammogram. *Breast Dis* 1989;**1**:261-7.
19. Baber CE, Libshitz HI. Bilateral fat necrosis of the breast following reduction mammoplasties. *AJR Am J Roentgenol* 1977;**128**:508-9.
20. Bassett LW, Gold RH, Cove HC. Mammographic spectrum of traumatic fat necrosis: The fallibility of "pathognomonic" signs of carcinoma. *AJR Am J Roentgenol* 1978;**130**:119-22.
21. Fajardo LL, Besson SC. Epidermal inclusion cyst after reduction mammoplasty. *Radiology* 1993;**186**:103-6.
22. Abboud M, Vadoud-Seyedi J, De May A, Cukierfajn M, Lejour M. Incidence of calcifications in the breast after surgical reduction and liposuction. *Plast Reconstr Surg* 1995;**96**:620-6.
23. Gray LN. Update on experience with liposuction breast reduction. *Plast Reconstr Surg* 2001;**108**:1006-10.
24. Habbema L. Breast reduction using liposuction with tumescent local anesthesia and powered cannulas. *Dermatol Surg* 2009;**35**:41-52.
25. Leibman AJ, Kruse BD. Imaging of breast cancer after reduction mammoplasty. *Breast Dis* 1991;**4**:261-70.

SECTION

NINE

Regulations in Breast Imaging

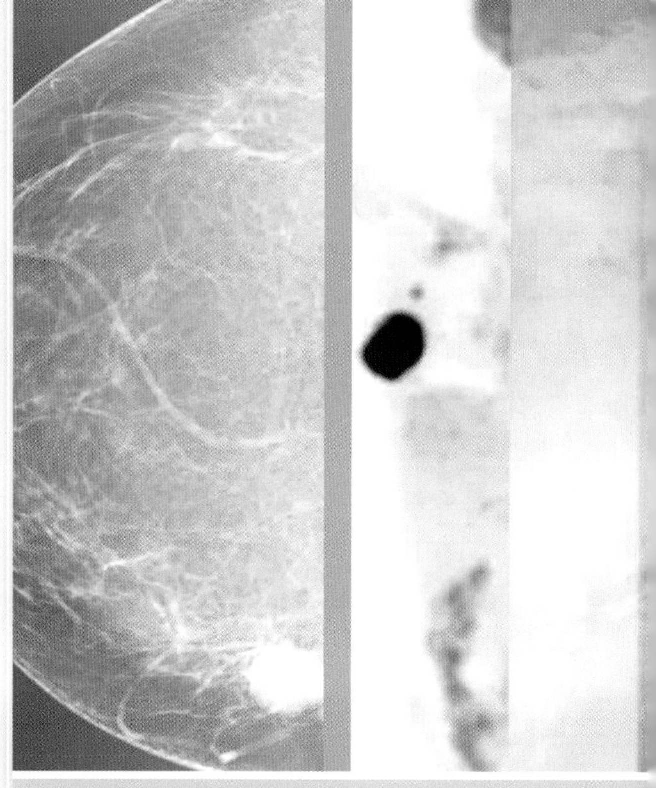

CHAPTER 37

The Mammography Quality Standards Act and Accreditation

Priscilla F. Butler

The technical quality of mammography improved during the 1980s as conventional x-ray units were replaced with dedicated mammography systems. Grids were integrated with these dedicated systems, screen-film image receptors designed specifically for mammography were used, and xeromammography was phased out. In the mid-1980s, however, it became apparent that despite these technical advances, image quality and breast radiation dose from mammography varied greatly. Significant evidence of those problems came from the 1985 Nationwide Evaluation of X-ray Trends (NEXT) study that was conducted by the U.S. Food and Drug Administration (FDA) and the Conference of Radiation Control Program Directors (CRCPD).[1] This recognition led to the establishment of voluntary mammography quality standards through the American College of Radiology (ACR) Mammography Accreditation Program in 1987.[2] The Mammography Accreditation Program required that a facility perform a number of quality assurance activities and its personnel meet certain qualification and continuing education standards. Furthermore, it required an evaluation of both phantom and clinical images produced in the facility by trained outside reviewers.

Several states passed legislation requiring mammography facilities to meet quality standards and submit to regular inspections by state radiation control inspectors.[3] In 1990, Congress passed legislation authorizing Medicare coverage of screening mammography; those facilities seeking Medicare reimbursement were required to register with the Health Care Financing Administration (HCFA) and meet quality standards similar to those of the ACR Mammography Accreditation Program.[4] Federal inspections of Medicare-registered screening facilities began in 1992.

THE MAMMOGRAPHY QUALITY STANDARDS ACT OF 1992

Recognizing the need for uniform national standards that would apply to both screening and diagnostic facilities, Congress passed the Mammography Quality Standards Act (MQSA) in 1992.[5] This Act, which became effective October 1, 1994, requires that all mammography facilities meet minimum quality standards for personnel, equipment, and record-keeping, and to be certified by the FDA (or an FDA-approved state certifying body) in order to legally operate in the United States.

Requirements

The Act specifies the following eight requirements:

1. All mammography facilities must be accredited by private, nonprofit organizations or state agencies that have met the standards established by the FDA for accreditation bodies and those that have been approved by the FDA. The MQSA requires a direct federal audit of the accreditation bodies through federal inspections by federal inspectors. It also requires that, as part of the overall accreditation process, actual clinical mammograms from each facility be evaluated for quality by the accreditation body.
2. A mammography facility physics survey, consultation, and evaluation must be performed annually by a qualified medical physicist.

3. An FDA-certified state or federal inspector must inspect mammography facilities annually. If state inspectors are used, the MQSA requires a federal audit of the state-inspected facilities.
4. Initial and continuing qualification standards for interpreting physicians, radiologic technologists, medical physicists, and inspectors must be established.
5. Boards or organizations eligible to certify the adequacy of training and experience of mammography personnel must be specified.
6. Quality standards for mammography equipment and practices, including quality assurance and quality control programs, must be established.
7. The Secretary of Health and Human Services (HHS) must establish a National Mammography Quality Assurance Advisory Committee (NMQAAC) to advise the FDA on issues including appropriate quality standards for mammography facilities and accreditation bodies.
8. Standards governing record-keeping for examinee files, requirements for mammography reporting, and examinee notification by physicians must be established.

In summary, from a mammography facility's point of view, MQSA requires three separate checks: certification by the FDA (or a state certifying body), accreditation by an approved body, and inspection by a state (or the FDA).

MAMMOGRAPHY QUALITY STANDARDS REAUTHORIZATION ACT OF 1998

Congress must periodically reauthorize the Act and its funding. The Mammography Quality Standards Reauthorization Act (MQSRA), signed by President Clinton in October 1998, made several significant changes that would affect mammography facilities.[6]

Firstly, it included a requirement that "a summary of the written [mammography] report be sent to the patient [by the mammography facility] in terms easily understood by a lay person." This applies to every patient who undergoes mammography, not just self-referred patients. The intent of this law was to address women's concerns about breakdowns in communication that prevent timely and appropriate diagnosis and treatment of breast disease. Failure to comply with this reporting requirement would result in a citation by MQSA inspectors. Although the lay report need only be a summary, it must be in writing. It is important that any summary of abnormal results provide clear direction about the appropriate steps to be taken by the patient.

Secondly, the Secretary of HHS was instructed to conduct a demonstration project to study the effect of reducing the inspection frequency for compliant mammography facilities from annual to every other year. The FDA, in collaboration with the CRCPD, conducted a program with 300 facilities to evaluate whether citation-free facilities can maintain their high standards without the scrutiny of annual inspections. They determined that facilities participating in every other year inspections did not maintain high quality (as determined by the follow-up inspections). Consequently, the pilot study was disbanded.

KEY PLAYERS IN THE MAMMOGRAPHY QUALITY STANDARDS ACT

The U.S. Food and Drug Administration

In 1993, the Secretary of HHS designated the FDA as the federal agency to implement the MQSA. The FDA's responsibilities are many; they include developing and promulgating the final standards, approving accrediting bodies, certifying all mammography facilities in the United States, training inspectors, inspecting facilities, evaluating the effectiveness of the program, and developing and implementing sanctions for noncompliant facilities. The MQSA program is administered by the Division of Mammography Quality and Radiation Programs of the FDA's Center for Devices and Radiological Health.

The State

A state's role can take many forms. The Act allows the Secretary of HHS to delegate inspections to a state agency, and most states have contracted with the FDA to do so. The Act also allows a state agency to apply to become an accrediting body. To date, three states are approved as accrediting bodies by the FDA: Arkansas, Iowa, and Texas. States may have stricter laws and regulations than the FDA, but if a state becomes an accrediting body, its regulations must be substantially similar to the MQSA regulations.

Finally, the Act allows the Secretary to authorize a state (upon application) to take on most of the FDA's roles in certifying mammography facilities within that state. In 2002, the FDA issued final regulations allowing states to become certifying bodies.[7] Currently there are four certifying states: Illinois, Iowa, South Carolina and Texas. Therefore, a state has the potential of serving not only as the inspecting organization but also as the accrediting body and certifying agency.

The Accrediting Body

Under MQSA, the accrediting body must have quality standards for both personnel and equipment that are equal to those established under MQSA. The accrediting body must review clinical images from each accredited facility not less than every 3 years and must conduct a random sample review of clinical images. It must ensure that these reviews are performed by qualified interpreting physicians who have no conflict of interest with the reviewed facility. The body must require an annual survey by a qualified medical physicist and must monitor and evaluate that survey.

The accrediting body must also make on-site visits annually to a sufficient number of facilities to evaluate the performance of its accreditation process. This body must develop a mechanism to investigate complaints, a system for reporting accreditation status to the FDA, and an adequate record-keeping system, and it must also maintain reasonable fees. The ACR is currently the only accrediting body that accredits mammography facilities nationwide. Arkansas, Iowa, and Texas currently perform accreditation only within their own jurisdictions.

The National Mammography Quality Assurance Advisory Committee

The NMQAAC was established for the following purposes: (1) to advise the FDA on appropriate standards and regulations for facilities, accrediting bodies, and sanctions; (2) to assist in developing procedures for monitoring compliance with MQSA quality standards; (3) to assist in developing a mechanism to investigate consumer complaints; and (4) to report on new developments in breast imaging that should be considered in the oversight of mammography facilities.

Furthermore, the Advisory Committee must determine the impact of the MQSA quality standards on access in rural areas and areas with a shortage of health professionals. It also must determine whether there will be an adequate number of qualified medical physicists after October 1, 1999, and assess the costs and benefits of compliance with MQSA. (The NMQAAC completed these studies prior to the implementation of the FDA's Final Rule and determined that MQSA would have little negative impact on access to mammography and that there were adequate qualified personnel to comply with MQSA.) The NMQAAC consists of 13 to 19 members, including radiologists, radiologic technologists, medical physicists, referring physicians, nurses, state radiation control personnel, and representatives from national breast cancer consumer health organizations.

THE INTERIM RULES

The Act required that all mammography facilities in the United States be certified before October 1, 1994. Recognizing the near impossibility of developing comprehensive regulations and providing initial certification of more than 10,000 mammography facilities within the same period, President Clinton signed legislation granting the FDA interim rule authority in 1993.

Because of the urgent public health need for national mammography standards, Congress decided to grant this interim rule authority rather than extend the deadline to develop standards. Under interim rule authority, the FDA could adopt appropriate existing standards from organizations such as the ACR and HCFA and from state regulations.

The FDA was not required to consult with the NMQAAC on the interim rules but was instructed to do so during the final rule-making process, as the Act stipulated. On December 21, 1993, the interim rules, entitled "Mammography Facilities-Requirements for Accrediting Bodies and Quality Standards and Certification Requirements," were published in the Federal Register.[8] The interim rules were divided into two subparts: the first dealt with accrediting bodies and the second with mammography facilities. They went into effect on February 22, 1994, and required that all facilities be certified by October 1, 1994.

MAMMOGRAPHY QUALITY STANDARDS: THE FINAL RULES

On April 3, 1996, the FDA published the proposed regulations for public comment.[9] Within the 90-day comment period, the FDA received approximately 1900 responses containing approximately 8000 individual comments from the health care community, state regulators, equipment manufacturers, and consumers. As a result, the FDA reworked the proposed rules to make them more performance based rather than proscriptive.

The final regulations for implementing the MQSA were released by the FDA on October 28, 1997.[10] In brief, the final rules established personnel requirements, clarified equipment standards, and shifted many of the proposed equipment requirements to performance outcomes in the quality assurance section of the regulations. Mammography facilities were also required to establish a system for communicating mammogram results and transferring the original mammograms at the request of the patient. The majority of the final regulations became effective on April 28, 1999. However, certain equipment regulations did not become effective until October 28, 2002. Some of the critical elements of the final rules are described in this section.

Requirements for Certification

To operate lawfully, a mammography facility must be MQSA certified as providing quality mammography services. In order to obtain an MQSA certificate, the facility must apply to an FDA-approved accrediting body. After the accrediting body decides to accredit the facility, the FDA (or state certifier) will issue a certificate to the facility or renew an existing certificate.

A new facility may apply for a provisional certificate. Effective for 6 months, the provisional certificate enables the facility to perform mammography and to obtain the clinical images needed to complete the accreditation process. A provisional certificate cannot be renewed, but a facility may apply for a 90-day extension of the provisional certificate.

To apply for a 90-day extension to a provisional certificate, a facility must submit to its accrediting body a statement of what the facility is doing to obtain certification as well as evidence that there would be a significant adverse impact on access to mammography in the geographic area served if such facility did not obtain an extension. The accrediting body forwards this request, with its recommendation, to the FDA (or state certifying body). If the FDA (or state certifying body) determines that the facility meets the criteria, a 90-day extension will be issued for a provisional certificate. A provisional certificate may not be renewed again beyond the 90 days.

A previously-certified facility whose certificate has expired, that the FDA (or state certifying body) has refused to renew, or that the FDA (or state certifying body) has suspended or revoked may apply to have the certificate reinstated. The facility must contact its accrediting body and fully document its history as a previously provisionally certified or certified mammography facility. The FDA may issue a provisional certificate to the facility if the accrediting body determines that the facility has adequately corrected pertinent deficiencies. After receiving the provisional certificate, the facility may lawfully resume performing mammography services while completing the requirements for accreditation and certification.

Personnel Standards

Requirements for initial qualification, continuing education, and continuing experience for interpreting physicians, medical physicists, and radiologic technologists were also codified in the final rules. These requirements are summarized in Table 8-2.

Equipment

The final rules followed the direction set by the interim regulations in defining the practice of mammography as "radiography of the breast" using specifically dedicated equipment for the detection of breast cancer. However, the FDA excluded from the final regulations stereotactic and all other radiographic invasive procedures for localization and biopsy. Also exempted from the final regulations were investigational devices with an FDA-approved investigational device exemption (IDE). Table 8-5 summarizes the equipment requirements.

Medical Records and Mammography Reports

The final rules incorporate specific requirements related to reporting and record-keeping. The interpreting physician must prepare a written report containing the results of each examination in addition to the following information: the name of the patient and an additional patient identifier, the date of the examination, the name of the examination's interpreting physician, and an overall final assessment. The final assessment must be categorized in the report into one of the following categories: "negative," "benign," "probably benign," "suspicious," or "highly suggestive of malignancy." In cases in which no final assessment can be assigned because of an incomplete evaluation, the assessment must be labeled "incomplete: need additional imaging evaluation"; the reasons why no assessments can be made must be stated. This approach was primarily based on the ACR's 1993 Breast Imaging Reporting and Data System (BI-RADS) for reporting and tracking of mammography outcomes.[11] In 2003, the FDA approved alternative standards to allow "incomplete: need additional imaging evaluation and/or prior mammograms for comparison" and a new final assessment category of "known biopsy-proven malignancy" as described in the 2003 BI-RADS atlas.[12]

This written report, signed by the interpreting physician, must be provided to the patient's health care provider within 30 days of the date of the examination. If the assessment is "suspicious" or "highly suggestive of malignancy," reasonable attempts must be made to communicate this news to the health care provider (or his or her designee) as soon as possible.

The final rules also required that the facility send a written summary of the mammography report to the patient in terms easily understood by a layperson. This applies to every patient who receives a mammogram, not only self-referred patients. If the patient is self-referred and has not named a health care provider, the facility must also send a copy of the written report to the patient.

Current mammograms and records must be kept by the facility for at least 5 years. For a patient who has not had additional mammograms at the facility, the mammograms and records must be retained at least 10 years (or longer if required by state or local law). The mammograms may be retained as either hard copy (film) or as soft copy (if originally obtained as a digital image). However, if a facility ceases performing mammography and closes its doors, the FDA continues to hold the facility responsible for ensuring that there is a mechanism to release the films to the appropriate entity when requested. Finally, original film mammograms and copies of the reports must be transferred to the patient, another medical institution, or the patient's health care provider if requested by the patient. The FDA requires facilities with full-field digital mammography units to have the capability of providing the original mammograms on film.

Quality Assurance Standards

The final rules address equipment quality control in great detail. These are described in Chapter 8. Additionally, the rules specify that each facility establish and maintain a mammography medical outcomes audit program to follow up positive mammogram assessments and to correlate pathology results with the interpreting physician's findings (see Chapter 38).

Mammographic Procedures and Techniques for Patients with Breast Implants

The final rules specify that facilities must have a procedure in place to inquire whether or not patients have breast implants and use appropriate views to maximize the visibility of breast tissues of patients who do.

Consumer Complaint Mechanisms

A serious complaint is defined by the FDA as "a report of a serious adverse event," which means an "adverse event that may significantly compromise clinical outcomes or an adverse event for which a facility fails to take appropriate corrective action in a timely manner." Examples of serious adverse events include: poor image quality, missed cancers, the use of personnel who do not meet the applicable requirements of the regulations, and failure to send to the appropriate person(s) mammography reports or lay summaries within 30 days.[10] Facilities must have a written system for collecting and resolving consumer complaints and must maintain records of each serious complaint for at least 3 years. If a facility cannot resolve a serious consumer complaint to the satisfaction of the patient, the facility must report the complaint to its accrediting body as soon as possible.

AMERICAN COLLEGE OF RADIOLOGY MAMMOGRAPHY ACCREDITATION PROGRAM

The ACR is a professional society whose purpose is to improve the health of patients and society by maximizing the value of radiology and radiologists by advancing the science of radiology, improving radiologic service to the patient, studying the socioeconomic aspects of the practice of radiology, and encouraging improved and continuing education for radiologists and allied professional fields. Through its professional committees, the ACR has developed and implemented nine modality-specific accreditation programs since 1987 to encourage the use of high-quality imaging and radiologic procedures in medicine.[13]

In 1994, the FDA approved the ACR as an accrediting body under MQSA. The ACR is the country's oldest and largest accrediting body for mammography and accredits more than 95% of the mammography units in the United States as well as a number of facilities in other countries. Initially developed in 1987 by the ACR Task Force on Breast Cancer, the ACR program is currently directed by the Committee on Mammography Accreditation of the Commission on Quality and Safety. The ACR Mammography Accreditation Program offers radiologists the opportunity for peer review and evaluation of their facility's staff qualifications, equipment, quality control and quality assurance programs, image quality, breast radiation dose, and processor quality control. The requirements for accreditation are identical or equivalent to those in the FDA final rules.

Application for Accreditation

A new mammography facility must apply for accreditation on all active mammography units. Furthermore, a new facility must apply for accreditation even if it is to be opened with a previously accredited unit from a sister facility. The ACR mammography accreditation procedure is summarized by the flow chart shown in Figure 37-1. The facility must first complete an entry application to provide basic facility, equipment, and personnel information and must submit a summary of the pass or fail results from their medical physicist's equipment evaluation along with an application fee. No clinical or phantom images are submitted at this time.

If a facility fulfills the criteria evaluated for the entry application, the FDA (or state certifying body) is notified, and a provisional certificate is issued. The ACR then sends a full application with the appropriate testing materials to the facility to obtain information on the qualifications of radiologists, medical physicists, and radiologic technologists; quality control results; and other requirements of the MQSA. Image quality and dose evaluations are an important part of the process and are evaluated through the use of a specially designed breast phantom and dosimeter. The facility must submit an image of the phantom as well as two sets of normal clinical films (one from a patient with fatty

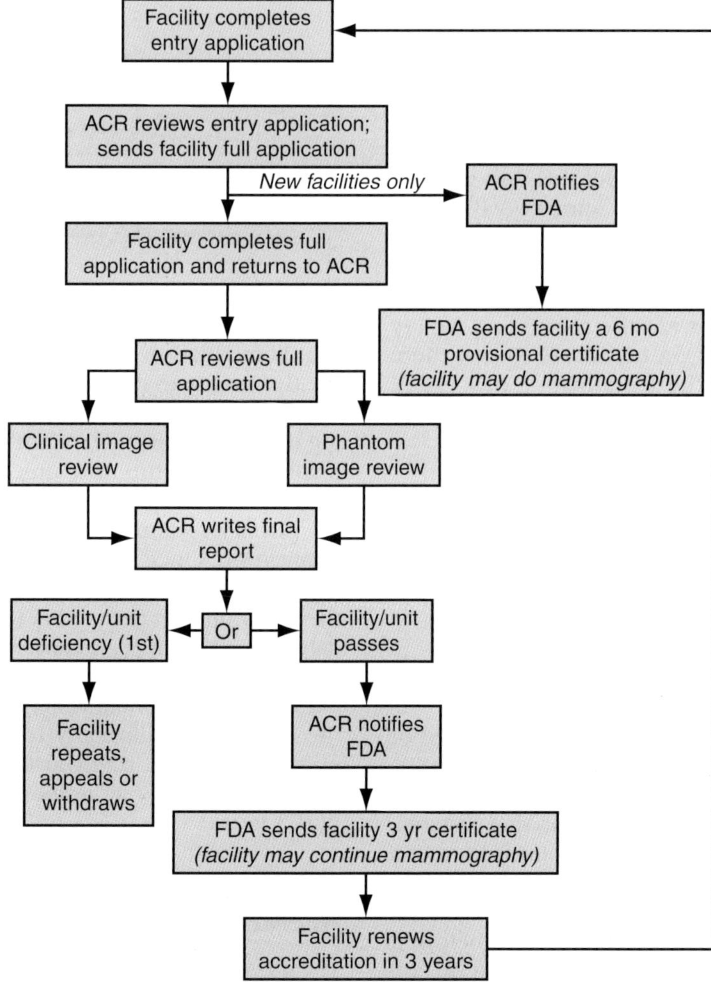

■ **FIGURE 37-1** Mammography accreditation process of the American College of Radiology (ACR). FDA, U.S. Food and Drug Administration.

breasts and one from a patient with dense breasts), which will be scored by a review panel of ACR-trained mammography medical physicists and radiologists. Finally, processor (or laser film printer) quality control for a 30-day period must also be submitted for evaluation. Facilities must send all application and testing materials to the ACR within 45 calendar days of the date the full application was mailed.

Final Reports

When all stages of the evaluation are completed, the ACR issues a final report to the lead interpreting physician that contains specific assessments and recommendations. (The facility's original images are also returned with the report.) Every facility that successfully meets all of the criteria is awarded a 3-year accreditation certificate and a unit decal for each approved mammography unit. The ACR notifies the FDA (or state certifying body) of each unit's accreditation approval so that the body may issue the facility a 3-year MQSA certificate. Because the FDA (and state certifying bodies) certify facilities rather than units, each accredited unit within the facility must have the same expiration date, regardless of when it was accredited. The MQSA certificate has the same expiration date as the ACR accreditation expiration. The ACR lists each accredited facility on its Web site (www.acr.org).

For those facilities that do not meet the ACR's accreditation criteria, specific recommendations for improvement are made. These recommendations provide guidance so that a facility can meet the criteria after corrective action and re-application. Facilities may appeal any denial of accreditation (Table 37-1). The ACR strongly recommends that facilities take out of service any unit that fails to meet all of the accreditation requirements after two consecutive attempts. The unit may reinstate only after the facility submits a corrective action plan to the ACR, the ACR approves it, and the facility completes it. The FDA (or state certifying body) will provide the reinstating facility with a 6-month provisional MQSA certificate so that there is adequate time to complete the accreditation process.

TABLE 37-1. How a Mammography Facility Should Proceed if Accreditation Is Not Granted

Attempt at Accreditation	Accreditation Result	Facility Options
First	*NOT GRANTED:* First deficiency Facility may continue performing mammography with the unit as long as facility has a valid MQSA certificate	*REPEAT* testing for unacceptable area(s) (only if more than 60 days on MQSA certificate), *APPLY FOR REINSTATEMENT* by retesting all areas (if 60 days or less on MQSA certificate), *APPEAL* decision on original images, or *WITHDRAW*
Second	*NOT GRANTED:* Second deficiency = first failure ACR strongly recommends that the facility cease performing mammography with the unit	*APPLY FOR REINSTATEMENT* (after corrective action) by retesting all areas, *APPEAL* decision on original images, or *WITHDRAW*
Third	*NOT GRANTED:* Third deficiency = second failure ACR strongly recommends that facility cease performing mammography with the unit	*APPLY FOR REINSTATEMENT* after participating in Scheduled On-Site Survey, *APPEAL* decision on original images, or *WITHDRAW*

ACR, American College of Radiology; FDA, U.S. Food and Drug Administration; MQSA, Mammography Quality Standards Act.

Renewal of Accreditation

The ACR sends a renewal application by mail to the accredited facility's lead interpreting physician approximately 8 months before the expiration of ACR accreditation. The renewal application process is the same as the process for new facilities.

New Units

When a facility installs a new unit (or a previously used or accredited unit that is new to the facility) after accreditation has been granted, the facility should contact the ACR for appropriate instructions. The FDA requires that all active mammography units be accredited. Furthermore, every facility must have an equipment evaluation performed by a qualified medical physicist and must submit the results to the ACR whenever a new unit is installed and before it is used for patient examination. All problems must be corrected, and documentation of correction provided to the ACR, before the new equipment is put into service.

If the facility has more than 13 months left on its current accreditation when the unit is installed, the ACR will ask the facility to complete a new unit addendum and submit a reduced fee. Facilities with new units that are applying in midcycle in this manner will need to submit testing results only for the new unit (phantom image, dosimeter, clinical images, processor quality control, and the medical physicist's annual survey report) rather than the full application. Once accreditation is approved for that unit, its expiration date is the same as the expiration date for the other units at the facility (or the same as the expiration date of the unit it replaced).

If the facility has less than 13 months left on its accreditation when a new unit is installed, the ACR will instruct the facility to begin early renewal of accreditation on all units at the usual renewal fee. Once accredited, the new expiration date for all units will be the old expiration date plus 3 years.

Full-Field Digital Mammography Accreditation

The FDA first approved the ACR to accredit full-field digital mammography (FFDM) on February 15, 2003. The ACR is currently approved to accredit the General Electric

Senographe 2000D, DS, and Essential, the Fischer Senoscan, the Lorad Selenia, the Siemens Mammomat Novation DR and the Fuji FCRm (computed radiography). At this time, the ACR accepts only hard-copy images for accreditation. Once an accrediting body is approved for an FFDM unit, the FDA no longer accepts applications to extend existing MQSA certificates to include their use. All new applicants with such units must contact the ACR and apply for the accreditation of the units. Until FDA-approved accreditation is available for FFDM units other than the ones specified above, applicants must continue to apply to and be approved by the FDA for extension of their certificate in order to legally operate the digital units.

Quality Control

Each facility must submit documentation of compliance for all quality control tests as part of the application process. Documentation for the technologist testing must be provided on the Mammography Quality Control Checklist; documentation of the medical physicist annual survey results must be submitted on the Medical Physicist Mammography QC Test Summary (or in a similar format). These forms may be copied from the 1999 ACR Mammography Quality Control Manual[14] or downloaded from the ACR Web site. The radiologic technologist and medical physicist may use a different format for their in-house documentation of quality control, if they choose. Facilities must also submit processor (or laser film printer) quality control records for a 30-day period for evaluation with the clinical and phantom images.

Phantom Images and Radiation Dose

Image quality, radiation dose, and half-value layer are evaluated using dosimeters and a specially designed breast phantom. The Lucite breast phantom with a wax insert containing fibers, specks, and masses simulates a 4.2-cm-thick compressed breast (Table 37-2).

A review panel of ACR-trained medical physicists scores the phantom image, which must meet the standards set by the Committee on Mammography Accreditation for the visualization of fibers, specks, masses, and artifacts. The four largest fibers, the three largest speck groups, and the three largest masses must be visualized for the image to pass. The ACR evaluation criteria are outlined in the 1999 ACR Mammography Quality Control Manual.

TABLE 37-2. Sizes for Phantom Test Object of Mammography Unit

Fibers (mm diameter)	Specks (mm diameter)	Masses (mm thick)
1.56	0.54	2.00
1.12	0.40	1.00
0.89	0.32	0.75
0.75	0.24	0.50
0.54	0.16	0.25
0.40		

Facility mammography personnel must expose the dosimeter on the phantom at the same time the accreditation image is produced. The dosimeter data are used to determine the average glandular dose for a breast of average size and density. The average glandular radiation dose may not exceed 300 mrad (3 mGy) per view.

Clinical Images

The facility must submit two sets of negative clinical images (one from a patient with fatty breasts and one from a patient with dense breasts), which are scored by a review panel of ACR-trained radiologists. Each set of four clinical images must consist of two views, a craniocaudal (CC) view and a mediolateral oblique (MLO) view of the left and right breast of each patient. The parameters that are scored on the clinical images are positioning, compression, exposure level, sharpness, contrast, noise, exam identification, and artifacts. Clinical images should be examples of the facility's best work and are judged accordingly by the review panel. A clinical image evaluation guide describing these eight parameters is available in the 1999 ACR Mammography Quality Control Manual. Facilities may not submit images from models or volunteers.

Validation Procedures

Annual Updates

The ACR mails each accredited facility an annual update package to complete and return to verify that the facility is maintaining consistent quality during the 3-year accreditation period. Each accredited facility is required to submit a recent medical physicist's annual survey report summary for each unit and an update of the application data, identifying changes in address or certain personnel as part of this annual update.

Validation Film Checks

Under MQSA, the ACR is required to conduct "random clinical image reviews of a sample of facilities to monitor and assess their compliance with standards established by the body for accreditation." The ACR Committee on Mammography Accreditation has also specified that this accreditation program validation provide facilities with midcycle educational feedback on image quality.

The ACR recognizes that clinical images selected for this evaluation may be drawn from a relatively small sample of films in relation to the total number of mammograms performed at the facility. Furthermore, variations in clinical image quality may be attributed to the natural anatomical differences present in the female population. The ACR reviewers take these issues into consideration during their evaluation of validation film check images. The ACR provides a written report when the review is complete.

On-Site Surveys

The ACR Mammography Accreditation Program is required to conduct on-site surveys on a random sample of accredited facilities. These surveys validate information submitted for accreditation and give facilities an

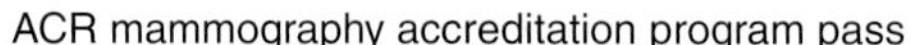

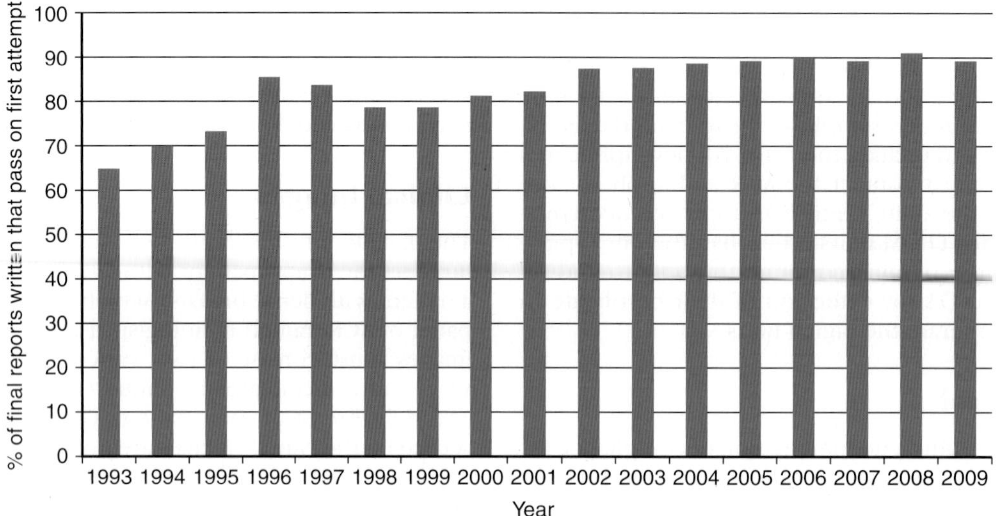

FIGURE 37-2 Pass rates for facilities participating in the American College of Radiology's Mammography Accreditation Program.

educational opportunity through constructive criticism for quality improvement from direct interaction with the ACR reviewers. Any facility chosen for an on-site survey is notified in advance. Radiologist and medical physicist reviewers from the Mammography Accreditation Program serve as members of the survey team along with an ACR staff person. During this survey, the site visit team performs the following acts: (1) reviews the quality assurance program; (2) reviews mammography policies and procedures; (3) reviews personnel qualifications; (4) reviews the facility's clinical images and mammography reports; and (5) works with the facility's staff to acquire and evaluate a phantom image along with a dose assessment of the x-ray unit.

SUMMARY

The quality of mammography performed in the United States has significantly improved since the ACR's accreditation program began in 1987 and Congress passed MQSA in 1992. In 1993, only 64.5% of mammography units applying for accreditation passed on their first attempt. Ten years later, 88.3% of units applying for (or renewing) accreditation passed on their first attempt.[15] Currently, more than 90% of mammography facilities pass accreditation on their first attempt (Fig. 37-2). This finding clearly illustrates the positive effects of the ACR Mammography Accreditation Program and the MQSA on the public health.

KEY POINTS

- A mammography facility must be accredited and certified in order to legally perform mammography in the United States.
- State radiation control programs inspect mammography facilities for MQSA annually.
- In order to accredit with the ACR, facilities must pass phantom and clinical image review.
- Under MQSA, facilities are required to renew their accreditation and certification every 3 years.
- The mammography accreditation pass rate has increased from 65% in 1993 to 90% in 2009 indicating that mammography quality in the United States has significantly improved.

REFERENCES

1. Conway BJ, McCrohan JL, Rueter FG, Suleiman OH. Mammography in the eighties. *Radiology* 1990;**177**:335-9.
2. Hendrick RE. Standardization of image quality and radiation dose in mammography. *Radiology* 1990;**174**:648-54.
3. Hendrick RE. Quality assurance in mammography. Accreditation, legislation and compliance with quality assurance standards. *Radiol Clin North Am* 1992;**30**:243-55.
4. US Department of Health and Human Services (DHHS), Health Care Financing Administration, Medicare Program. Medicare coverage of screening mammography. 42 CFR Parts 405, 410, 413, and 494; *Fed Regist* 1990;**55**:53510-25.
5. The Mammography Quality Standards Act. Public Law 102-539. 1992.
6. The Mammography Quality Standards Reauthorization Act. Public Law 105-248. 1998.
7. US Department of Health and Human Services, Food and Drug Administration. State certification of mammography facilities. *Fed Regist* 2002;**67**:5446-69.
8. US Department of Health and Human Services, Food and Drug Administration. Mammography facilities-requirements for accrediting bodies and quality standards and certification requirements: Interim rules. *Fed Regist* 1993;**58**:6765-72.
9. US Department of Health and Human Services, Food and Drug Administration. Mammography quality standards: Proposed rules. *Fed Regist* 1996;**61**:14855-920.
10. US Department of Health and Human Services, Food and Drug Administration. Quality mammography standards: Final rule. *Fed Regist* 1997;**62**:55852-994.

11. American College of Radiology. *Breast imaging reporting and data system (BI-RADS)*. Reston, Va.: American College of Radiology; 1993.
12. American College of Radiology. *Breast imaging reporting and data system (BI-RADS)*. Reston, Va.: American College of Radiology; 2003.
13. American College of Radiology. *Digest of Council Actions*. Reston, Va.: American College of Radiology; 2001.
14. American College of Radiology. *Mammography Quality Control Manual*. Reston, Va.: American College of Radiology; 1999.
15. Destouet JM, Bassett LW, Yaffe MJ, Butler PF, Wilcox PA. The ACR's Mammography Accreditation Program: ten years of experience since MQSA. *J Am Coll Radiol* 2005;**2**:585-94.

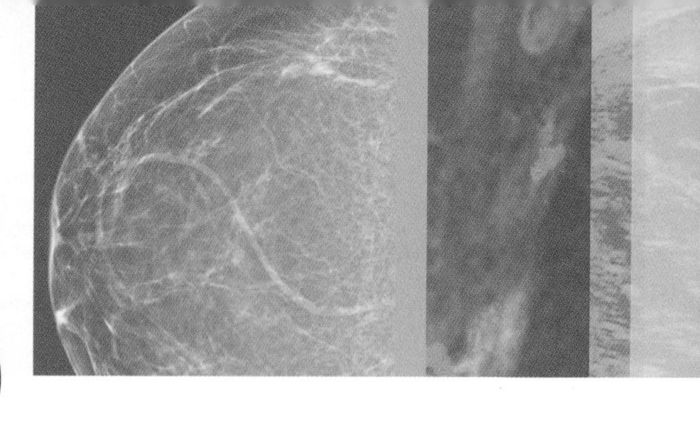

CHAPTER 38

The Medical Audit: Statistical Basis of Clinical Outcomes Analysis

Michael N. Linver

Medicine is the art of dealing with uncertainty.
The practice of breast screening is the acme of that art.
Myron Moskowitz, 1988

The *Mammography medical audit* can be defined in broad terms as a retrospective evaluation of the appropriateness and accuracy of mammographic image interpretation. The medical audit has been recognized by numerous experts in mammographic interpretation as the ultimate indicator of mammography performance.[1-4] It is the distillation of all of the quality assurance and quality control aspects addressed in mammography. It is the best measure of the interpretive ability of the interpreting physician. The medical audit removes the mystique and uncertainty of mammography and replaces them with a means to quantify and verify the value of the interpreting physician's work. It should therefore be an integral part of every practice.

As a member of the multidisciplinary Clinical Practice Guideline Panel on Quality Determinants of Mammography, convened by the Agency for Health Care Policy and Research (AHCPR, now called the Agency for Healthcare Research and Quality [AHRQ]) of the U.S. Department of Health and Human Services, I participated in the development of much of the material on the medical audit presented in this chapter. The material was published by AHCPR as part of its Clinical Practice Guideline series.[5]

The medical audit of a mammography practice has numerous benefits. It evaluates the ability of mammography to detect very small cancers at the desirable rate, one of the most important measures of success of any mammography practice.[2-4,6] In addition, radiologists receive individualized feedback regarding their performance. This feedback provides confidence, if the results are within expectations, or identifies the need for additional training in interpretive skills for the physician or for the radiologic technologist.[3,4,6-8] Longitudinal audits may detect the causes of false-negative errors, allowing for identification and correction of interpretive or technical shortcomings.[4,6,9-11] When audit data are reviewed and acted on appropriately, they become a powerful source of education for the interpreting physician.[9] Medical audit results within expected values can also be used to improve the compliance of both referring physicians and patients with screening mammography guidelines. Additionally, these results can provide evidence of acceptable levels of performance to third-party payers and government agencies.[3,6]

Individual audit data may be useful for a medicolegal defense.[3,4,8,12] As a part of a risk management program, timely audits of abnormal mammograms promote optimal follow-up of patients.[2] Audit data such as the number of screening cases recalled for additional evaluation have been valuable for calculating costs per patient screened.[1] As capitation arrangements become more prevalent throughout the medical community, radiologists seeking to contain costs when vying for capitation contracts with health care organizations should find such information useful. A final benefit of the audit process is that pooling of the data may allow universal outcomes analysis to be performed through a national database.[3,4,13]

Another compelling reason to perform a mammography audit relates to federal law. In 1992, Congress passed the Mammography Quality Standards Act (MQSA). This legislation regulates the practice of mammography. Subpart 3 Section 354f21A calls for "standards that require establishment and maintenance of a quality assurance and quality control program at the facility that is adequate and appropriate to ensure the reliability, clarity, and accurate interpretation of mammograms." The final rule of MQSA, which went into effect in 1999, mandates a limited form of the audit.[14] The specific audit requirements under MQSA are elaborated in more detail later.

Other regulatory organizations have also recognized the value of the medical audit. The Joint Commission (TJC) requires "periodic assessment by the radiology department/service of the collected information in order to identify important problems in patient care."[15] For compliance with its voluntary practice guidelines and technical standards, the American College of Radiology (ACR), in its document titled *ACR Practice Guideline for the Performance of Screening Mammography*, specifies the following: "Each facility shall establish and maintain a mammography medical outcomes audit program to follow up positive mammographic assessments (BI-RADS [ACR Breast Imaging Reporting and Data System] categories 4 and 5). In addition, follow-up of category 0 assessments is encouraged to correlate pathology results with the interpreting physician's findings. This program must be designed to ensure reliability, clarity, and accuracy for the interpretation of mammograms. Analysis of these outcome data must be performed for all interpreting physicians at a facility, individually and collectively, at least annually. It is understood that in most practice situations it will not be possible to obtain follow-up information on all positive mammograms."[16] In the fourth edition of the ACR BI-RADS Atlas, a major chapter is devoted to follow-up and outcomes monitoring, describing the performance of the audit in detail.[17]

COLLECTION OF AUDIT DATA: WHAT SYSTEM SHOULD BE USED?

When one undertakes a medical audit, the volume of data that must be acquired for analysis can present an imposing challenge. Although the data can be gleaned manually,[3,4] specially designed computer software programs have been created to make these tasks easier.[3,7,18-22] A variety of commercial software products are efficient, effective, and widely available. Most practices currently performing audits find these programs user friendly and affordable. These programs may include all the information recommended in "Follow-up and Outcomes Monitoring" chapter in the ACR BI-RADS Atlas,[17] or less information if only a limited audit is possible. A computer data collection program can be incorporated into a complete computerized reporting system.[17,20]

Computerized or manual collection of audit data has been greatly aided by use of the BI-RADS categories 0 through 6, which provide an already established number code for each report to be entered into the breast imaging database. The codes are as follows: BI-RADS category 0—Needs additional imaging evaluation and/or prior mammograms for comparison; BI-RADS category 1—Negative; BI-RADS category 2—Benign; BI-RADS category 3—Probably benign; BI-RADS category 4—Suspicious; BI-RADS category 5—Highly suggestive of malignancy; BI-RADS category 6—Known biopsy-proven malignancy. Because these category designations are required by law under MQSA for every mammography report,[14] they provide the consistency and uniformity required for accurate audit collection and analysis.

In deciding how best to collect audit data, one must consider the real cost of an audit in dollars and in time. Initiating and maintaining an audit requires a significant time commitment by at least one member of a mammography practice. For a small practice, use of a computer program to handle modest amounts of data is not essential, but for a large practice, it is a necessity. Careful assessment of needs before initiation of an audit can turn a data collection nightmare into a task that is manageable both fiscally and physically as well as one that is a rewarding educational experience.

THE DATA: WHAT SHOULD BE COLLECTED? WHAT SHOULD BE CALCULATED?

A variety of data can be collected that reflect the quality of performance of a mammography practice. To decide what data are most essential, one must consider the following three major questions, which directly measure an interpreting physician's performance:[23]

1. Does the practice meet the primary goal of an effective screening program? In other words, is a high percentage of cancers being detected in the screened population? What are the detection rates and sensitivity for asymptomatic cancers?
2. Does a large percentage of cancers being found have a favorable prognosis? That is, are the majority of mammography-detected cancers small and confined to the breast? What are the percentages of minimal cancers and lymph node-negative cancers being found?
3. Are other important parameters reflecting screening and diagnostic success equivalent to those demonstrated in other screening programs? In other words, are recommendations for further imaging evaluation or a biopsy in the acceptable range? What is the recall rate, and what is the positive predictive value (PPV) for recalls and recommended biopsies?

These questions require appropriate data to be properly answered quantitatively. The required data, in turn, provide surrogate markers for the lowering of breast cancer deaths, the ultimate goal of breast imaging. Demonstration of adequate values for these surrogate markers can then be considered strong supportive evidence that the ultimate goal of lowering breast cancer deaths through mammography and other breast imaging modalities is being achieved. The latter has been richly supported by the results of randomized screening trials.[23] Table 38-1 lists the essential raw and derived data that are required to answer the above questions (an exception is sensitivity, which is discussed later). *Raw data* refers to specific items of

TABLE 38-1. The Essential or Basic Mammography Audit: Minimum Desired Raw and Derived Data

A. Raw data:
1. Dates of audit period and total number of examinations in that period.
2. Number of screened examinations; number of diagnostic examinations.*
3. Number of recommendations for further imaging evaluation (recalls) (ACR BI-RADS Category 0—Needs further evaluation).
4. Number of recommendations for biopsy or surgical consultation (ACR BI-RADS Categories 4 and 5—Suspicious findings and Highly suggestive of malignancy).†
5. Biopsy results: malignant or benign (keep separate data for FNA or core biopsy cases).†
6. Tumor staging: histologic type (in situ [ductal] or invasive [ductal or lobular]), grade, size, and nodal status.

B. Derived data (calculated from the raw data):
1. True-positive results.
2. False-positive results—three sub-definitions: FP_1, FP_2, FP_3 (see text).
3. Positive predictive value:
   a. If a screening/diagnostic facility, can define any of three ways:
      (1) Based on abnormal screening examination (PPV_1).
      (2) Based on recommendation for biopsy or surgical consultation (PPV_2).
      (3) Based on result of biopsy (PPV_3 or positive biopsy rate).
   b. If screening facility only, can define only one way, based on abnormal screening examination (PPV_1).
4. Cancer detection rate for asymptomatic (true screening) cases.
5. Percentage of minimal cancers‡ found.
6. Percentage of node-negative invasive cancers found.
7. Recall rate.
8. Analysis of any known false-negative examinations.†

*Separate audit statistics should be maintained for asymptomatic and symptomatic patients.
†Collection of these data is required under Mammography Quality Standards Act (MQSA) final rules.
‡Minimal cancer: invasive cancer ≤1cm or in-situ ductal cancer.
ACR BI-RADS, American College of Radiology Breast Imaging Reporting and Data System; FNA, fine-needle aspiration.

information, interpretive results and recommendations, and pathology findings collected directly from the mammography and pathology reports. *Derived data* refers to calculated measures of various mammographic and pathologic parameters based on the collected raw data. The raw data that are listed in Table 38-1 have been collected in most major audits reported in the literature.[1-4,6,7,18,24-26] They are all readily accessible and relatively easy to collect, regardless of the method used. Sources of these data are discussed later.

Of the raw data to be collected for an audit of screening mammography, cases assigned BI-RADS categories 0, 4, or 5 are considered "positive," and those assigned BI-RADS categories 1 or 2 are considered "negative." (BI-RADS category 3 should never be assigned to a screening examination and many facilities do not assign a 4 or 5 to a screening examination.) Of the raw data to be collected for an audit of diagnostic mammography, cases assigned a final assessment of BI-RADS categories 4 or 5 are considered "positive," and those assigned BI-RADS 1, 2, or 3 are considered "negative."

Additional data are listed as part of the more complete raw data list in Table 38-2. They are also of great value, although they can add considerable time and complexity to the audit process. These data have been useful in many studies as determinants of prevalent versus incident cancer rates (*prevalent cancers* are those found on the patients first screening mammogram; *incident cancers* are those found on a later regular screening mammogram), predictive value of various mammographic findings, and significance of various risk factors.[1-3,6,7,18,24,25]

Although not required for calculation of the essential derived data listed in Table 38-1, the additional raw data listed in Table 38-2 are still worthwhile to collect because they provide information about certain variables that can cause marked fluctuation in audit results. For instance, if a large proportion of mammography examinations was performed on patients screened for the first time (those with prevalent cancers), the rate of cancers detected should be much higher than in a population that has been screened previously (incident cancers). Thus, knowledge of the proportion of initial screening mammograms to follow-up screening mammograms can be extremely useful in fine-tuning and interpreting the audit results.[3,7]

As with the raw data, the essential derived data can be supplemented with additional derived data of great value, as noted in Table 38-3. These additional data are also highly desirable, but time constraints and lack of accessibility of certain raw data, especially false-negative results (see the following list), may preclude their being calculated.

Before calculating any of the derived data in Table 38-1 or Table 38-3, one should categorize every mammographic examination result into one of four groups according to the following definitions (based on major audit studies in the literature):

1. True-positive (TP): Cancer diagnosed within 1 year after biopsy recommendation based on an abnormal mammogram (consensus).
2. True-negative (TN): No known cancer diagnosis within 1 year of a normal mammogram (consensus).
3. False-negative (FN): Diagnosis of cancer within 1 year of a normal mammogram result.[1,7,10,11,24,26,27] (Although numerous other definitions of false-negative results exist, this definition historically has been the one most widely applied.)
4. False-positive (FP): The literature supplies the following three different definitions:
   a. No known cancer diagnosed within 1 year of an abnormal screening mammogram result (i.e., a

TABLE 38-2. More Complete Mammography Audit: Raw Data to Be Collected*

A. Dates of audit period and total number of examinations in that period (usually a 6- or 12-month period).

B. Risk factors:
1. Patient age at the time of the examination.
2. Breast cancer history: personal or family (especially premenopausal cancer in first-degree relative—mother, sister, or daughter).
3. Hormone replacement therapy.
4. Previous biopsy-proven lobular carcinoma in situ or atypia.

C. Number and type of mammograms: screening (asymptomatic) or diagnostic (clinical breast signs or symptoms of possible abnormality or abnormal screening mammogram)†

D. First-time examination or follow-up (repeat) study.

E. Mammographic interpretation and recommendation (try to conform to ACR lexicon).
1. **Further imaging evaluation (recall) (ACR BI-RADS Category 0—Needs further evaluation).**
2. Routine follow-up (ACR BI-RADS Categories 1 and 2—Negative and Benign findings).
3. Early follow-up (ACR BI-RADS Category 3—Short-term follow-up).
4. **Biopsy or surgical consultation (ACR BI-RADS Categories 4 and 5—Suspicious findings and Highly suggestive of malignancy)‡**

F. Biopsy results: benign or malignant (keep separate data for FNA or core biopsy cases).‡

G. Cancer data:
1. Mammographic findings: mass, calcifications, indirect signs of malignancy, no mammographic signs of malignancy.
2. **Palpable or nonpalpable tumor.**
3. **Tumor staging (pathologic): histologic type, grade, size, and nodal status.**

*Bold type indicates data desired for the essential mammography audit.
†Separate audit statistics should be maintained for asymptomatic and symptomatic patients.
‡Collection of these data required under final rules of the Mammography Quality Standards Act (MQSA).
ACR BI-RADS, American College of Radiology Breast Imaging Reporting and Data System.
FNA, fine-needle aspiration.

TABLE 38-3. The More Complete Mammography Audit: Derived Data to Be Calculated*

A. True-positives, false-positives (three subdefinitions: FP_1, FP_2, FP_3), true-negative, false-negative results (MQSA final rules require analysis of any known false-negative results)†

B. Sensitivity.

C. Positive predictive value:
1. **Based on abnormal screening exam result (PPV_1).**
2. **Based on recommendation for biopsy or surgical consultation (PPV_2).**
3. **Based on results of biopsy (PPV_3).**

D. Specificity.

E. Cancer detection rate:
1. **Cancer detection rate for asymptomatic (true screening) cases.**
2. Prevalent vs incident.
3. Overall.
4. Rates within various age groups.

F. Percentage of minimal cancers‡ found.

G. Percentage of node-negative invasive cancers found.

H. Recall rate.

I. Analysis of any known false-negative examinations.†

*Bold type indicates data desired for the essential mammography audit analysis.
†Collection of these data required under MQSA final rules.
‡Minimal cancer: invasive cancer ≤1cm or in-situ ductal cancer.
FNA, fine-needle aspiration; MQSA, Mammography Quality Standards Act.

mammogram for which further imaging evaluation or biopsy is recommended) (FP_1).[1-3,24,26]

b. No known cancer diagnosed within 1 year after recommendation for biopsy or surgical consultation on the basis of an abnormal mammogram (FP_2).[1,7]
c. Benign disease found at biopsy within 1 year after recommendation for biopsy or surgical consultation on the basis of an abnormal mammogram result (FP_3).[3,7,24]

Another way to conceptualize the relationship among these four groups of results is expressed graphically in Figure 38-1.[28] Women screened for breast cancer with mammography were assigned to the top (positive) group when the result indicated a suspicion of breast cancer or in the bottom (negative) group if the result was judged to be normal. Each group was then subdivided according to whether patients were

Screening test for cancer	Biopsy results: Positive	Biopsy results: Negative
Positive	True positive (TP)	False positive (FP)
Negative	False negative (FN)	True negative (TN)

■ **FIGURE 38-1** Graphic representation of relationship among true-positive (TP), false-positive (FP), false-negative (FN), and true- negative (TN) screening mammogram results. TP and FP results derive from "positive" screening mammograms assessed as American College of Radiology Breast Imaging Reporting and Data System (BI-RADS) categories 0, 4, or 5. FN and TN results derive from "negative" screening mammograms assessed as BI-RADS categories 1 or 2. (See text for explanation.)

subsequently found to have breast cancer (left columns) or not (right columns). There are then four possible combinations:

1. If results of both mammogram and biopsy are positive for cancer, the mammogram result is designated true-positive (TP).
2. If both mammogram and biopsy results are negative for breast cancer, or if the mammogram result is negative and no clinical evidence of breast cancer is found in the absence of a biopsy, the mammogram result is designated true-negative (TN).
3. If the mammogram result is positive and either the biopsy result is negative or no clinical evidence of breast cancer is seen within 1 year, the mammogram result is designated false-positive (FP).
4. Conversely, if the mammogram interpretation is negative for cancer and the biopsy result is positive, the mammography interpretation is designated as a false-negative (FN).

Given these four definitions and the raw data, one can now calculate the following derived data on the basis of major audit studies in the literature.

Sensitivity

Sensitivity is defined as the probability of detecting a cancer when a cancer exists or, alternatively, as the percentage of all patients found to have breast cancer within 1 year of screening whose mammograms were correctly diagnosed as suspicious for breast cancer.[2,6,7,9,18,24,26,29,30] Sensitivity can be calculated as follows:

$$Sensitivity = \frac{TP}{TP + FN}$$

Positive Predictive Value

The following three separate definitions of PPV may be applied on the basis of the three definitions of false-positive results given previously:

1. PPV_1 (abnormal screening):The percent of *all abnormal screening examination results* that lead to a diagnosis of cancer.[2,3,18,26,29]

$$PPV_1 = \frac{TP}{\text{number of abnormal screening examinations}}$$

Or

$$PPV_1 = \frac{TP}{TP + FP_1}$$

2. PPV_2 (biopsy recommended): The percentage of *all cases recommended for biopsy or surgical consultation* as a result of screening that resulted in the diagnosis of cancer.[1,7] PPV_2 can therefore be expressed as:

$$PPV_2 = \frac{TP}{\text{number of cases recommended for biopsy after abnormal screening examinations}}$$

Or

$$PPV_2 = \frac{TP}{TP + FP_2}$$

3. PPV_3 (biopsy performed): The percentage of *all biopsies actually performed* as a result of screening that resulted in the diagnosis of cancer. This is also known as the *biopsy yield of malignancy*, or the *positive biopsy rate*.[3,7,18,31] PPV_3 can therefore be expressed as:

$$PPV_3 = \frac{TP}{\text{number of biopsies}}$$

Or

$$PPV_3 = \frac{TP}{TP + FP_3}$$

It should be noted that the various types of PPV just described are measures of completely different skills utilized by the breast imager. PPV_1 is considered a measure of one's perceptive skills at screening, whereas PPV_2 and PPV_3 are deemed measures of analytical skills utilized in diagnostic mammographic evaluation. Further, for interpretation and comparison of audit data from a particular mammography practice with published data to be accurate, it is important to know which definition of PPV is being used. For practices performing only screening mammography, only PPV_1 is of value in evaluating data. For practices performing both screening and diagnostic mammography, all three definitions of PPV can be applied.

Specificity

Specificity is defined as the probability of a normal mammogram report when no cancer exists or, alternatively, as the percentage of all patients with no evidence of breast cancer within 1 year of screening who were correctly identified as having normal mammograms at the time of screening.[1-3,18,24,26,29] Specificity can therefore be expressed as:

$$Specificity = \frac{TN}{FP + TN}$$

Some variation in the range of specificity exists, depending on the definition of false-positive results being applied, but the variations are small and probably insignificant because of the very small number of false-positive results and the very large number of true-negative results in screening populations evaluated in most audit series. In other words, the great majority of screening mammograms will be negative and the majority called abnormal will be very small.

Overall Cancer Detection Rate

Defined as the overall number of cancers detected per 1000 patients screened. the *overall cancer detection rate* should be available in all basic audits.[1-3,7,10,18,24,29-31] Of even greater value is the cancer detection rate in asymptomatic patients, as this group represents the true screening population.[2,3,7,32] Therefore, all mammograms should be classified as screening or diagnostic so that the cancer detection rate in the asymptomatic group can be calculated.

The following cancer detection rates can be calculated only if the appropriate raw data are collected. Although not essential to a basic audit, such rates provide valuable audit information and should be calculated when possible.

- Prevalent versus incident cancer rates (i.e., rates of cancer in first-time versus routine follow-up examinations).[3,5,7,18]
- Cancer detection rates by age group.[3,9,18]

In addition, separate sensitivities, PPVs, and specificities can be calculated for each of these subgroups, yielding yet another level of useful audit information. A summary of major articles that include medical audit data on mammography screening is shown in Table 38-4.

ANALYZING THE DATA: WHAT DO THE NUMBERS TELL YOU?

The real value of calculating the derived data as described in the previous section lies in creating quantitative measures of the six pieces of derived data that can address the three questions one must answer if mammography of high quality is to be achieved. By quantifying sensitivity and cancer detection rate, one can assess whether a desirable percentage of cancers are being detected in the screened population. By quantifying tumor size and node positivity, one can evaluate whether a high percentage of those cancers found at screening have a favorable prognosis. By quantifying recall rates and PPVs, one can determine whether those cancers are being found through the use of acceptably efficient and appropriate performance criteria.

The relationship among these data can best be conceptualized using a representative receiver operating characteristic (ROC) curve for mammography,[28,33] as shown in Figure 38-2. An ROC curve for individual interpreting physicians can be generated by assessing their interpretive skills in predicting the likelihood of malignancy in a mixed set of positive and negative mammogram examinations with proven outcomes. The interpreting physician plots his or her performance as a series of graph points based on his or her answers to such an assessment, with each point representing the physician's perceived likelihood of malignancy plotted against the actual findings. The resulting series of plotted points defines the ROC curve for that individual. Each interpreting physician's ROC curve is slightly different but should always be above the diagonal line in Figure 38-2 spanning the curve from lower left to upper right, which represents chance performance. Interpreting physicians with better mammography interpretative skills generate ROC curves whose arcs span higher above that line (showing a higher percentage of true-positive and true-negative interpretations), and those with lesser skills generate curves coming closer to the line. Regardless of the height of the arc of an interpreting physician's ROC curve, if he or she starts from a point in the middle of the curve (point A) and then increases his or her false-positive fraction to point B on the curve (which would be reflected in a relatively lower value for PPV or a higher recall rate), the interpreting physician would experience an obligatory decrease in the false-negative fraction; this change would be reflected in a higher sensitivity and a higher cancer detection rate. Conversely, if the interpreting physician decreases his or her false-positive fraction to point C on the curve (as reflected in an increase in PPV and a decrease in the recall rate), he or she would find an increase in the false-negative fraction; this would be reflected in a decrease in sensitivity and a lower cancer detection rate.

What the preceding discussion means, very simply, is that what we do in mammographic interpretation is a tradeoff: To find every cancer present and have *no* false-negative results, we would necessarily have to recall virtually every patient and request surgery on a large majority of these. These are unacceptable scenarios if screening mammography is to be cost-effective and psychologically accepted by the women being screened. Indeed, if one is operating too close to the high end of the ROC curve, where the slope is

TABLE 38-4. Summary of Medical Audit Data from Mammography Screening Studies in The Medical Literature, 1987–1993

	Population Screened					Results									Tumor Data			
Study*	**Total Patients**	**Asymptomatic (%)**	**Symptomatic (%)**	**Baseline (%)**	**F/U (%)**	**TN**	**FP†**	**TP**	**FN**	**PPV‡§**	**Sensitivity‡**	**Specificity‡**	**Recall Rate (%)**	**Cancer Detection Rate/1000**	**Median Size (cm)**	**Mean Size (cm)**	**Lymph Node Positivity (%)**
Spring and Kimbrell-Willmot, 1987[4]	6430	NG	NG	NG	NG	5960	338 (3)	117	15	0.257_C (0.218, 0.300)	0.886 (0.820 0.935),	0.946 (0.940, 0.952)	NG	18.19	NG	2.2	32.3
Bird, 1989[1]	21,716	NG	NG	NG	NG	19,402	2172 (1)	130	12	0.056_A (0.048, 0.067)	0.915 (0.857, 0.956)	0.900 (0.895, 0.903)	9.27	5.99	NG	1.7	29
Sickles, 1992[3]	37,093	94	6	61	39	36,399	456 (3)	220	18‖	0.325_C (0.290, 0.363)	0.924 (0.883, 0.955)	0.988 (0.986, 0.989)	5.66	5.93	1.2	1.5	11.2
Linver et al, 1992[7]																	
First year	18,706	86	14	39	61	18,215	340 (2)	121	30	0.263_B (0.223, 0.306)	0.801 (0.726, 0.860)	0.982 (0.980, 0.984)	5.34	6.47	1.5	1.7	2.6
Second year	19,927	88	12	29	71	19,232	487 (2)	181	27	0.271_B (0.238, 0.307)	0.870 (0.815, 0.912)	0.975 (0.973, 0.977)	8.12	9.08	1.2	1.6	18.5
Burhenne, 1992[18]	11,824	100	0	NG	NG	10,786	984 (1)	47	7	0.045_A (0.034, 0.061)	0.870 (0.751, 0.946)	0.916 (0.911, 0.921)	8.27	3.97	NG	NG¶	11
Lynde, 1993[30]	21,141	NG	NG	NG	NG	19,771	1263 (1)	98	7	0.072_A (0.059, 0.087)	0.933 (0.868 0.973)	0.940 (0.937, 0.943)	6.44	4.64	NG	1.2	2.0
Robertson, 1993[2]	25,788	100	0	NG	NG	24,061	1539 (1)	170	18	0.099_A (0.086, 0.115)	0.904 (0.853, 0.942)	0.940 (0.938, 0.943)	6.63	6.59	NG	NG**	NG

*Superscript numbers indicate chapter references.
†Numbers in parentheses represent type 1, 2, or 3 FP, as defined in text.
‡For PPV, sensitivity, and specificity, the two sets of numbers in parentheses represent the confidence intervals for each.
§Subscripts A, B, and C represent PPV_1, PPV_2, and PPV_3, respectively, as defined in text.
‖Estimated from partial sample.
¶85% were stage 0 or stage 1.
**66% were stage 0 or stage 1.
FN, false-negative mammogram results; FP, false-positive mammogram results; F/U, patients receiving a follow-up mammogram, screening or diagnostic, at any time after their baseline mammogram; NG, not given; PPV, positive predictive value; TN, true-negative examination results; TP, true-positive examination results.

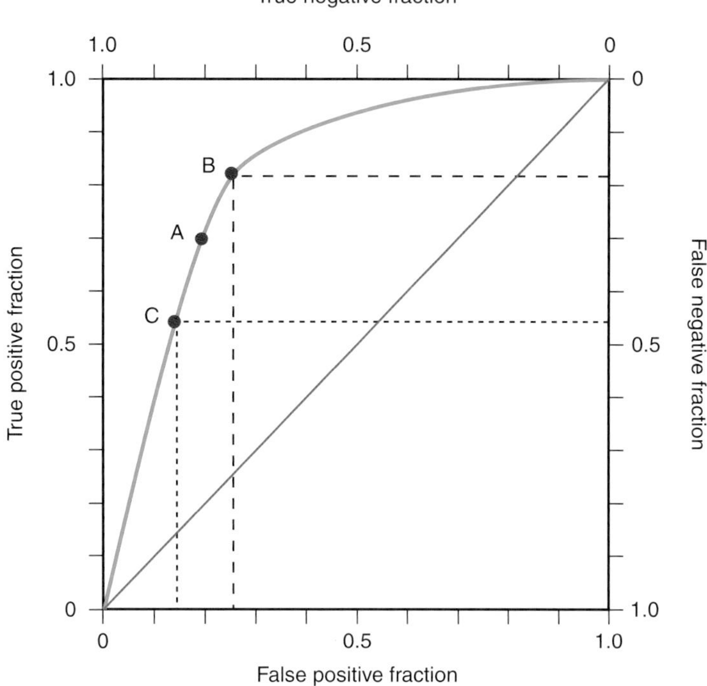

■ **FIGURE 38-2** Representative receiver operation characteristics (ROC) curve for mammography. (See text for explanation.)

shallow (e.g., to the right of point B in Fig. 38-2), the inefficiency is apparent: One can decrease the false-negative rate only minimally, while increasing the false-positive rate to an unacceptably high level. Therefore, one should operate closer to the middle of the ROC curve, where one can be the most efficient and yet still effective in detecting early breast cancer. By calculating and comparing the derived data described earlier, an interpreting physician can determine where he or she is operating on a representative ROC curve (or even on their own ROC curve, if known), and adjust their approach to mammographic interpretation accordingly.

It should be noted that those valuable parameters related to tumor size and node positivity are not reflected in this model of the ROC curve. However, the ROC curve still serves as a useful construct for understanding and utilizing the interrelationships among the other stated measures of interpretative quality. Desirable numerical goals designed to keep the interpreting physician operating near the middle of the ROC curve (those toward which the interpreting physician should strive) are as listed in Table 38-5. These numbers are based on a review of all major audits in the literature (most of which are listed in Table 38-4); they are discussed separately in this section.

Sensitivity

The published range of sensitivity in most mammography audits is between 85% and 90%, using the definition given in the previous section.[1,4,7,10,24,26,30,34,35] This range is therefore believed to be a desirable goal (see Tables 38-4 and 38-5). Sensitivity may vary with patient age, appearing to decrease in younger populations with denser breast tissue,[18] but nonetheless remains an extremely valuable parameter. Unfortunately, sensitivity is often among the most difficult data to obtain, because it requires knowledge of the actual number of false-negative results for accurate calculation (see previous section). It is usually necessary to establish a direct link with a complete tumor registry to find the actual number of false-negative results.[2,7,10,18] Thus, it may not be possible to calculate "true" sensitivity. One may be forced instead to estimate the number of false-negative results so as to obtain an approximation of sensitivity. However, it is still desirable to make such an estimate.[3]

Positive Predictive Value

The PPV is virtually always measurable, through the use of one or more of the definitions described previously. As already shown, definitions in the literature vary considerably, but the most often quoted is the PPV for all cases recommended for biopsy (PPV_2). This number is greater than 25% and less than 40% in most reported series (see Tables 38-4 and 38-5).[3,6,7,34] This range is considered an achievable goal for which to strive. If a facility performs only screening mammography, then the PPV based on the number of abnormal screening examination results (PPV_1) is more relevant and should be applied instead. The desirable goal is greater than 5% and less than 10% in most reported series.[2,3,18,26,29,34] For screening examinations, this range is considered an achievable goal for which to strive. Facilities performing both screening and diagnostic mammography may also find this number of value, in addition to PPV_2. For cases in which core, fine-needle aspiration (FNA), or vacuum-assisted needle biopsy is recommended and performed, separate PPV statistics should also be maintained for each of these biopsy groups.

TABLE 38-5. Screening Mammography Analysis of Medical Audit Data: Agency for Health Care Policy and Research Desirable Goals vs. Breast Cancer Surveillance Consortium Performance Results

Parameter	AHCPR Goals	BCSC Results
PPV based on abnormal screening examinations (PPV_1)*	5%-10%	4.5%
PPV for recommended biopsies† (PPV_2)	25%-40%	25%
Tumors found—stage 0 or 1	>50%	76%
Tumors found—minimal cancers£	>30%	51.8%
Node positivity	<25%	18.8%
Cancers found/1000 cases	2-10	4.4
Prevalent cancers found/1000 (first-time examination)	6-10	4.4
Incident cancers found/1000 (follow-up examination)	2-4	4.3
Recall rate	≤10%	9.7%
Sensitivity (if measurable)	>85%	80%
Specificity (if measurable)	>90%	—

*PPV = Positive predictive value. PPV_1, the percent of all abnormal screening examination results that lead to a diagnosis of cancer; PPV_2, the percentage of all cases recommended for biopsy or surgical consultation as a result of screening that resulted in the diagnosis of cancer.

$$PPV_1 = \frac{TP}{\text{number of abnormal screening examinations}}$$

$$PPV_2 = \frac{TP}{\text{number of cases recommended for biopsy after abnormal screening examinations}}$$

†FNA, fine-needle aspiration, or core needle biopsy
£Minimal cancer: invasive cancer ≤1cm or in-situ ductal cancer.
AHCPR, Agency for Health Care Policy and Research, now Agency for Healthcare Research and Quality (AHRQ); BCSC, Breast Cancer Surveillance Consortium.

In addition to measuring PPV_2 and PPV_3 for all positive (BI-RADS 4 and BI-RADS 5) studies for which biopsy is recommended and performed, PPV_2 and PPV_3 should also be evaluated for those lesions placed into BI-RADS category 3—Probably benign. Lesions meeting the criteria established for this category should have a PPV of less than 2%.[17] If the PPV is found to be greater than 2%, then an evaluation of the criteria being applied to such lesions should be undertaken, with assignment of lesions with features not meeting those criteria to BI-RADS category 4 in future interpretations.

As with sensitivity, the PPV in an individual practice is subject to many variables. Among these variables are the age distribution of patients with cancers in the population served, percentage of palpable cancers, cancer detection rate, the size and lymph node positivity of cancers found, and the sensitivity.[25,27,33,36-38] The obligatory relationship of cancer detection rate, sensitivity, and PPV to an individual interpreting physician's ROC curves was discussed earlier. The effect of the age distribution on PPV relates to findings by some researchers that PPV is directly proportional to the age of the population being screened and to the prior probability of disease within each age group.[3,27,37] The older the screened population, the higher the PPV will be. PPV varies directly with the size of tumors found in a screening mammography program: When most tumors are large, PPV tends to be higher; finding a greater number of small tumors can usually be accomplished only at the expense of a lower PPV.[27,34,35]

Tumor Size

In most reported series, more than 50% of tumors diagnosed through screening mammography are stage 0 or stage 1.[2,4,18,34] Even more importantly, most series have shown that more than 30% of cancers detected by mammography were minimal cancers (i.e., an invasive cancer ≤ 1cm or in situ ductal carcinomas).[1,3,7,10,18,26,30,31] Because it has been well established that mortality from breast cancer is directly related to tumor size, the preceding percentages for small and early-stage tumors found by mammography should be considered desirable goals for which to strive (see Tables 38-4 and 38-5). Later published audit data from my practice, and from other practices, show that tumors detected at screening that are stage 0 or stage 1 account for as many as 80% of all screening-detected tumors, and minimal cancers for as many as 60%.[34,34,37]

By reaching these goals, one can achieve the greatest impact on ultimate patient outcomes. Tumor size varies with the ratio of screening and diagnostic examinations in a mammography practice. Diagnostic examinations of symptomatic patients invariably yields larger tumors than those found in a screening population.[4,7,18,34-36]

Lymph Node Positivity

Tumor size should also be correlated with the rate of lymph node positivity, which in most reported series has been less than 25% in a screening population.[1,3,4,7,18,26,31,34] Because it has also been well established that mortality from breast cancer is directly proportional to node positivity, this rate for node positivity must also be considered a desirable goal for which to strive in one's practice (see Tables 38-4 and 38-5).

Cancer Detection Rate

The cancer detection rate is quite variable, with rates of 2 to 10 cancers per 1000 reported in most screening series (see Tables 38-4 and 38-5).[1-4,7,18,24-26,31,34,36,37] Variability in this rate is due to differing rates of detection in first-time screened women versus previously screened women (i.e., prevalent vs. incident cancers). In most screening populations, prevalent cancer rates vary from 6 to 10 per 1000, and incident cancer rates from 2 to 4 per 1000.[7,18,24,34] The cancer detection rate also varies with age.[3,7,18,24,37,39] Despite these variables, the cancer detection rate serves as a measure of the relative threshold for abnormal that is being achieved. For example, even if an audit shows that sensitivity and PPV are both high, but the number of cancers found is less than 2 per 1000 asymptomatic patients, then the sensitivity value is suspect. The number of cancers eluding detection in that particular population is probably too great, and the overall quality of the mammography being practiced should be further evaluated.[25,38]

Recall Rate

It is important to audit your *recall rate*—the percentage of patients for whom further imaging evaluation (e.g., coned compression views, magnification views, ultrasonography) is recommended after a screening mammography, for two reasons: Firstly, the recall rate can be used to calculate one of the commonly used definitions of false-positive results (FP_1) and one of the definitions of PPV (PPV_1) (see previous section on derived data). Accordingly, the recall rate is of value to all facilities, but especially to those performing only screening mammography. Secondly, the cost-effectiveness and credibility of mammography can be negatively affected by a disproportionately high recall rate.[1]

In most large reported series, the percentage of patients recalled for further imaging evaluation is 10% or less.[1-3,18,26,34,36] This value is therefore believed to be a desirable number for which to strive (see Tables 38-4 and 38-5). However, later data derived from more than 30 practices in North Carolina indicate that a rise in recall rates beyond 4.8% resulted in very little improvement in sensitivity, and that increasing recall rates beyond 5.8% was accompanied by a significant decrease in PPV_1. Therefore, it appears that the best trade-off between relatively high sensitivity and PPV_1 values may be accomplished with a recall rate of approximately 5% to 6%.[40] Many investigators have also noted that the recall rate decreases with the interpreting physician's experience over time.[1,3]

Specificity

Specificity is a measure of quality that is difficult to acquire. In fact, in many large screening studies, it is not even calculated.[1,2,4,7] When calculated, specificity is usually found to be greater than 90% (see Tables 38-4 and 38-5).[2,18,26] However, it is often difficult to obtain an accurate measure of specificity because its calculation requires knowledge of all true-negative results, a number that in turn is based on the number of false-negative results, the least accessible information in any audit. Consequently, specificity is not considered essential to a routine screening mammography audit.

ANALYZING THE RECENT BENCHMARK DATA: TAKING YOUR AUDIT DATA TO THE NEXT LEVEL

Until very recently, the only data with which radiologists could compare their own audit data were those desirable goals put forth by the AHCPR (now AHRQ) document[5] based on published data from a handful of relatively elite practices. However, in 2005 and 2006, the Breast Cancer Surveillance Consortium (BCSC) published two landmark articles summarizing the derived data outcomes from 2.5 million screening mammograms and 330,000 diagnostic mammograms performed in a broadly representative group of almost 200 primarily community-based practices throughout the country between 1996 and 2001.[34,35] The results for screening mammography are shown in Table 38-5, comparing the AHCPR desirable goals for the screening outcome parameters outlined above with the mean outcome values for the largely community-based radiologists studied by the BCSC. The BCSC values fell remarkably close to the "desirable" range of values proposed by AHCPR more than 10 years earlier. Thus, the average radiologist in the community-based BCSC study in 2006 was performing at the same or slightly greater level as the interpreting physicians in the more elite practices used as the models for the AHCPR document in 1994. From these data, one can glean a great deal of enlightening information. Firstly, it appears that the overall quality of mammography as practiced in the United States increased significantly between 1994 and 2006. Indeed, the median size of invasive cancers detected at screening in the BCSC study was 1.3 cm, in a range that correlates closely with decreased breast cancer deaths.[34]. This fact is borne out further by the steady drop in breast cancer deaths nationally during that same period.[41] Secondly, community-based radiologists now have "real world" data by which to measure their own performance. The BCSC outcome data were also presented as frequency plots, so that the range of values for 50% of interpreting physicians (those performing between 25% and 75%) and 80% of interpreting physicians (those performing between 10% and 90%) can easily be tracked for comparison purposes. Therefore, radiologists performing their own audits may now compare their screening performance to data truly representative of their colleagues throughout the country, thereby obtaining a much more realistic assessment of the quality of their own work.

As mentioned above, benchmarks for performance in diagnostic mammography were also published by BCSC.[35] These are displayed in Table 38-6. As one can see, the median cancer detection rate for each of the four indications listed for diagnostic mammography is between two times and ten times greater than for screening mammography. The cancer detection rate is especially high (49 cancers detected per 1000 examinations) in women presenting with a palpable lump. These numbers provide interpreting physicians with valid comparisons of diagnostic mammography outcomes to use for their own practices, for the first time. They show in dramatic fashion the special attention that interpreting physicians must pay to women presenting with symptoms, particularly a palpable lump, due to the relatively high incidence of breast cancer in this patient population. These benchmarks also demonstrate the importance of separating screening mammography data from diagnostic mammography, as the outcome data are vastly different. Clearly, if the screening and diagnostic data were combined, the analysis of the resulting outcome data would be largely meaningless.

ANALYZING THE DATA: WHEN SCREENING AND DIAGNOSTIC OUTCOMES ARE COMBINED

Many mammography practices cannot easily segregate screening and diagnostic mammography data to correctly and accurately calculate the requisite derived data for evaluating mammography performance outcomes. If the screening and diagnostic mammography cases remain

TABLE 38-6. Abnormal Interpretation Rates, PPV_3, Cancer Detection Rates, Histology, and Size According to Indication for Diagnostic Mammography Examination*

Parameter	Screen-detected Abnormality (%)	Short-interval Follow-up (%)	Symptomatic but no Lump (%)	Palpable Lump (%)	Total (%)
Abnormal interpretation rate	12.3	3.4	5.7	10.5	8.0
PPV_3	30.3	32.3	43.2	59.4	39.5
Cancer diagnosis rate per 1000 examinations[†]	30.8	8.4	18.1	49.0	25.3
Ductal carcinoma in situ	26.9	30.7	16.0	5.5	17.5
Invasive cancer	73.1	69.3	84.0	94.5	82.5
Minimal cancer	62.0	64.7	37.2	17.5	42.0

*Breast Cancer Surveillance Consortium performance results.
[†]Cancers per 1000 women screened.
From Sickles EA, Miglioretti DL, Ballard-Barbash R, Geller BM, Leung JW, Rosenberg RD, et al. Performance benchmarks for diagnostic mammography. *Radiology* 2005;**235**:775-790. PPV_3 (biopsy performed): The percentage of all biopsies actually performed as a result of screening that resulted in the diagnosis of cancer.

mixed, the calculated derived data cannot be properly analyzed, because of the confounding effects of combining screening and diagnosis. For this reason, Sohlich and colleagues[42] have developed mathematical models based on comprehensive audit data from their own practice. These outcomes tables give approximate values for recall rate, PPV, cancer detection rate, tumor size, and lymph node positivity for screening-to-diagnostic case mix ratios ranging from 90:10 to 10:90, and are summarized in Table 38-7. In this table, "diagnostic mammograms" are defined as those performed because of the following: (1) abnormal findings at screening; (2) 6-month follow-up for probably benign findings; (3) follow-up in patients with previous lumpectomy for breast cancer; (4) presentation of a patient with a palpable lump; and (5) "other."

Another outcomes table, Table 38-8, was created for practices that do not separate screening and diagnostic examinations to any extent during auditing. In Table 38-8, comparison is made between screening mammogram cases and cases in which the diagnostic examination is performed solely to evaluate a palpable lump, again giving approximate values for the same derived data as in Table 38-7 over a spectrum of screening-to-palpable lump proportions, from 2% palpable lumps, to 50% palpable lumps. Sohlich and colleagues[42] constructed several other tables for additional specific situations, consideration of which is beyond the scope of this discussion.

Once individuals in a practice have estimated their own mix of cases, they can use the appropriate derived data numbers in these tables as benchmarks to compare with their observed outcomes.

It should be understood that the data in these tables are from an academic institution with full-time breast imaging specialists and therefore may not be achievable in the community practice setting. Nonetheless, they provide approximate goals for which practices that cannot separate their screening and diagnostic mammography data should strive. They also provide the means by which further comparison to the national benchmarks for both screening and diagnostic mammography published by the BCSC can be made.[34,35]

TABLE 38-7. Outcomes Data for Case Mixes of Screening plus Diagnostic Mammography Examinations

	Rate of					
Screening-to-Diagnostic Case Mix	Abnormal Findings (%)	Positive Biopsy Findings (%)	Cancer Detection Per 1000	Nodal Metastasis (%)	Stage 0 & Stage 1 Cancer (%)	Mean Size of Invasive Cancer (mm)
90:10	6	38	10	8	87	14.4
80:20	7	40	15	9	86	14.8
70:30	8	41	20	9	85	15.2
60:40	10	41	25	9	83	15.6
50:50	11	42	30	11	82	16.0
40:60	12	43	35	11	80	16.4
30:70	13	44	39	12	79	16.8
20:80	14	45	44	13	78	17.2
10:90	15	45	49	13	76	17.6

From Sohlich RE, Sickles EA, Burnside ES, Dee KE. Interpreting data from audits when screening and diagnostic mammography outcomes are combined. *AJR Am J Roentgenol* 2002;**178**:681-686.

TABLE 38-8. Outcomes Data for Screening plus Diagnostic Mammography for Case Mixes Based on Percentage of Cases Evaluated for Palpable Masses

	Rate of					
Palpable Mass (%)	Abnormal Findings (%)	Positive Biopsy Findings (%)	Cancer Detection per 1000	Nodal Metastasis (%)	Stage 0 & Stage 1 Cancer (%)	Mean Size of Invasive Cancer (mm)
2	7	40	15	8	86	14.3
5	8	41	18	10	83	15.4
10	9	43	24	12	79	17.0
15	9	44	29	14	76	18.3
20	10	44	35	16	73	19.3
30	12	46	46	19	68	21.0
50	15	51	68	23	61	23.1

From Sohlich RE, Sickles EA, Burnside ES, Dee KE. Interpreting data from audits when screening and diagnostic mammography outcomes are combined. *AJR Am J Roentgenol* 2002;**178**:681-686.

AUDITING THE REST OF YOUR BREAST IMAGING PRACTICE: ULTRASOUND AND MAGNETIC RESONANCE IMAGING

Performance of an audit of screening breast ultrasound and screening breast magnetic resonance imaging (MRI) studies can be just as useful as it is for screening mammography. For breast ultrasound, such an audit is not clinically useful for most practices, as screening ultrasound is rarely performed in the United States at this time. However, breast MRI in both the screening and diagnostic setting has undergone a dramatic explosion in growth, and is now a common procedure in most practices. As such, an audit of one's breast MRI practice is essential in achieving a high level of performance with this modality. In view of the relatively recent advent of breast MRI, performance of an audit is perhaps even more critical for breast MRI than it is for mammography in even the most established breast imaging practices. With the recent recommendations for the performance of screening breast MRI in high-risk women by the American Cancer Society (ACS) in 2007,[43] there is now a pressing need for such a practice audit.

The goals of breast imagers performing screening MRI in high risk women are threefold and similar, but not identical, to those for mammography. Firstly, one should find a high percentage of small and node-negative breast cancers. Secondly, these cancers should be found at an acceptable "cost" (measured by recall rate and biopsy recommendations). Thirdly, one should expect a higher cancer yield than with mammography and ultrasound alone.

What should the audit numbers be to demonstrate that the above goals are being met? Given the short history of breast MRI in the United States, there is currently a paucity of breast MRI audit data in the literature by which to assess the ability of screening breast MRI to achieve these goals. There are some data for screening MRI in a cohort of high risk women.[44,45,46] In combining the data from the published studies, there were a total of 4443 screening MRI examinations performed in the cohort. Within this group, 150 breast cancers were detected on MRI for a cancer detection rate of 34 per 1000, as compared with 58 cancers detected on mammography in these same patients for a cancer detection rate of 14 per 1000. Sensitivity for MRI was 81%, as compared with the sensitivity of mammography of 35%. These audit data were compelling enough to lead to the 2007 ACS recommendations mentioned above.[43] The PPV_3 for breast MRI in these patients was 23% overall, not very different from the median PPV_3 for screening mammography in the benchmark data from the BCSC. Recall rates varied, but were between 10% and 15%, slightly higher than the median recall rate of 9.7% for screening mammography in the BCSC study. Data on tumor size was not available in these studies. However, a study by Kriege and colleagues[44] showed that another surrogate marker for predicting mortality reduction, the lymph node positivity rate, was less than half the rate expected in the patients with cancers detected on screening MR when compared with age-matched controls (18% vs. 42%).

The above audit numbers for screening MRI are based on a relatively small patient base, and therefore are subject to some variation and adjustment as more audit data are published. However, these do represent desirable goals toward which breast imaging practices performing screening MRI in high-risk women presently should strive. Recommended derived data to be calculated for audit analysis should therefore include: cancer detection rate, recall rate, short interval follow-up rate, biopsy rate, and positive predictive value at biopsy/surgery (PPV_3).

Diagnostic breast MRI is also now becoming widely accepted, particularly to better demonstrate extent of disease prior to definitive surgery for patients diagnosed with breast cancer by mammography, ultrasound, or both. For diagnostic breast MRI, the above data should also be calculated, but primarily for suspicious lesions found in addition to the known index cancer that initiated the MRI. Another parameter unique to the category of diagnostic breast MRI is the frequency with which the MRI significantly changed patient management by showing a greater or lesser extent of disease than expected, based on the initial mammographic and/or ultrasound evaluation. For instance, if a cancer found to be unifocal or multifocal on initial breast imaging evaluation is then found by MRI to be multicentric or bilateral, patient management will be affected greatly. A desirable goal for the percentage of cases in which management is changed has not been established in the literature at this time. Due to the subjective nature of this metric, attempts to establish such a goal will be somewhat arbitrary at best. However, it is still worthwhile to evaluate the effectiveness of diagnostic breast MRI when used in this setting. In a recent audit of 363 consecutive breast MRI examinations in my practice, patient management was changed in 40% of cases in which MRI was performed for preoperative evaluation of extent of a known cancer. The majority of these management changes were those leading to more accurate initial surgical excision, usually obviating the need for a second surgical resection for what would have been positive margins for residual tumor in the initial excised surgical specimen based on mammography and/or ultrasound imaging alone. This information provided more objective confirmatory evidence to our surgeons and the rest of the breast cancer community that MRI had a valuable role in the evaluation of the newly diagnosed breast cancer patient.

For lesions found in diagnostic MRI evaluations performed for reasons other than to show extent of disease in patients newly diagnosed with breast cancer by mammography and/or ultrasound, the audit should be performed in the same way as the audit for diagnostic mammography.

Separate practice audits for diagnostic ultrasound alone are usually not performed, as most diagnostic ultrasound studies are performed on patients undergoing diagnostic mammography and are reported in conjunction with the mammogram. Therefore, the audit results for diagnostic mammography will include the input provided by the supplemental diagnostic ultrasound in most cases. Separating out the diagnostic ultrasound data alone for audit purposes is possible, but is an arduous process. The present paucity of comparison audit data on diagnostic ultrasound in the literature also diminishes the value of such an audit at this time.

FURTHER BENEFITS: THE AUDIT AS A TEACHING TOOL

The audit is an important teaching tool. The *group* audit is important because it provides great statistical power, which in turn allows for comparison with overall expected rates in the audits of other groups, such as those listed in Table 38-5.[3,7] However, the multiple variables described previously (e.g., prevalent versus incident cancer rates, age of a population, ratio of screening to diagnostic mammograms) that markedly influence the results of a group audit may render comparisons with audits of other groups less valuable than a comparison of individual audits within one's own group practice.

A major advantage of an *individual* interpreting physician's audit is in providing a valid relative comparison among other practice group members. If certain facility members show considerable variation in sensitivity and other performance standards, measures can be taken to improve the performance of those at variance and thus improve future outcomes.[3,7] Even so, individual audit data can still be unclear, especially when the numbers involved are so small as to show large statistical variation. For example, a very competent interpreting physician with a low volume of cases might find 10 cases of breast cancer one year and only 2 cases the next year, strictly on the basis of random chance. This problem can be remedied in part as further data and larger numbers of cases for each individual accrue over the years, but should never be ignored when comparisons of audit data among the individual interpreting physicians are obtained.

As mentioned previously, false-negative results may be difficult to identify without access to a complete tumor registry.[3] However, if cases with false-negative results are available for review, they should be evaluated thoroughly to assess the reason for the false negatives (technical vs. interpretive error).[4,9-11] A critical review of such cases allows a facility to take action to improve overall quality and improve future outcomes.

THE AUDIT AS REQUIRED BY THE MAMMOGRAPHY QUALITY STANDARDS ACT

As mentioned earlier, all breast imaging facilities are now mandated to perform an audit under MQSA, as outlined under the final rules effective April 28, 1999.[14] However, the final rules require only that all "positive" mammogram results (BI-RADS final assessment categories 4 and 5) be tracked for pathologic outcome at biopsy, either a cancer (TP) or benign (FP). This requirement, although admirable, falls woefully short of measuring actual practice quality and efficiency as outlined in the preceding discussion. In fact, it allows for calculation of only one (PPV of recommended biopsies) of the six vital pieces of derived data required an effective medical audit.

The MQSA Final Rules suggest, but do not mandate, that false-negative cases be reviewed. In addition, a lead physician should be assigned to oversee the quality assurance process, assess the medical audit data at least yearly, take corrective actions when needed, and review data collectively for the practice overall and by the individual interpreting physicians.

The Final Rules further encourage, but do not require, mammography facilities to perform a more extensive medical audit. It is hoped that interpreting physicians truly serious about measuring their mammographic skills would do so through the collection and calculation of the more extensive parameters of practice quality and efficiency described in this chapter. In the near future, a more extensive medical audit may well be mandated. In the Institute of Medicine (IOM) 2005 report "Improving Breast Imaging Quality Standards," strong recommendations were made for a more stringent audit under the MQSA.[47] Some of the proposed derived data to be added include recording of results for all recommended biopsies, calculation of cancer detection rate for screening mammography, required tracking of BI-RADS 4, BI-RADS 5, and BI-RADS 0 cases, and separate audits for screening and diagnostic mammography. To its credit, the IOM also recommended that reimbursement rates be increased to cover a portion of the costs of performing these additional audit procedures. Thus far, the U.S. Food and Drug Administration (FDA) has not moved to recommend expansion of the current audit requirements under MQSA, but given the pressure to do so by the IOM and others, such action may well be put in place in the near future.

It should be emphasized that the mandates of MQSA pertain only to mammography. Therefore, although audits of the performance of other modalities utilized in breast imaging, such as breast ultrasound and breast MRI, are useful and are recommended, they are not required under the legislative mandates of MQSA at this time.

SOURCES FOR MEDICAL AUDIT DATA

Much of the patient demographic information and all of the pertinent mammographic findings should be readily available from a well-designed mammography reports record, especially if the reports are computerized.[3,7,18,22] Biopsy results are available from a variety of sources, as follows:[1–4,7,18,26,31]

1. If malignant, the results can be found through a complete regional or state-wide tumor registry. If such a registry does not exist, or access to its data is not possible; a definitive diagnosis of cancer can be obtained from one or more of the following (in order of preference):
   a. The pathology report.
   b. The surgical report (if a frozen-section analysis was done).
   c. The referring physician or surgeon by phone or letter.
   d. The patient herself (last resort), by phone or letter.
2. If benign, the results can be obtained from the pathology report.

   Patients often receive care at outside institutions, making data collection even more difficult. If hospital reports are not available, the diagnosis can usually be obtained by phone or letter from the referring physician or the surgeon. The patient herself should be considered as a possible last source. The importance of obtaining complete follow-up on every patient with suspicious imaging findings cannot be stressed enough. Every effort should be made to obtain this data.

THE VALUE OF THE MEDICAL AUDIT IN EVERYDAY PRACTICE: PERSONAL EXPERIENCE

In 1987, our group of 12 private practice radiologists elected to take measures to improve the overall quality and efficiency of mammography in our practice. To do so, we obtained additional mammographic training, developed our own computerized mammography reporting system, and began to evaluate our ongoing performance by conducting an audit of mammography results. The first 2 years of our audit experience have been previously reported[7] and are summarized in Table 38-4, along with other mammography audits in the literature. In the second year of our audit, the number of cancers diagnosed increased 50% (from 121 to 181), our sensitivity increased from 80% to 87%, and our PPV_3 and PPV_2 values remained essentially unchanged at 32% and 27%, respectively. Median tumor size decreased from 1.5 cm to 1.2 cm, and the rate of node positivity decreased from 26% to 18.5%. Our recall rate rose 50%, from 5.3% to 8.1%. We attributed the overall improvement in performance seen in the second year to, among other factors, an alteration in our overall interpretive approach learned through attendance at dedicated teaching courses during the first year of the audit. It was only through the audit process that we were able to assess our performance and obtain quantitative proof to support our belief that the quality of our mammography practice was improving.

Once its value to our practice was established, we continued to perform an extensive annual medical audit. Because of the unique combination of our computerized program and an accessible state-wide tumor registry, we have been able to obtain complete audit data on the more than 500,000 mammograms interpreted since the initiation of our computer program in 1988. In addition to the findings reported for the first 2 years, we have since identified several other trends of great value to our individual interpreting physicians and our group as a whole, some of which are worthy of mention here:

Firstly, in evaluating our raw data, we found that the proportion of initial screening (patients having their first screening mammography) to subsequent annual screening mammography examinations has progressively diminished since 1988 (Table 38-8).

Because a lower number of cancers is found in the follow-up group (incident cancers) than in the first-screened group (prevalent cancers) in screening populations, we therefore would have expected a slight decrease in the rate of screening-detected cancers over the years. This is indeed what we found. In 1989, we detected 6.24 cancers per 1000 screened patients. This value fell to 4.75 by 1992 (Table 38-10). Knowing that we were seeing a higher percentage of routine annual screening patients

TABLE 38-9. Summary by Year of Comparison of Initial vs. Routine Screening Follow-Up Examinations, Screening Cases Only, 1988–1992

Parameter	1988	1989	1990	1991	1992	5-Year Total
Total screening examinations	16,067	17,627	20,415	25,180	31,164	110,453
Initial examinations	6185	5059	4981	5741	8682*	30,648
	38.5%	28.7%	24.4%	22.8%	27.9%	27.7%
Follow-up examinations	9882	12,568	15,434	19,439	22,482	79,805
	61.5%	71.3%	75.6%	77.2%	72.1%	72.3%

*Reason for slight increase in 1992 was that we began screening in remote rural areas with two mammography vans, performing approximately 5000 mammograms, virtually all of which were initial screening studies. X-ray Associates of New Mexico, Albuquerque, New Mexico.

TABLE 38-10. Summary by Year of Surgical Consults Recommended, Number and Rate of Cancers Found, and PPV—Screening Cases Only, 1988–1992

Parameter	1988	1989	1990	1991	1992	5-Year Total or Average
Total screening examinations	16,067	17,627	20,415	25,180	31,164	110,453
Total surgical consults recommended	282	433	446	542	513	2216 (2.0%)
Cancers found at biopsy	77	110	111	149	148	595 (0.54%)
PPV based on recommended biopsy or surgical consults (PPV_2) (%)	27	25	25	27	29	27
Cancers found/1000 patients	4.79	6.24	5.44	5.92	4.75	5.43

PPV_2, the percentage of all cases recommended for biopsy or surgical consultation as a result of screening that resulted in the diagnosis of cancer.

each year, we therefore had a ready explanation for the gradual drop in rate of screening-detected cancers we had observed.

A second trend we identified relates to four of the other major parameters of mammographic screening performance: tumor size, node positivity, percentage of minimal cancers, and PPV (Tables 38-10 through 38-12). As mentioned earlier, we noticed a significant decrease in tumor size and node positivity between 1988 and 1989 in both the combined (symptomatic and asymptomatic) tumor group and the asymptomatic tumor group. We attributed this decrease to an overall improvement in our interpretive skills during that time related to attendance at dedicated mammography continuing medical education courses.[7] Since then, we have noted a continued slight downward trend in tumor size and node positivity in both groups as well as a progressive rise in the percentage of minimal cancers (see Tables 38-10 and 38-11). These data added further support to our original hypothesis and boosted our conviction that we were continuing to achieve a measurable level of success in detecting early breast cancer. Moreover, we found that we accomplished these goals without requesting a greater percentage of unnecessary biopsies: The PPV_3 remained between 31% and 35%, and the PPV_2 between 26% and 29% (see Tables 38-12 and 38-13).

Review of individual audit data has also proved helpful. We have observed some variation in sensitivity and PPV_3 in our group. Some members with acceptable sensitivity (cancer detection rates) have shown an inordinately low PPV_3. This would suggest that the threshold for the criteria for biopsy that they were using was set too low. By reviewing their audit numbers, they have taken measures to slide a bit more toward the middle of the ROC curve, with considerable success.

Another audit activity that has proven extremely useful, as shown previously in other audit reports, has been the review of the imaging of all identified cases with false-negative results.[4,9,10] We hold a group conference every 6 to 12 months to review each false-negative interpretation case in detail to establish the cause of its false-negative status. This non-threatening team approach has been highly

TABLE 38-11. Summary by Year of Size and Nodal Status of All Cancers Found by Mammography, 1988–1992

Parameter	1988	1989	1990	1991	1992
Average tumor size (cm)	1.72	1.57	1.50	1.37	1.49
Median tumor size (cm)	1.5	1.2	1.3	1.0	1.1
Minimal tumors* (%)	36	41	43	47	50
Node-positive tumors (%)	26	18.5	23	21	16

*Minimal tumors: invasive cancer ≤1cm or in-situ ductal cancer.

TABLE 38-12. Summary by Year of Size and Nodal Status of All Asymptomatic (Screening-Detected) Cancers Found, 1988–1992

Parameter	1988	1989	1990	1991	1992
Average tumor size (cm)	1.32	0.95	1.30	0.89	1.09
Median tumor size (cm)	1.2	0.9	1.0	0.8	0.8
Minimal tumors* (%)	50	62	55	60	63
Carcinoma in situ (%)	23	25	23	41	31
Node-positive tumors (%)	12.5	5.7	17	13	12

*Minimal tumors: invasive cancer ≤1cm or in-situ ductal cancer.

TABLE 38-13. Summary by Year of PPV_2 and Positive Biopsy Rate (PPV_3) for All Tumors Found by Mammography, 1988–1992

Parameter	1988	1989	1990	1991	1992	5-Year Total or Average
Surgical consultations requested	461	668	651	817	749	3346
Biopsies done in this group	368	570	526	704	670	2838
Benign results	247	389	341	485	456	1918
Malignant results	121	181	185	219	214	920
PPV_3 (positive biopsy rate) (%)	33	32	35	31	32	33
PPV_2 (all cases recommended for biopsy) (%)	26	27	28	27	29	27

successful and has firmly established the role of the mammography medical audit in our practice as a sophisticated and invaluable teaching tool.

We are now undertaking a separate audit of our performance in breast MRI. We expect this to further enhance our skills in interpreting this exciting new breast imaging modality, just as our mammography medical audit has done for us.

MEDICOLEGAL CONSIDERATIONS

At this time, all states have statutes that protect all peer review records generated by a structured peer review committee in the hospital setting from legal discovery.[32,38] However, virtually no statutes exist to protect from discovery all other information generated in the hospital under the auspices of organized quality review activities or quality review information obtained in the outpatient setting.[48] Therefore, it is recommended that complete mammography audits be maintained primarily as "internal audits." Interpreting physicians should not disseminate the audit data without being aware of confidentiality legislation in their state.

Model legislation does exist: Congress provided protection to participants of quality control programs and created a qualified immunity for the medical quality assurance records generated by the programs within the military health care system (10 USC 1102) and the Department of Veteran Affairs (38 USC 5705). Efforts have been made to enact legislation to protect audit material generated outside the military setting but have so far been unsuccessful.[48] Such legislation, if enacted, would encourage all mammography facilities to participate in the medical audit process without fear of increasing their medicolegal liability, allowing the facilities to more completely fulfill the quality assessment standards required by TJC, ACR, and MQSA and to provide audit information to benefit their interpreting physicians and, if released publicly, the medical community and patients they serve. At this time, however, such broadly drawn legislation does not exist.

THE EXPANDING ROLE OF THE MEDICAL AUDIT: PROBLEMS AND PROMISE

With the promulgation of the MQSA Final Regulations, some limited mammography audit activities are now required components of each mammography practice. Many interpreting physicians consider this development a mixed blessing. Although the virtues of the audit process are readily evident, the difficulties in collecting the necessary data, especially in smaller and rural practices, are just as obvious. The added time and cost required to perform an audit and other quality assurance activities mandated under MQSA for the interpreting physician, radiologic technologist, and other personnel may discourage some facilities to the extent that they will discontinue performing mammography. Such an outcome would undermine the very purpose of MQSA, that of improving access to high-quality mammography for women in all socioeconomic settings. Indeed, those women in greatest jeopardy of losing mammography services are the ones in rural and low-income areas that are already underserved. It is hoped that the FDA and other empowered regulatory agencies will take the necessary measures to avoid such an outcome.

The recent federal legislative initiatives tying reimbursement for medical services to performance outcomes cast an entirely new light on the role of the audit in breast imaging practices. This process has already begun: beginning in 2009, the Centers for Medicare & Medicaid Services (CMS) is offering bonus payments equaling 2% of a physician's Medicare reimbursement for reporting the use or lack of use of BI-RADS Category 3 in screening mammography reports. [49] Although this measure is more "pay for compliance" than it is "pay-for-performance," the message is clear: interpreting physicians must now look to the well-designed and well-maintained mammography audit to provide much-needed information for maximum reimbursement, especially if their performance outcomes are good. Given the current legislative climate, interpreting physicians would be ill-advised to continue to resist performing a complete mammography audit, despite the difficulties enumerated here.

If mammography audits can be successfully established in all practices, if federal legislation is passed protecting audit data from discovery, and if patient confidentiality can be ensured,[50] then the promise these data offer can be realized. We are now reaping some of the benefits of the invaluable information provided by the benchmark data published by the BCSC. By pooling and entering these data in a fully comprehensive national mammography database, we could provide even more accurate answers to many of the vital questions concerning mammography today.[3,13,51] We must improve screening compliance and tumor detection regionally and within various age and ethnic groups; we need more accurate and more complete feedback of data results to individual mammography facilities; and we need to achieve the ultimate goal of screening mammography: the reduction of mortality from breast cancer in all age groups. Through the efforts of the BCSC, we are well on our way to achieving some of these goals, but the challenge still remains for us to bring the highest quality breast imaging to every eligible woman in this country, whoever and wherever she may be.

CONCLUSIONS

The mammography medical audit is currently the only objective measure of the interpretive ability of physicians interpreting mammograms. It also offers a means of quantifying the success of mammography in detecting early breast cancer. Because it is such a vital component of mammography quality assurance, a limited form of the audit is now federally mandated by MQSA.

The appropriate collection, calculation, and analysis of raw and derived data for either a basic or a more complete audit should be performed to answer the following three essential questions that determine an interpreting physician's success: (1) Are the cancers that exist being found? (2) are a large proportion of these cancers small and node negative? and (3) are these cancers being found with an acceptable number of patient recalls and biopsies?

Answering these questions with quantitative data provides the means for assessing the surrogate markers for decreasing the number of breast cancer deaths, the ultimate goal of mammography. These quantitative performance data allow comparison with the range of desirable values found in other audits throughout the medical literature, and now with the benchmark performance data of other community radiologists nationwide published by the BCSC. By so doing, each interpreting physician can estimate where he or she is operating on the ROC curve and adjust his or her approach to mammographic interpretation accordingly. Additional audit activities, such as evaluating the group audit versus the individual audit statistics and reviewing false-negative results, can offer the further benefit of a teaching tool that can improve clinical outcomes. In view of the current legislative initiatives to tie reimbursement to medical outcomes, the performance of a complete audit may well offer the breast imaging facility remunerative value in the near future.

With the publication of benchmarks for diagnostic mammography by the BCSC, mammographers now have the ability to compare their diagnostic mammography audit data to those of their peers, and they should therefore be performing a diagnostic audit as well. If possible, these diagnostic data should be strictly separated from screening data, so as to preserve the value of both data sets. In addition, the recent ascent of breast MRI in both the screening sphere for high risk patients and the diagnostic realm have generated the need for facilities to be performing practice audits for breast MRI.

Certain medicolegal concerns regarding discoverability of audit records, particularly in the outpatient setting, must be kept in mind. These concerns, together with the difficulty and cost of performing an audit in many practices, currently impede widespread collection of audit data. If these problems can be remedied and the data pooled in a more complete national mammography database, ideally in collaboration with the BCSC, the full potential for using audit data to answer unresolved questions about the early detection of breast cancer can be realized.

ACKNOWLEDGMENTS

I thank Richard Bird, Peter Dempsey, Robert D. Rosenberg, and Charles Kelsey for their help in preparing the manuscript. I also thank the following fellow members and consultants on the AHCPR Panel on Quality Determinants of Mammography who helped me develop the section of the Clinical Practice Guideline on the medical audit: R. James Brenner, Janet R. Osuch, Robert Smith, Victor Hasselblad, and Darryl Carter.

KEY POINTS

- Performance of a mammography audit is the only means to objectively measure one's interpretive ability in mammography.
- Although only a minimal audit is mandated by MQSA, performance of a more complete audit with strict separation of screening and diagnostic mammography data is urged to obtain a truly accurate assessment of one's mammography skills.
- Comparison of complete audit data to published benchmark screening and diagnostic mammography performance data of other community interpreting physicians nationally offers great potential to improve one's outcomes.
- Current legislative initiatives attempting to tie reimbursement to medical outcomes may require collection of more complete mammography audit data for remuneration purposes.
- Although not mandated by MQSA, performance of an audit of one's breast MR practice is strongly recommended.

SUGGESTED READINGS

Feig SA. Auditing and benchmarks in screening and diagnostic mammography. *Radiol Clin N Am* 2007;**45**:791-800.

Linver MN. The expanded mammography audit: its value in measuring and improving your performance. *Semin Breast Dis* 2005;**8**:35-42.

Linver MN, Osuch JR, Brenner RJ, Smith RA. The Mammography Audit: a primer for the Mammography Quality Standards Act (MQSA). *Am J Roentgenol* 1995;**165**:19-25.

Sickles EA. Auditing your breast imaging practice: an evidence-based approach. *Semin Roentgenol* 2007;**42**:211-7.

REFERENCES

1. Bird RE. Low-cost screening mammography: report on finances and review of 21,716 cases. *Radiology* 1989;**171**:87-90.
2. Robertson CL A private breast imaging practice: medical audit of 25,788 screening and 1,077 diagnostic exams. *Radiology* 1993;**187**:75-9.
3. Sickles EA. Quality assurance: how to audit your own mammography practice. *Radiol Clin North Am* 1992;**30**:265-75.
4. Spring DB, Kimbrell-Wilmot K. Evaluating the success of mammography at the local level: how to conduct an audit of your practice. *Radiol Clin North Am* 1987;**25**:983-92.
5. Bassett LW, Hendrick RE, Bassford TL, et al. *Quality Determinants of Mammography* (Clinical Practice Guideline No. 13. AHCPR Publication No. 95-0632.) Rockville, Md: Agency for Health Care Policy and Research, Public Health Service, US Department of Health and Human Services; October 1994.
6. Sickles EA, Ominsky SH, Sollitto RA, Galvin HB, Monticciolo DL. Medical audit of a rapid-throughput mammography screening practice: methodology and results of 27,114 examinations. *Radiology* 1990;**175**:323-7.
7. Linver MN, Paster SB, Rosenberg RD, Key CR, Stidley CA, King WV. Improvement in mammography interpretation skills in a community radiology practice after dedicated teaching courses: 2-year medical audit of 38,633 cases. *Radiology* 1992;**184**:39-43.
8. Reinig JW, Strait CJ. Professional mammographic quality assessment program for a community hospital. *Radiology* 1991;**180**:393-6.
9. Bird RE, Wallace TW, Yankaskas BC. Analysis of cancers missed at screening mammography. *Radiology* 1992;**184**:613-7.
10. Burhenne HJ, Burhenne LW, Goldberg F, Hislop TG, Worth AJ, Rebbeck PM, et al. Interval breast cancers in the Screening

Mammography Program of British Columbia: analysis and classification. *AJR Am J Roentgenol* 1994;**162**:1067-71.
11. Moskowitz M. Interval cancers and screening for breast cancer in British Columbia [commentary]. *AJR Am J Roentgenol* 1994;**162**: 1072-5.
12. Brenner RJ. Medicolegal aspects of breast imaging. *Radiol Clin North Am* 1992;**30**:277-86.
13. Clark RA, King PS, Worden JK. Mammography registry: considerations and options. *Radiology* 1989;**171**:91-3.
14. US Department of Health and Human Services, Food and Drug Administration. Mammography quality standards: Final rule. *Fed Regist* 1997;**62**:55851-994.
15. *Joint Commission 1990 Accreditation Manual for Hospitals*. Chicago: Joint Commission on Accreditation of Healthcare Organizations; 1989.
16. American College of Radiology. ACR Practice Guideline for Performance of Screening Mammography [adopted by the ACR Council, 2008]. In: *ACR Practice Guidelines and Technical Standards*. Reston, Va: American College of Radiology; 2009.
17. D'Orsi CJ, Bassett LW, Berg WA, et al. *Illustrated Breast Imaging Reporting and Data System (BI-RADS); Mammography*, 4th ed. Reston, Va: American College of Radiology, 2003.
18. Burhenne LW, Hislop TG, Burhenne HJ. The British Columbia mammography screening program: Evaluation of the first 15 months. *AJR Am J Roentgenol* 1992;**158**:45-9.
19. Haug PJ, Tocino IM, Clayton PD, Bair TL. Automated management of screening and diagnostic mammography. *Radiology* 1987;**164**:747-52.
20. Heilbrunn K, Graves RE. *Increasing compliance with breast cancer screening guidelines: a clinician-oriented approach*. Presented at American College of Radiology 24th National Conference on Breast Cancer, New Orleans, March 12-18, 1990.
21. Monticciolo DL, Sickles EA. Computerized follow-up of abnormalities detected at mammography screening. *AJR Am J Roentgenol* 1990;**155**:751-3.
22. Sickles EA. The use of computers in mammography screening. *Radiol Clin North Am* 1987;**25**:1015-30.
23. Tabar L, Fagerberg G, Duffy SW, Day NE, Gad A, Grontoft O. Update of the Swedish two-county program of mammographic screening for breast cancer. *Radiol Clin North Am* 1992;**30**:187-210.
24. Braman DM, Williams HD. ACR accredited suburban mammography center: three year results. *J Fla Med Assoc* 1989;**76**:1031-40.
25. Ciatto S, Cataliotti L, Distante V. Nonpalpable lesions detected with mammography: review of 512 consecutive cases. *Radiology* 1987;**165**:99-102.
26. Lynde JL. A community program of low-cost screening mammography: the results of 21,141 consecutive examinations. *South Med J* 1993;**86**:338-43.
27. Kopans D. The positive predictive value of mammography. *AJR Am J Roentgenol* 1992;**158**:521-6.
28. D'Orsi CJ. Screening mammography pits cost against quality. *Diagn Imaging* 1994;**16**:73-6.
29. Baines CJ, Miller AB, Wall C, McFarlane DV, Simor IS, Jong R, et al. Sensitivity and specificity of first screen mammography in the Canadian National Breast Screening Study: a preliminary report from five centers. *Radiology* 1986;**160**:295-8.
30. Margolin FR, Lagios MD. Development of mammography and breast services in a community hospital. *Radiol Clin North Am* 1987;**25**:973-82.
31. Moseson D. Audit of mammography in a community setting. *Am J Surg* 1992;**163**:544-6.
32. American Medical Association. *A Compendium of State Peer Review Immunity Laws*. Chicago: American Medical Association; 1988.
33. D'Orsi CJ. To follow or not to follow, that is the question. *Radiology* 1992;**184**:306.
34. Rosenberg RD, Yankaskas BC, Abraham LA, Sickles EA, Lehman CD, Geller BM, et al. Performance benchmarks for screening mammography. *Radiology* 2006;**241**:55-66.
35. Sickles EA, Miglioretti DL, Ballard-Barbash R, Geller BM, Leung JW, Rosenberg RD, et al. Performance benchmarks for diagnostic mammography. *Radiology* 2005;**235**:775-90.
36. Dee KE, Sickles EA. Medical audit of diagnostic mammographic examinations: comparison with screening outcomes obtained concurrently. *AJR Am J Roentgenol* 2001;**176**:729-33.
37. Linver MN, Paster SB. Mammography outcomes in a practice setting by age: prognostic factors, sensitivity, and positive biopsy rate. *Monogr Natl Cancer Inst* 1997;**22**:113-7.
38. Moskowitz M. Predictive value, sensitivity and specificity in breast cancer screening. *Radiology* 1988;**167**:576-8.
39. Moskowitz M. Breast cancer: Age-specific growth rates and screening strategies. *Radiology* 1986;**161**:37-41.
40. Yankaskas BC, Cleveland RJ, Schell MJ, Kozar R. Association of recall rates with sensitivity and positive predictive values of screening mammography. *AJR Am J Roentgenol* 2001;**177**:543-9.
41. American Cancer Society. *Cancer Facts and Figures, 2009*. Atlanta Ga: American Cancer Society; 2009.
42. Sohlich RE, Sickles EA, Burnside ES, Dee KE. Interpreting data from audits when screening and diagnostic mammography outcomes are combined. *AJR Am J Roentgenol* 2002;**178**:681-6.
43. Saslow D, Boetes C, Burke W, Harms S, Leach MO, Lehman CD, et al. American Cancer Society guidelines for breast cancer screening with MRI as an adjunct to mammography. *CA Cancer J Clin* 2007;**57**:75-89.
44. Kriege M, Brekelmans CT, Boetes C, Besnard PE, Zonderland HM, Obdeijn IM, et al. Efficacy of MRI and mammography for breast cancer screening in women with a familial or genetic predisposition. *N Engl J Med* 2004;**351**:427-37.
45. Warner E, Blewes DB, Hill KA, Causer PA, Zubovits JT, Jong RA, et al. Surveillance of BRCA1 and BRCA2 mutation carriers with magnetic resonance imaging, ultrasound, mammography, and clinical breast examination. *JAMA* 2004;**292**:1317-25.
46. Lehman CD, Isaacs C, Schnall MD, Pisano ED, Ascher SM, Weatherall PT, et al. Cancer yield of mammography, MR, and US in high-risk women: prospective multi-institution breast cancer screening study. *Radiology* 2007;**244**:381-8.
47. Nass S, Ball J, editors. In: *Improving breast imaging quality standards. Committee on Improving Mammography Quality Standards, National Research Council*. Washington DC: National Academics Press; 2005.
48. American Medical Association. *Report of AMA reference committee G, substitute resolution 722, "Medical peer review outside hospital settings"*. Chicago: American Medical Association; June, 1992.
49. American College of Radiology. *New 2009 PQRI measure proposed to track inappropriate use of "probably benign" BI-RADS 3*. Available at: www.acr.org/Hidden/Economics/FeaturedCategories/Pubs/coding_source/archives/JulyAugust2008/New2009PQRIMeasureProposed.aspx.
50. Linver MN, Rosenberg RD, Smith RA. Mammography outcome analysis: potential panacea or Pandora's box? [commentary]. *Am J Roentgenol* 1996;**167**:373-5.
51. Hurley SF. Screening: The need for a population register. *Med J Austr* 1989;**153**:310-1.

CHAPTER 39

Coding and Billing in Breast Imaging

Michael N. Linver

The dramatic success of mammography in bringing about a 30% decrease in breast cancer deaths in the United States since the mid-1980s[1] has been accompanied by a precipitous drop in mammography reimbursement. The latter development has resulted in the curtailment and even elimination of mammography services in many radiology practices.[2] Those radiologists who perform breast imaging studies have become increasingly frustrated as fiscal disaster becomes the reward for their diligent effort and success in effectively changing the natural history of this disease. Even those most committed to the goal of driving down deaths from breast cancer through high-quality mammography now find that goal increasingly difficult to attain, owing to inadequate reimbursement.

It is therefore incumbent upon the radiologist to understand the workings of the reimbursement system as comprehensively as possible. With such an understanding, the radiologist can construct a strategic plan for financial survival in the breast imaging arena. Much of the following discussion centers on Medicare reimbursement, because Medicare sets the reimbursement precedents that most private payers follow.

CODING AND BILLING TERMINOLOGY: THE "LANGUAGE" OF REIMBURSEMENT

One must first have a thorough understanding of coding terminology. The code specified by the *International Classification of Diseases, 9th Revision: Clinical Modification*[3] (ICD-9-CM) for a service provided by the radiologist defines the medical indication for that service. This classification was begun and is overseen by the World Health Organization (WHO). With the receipt of a claim for payment, all payers initially evaluate the ICD-9-CM code to establish whether the service provided was appropriate for the medical condition being evaluated. For example, most providers consider ICD code 174.0 ("malignant neoplasm of the female breast") as an appropriate coding for performance and interpretation of a "diagnostic mammogram" and would allow coverage. More recently, the Centers for Medicare & Medicaid Services (CMS) has allowed radiologists to code certain findings from the radiology examination as the primary diagnosis on the CMS claim form (CMS Program Memorandum AB-01-144). Radiologists may now use, for example, ICD code 793.80, for "abnormal mammogram, unspecified," or ICD code 793.81, for "mammographic calcifications." Appropriate submission of the procedure code (CPT/HCPCS [see next paragraph]) would still be required before payment would be forthcoming for a covered diagnosis, however.

The Current Procedural Terminology (CPT) system was originally established by the American Medical Association (AMA) to identify procedures performed by physicians (CPT codes and descriptions only are copyrighted by the AMA; all rights reserved).[4] For more specificity, three additional modifying levels of CPT codes were added by HCFA (Health Care Financing Administration, the government body, now called CMS, that is responsible for overseeing Medicare payment).[5] These modifying codes are known as the CPT/HFCA Common Procedures Coding System CPT/HCPCS) codes and are divided into three levels: level I HCPCS codes, which are listed in the AMA CPT codebook, and two lower levels—level II alpha-numeric codes (primarily nonphysician codes, or new technology) and level III local or regional codes. These three levels of modifying codes allow for more detailed reporting of various health care services. Selected codes, primarily diagnostic, are further divided into the global procedure (combined professional and technical component) and the separate professional and technical components of a procedure. For instance, for the performance and interpretation of a bilateral digital diagnostic mammogram of a Medicare patient (performed under ICD code 174.0, "malignant neoplasm of the female breast," as its indication), a CPT/HCPCS code of G0204 should be applied, with a current global reimbursement under the 2009 Medicare Fee Schedule of $152.56, representing a summation of the professional fee of $43.28 and the technical fee of $109.28.

MEDICARE REIMBURSEMENT: SETTING THE PRECEDENT. BACKGROUND AND PRESENT STATUS

First and foremost, one must have a complete understanding of the precedent-setting Medicare reimbursement system. Medicare reimbursement underwent a major overhaul in the early 1990s, when Congress directed the HCFA to study physician payment reform. The system that resulted, initiated by Medicare in 1992, became known as the Resource-Based Relative Value System (RBRVS).[6]

The RBRVS was created when the existing CPT codes were wed to a weighted system assigning a relative value to each physician procedure under what was to be known as the Medicare Fee Schedule (MFS). The MFS is regarded as resource-based, because the fee for a physician's service is based on the resources needed to provide that service: physician work, practice expenses, and professional liability insurance costs. All three components for a particular service are assigned a numerical value called a Resource Value Unit (RVU). These values then undergo regional adjustment for local differences in resource costs.[7]

To determine dollar reimbursement, one multiplies the respective geographic adjustments by the three RVU values assigned the service, adds them, and then multiplies the sum times the conversion factor. The conversion factor is in turn determined by five factors: the prior year's conversion factor, the Medical Economic Index, the update adjustment factor, legislation changes, and a budget neutrality factor. For 2009, the Medicare Fee Schedule conversion factor (as modified by the Medicare Improvements for Patients and Providers Act of 2008 and by a budget neutrality factor mandated under the Deficit Reduction Act of 2005) is $36.07, a decrease of 5.31% compared with 2008. For current updates on the Physician Fee Schedule, one can consult the CMS Web site, at www.cms.hhs.gov/PhysicianFeeSched/01_overview.asp.

In April 2000, the HCFA published the final rules for a hospital outpatient prospective payment system (HOPPS) for hospital outpatient services.[8,9] The HOPPS standardized Medicare reimbursement for procedures (technical component only) performed in outpatient facilities within a hospital and reduced patient out-of-pocket expenses as well. By prohibiting the "unbundling" of non-physician outpatient services, the HCFA created instead 451 "bundled" Ambulatory Payment Classifications (APCs). The HCFA assigned a payment weight based on the factors for each APC. Payment is then determined through the use of a conversion factor and geographic adjustment factors. In general, the APC payment scale is similar to what existed before. The APC codes apply only to the technical components of radiology services for Medicare patients in a hospital setting. Professional fees are determined by the usual MFS based on the RBRVS.[10] For current updates on HOPPS, one can consult the CMS Web site, at www.cms.gov/HospitalOutpatientPPS/.

Medicare payment rates do change on a regular basis: The CMS seeks input from the Resource Value System Update Committee (RUC) of representatives from the AMA and 22 specialty organizations, including the American College of Radiology (ACR), in order to update the physician work component of the RVU scale each year, and uses this information to conduct a comprehensive review of all relative values every 5 years. In its 2002 and 2007 reviews, the HCFA accepted approximately 80% of RUC recommendations.[11] It is through the RUC that the greatest opportunity exists for an increase in reimbursement for breast imaging procedures in the near future.

The Medicare fee that is most critical to the success of every breast imaging facility is the reimbursement for screening mammography, originally set by congressional mandate in the Omnibus Budget Reconciliation Act of 1990.[12] Unfortunately for all financially struggling breast imagers, the initial reimbursement rate was set artificially low, at $55, and remained artificially low over the next decade. Congress did enlarge the pool of eligible women by extending yearly coverage to all Medicare-eligible women 40 years and older via the Balanced Budget Act of 1997[13] but did nothing to significantly improve reimbursement.

However, in December 2000, HR4577, the Medicare, Medicaid, and SCHIP Benefits Improvement and Protection Act (BIPA) was passed, returning screening mammography to the purview of the MFS.[14] The global rate for screening mammography for 2009 under the MFS was $81.51 for screen-film technique, and $129.84 for digital technique.

The entire medical climate in the United States has been, and continues to be, in the throes of radical change. The Deficit Reduction Act (DRA) of 2005 has had a dramatic effect on reimbursement for all of radiology, as reimbursement was slashed for all imaging by $2.8 billion over a 5-year span.[15] Radiology absorbed 40% of this reduction. Among other provisions of the DRA, the technical component reimbursement for non-hospital outpatient imaging was reduced to the lesser of the HOPPS or the MFS payment. Although screening and diagnostic mammography examinations were specifically excluded from the DRA, reduction among other breast imaging procedures varied from 4% to 37% initially, with reimbursement for computer-aided detection (CAD) scheduled to drop 48% and stereotactic biopsy reimbursement scheduled to fall 61% by 2010.

Another legislative initiative destined to affect reimbursement in breast imaging is the "pay-for-performance" movement, whereby reimbursement for medical services is tied to performance outcomes. This process has already begun: beginning in 2009, CMS is offering bonus payments equaling 2% of a physician's Medicare reimbursement for reporting the use or lack of use of ACR Breast Imaging Reporting and Data System (BI-RADS) Category 3 in screening mammography reports.[16] Although this measure is more "pay for compliance" than it is "pay-for-performance," the message is clear: the days of more traditional reimbursement in health care are numbered.[17] Mammographers must now look to the well-designed and well-maintained mammography audit to provide much-needed information for maximum reimbursement, as was discussed in more detail in Chapter 8 of this text. In addition, mammographers must adopt other new strategies for improving reimbursement. These will be enumerated later in the present chapter.

CURRENT MEDICARE REIMBURSEMENT: ACCEPTABLE CODES FOR MAMMOGRAPHY, AND PAYMENT RATES

The ICD-9-CM code for a screening mammogram, V76.12 ("special screening examination for malignant neoplasm, breast"), has been universally accepted by all regional Medicare carriers. However, acceptable reimbursement codes for diagnostic mammography vary tremendously from one Medicare carrier to the next. Although most payers adhere to the concept that "diagnostic mammography is generally indicated when there are signs or symptoms suggestive of malignancy,"[18] their individual interpretation of acceptable diagnosis codes is surprisingly diverse. Table 39-1 presents the ICD-9 codes for diagnostic mammography accepted for reimbursement by two large Medicare carriers, one in the Northeast and one in the Southwest.[18,19] As one can see, surprisingly few codes are accepted and reimbursed by both carriers, and a sizable number are reimbursed by only one of the two. It is therefore important to communicate with one's own Medicare carrier as to the acceptability of these or other ICD-9-CM codes for diagnostic mammography.

Table 39-2 lists examples of breast imaging-related procedural CPT codes and the corresponding reimbursement by Medicare for 2009 (Hayek D, personal communication, 2009).

In assessing the Medicare payment rates in Table 9-2, one must keep in mind that these are national averages. They do not reflect geographic adjustments made by individual regional carriers. Reimbursement by local Medicare carriers may vary by as much as 30%.[20] CMS does provide a means of computing Medicare reimbursements nationally or by region on its Web site at www.cms.hhs.gov/PFSlookup/01_Overview.asp#TopOfPage. By entering the CPT Category I or HCPCS Level II code desired, one can easily access the reimbursement rate for that code.

MEDICARE'S SPECIAL RULES RELATING TO MAMMOGRAPHY REIMBURSEMENT

Under Medicare, a screening mammogram is defined as a "preventive measure when a person has no history or personal history of breast cancer." It is "for routine screening of asymptomatic women, with or without a family history, and with or without a physician's recommendation." Thus, a Medicare-eligible woman does not need a written requisition to receive a screening mammogram. In essence, the screening mammogram for a Medicare-eligible woman has become a self-referred examination. If a woman needs a diagnostic mammogram because of clinical signs or symptoms of

TABLE 39-1. Regional Differences in Acceptance of Various ICD-9 Codes for Diagnostic Mammography

ICD-9 Codes for Diagnostic Mammography		Accepted by Medicare Carrier in Northeast United States	Accepted by Medicare Carrier in Southwest United States
172.5:	Malignant melanoma of skin of breast	Yes	No
173.5, 173.9:	Other malignant neoplasm	Yes	No
174.0-174.9:	Malignant neoplasm of female breast	Yes	Yes
175.0-175.9:	Malignant neoplasm of male breast	Yes	Yes
198.81:	Secondary neoplasm of breast	Yes	No
217.0:	Benign neoplasm of breast	Yes	No
232.5:	Carcinoma in situ of breast	Yes	No
233.0:	Carcinoma in situ of breast	Yes	Yes
238.3:	Neoplasm of breast soft tissue	Yes	Yes
239.2:	Neoplasm of uncertain behavior	Yes	No
239.3:	Neoplasm of unspecified nature of breast	Yes	Yes
451.89:	Thrombophlebitis of breast	Yes	No
610.0-611.9:	Other disorders of breast	Yes	Yes
793.8:	Nonspecific abnormal findings on radiological and other examination of body structure, breast	Yes	Yes
V10.3:	Personal history of malignant neoplasm, breast	Yes	Yes
V42.81-V42.9:	Organ or tissue replaced by transplant	No	Yes
V51.0:	Aftercare involving use of plastic surgery	No	Yes

TABLE 39-2. Selected Examples of Procedural Codes and Medicare Reimbursements for 2009: National Average Fees, Unadjusted for Geography*

		2009 Fees		
	Services	Global (Nonfacility) ($)	Professional (Facility 26) ($)	Technical (Facility TC) ($)
1. Screening Mammogram				
77057	Bilateral	81.51	36.07	45.80
Diagnostic Mammograms				
77055	Unilateral	84.76	35.71	49.05
77056	Bilateral	107.48	44.36	63.12
2. Breast Biopsy: Stereotactic				
99241	E & M consultation code (i.e., provide opinion or advise on treatment to referring physician)	48.69	33.18	—
77031	Stereotactic localization code	194.76	81.15	113.61
19102	Core needle biopsy with imaging guidance	206.30	103.51	—
19103	Automated vacuum-assisted biopsy	519.72	190.43	—
76098	Specimen radiograph	19.84	8.30	11.54
19295	Placement of titanium clip for possible follow-up surgery or localized radiation	85.12	NA	—
99211	E & M code (post-procedure, follow-up of patient, may not require presence of a physician)	18.75	8.66	—
99212	E & M brief physician visit with exam or counseling	37.15	23.08	—
3. Breast Biopsy: Ultrasound-Guided				
99241	E & M consultation code	48.69	33.18	—
76942	Ultrasound localization code	183.94	—	—
19102	Core needle biopsy with imaging guidance	206.30	103.51	—
76645	Echography, breast, with image documentation	90.53	27.41	63.12
99211	E & M code, post-procedure	18.75	8.66	—
4. Wire Needle Localization				
77032	Preoperative placement of needle localization wire (radiologist supervision and interpretation)	59.87	28.49	31.38
19290	Preoperative placement of needle localization wire	152.56	65.28	—
19291	Each additional lesion	66.00	32.46	
76098	Radiographic examination of surgical specimen	19.84	8.30	11.54
5. Ductography				
77053	Supervision and interpretation, single duct	76.82	18.39	58.43
77054	Supervision and interpretation, multiple ducts	103.51	23.08	80.43
19030	Ductogram/galactogram inj. of contrast	157.25	—	—
6. Full-Field Digital Mammograms				
G0202	Screening mammogram, bilateral	129.84	34.98	94.85
G0204	Diagnostic mammogram, bilateral	152.56	43.28	109.28
G0206	Diagnostic mammogram, unilateral	121.18	34.98	86.20
7. Computer-Assisted Detection (CAD)				
77052	Screening mammogram—use with 76092	12.26	3.25	9.02
77051	Diagnostic mammogram—use with 76090-76091 (76085 has been deleted)	12.26	3.25	9.02
8. Breast Magnetic Resonance Imaging (MRI)				
77058	Breast MRI, unilateral	839.98	82.95	757.03
77059	Breast MRI, bilateral	904.90	82.95	821.94
77021	MR guidance for needle placement	447.95	NA	—

*Medicare reimbursement rates do not contain local geographic adjustments for any of the fees noted in this outline. Current procedural terminology (CPT) codes. E & M, evaluation and management; facility, hospital-outpatient; Facility 26, Medicare modifier code for the professional component; Facility TC, Medicare modifier code for the technical component; non-facility, physician office.

possible breast cancer, Medicare does require a written, telephone, or e-mail referral from the clinician, under Medicare Carrier Memorandum (MCM) #1725, section 15021(A)(5)(a-3). However, if a diagnostic mammogram is required for further evaluation of a screening-detected abnormality, no physician request is required.

As of 2002, Medicare allows reimbursement for both a screening mammogram and a diagnostic mammogram for the same patient, even if both are performed on the same day, with the proviso that the diagnostic mammogram was precipitated by an abnormal screening mammogram. Before 2002, Medicare would reimburse only for the diagnostic mammogram under these circumstances. Medicare does require the modifier "GG" to be attached to diagnostic mammogram CPT codes to ensure reimbursement in this situation.

Medicare reimburses for one baseline screening mammogram between ages 35 and 40 years, and for yearly screening mammograms beginning at age 40, in Medicare-eligible women. Under the "Lapsed Time Rule," a screening mammogram performed for a Medicare-eligible patient is not covered unless at least 11 months have elapsed since the last screening. Another Medicare rule relates to the "Advance Beneficiary Notice." Under this rule, the facility must notify the patient before the mammogram if the facility believes that Medicare may not pay for the mammogram and must explain to the patient the specific reason why Medicare may not pay (not enough time elapsed since last screening, patient does not meet Medicare age requirements, etc.). Further, the facility is required to obtain acknowledgment of this notice, in writing, from the patient. If a facility fails to meet these requirements, any charges denied reimbursement by Medicare cannot be passed on to the patient; if the patient in such a case is "erroneously" billed, the action may constitute fraud and may subject the facility to heavy penalties.[21] Also, the mammography center must be certified by the U.S. Food and Drug Administration (FDA) to be eligible for Medicare reimbursement.

FOLLOWING MEDICARE'S EXAMPLE: THE REST OF THE PAYERS

Virtually all payers currently reimburse physicians using the same CPT coding for procedures that CMS (formerly HCFA) uses for Medicare reimbursement. However, there is considerable variability by payer group in the amount of reimbursement. For instance, many private payers are reimbursing full-field digital mammography at the same rate as film mammography, even though Medicare global reimbursement rates for full-field digital mammography are almost 50% higher than those for film mammography. Even the conditions under which reimbursement is distributed vary considerably by payer. Each private company has its own interpretation of the "Elapsed Time Rule" and holds each patient responsible for establishing her own eligibility for a mammogram. However, like the Medicare carriers, the private insurers inevitably deny and delay payment for claims if they believe that their particular "rules" for reimbursement have not been strictly followed.

Health Maintenance Organizations (HMOs) usually reimburse at rates arrived at through negotiation with individual facilities. These rates are usually calculated as a percentage of Medicare rates and vary from one extreme to the other, depending on local competition. In general, the HMO rules for reimbursement are more convoluted than those of private insurers; one might be tempted to wonder whether the intent of such complications is to delay and deny payment for even the most legitimate claim for reimbursement.

Both HMOs and private payers often require pre-authorization for certain breast imaging procedures, especially interventional procedures. If pre-authorization is not requested and not granted, most payers do not reimburse the costs, regardless of other circumstances. (Under Medicare rules, CMS does not require pre-authorization for interventional breast imaging procedures, but Medicare carriers reserve the right to deny claims for payment later if they deem the procedures inappropriate for any reason.) At present, virtually no payers are reimbursing costs on a routine basis for screening breast ultrasonography. However, with the publication of the recommendations for the performance of screening breast MRI in high risk women by the American Cancer Society (ACS) in 2007,[22] Medicare and most other carriers are now reimbursing for screening breast MRI in women who meet the ACS criteria for being at "high risk" for contracting breast cancer. Pre-authorization is still required on a case-by-case basis.

In an effort to create stronger relations with private payers, and resolve many of the contentious reimbursement issues, the ACR has established the ACR Managed Care Committee. This committee acts as a liaison to the radiology community at large, bringing radiologists' concerns to the private payers, and providing useful information and resources as needed. If radiologists have concerns or problems regarding reimbursement issues with private payers, they would do well to use this valuable resource.[23]

The last significant, but nearly extinct, payer group is the cash-paying customer. Some states require that even a self-paying patient must present a signed referral from the clinician before a facility performs the examination. Aside from this minor exception, the facility dictates the rules for payment from self-paying patients.

REIMBURSEMENT: STRATEGIES FOR SUCCESS

Faced with the current woefully low levels of reimbursement for most mammographic procedures, and the impending changes in the Medicare reimbursement system mentioned above, each mammography facility must adopt an aggressive and vigilant attitude to avoid financial loss. The strategy for success should focus on implementation of the following measures:

1. Know and diligently apply the preceding rules for reimbursement.
2. Appropriately combine the identification of the patient, the indication for the examination, and all applicable procedural codes with the report of the procedure itself.
3. Pay close attention to coding and billing habits.
4. Solicit and cultivate the cooperation of the clinicians.
5. Train all facility personnel to be knowledgeable regarding these same billing issues and to be fastidious in collecting all patient information relevant to billing.
6. Perform periodic internal data-quality audits.

7. Challenge payer denials and underpayments if they appear inappropriate or contradictory.
8. When negotiating with HMOs, use the facility's own mammography outcome data to demonstrate that finding earlier, smaller cancers with mammography translates into dollar savings for the HMO.
9. Do not forget about making services attractive for the cash-paying customers by offering a "discount."
10. Get involved politically by mobilizing patients and women's advocacy groups to support legislation increasing mammography reimbursement.

Knowing and Applying the Rules

According to a Medical Group Management Association survey conducted in 2001, more than one third of all claims submitted to payers are rejected or ignored, most often because of submission errors.[24] Therefore, one must do everything possible to beat the insurance carriers at their own game by preempting their anticipated denial of a claim. A basic but extremely effective first step is to identify and correct the most common causes of delay and denial:[25,26]

- Incorrect procedure ordered by the clinician
- Application of incorrect ICD-9-CM and/or CPT code(s) for the procedure
- Failure to obtain pre-authorization from the payer before the desired procedure
- Improper documentation for the procedure provided by the radiologist in his or her dictated report
- Provision of inadequate written documentation and/or incorrect billing information

Appropriate Combination of Information and Report and Applicable Procedural Codes

Verify that all the relevant information—patient identification, examination indications, and procedure codes—is accurately reflected in the dictated report.[27] The report should have clear findings and conclusions and should include the following: (1) correct identification of the mammogram as either screening or diagnostic; (2) listing of all views performed; and (3) the clinical history, because payment is based on the correct ICD-9-CM code in addition to all applicable CPT codes. For interventional breast procedures, it is important to include all applicable CPT codes, because these procedures always have more than one code (see Table 9-2). In addition, Medicare has assigned the interventional codes 19102 and 19103 a global period of 0 days. This means that other biopsy-related preprocedure or postprocedure examinations, as well as any consultations with the patient before or after the procedure—E and M codes (see Table 9-2)—are not "bundled" with the original procedural code and may be billed separately. Although controversial, E and M codes can be successfully billed by breast imagers, provided that proper and complete documentation is performed.[28] Because E and M codes have been "unbundled" from the interventional procedures, one should be successful in billing for CPT codes 9924x and 992xx. However, one must meet the E and M Documentation Guidelines to do so. Additional documentation criteria for consultations (9924x) include a physician's request for an opinion or advice and a separate written report to the referring physician.

The 1995 and 1997 E and M Documentation Guidelines, as well as the proposed 2000 Guidelines released by HCFA, can be obtained from the CMS Web site, at www.cms.hhs.gov/MLNEdwebGuide/25_EMDOC.asp (the 1995 guidelines are preferred by most providers at this time). A strong word of caution is in order: If one does choose to bill the CPT E and M codes, one should be fastidious in following and documenting all the necessary steps required by the E and M Documentation Guidelines, including the appropriate history, mini-physical examination, and recommendations.[28] Failure to do so, if detected on Medicare review, may lead to charges of fraud and abuse.[21]

Proper Coding and Billing Habits

If the radiologist is doing the coding and using a short list of CPT codes (a cheat sheet), the listing must be verified as accurate and current, including all the newest codes. Otherwise, coding should be left in the hands of dedicated and well-trained staff personnel. One should monitor the local Medicare Review Policy (LMRP) portion of Medicare Part B bulletins for any local policy change.

Certain coding and billing practices should be avoided. In particular, one should not *up-code* (i.e., change a code to one with higher reimbursement) inappropriately, and one should try not to re-bill a patient for a procedure. If done too frequently, these actions create a suspicious situation that payers will target, setting up a potential adverse profile for the entire practice.[29]

Clinician Cooperation

One may have to educate clinicians and their staffs as to their contribution to proper reimbursement procedures. Firstly, they should send or fax a signed referral before the examination is performed. Secondly, the clinician must provide the appropriate clinical diagnosis for each examination. For example, "fibrocystic disease" cannot be listed as the reason for a diagnostic mammogram if this diagnosis is not biopsy proven. Thirdly, the clinician must fill out the requisition as correctly and completely as possible. This can best be accomplished with the help of a well-designed, user-friendly order form provided by the facility. Such a form should include: a checklist of possible procedures to be performed (screening mammogram, diagnostic mammogram, breast ultrasonogram, ultrasound-guided core biopsy, ductogram, etc.), a checklist of the patient's symptoms, if any (pain, lump, thickening, etc.), and a diagram of the breasts for the purpose of marking the location of pertinent physical findings. It is also useful for the form to contain all the facility's office phone numbers, including a fax number. Meeting regularly with all major clinician referrers, their respective staffs, or both, and apprising them of the importance of complying with the preceding conditions, enables one to avoid many reimbursement problems.[25]

Facility Personnel Training

If possible, designate one or two billing staff members as specialists in billing breast imaging procedures. The contributions of such individuals are invaluable. Not only are 35% of claims denied by payers, but a further 5% to 10% of claims are reimbursed at an inappropriately reduced rate.[24] Only through careful monitoring of claims by well-trained, specialized billing staff members can such situations be discovered in one's own practice. Important billing benchmarks, such as total charges, collections, number of days claims remain in Accounts Receivable, the distribution of the Accounts Receivable, and payer mix, should be monitored monthly for unexpected changes and trends. For instance, if a large and growing number of claims are suddenly remaining in Accounts Receivable and are not being resolved in 60 days or less, a more serious look at the entire billing system is in order. This kind of analysis can best be performed by billing specialists. If a practice does not allow for such individuals in-house, consideration should be given to using a competent and proven outside billing service.[24]

Periodic Internal Audits of Data Quality

Every facility should compile and subdivide the causes for denials and delays of claims. Persons responsible for such problems, be they physicians or other staff members, should be identified and trained to minimize recurrences. Although time-consuming, this approach offers obvious and immediate benefits.[29]

Challenging Denials and Underpayments

A facility should make a habit of challenging denials of payments and underpayments. If necessary, one should arrange to meet with key payer personnel to review one's legitimate claims. A well-placed explanation and demonstration of what one actually does for customers (i.e., patients) may go a long way toward increasing reimbursement.[30]

Using Outcome Data in HMO Negotiations

In negotiations with HMOs, a facility should use its own mammography outcomes data to demonstrate the savings to the HMOs of finding cancers at earlier stages, while they are smaller.[30] Further, if one's call-back rate is low and positive biopsy rate appropriately high, one can argue even more effectively about the savings to the HMO. Through such demonstrations, one may be able to negotiate a "carve-out" for proportionally higher reimbursement from the HMO for breast imaging procedures than for other imaging modalities.

Discounts for Cash Payments

A facility can make its service more attractive to cash-paying customers by offering discounts. If not participating with Medicare, one can even negotiate individual contracts with patients (usually discounting 20% for cash payment). In doing so, one must also treat all patients the same, so the discount rate chosen must be consistent. Additionally, a facility cannot waive copays and must bill at least once. Professional courtesy discounts should not be offered.

Political Involvement

Mammographers should mobilize patients and women's advocacy groups to support legislation to increase reimbursement for mammography. Such groups potentially represent the single most powerful weapon in the battle for better reimbursement. However, in today's political environment of shifting initiatives and wildly varying proposals for national health care reform, mobilization of patients and other women's advocacy groups may prove difficult. Nonetheless, such efforts should still be strongly pursued, once the political stage has stabilized. At the same time, radiologists should continue to work through the ACR and other professional groups to maintain political pressure on Congress to consider legislation providing more reasonable reimbursement for the many presently undervalued breast imaging procedures.

SUMMARY

Through high-quality breast imaging services, radiologists have contributed mightily to the dramatic drop in breast cancer deaths observed since the mid-1980s in the United States. Despite their medical success, however, breast imagers face the continuing problems of rising costs and falling reimbursement. They also face new challenges with the impending seismic shift in reimbursement based on performance outcomes. Therefore, their understanding of coding and billing under the current and any subsequent reimbursement system is critical to the very survival of breast imaging services within their practices. By effectively transforming reimbursement information into a careful coding and billing strategy for success, radiologists can more realistically anticipate the day when their breast imaging facilities evolve from their present status as lifesaving "loss leaders" to true financial "profit centers."

KEY POINTS

- As reimbursement for breast imaging continues to fall, radiologists must understand and improve their coding and billing of breast imaging procedures in order to survive financially.
- After mastering the payers' rules for breast imaging reimbursement, radiologists should devise a carefully constructed coding and billing strategy to preempt delays and denials of claims.
- A reimbursement improvement strategy should include such steps as an internal audit, specialized training of billing personnel, and direct contact with payers and referring physicians.
- Radiologists should be aware of the impending radical changes in reimbursement methodology based on performance outcomes, some of which are now being implemented.

SUGGESTED READINGS

Allen B. Valuing the professional work of diagnostic radiologic services. *J Am Coll Radiol* 2007;**4**:106-14.

Lee RK. A resident's primer of Medicare reimbursement in radiology. *J Am Coll Radiol* 2006;**3**:58-63.

Linver MN. Coding and billing of breast imaging procedures. *Sem Br Dis* 2001;**4**:78-87.

Petrey WB, Allen B, Thorwarth WT. Radiology coding, reimbursement, and economics: a practical playbook for housestaff. *J Am Coll Radiol* 2009;**6**:643-8.

Thorwarth WT, Borgstede JP. Mammography reimbursement: components and strategies for change. *Sem Br Dis* 2001;**4**:46-53.

REFERENCES

1. American Cancer Society. *Cancer Facts and Figures, 2009*. Atlanta Ga:American Cancer Society; 2009.
2. Brice J. Mammography in jeopardy. *Diagn Imaging* 2001;**23**:50-5.
3. *International Classification of Diseases, Ninth Revision: Clinical Modification*. 6th ed. Salt Lake City, Utah: Ingenix Publishing Group; 2000.
4. *Current Procedural Terminology: CPT 2009 Professional Edition*. Chicago, Il:American Medical Association; 2008.
5. *HCPCS National Level II Codes 2009*. Salt Lake City, Utah: Ingenix Publishing Group; 2008.
6. Mitchell JB. Physician DRGs. *N Engl J Med* 1985;**313**:670-5.
7. U.S. Department of Health and Human Services, Health Care Financing Administration. Medicare Program: revisions to payment policies and adjustments to the relative value units under the physician fee schedule for calendar year 1999: final rule and notice. *Fed Regist* 1999;**63**:211.
8. U.S. Department of Health and Human Services, Health Care Financing Administration. Prospective payment system for hospital outpatient services. *Fed Regist* 2000;**65**:18433-82.
9. Rawson JV, Kassing P. HOPPS: evolution of a CMS process. *J Am Coll Radiol* 2007;**4**:102-5.
10. Farria DM. The Hospital Outpatient Prospective Payment System. An overview. *Semin Breast Disease* 2001;**4**:21-6.
11. Allen B. Valuing the professional work of diagnostic radiologic services. *J Am Coll Radiol* 2007;**4**:106-14.
12. U.S. Department of Health and Human Services. Interim final rules on conditions for Medicare coverage of screening mammograms. *Fed Regist* 1990;53511-25.
13. Balanced Budget Act of 1997 (Medicare revisions), Section 4104. Public Law 105-33. August 5, 1997.
14. Medicare, Medicaid, and SCHIP Benefits Improvement and Protection Act (BIPA) of 2000. Public Law 106-554. December 21, 2000.
15. Deficit Reduction Act of 2005. Public Law 109-171. Enacted February 8, 2006.
16. American College of Radiology. *New 2009 PQRI measure proposed to track inappropriate use of "probably benign" BI-RADS 3*. Available at: www.acr.org/Hidden/Economics/FeaturedCategories/Pubs/coding_source/archives/JulyAugust2008/New2009PQRIMeasureProposed.aspx. Accessed Jan. 25, 2010.
17. Thrall JH. The emerging role of pay-for-performance contracting for health care services. *Radiology* 2004;**233**:637-40.
18. *Medicare Providers' News. Part B*. Oklahoma/New Mexico, November 1997.
19. Radiology Coding Alert, sample issue, 1999;1-3.
20. Brice J. Small change for big medicine. *Diagn Imaging* 2000;**22**:42-9.
21. Lucey LL, Hoffman TR. Fraud and abuse in breast imaging coding and billing. *Sem Br Dis* 2001;**4**:94-8.
22. Saslow D, Boetes C, Burke W, Harms S, Leach MO, Lehman CD, et al. American Cancer Society guidelines for breast cancer screening with MRI as an adjunct to mammography. *CA Cancer J Clin* 2007;**57**:75-89.
23. Ullrich CG, Keysor KJ. The ACR Managed Care Committee: focusing private payers on radiology issues. *J Am Coll Radiol* 2007;**4**:115-8.
24. Cassel D, Brant-Zawadzke M, Dwyer C. Learn importance of billing carefully. *Diagn Imaging* 2003;**25**:49-55.
25. Ikeda DM, Linver MN. ICD-9-CM codes, CPT codes, billing and collection. *SBI News* October 2000;**1**:7-9.
26. Chicoine J. Know the codes. *Imaging Economics*, May 2009, 36-9.
27. Thorwarth WT. Get paid for what you do: dictation patterns and impact on billing accuracy. *J Am Coll Radiol* 2005;**2**:665-9.
28. Linver MN, Poller WR, Granucci S. E & M Codes: to bill or not to bill. *SBI News* Summer, 2006;5-8.
29. Yoder L, Anderson R. Assess your practice's coding intelligence. *Imaging Economics* July-August 1999;74-80.
30. Wade T, Seifert P. Preparing to negotiate with payers. *Sem Breast Dis* 2008;**11**:195-7.

CHAPTER 40

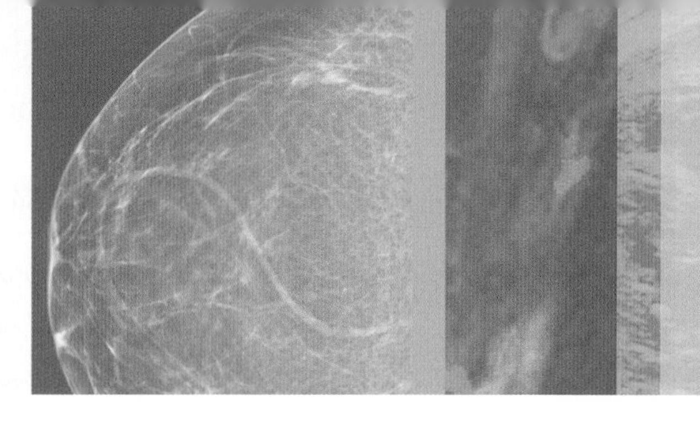

Medical-Legal Aspects of Breast Imaging and Intervention

R. James Brenner

Accountability for medical practice may be found in different forms and associated with a variety of purposes. Quality assurance programs and initiatives are often designed to assess current patterns of care and to determine potential interventions that may improve outcomes. Such interventions can then be reassessed to evaluate quality improvement. Peer review conferences and "tumor board" discussions provide an opportunity to review prior and intended health care, with one of the goals being a determination, albeit in retrospect, of what might have led to a more successful outcome. Beyond the medical environment, accountability may sometimes be determined in a civil forum, namely, a court of law. When a woman believes that her care with respect to breast cancer evaluation has been insufficient, she may seek legal redress to help determine whether her care providers have met with a standard of care that should be and is expected.

The concept of medical legal consequences of medical practice often evokes a negative reaction from health care providers who sometimes feel that they are being unfairly "second-guessed" for what they consider bona fide efforts in a difficult medical-economic environment to provide service. Some consider rising medical liability insurance rates as a disincentive to enter certain professional endeavors, assigning fault to litigious patients and aggressive plaintiff attorneys. This situation, for breast cancer, may be even more severe when encouraging published results from breast cancer screening studies and ambitious advertisements create expectations among women that all malignancies can be found at a curable stage. More often than not, a misunderstanding of the purpose and function of the legal system accounts for unmeasured responses to that system by medical providers.

According to the Physician Insurers Association of America (PIAA), a consortium of physician-owned liability carriers that pool claims data and dispositions, delay in the diagnosis of breast cancer was the second most common reason for malpractice claims against physicians in their 1990 report.[1] In 1995, after again studying the issue, the PIAA concluded that this claim was the most common reason for such lawsuits.[2] In a follow-up report in 2002, this allegation remained the most common reason for such lawsuits and—in part because among women bringing legal action, most have had at least one mammogram —the radiologist was the most commonly named defendant.[3]

Given these circumstances, breast imagers—most of whom are radiologists— have reason for concern. Such legal exposure has been cited as one of the reasons that radiologists-in-training have sought to avoid breast imaging as a subspecialty.[4] The response from practicing radiologists has been studied as well. Indeed, without discounting the relatively higher legal exposure, surveyed radiologists report a clear overestimate of the likelihood of being sued for delay in diagnosis of breast cancer.[5]

As a complement to the multiple discussions that have taken place in this text, it is worth understanding the legal system within which breast imaging is practiced, not only as an exercise in edification but also as a tool to better address what is and is not expected in daily medical practice that serves both medical and legal directives.

MEDICAL MALPRACTICE: WHAT DOES IT MEAN?

The practice of law, like medicine, encompasses many different types of fields. Corporate law, navigation law, constitutional law, and environmental law all constitute specialized fields that do not usually relate to the actual practice of breast imaging. Some peripheral fields such as regulatory law may impact practices when, for example, fraud and abuse laws are violated from improper medical billing procedures. Civil law governs relationships between and among individuals and one field of civil law, the law of negligence, generally applies to the practice of medicine. Such civil actions are often referred to as "torts." Rarely, criminal law sanctions may be imposed for reckless disregard in the practice of medicine. Criminal law, however, defines the relationship of society to an individual, with higher standards of proof and potential severe consequences, such as incarceration. Thus, actions brought against individuals in criminal courts involve the "state" as the offended party, which seeks to protect the citizenry from offensive conduct.

When an individual (in the field of breast imaging this is usually a female patient) believes that her care has been substandard, she may hold her caregivers accountable. As mentioned, the law of negligence governs the analysis of such situations. This law, derived from 18th century English legal concepts, originally was construed to define considered relationships that exist in society, such as special duties that innkeepers had to guests. This rationale was incorporated into the medical field where physicians were held to have special relationships to patients.

Although the law of negligence carries negative connotations, it is, in the legal field, a term of art defining certain elements that must be satisfied for a legal action—often referred to as medical malpractice—to prevail. Although an adverse consequence of care usually triggers a consideration of malpractice, it is the conduct of the physician, not the consequences of that conduct, that determines liability. Only when liability can be shown will consequences be considered.

The law of negligence involves the showing of four elements: duty, breach of duty, causation, and damages.[6] Each claim, or *cause of action* must satisfy all four elements to establish legal harm. The duty of the breast imager involves three directives: the production and approval of satisfactory images, the rendering of a reasonable interpretation, and the effective communication of that information. This is often referred to as the *standard of care*, which has been the variable defined by most courts as what "a reasonable and prudent physician would do under similar circumstances."[7] The breach of any of these duties, if it bears a substantial causative relationship to injury (often defined as *cause-in-fact* and *proximate cause*), constitutes potential negligence. Sometimes, duty and breach of duty are referred to as a *liability issue*, distinguished from causation issues. The analysis of causation is usually reserved to nonimaging oncologists (medical, surgical, radiation) because the considerations are often beyond the customary purview of the imager.

The law is not focused on assigning blame or punishment, although defendants often perceive the consequences of the law as resulting in both. Rather, civil law is aimed at restitution, or attempting to "make the plaintiff whole." Essentially, this remedy is expressed in money damages, because the law cannot redo suboptimal care, replace potential years of life lost, or mitigate future anxiety. Thus, where actual damages cannot be assigned as consequences of liability, courts will not customarily be interested in hearing the case. Such cases are often dismissed subsequent to legal requests referred to as actions for *demurer* or *motion for summary judgment*.

An example of this interrelationship may be understood by considering the mammographic examination of a woman when a highly suspicious lesion such as a spiculated mass is not detected, circumstances that might be indicative of a breach of the standard of care. However, if the woman is examined by her physician within the next week and a palpable lump corresponding to the spiculated mass is found and sampled within a week, then the misinterpretation of the mammogram does not ripen into a cause of action in negligence because it fails to satisfy the elements of causation and damages. One might posit that future anxiety and lack of confidence in the medical system are the consequent damages, often conveyed in legal terms as *mental distress*, and thus should be compensated. Most states regard damages of mental distress as a separate cause of action but a derivative tort that may be considered only if the tort of negligence can be established. Medical malpractice law is, for the most part, governed by state—not federal or local—law and found in published state business and professional codes.

When the conduct of a provider is called into question, a legal process is instituted.[8] Some states require different forms of screening a legal complaint, which may result in notices of intent to sue (e.g., California) or affidavits of legal merit by a preliminary reviewer (e.g., Florida) as an attempt to either prevent unmeritorious claims from proceeding (and unnecessarily imposing on restricted legal resources) or inviting opportunities to address matters that may result in clarification of facts without resorting to the further legal process.

Once a formal complaint is filed listing one or more causes of action a deliberate process is triggered. Under such circumstances, defendants are advised to "freeze the case in time and place."[8] In other words, imaging studies should be sequestered because the sudden disappearance of relevant images may be considered as *spoilation of evidence* for which a special jury instruction may be requested, often with an adverse impact on the defendant. Defendants are advised to not discuss the case with others and to resist the urge to show the case to a colleague in an attempt to gain reassurance that the interpretation was correct. All actions by defendants, beyond the protected conferences between a defendant and assigned attorney, are considered *discoverable*, meaning that the results of such conversations—even if adverse to the defendant's intended goals—can be probed and exposed by the opposing party. Opposing parties will seek to clarify facts through legal mechanisms such as interrogatories (series of written questions and responses) and depositions, in which responses to oral questions under oath are obtained that can be used to corroborate or impugn testimony during a court trial. The legal process that dictates actions before a trial is called *discovery*, where information is exchanged with an intent to informally settle such disputes without trial. Not every state invites such discovery depositions from all participants in the case. Indeed, most legal complaints do not proceed to trial, although any exchange of monies in settlement of a complaint must be reported to the National Practitioner Data Bank and often to state medical boards.

A trial is the final civil manner in which to resolve legal conflicts. A trial, governed by a single judge or more often a jury, is an attempt to resolve issues of fact, not law. Specifically, the fact in dispute relates to whether the defendant comported to a standard of care that reflects reasonable care, as well as the consequences of that conduct. Specific standards of proof, evidence, and testimony are governed by established legal procedure. A trial has no precedent-setting value, because it relates to the particular facts of a given case. Thus, defendants who believe a verdict is unjustified are unlikely to succeed in appealing their case to a higher court, because appellate courts are neither inclined to review every trial decision nor focused on issues of fact.

Appellate court decisions, unlike trial court decisions, do have precedent-setting value, so that legal principles that are rendered are expected to be followed by other courts within that jurisdiction (a principle called *stare decisis*), and such decisions are usually published. Indeed, courts outside that jurisdiction often borrow such logic in rendering their own opinions. As mentioned, appellate courts are interested in issues of law, rather than fact. If a trial verdict is accepted by an appellate court for review—related to issues such as jury instructions, statute of limitations, or other questions of law, not fact—the court may nonetheless take the opportunity to review the facts of the case and make comment or *dicta* that has bearing on future conduct. Through this mechanism, some appellate principles of breast imaging practice have been developed, although the number of directives is relatively small.[9]

The initiation of a lawsuit usually follows an adverse event, such as the diagnosis of cancer at a point in its natural history when the patient believes it should have been discovered earlier. However, a lawsuit is, as may be inferred from the previous discussion, not about outcome but rather about conduct, namely, was the conduct that of a reasonable and prudent physician under the circumstances of the case. Inherent within this analysis are two fundamental principles. The first is the legal benchmark of reasonableness. Reasonable image quality is required of the standard of care, not perfection. Likewise, the reasonableness of recall from screening or of a diagnostic interpretation, correct or incorrect, will often be determined with the assistance of experts. The second principle is that of foreseeability, which is related to reasonableness. The court is often asked to determine, in assessing compliance with the standard of care, if a patient is not recalled for re-imaging of a lesion or the lesion is not diagnosed as suggestive of malignancy was sufficiently foreseeable as being a potential cancer to have prompted conduct other than that exhibited by the defendant. Again, expert testimony is usually required.

Different legal standards may impact the disposition of a given case. Recall that it is the showing of *legal harm* that determines the outcome of a trial decision. Although breast imagers are primarily involved in a liability determination—should the imaged lesion have been recommended for biopsy?—the individual state determinations of the consequences of their actions (causation) may impact whether or not legal redress is sought. Some states maintain a traditional legal approach called *the 50% rule* in which the defendant's action must be shown with greater than 50% likelihood to have altered the patient's course to prevail in court. Thus, the delay in diagnosis of a 2.1-cm cancer (stage 2) that becomes 2.4 cm before biopsy (remember volume is a function of the radius cubed) may not be considered sufficient legal harm for recovery. Other state jurisdictions follow the *loss of chance* doctrine in which any delay may invite recovery (the previous example might invite a different legal result under such circumstances). Finally, some states have adopted by statute or legal precedent a formula that is somewhat a hybrid between the two approaches.

STANDARDS OF CARE

Standards of care are usually established during a trial for medical malpractice from two sources: statutory and common law. Statutes are expressed forms of law passed by legislative bodies and often applied through regulatory agencies that indicate a societal determination of what is expected from providers. The Mammography Quality Standards Act (MQSA), originally implemented in 1997, and its reauthorized implementation, is an unusual federal law that applies to some of the practice of mammography, and aspects of this statute will be considered later.[10] It should be noted that violation of such statutory provisions may not require or necessarily invite expert testimony when the language and therefore criteria establishing society's determination of a standard of care can be interpreted by lay juries.

Guidelines or practice patterns propagated from different societies are not tantamount to standards of care. There are more than 300 published guidelines, including those issued by the American College of Radiology (ACR). Most current guidelines are consensus based, rather than evidence based; when different deliberative processes lead to different results by reputable organizations, the courts will avoid favoring one over another. This is an application of the legal principle of the *alternative school of thought* doctrine, which permits introduction of evidence contrary to one posited so long as there is a rational basis. For example, the ACR may recommend annual mammography for all women older than 40 years of age, whereas the American College of Physicians/Academy of Family Practitioners or American College of Obstetrics and Gynecology have less-specific recommendations for women between the ages of 40 and 50. Guidelines are not permitted per se into evidence but may be presented as a basis or foundation for a given expert's opinion and testimony. This restriction occurs because the opposing attorney cannot cross-examine the committee that developed such positions. Rather, an expert who cites such standards can be interrogated regarding the substance of such positions. Because certain local or national guidelines may have widespread endorsement, radiologists are encouraged to be familiar with such recommendations and be prepared to establish a rational basis for departing from these endorsed patterns of practice, if applicable.

Most cases that are litigated are, as stated earlier, fact specific. Certain basic principles apply to the analysis of most cases that involve the allegation of delay in diagnosis of breast cancer, which is the most common legal redress cited by the PIAA. As mentioned, the first duty is the production and supervision of reasonable images. Whereas certain personnel may be subject to institutional (e.g., hospital) accountability, the interpreting radiologist—even as an independent contractor working with the institution—is charged by MQSA as responsible for the final approval of the image. Historical benchmarks for quality control of analogue images have been propagated related to proper exposure, film processing, positioning, labeling, and so on. Current quality control (QC) procedures for full-field digital mammography (FFDM) have been delegated by the U.S. Food and Drug Administration (FDA), which is responsible for implementing MQSA provision to individual manufacturer's specifications. Although radiologists are therefore less involved with QC performance, they are as supervising radiologists under MQSA responsible for proper oversight of the program. Indeed, designated radiologists are asked to sign a verification of such oversight.[11] Moreover, certain QC aspects of FFDM may be more difficult to appreciate than in the past. For example, FFDM provides during the imaging processing phase compensating mechanisms that seek to provide a similar darkness to the image through a series of proprietary algorithms. Whereas technique issues such as too low a kilovolts (peak) (kVp) may cause underexposure more readily recognized on analogue images as whiter fat (instead of blacker fat), compensatory processing can partially mask the problem by producing a relatively darker-appearing image. However, when the underexposure is significant, the image will demonstrate insufficient contrast ("flatter image"), which can be recognized by comparison with other images. Thus, some of the paradigms that radiologists employ to evaluate image quality in an FFDM environment vary from historic analogue image analysis.

Positioning may be more challenging with FFDM, when a thicker detector plate requires adaptation to position the inferior mammary fold properly. Obtaining a sufficient amount of tissue on the image remains a directive for mammography, FFDM, or analogue. One measure of sufficient positioning may be recognized by comparing current examinations to prior ones, ensuring at least as much tissue. Often, internal landmarks on the image such as calcifications can assist in this determination. Other benchmarks, such as the amount of tissue on a craniocaudal (CC) projection as measured from the nipple to the edge of the film being within 1 cm of the amount of tissue imaged on the mediolateral oblique (MLO), have been prescribed by the ACR.[12] Because "you can't call what you can't see," imaging a reasonable amount of breast tissue on the mammogram is an important component of fulfilling the standard of care.

There are a host of QC measures that are beyond the scope of this discussion. Because one cannot foresee from an otherwise negative mammographic study that a woman might develop radiographic findings of breast cancer within a year, attention to QC is important. Motion blurriness is an example of an imaging problem that is common to both screen-film and FFDM environments. For example, if an image suffers from substantial motion blurriness, it should be repeated, even if no lesion is suspected, because if a malignant lesion is seen at this focus next year, aggrieved patients may legitimately speculate that the lesion would have been visible with a properly conducted examination during the prior year.

Screening mammography, a quasi-public health effort, is primarily concerned with the detection of abnormalities among women who are asymptomatic with respect to the breasts; in other words, they have no physical signs or symptoms of breast cancer. As discussed, one element of such detection is image quality and so liability may be found when detection is not possible because of too little breast tissue on the image or motion blurriness that has occurred. Beyond image quality, judgment is exercised in deciding whom to recall, and so prescriptive formulas do not apply necessarily to any given case. Benchmarks have been studied regarding the current practice of recall, but the relationship to outcome is not established. For example, in the large National Cancer Institute (NCI)-sponsored Breast Cancer Surveillance Consortium (BCSC) report, the median recall rate was 10%, a number that has been criticized as being substantially higher than in some European countries where there are national screening programs (as opposed to more tailored service screening programs in the United States).[13,14] In part, such determinations are made by available resources and goals (what is the acceptable mean tumor size at time of diagnosis), as well as different patient populations studied (e.g., high-risk patients may have a higher predisposing probability of cancer for a given examination). However, benchmarks are often not directly germane in an individual case at trial but rather a specific lesion. Imagers struggle with balancing the primary effort of detecting early breast cancer with defeating a medical system not designed to embrace unnecessarily high recall rates.[13,14] For example, the presence of a one-view mammographic asymmetric density or three round calcifications is so unlikely to represent early breast cancer that such features are not usually subject to recall.[15,16] In any given case, however, cancer may indeed be associated with such signs. This is where the legal principles of foreseeability and reasonableness apply. Because it may not be unreasonable to avoid recall for the presence of three round calcifications owing to empirical data suggesting that such a finding is not sufficiently foreseeable as representing malignancy, a decision to consider such findings as a normal variant may be in a particular case incorrect but not negligent. The law does not require a "warranty of certainty" as a standard of care.[17]

Image quality and reasonableness of interpretation also apply to the diagnostic environment. In evaluating a cluster of microcalcifications, radiologists will often employ microfocal spot physical magnification techniques, which often lengthen the time of radiographic exposure and invite the risk, therefore, of introducing motion unsharpness or blur. If this is not recognized and repeated, a misinterpretation may result and the approval of such an image, as mentioned earlier regarding MQSA, is the responsibility of the interpreting physician.

Generally accepted criteria for suspect lesions that warrant recall for further evaluation have been discussed elsewhere in this text. The non-recall of a large cluster of fine pleomorphic calcifications is not likely to survive challenge and usually reflects the overlooking of such a sign or film quality impairing one's ability to identify the lesion. Causes for "missed cancer" have been addressed elsewhere.[18] Less obvious lesions such as several amorphous calcifications or an ill-defined mass invite contested testimony as to the foreseeability of the lesion representing cancer, assuming it has in fact been detected. As mentioned earlier, each situation that is brought to legal attention is case specific.

Because diagnostic radiology seeks to arrive at a specific impression that is intended to prompt management considerations, the reasonableness of such interpretation is often at issue. An analogous situation to the non-recall of the three round calcifications discussed earlier can be applied to diagnostic circumstances. Consider a focal asymmetry found on a first prevalent mammographic study that fails, after proper mammographic and sonographic evaluation, to show signs of a mass. The likelihood of such a mammographic sign representing cancer is less than 1%.[19] Nonetheless, it is a finite number, not 0%, so that, on occasion, focal asymmetry does indeed represent the earliest imaging manifestations of malignancy. The failure to assign a suspicious impression to this finding may be incorrect but not necessarily be negligent. On the other hand, the development of a solid (by ultrasound) mass with irregular margins, absent a history of trauma or inflammation, is sufficiently foreseeable as representing malignancy—again by empirical observation and reported studies—that the failure to recommend biopsy does likely represent a departure from an acceptable standard of care.[20]

The range of lesions to which this analysis applies is myriad and beyond the purview of this discussion. As in the decision to recall or not recall a given patient for a finding on a screening mammogram, a defensible—or in legal context, a reasonable—decision regarding either a recalled screening detected lesion or a finding associated with clinical symptoms will be case specific, and reference to discussions elsewhere in this text is suggested.

The medical field, especially one as technologically oriented as breast imaging, continues to invite new methods of detection and diagnosis. Such tools are introduced into practice and the legal implications are sometimes difficult to determine. A later discussion in this chapter, as it relates to computer aided detection (CAD), will illustrate the relationship between the advances in law and medicine and how this relationship may impact contested legal outcomes. However, at this point, it is worth considering certain advances and how they relate to the standard of care.

Ongoing investigations have indicated that magnetic resonance imaging (MRI) of the breast can detect cancers that would not have been identified by standard mammographic techniques. In the focal asymmetry case discussed previously, in which the likelihood of malignancy is less than 1% but for a given circumstance might, in fact, represent cancer, one might contend that MRI should have been recommended. MRI has repeatedly been found to be more sensitive than mammography to the detection of breast cancer.[21] Such an approach represents a potential for earlier diagnosis but not necessarily a standard of care. Based on the very low likelihood of malignancy, as mentioned, the foreseeability issue fails to support a claim of negligence because the assertion that MRI should have been performed under such circumstances does not reflect what a reasonable and prudent imager would do under certain circumstances. On the other hand, the development of a lump in a postmenopausal woman requires appropriate evaluation even if an MRI does not show a specific lesion; MRI has a finite false-negative rate.[22] Thus, new technology may advance the diagnostic capability of a given imaging facility without necessarily rising to a standard of care.

That the application of certain technologies does not constitute in a legal sense the standard of care does not imply that they should be discouraged. Perhaps one manner of understanding this situation is to distinguish preferred approaches to standard of care thresholds. In a sense, this is an application of the *alternative school of thought* doctrine. In like manner, although screening ultrasonography has been advocated for several circumstances, including the mammographically dense breast or high risk patients, or both,[23] it does not currently represent the standard of care. Contrast this consideration to that of screening mammography, which has not only been validated by common use and evidence-based clinical trials but also guideline recommendations from several professional societies. In this context, one may wonder if FFDM has emerged as the standard of care, especially in women with dense breasts, because improved outcomes were reported during the American College of Radiology Imaging Network Digital Mammography In Screening Trial (ACRIN DMIST) study.[24] Rather, because that study using the new technology available at the time showed a strong (but not statistically significant) trend toward superiority in the fatty replaced breast for cancer detection for analogue images, it is difficult to advocate a required change in the global paradigm. In like manner, CAD has shown a positive impact on cancer detection in many situations, although conflicting results from other studies mitigate against arguments that this is a standard of care.[25-27]

ADMINISTRATIVE ISSUES IN LIABILITY

The previous discussion assumes a working familiarity with the difference between screening and diagnostic or problem-solving imaging. Because the likelihood or pretest probability of malignancy is higher in a symptomatic population and because other conventional techniques employed during diagnostic studies have been demonstrated repeatedly to influence final management decisions, it is important to triage a patient correctly into one of the two groups.[28] This can be challenging at times when the clinical history is ambiguous. Such ambiguity should to the extent possible be clarified before the examination. A dominant lump for which there are no specific associated mammographic features may be readily diagnosed as a cyst or a suspicious lesion with ultrasonography performed at the site of clinical concern, but if a proper history is not even sought and the study treated as a screening mammogram, diagnosis might be delayed. Although the clinician may bear responsibility for the management of such an abnormality, any delay that is attributed to the mis-triaging of the patient at the radiology facility invites legal redress for the latter.

As a standard of care, facilities should document the patient's history, which serves as a basis for such triaging. A woman with multiple lumps bilaterally and diffusely with no dominant area may indeed be a candidate for screening whereas a woman with specific dominant and limited lumps on each side may not. This history may be obscured because of insufficient clinical breast examination when thickening in both upper outer quadrants, often a normal variant, is confused with a more specific clinical index of suspicion. Facilities are advised to develop and promote compliance with policies and procedures that reasonably attempt to reconcile such histories. To validate the final assignment, it is advisable for the patient to sign or initial the history (which in paperless environments may be scanned into a computer), a concept sometimes referred to as ratification. Tantamount in importance, if there develops a need to correct the intake information subsequent to such signature, the patient, not facility personnel, should initial such changes to avoid conflicting recollections should cancer develop subsequently at a suspect site.

The more specific the designation of an area subject to evaluation, the more defensible the examination should malignancy arise near but not at the site undergoing study. For example, although quadrants of the breast represent a functional and not anatomic designation, the evaluation of a lesion near the nipple in the upper outer quadrant may be negative. If the patient presents with another area of concern that results in a malignant diagnosis in the same quadrant but near the axillary tail, reference to the prior examination will likely be undertaken. Whether by specified description or even film marker, indicating the site of each evaluation has far-reaching risk management implications that have been supported by appellate court decisions.[9] Additionally, because most breast cancers are not fatal, it may be important for both the facility and the woman to understand that the care rendered at the time was appropriate and deliberate because breast cancer survivors will need to avail themselves of future medical and imaging surveillance and confidence in that system will encourage such participation.

In this respect, histories can sometimes be misleading. If a facility has never evaluated a given clinical complaint such as a lump, reliance on the chronicity of the finding may be ill founded. A woman who had a lump in a similar region years ago might have developed a new abnormality. Image verification of the site of complaint and evaluation help to clarify what has and has not been studied. Indeed, satisfactory evaluation of a sign or symptom that is associated with breast cancer that has been anatomically assigned on the study may permit less intensive imaging within a short proximate time if the patient returns with the same complaint. As has been recognized for decades, a negative imaging examination will not obviate the need for biopsy of a clinically suspicious abnormality, when, for example, both ultrasonography and mammography have not demonstrated suspicious findings, because a small percentage of such cases are associated with malignancy.[29]

Because developing densities have a relatively high association with malignancy when they are not associated with a history of trauma, inflammation, or exogenous hormones and are not found to represent cysts or lymph nodes, prior films for comparison will provide a basis for identifying such "neodensities."[8] Controversy exists as to the advisability of procuring old films, given the attendant costs.[30] However, as was observed in a California appellate court, costs may be considered but will not prevent potential exposure to tort liability.[31] Uniform approaches to requesting old films provides a more defensible position should a developing density appear and should be compliant with the Health Insurance Portability and Accountability Act (HIPAA). Of note, studies have shown that requests for prior studies are frequently not successful[30]; it is unlikely that extraordinary efforts need be extended, but it is equally likely that the absence of any attempt may be considered unreasonable.

Other requirements of MQSA have been addressed elsewhere. It should be recalled that this is a statutory standard of care and leaves relatively little latitude for variations.

COMMUNICATION OF RESULTS

Beyond the issues of production of reasonable image production and reasonable interpretation, the process of communication completes the third duty attendant to the satisfactory completion of the breast imaging examination. Communication of information to the referring physician has been a longstanding directive in medicine,[32] but communication of results to the patient, as prescribed by MQSA, is a departure from customary medical imaging practice. The customary practice in all of imaging of issuing an interpretive report applies, of course, to breast imaging. However, given the dual goals of both screening and diagnostic studies, certain principles should be both emphasized and distinguished.

When there is a suspicion of malignancy, especially in an asymptomatic woman who has been recalled from screening and further evaluated, there is a generally recognized duty to directly communicate the information to the referring physician or identifiable designate. Both ACR guidelines and longstanding appellate court reasoning emphasize this effort because the receipt of the results by the appropriate party are of tantamount importance to the results themselves.[33] The emphasis on receipt rather than transmission of information is the operative directive because it is "foreseeable" that a simple mailed or faxed report may not reach the intended party; usually direct speaking to the referring physician or authorized designate (or patient for self-referred patients, see later) will satisfy the duty, and such discussions should be documented as specifically as possible (e.g., date and time as well as person receiving results) in the report. In fact, the facility's or imager's medical record is in large measure the interpretative report.[34] Although a negative report should be sent, the failure to verify its receipt is an example of a potential allegation of breach of duty, but because there is no causation issue with respect to delay in diagnosis (or other adverse consequence) as in the case of a suspicious finding, there is no legal harm that can be shown. Administrative remedies related to MQSA may be imposed for the regular failure to properly issue reports, but this is not generally an issue in tort law.

Because the interpretative report is the medical record of the imaging facility,[34] it is reviewed in detail when legal issues arise. Structured reporting systems have been developed that address most issues. However, when unusual circumstances or conditions apply to the examination (e.g., the patient declined repeat view of a blurry image) that may not be part of the standard selection text, this information should be included nonetheless in the report. Virtually all systems permit free text where appropriate, even if such data cannot always been captured in audit summaries.

A conclusive statement with regard to a lesion is sometimes employed for purposes of expediency. When no significant abnormality exists, it is unlikely that negligence will be found. However, if the conclusion is not correct, and there is no description of the abnormality on which to find a reasonable or rational (albeit incorrect) basis for that conclusion, defense of such an interpretation becomes difficult.

In this regard, it is important that consistency exist between the description of an abnormality and the conclusion that is drawn. A cluster of amorphous calcifications in a 42-year-old woman is unlikely to be associated with, for example, an early calcifying fibroadenoma. There is in this case a discordance between such description and conclusion, a result that in general should be avoided. In other words, the description of a lesion should reasonably lead to a defensible conclusion, even if incorrect. Remember that the finding of negligence is not based on correct evaluation but rather a reasonable one, because medical diagnoses have not been held to a warranty of certainty by the courts.[17]

The development of the ACR Breast Imaging Reporting and Data System (BI-RADS) with its first publication in 1992 was an attempt to provide a consensus-based road map for descriptive terms of art and reproducibly understandable conclusions.[35] The MQSA incorporated the conclusion categories of BI-RADS into its statutory language, indicating its importance as a standard of care. The FDA, which is the regulatory body charged with implementing MQSA, adopted the language associated with BI-RADS categories 0 to 5, but the statute did not, unlike the intended implementation, specify that category 0 was to be used for screening while desired final categories were to be used for diagnostic studies. In the fourth edition of BI-RADS,[36] an advisory suggested that category 0 could be applied in a restricted number of cases for diagnostic cases awaiting prior films. Some imagers have applied this reasoning to studies for which MRI or other imaging technique is sought. Unless a facility can virtually ensure that such diagnostic category 0 designations (or the statutory equivalent language) will be amended, the facility runs the risk, both medically and legally, of inviting mismanagement from such ambiguity; the development of a uniform reporting system was intended to avoid this predicament. Laudable intentions are not relevant to the law of negligence. Because it is foreseeable that old films may not be recovered[30] or that MRI studies may be performed at other institutions that will not necessarily inform the index institution of the findings, the diagnostic category of "indeterminate, needs further evaluation" creates a situation that is vulnerable to legal redress under many circumstances. To rely on the ambiguity of MQSA as a defense to such practice is to ignore the legislative history of MQSA, a history that can be introduced at trial. ACR endorsement of this approach may not be sufficient to defeat basic responsibility in tort law, and thus the caution exerted by the ACR in its advisory should be carefully considered.

An alternative to the "indeterminate" category is to issue a final conclusion and, in the report, indicate that the subsequent performance of MRI or prior films being recovered may invite an amended report. This should not be construed to change the imaging findings on the initial mammogram or ultrasound image; indeed, the usefulness of an audit is derived specifically from such findings that ordinarily should not be influenced, for example, by MRI. Consider a focal asymmetry for which prior films were performed but are not available. A BI-RADS 3, for example, may be amended to a BI-RADS 2—Benign finding, if prior films show no change; whereas the same finding may be amended to a BI-RADS 4—Suspicious finding, if prior films indicate this is a new finding that is not associated with a cyst or lymph node and without an associated explanatory history of, for example, trauma.

A certain percentage of patients who are recalled from screening will not return to the index facility for different reasons, which include seeking care elsewhere. In like manner, a percentage of patients for whom a biopsy recommendation is made will not respond accordingly to this medical directive. MQSA requires a bona fide attempt to follow up on cases for which biopsy is recommended, but risk management principles encourage the follow-up of all patients not returning for recall or biopsy after a finite period of time. This may not reach an absolute requirement, assuming the proper communication has already been completed. However, it may serve to defeat allegations of miscommunication if there is a subsequent delay in diagnosis that is a result of the referring physician failing to inform the patient.[37] Both the interpreting breast imager and facility may benefit by such documented follow-up.

The wording of the interpretative report is often conditioned on the type of reporting system and style particular to the facility. However, issues regarding fraud or other legal repercussion may arise consequent to the report.

BEYOND NEGLIGENCE: OTHER TORTS RELATED TO BREAST IMAGING

Consent

A number of circumstances arise in the clinical practice of breast imaging that invite familiarity with other legal principles. Although this discussion will not exhaust the application of such concepts, illustrative situations should help to identify the importance of other expected modes of conduct.[38]

Interventional procedures have become a growing aspect of breast imaging clinical practices.[39] Previously related only to preoperative radiographic localizations, such procedures now apply to lesions identified by, among other imaging modalities, ultrasonography and MRI. Informed consent plays an integral role in such procedures.

The "intentional" tort of battery may be claimed when an intervention is conducted without affirmative consent by the patient. Indeed, intentional torts are often not covered by liability insurance policies and invite punitive damage claims, beyond the concept of restitution discussed earlier. Although one might consider the presentation of a patient for a procedure is sufficient to obviate the claim of battery, "assent" is not tantamount to consent, because the patient may not recognize the potential adverse consequences of a procedure.

Rather, when consent is an issue for the breast imager, it more often is claimed as the negligent obtaining of such consent. General consent principles require a reasonable discussion of the advantages and potential complications of a procedure, as well as alternatives. The signing of a consent form is evidence, not proof, of a meaningful discussion, the latter being the essence of informed consent. Although the discussion may be preceded by other health care personnel informing the patient about the procedure, the operator—or person doing the procedure—is generally held responsible for satisfying the requirements. Thus, at least a short readdressing of the issues by the operator is warranted. This may require, for example, not only the risks of a given biopsy but also the intent to recommend surgery if certain results (e.g., large area of atypical ductal hyperplasia) are recovered, even though specific evidence of malignancy is not present, based on published studies.[40]

When patients have been premedicated before consent (a situation that is preferably avoided), then additional efforts need to be made to ensure that the patient understands the consent process. For example, additional efforts to establish orientation and comprehension should be considered. The successful claim of duress or lack of comprehension may serve to defeat the process of informed consent. Consent parameters should include both frequent if only minor consequences and severe consequences even if infrequent, so long as they are reasonably foreseeable.

Agency

Those personnel who work for the benefit of or under the control of another, such as a radiologist, are considered agents. In this context, error of omission and commission are attributed to the radiologist under legal doctrines sometimes referred to as respondeat superior or, in more colloquial terms, *captain of the ship*. In this respect, it is helpful to have an institutional policy and procedure that defines expected conduct. Thus, when personnel act outside of such parameters, the consideration of agency may be defeated. On the other hand, as long as such persons are indeed working within established frameworks, both the supervising physician and the facility are exposed to errors committed by these individuals. Orientation of new personnel should help to mitigate the adverse consequences of these relationships.

For example, a technologist who repeatedly achieves suboptimal patient imaging is more likely to incur liability for the radiologist and institution than herself, under the law of agency. The MQSA charges the supervising radiologist with responsibility for approving the final images. Improper relationships of the technologist and patient may expose the facility to legal redress. In part, this is a consequence of offended parties seeking damages from defendants with larger liability insurance coverage, sometimes referred to as *deep pockets*.

Duty to Refer, Negligent Referral, and Abandonment

When a health care worker or facility is faced with a situation for which either experience or facilities is insufficient to attend to a proper standard of care, there exists a recognized duty to refer. Economic disincentives sometimes encourage circumvention of this approach but nonetheless incur potential legal exposure. For example, if a facility does not have the capabilities of performing stereotactic biopsy of a cluster of calcifications that have been interpreted as suspicious, and ultrasonography fails to demonstrate such findings, a duty to refer the patient for a successful biopsy procedure is recognized.

If a referring physician knows or has reason to know that the consultant or institution to which he or she refers a patient is not reasonably capable of attending to the issue, and if an adverse event occurs, then the referring physician may be liable for the tort of negligent referral. Collegial relationships should not interfere with proper referral patterns. For example, if a lesion requires excisional biopsy and the patient also seeks reconstructive surgery, a situation may arise in which the patient is referred to a plastic surgeon who although during training may have been performed breast surgery but has not performed such procedures for many years and thus may not be a suitable clinician to perform a proper excision. If untoward results occur, that plastic surgeon may be exposed to legal repercussions and the referring radiologist may also be exposed to the claim of negligent referral.

Patient relations may from time to time suffer for a variety of reasons. The law does not view patients and their health care providers on a par scale. Rather, physicians are charged with superior knowledge that must be taken into account depending on the circumstances. A patient may elect to leave the care of a physician at her own election. But when a physician chooses to discontinue care, depending on the exigencies of the situation, remedial measure need be applied. Otherwise the physician may be charged with the tort of "abandonment."

For example, after a percutaneous biopsy that demonstrates a radial scar with associated cellular atypia that may be an indication for surgical referral,[41] a breakdown in physician patient relations does not excuse the radiologist from providing for a reasonable transfer of care that might include direct communication with the initial referring physician. For self-referred patients (see later), reasonable and documented attempts to provide transfer of care, even under adversarial circumstances, need be undertaken. The tort of abandonment may otherwise be advanced, a liability applicable to the responsible physician but one that is not reciprocal.

Fraud

From a regulatory perspective, issues in "fraud and abuse" usually apply to economic aspects of practice, such as submitting false claims or violating prohibited relationships in referral patterns.

However, in the current discussion, the civil concern regarding fraud relates to the withholding of material information from a patient or the intentional misrepresentation of information. The consequence of fraud is that it *tolls* or indefinitely extends what is called the *statute of limitations* regarding the filing of lawsuits.

When a patient discovers or should discover that possible negligent care has been committed, there is a period of time in which a legal complaint may be filed. Beyond such a time frame, or statute of limitations, such a filing will be denied. The rationale for this jurisprudential doctrine is beyond the scope of this chapter but relates to the difficulty in obtaining reliable recollections and medical records.

If civil fraud is found relating to the accessing of information regarding a woman's clinical condition, then the time frame for filing legal actions is considered virtually indefinite. Consider, for example, the missed diagnosis of a cluster of suspicious calcifications that, when subsequently sampled, demonstrates ductal carcinoma in situ (DCIS). A very small, but finite number of cases initially diagnosed as DCIS demonstrate delayed recurrence and possible metastatic disease. If information is not misrepresented to a patient regarding this diagnosis, then unusual delayed adverse consequences from this diagnosis will not be subject to legal action if recurrence develops after several years, as provided by statutes of limitation barring such claims as a matter of law.

The situation in which this issue sometimes arises relates to representations made to the patient who inquires as to possible earlier mammographic signs relating to the currently suspicious mammogram (or other imaging study). Once one has determined that lesion is suspicious, the bias of retrospective review of prior studies may influence the discussion.[42-44] In one sense, the current interpreter has a natural bias in that a conclusion of current suspicion has been proven. Frequently, imaging findings are present previously but the issue of whether the lesion *should* have been diagnosed earlier is difficult to determine because the fundamental concept of foreseeability is obviated by the current findings. A woman has a right to reconcile this question, but it is best addressed by an independent prospective review of the images by a different party. What is essential under such circumstances is to avoid misrepresenting or withholding material or important information; the consequences of such conduct may relate to fraud.

Because breast cancer is treated at the stage it is diagnosed, the question arises as to whether comment in the interpretative report should be made regarding possible prior findings or even avoiding a comparison entirely. Firstly, comparison is part of the standard of care and assists in corroborating that no other areas except the ones in question have either changed or are suspicious. Secondly, commenting on the prior findings does not impact management. However, as mentioned, if directly asked, information should be neither withheld nor misrepresented.

Such circumstances illustrate the difficulty in navigating an appropriate response in a field that, as previously discussed, maintains a high profile for legal exposure. One confronts the ethical dilemma of affirmatively reporting to the patient information that may be sought while trying to contain an inherent bias. Indeed, reporting an erroneous conclusion due to such bias may itself pose ethical challenges. This situation is not restricted to mammography. As is discussed later, emerging technologies introduce this dilemma almost by definition. Nonspecific MRI findings, especially if multiple, may, in fact, represent at certain anatomic foci actual malignancy and retrospective review will likely be influenced by an established diagnosis.

There are developing efforts to seek a middle ground to such encounters that relate to the use of a bona fide apology that is attended by legal protections against what are referred to as legal *admissions*. In other words, constructive relationships among physicians and patients may be better served by frank discussions in such a manner that, if a grievance is sought in a legal context, such comments do not hinder the proper discovery of facts related to a proper resolution of conduct subject to judicial accountability. Whether this promotes more favorable and less costly legal resolutions is controversial.[45,46]

TECHNOLOGY DEVELOPMENT AND THE LAW

In all fields of imaging, including breast imaging, new technologies are under continual development. When they rise to a level of reliability and acceptability, they begin to influence the determination of the standard of care. Whether it be new radiopharmaceuticals or new applications of prior isotopes or molecular imaging agents, such technology requires both clinical validation and acceptance for the purpose to which it is applied. This remains an ongoing issue for imagers. Unreasonable reliance on unproven but commercially reliable techniques may invite legal redress. Thus, introduction or implementation of new technology is best predicated on evidence-based studies, perhaps attended by informed consent.

The introduction of CAD programs into clinical practice has found a welcomed reception, especially in a digital environment, where the formidable challenge of reviewing large numbers of cases for a small number of prevalent cancers may be assisted by such technology. Controversy regarding the current status and reliability of CAD has been addressed elsewhere in this text. But this technology provides an illustration of how new developments are considered in a legal context.

There has been at least one appellate court decision that considered the introduction of CAD technology into trial.[47] The court struggled with the issues associated with any new technology, incorporating both court opinion and rules of evidence in making its determination. If a new technology is permitted to be introduced into evidence through the testimony of an expert witness, then its reliability must be sufficiently established to outweigh the potential prejudicial value it may have on a jury. For example, during a contested case, experts for both plaintiff and defendant will argue different positions. If a new technology is introduced to support one side or the other, this may influence the substance of the discussion.

In a case involving the non-recall of faint microcalcifications, an Ohio appellate court permitted CAD findings to be introduced for the defense.[48] This was based in part on the relatively superior performance of CAD for detection of calcifications as opposed to detection of masses or architectural distortions (or developing densities). The absence of a CAD mark on the anatomic focus in question was considered sufficiently reliable not as proof, but evidence of the reasonableness of non-recall. This may have represented a best case scenario of the introduction of CAD and, even under these circumstances, substantive issues regarding its introduction were not raised. For example, many studies show relatively high sensitivity for CAD detection of calcifications but not as high sensitivity for amorphous calcifications, which were suggested in this case.[49]

The importance of the trial decision is, of course, fact specific, but as a matter of law the appellate court decision reflects the kinds of concerns that relate not only to the legal arena but also to the medical arena when considering new technologies. Reliability, common usage, and corroborative studies help to establish any new medical development as part of the standard of care. Indeed, these same principles interestingly apply to the development of policies for reimbursement as well.

The use of CAD, like double reading,[50] may be considered a standard of care but not necessarily *the* standard of care. This concept is advanced to clarify that the employment of certain different approaches (recall the *alternative school of thought* doctrine) may all fall within the scope of reasonable practice, whereas others simply do not. The rapid development of new technologies and their employment in clinical practice are well served by considering such issues in the context of foreseeability and reasonableness, which remain the cornerstones for analysis of standard of care.

CONCLUSION

Although there have been both calls and proposals for alternatives to the current legal method of reconciling expected and actual conduct by physicians, current resolution of tortuous disputes involves an adversarial system in which advocates for both parties to the action seek to establish that facts in the case that support each respective position. Such alternative dispute resolutions (ADRs) have taken many forms, and such initiatives have been incorporated into different state systems to a variable extent.[51,52] Although the motivation for filing lawsuits are manifold, most studies converge on notions related to patients seeking both facts that are not forthcoming and acknowledgment by health care providers of mistakes.[53,54]

The practice of defensive medicine in which examinations are recommended without a rational basis under the mistaken notion that such an approach will shield health care providers against lawsuits may be a source of wasted resources and little liability protection. Rather, defensible medicine is the primary directive when caring for patients, whereby each examination incurs a separate duty for which reasonable care is required.

Identifying problems in delivering care requires both a systems approach and proper individual judgment. The former is exemplified by the triaging of patients to appropriate studies and the latter by reasonable imaging and interpretation of the study.

Although the large number of issues raised in this chapter may appear onerous, none requires extraordinary efforts and all are extensions of reasonable care directed to fulfilling the mission of breast imaging. In fact, virtually all of the basic principles here apply not only to every radiology consultation (beyond breast imaging) but also to the entire practice of medicine. Recognizing such responsibilities is fundamental to attempting to complete them successfully. This discussion has been an attempt to alert practitioners to such responsibilities so that they may apply their skills in a manner expected by their patients, their colleagues, and the courts.

KEY POINTS

- Most medical practice is subject to the law of negligence that defines departures of conduct below a standard of care regarding what a reasonable and prudent physician would do under similar circumstances.
- Liability for radiologists for image interpretation relates to the approval of satisfactory images and reasonable, although not necessarily accurate, interpretation.
- Reporting of results should avoid, to the extent possible, ambiguity that may invite mismanagement.
- Communication of interpretative or biopsy results that should prompt further management should be aimed at the receipt, rather than transmission, of information.
- Triaging of patients between screening and diagnostic settings should be deliberate and based on presenting signs and symptoms, or lack thereof, a process that should be documented,
- The implementation of evolving technology should be predicated on evidence-based platforms, sometimes supplemented with informed consent.

SUGGESTED READINGS

Brenner RJ. Breast cancer and malpractice: a guide to the clinician. *Sem Breast Dis* 1998;**1**:3-14.

Brenner RJ. False negative mammograms: medical, legal, and risk management implications. *Radiol Clin North Am* 2000;**38**:741-57.

Brenner RJ. Interventional procedures of the breast: medical legal considerations. *Radiology* 1995;**195**:611-5.

Brenner RJ. Medical legal aspects of breast imaging: variable standards of care relating to different types of practice. *AJR Am J Roentgenol* 1991;**156**:719-23.

Brenner RJ, Lucey LL, Smith JJ, Saunders R. Radiology and medical malpractice claims: a report on the practice standards survey of the Physician Insurers Association of America and the America College of Radiology. *AJR Am J Roentgenol* 1996;**171**:19-22.

Brenner RJ, Ulissey M, Witt R. Role of Computer Aided Detection in the Courtroom: implications for radiologists. *AJR Am J Roentgenol* 2006;**186**:48-51.

REFERENCES

1. Physician Insurers Association of America. *Breast Cancer Study*. Washington, D.C: Physicians Insurers Association of America; 1990.
2. Physicians Insurers Association of America. *Breast Cancer Study*. Rockville, Md.: Physician Insurers Association of America; 1995.
3. Physicians Insurers Association of America. *Breast Cancer Study*. Rockville, Md.: Physicians Insurers Association of America; 2002.
4. Bassett LW, Monsees BS, Smith RA, Wang L, Hooshi P, Farria DM, et al. Survey of radiology residents: breast imaging training and attitudes. *Radiology* 2003;**227**:862-9.
5. Elmore JG, Taplin SH, Barloa WE, Cutter GR, D'Orsi CJ, Hendrick RE, et al. Does litigation influence medical practice? The influence of community radiologists' medical malpractice perceptions and experiences on screening mammography. *Radiology* 2005;**236**:37-9.
6. Brenner RJ. Medical legal aspects of breast imaging: variable standards of care relating to different types of practice. *AJR Am J Roentgenol* 1991;**156**:719-23.
7. Skettington v Bradley, 366 Mich 552, 115 N.W. 2d 303 1962.
8. Brenner RJ. Mammography and malpractice litigation: current status, lessons, and admonitions. *AJR Am J Roentgenol* 1993;**161**:931-5.
9. Brenner RJ. Breast cancer and malpractice: a guide to the clinician. *Sem Breast Dis* 1998;**1**:3-14.
10. Mammography Quality Standards Reauthorization Act 1998, Public Law No 105-248 1998.
11. Brenner RJ, Lucey LL, Smith JJ, Saunders R. Radiology and medical malpractice claims: a report on the practice standards survey of the Physician Insurers Association of America and the American College of Radiology. *AJR Am J Roentgenol* 1996;**171**:19-22.
12. American College of Radiology. *Mammography Quality Control Manual*. Reston, Va: American College of Radiology; 1999 revised 2004, 2007.
13. Smith-Bindman R, Chu PW, Miglioretti DL, Sickles EA, Blanks R, Ballard-Barbash R, et al. Comparison of screening mammography in the United States and the United Kingdom. *JAMA* 2003;**290**:2129-937.
14. Schell MJ, Yankaskas BC, Ballard-Barbash R, Qaqish BF, Barlow WE, Rosenberg RD, et al. Evidence-based target recall rates for screening mammography. *Radiology* 2007;**243**:681-9.
15. Sickles EA. Findings at mammographic screening on only one standard projection: outcomes analysis. *Radiology* 1998;**208**:471-5.
16. Brenner RJ. Asymmetric densities of the breast: strategies for imaging evaluation. *Semin Roentgenol* 2001;**36**:201-16.
17. Todd v Eitel Hospital 237 NW 2d 357, 79 ALR 3d 907 (Minn 1975).
18. Brenner RJ. False negative mammograms: medical, legal, and risk management implications. *Radiol Clin North Am* 2000;**38**:741-57.
19. Sickles EA. Successful methods to reduce false-positive mammography interpretations. *Radiol Clin North Am* 2000; **38**:693-700.
20. Leung JW, Sickles EA. Developing asymmetry identified on mammography: correlation with imaging outcome and pathologic findings. *AJR Am J Roentgenol* 2007;**188**:667-75.
21. Kriege M, Brekelmans CT, Boetes C, Besnard PE, Zonderland HM, Obdeijn IM, et al. Efficacy of MRI and mammography for breast cancer screening in women with a familiar or genetic predisposition. *N Engl J Med* 2004;**351**:427-37.
22. Kuhl CK, Schmutzler RK, Leutner CC, Kempe A, Wardelmann E, Hocke A, et al. Breast MR imaging screening in 192 women proved or suspected to be carriers of a breast cancer susceptibility gene: preliminary results. *Radiology* 2000;**215**:267-79.
23. Berg WA. Rationale for a trial of screening breast ultrasound: American College of Radiology Imaging Network (ACRIN) 6666. *AJR Am J Roentgenol* 2003;**180**:1225-8.
24. Pisano ED, Gatsonis C, Hendrick E, Yaffe M, Baum JK, Acharyya S, et al. Diagnostic performance of digital versus film mammography for breast-cancer screening. *N Engl J Med* 2005;**353**:1773-83.
25. Warren Burhenne LJ, Wood SA, D'Orsi CJ, Feig SA, Kopans DB, O'Shaughnessy KF, et al. Potential contribution of computer-aided detection to the sensitivity of screening mammography. *Radiology* 2000;**215**:554-62.
26. Freer TW, Ulissey MJ. Screening mammography with computer aided detection: prospective study of 12,860 patients in a community breast center. *Radiology* 2001;**220**:781-6.
27. Fenton JJ, Taplin SH, Carney PA, Abraham L, Sickles EA, D'Orsi C, et al. Influence of computer-aided detection on performance of screening mammography. *N Engl J Med* 2007;**356**:1399-409.
28. Feig SA. Auditing and benchmarks in screening and diagnostic mammography. *Radiol Clinics North Am* 2007;**45**:793-800.
29. Moy L, Slanetz PJ, Moore R, Satija S, Yeh ED, McCarthy KA, et al. Specificity of mammography and US in the evaluation of a palpable abnormality: retrospective review. *Radiology* 2002;**225**:176-81.
30. Farria DM, Monsees B. Screening mammography practice essentials. *Radiol Clin North Am* 2004;**42**:831-43.
31. Wickline v State of California 183 Cal App 1064, 118 Cal Rptr 661 1986.
32. Townsend v Turk 218 Cal App 3d 278, 266 Cal Rptr 821 1990.
33. Phillips v Good Samaritan Hospital 416 NE 2d 640 (Ohio 1979).
34. Brenner RJ, Westenberg L. Film management and custody: current and future medicolegal issues. *AJR Am J Roentgenol* 1996;**167**:1371-5.
35. American College of Radiology. *Breast Imaging Reporting and Data System (BI-RADS)*. Reston, Va: American College of Radiology; 1995.
36. D'Orsi CJ, Bassett LW, Berg WA, et al. *Illustrated Breast Imaging Reporting and Data System (BI-RADS): Mammography,* 4th ed. Reston, Va: American College of Radiology, 2003.
37. Brenner RJ, Bartholomew L. Communication errors in radiology: liability and cost assessment. *J Am Coll Radiol* 2005;**2**:428-31.
38. Brenner JW. Medical legal aspects of breast imaging. *Radiol Clin North Am* 1992; **30**:277-86.
39. Brenner RJ. Interventional procedures of the breast: medical legal considerations. *Radiology* 1995;**195**:611-5.
40. Brenner RJ, Bassett LW, Fajardo L, Dershaw DD, Evans WP, Hunt R, et al. Stereotactic core breast biopsy: a multiinstitutional prospective trial. *Radiology* 2001;**218**:866-72.
41. Brenner RJ, Jackman R, Parker SH, Evans WP, Philpotts L, Deutch BM, et al. Percutaneous core needle biopsy of radial scars: When is excision necessary? *AJR Am J Roentgenol* 2002;**179**:1179-84.
42. Harvey JA, Fajardo LL, Innis CA. Previous mammograms in patients with impalpable breast carcinoma: retrospective vs blinded interpretation. *AJR Am J Roentgenol* 1993;**161**:1167-72.
43. Ikeda DM, Birdwell RL, O'Shaughnessy KF, Brenner RJ, Sickles EA. Analysis of 172 subtle findings on prior "negative" mammograms in women with screening detected cancer. *Radiology* 2003;**226**:494-503.

44. Gordon PB, Rorugian MJ, Warren Burhenne LJ. A true screening environment for review of interval breast cancers: pilot study to reduce bias. *Radiology* 2007;**245**:411-5.
45. Studdert DM, Mello MM, Brennan TA. Medical Malpractice: health policy report. *N Engl J Med* 2004;**350**:283-92.
46. Gallagher TH, Studdert D, Levinson W. Disclosing harmful medical errors to patients. *N Engl J Med* 2007;**356**:2713-9.
47. Brenner RJ, Ulissey M, Witt R. Role of computer aided detection in the courtroom: implications for radiologists. *AJR Am J Roentgenol* 2006;**186**:48-51.
48. Gray v Fairview General Hospital, 8th Dist no 82318, 2004-Ohio-1244, app LEXIS 1099 (civil appeal from Cuyahoga County Common Pleas Court, case no CV443871, decided on December 5, 2003).
49. Berg WA, Arnoldus CL, Teferra E, Bhargavan M. Biopsy of amorphous breast calcifications: pathologic and yield at stereotactic biopsy. *Radiology* 2001;**221**:495-503.
50. Gilbert FJ, Astley SM, Gillan MG, Agbaje OF, Wallis MG, James J, et al. Single reading with computer-aided detection for screening mammography. *N Engl J Med* 2008;**359**:1675-84.
51. Smith JJ, Brenner RJ. The malpractice liability crisis: potential solutions. *J Am Coll Radiol* 2004;**1**:249-54.
52. Meruelo NC. Mediation and medical malpractice. The need to understand why patients sue and a proposal for a specific model of mediation. *J Legal Med* 2008;**29**:285-306.
53. Hickson GB, Clayton EW, Githens PB, Sloan FA. Factors that prompted families to file medical malpractice claims following perinatal injuries. *JAMA* 1992;**267**:1359-63.
54. Levinson W, Roter DI, Mullooly JP, Dull VT, Frankel RM. Physician-patient communications: the relationship with malpractice claims among primary care physicians and surgeons. *JAMA* 1997;**277**:553-9.

SECTION

TEN

Emerging Technologies

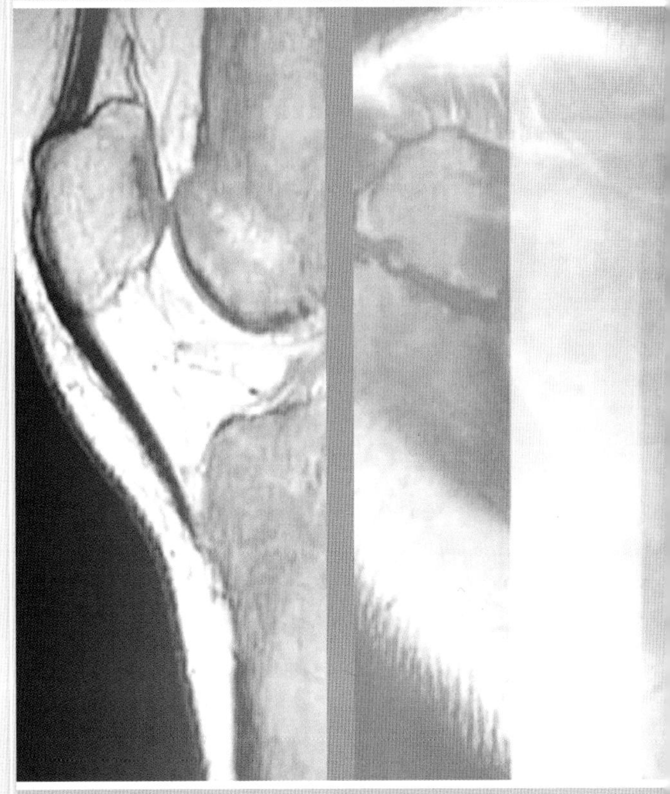

CHAPTER 41

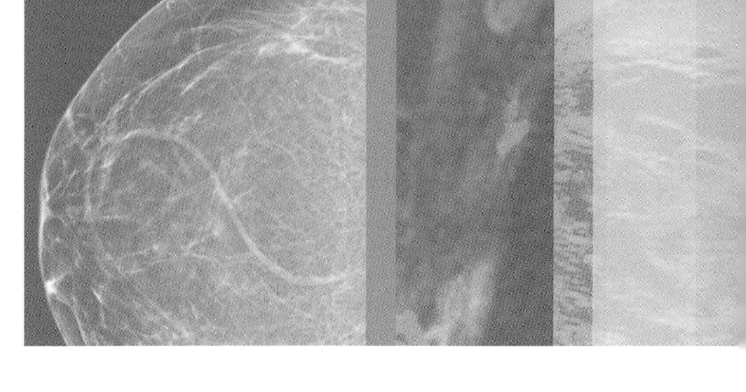

Emerging X-Ray-Based and Nuclear Technologies

Carl J. D'Orsi

There are many technologies we hear about that claim to correct the deficiencies in mammography, either for detection, analysis or both. In order to evaluate these technologies and determine when they will be useful, if at all, we must understand current limitations of mammography in both a screening and diagnostic setting. For convenience, the newer technologies can be divided into those that are based on morphology, those exploiting the physiology of malignancy, and those based on the metabolic properties of malignancies.

The first major technique change in mammography occurred with the introduction of digital mammography. This allowed the processes of image acquisition, display and storage to be separated, with the ability to optimize each one independently of the others. Digital technique has also allowed the development of novel new technologies such as stereo digital mammography (SDM), tomosynthesis, and dedicated breast computed tomography (CT) for volumetric morphologic breast interpretation. Magnetic resonance imaging (MRI) has added a new blood flow dynamic to morphology, and dedicated breast nuclear medicine studies have helped determine metabolic features of findings suggestive of malignancy. Because these studies tend to investigate different aspects of suspicious findings, some of these newer technologies have been synchronized into single units to register morphology with other aspects of tumor profiles.

STEREO DIGITAL MAMMOGRAPHY

With the advent of SDM,[1-3] high quality stereoscopic digital mammography is now a practical possibility, providing direct in-depth views of the internal structure of the breast and a potentially improved technique for breast cancer screening.[4-6] Two-dimensional (2D) x-ray mammography is currently the primary screening approach for the early detection of breast cancer in women. However, it suffers from three basic limitations that stereo mammography may overcome.

In a standard mammographic screening exam, the tissue of the breast volume is captured as a 2D projected image from two different points of view, one vertical (a craniocaudal, or CC, view) and the other approximately horizontal (a mediolateral oblique, or MLO, view). The first limitation with standard mammography is that a true focal abnormality may often be undetected when masked in the 2D projections by overlying or underlying normal tissue.[7,8] Masking may affect the detection of both focal soft tissue abnormalities and microcalcifications. The probability of false negatives caused by masking may be reduced with stereo mammography because the lesion may be seen in the stereo image as separated from normal tissue aligned with it on 2D images at different depths in the breast volume.

The second limitation with standard mammography is the chance alignment of normal tissue, or isolated elements of calcium, at different depths within the breast, which in the 2D projected image may mimic a true focal lesion.[9] Many of the false-positive detections that arise in this way with standard mammography have potential to be eliminated with stereo mammography because the superimposed tissue or calcification particles can be seen in the stereo mammogram as separated in depth.

The third limitation is in regard to the ability to derive information about the volumetric structure of a detected lesion, information particularly important in suggesting the presence of architectural distortion, and the significance of calcification distribution. For standard mammography, volumetric information can be obtained only in a limited way by cognitive merging of information taken separately from the two orthogonal 2D images. With stereo mammography, a lesion's volumetric structure is immediately and directly visualized.

SDM offers the potential to produce a three-dimensional (3D) image of the breast that is directly interpreted in three dimensions without reconstruction. The acquisition of a stereo mammogram requires the capture of two x-ray mammograms with the x-ray tube shifted by 5 to 10 degrees between the two image captures (−3 to −5 degrees from 0 and +3 to +5 degrees from straight 0). This must be done with the digital receptor at 180 degrees for each of the images. This technique can be done both in the CC and MLO projections. These images are then stored on a hard disk in the imaging system. The stereo mammograms may then be viewed on a prototype medical stereo display (StereoMirror SD2250, Planar Systems Inc, Beaverton, Ore). This stereo display, shown in Figure 41-1, consists of two 5 megapixel, gray-scale monitors mounted one above the other with an angular separation of 110 degrees between the two faces. The two images, each displayed on one of the two monitors, are cross-polarized. A glass plate with a half-silvered coating is placed between the two monitor faces, bisecting the angle between them. The image presented on the lower (vertical) monitor is transmitted through the glass plate, while the image presented on the upper (angled) monitor is reflected from the top surface of the glass plate. The radiologist wears lightweight passive cross-polarized glasses with the result that each eye sees only one of the two images. The radiologist's visual system fuses the two images into a single in-depth image of the internal structure of the breast.

A recent study designed to determine the true positive lesion detection, accrued 850 women at high risk for breast cancer who had 1458 exams over a 3-year period. These women served as their own control and each exam consisted of the standard 2D digital mammogram and the two-view stereo mammogram.[10] Every reported finding on stereo, standard mammography, or both, was recalled for workup whether concordant or not. All patients with reported findings requiring recall received standard (non-stereo) clinical diagnostic workup examinations. For each worked up finding, a final American College of Radiology Breast Imaging Reporting and Data System (ACR BI-RADS)[11] assessment of category 1, or 2 was truth for absence of an actionable lesion (i.e., negative), while a workup assessment of categories 3, 4, or 5 constituted truth that the finding of concern was a true lesion. Truth about the presence of cancer was determined from subsequent biopsy, if performed.

Three hundred and thirty-two lesions were classified as category 0[11] from the findings reported by one or both modalities and sent for diagnostic workup. At workup, 140 were true findings (category 3, 4, and 5) and 192 did not result in an actionable finding (category 1 or 2). Of the 140 true findings standard mammography detected 86, while stereo mammography detected 106. The positive predictive value of SDM was 32% while standard was 26%. There were 18 cancers found among the 854 patients for a cancer detection rate for both modalities of 12.4 per 1000. Each of the modalities (standard 2D and SDM) detected 15 of the 18 cancers for an equal cancer detection rate of 10.3 per 1000. Thus, from this update of preliminary data it appears that SDM has the potential to significantly increase the accuracy of screening mammography for true lesion detection by decreasing the false positives. Results are still being collected for determination of sensitivity and specificity for detection of actionable findings.

TOMOSYNTHESIS

Digital tomosynthesis[12,13] of the breast is a novel x-ray-based imaging technique that is being investigated as an adjunct to or as a replacement for mammography in the detection and diagnosis of breast cancer. The geometry involved in tomosynthesis imaging is very similar to that used in mammography. The difference is that the x-ray tube is rotated around the static compressed breast or the detector is angled and a series of images is acquired, one at each x-ray tube or detector position, at a fraction

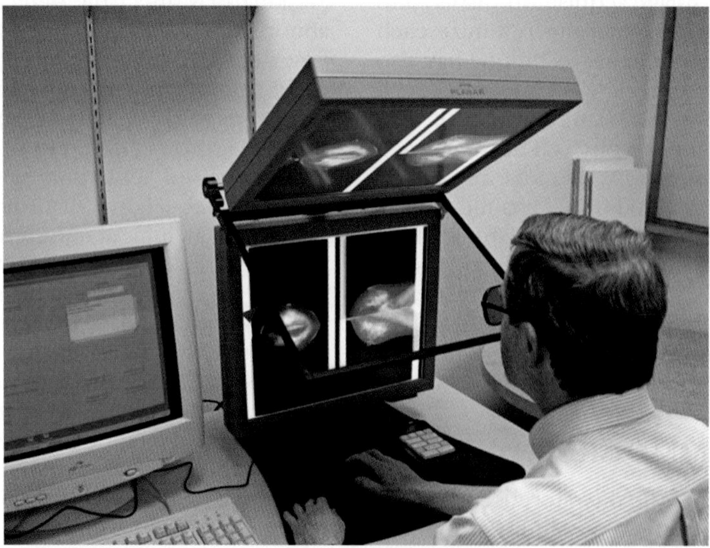

■ **FIGURE 41-1** Stereo workstation with two monitors each displaying cross-polarized images, each of which can be seen independently by the reader who is also wearing polarizing lenses.

of the dose required for a standard projection. Thus if 11 projections are obtained, the dose for each angle acquisition would be approximately 1/11 of the full standard dose. The series of images acquired denotes the tomosynthesis projection set, and is then processed by a reconstruction program that uses the different locations of the same tissues in the projections to compute their vertical position, thereby reconstructing the 3D volume (Fig. 41-2). Several tomosynthesis reconstruction methods have been compared with mammography and significantly better contrast-detail characteristics were found in the tomosynthesis phantom images.[14,15]

Several studies that investigated the performance of breast tomosynthesis compared with standard mammography have been reported.[16-20] Helvie and colleagues presented the results of a retrospective clinical study in which 30 cases with suspicious masses were analyzed by three radiologists. They determined that all six malignant masses were detected with tomosynthesis, while with mammography one was missed. In all other visibility ratings recorded (visibility, percent of margin depicted, etc.), tomosynthesis yielded better results than mammography. Poplack and associates performed a retrospective study that included 98 cases of abnormal screens. The observers subjectively compared the tomosynthesis images to the mammogram and provided a rating (better, equivalent, or worse) and recorded whether the additional information from the tomosynthesis images would reverse the decision to recall the patient due to the 2D mammogram interpretation. The investigators reported that the addition of tomosynthesis would have reduced the recall rate by 52%. Moore and coworkers reported the callback rate resulting from mammography interpreted by one of ten mammographers (4-33 years of experience) and from single-view (MLO view) tomosynthesis interpreted by one of two mammographers (10-33 years of experience). A total of 1957 cases were included in the study. They determined that the tomosynthesis images would have resulted in a callback rate 43% lower than that of mammography. Andersson and colleagues performed a retrospective study comparing single-view (MLO) tomosynthesis to single-and two-view mammography for 36 cases using two radiologists. In 55% of the cases, the radiologists determined that the lesions were more visible in the tomosynthesis images. Smith and colleagues reported a higher area (accuracy) under the receiver operating characteristic (ROC) curve with the addition of tomosynthesis when 12 radiologists of varying experience interpreted 316 images retrospectively. This study involved having the radiologists score the mammography images first, and then the mammography and tomosynthesis images together. Gennaro and associates[21] reported on a retrospective study comparing single-view (MLO) tomosynthesis to two-view mammography. The investigators report an increase in lesion conspicuity and area under the ROC curve for the tomosynthesis images compared with the mammograms. Finally, Gur and coworkers[22] performed a retrospective reader study including 125 cases and 8 radiologists and showed a 30% decrease in recall rate when mammograms and tomosynthesis images were interpreted together, versus only a 10% decrease when tomosynthesis images were interpreted alone. However the investigators were not able to detect a significant increase in sensitivity with the use of tomosynthesis.

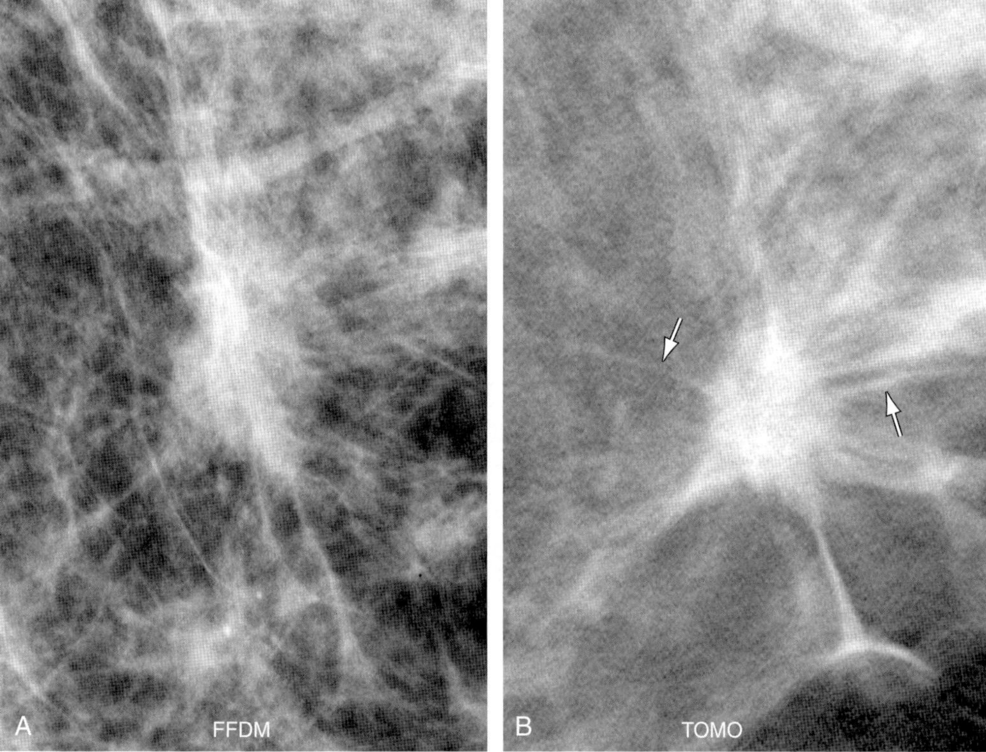

■ **FIGURE 41-2** A, Full-field digital mammography spot compression view of irregular, spiculated mass. **B,** Same mass as depicted on one of the tomographic images. Note the increased clarity of the spiculations (*arrows*) and of the mass itself. *(Courtesy of Hologic Corp)*

As can be seen, all but one of these studies has shown that tomosynthesis, using various metrics, has the potential to be an improvement over standard mammography, especially for decrease of false-positive interpretations and could have a marked effect by increasing specificity. But it underscores the need for further research. Most of the studies discussed here are retrospective, limiting the ability to determine the true sensitivity of tomosynthesis as a screening test. Additionally, most of the studies were performed acquiring a single tomosynthesis view, or with the tomosynthesis images being read by a different group of radiologists than those reading the mammography images, or both. It is unclear whether tomosynthesis will have its greatest use in screening or diagnostic exams and if one-view or two-view tomosynthesis is adequate to replace the two-view 2D mammogram. Indeed, some studies suggest that tomosynthesis should be used with 2D mammography. When these various scenarios are considered, dose must also be evaluated. Certainly a combination of 2D mammography and tomosynthesis will result in a dose higher than either alone.

DEDICATED BREAST COMPUTED TOMOGRAPHY

Dedicated breast computed tomography (DBCT) is being developed as either an adjunct to or replacement for mammography for the detection and diagnosis of breast cancer. This technology results in isotropic high resolution 3D images with very high contrast. Thus, once this data is obtained, reconstruction in any plane can be accomplished while experiencing any loss of spatial or contrast resolution. During acquisition, the patient lies prone on a table with an aperture through which the breast is pendant. Under the table, a vertically placed, full-field flat panel detector and an x-ray tube rotate around a vertical axis located approximately at the center of the breast (Fig. 41-3). During one full 360-degree rotation, the system acquires multiple individual projections, each covering the entire breast. To achieve this, the x-ray field is shaped as a half-cone, with the central ray at the patient's chest wall. To date, there are two clinical systems available for research purposes. The first unit was fabricated by John Boone and colleagues at the University of California, Davis.[23] His unit is operated at 80 kilovolts peak (kVp) from 50 to 120 milliampere seconds (mAs) producing 500 projection images acquired in 16.6 seconds. The dose delivered is approximately the same as a two-view standard mammogram compressed to 5 cm. A second clinical prototype system is manufactured by the Konig Corp., West Henrietta, N.Y.[24] This unit operates at 49 kVp acquiring 300 projection images over a 10 second scan time. The system developed by Konig operates at a lower energy (49 kVp and mean energy of 30.3 kVp). This produces a dose to glandular tissue of one to five times the dose of a standard two-view mammogram. The tradeoff with the higher kVp is a loss of contrast resolution, potentially making the detection of microcalcifications more difficult. These issues are of special concern if DBCT is to be used in a screening scenario. However, the very high spatial resolution in all three directions minimizes partial volume effects that could degrade resolution and also allows novel isotropic image reconstructions (Fig. 41-4).

The only clinical study to date was reported by Lindfors and coworkers.[25] A breast CT prototype[23] was used to scan 65 women with a BI-RADS score of 4 or 5 who subsequently had a biopsy and a pathologic diagnosis. Twenty-eight were benign findings and 37 were malignant. Breast CT images were compared with screen-film mammograms using a scale of 1 to 10. One indicates excellent CT visualization and poor visualization with standard mammography while the opposite is true for a score of 10, indicating excellent visualization with standard mammography and poor visualization with CT. Thus, a score of 5.5 would indicate visualization equivalency. For all lesions combined the mean score was 5.4, which is equal visualization with standard mammography and dedicated breast CT. For masses the score was 4.9, which was significance for lesion visualization in favor of CT but 7.8 for calcifications, indicating significance for standard mammography .Taking into account benign versus malignant and breast density, no difference in lesion visualization based on these variables was noted. Eighty-two women were also asked to compare the CT experience to the standard mammogram experience. A significant majority voiced a strong preference for CT, on a comfort level, compared with standard mammography. Some

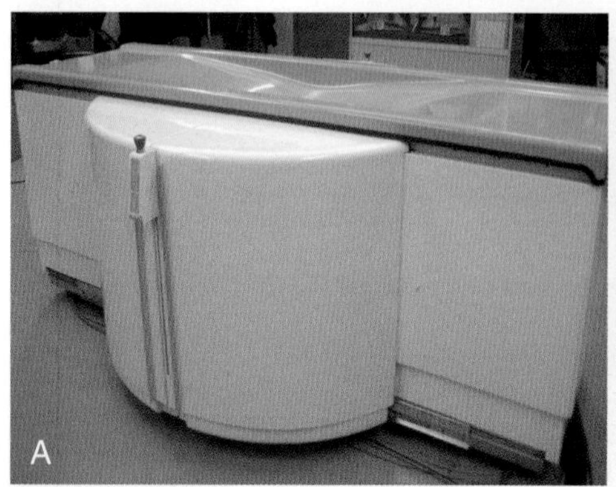

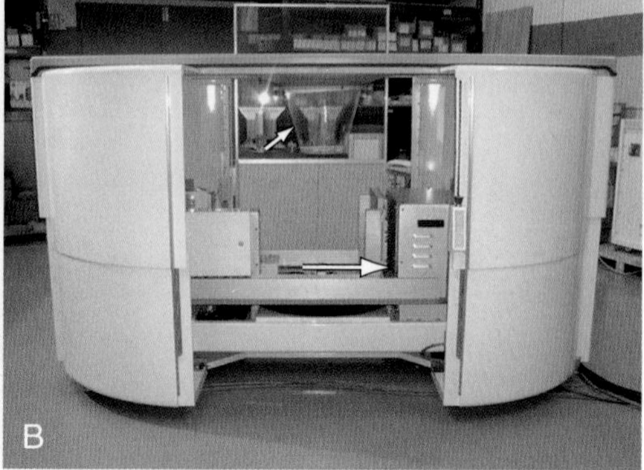

■ **FIGURE 41-3** The dedicated table is shown in **A** with a design similar to the stereotactic biopsy tables. The table in an open and elevated position (**B**), allows visualization of the dependent breast within the cone (*small arrow*) and the detector (*large arrow*), which will rotate around the cone in a full circle.

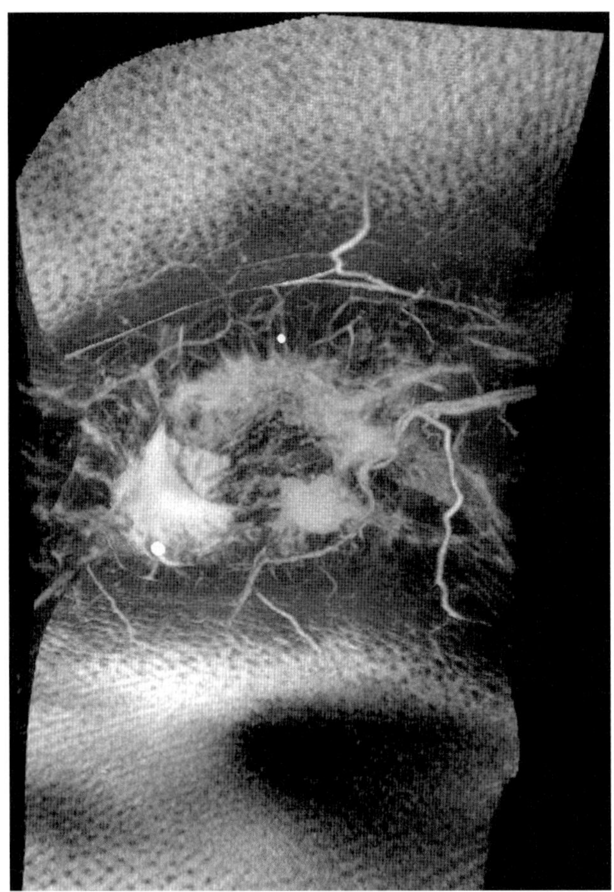

■ **FIGURE 41-4** Three dimensional (3D) reconstruction of the breast as viewed from posterior (chest wall aspect) to anterior (nipple aspect).This image may be rotated either manually or with a continuous cine loop.

women did, however, mention the firmness of the table top and difficulty maintaining their neck in a position needed to complete the CT scan.

The use of intravenous contrast in other breast imaging modalities, particularly in MRI, has been successful in improving lesion conspicuity. Because iodinated contrast material would behave in a manner similar to gadolinium agents for MRI, improvements would also be expected in contrast enhanced dedicated breast CT (CE-DBCT). Additionally, in CT the Hounsfield unit (HU) is directly proportional to attenuation and may serve as a tool for quantification of differential capillary permeability between normal and malignant tissues

In a pilot study, 46 women with 54 BI-RADS category 4 or 5 lesions underwent both DBCT and CE-DBCT prior to image guided biopsy,[26] and lesion conspicuity on CE-DBCT was compared with MLO and CC mammograms.

All 29 malignant lesions were significantly more conspicuous on CE-DBCT than on mammography. When divided by lesion type, malignant masses were significantly more conspicuous on CE-DBCT than on mammography. The conspicuity of the seven malignant calcification lesions was slightly better on CE-DBCT than on mammography, but the difference was not statistically significant. On CE-DBCT the conspicuity of the 25 benign lesions was similar to that on mammography; however, benign calcifications were significantly better seen on mammography. This diminished visualization on CE-DBCT of calcifications associated with benign lesions may provide improved specificity for calcifications.

The use of intravenous contrast in DBCT clearly improves visualization of malignant lesions, including ductal carcinoma in situ (DCIS), in a manner similar to contrast enhanced MRI. The ability to improve temporal resolution with CE-DBCT may provide information not previously available with contrast enhanced MRI. Additionally, the ability to perform subtraction of pre and post CE-DBCT may allow detection of suspicious findings in a manner similar to MRI but with much better spatial resolution.

Dedicated breast CT is a very promising technology offering true isotropic 3D visualization of the breast allowing for exquisite soft tissue detail.There are problems that must still be resolved. One of the major issues is the inclusion of axillary breast tissue. This may be solved by better table-top ergonomics. Visualization of calcifications is a problem. In the clinical trial described, a dose equivalent to a standard mammogram was used.This may have a negative effect on contrast and possibly hinder visualization of fine pleomorphic or amorphous calcifications. If the dose were increased, contrast resolution would also improve but the dose might be prohibitive, especially in a screening situation.

NUCLEAR MEDICINE BREAST IMAGING TECHNOLOGY

The introduction of radionuclides as possible agents for breast cancer detection had its start with the observation that technetium Tc 99m sestamibi (^{99}Tc-sestamibi), an energy emitter centered at 140 kiloelectron volt (KeV) and evaluated as a cardiac agent, was also seen to concentrate in women with suspected breast cancers. This increased uptake is thought to be due to increased vascularity and mitochondrial activity in and around malignancies. A 2005 review reported on 5660 cases of ^{99m} Tc-sestamibi scintimammography.[27] The sensitivity for detection of breast cancer ranged anywhere from 80% to 90% with a mean of 84%. However, the sensitivity for lesions measuring less than 10 mm was low and nonexistent for those less than 5 mm. The specificity averaged 86%.The size limitations for breast cancer detection in these earlier studies was related to the use of traditional gamma cameras that were not breast specific and did not allow projections similar to those used in mammography.

Using modern breast-specific gamma imaging (BSGI) with a detector mounted so the breast can be imaged in all directions, including those specific for mammography, markedly reducing background noise from other organs, Brem and associates[28] retrospectively reviewed 146 women who had BSGI and breast biopsy. The indications for BSGI were broad and included palpable lesions with negative mammograms and women diagnosed with multi focal, or multicentric breast cancer, or both. Uptake of the radiotracer was scored from 1 to 5 ranging from

1 indicating no focal uptake to 5 indicating intense focal uptake. A score of 1, 2, or 3 was considered a negative exam and 4 or 5, a positive exam. One hundred and sixty-seven lesions were biopsied yielding 16 DCIS, 67 invasive ductal carcinoma and 84 benign results. The sensitivity was reported as 96.4% and specificity of 59.5%. The smallest malignancy discovered was 1 mm. Interestingly, the average tumor size was 20 mm and sensitivity of BSGI was directly tied to size with a sensitivity of 83.3% for tumors 0 to 5 mm and 100% for those larger than 11 mm. When we compare these results to the era before specific units dedicated for breast imaging were available, the sensitivity has increased but the false positives have also increased, as reflected in the decreased specificity.

A second popular technology to detect malignancy uses a radiolabelled glucose analog [2-(flourine-18)-fluoro-2-deoxy-D-glucose] designated FDG. The F^{18} decays by an annihilation reaction between a positron and electron which results in two 511 KeV photons directed 180 degrees from each other. Thus, this event requires that the 511 KeV photons, 180 degrees apart be detected simultaneously. Since FDG is an analog of glucose it is handled by the body in a similar manner. While taken up by metabolizing cells in a normal manner, its byproducts are trapped within the cell. Thus, the more actively metabolizing cells, as one would expect with malignancy, trap more FDG than normal cells and, thus, potentially can distinguish malignant from normal tissue. There are also benign lesions that will produce false positives such as fibroadenomas and dysplastic tissue.

Employing whole body positron emission tomography (PET), Avril and associates[29] analyzed 185 suspicious breast masses in 144 women. Pathology was returned as malignant in 132 masses and benign in 53. Three levels of concern for malignancy were used by the interpreters. Grade I (regional uptake) was unlikely to represent malignancy while grade II (moderate focal uptake of FDG) and grade III (marked focal increase of FDG) were considered probable and definite for malignancy, respectively. The metrics were calculated using grade III only as a positive exam and also using grade II and III as positive exams. When only grade III was considered a positive exam, sensitivity was found to be 64.4% and specificity 94.3%. Using more lenient guidelines defining grades II and III as positive, a sensitivity of 80.3% was found, but specificity decreased to 75.5%, which is to be expected because sensitivity and specificity are frequently inversely related. When size of tumor detection was related to sensitivity, those breast cancers smaller than 1 cm had a sensitivity of 57%, while those larger than 1 cm had a sensitivity of 91%. Clearly this is not optimal for early breast cancer detection. These metrics become understandable because the spatial resolution of whole body PET scanners is on the order of 5 mm.

The low detection sensitivity of whole body PET scanners used for detection of breast malignancy relate to spatial resolution and volume averaging of tumors smaller than 1 cm diminishing the signal-to-noise ratio. In an effort to improve the capability of PET technology for breast cancer detection, units devised solely to view the breast have been developed (PEM Flex, Naviscan Pet Systems Inc, Rockville, Md). The major factor determining spatial resolution is the size of the detector. By using thin detectors and controlling for cardiac and respiratory motion, spatial resolution of PET scans can approach the technology limit of 1.5 mm.[30] Using this dedicated breast PET scan (PEM), Berg and coworkers studied 92 pathologically verified lesions, 48 of which were malignant, in 77 women with either known breast cancers or findings suggestive for breast cancer. The overall sensitivity of PEM for cancers was 90% with a specificity of 86%. Of particular interest is the 91% sensitivity for detection of DCIS and the 80% sensitivity for T1 lesions. Three additional foci of otherwise occult malignancy were also detected with PEM. These metrics represent a marked improvement over whole body PET scanners used for breast cancer detection.

Since both PET and MRI add new dimensions to the exquisite morphologic information supplied by mammography, their utilization is similar. MRI demonstrates the increased vessel density and permeability of tumor vessels for detection and analysis while PET is an indicator of increased glucose metabolism by malignancies. It is unlikely that MRI or PET will be used for routine screening, because both require injection of agents to highlight vascular and metabolic information, are costly, require a much longer period of time to perform compared with mammography and in the case of PET technology, there is need for patient preparation prior to the exam.

A complete response to chemotherapy is important as a prognostic indicator of overall survival. Early positive response to chemotherapy will allow either continuation of the successful treatment or if a less than optimal response to chemotherapy is determined the patient can have the therapy altered and not undergo the side effects of inadequate therapy. Using a whole body PET/CT scanner, Duch and colleagues[31] evaluated 50 women with newly diagnosed breast cancers placed on neoadjuvant chemotherapy. In women who were ultimately considered to be nonresponders at the end of chemotherapy, PET demonstrated findings at mid cycle of chemotherapy that corroborated this final pathologic evaluation. The same was true for complete responders and the difference in the PET results between nonresponders and responders was significant.

It becomes clear that a combination of high resolution morphologic criteria for breast cancer coupled with a second technology that has strengths in other parameters indicating the possible presence of breast cancer would be a very powerful tool. Bowen and associates[32] have recently constructed a dedicated breast PET/CT scanner. Average registration error was determined to be 0.18 mm, indicative of excellent lesion position concordance between the combined dedicated PET and CT scanners. Four patients with five lesions were imaged prior to breast biopsy who had category five findings by BI-RADS. A CT scan was first done, followed by a 12.5 minute PET scan. One patient also had iodinated contrast administered with a PET scan obtained first then a pre contrast/post contrast CT scan. All four patients had malignancy. Both PET and CT were positive on two of four women and two of five findings; CT was positive on three of four women and three of five findings; and PET was positive on all four women and four out of five findings. Two Findings of DCIS were present, one positive on PET and one on CT.

CONCLUSION

Although standard screen-film and now digital mammography have been shown to have a significant effect on decreasing the mortality from breast cancer there are still issues concerning false-positive exams and biopsies, and a need to increase the sensitivity for breast cancer detection at an early stage. Because of the development of digital mammography novel x-ray technologies are now possible. The addition of molecular imaging with dedicated breast PET technology promises to allow very specific probes for the detection of breast cancer with the promise of increased accuracy. As can be seen from this brief overview of the technologies, there is a great need for research ranging from mode of usage to dose to improved sensitivity and specificity.

KEY POINTS

- Stereo digital mammography has the potential to decrease recall rates and maintain sensitivity.
- Tomosynthesis has excellent soft tissue detection capabilities but the exact format of usage is under investigation.
- Dedicated breast CT produces true isotropic 3D information but calcification detection and full breast coverage are problematic.
- Dedicated breast PET scans can detect subcentimeter malignancies, may be useful to determine early response to breast cancer, and can be united with dedicated breast CT in one unit.

SUGGESTED READINGS

Eubank WB, Mankoff DA. Evolving role of positron emission tomography in breast cancer imaging. *Semin Nucl Med* 2005;**35**:84-99.

Karellas A, Vedantham S. Breast cancer imaging: a perspective for the next decade. *Med Phys* 2008;**35**:4878-97.

O'Connor M, Rhodes D, Hruska C. Molecular breast imaging. *Expert Rev Anticancer Ther* 2009;**9**:1073-80.

REFERENCES

1. Lewin JM, D'Orsi CJ, Hendrick RE, Moss LJ, Isaacs PK, Karellas A, et al. Clinical comparison of full-field digital mammography for detection of breast cancer. *AJR Am J Radiology* 2002;**179**:671-7.
2. Skaane P, Skjennald A. Screen-film mammography versus full-field digital mammography with soft-copy reading: randomized trial in a population-based screening program-the Oslo II study. *Radiology* 2004;**232**:197-204.
3. Pisano ED, Gatsonis CA, Hendrick RE, Yaffe M, Baum JK, Acharyya S, et al. Diagnostic performance of digital versus film mammography for breast-cancer screening. *N Engl J Med* 2005;**353**:1773-83.
4. Getty DJ. Stereoscopic digital mammography. In: *Proceedings of 1st Americas display engineering and applications conference (ADEAC 2004)*. Fort Worth, Texas: Society for Information Display (SID); 2004. Chapter 2.3.
5. Chan HP, Goodsitt MM, Helvie MA, Hadjiiski LM, Lydick JT, Roubidoux MA, et al. ROC study of the effect of stereoscopic imaging on assessment of breast lesions. *Med Phys* 2005;**32**:1001-9.
6. Getty DJ, Green PJ. Clinical medical applications for stereoscopic 3D displays. *J Soc Inf Dis* 2007;**15**:377-84.
7. Meeson S, Young KC, Wallis MG, Cooke J, Cummin A, Ramsdale ML. Image features of true positive and false negative cancers in screening mammograms. *Br J Radiol* 2003;**76**:13-21.
8. Van Gils CH, Otten JD, Verbeek AL, Hendriks JH. Mammographic breast density and risk of breast cancer: masking bias or causality? *Eur J Epidemiol* 2004;**14**:315-20.
9. Blanchard K, Colbert JA, Kopans DB, Moore R, Halpern EF, Hughes KS, et al. Long-term risk of false-positive screening results and subsequent biopsy as a function of mammography use. *Radiology* 2006;**240**:335-42.
10. Getty DJ, D'Orsi CJ, Newell MS, et al. Improved accuracy of lesion detection in breast cancer screening with stereoscopic digital mammography (abstract). In: *RSNA Scientific Assembly and Annual Meeting Program*. 2007. p. 381-2.
11. D'Orsi CJ, Bassett LW, Berg WA, et al. *Illustrated Breast Imaging Reporting and Data System (BI-RADS): Mammography*. 4th ed. Reston, Va: American College of Radiology; 2003.
12. Kolitsi Z, Panayiotakis G, Anastassopoulos V, Scodras A, Pallikarakis N. A multiple projection method for digital tomosynthesis. *Med Phys* 1992;**19**:1045-50.
13. Niklason LT, Christian BT, Niklason LE, Kopans DB, Castleberry DE, Opsahl-Ong BH, et al. Digital tomosynthesis in breast imaging. *Radiology* 1997;**205**:399-406.
14. Suryanarayanan S, Karellas A, Vedantham S, Glick SJ, D'Orsi CJ, Baker SP, et al. Comparison of tomosynthesis methods used with digital mammography. *Acad Radiol* 2000;**7**:1085-97.
15. Suryanarayanan S, Karellas A, Vedantham S, Baker SP, Glick SJ, D'Orsi CJ, et al. Evaluation of linear and nonlinear tomosynthetic reconstruction methods in digital mammography. *Acad Radiol* 2001;**8**:219-24.
16. Moore RH, Kopans DB, Rafferty EA, Georgian-Smith D, Hitt RA, Yeh ED. Initial callback rates for conventional and digital breast tomosynthesis mammography comparison in the screening setting. In: *Radiological Society of North America 93rd Scientific Assembly and Annual Meeting Program*. Chicago, Ill: Radiological Society of North America; 2007.
17. Helvie MA, Roubidoux MA, Hadjiiski LM, Zhang Y, Carson PL, Chan HP. Tomosynthesis mammography versus conventional mammography: comparison of breast masses detection and characterization. In: *Radiological Society of North America 93rd Scientific Assembly and Annual Meeting Program*. Chicago, Ill: Radiological Society of North America; 2007.
18. Poplack SP, Tosteson TD, Kogel CA, Nagy HM. Digital breast tomosynthesis: initial experience in 98 women with abnormal digital screening mammography. *AJR Am J Roentgenol.* 2007;**189**:616-23.
19. Andersson I, Ikeda D, Zackrisson S, Ruschin M, Svahn T, Timberg P, et al. Breast tomosynthesis and digital mammography: a comparison of breast cancer visibility and BIRADS classification in a population of cancers with subtle mammographic findings. *Eur Radiol* 2008;**18**:2817-25.
20. Smith A, Rafferty E, Niklason L. Clinical performance of breast tomosynthesis as a function of radiologist experience level. In: *9th International Workshop on Digital Mammography*. 2008.
21. Gennaro G, Baldan E, Bezzon E, La Grassa M, Pescarini L, di Maggio C. Clinical performance of digital breast tomosynthesis versus full-field digital mammography: preliminary results. In: *9th International Workshop on Digital Mammography*. 2008. p. 477-82.
22. Gur D, Abrams GS, Chough DM, Ganott MA, Hakim CM, Perrin RL. Digital breast tomosynthesis: observer performance study. *AJR Am J Roentgenol* 2009;**193**:586-91.

23. Boone JM, Nelson KK, Lindfors, Seibert JA. Dedicated breast CT: radiation dose and image quality evaluation. *Radiology* 2001;**221**:657-67.
24. Ning R, et al. *Proc SPIE* 2007;**6510**:651030-9.
25. Lindfors KK, Boone JM, Nelson TR, Yang K, Kwan AL, Miller DF. Dedicated breast CT: initial clinical experience. *Radiology* 2008;**246**:725-33.
26. Prionas ND, Lindfors KK, Ray, et al. Contrast-enhanced dedicated breast computed tomography: initial clinical experience. *Radiology* (in press).
27. Taillefer R. Clinical applications of ^{99m}Tc-sestamibi scintimammography. *Semin Nucl Med* 2005;**35**:100-15.
28. Brem RF, Floerke AC, Rapelyea JA, Teal C, Kelly T, Mathur V. Breast-specific gamma imaging as an adjunct imaging modality for the diagnosis of breast cancer. *Radiology* 2008;**247**:651-7.
29. Avril N, Rose CA, Schilling M, Dose J, Kuhn W, Bense S, et al. Breast imaging with positron emission tomography and fluorine-18 fluorodeoxyglucose: use and limitations. *J Clin Oncol* 2000;**18**:3495-3502.
30. Budinger TF. PET instrumentation: what are the limits? *Semin Nuc Med* 1998;**28**:247-67.
31. Duch J, Fuster D, Muñoz M, Fernández PL, Paredes P, Fontanillas M, et al. 18 F-FDG PET/CT for early prediction of response to neoadjuvant chemotherapy in breast cancer. *Eur J Nucl Med Mol Imaging* 2009;**36**:1551-7.
32. Bowen SL, Wu Y, Chaudhari AJ, Fu L, Packard NJ, Burkett GW, et al. Initial characterization of a dedicated breast PET/CT scanner during human imaging. *J Nucl Med* 2009;**50**:1401-1408.

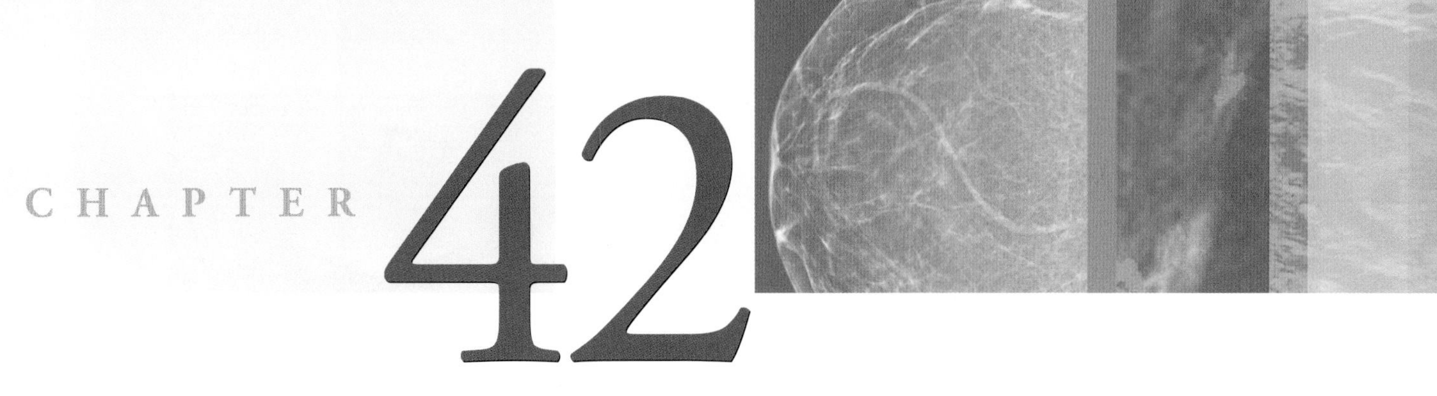

CHAPTER 42

Ultrasound-Based Technologies Including Elastography and Automated Whole Breast Scanning

Christopher Comstock

The foundation of ultrasound (US) applications in medicine can be traced back to the development in the late 1800s of techniques to measure distances under water using sound waves.[1] The first patent for SONAR (sound navigation and ranging) came one month after the sinking of the Titanic and was designed to aid in underwater navigation. A major breakthrough in the evolution high-frequency echo-sounding techniques was the discovery of the piezoelectric effect by Pierre and Jacques Curie in 1880. They observed that certain quartz crystals could be used to generate and receive "ultrasound" that is in the frequency range of millions of cycles per second (MHz). Further refinements in US technology came with the development of US equipment to detect flaws in metal during World War II. Current US scanners can be regarded as a form of medical sonar. The initial uses of US in medicine were applications in therapy rather than diagnosis. Its heating and disruptive effects were employed in neurosurgical tools and therapies for rheumatoid arthritis. The use of US for medical imaging and diagnosis began in the 1940s. Developments including gray-scaling and beam focusing, as well as the emergence of microprocessors and digital signal processing in the 1980s and 1990s, brought about vast improvements in spatial and contrast resolution, background noise reduction, dynamic range, and near and far field visualization. Further advances in US imaging have included real-time color and power Doppler, tissue harmonic imaging, speckle reduction, spatial compounding and three-dimensional (3D) imaging.

In 1951 Wild and Neal described the acoustic characteristics of 2 breast tumors in vivo using a 15-MHz A-mode device, and in 1952 Wild and Reid published the results of US examinations in 21 breast tumors, 9 benign and 12 malignant, using one of the first two-dimensional (2D) B-mode scanners.[2,3] These early studies of breast US aimed at distinguishing between benign and malignant lesions; however, in the 1960s and 1970s, hopes of replacing x-ray mammography briefly pushed the development of automated whole breast US systems for screening purposes.[4] It is interesting that more than 40 years later, we have come full circle and automated whole breast US is again being explored as a breast cancer screening tool. Advances in computer processing and computational power have also allowed the emergence of other US-based technologies such as elastography and computer aided diagnosis. In addition, photoacoustic imaging and US mediated drug delivery are also under investigation.

AUTOMATED WHOLE BREAST ULTRASOUND

During the early application of US for breast imaging in the 1960s and 1970s, several automated whole breast systems were developed (Fig. 42-1). These systems employed various methods including prone water-bath type scanning as well as supine water-coupled scanning using 4 to 7 megahertz transducers.[5,6] However, the low resolution

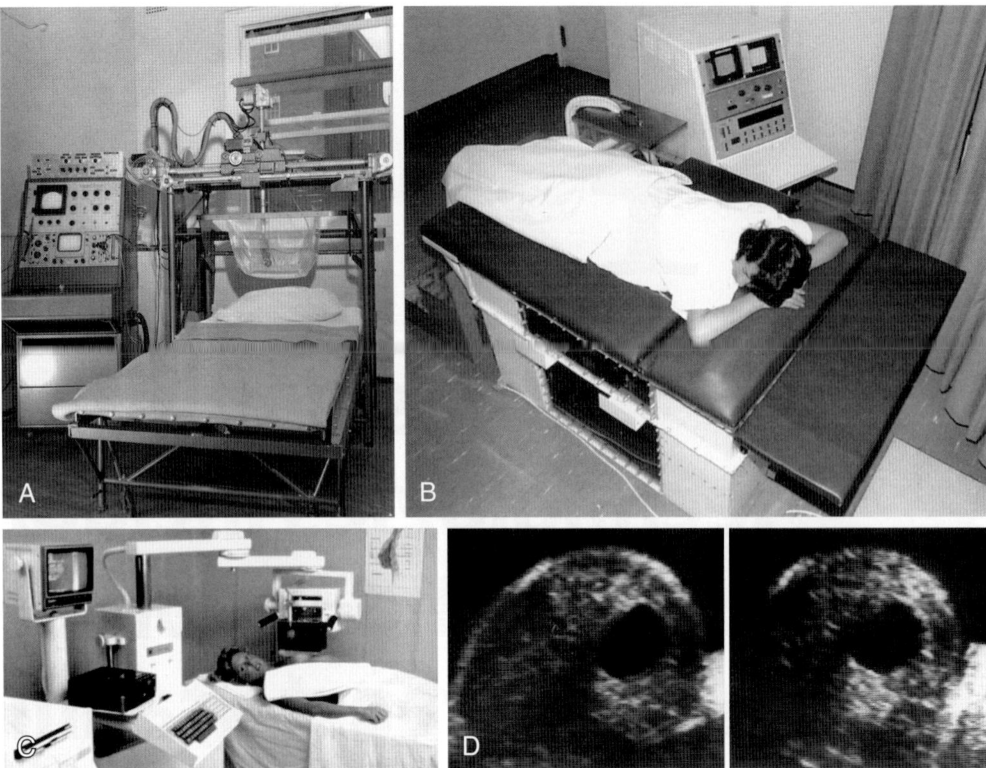

■ **FIGURE 42-1** Early whole breast ultrasound. **A,** Early breast ultrasound scanner, developed by Jellins and Kossoff at Australia's Ultrasonics Institute in1969, showing the enclosed water bath that was lowered across the patient's chest; the transducer mechanism is visible within the water bath. **B,** The original Australian-developed Octoson whole breast ultrasound scanner, 1975. The patient is lying prone with her breasts in a water bath below. **C,** The commercially produced Labsonics water-coupled breast ultrasound scanner with patient lying supine, 1986. **D,** Early automated breast ultrasound images demonstrating a cyst, 1980. *(A, B, and C, from Dempsey PJ. The history of breast ultrasound. J Ultrasound Med 2004;23:887–894; D, from Maturo VG, Zusmer NR, Gilson AJ, Smoak WM, Janowitz WR, Bear BE, et al. Ultrasound of the whole breast utilizing a dedicated automated breast scanner. Radiology 1980;137:457–463.)*

transducer technology and limited computer processing at the time restricted their accuracy. Initial studies of breast US for cancer screening were disappointing, because of excessive false-positive rates and poor detection of small cancers.[7-12] With the advent in the early 1990s of technological improvements in US, including higher frequency transducers (7–14 MHz) allowing improved spatial and contrast resolution, the potential of whole breast US as a screening tool is again being explored. Several more recent single-institution studies using hand-held scanning have demonstrated a prevalence detection rate of 3 to 4 mammographically occult cancers per 1000 women screened.[13-22] These initial studies have focused mainly on women with mammographically dense breasts and evaluated prevalence (initial) detection rates rather than incidence (subsequent) detection rates. Screening US appears to be more sensitive in detecting early invasive cancer, particularly invasive lobular carcinoma, whereas mammography is more sensitive in the detection of ductal carcinoma in situ (DCIS). Therefore, whole breast US is intended as a supplement to mammographic screening rather than a replacement. However, the biopsy positive predictive value (PPV_2) of hand-held whole breast US has shown to be considerably lower than that accepted for mammography.[23,24] The American College of Radiology Imaging Network (ACRIN) is currently conducting a randomized multicenter trial evaluating hand-held whole-breast bilateral screening US in high-risk asymptomatic women with dense breasts. The initial results of the prevalence screen demonstrated that adding a single screening US to mammography yielded an additional 1.1 to 7.2 cancers per 1000 high-risk women; however this generated a significant number of false positives (PPV_2 of 8.9%).[25] In addition, US-guided needle aspiration procedures, performed to exclude solid masses in cases of questionable complicated cysts, were not counted in the PPV_2 as false positives.

Despite the recent studies and current public attention on the benefits of hand-held whole breast US, its practicality has been questioned, because of the lack of standardized techniques, operator dependence, nonreproducibility and time required by the radiologist to perform the exams, in addition to the false positives.[26] In the recent ACRIN whole breast screening US study, the median time to perform bilateral hand-held screening US was 19 minutes. Another hurdle to whole breast screening US lies in the fact that there is currently no designated Medicare (Centers for Medicare & Medicaid Services [CMS]) reimbursement. Because of these challenges, manufactures are exploring automated whole breast ultrasound (AWBU) methods to help streamline and standardize whole breast screening US. One manufacturer, SonoCine Inc., has developed a hybrid type system (Fig. 42-2)

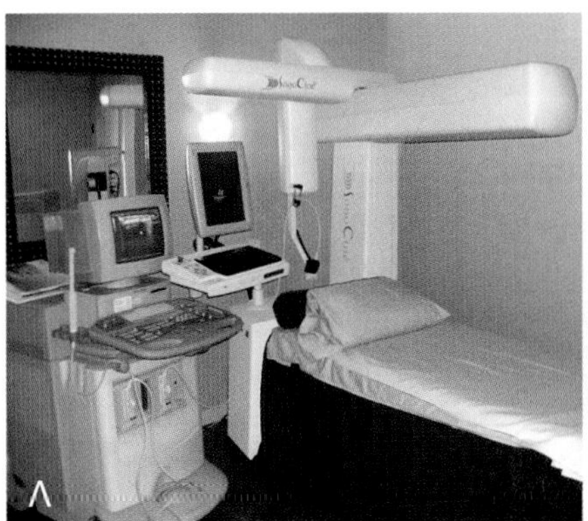

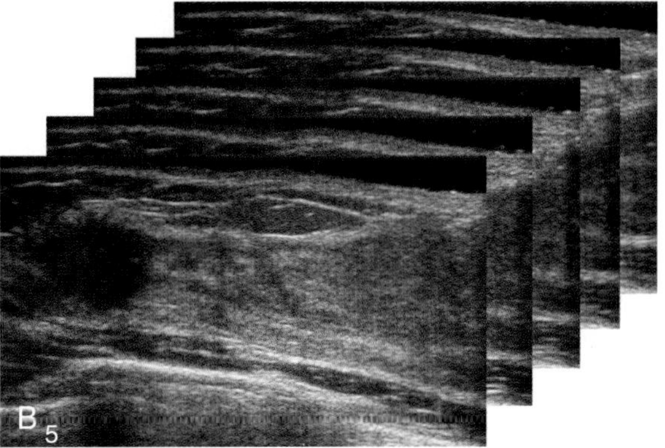

■ **FIGURE 42-2** Automated whole breast ultrasound (AWBU). **A,** Automated whole breast scanning system by SonoCine, 2010. Imaging is performed using a conventional 2D ultrasound transducer coupled to an automated scanning system. **B,** Sequential automated whole breast images showing a small invasive ductal carcinoma. *(Courtesy of SonoCine Inc.)*

that combines a conventional high-resolution 2D hand-held transducer with an automated scanning arm to perform automated scanning across the breasts.[27] Siemens AG and U-Systems, Inc., currently offer AWBU systems that use a wide field of view large footprint (on the order of 15 × 17 cm) high-frequency transducer (Fig. 42-3). After the application of a coupling medium, the transducer is placed on the breast and a series of 2D images is acquired that can be viewed in 2D or processed and viewed in a 3D format (Fig. 42-4). Depending on the size of the breast, the US transducer plate might have to be repositioned and might require more than one scan to cover the breast. Another approach currently under investigation uses a prone water-bath type platform similar to those used in the 1970s. However, instead of scanning across the breast, equipment made by TechniScan Medical Systems, Inc., incorporates two opposing transducers in the water bath, to send and receive the sound transmission information, as well as a third arm containing a reflection transceiver that rotates around the breast. Similar to CT, scanning is performed in a tomographic manner with the rotating array moving up to obtain a series of coronal slices of the breast (Fig. 42-5). These images may be processed in 2D and 3D formats to display not only standard reflection images but also inverse scattered, attenuation and speed of sound information. In additional to stand-alone AWBU, research is also being conducted to develop dual modality systems combining automated breast US with full-field digital mammography and digital tomosynthesis (Fig. 42-6).[28] It is hoped that mammography with the combined US information will have improved specificity and sensitivity.

US based screening technologies may offer lower cost and wider availability than magnetic resonance imaging (MRI). However recent results from the ACRIN whole breast hand-held US screening trial indicate that supplemental MRI, even after 3 years of combined mammography and US screening, can detect a significant number of occult carcinomas.[29] Therefore, without continued improvements in US technology, the role of whole breast US as a supplemental screening tool may be limited by the expanding use of MRI.

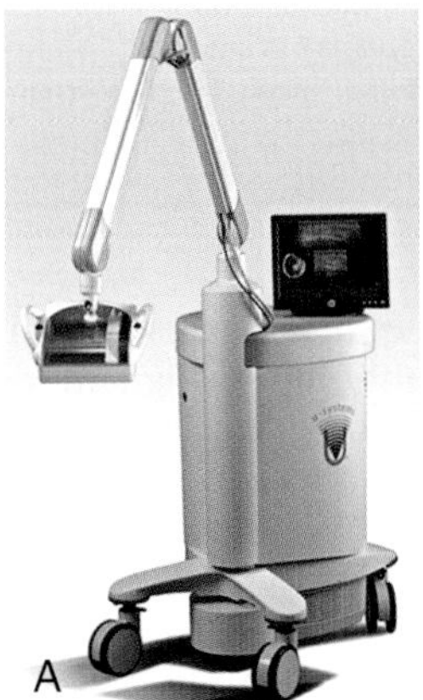

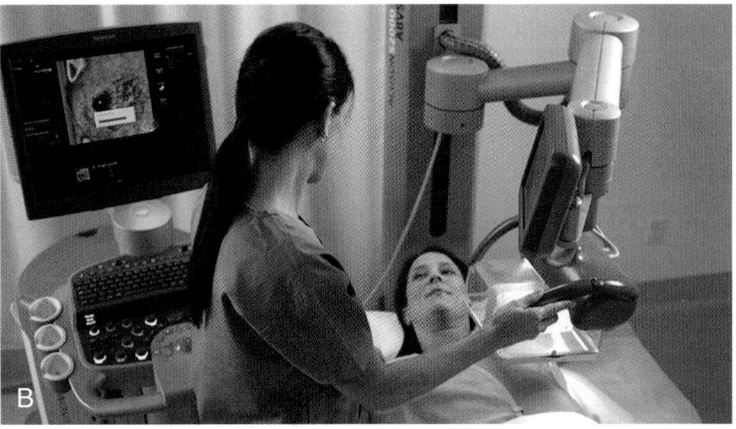

■ **FIGURE 42-3** Large transducer plate whole breast ultrasound. **A,** SomoVu automated whole breast ultrasound system. **B,** The ACUSON S2000 ABVS automated breast volume scanning system. The transducer plate is positioned over the breast and an automated scan is performed to obtain a series of 2D images. Depending on the breast size, more than one scan per breast may be required. *(A, Courtesy of U-Systems Inc.; B, Courtesy of Siemens AG.)*

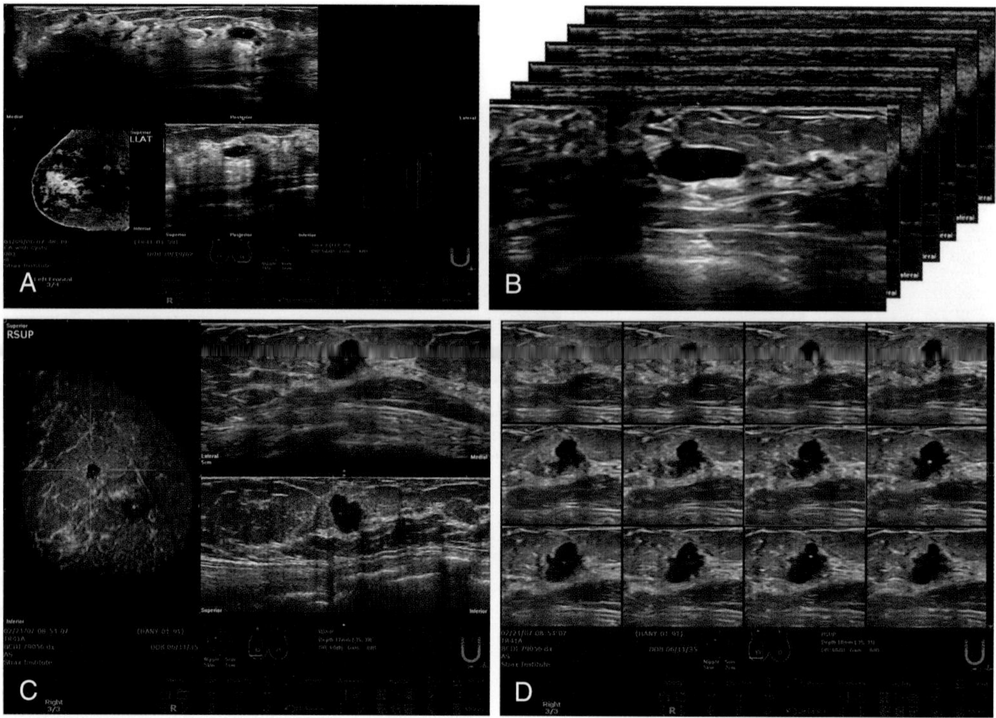

■ **FIGURE 42-4** Automated whole breast ultrasound (AWBU) clinical images. Images acquired using U-Systems' SomoVu whole breast ultrasound scanner demonstrating a cyst (**A** and **B**) and an invasive ductal carcinoma (**C** and **D**). The user interface allows the images to be viewed as a 3D data set with coronal reconstruction or as a set of conventional 2D ultrasound images. *(Courtesy of Dr. Stuart S. Kaplan, Mt. Sinai Medical Center, Miami Beach, FL.)*

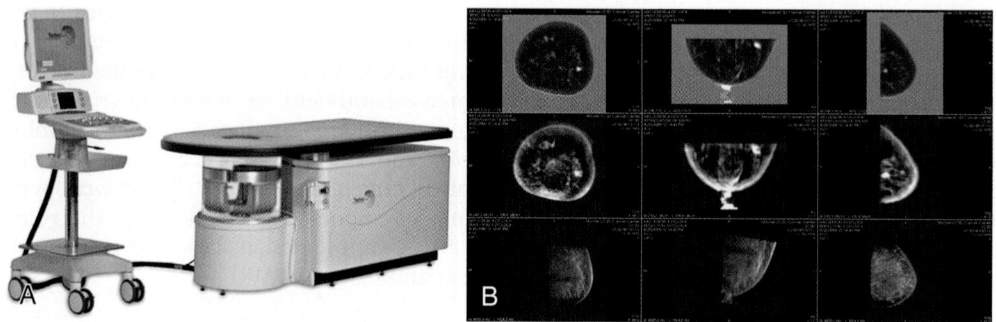

■ **FIGURE 42-5** Prone water-bath type whole breast tomographic breast ultrasound scanner. **A,** TechniScan automated whole breast scanning system. **B,** Three-plane presentation of left breast tomographic data demonstrating speed of sound (***top***), attenuation (***middle***) and reflection information (***bottom***). A small fibroadenoma is seen in the lateral aspect of the left breast *(A, Courtesy of TechniScan Medical Images, Inc.; B, courtesy of Dr Michael Andre, University of California, San Diego, San Diego, CA.)*

ELASTOGRAPHY

Evaluation of tissue stiffness has been part of physical exam for many centuries. The premise being that malignant conditions tend to be hard or firm where as benign processes are more often soft and mobile. An emerging technology to assess stiffness (or elasticity) of palpable breast masses as well as nonpalpable lesions detected on US is called *elastography* or strain imaging. Although this application of breast US has been explored for longer than 15 years, recent advances in technology and computer processing have allowed elastography to begin to appear in clinical practice.[30] The main objective is to provide an imaging representation of lesion stiffness to improve diagnostic confidence and increase specificity of the US exam.[31-37] However, although malignant lesions tend to be stiffer than benign lesions, exceptions such as mucinous carcinomas, necrotic tumors and high-grade carcinomas can lead to false negatives. The most useful application of elastography may be in reducing the number of short-term follow ups (American College of Radiology Breast Imaging Reporting and Data System [BI-RADS] 3) of probably benign masses and aspirations of borderline or complicated cysts.[38,39] Further prospective clinical trials are needed to determine its optimal use.

Tissue stiffness can be measured by a physical quantity called the Young modulus and expressed in pressure

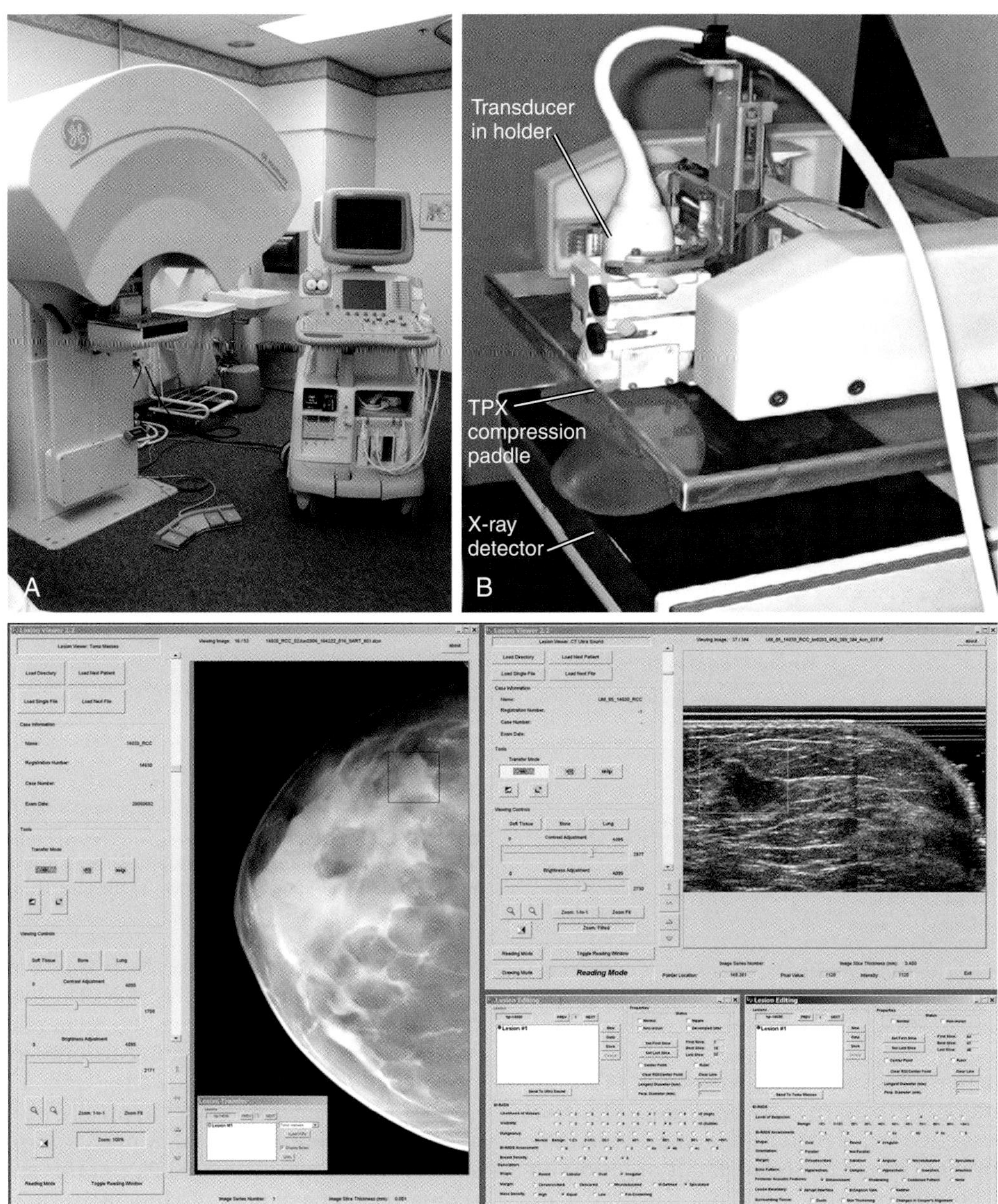

■ FIGURE 42-6 Dual modality imaging. GE prototype dual modality system combining digital tomosynthesis with automated breast ultrasound. **A,** Digital tomographic unit with adjacent ultrasound system. **B,** Close-up of the automated ultrasound system housing a conventional ultrasound transducer. Digital tomographic images are obtained, then the ultrasound system is attached and a series of matching ultrasound images is acquired. **C,** Image of the user interface demonstrating correlation of the tomographic image with ultrasound demonstrating a solid mass in the lateral right breast. *(A and B, Courtesy of GE; C, Courtesy of the University of Michigan.)*

units—Pascals, or more commonly kilo Pascals (kPa). The relationship between stress and strain is expressed in the Young modulus and is defined simply as the ratio between the applied stress and the induced strain (Fig. 42-7). Typical values of elasticity in various tissue types have been reported in the literature (Table 42-1).

The basic process of elastography involves inducing some form stress in tissue (low frequency vibration), imaging the tissue and then analyzing the deformation (strain) of lesions. Elastography techniques can be classified according to the type of stress or vibration applied to the tissue.

Static or compressive elastography employs manual compression using the transducer on the breast surface to cause deformation of the tissue (Fig. 42-8). With static elastography, because the compression applied by the user cannot be quantified, the Young modulus cannot be calculated. The amount of lesion deformation can only be depicted as a ratio to normal tissues or displayed in relative terms in gray scale (Fig. 42-9) or in color. Unfortunately, there are currently no standards between vendors for the colors used to depict degrees of relative tissue stiffness. Although various lesion patterns can be indentified during elastography, in general they can be categorized into the

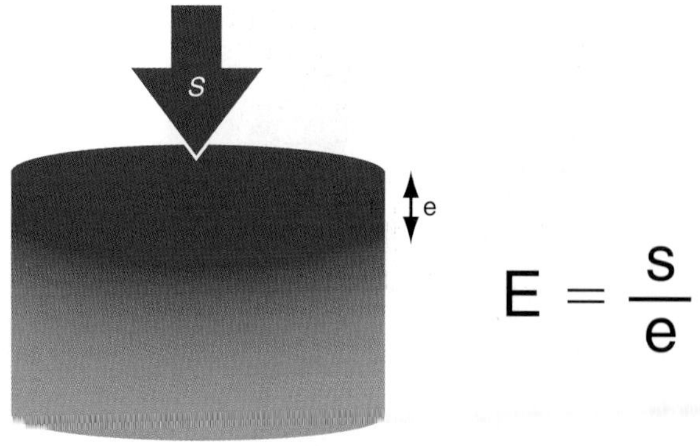

$$E = \frac{S}{e}$$

■ **FIGURE 42-7** The Young modulus. Deformation (strain) of a solid under an external stress. Young modulus or elasticity (E) can be described by the ratio between the applied stress (S) and the induced strain (e). Hard tissue has a higher elasticity than softer tissue.

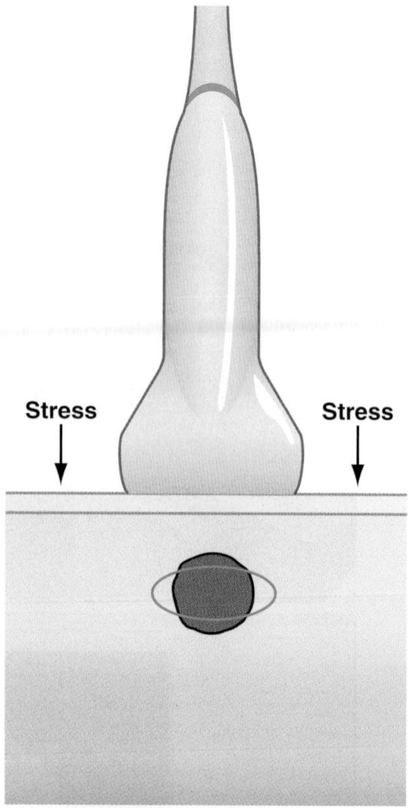

■ **FIGURE 42-8** Static or compression elastography. Stress is applied by repeated light manual compression of the transducer on the breast surface resulting in mild deformation of the underlying lesion.

TABLE 42-1. Relative Values of Elasticity in Different Types of Tissues

Types of Soft Tissue		Young Modulus (E in kPa)
Breast	Normal fat	18–24
	Normal glandular	28–66
	Fibrous tissue	96–244
	Carcinoma	22–560
Prostate	Normal gland	55–71
	BPH	36–41
	Carcinoma	96–241
Liver	Normal	0.4–6
	Cirrhosis	15–100

BPH, Benign prostatic hyperplasia; E, elasticity; kPa, kilo Pascals.

following five patterns of increasing suspicion: (1) fluid pattern (trilaminar color pattern); (2) predominantly soft; (3) mixed stiffness (two color pattern); (4) predominantly firm; and (5) firm with apparent enlargement of lesion on elastography as compared with conventional gray-scale image (Fig. 42-10). Examples of various lesions and their corresponding elastograms are shown in Figure 42-11.

Another form of elastography being used in the breast is called shear wave elastography or shear wave imaging. Unlike compression elastography, where the stress is applied by the user, shear wave elastography uses the acoustic radiation force induced by the US beam itself to perturb the underlying tissue. This force induces mechanical waves including shear waves which propagate transversely in the tissue (Fig. 42-12). Due to limitation of possible transducer heating, US generated shear waves must be very weak, amounting to only a few microns of displacement that dissipates after only a few millimeters of propagation. Shear waves typically propagate in tissue at speeds between 1 and 10 mm/sec (corresponding to tissue elasticity from 1 to 300 kPa). At this speed they cross a standard US image field of view in 10 to 20 msec. In order to capture shear waves in sufficient detail, imaging frame rates on the order of several thousand frames per second are required. Recent advances in computer and graphics processing have made possible shear wave imaging by allowing imaging frame rates as high as 20,000 Hz. Because the amount of applied stress is known, shear-wave based elastography is able to provide quantitative elastic information in real time (although currently only approved by

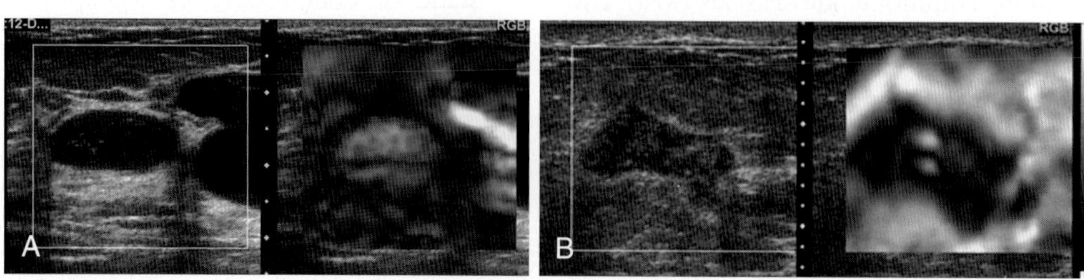

■ **FIGURE 42-9** Gray scale elastography. **A,** Typical *bull's-eye* pattern of a benign cyst. A rim of high elasticity is seen surrounding an area of central low elasticity. **B,** Ductal carcinoma demonstrating high elasticity as compared to the surrounding tissue. *(Courtesy of Siemens AG.)*

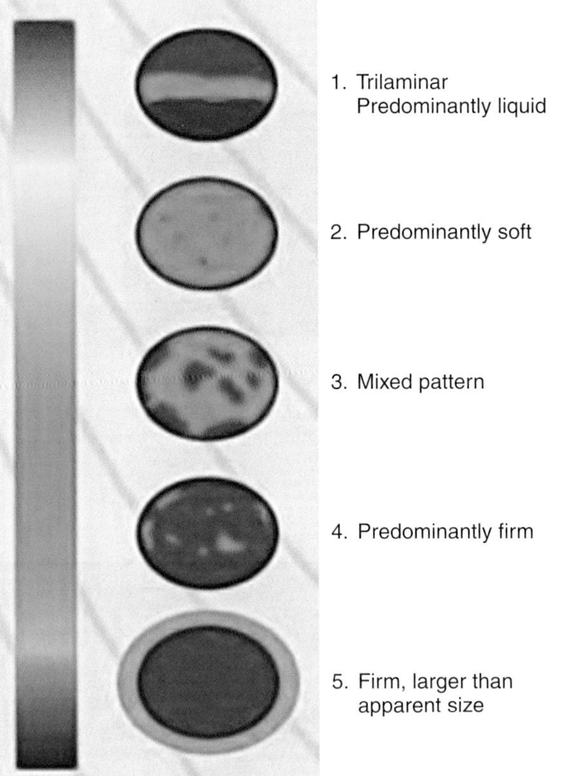

■ **FIGURE 42-10** Elastography color patterns. Five general categories of color patterns seen on elastography, with 1 being the most benign and 5 being the most suspicious. *(Modified from Scaperrotta G, Ferranti C, Costa C, Mariani L, Marchesini M, Suman L, et al. Role of sonoelastography in non-palpable breast lesions. Eu Radiol 2008.18:2381–2389.)*

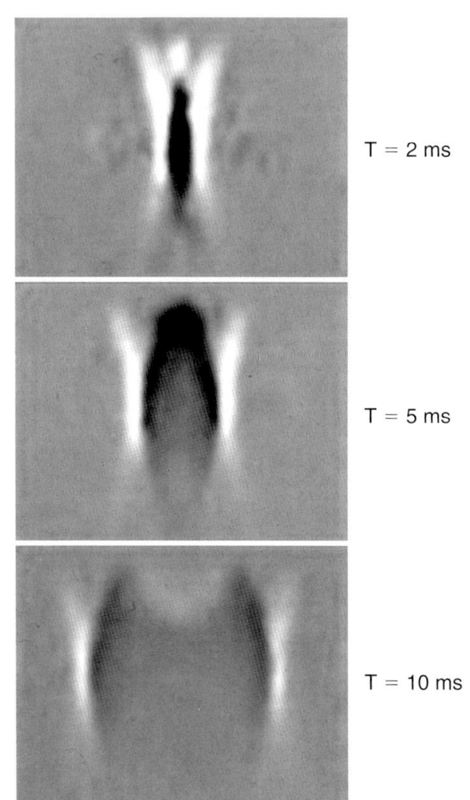

■ **FIGURE 42-12** Shear wave generation. Induced by an ultrasound beam focused in the center of the image, the shear wave can be seen expanding laterally. *(Courtesy of SuperSonic Imagine.)*

the U.S. Food and Drug Administration [FDA] for display of non-quantitative scale). The stiffer the tissue, the faster the shear wave propagates (Fig. 42-13). As with compression elastography, depending on the nature of the lesion, various stiffness patterns can be seen with shear wave imaging. However, these may be somewhat different from that of manual compression elastography because of the different forces being measured and differences in imaging methods (Fig. 42-14).

The clinical use of elastography will undoubtedly continue to grow as several vendors now offer US units with elastography as an option. The addition of stiffness as a lesion feature, in combination with other lesion parameters, may help to increase the diagnostic confidence and accuracy of breast US. Further studies are needed to better define its usefulness and optimal incorporation into current practice.

ULTRASOUND COMPUTER AIDED DIAGNOSIS

Besides hardware-based US technologies, advances in post processing and interpretation software are also emerging. Ultrasound-based computer aided diagnosis (CAD) programs that analyze combinations of lesion features, such as margin and echogenicity, as well as programs using lesion-matching functions are currently being developed (Fig. 42-15). After the lesion has been identified by the radiolo-

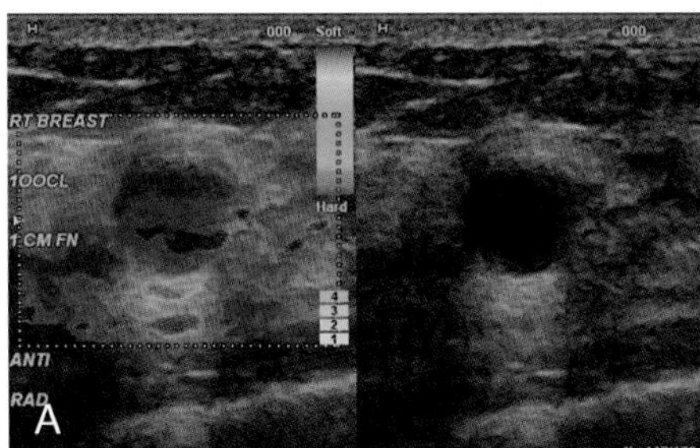

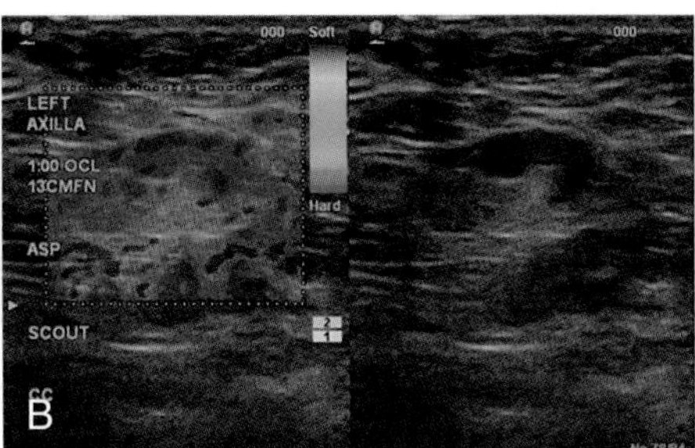

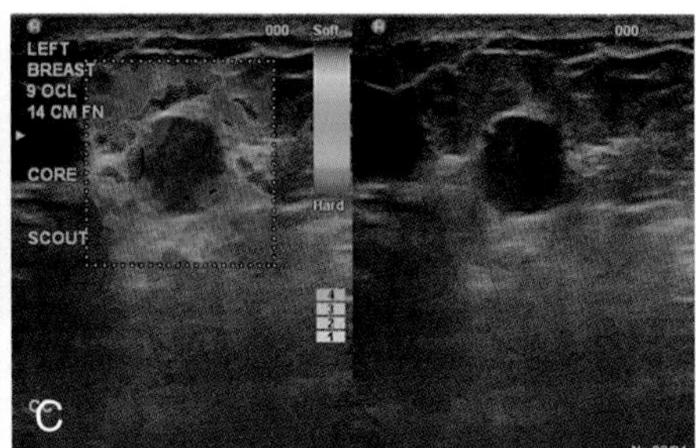

■ **FIGURE 42-11** Static elastography clinical images obtained using Hitachi's Vision 8500 Sonoelastography. **A,** Typical trilaminar color pattern of a benign cyst. **B,** Normal axillary lymph node showing a mixed stiffness two-color pattern. **C,** Invasive ductal carcinoma demonstrating a predominately firm color pattern.

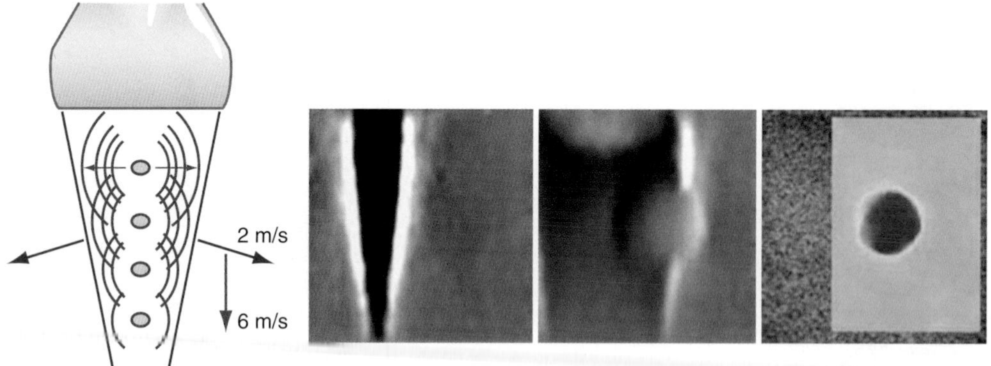

■ **FIGURE 42-13** Propagation of shear waves. Images capturing the shear wave, moving lateral to the direction of the applied compression, which is seen to speed up when it encounters a firm inclusion (high elasticity). On the color overlay of relative elasticity (*right*), the inclusion is colored red denoting high elasticity. *(Courtesy of SuperSonic Imagine.)*

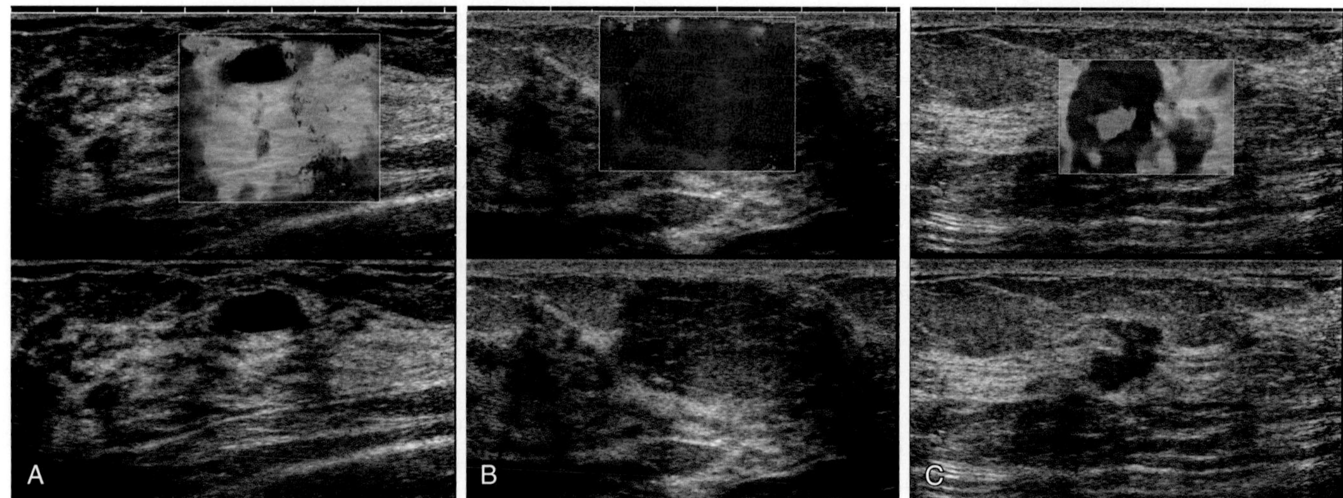

■ **FIGURE 42-14** Shear wave imaging. **A,** Gray scale and corresponding shear wave image of a simple cyst. The cyst is seen to have a black void on the elasticity image. **B,** A benign fibroadenoma demonstrates a predominately soft pattern on the elasticity image. **C,** Invasive ductal carcinoma demonstrating a firm, high elasticity pattern that is larger than its corresponding gray-scale size. This is a suspicious pattern and may relate to desmoplastic reaction in the surrounding tissue. *(Courtesy of SuperSonic Imagine.)*

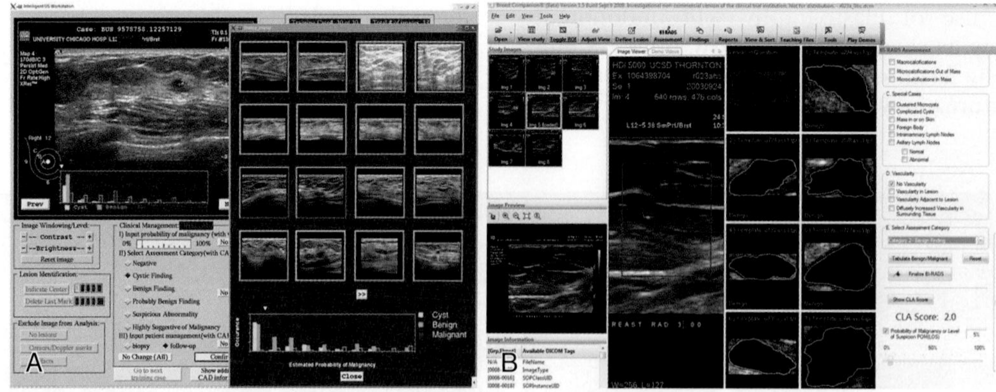

■ **FIGURE 42-15** Ultrasound CAD. **A,** Ultrasound computer aided diagnosis, performed after a lesion is identified by the radiologist, can analyze lesion features and estimate the probability of malignancy. **B,** User interface from the Image Companion. In addition to assisting BI-RADS US lexicon descriptor analysis, similarity indexing can be performed from a library of known lesions. *(A, Courtesy of the University of Chicago; B, Courtesy of Almen Laboratories Inc.)*

gist, some form of manual or automatic segmentation is applied and the lesion features are analyzed. The main goal is to assist in diagnostic interpretation and improve specificity. Additionally, these programs may provide applications to perform automatic extraction of BI-RADS lexicon descriptors for importation into reporting software. Future application may also include multi-modality CAD in which mammographic, and US, as well as MRI CAD features of a lesion are combined to further improve accuracy.

FUTURE DIRECTIONS

With further advances, particularly in transducer technology and processing, breast US will continue to evolve. Image resolutions of less than 20 microns may be possible. Emerging US-based technologies on the horizon also include hybrid modalities, such as photoacoustic imaging. Based on the photoacoustic effect, photoacoustic imaging involves the delivery of nonionizing laser pulses into tissue (when radio frequency pulses are used, the technology is referred to as thermoacoustic imaging). Some of the delivered energy will be absorbed and converted into heat, causing transient thermoelastic expansion and resulting in wide-band ultrasonic emission. These generated ultrasonic waves can then be detected by US transducers to form images. In photoacoustic imaging, because of its direct relationship to tissue optical absorption, properties such as hemoglobin concentration and oxygen saturation can also be evaluated. Other uses of US currently being explored include US-ablation techniques for tumor destruction, and US-activated nanoemulsions or microbubbles for targeted drug delivery (Fig. 42-16).[40] Radiologists performing breast US in the future will undoubtedly play an expanding role not only in diagnosis but also in cancer therapy.

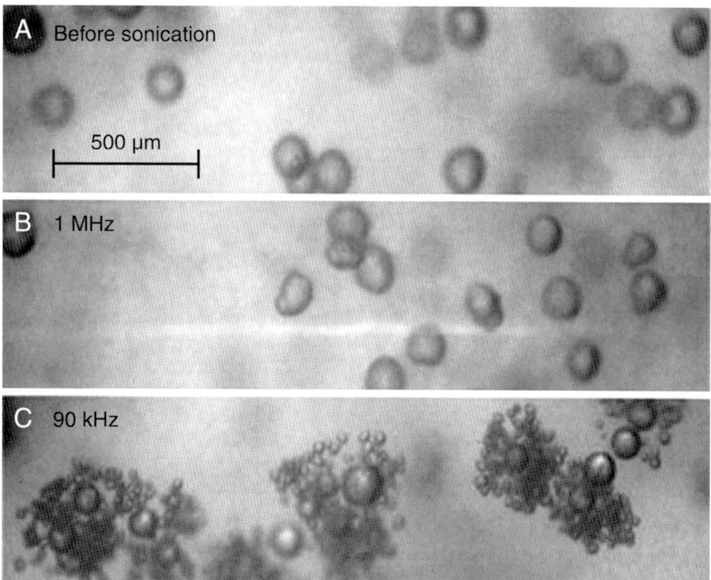

■ **FIGURE 42-16** Ultrasound activated microbubble drug delivery. Microbubbles containing cytotoxic agents that are stable unless activated (cavitated) by US, may allow targeted drug delivery to breast cancers. PFP microbubbles before (**A**) and after (**B**) sonication for 1 minute by 1-MHz, 3.4 W/cm^2, and 90-kHz, 2.8 W/cm^2 ultrasound (**C**) at room. *(Adapted from Rapoport NY, Kennedy AM, Shea JE, Scaife CL, Nam KH. Controlled and targeted tumor chemotherapy by ultrasound-activated nanoemulsions/microbubbles. J Control Release 2009;138:268–276.)*

SUGGESTED READINGS

Weinstein SP, Conant EF, Sehgal C. Technical advances in breast ultrasound imaging. Semin Utlrasound CT MR. 2006; 27(4):273–83.

REFERENCES

1. Woo J. A short history of the development of ultrasound in obstetrics and gynecology. *Obstetric Ultrasound–A Comprehensive Guide* Available at: www.ob-ultrasound.net/history1.html. [Accessed May 12, 2010.]
2. Wild JJ, Neal D. Use of high-frequency ultrasonic waves for detecting changes of texture in living tissue. *Lancet* 1951;**1**:655–7.
3. Wild JJ, Reid JH. Further pilot echographic studies on the histologic structure of tumors of the living intact breast. *Am J Pathol* 1952;**28**:839–61.
4. Dempsey PJ. The history of breast ultrasound. *J Ultrasound Med* 2004;**23**:887–94.
5. Jackson VP, Kelly-Fry E, Rothschild PA, Holden RW, Clark SA. Automated breast sonography using a 7.5-MHz PVDF transducer: preliminary clinical evaluation. Work in progress. *Radiology* 1986;**159**:679–84.
6. Maturo VG, Zusmer NR, Gilson AJ, Smoak WM, Janowitz WR, Bear BE, et al. Ultrasound of the whole breast utilizing a dedicated automated breast scanner. *Radiology* 1980;**137**:457–63.
7. Cole-Beuglet C, Goldberg BB, Kurtz AB, Patchefsky AS, Rubin CS. Clinical experience with a prototype real-time dedicated breast scanner. *AJR Am J Roentgenol* 1982;**139**:905–11.
8. Sickles EA, Filly RA, Callen PW. Breast cancer detection with sonography and mammography: comparison using state-of-the-art equipment. *AJR Am J Roentgenol* 1983;**140**:843–5.
9. Egan RL, Egan KL. Detection of breast carcinoma: comparison of automated water-path whole-breast sonography, mammography, and physical examination. *AJR Am J Roentgenol* 1984;**143**:493–7.
10. Egan RL, Egan KL. Automated water-path full-breast sonography: correlation with histology of 176 solid lesions. *AJR Am J Roentgenol* 1984;**143**:499–507.
11. Egan RL, McSweeney MB, Murphy FB. Breast sonography and the detection of breast cancer. *Recent Results Cancer Res* 1984;**90**:90–100.
12. Kopans DB, Meyer JE, Lindfors KK. Whole-breast US imaging: four-year follow-up. *Radiology* 1985;**157**:505–7.
13. Gordon PB, Goldenberg SL. Malignant breast masses detected only by ultrasound. *Cancer* 1995;**76**:626–30.
14. Kolb TM, Lichy J, Newhouse JH. Occult cancer in women with dense breasts: detection with screening US-diagnostic yield and tumor characteristics. *Radiology* 1998;**207**:191–9.
15. Buchberger W, DeKoekkoek-Doll P, Springer P, Obrist P, Dunser M. Incidental findings on sonography of the breast: clinical significance and diagnostic workup. *AJR Am J Roentgenol* 1999;**173**:921–7.
16. Buchberger W, Niehoff A, Obrist A, DeKoekkoek-Doll M, Dunser M. Clinically and mammographically occult breast lesions: detection and classification with high-resolution sonography. *Semin Ultrasound CT MR* 2000;**21**:325–36.
17. Kaplan SS. Clinical utility of bilateral whole-breast US in the evaluation of women with dense breast tissue. *Radiology* 2001;**221**:641–9.
18. Kolb TM, Lichy J, Newhouse JH. Comparison of the performance of screening mammography, physical examination, and breast US and evaluation of factors that influence them: an analysis of 27,825 patient evaluations. *Radiology* 2002;**225**:165–75.
19. Leconte I, Feger C, Galant C, Berlière M, Berg BV, D'Hoore W, et al. Mammography and subsequent whole-breast sonography of nonpalpable breast cancers: the importance of radiologic breast density. *AJR Am J Roentgenol* 2003;**180**:1675–9.
20. Crystal P, Strano S, Shcharynski S, Koretz MJ. Using sonography to screen women with mammographically dense breasts. *AJR Am J Roentgenol* 2003;**181**:177–82.
21. Cortesi L, Turchetti D, Marchi I, Fracca A, Canossi B, Rachele B, et al. Breast cancer screening in women at increased risk according to different family histories: an update of the Modena Study Group experience. *BMC Cancer* 2006;**6**:210.
22. Corsetti V, Ferrari A, Ghirardi M, Bergonzini R, Bellarosa S, Angelini O, et al. Role of ultrasonography in detecting mammographically occult breast carcinoma in women with dense breasts. *Radiol Med* 2006;**111**:440–8.
23. Quality Determinants of Mammography Guideline Panel. *Quality determinants of mammography*. AHCPR Publication no. 95-0632. Rockville, Md: U.S. Department of Health and Human Services, Public Health Service; 1994.
24 Rosenberg RD, Yankaskas BC, Abraham LA, Sickles EA, Lehman CD, Geller BM, et al. Performance benchmarks for screening mammography. *Radiology* 2006;**241**:55–66.
25. Berg WA, Blume JD, Cormack JB, Mendelson EB, Lehrer D, Böhm-Vélez M, et al, ACRIN 6666 Investigators. Combined screening with ultrasound and mammography vs mammography alone in women at elevated risk of breast cancer. *JAMA* 2008;**299**:2151–63.
26. Berg WA, Blume JD, Cormack JB, Mendelson EB. Operator dependence of physician-performed whole-breast US: lesion detection and characterization. *Radiology* 2006;**241**:355–65.
27. Kelly KM, Dean J, Comulada WS, Lee SJ. Breast cancer detection using automated whole breast ultrasound and mammography in radiographically dense breasts. *Eur Radiol* 2010;**20**:734–42.
28 Sinha SP, Roubidoux MA, Helvie MA, Nees AV, Goodsitt MM, LeCarpentier GL, et al. Multi-modality 3D breast imaging with X-Ray tomosynthesis and automated ultrasound. *Conf Proc IEEE Eng Med Biol Soc* 2007;**2007**:1335–8.
29. Zhang Z, Cormack JB, Jong RA, Barr RG, Lehrer DE, ACRIN 6666 investigators. Supplemental yield and performance characteristics of screening MRI after combined ultrasound and mammography: ACRIN* 6666 *American College of Radiology Imaging Network. In: *RSNA 2009 annual meeting, Chicago, Il.* Dec 1, 2009.
30. Garra BS, Cespedes EI, Ophir J, Spratt SR, Zuurbier RA, Magnant CM, et al. Elastography of breast lesions: initial clinical results. *Radiology* 1997;**202**:79–86.
31. Burnside ES, Hall TJ, Sommer AM, Hesley GK, Sisney GA, Svensson WE, et al. Differentiating benign from malignant solid breast masses with US strain imaging. *Radiology* 2007;**245**:401–10.
32. Fleury Ede F, Fleury JC, Piato S, Roveda Jr D. New elastographic classification of breast lesions during and after compression. *Diagn Interv Radiol* 2009;**15**:96–103.
33. Itoh A, Ueno E, Tohno E, Kamma H, Takahashi H, Shiina T, et al. Breast disease: clinical application of US elastography for diagnosis. *Radiology* 2006;**239**:341–50.
34. Tardivon A, El Khoury C, Thibault F, Wyler A, Barreau B, Neuenschwander S. [Elastography of the breast: a prospective study of 122 lesions]. *J Radiol* 2007;**88**(5 Pt 1):657–62.
35. Zhi H, Ou B, Luo BM, Feng X, Wen YL, Yang HY. Comparison of ultrasound elastography, mammography, and sonography in the diagnosis of solid breast lesions. *J Ultrasound Med* 2007;**26**:807–15.
36. Schaefer FK, Heer I, Schaefer PJ, Mundhenke C, Osterholz S, Order BM, et al. Breast ultrasound elastography-results of 193 breast lesions in a prospective study with histopathologic correlation. *Eur J Radiol* Sep 19 2009 Epub ahead of print.
37. Regini E, Bagnera S, Tota D, Campanino P, Luparia A, Barisone F, et al. Role of sonoelastography in characterising breast nodules. Preliminary experience with 120 lesions. *Radiol Med* Feb 22 2010 Epub ahead of print.
38. Booi RC, Carson PL, O'Donnell M, Roubidoux MA, Hall AL, Rubin JM. Characterization of cysts using differential correlation coefficient values from two dimensional breast elastography: preliminary study. *Ultrasound Med Biol* 2008;**34**:12–21.
39. Scaperrotta G, Ferranti C, Costa C, Mariani L, Marchesini M, Suman L, et al. Role of sonoelastography in non-palpable breast lesions. *Eur Radiol* 2008;**18**:2381–9.
40. Rapoport NY, Kennedy AM, Shea JE, Scaife CL, Nam KH. Controlled and targeted tumor chemotherapy by ultrasound-activated nanoemulsions/microbubbles. *J Control Release* 2009;**138**:268–76.

CHAPTER 43

Recent Advances in Magnetic Resonance Spectroscopy in the Breast

Xiaoyu Liu, Scott Lipnick, Shida Banakar, James W. Sayre, Nanette D. DeBruhl, Lawrence W. Bassett, and M. Albert Thomas

Conventional diagnostic methods such as x-ray mammography, ultrasound (US) and clinical examinations are limited in their sensitivity for detecting disease and their specificity for distinguishing between benign and malignant lesions. Magnetic resonance imaging (MRI) of the breast is increasingly being used because of its high sensitivity.[1] The most sensitive technique for locating lesions uses contrast enhancement characteristics and is known as dynamic contrast enhanced (DCE) MRI,[2] which can detect not only information on lesion morphology but also on tissue enhancement kinetics. Although DCE-MRI has the highest sensitivity (>95%) for invasive breast cancer detection, the specificity has been reported between about 37% and 97%.[3] The final diagnosis of breast cancer is still based on a biopsy of the breast lesion and has a positive predictive value of only 20% to 40%. Finding a noninvasive method with high specificity and sensitivity to detect breast cancer is still a major goal for breast cancer diagnostic research.[4]

Magnetic resonance spectroscopy (MRS) can be performed as an adjunct to any MRI examination to increase breast cancer detection specificity. The noninvasive nature of this technique makes it an ideal diagnostic tool in breast cancer detection. A number of prior investigators have applied one-dimensional (1D) MRS to characterize breast tissue with promising results. MRS of human breast tissue detects resonances due to water, choline (Cho), nucleotides, and saturated and unsaturated fatty acids.[5,6] Cancer tissue demonstrates altered metabolic concentrations that are detectable using MRS compared with normal tissue. Cho (at ~3.2 ppm) has been highlighted as a biomarker to distinguish between benign and malignant breast tumors in vivo. In addition, the water-to-fat ratio[7] has also been shown to enable differentiation of malignant breast tumors from other breast tissues. Consecutive DCE-MRI and 1D MRS images have been used for the diagnosis of breast cancer in several studies with promising results,[8] which suggest MRS may be a promising technique for improved classification of breast lesions when structural and enhancement characteristics alone cannot provide a differential diagnosis. While potentially beneficial, 1D MRS suffers from severe overlap of spectral peaks, limiting the complexity of its analysis given in vivo conditions. Two-dimensional (2D) MRS overcomes this problem with the addition of a second spectral dimension to each spectrum that facilitates discrimination of overlapping resonances.

A study by Thomas and colleagues[9] used 2D localized shift correlated spectroscopy (L-COSY) MRS and showed an elevated water-to-fat ratio and a detectable Cho resonance in spectra of breast cancer patients and not in healthy breast tissues. In another study, Thomas and colleagues[10] used the classification and regression tree analysis (CART) of 2D L-COSY spectra to characterize invasive ductal carcinoma and healthy fatty breast tissue with 92.4% sensitivity and 92.7% specificity. Liu and associates[11] used CART analysis to classify four different breast tissues (malignant, benign, healthy fatty and healthy glandular) by analyzing 2D MRS data acquired from breast tissues in vivo. The results showed that CART analysis can reach an overall correct rate of 82.0% in cross validated cases, and in original cases, CART can reach an overall correct rate of 96.0%. This is the first report on the statistical classification of 2D L-COSY in four human breast tissues in vivo. Lipnick and coworkers[12] combined DCE MRI with 2D L-COSY to detect breast cancer; the overall sensitivity and specificity were 89% and 100%, respectively.

Single voxel (SV)-based 1D and 2D MRS studies have shown altered metabolite concentrations in abnormal breast lesions; SV MRS cannot provide information on the regional distribution of the metabolites within the breast, but its clinical usefulness could be improved through increased breast coverage. Multidimensional magnetic resonance spectroscopic imaging (MRSI) can be used to provide higher spatial resolution and generate metabolic images of fat, water and other metabolites.[13] The clinical value of MRSI has been demonstrated for breast cancer.[14] 1D MR spectra extracted from the MRSI data show severe overlap of metabolite resonances due to J-coupling and co-resonant chemicals; 2D spatial encoding based MRSI combined with 2D MRS has been applied to overcome this problem. Due to the added second dimension, four-dimensional (4D) MRSI (two spatial + two spectral dimensions) of breast tissue has potential to offer better spectral dispersion and enables better identification of several J-coupled metabolites.[15]

There are two main research areas in MRS very much similar to MRI[16]; one is how to acquire high quality spectra, the other one is how to perform MRS postprocessing, including MRS quantification, which is performed to obtain specific metabolic concentrations. A variety of approaches have been used for quantifying MRS; however, each method has its own limitations.

In this chapter, we will introduce basic theories of MRS, 1D MRS of breast tissues, 2D MRS of breast tissues, 4D MRSI of breast tissues, MRS quantification, and high field MRS techniques.

PRINCIPLES OF SPECTROSCOPY

MRS, like MRI, is based on the principles of nuclear magnetic resonance (NMR). According to the basic laws of physics, protons (^{1}H) possess inherent spin. In the absence of an external magnetic field, these spins are oriented randomly; however, if a magnetic field is applied, the spins align either parallel or anti-parallel to the field and the energy levels split into lower and higher energy states. It is possible to excite the nuclei in the lower energy levels into the higher levels with electromagnetic radiation. The frequency of the needed radiation is determined by the difference in energy between the levels. MRS examines the fine splitting of the energy levels by detecting the small variations in resonance frequencies, which are displayed with the intensity along one axis and the frequency along the other axis.

Localized MRS techniques are very useful for in vivo studies because they enable detection of metabolic concentrations within a specific volume of interest (VOI). Rather than acquiring signal from the entire volume, we need to specify the desired VOI. This can be achieved by applying three slice-selective radiofrequency (RF) pulses to select the desired VOI. Clinical MRS protocols include either point resolved spectroscopy (PRESS) or stimulated echo acquisition mode (STEAM) sequence along with outer volume suppression (OVS) of signals from outside the VOI, elimination of the effects of motion, and reduction of susceptibility to changes in spin lattice relaxation time (T1) and spin spin relaxation time (T2). It is also critical to achieve a VOI over which Static magnetic field B_0-field homogeneity is excellent or well-shimmed and to obtain reliably good water suppression.

STEAM has three slice selective 90-degree RF pulses whereas PRESS has one 90-degree and two 180-degree slice selective RF pulses.[17] The double-echo PRESS technique is favored over STEAM method for its advantage of two times more signal-to-noise ratio (SNR) given identical echo times (TE). The best choice of TE for quantitative ^{1}H MRS is still controversial. Evidently, the shortest possible TE gives rise to the smallest T2 losses and therefore to the best SNR and also to the smallest susceptibility to T2 changes in pathology.

Most studies based on PRESS or STEAM localization have applied water saturation using multiple chemical shift selective RF pulses with narrow bandwidth (typically 50–100 Hz at 1.5 Tesla [T]) followed by gradient dephasing.[18] A well-shimmed VOI is crucial for quantitative[1] MRS, as resolution and line shape influence accuracy of data fitting. Other automated steps in setting up an MRS scan include adjustment of the RF pulse.

ONE-DIMENSIONAL MAGNETIC RESONANCE SPECTROSCOPY

Cancer tissue demonstrates altered metabolism compared with normal tissue. MRS is a powerful tool for exploring the cellular chemistry of human tissues. It can be used to identify specific metabolic patterns that may be used as markers for cancer. Proton MRS of surgically excised breast tumors was first performed by Chu and coworkers with differences between the malignant and uninvolved healthy tissues detected. Unfortunately, spectra from benign and malignant tissues appeared indistinguishable.[19] However, a study using breast cancer cell line MCF7 as well as human mammary epithelial cell lines with similar proliferation rate demonstrated that in both the perfused malignant cells and water soluble cellular extracts of such cells, the levels of phosphocholine (PCh) were significantly higher than in nonmalignant cells,[20] which indicated that malignancy is associated with the induction of phospholipid biosynthesis and breakdown.[21]

A study by Mountford and coworkers concluded that the peak intensity ratios of water and fat to the Cho group—which includes Cho, PCh, and glycerophosphocholine (GPC)—has a sensitivity and specificity for the discrimination of invasive carcinoma from benign breast lesions of 95% and 96%, respectively in MRS of fine-needle biopsy specimens.[22] Mackinnon and associates used 1D MRS to distinguish 102 of 106 fine-needle biopsy samples of benign and normal tissue from samples of breast carcinomas.[5] Kvistad and colleagues using in vivo 1D MRS identified Cho-containing compounds in 9 of 11 patients with breast carcinomas, 2 of 11 benign breast lesions and 5 of 7 healthy breast-feeding volunteers.[6]

Limitations of One-Dimensional Magnetic Resonance Spectroscopy in Breast Cancer Detection

1D MRS used in vivo, while potentially beneficial, suffers from the severe overlap of spectral peaks at clinical magnetic field strengths, mainly 1.5T and 3.0T. The overlap is caused by many features, some of which modulate periodically with TE, and can be resolved using 2D MRS.

Previous reports on 1D MRS of breast cancer have discussed the role of three major resonances: water, lipids and total choline (tCho). In addition to water, two other major resonances at 1.4 ppm and 3.2 ppm are produced from the multiple methylene protons of lipids and the trimethyl amines of choline groups, respectively. 1D MRS of breast cancer is complicated due to overlapping multiplets from methyl, methylene and olefenic groups of saturated and unsaturated fatty acids. Similarly, the Cho groups contain methylene protons giving rise to J-coupled multiplets in the 3 to 4 ppm region. Due to significant overlap of these J-coupled multiplets, there is a hindrance to reliably assigning these peaks using 1D MRS.

Another complication in 1D MRS is that the strong signal from adipose tissue mobile lipids can introduce sidebands that may be indistinguishable from the Cho peak. The source of the sideband artifacts is a modulation in the B_0 field caused by the pulsed gradients. The sidebands are coherent and modulate periodically with TE.

THE BENEFITS OF TWO-DIMENSIONAL MAGNETIC RESONANCE SPECTROSCOPY

2D MRS overcomes the problem of sidebands by adding a second frequency dimension to each spectrum. In general, in a 2D MRS acquisition, a 1D sequence is repeated with the evolution period (t_1) incremented in small steps and the final pulse altered to create a difference between the state of the spins during the evolution and detection period. Hence, the raw 2D MRS data is a function of two temporal variables: t_1 represents the evolution dimension and t_2 represents the acquisition dimension. Double Fourier transform applied on the raw 2D time domain data will produce a 2D spectrum.[23] The result is a 2D data set that is characterized by the frequencies of modulation in the acquired signal with respect to both evolution (F_1) and detection (F_2) periods.

The peaks in the 2D spectrum can be defined as diagonal peaks ($F_1 = F_2$) and cross peaks that do not lie on the diagonal ($F_1 \neq F_2$). Coupled spin systems produce the cross peaks detailing the connectivities of resonances along the diagonal. The cross peaks give information as to which resonances have contributions that are J-coupled and originate from the same molecule, and they are undetectable in 1D MRS. The cross peaks provide information that can be used to improve evaluation of molecular contributions to spectra. Unlike the spectral editing techniques, which target one metabolite at a time, 2D MRS can unambiguously resolve many overlapping peaks nonselectively as demonstrated by Ernst and coworkers more than two decades ago.[23] Better dispersion of several metabolite peaks and improved spectral assignment make 2D MRS techniques more attractive.

Localized Two-Dimensional Magnetic Resonance Spectroscopy Sequences

In 2D MRS acquisition schemes, a 1D MRS sequence is repeated with the t_1 incremented in small steps, with the final pulse facilitating different spin energy states during evolution and detection. The additional spectral dimension (indirect dimension) facilitates the separation of overlapping multiplets by detecting the coupled spin systems. A 2D spectrum has resonances located along the diagonal that contain signals from both uncoupled spins and coupled spins, much like a 1D spectrum ($F_2 = F_1$). Coupled spin systems produce off diagonal peaks detailing the connectivities of resonances along the diagonal. Typically, up to now, the efforts in multidimensional MRS have been with sequences such as JPRESS (J-resolved spectroscopy)[24] and L-COSY.[25]

Localized 2D JPRESS is a simple double spin-echo experiment with different echo times encoding the J coupling in the indirect t_1 dimension consisting of three slice-selective RF pulses (90 degree-180 degree-180 degree). The echo top is used as reference point for the reconstruction along t_1 so that no chemical shift (CS) evolution is present in that dimension. The J evolution is not influenced by the 180 degree pulses and is resolved along t_1. The acquisition is encoded along the direct t_2 dimension, which contains both CS and J evolution. After a Fourier transformation of the data in two dimensions, a spectrum is obtained with its resonances aligned on the horizontal axis. J-coupled spin systems are split up into multiplets tilted by 45 degrees. As a result, the original 1D MR spectral resonances are better separated.

Although JPRESS is able to distinguish coupled metabolites, there are complex 2D cross-peak patterns for some metabolites. Compared to JPRESS, a 2D L-COSY spectrum produces a better dispersion of J-cross peaks, although it requires a larger spectral window to be sampled during the evolution time. The VOI can be localized in one shot by a combination of three slice-selective RF (90 degree-180 degree-90 degree), a MRS volume localization sequence called CABINET (coherence transfer based spin-echo) spectroscopy. The last slice-selective 90 degree RF pulse acts also as a coherence transfer pulse for the 2D spectrum. An incremental period for the second dimension is inserted immediately after the formation of the Hahn spin-echo.

Phantom Study Using Two-Dimensional Magnetic Resonance Spectroscopy

Figure 43-1 shows the 2D L-COSY spectrum of corn oil.[26] This phantom was developed to mimic healthy breast fatty tissue. The dominant diagonal peaks ($F_2 = F_1$) in the corn oil phantom spectrum were due to the olefinic protons (UFD) (−CH = CH−), the polymethylene protons ($(CH_2)_n$) (fat), and methyl protons (CH_3) (FMETD). In addition, the 2D L-COSY spectra showed several pairs of cross peaks. The cross peaks labeled UFR and UFL are due to the scalar coupling (J) between olefinic with allylic $CH_2CH{=}CH-$ and diallylic $-CH{=}CH{-}CH_2{-}CH{=}CH-$ methylene protons of unsaturated lipids. The cross peaks

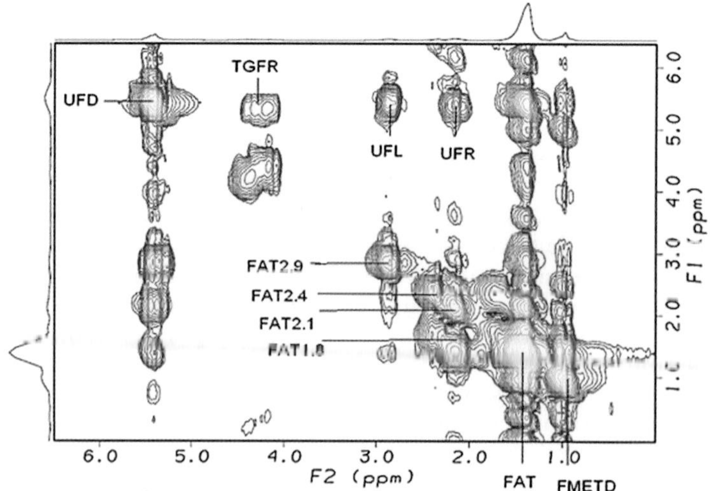

■ **FIGURE 43-1** Two-dimensional localized shift correlated spectroscopy (2D L-COSY) spectrum recorded in corn oil using the Siemens 3.0T MRI scanner equipped with a dedicated breast coil. The 2D L-COSY sequence was compiled on the Siemens VB13 platform using a VC++ based IDEA compiler. The voxel size was 1 cm^3 and WET method for global water saturation. Parameters were TR of 2 seconds, TE of 30 msec, 1024 complex points and 2000 Hz along t_2, and 45 increments and 1250 Hz along t_1. Before zero filling of the data to 2048 and 128 complex points, the raw 2D data were apodized using skewed and squared sine-bell filter along the t_2 dimensions and squared sine-bell filter along the t_1 dimensions.

labeled TGFR are due to the triglyceryl back-bone protons and the corresponding cross peaks below the diagonal of the 2D spectrum.

The assignments of the diagonal and cross peaks are (1) Fat (FAT) at (1.4, 1.4) ppm; (2) fat 2.1 at (2.1, 2.1) ppm; (3) fat 2.9 at (2.9, 2.9) ppm; (4) methyl fat (FMETD) at (0.9,0.9) ppm; (5) unsaturated fatty acid cross peaks right (UFR) at (2.1,5.4) ppm; (6) unsaturated fatty acid cross peak left (UFL) at (2.9, 5.4) ppm, (7) olefinic fat (UFD) at (5.4, 5.4) ppm; and (8) triglyceryl fat cross peak (TGFR) at (4.3, 5.3) ppm.

Two-Dimensional Localized Shift Correlated Spectroscopy Spectra of Different Breast Tissues

Figures 43-2 to 43-5 show 2D L-COSY spectra of healthy breast fatty tissue, healthy glandular tissue, malignant tumor tissue, and benign tumor tissue.[26] 2D L-COSY spectra were recorded using the following parameters: Repetition time (TR) of 2 seconds, TE of 30 msec, 45 increments of Δt_1, and 8 excitations per Δt_1. Δt_1 is 1.6 msec. The raw data were acquired using 1024

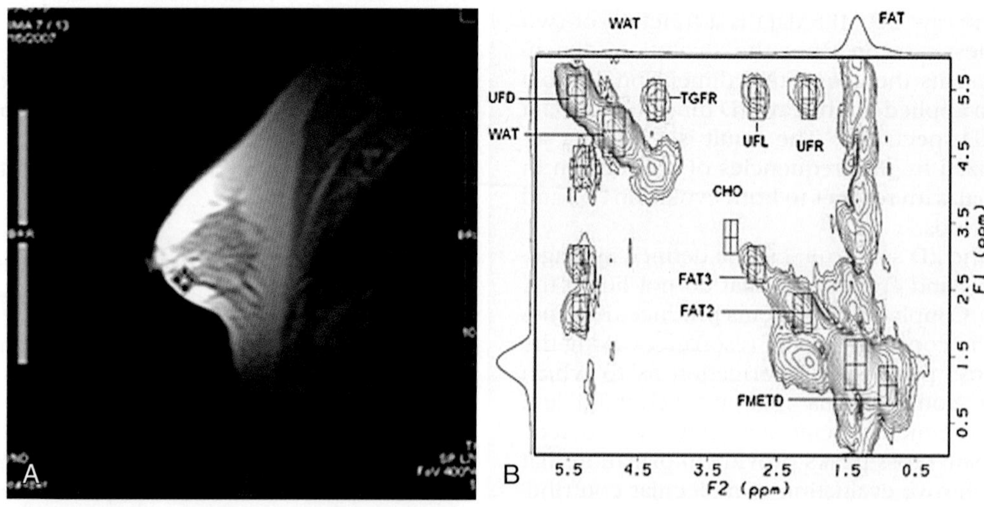

■ **FIGURE 43-2** **A,** Sagittal T_1-weighted breast image of a 36-year-old healthy woman. The yellow box indicates the location of the MRS voxel (1 × 1 × 1 cm^3) in the fatty tissue. **B,** The 2D MR spectrum recorded from the same fatty location. The rectangular boxes are the areas of volume integration for different metabolites. 2D L-COSY spectra were recorded using the following parameters: TR of 2 seconds, TE of 30 msec, 45 increments of Δt_1, and 8 excitations per Δt_1. Δt_1 is 1.6 ms. The raw data were acquired using 1024 complex points and 2000 Hz spectral width along the first dimension (F_2) and 625 Hz along the second dimension (F_1).The fat signals were more than water in the fatty tissue.

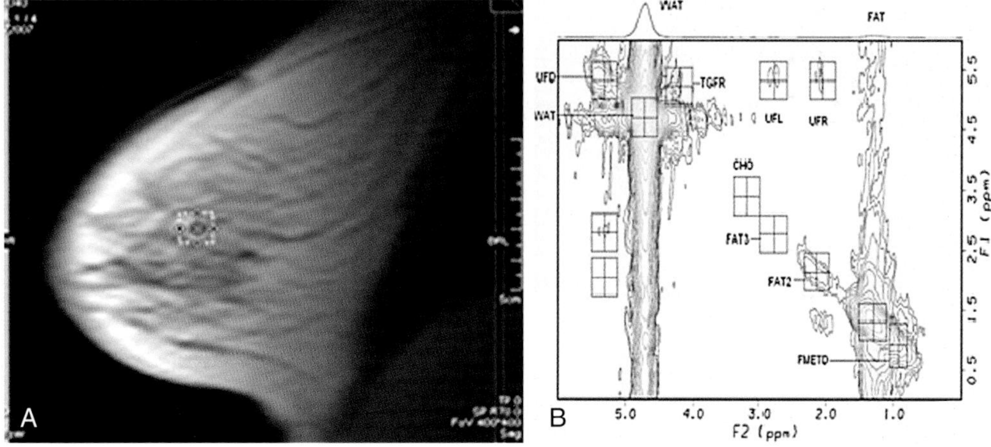

■ **FIGURE 43-3** **A,** Sagittal T_1-weighted MR image of a 38-year-old healthy volunteer. The yellow box indicates the location of the MRS voxel (1× 1× 1 cm³) in the glandular tissue. **B,** The 2D spectrum recorded from the same glandular location. The rectangular boxes are the areas of volume integration for different metabolites. 2D L-COSY spectra were recorded using the following parameters: TR of 2 seconds, TE of 30 msec, 45 increments of Δt_1, and 8 excitations per Δt_1. Δt_1 is 1.6 msec. The raw data were acquired using 1024 complex points and 2000 Hz spectral width along the first dimension (F_2) and 625 Hz along the second dimension (F_1). There is more water than fat in the glandular tissue.

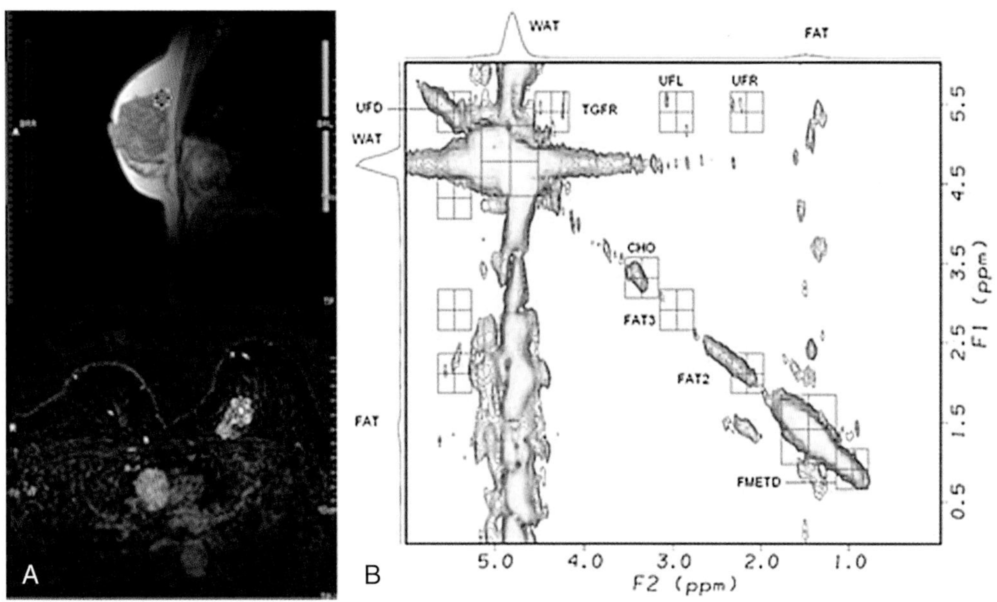

■ **FIGURE 43-4** **A,** Dynamic contrast enhanced (DCE) MR image of a 55-year-old patient with malignant breast tumor. The yellow box indicates the location of the MRS voxel (1 × 1 × 1 cm³) in the malignant tumor. **B,** The 2D spectrum recorded from the same malignant tumor location. The rectangular boxes are the areas of volume integration for different metabolites. 2D L-COSY spectra were recorded using the following parameters: TR of 2 seconds, TE of 30 msec, 45 increments of Δt_1, and 8 excitations per Δt_1. Δt_1 is 1.6 msec. The raw data were acquired using 1024 complex points and 2000 Hz spectral width along the first dimension (F_2) and 625 Hz along the second dimension (F_1). There was a choline peak appearing at 3.3, 3.3 ppm diagonal peak, which is the biomarker for malignant breast tumor.

complex points and 2000 Hz spectral width along the first dimension (F_2) and 625 Hz along the second dimension (F_1). Spectra were acquired from selected VOIs in each subject's breast tissue. For breasts with malignant and benign tumors, at least one voxel was acquired from the malignant and benign tumor, respectively, and from one healthy tissue. The size of each VOI was 1 × 1 × 1 cm³ for each acquisition; the total scan time was 12 minutes.

All 2D MRS data files were processed using a Felix2000 software package (Accelerys Inc., San Diego, Calif). The data were zero-filled to 2048 × 96 points, filtered and Fourier-transformed along both dimensions. The 2D L-COSY spectral peaks were displayed using contour plots in the magnitude mode, which were used to evaluate the spectra and to calculate the volume under each detectable peak.

Each 2D spectrum contains contributions from the following proton resonances: water (WAT; 4.8 ppm), poly methylene group (FATs; 1.4 ppm, 2.1 ppm, 2.4 ppm, 2.9 ppm), methyl group (FMETD, 0.9 ppm), olefinic group (UFD; 5.4 ppm). In addition to the peaks that lie on the diagonal (F_1=F_2) of the spectrum, off diagonal cross-peaks occur due to the J-coupled resonances. There are two distinct sets of cross peaks detectable at 1.5T in breast lesions connecting the olefinic and methylene protons of unsaturated lipids (UFR: F_2=2.4 ppm, wF_1=5.4 ppm, and

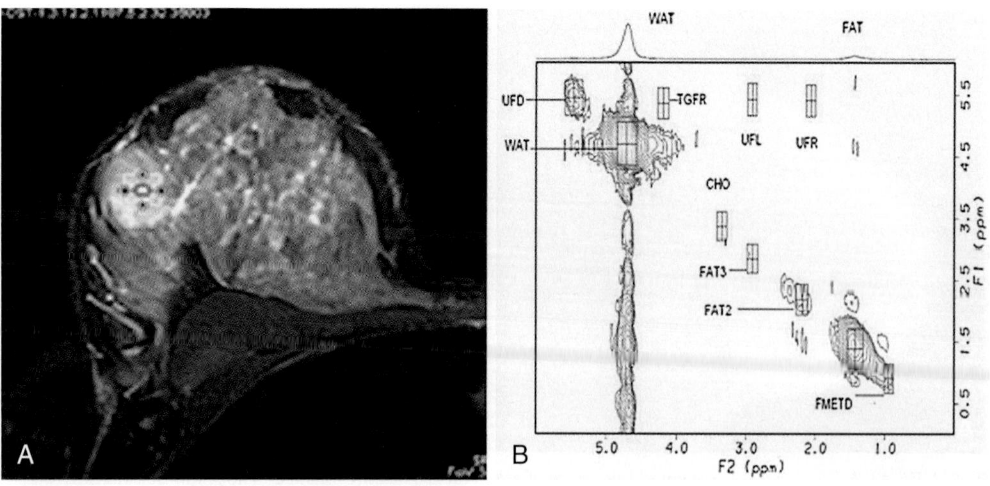

■ **FIGURE 43-5** **A,** Dynamic contrast enhanced (DCE) MR image of a 28-year-old patient with benign breast tumor. The yellow box indicates the location of the MRS voxel ($1 \times 1 \times 1$ cm^3) in the benign tumor. **B,** The 2D spectrum recorded from the same benign tumor location. The rectangular boxes are the areas of volume integration for different metabolites. Two-dimensional (2D) L-COSY spectra were recorded using the following parameters: TR of 2 seconds, TE of 30 msec, 45 increments of Δt_1, and 8 excitations per Δt_1. Δt_1 is 1.6 msec. The raw data were acquired using 1024 complex points and 2000 Hz spectral width along the first dimension (F_2) and 625 Hz along the second dimension (F_1). Only diagonal peaks (FMETD, FAT, WATER, UFD) appear in the 2D spectrum, the cross peaks concentrations are too small to be seen on the contoured spectrum.

TABLE 43-1. Metabolites Identified in the Two-Dimensional Localized Shift Correlated Spectroscopy Spectra of Breast Tissues

Spectral Peaks Locations (F_2, F_1) ppm
Water (WAT) (4.8, 4.8)
Fat (FAT) (1.4, 1.4)
Methyl fat (FMETD) (0.9, 0.9)
Olefinic fat (UFD) (5.4, 5.4)
Choline (CHO) (3.3, 3.3)
Unsaturated fatty acid cross peaks, right (UFR) (2.1, 5.4)
Unsaturated fatty acid cross peak left (UFL) (2.9, 5.4)
Triglyceryl fat cross peak (TGFR) (4.3, 5.3)

UFL; F_2= 2.9 ppm, F_1= 5.4 ppm), and the corresponding peaks below the diagonal. Table 43-1 shows the list of all the spectral resonances analyzed in this study. The volume under each resonance was calculated to estimate the respective contribution to the overall spectrum by integrating the signal within a set region. Metabolite ratios were computed by dividing these volume integrals.

CLASSIFICATION AND REGRESSION TREE ANALYSIS RESULTS

To distinguish among malignant tumor (M), benign tumor (B), healthy fatty (F) and glandular (G) breast tissues, Liu and associates[11] used a statistical method called classification and regression tree analysis (CART) to analyze four different 2D MR spectra. A total of 31 women participated in this study, including 13 healthy women, 9 subjects with malignant tumor, 9 women with benign tumor. For healthy volunteers, T1-weighted or T2-weighted MRI images were used for 2D COSY localization; for malignant and benign patients, DCE MRI was used for 2D COSY localization. All scans were performed on a 1.5T Avanto whole body MRI/MRS scanner with a dedicated Siemens phased arrayed breast coil. Manual shimming was done before acquiring each 2D L-COSY data.

CART is a tree-building technique that is unlike traditional data analysis methods. It is ideally suited to the generation of clinical decision rules.[27] Using CART version 6.0 (Salford Systems, San Diego, Calif), a recursive partitioning analysis was investigated to divide the cohort into malignant, benign, healthy fatty and glandular breast tissues. Variables entered into the model included all the peak volumes (Table 43-1) calculated from the 2D COSY spectra and a total of 18 cross and diagonal peak ratios.

The Gini method for classification trees was used. The Gini method is the measure of impurity of a node and is commonly used when the dependent variable is a categorical variable, defined as:

$$g(t) = \sum C(i/j)p(i/t)p(j/t)$$

where the sum extends over all k categories. $p(j/t)$ is the probability of category j at the node t and $C(i/j)$ is the probability of misclassifying a category j case as category i. The Gini method was used to select the best classification model. CART automatically searches for important patterns and relationships in complex data without rigid assumptions. The results are shown in Table 43-2 A and B.

The difference between A and B in Table 43-2 is discussed as follows: Table A is from the original cases method, while Table B is cross-validated method. In the

TABLE 43-2. Classification and Regression Tree Analysis of Two-Dimensional Localized Shift Correlated Spectroscopy Spectral Data Recorded from Four Types of Tissues*

A. Original method: Selecting combination of three diagonal and cross peak ratios: WAT/FAT, FAT/UFR, CHO/UFD; Total = 50, Overall % Correct = 96.00%

Tissue	Predicted B	Predicted F	Predicted G	Predicted M	Total
Actual benign tissue	11(100%)	0	0	0	11(100%)
Actual fatty tissue	0	18	0	0	18(100%)
Actual glandular tissue	0	0	7(87.5%)	1(12.5%)	8(100%)
Actual malignant tissue	0	0	1(7.7%)	12(92.3%)	13(100%)

B. Cross-Validated method: Selecting combination of three diagonal and cross peak ratios: WAT/FAT, FAT/UFR, CHO/UFD; Total=50, Overall % Correct = 82.00%

Tissue	Predicted B	Predicted F	Predicted G	Predicted M	Total
Actual benign tissue	8(72.7%)	0	2(18.2%)	1(9.1%)	11(100%)
Actual fatty tissue	0	18	0	0	18(100%)
Actual glandular tissue	1(12.5%)	0	6(75%)	1(12.5%)	8(100%)
Actual malignant tissue	0	0	4(30.8%)	9(69.2%)	13(100%)

*Invasive breast carcinoma and healthy fatty breast tissues: malignant (M) vs. benign (B) vs. glandular (G) vs. fatty (F) tissues
CHO, choline, FAT, fat; UFD, olefinic fat; UFR, unsaturated fatty acid cross peaks, right; WAT, water.

original cases method, each case is classified by the functions derived from the group cases, including that case, so it is a biased result and the overall correct rate of Table 43-2A is 96.0%. In cross validation, each case is classified by the functions derived from all cases other than that case, so it is an unbiased result, the overall correct rate of Table 43-2B is 82.0%. 2D L-COSY spectrum of breast tissue shows the diagonal peaks of water, FAT, Cho, UFD, and FMETD. Additionally, three well resolved cross peaks due to UFR, UFL and TGFR were also recorded. These cross peak ratios are significant in classifying between malignant tumor and other breast tissues, which cannot be detected using 1D MRS. The WAT/FAT ratios are used in 1D MRS to classify between healthy woman and woman in breast cancer. In this study, 18 metabolite ratios including diagonal and cross peaks were input to CART statistical software; CART can select the optimum combinations of different metabolite ratios to classify the breast tissues.

A number of 1D MRS studies using biopsy specimens and tissue extracts have attempted to distinguish biochemical features of breast tumors, and have focused on the presence of Cho predominantly in malignant tumors. In the current work, the diagonal peak of Cho was identified reliably in the 2D L-COSY spectra. The Cho-to-noise ratio was measured in the four different breast tissues in 13 malignant lesions, 11 benign tumors, 8 healthy glandular and 18 healthy fatty breast; STUDENT t-test and p values were calculated for each pair of breast tissues, The p value shows that the Cho-to-noise ratio in malignant tumor is significantly different from the ratio in the other three breast tissues; this is the same conclusion derived from 1D MRS. CART analysis picks up three ratios WAT/FAT, FAT/UFR, CHO/UFD, in which Cho was selected as a classification function, this shows that Cho is important in classifying different breast tissues.

These statistic analysis results were verified in a previous study by Thomas and colleagues using a GE 1.5-T MRI/MRS scanner (General Electric Healthcare Technologies, Waukesha, Wis) equipped with a two-channel phased-array breast MR coil.[10] A body RF coil was employed for RF transmission and a phased-array breast coil for reception. The following parameters were used to acquire each 2D L-COSY spectrum: TR of 2 seconds, along the first and 625 Hz along the second dimensions, 8–12 excitations per Δt_1, and 40 increments of Δt_1. Total duration for recording a 2D L-COSY was approximately 10 to 16 minutes after 3 to 5 minutes of optimization of transmitter and receiver, and the B_0 homogeneity. The pulse sequence included a combination of three slice-selective RF pulses (90 degree-180 degree-90 degree) to localize a VOI and the second 90 degree RF pulse also acted as a coherence transfer pulse in L-COSY. A two steps phase cycling was imposed on each RF pulse with receiver cycled through addition/subtraction. No water suppression was used while recording the 2D L-COSY spectra.

Each 2D spectrum was recorded in approximately 10 to 16 minutes. The MRS voxel size varied from $1 \times 1 \times 1\,cm^3$ to $2 \times 2 \times 2\,cm^3$ without any water suppression technique. For healthy breasts, spectra were acquired from at least one fatty region. 2D L-COSY spectra were recorded in a total of 43 voxels.

Five diagonal and six cross peak volumes were integrated and eighteen ratios were selected as potential features for the statistical method CART to characterize invasive ductal carcinoma and healthy fatty breast tissues noninvasively using CART analysis of 2D MR spectral data. The results are shown in Table 43-3.

TABLE 43-3. Classification and Regression Tree Analysis of Two-Dimensional Localized Shift Correlated Spectroscopy Spectral Data Recorded from Two Types of Tissues

A. Combination of three diagonal peak ratios: WAT/FAT, WAT/CHO and CHO/FAT

Tissue	Predicted Fatty Tissue	Predicted Invasive Carcinoma	Total
Actual fatty tissue	28 (93.3%)	2 (6.7%)	30 (100.0%)
Actual invasive carcinoma	2 (15.4%)	11 (84.6%)	13 (100.0%)

B. Combination of three cross peak ratios: WAT/UFR, WAT/UFL and WAT/TGFR

Tissue	Predicted Fatty Tissue	Predicted Invasive Carcinoma	Total
Actual fatty tissue	28 (93.3%)	2 (6.7%)	30 (100.0%)
Actual invasive carcinoma	2 (15.4%)	11 (84.6%)	13 (100.0%)

C. Combination of six ratios: WAT/FAT, WAT/CHO, CHO/FAT, WAT/UFR, WAT/UFL and WAT/TGFR

Tissue	Predicted Fatty Tissue	Predicted Invasive Carcinoma	Total
Actual fatty tissue	29 (96.7%)	1 (3.3%)	30 (100.0%)
Actual invasive carcinoma	2 (15.4%)	11 (84.6%)	13 (100.0%)

CHO, choline; FAT, fat; UFL, unsaturated fatty acid cross peak left; UFR, unsaturated fatty acid cross peaks, right; TGFR, triglyceryl fat cross peak; WAT, water.

MAGNETIC RESONANCE SPECTROSCOPY IMAGING OF BREAST TISSUE

Magnetic resonance spectroscopy (MRS) can provide important information about metabolism noninvasively in vivo. MRS studies have shown that the metabolites change in abnormal breast lesions. However, SV MRS has significant limitations in terms of breast coverage, because it cannot provide information on the regional distribution of the metabolite within the breast. MRSI can solve the problem by providing spatially resolved spectra from which metabolic images of fat, water and other metabolites can be generated.

The majority of MRSI implementations in vivo are resolved in two spatial dimensions of and one spectral dimension of MRS (2D spatial + 1D spectral). MRSI generates maps of the spatial distribution of a limited set of high-concentration metabolites within a slab or volume material. The clinical value of MRSI has been demonstrated for focal diseases such as brain tumors, prostate cancer and breast cancer. 1D spectra extracted from the MRSI data similarly suffer severe overlap of metabolite resonances as described previously for SV 1D MRS, and recent developments of MRSI involving two spectral dimension MRS has been studied in order to overcome this problem.

A study by Liu and associates[15] demonstrates the feasibility of implementing a four-echo based spatially resolved 2D L-COSY sequence on a Siemens 3T MRI scanner and evaluation in breast tissues in vivo. Seven volunteers (including six healthy subjects, one subject with a benign tumor) were scanned using SV based 2D L-COSY and four-echo based spatially resolved 2D COSY MRSI sequences, respectively. From the four-dimensional MRSI data (2D spatial+2D spectral) of each breast, six metabolite distribution images of the breast were generated. The metabolites are fat (1.4, 1.4 ppm), water (4.8 ppm, 4.8 ppm), unsaturated fatty acid (UFD; 5.4 ppm, 5.4 ppm), unsaturated fatty acid cross peak left (UFL; 2.9 ppm, 5.4 ppm), unsaturated fatty acid cross peak right (UFR; 2.1 ppm, 5.4 ppm), and triglyceryl fat cross peak (TGFR; 4.3 ppm, 5.3 ppm). The images between different healthy and benign subjects were compared. The metabolite spatial distribution patterns are different, and there was more water and less fat in the benign tumor area. The composition and distribution of metabolites are related to abnormal breast tissue changes, these metabolite distribution patterns may serve as the biomarkers for early diagnosis and therapeutic monitoring of breast disease. The pilot data needed a larger cohort of patients in order to more accurately characterize the potential benefits of utilizing 2D spatial and 2D spectral MRSI acquisitions for breast tissue differentiation.

MAGNETIC RESONANCE SPECTROSCOPY QUANTIFICATIONS

In the previous studies, metabolite contributions were detailed through the metabolite ratios for breast cancer detection. Quantifying each metabolite's concentration is an important research area in MRS and could provide more specific information for improved tissue characterization. MRS quantitation can be defined as a mathematical process to obtain numerical values that detail the concentration of each of the components (metabolites) contributing to the overall signal.[28] This is, in general, a very complex task because of the complexity of spectra of in-vivo tissue and because of the unpredictable forms of the line shape and baseline.

There are two main approaches for measuring metabolite concentrations using the MRS signals either in the time domain signal or the frequency domain signal. Although it may seem more natural to process the signal in the time domain, just because it is the original form, frequency processing has produced very good results. These approaches also can be classified depending on whether they use or do not use prior knowledge. In this context prior knowledge

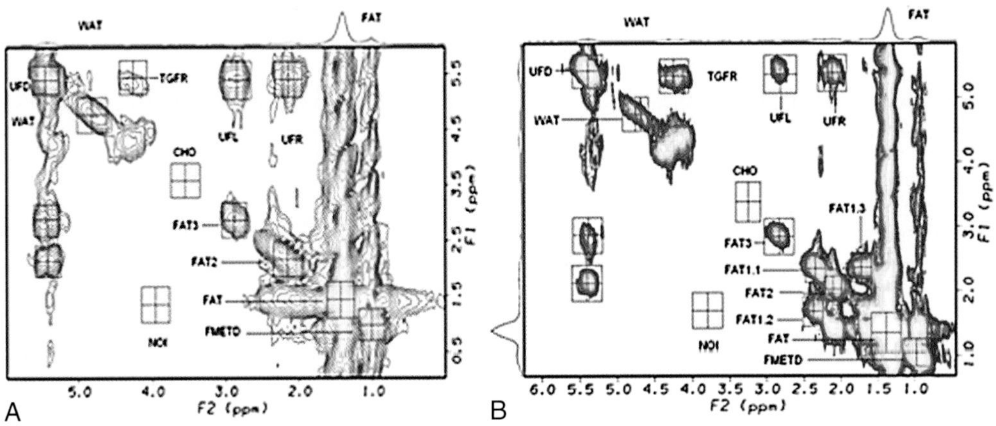

■ **FIGURE 43-6** **A,** 2D L-COSY spectra recorded in fatty breast tissue in a 38-year-old healthy woman at 1.5T MRI scanner. **B,** The corresponding 2D L-COSY spectra recorded in the fatty breast tissue in the 38-year-old healthy woman at 3.0 T MRI scanner. Volume of interest (VOI) is placed on the fatty tissue and the size is 1 × 1 × 1 cm^3. In each figure, the 2D MR spectrum shows peaks due to water, saturated and unsaturated fatty acids. The rectangular boxes are the areas of volume integration. 2D L-COSY spectra were recorded using the following parameters: TR of 2 seconds, TE of 30 msec, 45 increments of Δt_1, and 8 excitations per Δt_1. Δt_1 is 1.6 msec. The raw data were acquired using 1024 complex points and 2000 Hz spectral width along the first dimension (F_2) and 625 Hz along the second dimension (F_1).

is defined as any knowledge regarding the metabolites that are part of the spectrum to be fitted. Many studies both in time and frequency domain have shown that the inclusion of prior knowledge is essential for reliable quantification.

In 2D MRS, a quantifying method that analyzes spectral contributions in both the time and frequency domains and uses prior knowledge of expected signals is called prior-knowledge fitting (ProFit) and has showed promising results.[29] ProFit was developed to perform metabolic quantification in the brain using the 2D JPRESS MRS data. In the algorithm, two specific techniques are combined, namely, linear combination of model spectra (LC-model), which provides the maximal prior-knowledge constraint, and a variable projection (VARPRO) reduces the degrees of freedom of the fit by dividing it into a linear and a nonlinear part. ProFit combines several different strategies in order to approach the global minimum.

Future research in quantifying 2D MRS of breast tissue will require developing prior-knowledge basis-sets for breast lipids and metabolites, including saturated and unsaturated lipids, Cho groups (PCh, GPC and free Cho, etc.). Optimize the algorithm to process the breast 2D COSY spectra to quantify choline, water, lipids and other metabolites in breast tissues.

HIGH FIELD MAGNETIC RESONANCE SPECTROSCOPY IN BREAST TISSUES

With the integration of 3.0T MRI technology into standard clinical practice, there is growing interest in the diagnostic performance of proton MRS at 3.0T with respect to the established magnetic field strength of 1.5T. MR spectroscopy performed using a higher magnetic field strength provides higher SNR and improved spectral dispersion. However, these gains are partially lost because of the decrease in transverse relaxation times and the increase in magnetic susceptibility effects with increasing field strength.

1D MRS has been demonstrated in breast tissue in vivo using 1.5T, 3.0T and 4.0T MRI scanners. Results have shown that MRS can detect more metabolites in higher magnetic fields. Although theoretical advantages and disadvantages of MRS at higher field strengths are well documented, studies using 2D MRS in breast tissue in vivo have been limited to 1.5T. One study by Liu and colleagues showed the difference between 1.5T and 3.0T images of healthy breast tissues.[30] Data acquisition parameters were closely matched between the two field strengths, except two parameters. As shown in Figure 43-6, at 1.5T, Δt_1=1.6 msec; at 3.0T, Δt_1=0.8 msec; the spectra width are 625 Hz and 1250 Hz along the indirect spectral dimensions at 1.5T and 3T, respectively.

2D MRS images were compared in terms of metabolite SNRs, diagonal and cross peak volumetric ratios, water and fat full width at half maximum (FWHM) resolutions at both field strengths. The SNR increased from about 8.2% to 44.3% for 11 different metabolites at 1.5T versus 3.0T. Metabolite diagonal and cross peak ratios showed no significant difference between 1.5T and 3.0T. Some previously overlapping resonances of fat acquired at 1.5T can be identified in spectra acquired at 3.0T. The spectral resolutions at 1.5T and 3.0T measured using the FWHM of fat in the direct F_2 dimension were 0.218 ± 0.047 and 0.143 ± 0.02 ppm; in the indirect F_1 dimension were 0.388 ± 0.013 ppm and 0.368 ± 0.082 ppm, respectively.

CONCLUSIONS

MRS can detect the metabolite composition of breast tissues noninvasively. 1D MRS has been used in the clinical setting to increase breast cancer detection specificity recently. 2D MRS can provide more biochemical information than 1D MRS, which has the potential to improve the accuracy and precision of breast cancer detection. Further work should focus on technological developments, such as quantitative MRS methods and high-field MR systems. With the effort of MRS research scientists, manufacturers and clinicians, MRS may become a routine noninvasive breast cancer detection method in clinics in the future.

KEY POINTS

- Magnetic resonance spectroscopy (MRS) enables a noninvasive biochemical assay to quantify saturated and unsaturated lipids and metabolites such as choline groups.
- 2D MRS facilitates unambiguous assignment of metabolite and lipid resonances in patients with malignant and benign breast cancer and in healthy women.
- 2D MRS can be easily added to a clinical MRI protocol.
- When 2D MRS is added to DCE-MRI, the overall specificity of breast cancer detection is improved more than when DCE-MRI alone is used.

SUGGESTED READINGS

Bolan PJ, Nelson MT, Yee D, Garwood M. Imaging in breast cancer: Magnetic resonance spectroscopy. *Breast Cancer Res* 2005;**7**:149-52.

Haddadin IS, McIntosh A, Meisamy S, Corum C, Styczynski Snyder AL, et al. Metabolite quantification and high-field MRS in breast cancer. *NMR Biomed* 2009;**22**:65-76.

He QH, Xu RZ, Shkarin P, Pizzorno G, Lee-French CH, Rothman DL, et al. Magnetic resonance spectroscopic imaging of tumor metabolic markers for cancer diagnosis, metabolic phenotyping, and characterization of tumor microenvironment. *Dis Markers* 2003-2004;**19**:69-94.

Miersova S, Ala-Korpela M. MR spectroscopy quantitation: a review of frequency domain methods. *NMR Biomed* 2001;**14**:247-59.

Mountford C, Lean C, Malycha P, Russell P. Proton spectroscopy provides accurate pathology on biopsy and in vivo. *J Magn Reson Imaging* 2006;**24**:459-77.

Mountford C, Ramadan S, Stanwell P, Malycha P. Proton MRS of the breast in the clinical setting. *NMR Biomed* 2009;**22**:54-64.

Sardanelli F, Fausto A, Podo F. MR Spectroscopy of the breast. *Radiol Med* 2008;**113**:56-64.

Sinha S, Sinha U. Recent advances in breast MRI and MRS. *NMR Biomed* 2009;**22**:3-16.

Thomas MA, Lipnick S, Velan SS, Liu X, Banakar S, Binesh N, et al. Investigation of breast cancer using two-dimensional MRS. *NMR Biomed* 2009;**22**:77-91.

Vanhamme L, Sundin T, Van Hecke P, Huffel V. MR spectroscopy quantitation: a review of time-domain methods. *NMR Biomed* 2001;**14**:233-46.

REFERENCES

1. Morris EA. Diagnostic breast MR imaging: current status and future directions. *Radiol Clin North Am* 2007;**45**:863-80.
2. Kuhl CK, Mielcareck P, Klaschik S, Leutner C, Wardelmann E, Gieseke J, et al. Dynamic breast MR imaging: are signal intensity time course data useful for differential diagnosis of enhancing lesions? *Radiology* 1999;**211**:101-10.
3. Kvistad KA, Rydland J, Vainio J, Smethurst HB, Lundgren S, Fjosne HE, et al. Breast lesions: evaluation with dynamic contrast-enhanced T1 weighted MR Imaging and with T2* weighted first-pass perfusion MR imaging. *Radiology* 2000;**216**:545-53.
4. Kuhl CK. Current status of breast MR imaging. Part I. Choice of technique, image interpretation, diagnostic accuracy, and transfer to clinical practice. *Radiology* 2007;**244**:356-78.
5. Mackinnon WB, Barry PA, Malycha PL, Gillett DJ, Russell P, Lean CL, et al. Fine-needle biopsy specimens of benign breast lesions distinguished from invasive cancer ex vivo with proton MR spectroscopy. *Radiology* 1997;**204**:661-6.
6. Kvistad KA, Bakken IJ, Gribbestad IS, Ehrnholm B, Lundgren S, Fjosne HE, et al. Characterization of neoplastic and normal human breast tissues with in vivo (1)H MR spectroscopy. *J Magn Reson Imaging* 1999;**10**:159-64.
7. Cecil KM, Schnall MD, Siegelman ES, Lenkinski RE. The evaluation of human breast lesions with magnetic resonance imaging and proton magnetic resonance spectroscopy. *Breast Cancer Res Treat* 2001;**68**:45-54.
8. Huang W, Fisher PR, Dulaimy K, Tudorica LA, O'Hea B, Button TM. Detection of breast malignancy: diagnostic MR protocol for improved specificity. *Radiology* 2004;**232**:585-91.
9. Thomas MA, Binesh N, Yue K, DeBruhl N. Volume localized two-dimensional correlated magnetic resonance spectroscopy of human breast cancer. *J Magn Reson Imaging* 2001;**14**:181-6.
10. Thomas MA, Wyckoff N, Yue K, DeBruh N, Banakar S, Chung HK, et al. Two-dimensional MR spectroscopic characterization of breast cancer in vivo. *Technol Cancer Res Treat* 2005;**4**:99-106.
11. Liu X, Lipnick S, Debruhl N. *Breast lesion classification by statistical analysis of features from using two dimensional MR spectroscopy*. Honolulu, Hawaii: 17th ISMRM Scientific Meeting and Exhibition; April 18-24, 2009.
12. Lipnick S, Liu X, Debruhl N, et al. Combined 2D MR Spectroscopy and Dynamic Contrast Enhanced MRI for Breast Cancer Detection. May 3-9, 2008. Abstract#592.
13. Herigault G, Zoula S, Remy C, Decorps M, Ziegler A. Multi-spin-echo J-resolved spectroscopic imaging without water suppression: application to a rat glioma at 7 T. *MAGMA* 2004;**17**:140-8.
14. Jacobs MA, Barker PB, Bottomley PA, Bhujwalla Z, Bluemke DA. Proton magnetic resonance spectroscopic imaging of human breast cancer: A preliminary study. *J Magn Reson Imaging* 2004;**19**:68-75.
15. Liu X, Verma G, Lipnick S. Multi-dimensional spectroscopic imaging of breast in vivo. Honolulu, Hawaii: International Society for Magnetic Resonance in Medicine 17th Scientific Meeting and Exhibition; April 18-24, 2009.
16. Kuperman V. *Magnetic resonance imaging physical principles and applications*. San Diego, Calif: Academic Press; 2002.
17. Moonen CT. Comparison of single-shot localization methods (STEAM and PRESS) for in vivo proton NMR spectroscopy. *NMR Biomed* 1989;**2**:201-8.
18. Kreis R. Quantitative localized 1H MR spectroscopy for clinical use. *Prog Nucl Magn Reson Spectrosc* 1997;**31**:155-95.
19. Chu DZ, Yamanashi WS, Frazer J, Hazlewood CF, Gallager HS, Boddie AW, et al. Proton NMR of human breast tumors: correlation with clinical prognostic parameters. *J Surg Oncol* 1987;**36**:1-4.
20. Ting YL, Sherr D, Degani H. Variation in energy phospholipid metabolism in normal and cancer human mammary epithelial cells. *Anticancer Res* 1996;**16**:1381-8.
21. Tse GM, Yeung DK, King AD, Cheung HS, Yang WT. In vivo proton magnetic resonance spectroscopy of breast lesions: an update. *Breast Cancer Res Treat* 2007;**104**:249-55.
22. Mountford C, Lean C, Malycha P, Russell P. Proton spectroscopy provides accurate pathology on biopsy and in vivo. *J Magn Reson Imaging* 2006;**24**:459-77.
23. Ernst RR, Bodenhausen G, Wokaun A. *Principles of NMR Spectroscopy in one and two dimensions*. Oxford: Oxford Publications; 1987: 283-357.
24. Schulte R, Lange T, Beck J, Meier D, Boesiger P. Improved two-dimensional J-resolved spectroscopy. *NMR Biomed* 2006;**19**:264-70.
25. Thomas MA, Hattori N, Umeda M, Sawada T, Naruse S. Evaluation of two dimensional L-COSY and JPRESS using a 3T MRI scanner; from phantoms to human brain in vivo. *NMR Biomed* 2003;**16**:245-51.
26. Liu X. *Multi-dimensional MR spectroscopy of breast cancer in vivo*. Ph.D. dissertation, Los Angeles: University of California; 2008.

27. Breiman, L., J.H. Friedman R.A. Olshen, and C.J. Stone, 1984. Classification and Regression mes, Wadsworth International Group, Belmont, California, pp 358.
28. Van HP, Van HS. Editorial: NMR spectroscopy quantitation. *NMR Biomed* 2001;**14**:223.
29. Schulte RF, Boesiger P. ProFit: two-dimensional prior-knowledge fitting of J-resolved spectra. *NMR Biomed* 2006;**19**:255-63.
30. Liu X, Lipnick S, Debruhl N, et al. Using two-dimensional magnetic resonance spectroscopy in breast cancer detection: comparing 3.0T versus 1.5T. Toronto, Canada: 16th ISMRM Meeting; May 3-9, 2008.

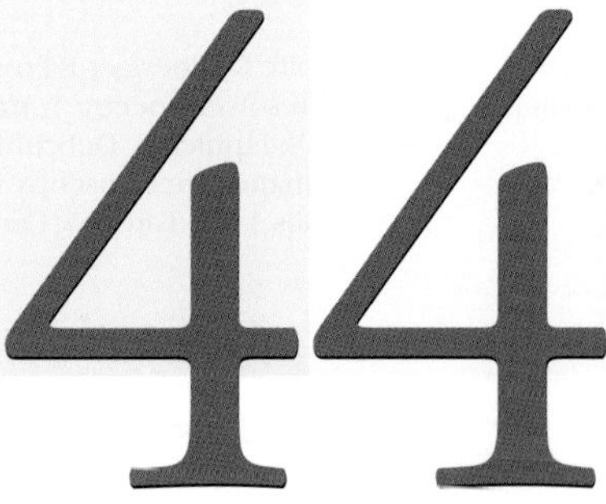
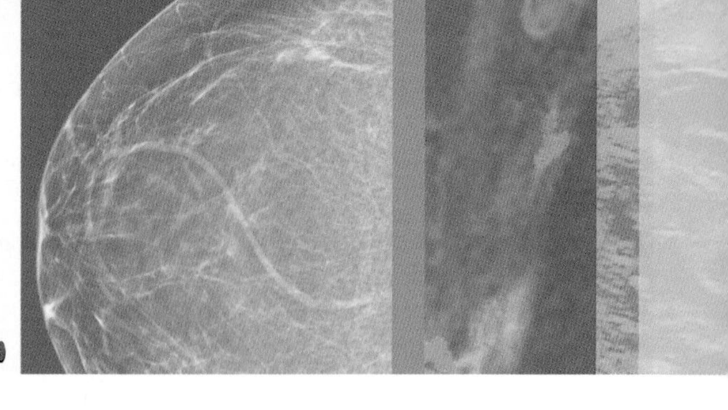

CHAPTER 44

Minimally Invasive Percutaneous Breast Cancer Ablation

Gary M. Levine and Steven P. Poplack

Widespread use of screening mammography over the past two decades has dramatically altered the clinical presentation of breast cancer. About 25% of breast carcinoma is now being discovered when still confined to the ducts (in situ) while invasive breast carcinomas are often being found when still small and non-palpable. Breast cancer is no longer a disease diagnosed through visual inspection and manual palpation; instead diagnosis now generally involves imaging. The median size of breast cancer at time of diagnosis is currently 15 mm and it has been predicted that in the near future half of all newly diagnosed breast cancers will be less than 10 mm in size.[1] This trend toward earlier diagnosis through screening has resulted in markedly improved breast cancer survival rates[2,3] (Fig.44-1).

In concert with earlier detection, there has been an evolution in the surgical management of breast carcinoma. This was prompted by the lack of a demonstrable survival difference in women with early stage breast carcinoma treated with breast conserving surgery as opposed to mastectomy.[4] The preferred surgical management of unifocal, localized breast cancer has evolved from radical mastectomy to modified radical mastectomy to partial mastectomy (lumpectomy) with radiation therapy. Similarly, less invasive sentinel node biopsy has largely replaced formal axillary node dissection.[5] This shift toward less invasive management of breast cancer has resulted in more favorable cosmetic and functional surgical outcomes. Still, even limited surgery has shortcomings, including: risk of anesthesia, margin involvement requiring re-excision, postoperative infection and morbidity, scarring with suboptimal cosmesis and the high cost associated with any visit to the operating room. In response, non-operative approaches to the local management of breast cancer have been proposed. Current research is investigating the feasibility of the percutaneous in-vivo ablation of small, unifocal invasive breast cancers with the hope of obviating the need for surgical intervention in a subset of cases.

All of the technologies being studied for ablation of benign and malignant breast tumors involve some form of thermal ablation. Extreme heat or cold is used to cause cell death. Clinical trials are studying cryoablation, radiofrequency ablation, focused ultrasound (US) ablation, laser ablation and microwave ablation. It is important to note that until now all clinical use of percutaneous tumor ablation, including for example cryoablation of liver tumors and radiofrequency ablation of bone metastases, has been intended for cancer palliation rather than for cure, as is now proposed. The goal of in-situ ablation of malignant breast tumors is to eradicate the tumor along with a margin of surrounding normal breast tissue. This is analogous to the strategy utilized in partial mastectomy.

CRYOABLATION

Cryoablation involves the in vivo freezing and devitalization of tumor tissue and has been used extensively in the treatment of benign and malignant tumors of the skin, liver, kidney and prostate. Cryoablation causes tissue necrosis through both direct and indirect means. Exposure of tissue to ultra cold temperatures results in intracellular and extracellular ice formation as well as osmotic fluid shifts, both resulting in rupture of the cellular membrane and

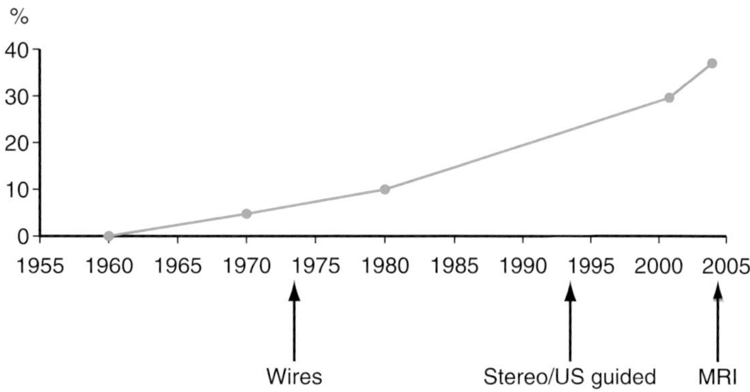

■ **FIGURE 44-1** Image detected breast cancer. Because of mammographic screening, breast cancer is increasingly being discovered when still small and nonpalpable.

cell death. Additionally, the microvasculature within the ablation zone is disrupted, resulting in vascular stasis and ischemic damage. Several studies have demonstrated that necrosis occurs reliably when tissue is exposed to temperatures of -40° C or lower.[6]

Interestingly, the use of cryoablation dates back to the mid 19th century.[7] Cryosurgery for breast cancer was first described in 1987 by Staren and colleagues.[8] In 2004, Sabel and coworkers reported on 29 patients with US visible invasive carcinomas, less than 2 cm in diameter.[9] Cryoablation successfully destroyed 100% of cancers less than 1 cm in size. For tumors between 1.0 and 1.5 cm in size 100% ablation was achieved only when there was no significant in situ component (<25%). For tumors greater than 2.0 cm in size cryoablation was not capable of complete ablation.

Either argon or liquid nitrogen are currently used as the cryogen (freezing agent) in commercially available cryoablation systems. Modern cryoprobes utilize the Joule-Thompson effect, in which gases rapidly cool or heat as they expand when going from high to low pressure. Argon, which rapidly cools at it expands, will reach –186° C at the probe tip. The cryoprobe is positioned in the center of the lesion, most commonly using direct US visualization. Time dependent or size dependant algorithms can be used to determine freezing time and ice-ball size. Generally at least one freeze-thaw-freeze cycle is utilized. Real-time US visualization of the developing ice ball can be used throughout the entire cryoablation procedure. Helium, which heats at it expands, is generally used at the conclusion of the cryoblation procedure to warm the probe and facilitate its removal from the breast.

When compared to the heat-based ablative modalities for treatment of breast lesions, cryoablation has some advantages. First, while increasing tissue temperature often causes pain both during and after heat based ablative techniques, cryoablation has an inherent, natural anesthetic effect. Generally, no additional anesthesia is required following local analgesia of the tissues to allow probe placement. Second, ice ball formation is well visualized with US, allowing the operator real time feedback of the treatment volume and the ability to inject room temperature saline between the developing ice ball and overlying skin to prevent thermal injury.

As with the other nonoperative ablation methods, there is a critical need to noninvasively determine the effectiveness of the cryoablation procedure, that is, to confirm nonviability of the malignant tissue, both at the target volume and surrounding margin. To this end, we conducted a two-site pilot study of US guided cryoablation of invasive breast carcinoma using contrast enhanced magnetic resonance imaging (CEMRI) as the non-invasive method to confirm eradication of the tumor volume (presented at the Scientific Session of 2008 International Radiological Sciences of North America Annual Meeting, November, 2008, Chicago). Based on the results from the study of Sabel and colleagues, we constrained the study population to small (≤ 15 mm) unifocal invasive ductal carcinoma without extensive ductal carcinoma in situ (DCIS). Maximum lesion size was confirmed with mammography/US and CEMRI prior to cryoablation (Fig. 44-2). A second CEMRI exam was performed about 4 weeks after cryoablation to assess for residual enhancement at or around the target lesion (Fig. 44-3). All lesions were subsequently excised surgically. Twenty subjects were accrued and post-surgical histopathology confirmed complete tumor kill within the ablation zone in every case (Fig. 44-4). In three cases (15%) unsuspected residual DCIS and/or small (<3 mm) satellite invasive lesions were discovered outside the central cryoablation zone but at the margin of the necrotic tissue and inflammatory response. Further study is needed to determine if ice-ball volume can be adjusted to ensure negative margins and if CEMRI can reliably detect residual viable tumor measuring 3 mm or less at the cryoablation margin. The American College of Surgeons Oncology Group (ACOSOG) is now beginning a National Institutes of Health (NIH)-supported multicenter clinical trial (Z1072) of percutaneous cryoablation with CEMRI confirmation based on a similar protocol.

RADIOFREQUENCY ABLATION

Radiofrequency ablation (RFA) is based on the destruction of tumor tissue with heat. A radiofrequency probe

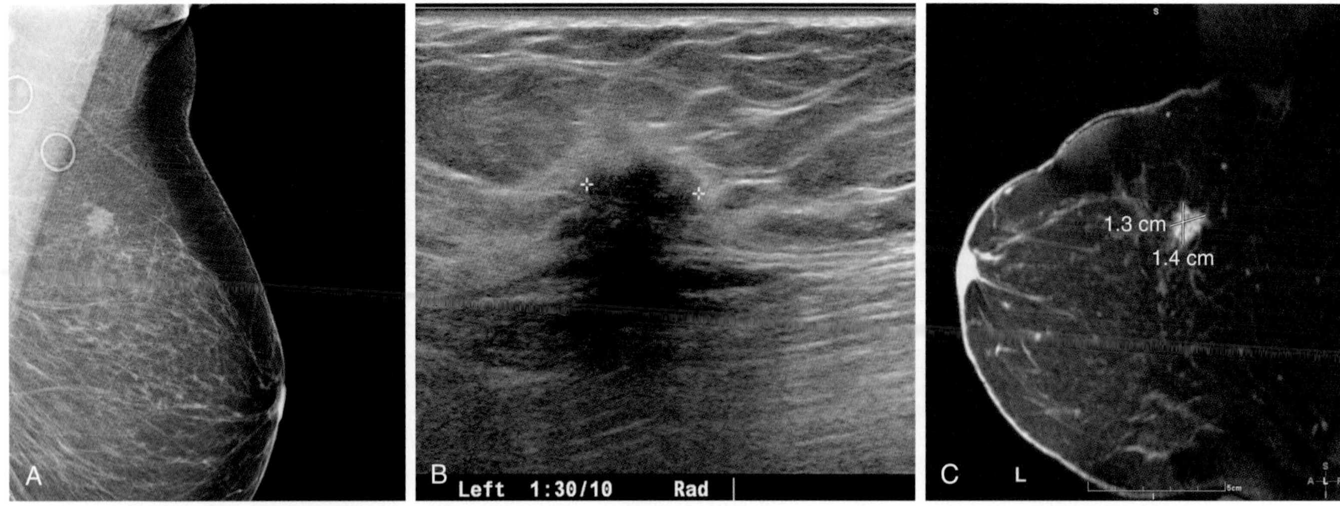

■ **FIGURE 44-2** Mammography, ultrasound (US), magnetic resonance imaging (MRI). An optimal lesion for percutaneous ablation should be small and solitary. The mammogram demonstrates a round, microlobulated mass (**A**), US of this mass shows a microlobulated hypoechoic shadowing mass with a partial echogenic collar (**B**), and contrast-enhanced MRI [(EMRI][**C**]) reveals a lobulated, homogeneously enhancing mass with a smooth margin with no associated calcifications and no evidence of in-situ disease.

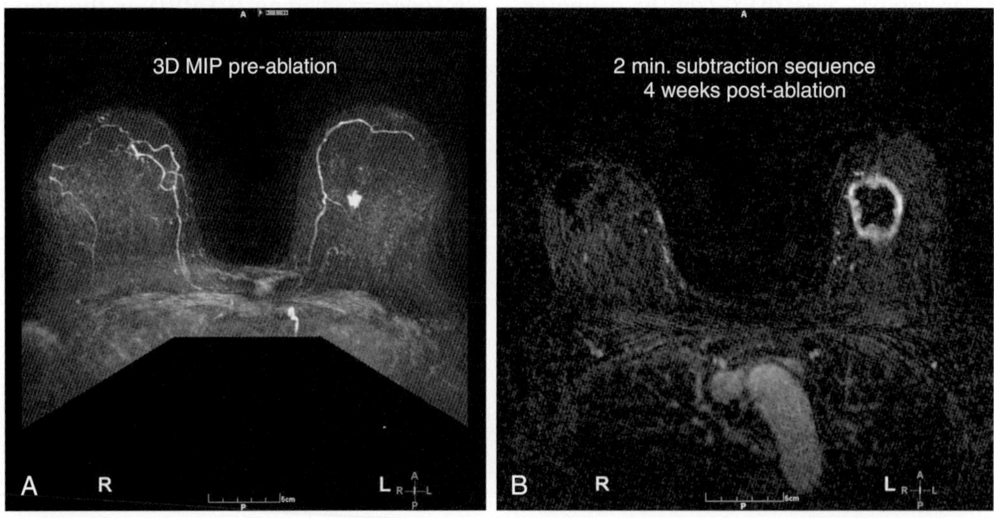

■ **FIGURE 44-3** Pre-ablation and post-ablation contrast enhanced magnetic resonance imaging (CEMRI). **A,** Pre-ablation CEMRI demonstrates a small, unifocal enhancing lesion. **B,** Post-ablation CEMRI demonstrates no residual enhancement in the cryo zone. There is a characteristic *black hole* and surrounding *cryo-halo*.

(15 gauge) is inserted percutaneously, generally using real time US for guidance. The probe is centered in the tumor and RFA electrodes are deployed from the probe tip extending throughout the tumor. An alternating high frequency electric current (400–500 kHz) is then applied. The resulting heat generated (target temperature 95° C) affects the cell membranes fluidity and the cytoskeleton proteins, eventually disrupting the nuclear structure resulting in the interruption of cell replication. Approximately 15 minutes is needed to achieve complete ablation. Temperature is monitored throughout the procedure by temperature sensors.

The first study of RFA for the treatment of breast cancer was reported by Jeffrey and coworkers in 1999.[10] Five patients with locally advanced invasive breast cancer were treated with RF ablation while under general anesthesia and just prior to standard surgical resection. Five patients with large, 4 to 7 cm breast cancers (4 of whom had undergone preoperative neoadjuvant chemotherapy) were treated with RFA. In four of the five patients complete tumor cell death was reported in a diameter of 0.8 to 1.8 cm around the probe. No complications were reported. Based on this initial limited study, several subsequent clinical trials have been undertaken.

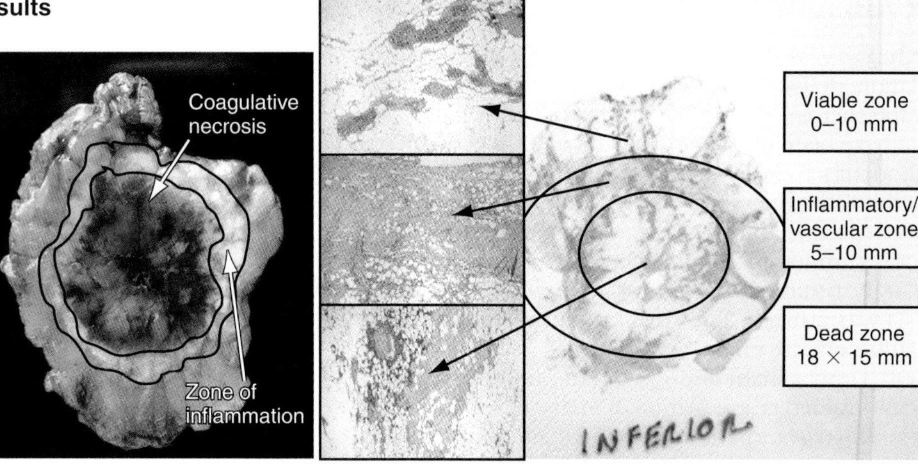
Results
• CEMRI "Black Hole" correlates with an area of coagulative necrosis at the cryoablation site
• CEMRI "Cryohalo" correlates with zone of inflammation at cryoablation margin
Coagulative necrosis
Zone of inflammation
Viable zone 0–10 mm
Inflammatory/ vascular zone 5–10 mm
Dead zone 18 × 15 mm
INFERIOR

■ **FIGURE 44-4** Gross and large section histology. Note a central zone of hemorrhagic necrosis correlating with the ablation zone. A thin yellow rim of tissue surrounding the ablation zone represents a zone of inflammatory infiltrate. CEMRI, contrast-enhanced magnetic resonance imaging.

Burak and colleagues in 2003[11] utilized pre-ablation and post-ablation MRI imaging to assess the efficacy of RF ablation in 10 women with breast cancer. All tumors were resected 1 to 3 weeks following the percutaneous ablation. On pre-ablation MRI, 90% of the lesions demonstrated contrast enhancement. Following ablation, 89% of lesions demonstrated no residual contrast enhancement. The single patient with residual enhancement at the treatment site indeed had residual disease at histology at the time of resection. It was suggested that MRI may represent a noninvasive method for evaluating the effectiveness of the ablation.

Hayashi et al in 2003[12] treated 22 patients with clinically T1N0 (tumor less than 2 cm, no lymph node involvement) breast carcinomas with US guided RFA with surgical resection 1 to 2 weeks later. Residual viable tumor was found in 5 of the 22 patients, all at a distance from the ablation zone.

Fornage and colleagues reported in 2004 on 20 patients with 21 lesions who were treated with RFA immediately before their scheduled lumpectomy or total mastectomy.[13] In all 21 cases complete ablation of the targeted tissue was noted at ultrasound. In one patient who had undergone preoperative chemotherapy the target lesion was ablated successfully but residual mammographically and sonographically occult tumor was found histologically in an area of 4 cm around the targeted lesion.

Finally, in 2008, Van den Bosch and colleagues reported on three patients treated with MRI guided RF ablation.[14] Magnetic resonance imaging (MRI) thermometry and contrast-enhanced post-ablation MRI were used to evaluate the ablation process. Patients underwent lumpectomy within 1 week of the ablation procedure. Histopathology confirmed 100% tumor ablation in one patient and only partial tumor ablation (33% and 50%) in two patients.

RFA is a promising technology for the in-situ treatment of breast cancer and warrants further investigation. A known limitation to the technique relates to the discomfort caused by the heating of breast tissue, at times dictating the use of general anesthesia. Additionally, the risk of thermal burn to the skin limits the treatment of superficial lesions.

HIGH-INTENSITY FOCUSED ULTRASOUND ABLATION

High-intensity focused ultrasound ablation (HIFU) uses focused US waves to rapidly heat local tissues up to 90° C, thereby achieving tissue necrosis. It is a truly non-invasive method of ablation as no probe is inserted into the breast and therefore no skin incision is required. In HIFU acoustic energy is converted to heat resulting in coagulative necrosis at the ablation site. Additionally, tumor vessels are damaged within the ablation zone, resulting in vascular disruption and vessel occlusion. HIFU utilizes a 1.5 MHz US source. Treatment time varies based on the volume of the tumor and the number of sonications required to treat the lesion. The procedure is monitored using skin monitors and temperature probes. The method has been used to ablate benign fibroadenomas and early studies report ablation of breast carcinoma.

In 2003, Gianfelice and colleagues[15] reported on 12 patients with invasive breast carcinoma treated with MRI guided focused US ablation. In three patients treated with an initial US system a mean of only 46.7% of the tumor was within the targeted zone and 43.3% of the cancer tissue was destroyed. An additional nine patients were treated with a second US system and a mean of 95.6% of the tumor was within the targeted zone and 88.3% of the malignant tissue was destroyed. Two patients suffered second degree skin burns.

Wu and colleagues in 2003[16] completed the largest study of focused US ablation of breast carcinomas. Forty-eight women were randomized into either total mastectomy or focused US ablation followed by total mastectomy 2 weeks later. Tumor cells within the ablation zone were reported to undergo complete coagulative necrosis. Patients reported transitory edema with spontaneous resolution 7 to 10 days later. No severe side effects were reported.

The major advantage of focused US ablation is that no skin incision is required. Patients do experience some discomfort during and after the procedure. Early results suggest that superficial tumors may be incompletely treated and there is the risk of thermal burn to the skin.

LASER ABLATION

Another heat-based thermal ablation technique, interstitial laser ablation, delivers laser energy to a tumor via a fiber-optic probe that is inserted under imaging guidance. Laser types that have been utilized include the YAG laser, semiconductor diode laser and argon laser. Laser ablation has been performed utilizing mammography, US and MRI guidance.

Harms treated 12 localized breast cancer patients using laser therapy under MRI guidance.[17] For tumors less than 3 cm in size, tumor ablation was complete. Only local anesthesia was utilized. The MRI findings were correlated with ablation effectiveness.

In 2000, Dowlatshahi and coworkers reported on stereotactically guided laser ablation of image detected breast tumors.[18] Thirty-six patients with mammographically detected well-defined breast tumors were treated using a 16 to 18 gauge laser probe. A multi-sensor thermal probe was inserted into the breast and positioned adjacent to the laser probe. Patients required light sedation administered by an anesthesiologist during the procedure. Complete tumor ablation was noted in 66% of patients who underwent surgical excision 1 to 8 weeks post-ablation. Minor skin burns were reported in two patients.

CONCLUSION

In selected "early breast cancers," minimally invasive percutaneous tumor ablation may prove to have the same therapeutic benefit as lumpectomy, but with less morbidity, improved cosmesis and less cost to society. The goal of in-situ ablation techniques is to kill the targeted breast tumor along with a margin of surrounding normal breast tissue. This is analogous to the strategy utilized in surgical lumpectomy. Percutaneous ablation may be especially suitable for an elderly patient, a patient with multiple comorbidities or a patient who is not a surgical candidate. However, for any of these minimally invasive ablative technologies to be adopted more widely they must first prove to be at least as efficacious as traditional surgical excision with pathology proven negative surgical margins.

Two additional obstacles need to be overcome. First, an imaging technology needs to be identified that is accurate in predicting complete tumor kill and which is able to identify any residual viable tumor present post-ablation. This could then serve as an imaging surrogate for histologic negative margins. Second, a percutaneous image guided method of sentinel node biopsy needs to be developed; otherwise the patient will still require operative intervention.

KEY POINTS

- Use of routine screening mammography has resulted in the earlier diagnosis of breast cancer.
- In selected "early breast cancers," minimally invasive percutaneous tumor ablation may prove to have the same therapeutic benefit as lumpectomy, but with less morbidity, improved cosmesis and less cost to society.
- Technologies currently being studied for percutaneous breast cancer ablation involve the application of extreme heat or cold to the tumor.
- For percutaneous ablation to gain wide acceptance, an imaging technology needs to be identified that can serve as an imaging surrogate for histologic negative margins.

SUGGESTED READINGS

Sabel MS, Edge SB. In-situ ablation of breast cancer. *Breast Dis* 2001; **12**:131-40.

Vlastos G, Verkooijen HM. Minimally invasive approaches for diagnosis and treatment of early-stage breast cancer. *Oncologist* 2007;**12**:1-10.

REFERENCES

1. Cady B, Stone MD, Schuler JG, Thakur R, Wanner MA, Lavin PT. The new era in breast cancer: invasion, size and nodal involvement dramatically decreasing as a result of mammographic screening. *Arch Surg* 1996;**131**:301-8.
2. Tabar L, Yen M, Vitak B, Chen HH, Smith RA, Duffy SW. Mammography service screening and mortality in breast cancer patients: 20 year follow-up before and after introduction of screening. *Lancet* 2003;**361**:1405-10.
3. Jatoi I, Chen BE, Anderson WF, Rosenberg PS. Breast cancer mortality trends in the United States according to estrogen receptor status and age at diagnosis. *J Clin Oncology* 2007;**25**:1683-90.
4. Fisher B, Redmond C, Poisson R, Margolese R, Wolmark N, Wickerham L, et al. Eight year results of a randomized clinical trial comparing total mastectomy and lumpectomy with or without irradiation in the treatment of breast cancer. *N Engl J Med* 1989;**320**:822-8.
5. Silverstein MJ, Recht A, Lagios MD, Levine GM, et al. "Image-detected breast cancer: state-of-the- art diagnosis and treatment." *J Am Coll Surg* 2009;**209**:504-520.
6. Farrant J, Walter CA. The cryobiological basis for cryosurgery. *J Dermatol Surg Oncol* 1977;**3**:403-407.
7. Arnott J. Practical illustrations of the remedial efficacy of a very low or anesthetic temperature. *Lancet* 1850;**(Vol. 56 No. 1409)**:257-9.
8. Staren E, Sabel M, Gianakakis LM, Wiener GA, Hart VM, Gorski M, et al. Cryosurgery of breast cancer. *Arch Surg* 1997;**132**:28-33.
9. Sabel M, Kaufman C, Whitworth P, Chang H, Stocks LH, Simmons R, et al. Cryoablation of early-stage breast cancer: work in progress report of a multi-institutional trial. *Ann Surg Oncol* 2004;**11**:542-9.
10. Jeffrey S, Birdwell R, Ikeda DM, Daniel BL, Nowels KW, Dirbas FM, et al. Radiofrequency ablation of breast cancer: first report of an emerging technology. *Arch Surg* 1999;**134**:1064-8.
11. Burak Jr WE, Agnese DM, Povoski SP, Yanssens TL, Bloom KJ, Wakely PE, et al. Radiofrequency ablation of invasive breast carcinoma followed by delayed surgical excision. *Cancer* 2003;**98**:1369-76.
12. Hayashi AH, Silver SF, van der Westhuizen NG, Donald JC, Parker C, Fraser S, et al. Treatment of invasive breast carcinoma with ultrasound guided radiofrequency ablation. *Am J Surg* 2003;**185**:429-35.
13. Fornage B, Sneige N, Ross MI, Mirza AN, Kuerer HM, Edeiken BS, et al. Small (< or = 2-cm) breast cancer treated with US guided radiofrequency ablation: feasibility study. *Radiology* 2004;**231**:215-24.
14. Van den Bosch M, Daniel B, Rieke V, Butts-Pauly K, Kermit E, Jeffrey S. MRI-guided radiofrequency ablation of breast cancer: preliminary clinical experience. *J Magn Reson Imaging* 2008;**27**:204-8.
15 Gianfelice D, Khiat A, Amara M, Belblidia A, Boulanger Y. MR imaging-guided focused US ablation of breast cancer: Histopathologic assessment of effectiveness–initial experience. *Radiology* 2003;**227**:849-55.
16. Wu F, Wang ZB, Cao YD, Chen WZ, Bai J, Zou JZ, et al. A randomised clinical trial of high-intensity focused ultrasound ablation for the treatment of patients with localised breast cancer. *Br J Cancer* 2003;**89**:2227-33.
17. Harms SE. MR guided minimally invasive procedures. *Magn Reson Imaging Clin N Amer* 2001;**9**:381-92.
18. Dowlatshahi K, Fan M, Gould VE, Bloom KJ, Ali A. Stereotactically guided laser therapy of occult breast tumors: work-in-progress report. *Arch Surg* 2000;**135**:1345-52.

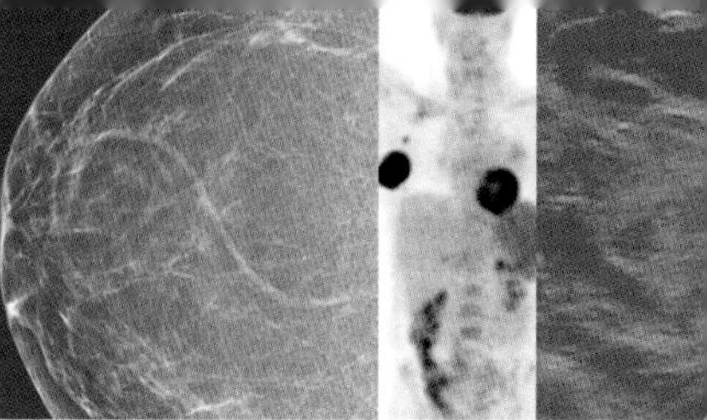

Index

Note: Page numbers followed by "*f*" indicate figures, "*t*" indicate tables, and "*b*" indicate boxes.

A

AAFP (American Academy of Family Physicians), on screening, 62
Abandonment, 735
Aberrations of normal development and involution (ANDIs), 168–171
Abscess, 379
  mammography of, 376, 377f
  pathology findings in, 379–380, 381*f*, 382*f*
  subareolar, 377*f*, 379–380, 382*f*
  ultrasonography of, 376–378, 379*f*, 380*f*, 381*f*
Absolute risk, 39–40
AC. *See* Appropriateness Criteria (AC).
Acceleration factor, in MRI, 189
Acceptance testing, for mammography equipment, 96–97
Accreditation
  ACR program of, 696–700
  application for, 697–698, 697*f*
  clinical images in, 699
  denial of, 698, 698*t*
  final reports on, 698
  for full-field digital mammography, 698–699
  Mammography Quality Standards Act on, 693, 694
  of new units, 698
  pass rate for, 700, 700*f*
  phantom image in, 699, 699*t*
  quality control in, 699
  radiation dose in, 699
  renewal of, 698
  validation procedures in, 699–700
    annual updates as, 699
    on-site surveys as, 699–700
    validation film checks as, 699
Accrediting body
  ACR as, 697
  Mammography Quality Standards Act on, 693, 694
Acini
  anatomy of, 224*f*
  histology of, 226*f*
ACOG (American College of Obstetricians and Gynecologists), on screening, 62
ACoS (American College of Surgeons), on screening, 62
ACP (American College of Physicians), on screening, 62
ACPM (American College of Preventive Medicine), on screening, 62
Acquisition console, 91, 92*f*
Acquisition workstation (AW), for mammography, 91, 91*f*, 92*f*
ACR. *See* American College of Radiology (ACR).
ACRIN DMIST (American College of Radiology Imaging Network Digital Mammography In Screening Trial), 732
ACS (American Cancer Society)
  on cancer statistics, 25
  on screening, 62
Actions for demurer, 729
ACUSON S2000 system, for automated whole breast ultrasound, 752–753, 753*f*
Adenoid cystic carcinoma, 453–455, 454*f*, 455*f*
  cribriform DCIS *vs.*, 401–402, 402*f*
Adenoma(s)
  apocrine, 276
  fibro- (*See* Fibroadenoma)
  lactating, 274–276
    clinical presentation of, 274
    defined, 274
    etiology and pathophysiology of, 274
    imaging indications and algorithm for, 274
    mammography of, 274
    MRI of, 274
    pathology findings with, 274–276, 276*f*, 277*f*
    prevalence and epidemiology of, 274
    treatment options for, 276
    ultrasonography of, 274, 275*f*
  nipple, 297–298, 409
    classic signs of, 297
    clinical presentation of, 297
    defined, 297
    etiology and pathophysiology of, 297
    imaging indications and algorithm for, 297
    mammography of, 297
    MRI of, 297
    pathology findings with, 297–298, 297*f*, 298*f*, 409, 409*f*
    prevalence and epidemiology of, 297
    treatment options for, 298
    ultrasonography of, 297
  tubular, 274–276
    clinical presentation of, 274
    defined, 274
    etiology and pathophysiology of, 274
    imaging indications and algorithm for, 274
    mammography of, 274
    MRI of, 274
Adenoma(s) *(Continued)*
    pathology findings with, 274, 275*f*
    prevalence and epidemiology of, 274
    treatment options for, 276
    ultrasonography of, 274, 275*f*
Adenomyoepithelioma, 295–297
  classic signs of, 295
  clinical presentation of, 295
  defined, 295
  etiology and pathophysiology of, 295
  imaging indications and algorithm for, 295
  mammography of, 295
  MRI of, 295
  pathology findings with, 295–296, 296*f*
  prevalence and epidemiology of, 295
  treatment options for, 296–297
  ultrasonography of, 295
Adenopathy. *See* Lymphadenopathy.
Adenosis, 274–276
  apocrine adenoma in, 276
  clinical presentation of, 274
  defined, 274
  etiology and pathophysiology of, 274
  imaging indications and algorithm for, 274
  lactating adenoma in, 274–276, 276*f*, 277*f*
  mammography of, 274
  microglandular, 318–319
    atypical, 318–319, 320*f*, 321*f*
    clinical presentation of, 318
    defined, 318
    etiology and pathophysiology of, 318
    imaging technique and findings with, 318–319
    pathology findings with, 318–319, 319*f*, 320*f*
    prevalence and epidemiology of, 318
    treatment options for, 319
  MRI of, 274
  pathology findings with, 274–276
  prevalence and epidemiology of, 274
  sclerosing, 300–304
    classic signs of, 302
    clinical presentation of, 300
    DCIS with
      mammography of, 395f
      microscopic findings in, 403–404, 407*f*, 408*f*
    defined, 300
    differential diagnosis of, 302–304
    etiology and pathophysiology of, 300

Adenoma(s) *(Continued)*
false positive core needle biopsy due to, 616-617, 616*f*
imaging indications and algorithm for, 300
mammography of, 300, 301*f*, 302*f*
MRI of, 302
nodular, 302-303
pathology findings with, 302-304, 302*f*, 303*f*
post-biopsy management of, 641-642, 643*f*
prevalence and epidemiology of, 300
ultrasonography of, 302
treatment options for, 276
tubular adenoma in, 274, 275*f*
ultrasonography of, 274, 275*f*
Adenosis tumor, 302-303
ADH. *See* Atypical ductal hyperplasia (ADH).
Administrative issues, in liability, 732-733
Admissions, legal, 736
"Advance Beneficiary Notice", 724
AEC. *See* Automatic exposure control (AEC).
African-American women
incidence of breast cancer in, 33-34, 33*f*
mortality rate in, 38, 39*f*
stage of diagnosis in, 34, 35, 35*f*, 36*f*
and survival rate, 35, 36*f*
tumor characteristics in, 35-37
tumor size in, 34, 34*f*
Age
incidence of breast cancer and, 32-33, 32*f*
as prognostic and predictive factor, 231
Age standardized rate, of breast cancer, 26-29
international comparisons of, 26, 26*f*, 27*f*, 28*f*
Age-adjusted rate, of breast cancer, 26-29
international comparisons of, 26, 26*f*, 27*f*, 28*f*
Agency, legal aspects of, 735
Agency for Health Care Policy and Research (AHCPR), on goals for screening mammography, 710*t*, 711
Air gap technique, in stereotactic-guided core needle biopsy, 582-583
Alaskan natives, incidence of breast cancer in, 33-34, 33*f*
Alcohol consumption, and breast cancer risk, 42-43
ALH. *See* Atypical lobular hyperplasia (ALH)
Allred Score, 626-627, 627*f*
Alternative school of thought doctrine, 730, 732, 737
Alveolar cell variant, of invasive lobular carcinoma, 491-493, 492*f*
AMA (American Medical Association), on screening, 62
Ambulatory Payment Classifications (APCs), 721
American Academy of Family Physicians (AAFP), on screening, 62
American Cancer Society (ACS)
on cancer statistics, 25
on screening, 62
American College of Obstetricians and Gynecologists (ACOG), on screening, 62
American College of Physicians (ACP), on screening, 62
American College of Preventive Medicine (ACPM), on screening, 62
American College of Radiology (ACR)
accreditation program of, 696-700
Appropriateness Criteria of, 539-541
background of, 539-540
current guidelines for, 540
defined, 539
discussion of, 540
methodology of, 540
purpose of, 539
and radiology benefits managers, 540
American College of Radiology (ACR) *(Continued)*
required attributes of, 539
underutilization by referring physicians of, 540
BI-RADS by (*See* Breast Imaging, Reporting, and Data System (BI-RADS))
on medical audit, 703
on quality control, 133-134, 144
on screening, 62
American College of Radiology Imaging Network Digital Mammography In Screening Trial (ACRIN DMIST), 732
American College of Surgeons (ACoS), on screening, 62
American Indians
incidence of breast cancer in, 33-34, 33*f*
mortality rate in, 39*f*
American Medical Association (AMA), on screening, 62
AMF (anterior mammary fascia), ultrasound of, 168-171, 170*f*, 171*f*
A-mode ultrasound technology, 13, 14*f*
Ampulla, 224*f*
Analytic epidemiology, 25
Anatomy, of breast
mammographic, 111, 224-226, 224*f*
ultrasonographic, 226, 228*f*
ANDIs (aberrations of normal development and involution), 168-171
Androgen deficiency, gynecomastia due to, 314*t*
Anesthesia, for core needle biopsy
MRI-guided, 590-591
epinephrine with, 591
expected route of, 591
injection site for, 591
minimizing pain of, 591
stereotactic-guided
epinephrine with, 581
injection tract of, 581
local, 581
site of, 581
topical, 581
ultrasound-guided
epinephrine with, 568-569
injection site for, 569, 569*f*
local, 568-569
topical, 569
Angiolipoma, 271*f*
Angiosarcoma
etiology of, 511
pathology of, 511, 512*f*
primary
mammography of, 509
MRI of, 509
prognosis of, 511
secondary
mammography of, 509
MRI of, 509
ultrasonography of, 509
Angled lateromedial (LM) view, 115-116
Angled mediolateral (ML) view, 115-116, 116*f*
Annual updates, in accreditation, 699
Anterior mammary fascia (AMF), ultrasound of, 168-171, 170*f*, 171*f*
Antiperspirant, calcifications due to, 325-326, 327*f*
Antiscatter grid assembly, 88-89, 88*f*
APCs (Ambulatory Payment Classifications), 721
Apocrine adenoma, 276
Apocrine carcinoma, 461-462, 462*f*
Apocrine metaplasia
calcifications with, 342*f*, 343*f*
columnar cell lesions with, 356, 358*f*
Apocrine-type DCIS, 402, 405*f*
Appellate courts, 730
Appropriateness Criteria (AC), of American College of Radiology, 539-541
background of, 539-540
current guidelines for, 540
defined, 539
discussion of, 540
methodology of, 540
purpose of, 539
and radiology benefits managers, 540
required attributes of, 539
underutilization by referring physicians of, 540
Architectural distortion
defined, [illegible]
in invasive ductal carcinoma, 432-434, 434*f*, 435*f*
spot compression view of, 432, 434*f*, 435*f*
after reduction mammoplasty, 685, 685*f*, 686-688, 686*f*
due to scar
postoperative, 434
radial, 434
Areola, anatomy of, 224*f*
Arterial calcifications, 327, 330*f*
Arthritis, rheumatoid, gold deposits in, 261, 262*f*
Artifact(s)
evaluation of
clinical image, 125-126, 128*f*, 129*f*
for quality control, 138*t*, 142-143
in mammography
full-field digital, 125, 128*f*
screen-film, 126, 129*f*
on MRI, 189-192
chemical shift, 190-191
due to fat saturation errors, 189-190, 190*f*
due to magnet and coil inhomogeneities, 190, 191*f*
due to metallic clips, 191-192, 191*f*
due to missed uptake of gadolinium contrast, 190
motion and misregistration, 189, 190*f*
reverberation, in ultrasonography of breast implants, 674, 677*f*
Asian-American women, incidence of breast cancer in, 33-34, 33*f*
Aspiration, of cyst, in ultrasound-guided core needle biopsy, 574
Assessment, BI-RADS on, 216-217
Associated findings, on ultrasonography, 218
Asymmetry(ies)
in axilla, 435, 437*f*
BI-RADS on, 215
defined, 215, 434
developing, 215
in invasive ductal carcinoma, 431-432, 433*f*, 434*f*
focal, 215, 434
global, 215, 434
in invasive ductal carcinoma
clinical presentation of, 425
developing, 431-432, 433*f*, 434*f*
mammography of, 434-435, 436*f*, 437*f*
vs. mass, 215
after reduction mammoplasty, 686-688
AT (axillary tail) view, 117-118, 119*f*
Ataxia-telangiectasia (AT), and breast cancer risk, 48
Ataxia-telangiectasia mutation *(ATM)* gene, and breast cancer risk, 48
Atypical ductal hyperplasia (ADH), 357-360
clinical presentation of, 358
vs. DCIS, 360, 361*f*, 415, 638, 639*f*

Atypical ductal hyperplasia (ADH) *(Continued)*
defined, 357
differential diagnosis of, 360
etiology and pathophysiology of, 358
imaging indications and algorithm for, 358–359
mammography of, 359, 359*f*
MRI of, 360
pathology findings with, 360, 361*f*, 362*f*
post-biopsy management of, 637–638, 639*f*
prevalence and epidemiology of, 358
treatment options for, 360
ultrasonography of, 360
Atypical hyperplasia, 226–228
Atypical lobular hyperplasia (ALH), 360–366
classic signs of, 361
clinical presentation of, 360
defined, 360
differential diagnosis of, 361–364
etiology and pathophysiology of, 360
mammography of, 361
MRI of, 361
pathology findings with, 362–364, 362*f*
post-biopsy management of, 640–641
prevalence and epidemiology of, 360
treatment options for, 365–366
ultrasonography of, 361
Audit, BI-RADS on, 217
Audit interpreting physician, in quality control, 134*t*
Augmented breast. *See* Breast augmentation; Breast implant(s).
Automated whole breast ultrasound (AWBU), 751–753
ACUSON S2000 system for, 752–753, 753*f*
digital tomosynthesis with, 752–753, 755*f*
history of, 751–752, 752*f*
SomoVu system for, 752–753, 753*f*
SonoCine system for, 752–753, 753*f*
TechniScan system for, 752–753, 754*f*
Automatic exposure control (AEC)
history of, 10
performance assessment of, 138*t*, 142
quality control test of, 139*t*
for reproducibility, 138*t*, 143
system for, 81, 89–90, 89*f*
Automatic film processor, 10–11, 11*f*, 80
Average glandular dose, quality control test of, 138*t*, 143
AW (acquisition workstation), for mammography, 91, 91*f*, 92*f*
AWBU. *See* Automated whole breast ultrasound (AWBU)
Axilla, asymmetrical breast tissue in, 435, 437*f*
Axillary adenopathy. *See* Axillary lymphadenopathy.
Axillary breast tissue, 224, 226, 227*f*
Axillary lymph node(s)
levels of, 467
MRI of, 199, 200*f*
ultrasound of, 165–166, 165*f*
Axillary lymph node metastases, 467
of DCIS, 411–415
vs. benign inclusion, 414*f*
vs. dendritic cells, 413*f*
vs. histiocyte aggregates, 412*f*
vs. intracapsular nevus, 413*f*
vs. nonspecific debris, 413*f*
of invasive ductal carcinoma, 429–431, 431*f*
calcified, 432*f*
and survival, 442–445, 445*t*, 467, 468*t*
tumor size and, 467, 468*t*
Axillary lymph node status, as prognostic and predictive factor, 231
Axillary lymphadenopathy
bilateral, 546
differential diagnosis of, 429–431
in invasive ductal carcinoma, 425
MRI of, 199, 200*f*
unilateral, 546
workup for, 546, 546*f*
Axillary sentinel lymph node biopsy, 623–625
isolated tumor cells in, 624–625, 625*f*
macrometastatic disease in, 624–625
micrometastatic disease in, 624–625, 625*f*
protocol for, 623–625, 624*f*
radiation therapy after positive, 625
Axillary tail (AT) view, 117–118, 119*f*

B

Background enhancement, on MRI, 218
Bailer, John C., III, 21
Basal-like DCIS, 403–404
Basophilic calcifications, 333–334, 341*f*, 342*f*
Batch reading, 66
Battery, 735
BCDDP (Breast Cancer Detection Demonstration Project), 16, 44, 56, 57
B-cell lymphoma, diffuse large
case study of, 520*b*
commentary in, 523
diagnosis in, 522
differential diagnosis in, 522, 523*f*
excisional biopsy in, 521, 522*f*
fine-needle aspiration findings in, 521, 521*f*
history in, 520
immunohistochemical stains in, 521
mammography in, 520, 520*f*
ultrasonography in, 520, 521*f*
differential diagnosis of, 502–503, 504*f*, 523*f*
pathology of, 502–503, 503*f*
prevalence and epidemiology of, 502
BCSC (Breast Cancer Surveillance Consortium)
on goals for screening mammography, 710*t*, 711, 712*t*
recall rates at, 66–67
Beam limitation, quality control test of, 139*t*
Beam quality assessment, 138*t*, 143
Benchmark data, 711, 712*t*
Benefits Improvement and Protection Act (BIPA), 721
Benign lesion(s)
cystic, 239–254
case study of, 250*b*
core needle biopsy in, 250, 253*f*
diagnosis in, 250
differential diagnosis in, 250
findings in, 250, 251*f*
fine needle aspiration in, 250, 252*f*
impression in, 250
patient history in, 250
duct ectasia as, 244–247
classic signs of, 245
clinical presentation of, 245
defined, 244
differential diagnosis of, 245–246, 247*f*
etiology and pathophysiology of, 244
imaging indications and algorithm for, 245
mammography of, 245, 246*f*
MRI of, 245
pathology of, 245–246, 247*f*
prevalence and epidemiology of, 244
treatment options for, 246–247
ultrasonography of, 245, 246*f*
epidermal inclusion cysts and sebaceous cysts as, 239–241
Benign lesion(s) *(Continued)*
clinical presentation of, 239
defined, 239, 240*f*
differential diagnosis of, 240–241, 242*f*, 243*f*
etiology and pathophysiology of, 239
imaging indications and algorithm for, 239
mammography of, 240, 241*f*
MRI of, 240
pathology of, 241, 242*f*, 243*f*
prevalence and epidemiology of, 239
treatment options for, 241
ultrasonography of, 240, 241*f*, 242*f*
fibrocystic change as, 247–249
and breast cancer risk, 247–248, 248*b*
clinical presentation of, 248–249
defined, 247
differential diagnosis of, 249
etiology and pathophysiology of, 248
imaging indications and algorithm for, 249
imaging technique and findings for, 249
pathology of, 248*f*, 249, 249*f*
prevalence and epidemiology of, 247–248, 248*b*
treatment options for, 249
galactocele as, 241–244
classic signs of, 244
clinical presentation of, 242–244
defined, 241
differential diagnosis of, 244, 245*f*
etiology and pathophysiology of, 242
imaging indications and algorithm for, 242
mammography of, 242–243, 243*f*
MRI of, 244
pathology of, 244, 245*f*
prevalence and epidemiology of, 241
treatment options for, 244
ultrasonography of, 243, 244*f*
high-risk, 349–372
atypical ductal hyperplasia as, 357–360
clinical presentation of, 358
defined, 357
differential diagnosis of, 360
etiology and pathophysiology of, 358
imaging indications and algorithm for, 358–359
mammography of, 359, 359*f*
MRI of, 360
pathology findings with, 360, 361*f*, 362*f*
prevalence and epidemiology of, 358
treatment options for, 360
ultrasonography of, 360
case study of, 370*b*
diagnosis in, 372, 372*f*, 373*f*
differential diagnosis in, 371
findings in, 370–371, 370*f*, 371*f*
history in, 370
flat epithelial atypia as, 355–357
and apocrine metaplasia, 356, 358*f*
with calcifications, 356, 357*f*
classic signs of, 356
clinical presentation of, 355
columnar cell change with, 356, 356*f*
columnar cell hyperplasia with, 356, 357*f*
cytologic atypia in, 356–357, 358*f*, 359*f*
defined, 355
differential diagnosis of, 356–357
etiology and pathophysiology of, 355
imaging indications and algorithm for, 355
mammography of, 355, 355*f*

Benign lesion(s) *(Continued)*
MRI of, 356
pathology findings with, 356-357
prevalence and epidemiology of, 355
treatment options for, 357
ultrasonography of, 355
lobular neoplasia as, 360-366
classic signs of, 361
clinical presentation of, 360
defined, 360
differential diagnosis of, 361-364
etiology and pathophysiology of, 360
mammography of, 361
MRI of, 361
pathology findings with, 362-364, 362*f*, 363*f*
prevalence and epidemiology of, 360
treatment options for, 365-366
ultrasonography of, 361
variants of, 364-365, 364*f*, 365*f*
papillary, 349-355
atypical papilloma as, 352-353, 354*f*
classic signs of, 351
clinical presentation of, 349
defined, 349
differential diagnosis of, 352-353
etiology and pathophysiology of, 349
imaging indications and algorithm for, 349
intraductal papilloma as, 352, 352*f*, 353*f*
mammography of, 349-351, 350*f*, 351*f*
MRI of, 351, 352*f*
papillomatosis as, 352, 353*f*
pathology findings with, 352-353
prevalence and epidemiology of, 349
treatment options for, 353-355
ultrasonography of, 351, 351*f*
phyllodes tumor as, 366-372
classic signs of, 367
clinical presentation of, 366
defined, 366
differential diagnosis of, 367-369
etiology and pathophysiology of, 366
imaging indications and algorithm for, 366
mammography of, 366, 366*f*
MRI of, 366-367
pathology findings with, 367-369, 368*f*
prevalence and epidemiology of, 366
treatment options for, 369-372
ultrasonography of, 366
infectious and inflammatory, 375-388
with abscess, 379
mammography of, 376, 377*f*
pathology findings in, 379-380, 381*f*, 382*f*
subareolar, 377*f*, 379-380, 382*f*
ultrasonography of, 376-378, 379*f*, 380*f*, 381*f*
case study on, 386*b*
commentary in, 388
diagnosis in, 388
differential diagnosis in, 386
findings in, 386, 386*f*, 387*f*
history in, 386
classic signs of, 379
clinical presentation of, 375
due to coccidioidomycosis, 380-381, 384*f*
defined, 375
differential diagnosis of, 379-385
due to echinococcosis, 380-381, 383*f*
etiology and pathophysiology of, 375
due to filariasis, 386*b*
commentary on, 388
diagnosis of, 388

Benign lesion(s) *(Continued)*
differential diagnosis of, 386
findings with, 386, 386*f*, 387*f*
history of, 386
granulomatous
mammography of, 376, 378*f*
pathology findings with, 380-381, 381*f*
imaging indications and algorithm for, 375-376
mammography of, 376
with abscess, 376, 377*f*
granulomatous, 376, 378*f*
with reactive lymph node, 376*f*
with skin and trabecular thickening, 376, 377*f*
with trichinosis, 376, 379*f*
MRI of, 378-379
pathology findings with, 379-385
acute inflammatory cells in, 382*f*
with breast abscess, 379
with coccidioidomycosis, 380-381, 384*f*
with echinococcosis, 380-381, 383*f*
granulomatous, 380-381, 381*f*
with subareolar abscess, 379-380, 382*f*
tuberculous, 384*f*, 385
prevalence and epidemiology of, 375
treatment options for, 385-388
due to trichinosis, 376, 379*f*
tuberculous, 384*f*, 385
ultrasonography of, 376-378, 379*f*, 380*f*, 381*f*
proliferative, 300-322
ductal hyperplasia of usual type as, 309-314
with central apocrine metaplasia, 312*f*
clinical presentation of, 309
with cribriform pattern, 313*f*
defined, 309
differential diagnosis of, 310-314
etiology and pathophysiology of, 309
with florid proliferation, 312*f*
with gynecomastia-like or micropapillary pattern, 313*f*
imaging indications and algorithm for, 310
mammography of, 310, 310*f*, 311*f*
MRI of, 310
normal terminal ductal lobular unit *vs.*, 310-314, 311*f*, 312*f*
with overlapping nuclei, 313*f*
pathology findings with, 310-314
prevalence and epidemiology of, 309
treatment options for, 314
ultrasonography of, 310
gynecomastia as, 314-318
asymmetric, 316*f*
classic signs of, 317
clinical presentation of, 315
defined, 314
dendritic pattern of, 315
differential diagnosis of, 317-318
diffuse glandular pattern of, 315
early nodular pattern of, 315, 315*f*
etiology and pathophysiology of, 314, 314*t*
imaging indications and algorithm for, 315-317
mammography of, 315, 315*f*, 316*f*
MRI of, 315-317
pathology findings with, 317-318, 317*f*, 318*f*
prevalence and epidemiology of, 314
pseudo-, 315, 316*f*
treatment options for, 318
ultrasonography of, 315, 317*f*

Benign lesion(s) *(Continued)*
microglandular adenosis as, 318-319
atypical, 318-319, 320*f*, 321*f*
clinical presentation of, 318
defined, 318
etiology and pathophysiology of, 318
imaging technique and findings with, 318-319
pathology findings with, 318-319, 319*f*, 320*f*
prevalence and epidemiology of, 318
treatment options for, 319
radial scar as, 304-309
clinical presentation of, 304
defined, 304
differential diagnosis of, 306-308
with ductal hyperplasia, 306-308, 308*f*
etiology and pathophysiology of, 304
imaging indications and algorithm for, 304
mammography of, 304, 304*f*, 305*f*
MRI of, 306
pathology findings with, 306-308, 306*f*, 307*f*
prevalence and epidemiology of, 304
treatment options for, 308-309
vs. tubular carcinoma, 306-308, 307*f*, 308*f*, 309*f*
ultrasonography of, 306, 306*f*
sclerosing adenosis as, 300-304
classic signs of, 302
clinical presentation of, 300
defined, 300
differential diagnosis of, 302-304
etiology and pathophysiology of, 300
imaging indications and algorithm for, 300
mammography of, 300, 301*f*, 302*f*
MRI of, 302
nodular, 302-303
pathology findings with, 302-304, 302*f*, 303*f*
prevalence and epidemiology of, 300
ultrasonography of, 302
solid, 255-299
adenomyoepithelioma as, 295-297
classic signs of, 295
clinical presentation of, 295
defined, 295
etiology and pathophysiology of, 295
imaging indications and algorithm for, 295
mammography of, 295
MRI of, 295
pathology findings with, 295-296, 296*f*
prevalence and epidemiology of, 295
treatment options for, 296-297
ultrasonography of, 295
adenosis as, 274-276
apocrine adenoma in, 276
clinical presentation of, 274
defined, 274
etiology and pathophysiology of, 274
imaging indications and algorithm for, 274
lactating adenoma in, 274-276, 276*f*, 277*f*
mammography of, 274
MRI of, 274
pathology findings with, 274-276
prevalence and epidemiology of, 274
treatment options for, 276
tubular adenoma in, 274, 275*f*
ultrasonography of, 274, 275*f*
diabetic mastopathy as, 276-280

Benign lesion(s) *(Continued)*
classic signs of, 278
clinical presentation of, 277
defined, 276
etiology and pathophysiology of, 277
imaging indications and algorithm for, 277
mammography of, 277-278, 277*f*
MRI of, 278, 278*f*, 279*f*
pathology findings in, 278, 279*f*
prevalence and epidemiology of, 277
treatment options for, 280
ultrasonography of, 278, 278*f*
fat necrosis as, 283-286
classic signs of, 286
clinical presentation of, 283
defined, 283
etiology and pathophysiology of, 283
imaging indications and algorithm for, 283
with lipid or oil cyst, 283, 284*f*
mammography of, 283, 283*f*, 284*f*, 285*f*
with microcalcifications and architectural distortion, 283, 284*f*, 285*f*
MRI of, 283-286
pathology findings with, 286, 286*f*
prevalence and epidemiology of, 283
treatment options for, 286
ultrasonography of, 283, 285*f*
fibroadenoma as, 255-260
classic signs of, 256
clinical presentation of, 255
complex, 256-259
defined, 255
with epithelial hyperplasia, 256-259, 259*f*
etiology and pathophysiology of, 255
fibrosed (old), 256-259, 258*f*, 259*f*
fine needle aspiration biopsy of, 256-259, 260*f*
imaging indications and algorithm for, 255
with intracanalicular growth pattern, 256-259, 258*f*
juvenile, 259-260, 261*f*
mammography of, 256, 256*f*
MRI of, 256
pathology findings with, 256-260
with pericanalicular growth pattern, 256-259, 258*f*
prevalence and epidemiology of, 255
treatment options for, 260
ultrasonography of, 256, 257*f*
fibromatosis as, 270-273
clinical presentation of, 271
defined, 270
etiology and pathophysiology of, 271
imaging indications and algorithm for, 271
mammography of, 271
MRI of, 272
pathology findings with, 272, 272*f*
prevalence and epidemiology of, 270
treatment options for, 273
ultrasonography of, 271, 271*f*
fibrosis as, 273-274
classic signs of, 274
clinical presentation of, 273
defined, 273
etiology and pathophysiology of, 273
imaging indications and algorithm for, 273
mammography of, 273, 273*f*
MRI of, 274
pathology findings with, 274

Benign lesion(s) *(Continued)*
prevalence and epidemiology of, 273
treatment options for, 274
ultrasonography of, 273-274
granular cell tumor as, 280-283
classic signs of, 281
clinical presentation of, 280
defined, 280
etiology and pathophysiology of, 280
imaging indications and algorithm for, 280
mammography of, 280, 280*f*
MRI of, 281
pathology findings with, 281, 282*f*
prevalence and epidemiology of, 280
treatment options for, 283
ultrasonography of, 281, 281*f*
hamartoma as, 265-268
classic signs of, 266
clinical presentation of, 265
defined, 265
etiology and pathophysiology of, 265
imaging indications and algorithm for, 265
mammography of, 265, 266*f*
MRI of, 265, 267*f*
pathology findings with, 266, 268*f*
prevalence and epidemiology of, 265
treatment options for, 266-268
ultrasonography of, 265, 266*f*
hemangioma as, 288-290
cavernous, 290-291, 291*f*
clinical presentation of, 289
defined, 288
etiology and pathophysiology of, 289
imaging indications and algorithm for, 289
mammography of, 289
MRI of, 289, 290*f*
pathology findings with, 289-290, 291*f*
perilobular, 290-291, 291*f*
prevalence and epidemiology of, 288-289
treatment options for, 290
ultrasonography of, 289
intramammary lymph node as, 260-264
classic signs of, 263
clinical presentation of, 262
defined, 260
differential diagnosis of, 263-264
etiology and pathophysiology of, 261, 261*f*, 262*f*
imaging indications and algorithm for, 262
mammography of, 262-263, 262*f*, 263*f*
MRI of, 263
pathology findings with, 264, 264*f*, 265*f*
prevalence and epidemiology of, 261
reactive inflammatory, 263, 263*f*, 264*f*
treatment options for, 264
ultrasonography of, 263, 263*f*, 264*f*
lipoma as, 268-270
classic signs of, 268
clinical presentation of, 268
defined, 268
etiology and pathophysiology of, 268
imaging indications and algorithm for, 268
mammography of, 268, 269*f*
MRI of, 268
pathology findings with, 269, 271*f*
prevalence and epidemiology of, 268
treatment options for, 270
ultrasonography of, 268, 269*f*, 270*f*
myofibroblastoma as, 293-295
clinical presentation of, 294

Benign lesion(s) *(Continued)*
defined, 293
etiology and pathophysiology of, 294
imaging indications and algorithm for, 294
mammography of, 294
MRI of, 294
pathology findings with, 294-295, 294*f*, 295*f*
prevalence and epidemiology of, 294
treatment options for, 295
ultrasonography of, 294
nipple adenoma as, 297-298
classic signs of, 297
clinical presentation of, 297
defined, 297
etiology and pathophysiology of, 297
imaging indications and algorithm for, 297
mammography of, 297
MRI of, 297
pathology of findings with, 297-298, 297*f*, 298*f*
prevalence and epidemiology of, 297
treatment options for, 298
ultrasonography of, 297
pseudoangiomatous stromal hyperplasia as, 290-293
classic signs of, 292
clinical presentation of, 291-292
defined, 290-291
etiology and pathophysiology of, 291
imaging indications and algorithm for, 292
mammography of, 292, 292*f*
MRI of, 292
pathology findings with, 292, 293*f*
prevalence and epidemiology of, 291
treatment options for, 293
ultrasonography of, 292, 293*f*
silicone breast implant rupture as, 286-288
classic signs of, 287
clinical presentation of, 287
defined, 286-287
etiology and pathophysiology of, 287
imaging indications and algorithm for, 287
mammography of, 287, 287*f*
MRI of, 288
pathology findings with, 287-288, 288*f*, 289*f*
prevalence and epidemiology of, 287
ultrasonography of, 288-290, 288*f*
Benign sclerosing ductal hyperplasia. *See* Radial scar.
Benign triplets, 635-637
BENT (Breast Exposure: Nationwide Trends), 20-21
Bias
lead-time, 57
length, 57
selection, 57
Bilateral carcinoma, 467
Billing, 720-727. *See also* Reimbursement.
proper habits for, 725
terminology for, 720-721
Biomarker(s), 626-629
Allred Score for, 626-627, 627*f*
estrogen receptor as, 626, 626*f*
for invasive ductal carcinoma, 449, 449*f*
HER-2/neu as, 627-629
chromosomal location of, 627-629, 627*f*
FISH testing for, 627-629, 629*f*
immunohistochemical testing (HercepTest) for, 450, 627-629

Biomarker(s) *(Continued)*
new standard protocol and guidelines for, 450
score 0 in, 450, 450*f*, 628*f*
score 1 on, 450, 451*f*, 628*f*
score 2 on, 450, 451*f*, 628*f*
score 3 on, 450, 451*f*, 629*f*
for invasive ductal carcinoma, 449–450
FISH for, 450, 452*f*
immunohistochemical stain for, 450, 450*f*, 451*f*
rationale for, 627–629
for invasive ductal carcinoma, 447–453
estrogen receptor as, 449, 449*f*
HER-2/neu as, 449–450
FISH for, 450, 452*f*
immunohistochemical stain for, 450, 450*f*, 451*f*
Ki-67 as, 453
progesterone receptor as, 453
for invasive lobular carcinoma, 495
Ki-67 as, 453
progesterone receptor as, 626
for invasive ductal carcinoma, 453
as prognostic *vs.* predictive indicators, 626
reports on, 629, 630*t*
Biopsy
axillary sentinel lymph node, 623–625
isolated tumor cells in, 624–625, 625*f*
macrometastatic disease in, 624–625
micrometastatic disease in, 624–625, 625*f*
protocol for, 623–625, 624*f*
radiation therapy after positive, 625
for calcifications, 552, 556, 557*f*
concordance with, 635–637, 636*f*, 637*f*
core needle (*See* Core needle biopsy (CNB))
directional vacuum-assisted, ultrasound-guided, 167–168, 565
of calcifications, 170*f*
confirmation of sampling adequacy with, 569–571, 572*f*
cutting mechanism of, 565, 566*f*
for cysts, 171–176, 176*f*
of fibroadenoma, 169*f*
for nipple discharge, 158–159, 159*f*
excisional, 618–619, 618*f*
false-positive results and, 67
fine-needle aspiration (*See* Fine-needle aspiration (FNA) biopsy)
image-guided percutaneous (*See* Image-guided percutaneous biopsy)
incisional, 618
management after, 635–645
assessing for concordance in, 635–637, 636*f*, 637*f*
with atypical ductal hyperplasia, 637–638, 639*f*
with columnar cell lesions, 641, 642*f*
communication responsibilities in, 642–643
for definite benign and concordant benign cases, 637, 638*f*
with false-negative results, 637, 638*f*
with false-positive results, 642
with lobular neoplasia, 640–641
with papillary lesions, 640, 640*f*
with radial scar, 638–640, 639*f*
with sclerosing adenosis, 641–642, 643*f*
MRI-guided (*See* Magnetic resonance imaging (MRI)-guided core needle biopsy)
re-excisional, 620–621
reimbursement for, 723*t*, 725
stereotactic-guided (*See* Stereotactic-guided core needle biopsy (SCNB))
ultrasound-guided (*See* Ultrasound-guided core needle biopsy (US CNB))
Biopsy tray, for core needle biopsy
MRI-guided, 587–588
stereotactic-guided, 579
ultrasound-guided, 564–565, 564*f*
BIPA (Benefits Improvement and Protection Act), 721
BI-RADS (*See* Breast Imaging, Reporting, and Data System (BI-RADS))
Black women
incidence of breast cancer in, 33–34, 33*f*
mortality rate in, 38, 39*f*
stage of diagnosis in, 34, 35, 35*f*, 36*f*
and survival rate, 35, 36*f*
tumor characteristics in, 35–37
tumor size in, 34, 34*f*
Bleeding, due to core needle biopsy
MRI-guided, 594
stereotactic-guided, 586
ultrasound-guided, 576
Blood cell invasion, as prognostic and predictive factor, 231
Bloom and Richardson grade, after neoadjuvant chemotherapy, 526–529
Blur, clinical image evaluation of, 125, 126*f*, 127*f*, 128*f*
B-mode ultrasound technology, 13, 14*f*
Body fat distribution, and breast cancer risk, 42
Body mass index (BMI), and breast cancer risk, 42
Body size, and breast cancer risk, 42
Boerhaave, Herman, 16
Boone, John, 746
BOPTA (gadopentetate dimeglumine), for contrast-enhanced MRI, 187
Bowen disease, *vs.* Paget's disease, 405–409
"Bracketing of the lesion", 394, 397*f*
Branch pattern, solid breast nodules with, 171, 172*f*
BRCA1 gene, 230–232
and breast cancer risk, 46–47
in men, 469
BRCA1 interacting protein C-terminal helicase 1 *(BRIP1)* gene, and breast cancer risk, 48
BRCA2 gene, 230–232
and breast cancer risk, 46–47
in men, 469
Breach of duty, 729
Breast
normal, 223–235
anatomy of
mammographic, 111, 224–226, 224*f*
ultrasonographic, 226, 228*f*
variations in, 226, 227*f*
embryology and development of, 223–224
histology of, 224–226, 225*f*, 226*f*
pathology of, 226–230
Breast abscess, 379, 380*f*
Breast augmentation, 662–681
methods of, 662–666
with implantable prostheses (*See* Breast implant(s))
with injectable materials, 662, 663*f*
MRI after, 201–202, 202*f*, 203*f*
Breast cancer
epidemiology of, 228
familial risk of, 230–232
genetic mutation(s) in, 229
gene expression patterns with, 229–230, 230*f*
due to loss of heterozygosity, 229
due to microsatellite instability, 229
due to tumor suppressor genes, 229
prognostic and predictive factor(s) for, 231–232
Breast cancer *(Continued)*
age as, 231
DNA amplification as, 232
expression profiling as, 232, 233*f*, 234*f*, 234*t*
extent of ductal carcinoma in situ as, 232
Her2 oncogene as, 232
histologic grade as, 231
histologic type as, 231
inflammatory cell infiltrates as, 231
lymph node status as, 231
lymphatic and blood cell invasion as, 231
perineural invasion as, 231
pregnancy as, 231
steroid hormone receptor status as, 232
TP53 mutation as, 232
tumor cell proliferation as, 231
tumor necrosis as, 231
tumor size as, 231
Breast Cancer Detection Demonstration Project (BCDDP), 16, 44, 56, 57
Breast Cancer Screening Consortium report, 731
Breast Cancer Surveillance Consortium (BCSC)
on goals for screening mammography, 710*t*, 711, 712*t*
recall rates at, 66–67
Breast coils, for MRI, 179, 179*f*, 180*f*
artifacts due to, 190, 191*f*
multi-channel bilateral, 188, 188*f*, 189*f*
Breast compression. *See* Compression
Breast contour, after reduction mammoplasty, 684, 684*f*
Breast density
BI-RADS on, 214–215
in ultrasound-guided core needle biopsy, 572
Breast development, 223–224
Breast exposure, quality control test of, 138*t*, 143
Breast Exposure: Nationwide Trends (BENT), 20–21
Breast imaging, history of. *See* History, of breast imaging
Breast Imaging Accreditation Information Line, 144
Breast Imaging, Reporting, and Data System (BI-RADS), 213–220
history of, 213
and importance of communication process, 213–214
legal aspects of, 734
for mammography, 214–217
assessment and management in, 216–217
audit in, 217
breast density in, 214–215
calcifications in, 215–216
masses and asymmetries in, 215
in medical audit, 703
for MRI, 218–219
background enhancement in, 218
dynamic contrast enhancement in, 218–219
focus or foci in, 218
for ultrasound, 153–154, 154*t*, 217–218
technical considerations in, 217–218
Breast implant(s), 662–681
alternatives to, 665
comparison of imaging modalities with, 680, 680*f*
complications of, 663–665
CT of, 680, 680*f*
demographics of, 663
dual chamber (double lumen), 663, 665*f*
MRI of, 670, 670*f*
encapsulation of, 666

Breast implant(s) *(Continued)*
FDA approval of, 666
fluid on periphery of, 673, 675*f*
gel bleed from, 666
history of, 662-666
imaging indications and algorithm for, 663-666
mammography of, 667-668
with rupture, 287, 287*f*, 667-668, 668*f*
with silicone adenopathy, 667, 667*f*
with silicone granulomas, 667-668, 668*f*
Mammography Quality Standards Act on, 696
MRI of, 201-202, 668-674
in evaluation for malignancy, 201-202
with gel fracture, 674
imaging protocols for, 669-670
normal appearance in, 670-671, 670*f*
with radial folds, 671, 671*f*
rat-tail sign in, 670*f*, 673
with rupture, 288
axial and sagittal inversion recovery water saturation images in, 201, 668*f*
contour deformities in, 673
extracapsular, 673-674, 676*f*
fluid on periphery of implant in, 673, 675*f*
inconclusive signs in, 673
intracapsular, 671-673
linguine sign in, 671, 672*f*
subscapular line sign in, 671, 672*f*, 673*f*
teardrop, keyhole, or noose sign in, 673, 673*f*
water droplets in, 673, 674*f*
with silicone granulomas, 202, 203*f*, 676*f*
technical factors in, 669, 669*f*, 669*t*
multi-compartment, 671, 673*f*
pathology findings with, 287-288, 288*f*, 289*f*
prevalence and epidemiology of, 287
with radial folds
MRI of, 671, 671*f*
ultrasonography of, 674, 677*f*
rupture of, 286-288, 666
classic signs of, 287
clinical presentation of, 287
CT of, 680, 680*f*
defined, 286-287
etiology and pathophysiology of, 287
etiology of, 666
extracapsular, 666
MRI of, 673-674, 676*f*
ultrasonography of, 677-678, 678*f*, 679*f*
imaging indications and algorithm for, 287
intracapsular, ultrasonography of, 677, 678*f*
mammography of, 287, 287*f*, 667-668, 668*f*
MRI of, 288
axial and sagittal inversion recovery water saturation images in, 201, 668*f*
contour deformities in, 673
extracapsular, 673-674, 676*f*
fluid on periphery of implant in, 673, 675*f*
inconclusive signs in, 673
intracapsular, 671-673
linguine sign in, 671, 672*f*
subscapular line sign in, 671, 672*f*, 673*f*
teardrop, keyhole, or noose sign in, 673, 673*f*
water droplets in, 673, 674*f*
pathology findings with, 287-288, 288*f*, 289*f*
prevalence and epidemiology of, 287
saline, 667
ultrasonography of, 674-678
extracapsular, 677-678, 678*f*, 679*f*
intracapsular, 677, 678*f*
with silicone granulomas, 287, 288*f*

Breast implant(s) *(Continued)*
saline, 663
rupture of, 667
with silicone adenopathy, 667, 667*f*
single chamber (single lumen), 663, 664*f*, 665*f*
MRI of, 670, 670*f*
stacked, 670
subglandular, 663, 664*f*
subpectoral, 663, 665*f*
ultrasonography of, 288-290, 674-679
limitations of, 678-679
normal findings in, 674, 676*f*, 677*f*
with radial folds, 674, 677*f*
with reverberation artifacts, 674, 677*f*
with rupture, 674-678
extracapsular, 677-678, 678*f*, 679*f*
intracapsular, 677, 678*f*
and silicone granulomas, 287, 288*f*
Breast nodules, ultrasound of, 171
with branch pattern, 171, 172*f*
with duct extension, 171, 172*f*
due to fibroadenoma, 171, 173*f*
hard finding in, 171, 172*f*
hypoechoic, 171, 173*f*
with microcalcifications, 171, 172*f*, 173*f*
with microlobulations, 171, 172*f*, 173*f*
nonspecific findings in, 171, 173*f*
soft findings in, 171, 172*f*, 173*f*
with spiculation, 171, 172*f*
terminal duct lobular unit in, 173*f*
Breast pain
in invasive ductal carcinoma, 425
ultrasound for, 157-158, 158*f*
Breast reduction
liposuction for, 688
reduction mammoplasty for (*See* Reduction mammoplasty)
Breast self-examination (BSE), for screening, 56-57
Breast tissue
axillary, 224, 226, 227*f*
ectopic, 223
Breast-conserving therapy, 649-661
calcifications after, 651-653, 652*f*, 656, 656*f*
clinical trials of, 649
contraindications to, 649-651
fat necrosis after, 327-329, 332*f*, 333*f*
imaging indications and algorithm for, 651, 651*t*
imaging technique and findings with, 651-653, 652*f*, 653*f*
mammography after, 653-656
calcifications in, 651-652, 652*f*, 656, 656*f*
diffuse changes in, 655, 655*f*
goals of, 653
indications and algorithm for, 651, 651*t*
parenchymal changes in, 656
scars in, 654-655, 655*f*
seromas and hematomas in, 653*f*, 654, 654*f*, 655*f*
skin changes in, 655
timing of, 653-654
views for, 653
microclips in specimen from, 347*f*
MRI with, 198
of positive margins, 653, 653*f*
post-treatment changes in, 656
uses for, 651*t*
patient selection for, 649-653, 650*f*
recurrence after, 656-658, 657*f*, 658*f*
benign sequela(e) mimicking, 658-660
calcifications as, 658, 659*f*
fat necrosis as, 658, 658*f*
on mammography, 658-660, 658*f*, 659*f*
on MRI, 659-660, 660*f*

Breast-conserving therapy *(Continued)*
re-excisional biopsy after, 620-621
specimen radiography in, 651, 652*f*
ultrasonography with, 660
Breastfeeding, and breast cancer risk, 41-42
Breast-specific gamma imaging (BSGI), 747-748
Breslow, Lester, 21
BRIP1 (*BRCA1* interacting protein C-terminal helicase 1) gene, and breast cancer risk, 48
BSE (breast self-examination), for screening, 56-57
Bucky factor, 89
Bullet fragments, calcifications due to, 332, 337*f*, 338*f*
Bush, George H.W., 22
Butler, P. D., 10

C

CABINET (coherence transfer based spin-echo spectroscopy), 763
CAD. *See* Computer-aided detection (CAD).
Cadherin 1, and breast cancer risk, 47-48
CADx (computer-aided diagnosis), 99
Calcifications
amorphous, indistinct, 216, 555, 555*f*
evaluation of, 555, 555*f*
due to milk of calcium, 323, 324*f*, 554*f*
with apocrine metaplasia, 342*f*, 343*f*
arrangement of, 216
of axillary node metastases, 432*f*
basophilic, 333-334, 341*f*, 342*f*
BI-RADS on, 215-216
branching
in DCIS, 392-394, 392*f*, 394*f*
fine, linear, 553*f*, 556
after breast-conserving therapy, 651-653, 652*f*, 656, 656*f*
calcium oxalate, 333-334, 342*f*, 343*f*
calcium phosphate, 333-334, 341*f*, 342*f*
clustered, 216
coarse
heterogeneous, 216, 555-556, 556*f*
in DCIS, 555-556, 556*f*
popcorn-like, 554*f*
within columnar cell lesions, 346*f*, 356, 357*f*
core needle biopsy of, 612-614, 614*f*, 615*f*
in DCIS, 392-394
biopsy for, 556, 557*f*
branching, 392-394, 392*f*, 394*f*
coarse heterogeneous, 555-556, 556*f*
in ductal distribution, 393*f*
in linear distribution, 392-394, 393*f*, 394*f*
micro-, 392
pathology of, 333-334, 343*f*
round and punctate, 553, 554*f*
in segmental distribution, 392-394, 392*f*, 393*f*, 394*f*
dermal, 323-325
grid compression paddle for, 323, 326*f*
mammography of, 323, 325*f*, 554*f*
parenchymal *vs.*, 323-325
in dermatomyositis, 325, 326*f*, 327*f*
diffuse (scattered), 216
with ductal hyperplasia, 344*f*
dystrophic, 216
evaluation of, 552-559
amorphous, indistinct, 555, 555*f*
biopsy for, 552
approach for, 556, 557*f*
coarse heterogeneous, 555-556, 556*f*
comparison with previous mammograms for, 552

Calcifications *(Continued)*
fine
linear branching, 553*f*, 556
pleomorphic, 553*f*, 556
intermediate risk, 555–556, 555*f*, 556*f*
magnification views *vs.* digital zoom for, 552–556, 553*f*
morphology, distribution, and change over time of, 552, 553*t*
MRI for, 556–557, 558*f*
round and punctate, 553–555, 554*f*
suspicious and malignant, 556
typically benign, 553, 553*b*, 554*f*
ultrasonography for, 556–557, 557*f*
due to fat necrosis, 327–329
clinical features of, 327
with lipid or oil cyst, 327–329, 330*f*, 331*f*
mammographic appearance of, 327–329, 330*f*, 331*f*, 332*f*
pathology of, 345*f*
post-lumpectomy, 327–329, 332*f*, 333*f*
post-mastectomy, 332*f*
post-surgical, 327–329, 331*f*
post-traumatic, 327–329, 331*f*
ultrasound appearance of, 329, 332*f*, 333*f*
fine
linear branching, 553*f*, 556
pleomorphic, 553*f*, 556
foreign body, 332–333
due to bullet or bullet fragments, 332, 337*f*, 338*f*
due to calcified sutures, 332, 340*f*
due to gold deposits, 333, 340*f*
parasitic, 333, 341*f*
due to retained Hickman catheter, 332, 339*f*
due to sewing needle or localizing wire, 332, 339*f*
historical background of, 5, 7*f*, 8*f*
intermediate risk, 555–556, 555*f*, 556*f*
in invasive ductal carcinoma
of axillary node metastases, 432*f*
micro-, 426–427, 428*f*, 429*f*
in involuting fibroadenomas, 329–331
clinical aspects of, 329
mammographic appearance of, 331, 334*f*
pathology of, 346*f*
popcorn shape of, 331, 333*f*, 335*f*, 554*f*
ultrasound of, 331, 335*f*
with lactational changes in pregnancy, 342*f*
linear, 216
in DCIS, 392–394, 393*f*, 394*f*
fine branching, 553*f*, 556
malignant, 556
due to milk of calcium, 323, 553
crescent shape (teacup sign) of, 323, 324*f*
on mammogram, 323, 324*f*, 554*f*
rounded or amorphous, 323, 324*f*, 554*f*
on ultrasound, 324*f*
popcorn-like
coarse, 554*f*
in involuting fibroadenomas, 331, 333*f*, 335*f*, 554*f*
positive predictive value for, 552
with radiation changes, 345*f*
after reduction mammoplasty, 686–688, 688*f*
regional distribution of, 216
rod-like, 554*f*
round and punctate, 553–555, 554*f*
in DCIS, 553, 554*f*
due to milk of calcium, 323, 324*f*, 554*f*
with sclerosing adenosis, 344*f*
secretory, duct ectasia with, 331–332
clinical aspects of, 331
imaging features of, 331–332, 336*f*

Calcifications *(Continued)*
segmental distribution of, 216
in DCIS, 392–394, 392*f*, 393*f*, 394*f*
with stroma, 344*f*
due to substances on skin, 325–326
antiperspirant as, 325–326, 327*f*
powders, creams, and ointments as, 325–326, 328*f*
tattoos as, 325–326, 328*f*
suspicious, 215–216, 556
typically benign, 323–348
BI-RADS on, 215–216
dermal, 323–325
grid compression paddle for, 323, 326*f*
mammography of, 323, 325*f*, 554*f*
parenchymal *vs.*, 323–325
in dermatomyositis, 325, 326*f*, 327*f*
duct ectasia with secretory, 331–332
clinical aspects of, 331
imaging features of, 331–332, 336*f*
evaluation of, 553, 553*b*, 554*f*
due to fat necrosis, 327–329
clinical features of, 327
with lipid or oil cyst, 327–329, 330*f*, 331*f*
mammographic appearance of, 327–329, 330*f*, 331*f*, 332*f*
pathology of, 345*f*
post-lumpectomy, 327–329, 332*f*, 333*f*
post-mastectomy, 332*f*
post-surgical, 327–329, 331*f*
post-traumatic, 327–329, 331*f*
ultrasound appearance of, 329, 332*f*, 333*f*
foreign body, 332–333
due to bullet or bullet fragments, 332, 337*f*, 338*f*
due to calcified sutures, 332, 340*f*
due to gold deposits, 333, 340*f*
parasitic, 333, 341*f*
due to retained Hickman catheter, 332, 339*f*
due to sewing needle or localizing wire, 332, 339*f*
in involuting fibroadenomas, 329–331
clinical aspects of, 329
mammographic appearance of, 331, 334*f*
pathology of, 346*f*
popcorn shape of, 331, 333*f*, 335*f*, 554*f*
ultrasound of, 331, 335*f*
due to milk of calcium, 323, 553
crescent shape (teacup sign) of, 323, 324*f*
on mammogram, 323, 324*f*, 554*f*
rounded or amorphous, 323, 324*f*, 554*f*
on ultrasound, 324*f*
pathology of, 333–337
with apocrine metaplasia, 342*f*, 343*f*
basophilic, 333–334, 341*f*, 342*f*
with benign terminal ductal-lobular unit, 341*f*
calcium oxalate, 333–334, 342*f*, 343*f*
calcium phosphate, 333–334, 341*f*, 342*f*
within columnar cell lesion, 346*f*
with ductal hyperplasia, 344*f*
with fat necrosis, 345*f*
in involuted and hyalinized fibroadenoma, 346*f*
with lactational changes in pregnancy, 342*f*
from lumpectomy specimen, 347*f*
Mönckeberg, 345*f*
with radiation changes, 345*f*
with sclerosing adenosis, 344*f*
with stroma, 344*f*

Calcifications *(Continued)*
due to substances on skin, 325–326
antiperspirant as, 325–326, 327*f*
powders, creams, and ointments as, 325–326, 328*f*
tattoos as, 325–326, 328*f*
vascular, 326–327
arterial, 327, 330*f*
Mönckeberg type, 326–327, 329*f*, 345*f*
tram-track appearance of, 326–327, 329*f*
ultrasound of, 157, 157*f*
vascular, 326–327
arterial, 327, 330*f*
Mönckeberg type, 326–327, 329*f*, 345*f*
tram-track appearance of, 326–327, 329*f*
Calcium, milk of, 323, 553
crescent shape (teacup sign) of, 323, 324*f*
on mammogram, 323, 324*f*, 554*f*
rounded or amorphous, 323, 324*f*, 554*f*
on ultrasound, 324*f*
Calcium oxalate calcifications, 333–334
with benign breast lesions, 333–334, 342*f*, 343*f*
core needle biopsy of, 612–614, 614*f*, 615*f*
in DCIS, 333–334, 343*f*
Calcium phosphate calcifications, 333–334, 341*f*, 342*f*
core needle biopsy of, 612–614, 614*f*
Canadian National Breast Screening Study (NBSS), 57–58, 58*t*
and screening guidelines, 62
on screening of women 40 to 49 years old, 59–60, 70–71
and underestimation of benefits from screening, 61
Cancer detection rate, in medical audit
analysis of, 710–711
defined, 707
goals for, 710*t*, 712*t*
in medical literature, 708*t*
with screening and diagnostic mammography data combined, 712*t*, 713*t*
value of, 715–716, 715*t*, 716*t*
Cancerization of lobules (COL), 391, 400–401, 401*f*
radiation atypia *vs.*, 531–533, 532*f*
CAPSS (columnar alteration with prominent apical snouts and secretions), 356
"Captain of the ship", 735
Carcinoma in situ (CIS), 228
ductal (*See* Ductal carcinoma in situ (DCIS))
intracystic, 175*f*
lobular (*See* Lobular carcinoma in situ (LCIS))
in medical audit
in medical literature, 712*t*
with screening and diagnostic mammography data combined, 712*t*, 713*t*
value of, 716, 716*t*
micropapillary, 175*f*
ultrasound of, 160–161, 161*f*
Care, standards of, legal aspects of, 729, 730–732
Carlsen, Ernest, 15
Carlson, Chester, 11
CART (classification and regression tree) analysis, for magnetic resonance spectroscopy, 761–762, 766–767, 767*t*, 768*t*
Case sensitivity, of computer-aided detection, 102
Cash-paying customers, 724, 726
Caucasian women
incidence of breast cancer in, 33–34, 33*f*
mortality rate in, 38, 39*f*
stage of diagnosis in, 34, 35, 35*f*, 36*f*
and survival rate, 35, 36*f*
tumor size in, 34, 34*f*

Causation, 729
Cause of action, 729
Cavernous hemangioma, 290-291, 291*f*
CC view. *See* Craniocaudal (CC) view.
CCC. *See* Columnar cell change (CCC).
CCD (charge-coupled device) system, for image detection, 94-95, 94*f*
CCH (columnar cell hyperplasia), 356, 357*f*
 post-biopsy management of, 641, 642*f*
CCLs. *See* Columnar cell lesions (CCLs).
CDH1 gene, 229
 and breast cancer risk, 47-48
CE-DBCT (contrast-enhanced dedicated breast CT), 747
Centers for Disease Control and Prevention (CDC), on cancer statistics, 25
Central venous catheter, retained, calcifications due to, 332, 339*f*
Certification
 Mammography Quality Standards Act on, 694, 695
 provisional, 695
 reinstatement of, 695
Cervical metastatic lymphadenopathy, 199, 200*f*
Cesium iodide (CsI) crystals, for image detection, 95-96, 96*f*
CGH (comparative genomic hybridization), 229
Charge-coupled device (CCD) system, for image detection, 94-95, 94*f*
CHEK2 (CHK2 checkpoint homolog) gene, and breast cancer risk, 47, 48
Chemical saturation, for fat suppression, in MRI, 184-185, 184*f*, 185*f*
Chemical shift artifacts, on MRI, 190-191
Chemotherapy
 MRI after, 205*t*
 neoadjuvant, 524-531
  advantages of, 524
  DCIS after, 526*f*, 527*f*
  effects on normal breast tissue of, 525
  indications for, 524
  invasive lobular carcinoma after, 528*f*, 529*f*
  lymph nodes after, 524, 527*f*, 528*f*, 529*f*
  tumor response to
   Bloom and Richardson grade for, 526-529
   cytoplasmic ballooning in, 526*f*
   in DCIS, 526*f*, 527*f*
   degenerated tumor cells in, 525*f*
   FDG-PET and PET/CT of, 531, 531*f*
   histologic changes in, 525
   in invasive lobular carcinoma, 528*f*, 529*f*
   in lymph nodes, 527*f*, 528*f*, 529*f*
   mammography of, 529-530, 529*f*
   MRI of, 201, 529-530, 530*f*
   and pathologic response, 525
   predictors of, 524-525
   residual tumor size in, 524, 525-526
   ultrasonography of, 529-530, 530*f*
Chest wall invasion, MRI of, 198, 198*f*
CHK2 checkpoint homolog *(CHEK2)* gene, and breast cancer risk, 47, 48
Chloromas, 502, 504-505, 505*f*
Choline (Cho), in magnetic resonance spectroscopy, 761-762
Chondroid element, metaplastic carcinoma with, 463-465, 464*f*
Chondrosarcoma, 510
Cicatrization, in invasive ductal carcinoma, 425, 428
CIF (contrast improvement factor), 89
CIS. *See* Carcinoma in situ (CIS).
Civil law, 729
Classification and regression tree (CART) analysis, for magnetic resonance spectroscopy, 761-762, 766-767, 767*t*, 768*t*
Claus model, 46
Claustrophobia, with MRI, 193
Claw sign, with epidermal inclusion cysts, 240
Clear cell intraductal carcinoma, 403, 406*f*
Cleavage (CV) view, 118
Clinging-type DCIS, 403, 405*f*
Clinical examination, for screening, 56-57
Clinical findings, MRI for difficult or equivocal, 201
Clinical image(s), in accreditation, 699
Clinical image evaluation, 121-132
 artifacts in, 125-126, 128*f*, 129*f*
 compression in, 123, 126*f*
 contrast in, 123
 exposure in, 123-124, 127*f*
 labeling in, 126-127, 129*f*, 130*f*, 131*f*
 noise in, 125
 overview of, 121-127, 122*t*
 positioning in, 121-122
  for CC view, 122-123, 124*f*, 125*f*
  for MLO view, 122, 122*f*, 123*f*, 124*f*
 sharpness in, 125, 127*f*, 128*f*
Close margins, 623
CNB. *See* Core needle biopsy (CNB).
Coaxial system, for ultrasound-guided core needle biopsy, 569, 570*f*
Coccidioidomycosis, mastitis due to, 380-381, 384*f*
Coding, 720-727
 appropriate combination of information and, 725
 current acceptable, 722, 722*t*, 723*t*
 proper habits for, 725
 terminology for, 720-721
 up-, 725
Coherence transfer based spin-echo spectroscopy (CABINET), 763
COL (cancerization of lobules), 391, 400-401, 401*f*
 radiation atypia *vs.*, 531-533, 532*f*
Collagenous spherulosis (CP), cribriform DCIS *vs.*, 401-402, 403*f*
Collimation assessment, in quality control, 138*t*, 142
Collimator, in mammography unit, 81, 82*f*, 85, 85*f*
Colloid carcinoma, 455-456, 456*f*
Colon carcinoma, with male breast cancer, 470
Color patterns, in elastography, 755-756, 757*f*
Columnar alteration with prominent apical snouts and secretions (CAPSS), 356
Columnar cell change (CCC), 356, 356*f*
 with apocrine metaplasia, 358*f*
 with microcalcifications, 357*f*
 post-biopsy management of, 641, 642*f*
Columnar cell hyperplasia (CCH), 356, 357*f*
 post-biopsy management of, 641, 642*f*
Columnar cell lesion(s) (CCLs), 355-357
 and apocrine metaplasia, 356, 358*f*
 calcifications within, 346*f*, 356, 357*f*
 classic signs of, 356
 clinical presentation of, 355
 columnar cell change as, 356, 356*f*
 columnar cell hyperplasia as, 356, 357*f*
 with cytologic atypia, 356-357, 358*f*, 359*f*
 defined, 355
 differential diagnosis of, 356-357
 etiology and pathophysiology of, 355
 imaging indications and algorithm for, 355
 mammography of, 355, 355*f*
 MRI of, 356
 pathology findings with, 356-357
 post-biopsy management of, 641, 642*f*
 prevalence and epidemiology of, 355
 treatment options for, 357
 ultrasonography of, 355
Comedocarcinoma, 392
 with cancerization of lobules, 400-401, 401*f*
 clinical presentation of, 392
 gross pathology of, 398-399
 microscopic findings in, 400-401, 401*f*
Comedomastitis, 244, 331
Comedo-type DCIS, 392
 with cancerization of lobules, 400-401, 401*f*
 case study on, 479, 479*f*
 clinical presentation of, 392
 gross pathology of, 398-399
 microscopic findings in, 400-401, 401*f*
Common law, 730
Communication
 BI-RADS and importance of, 213-214
 of results
  after core needle biopsy, 618, 642-643
  legal aspects of, 733-734
  of mammography, 213-214
Comparative genomic hybridization (CGH), 229
Complex mass, 239
Complicated cysts, 239, 240*f*
Compression
 advantages of, 87
 adverse consequences of, 66
 clinical image evaluation of, 123, 126*f*
 foot pedals and digital display for, 87, 87*f*, 88*f*
 inadequate, 123, 126*f*
 during mammography, history of, 5, 7*f*, 8*f*
 and positioning, 111-112, 112*f*
 quality control tests of, 137*t*, 139*t*, 142
Compression devices, 82*f*, 86-87, 86*f*, 87*f*
Compression paddles, 82*f*, 86-87, 86*f*, 87*f*
 quality control test of, 139*t*
Compressive elastography, 755-756, 756*f*
Computed radiography (CR) system, for image detection, 95-96, 96*f*
Computed tomography (CT)
 of breast implants, 680, 680*f*
 dedicated breast, 746-747, 746*f*, 747*f*
 with PET, 748
Computer-aided detection (CAD), 99-109
 algorithms for, 100
 basic principles of, 100-102
 and biopsy rate, 105*t*, 106*t*
 coding and billing for, 723*t*
 vs. computer-aided diagnosis, 99
 defined, 99
 and detection rate, 105*t*, 106*t*
 and digital mammography, 107
 vs. double-reading protocols, 99
 evaluation of, 102-107
  with double reading *vs.* single reader, 104-107
  historical controlled studies for, 104, 105*t*
  impact on missed cancers for, 102-104
  prospective, sequential read studies for, 104, 106*t*
  stand-alone performance studies for, 102, 103*f*
 false-positive marks with, 102, 103*f*, 107
 FDA approval of, 99
 learning curve for, 101-102
 legal aspects of, 732, 736-737
 mammographic image in, 100, 100*f*
 in MRI-guided core needle biopsy, 588-590, 590*f*
 rationale for, 99
 reading protocol for, 101
 and recall rates, 99, 105*t*, 106*t*, 107-108
 sensitivity and specificity of, 100-101, 101*f*
 ultrasound-guided, 757-759, 758*f*
Computer-aided diagnosis (CADx), 99
Concordance, with biopsy, 635-637, 636*f*, 637*f*
Conscious sedation, for MRI, 204

Consent
  for core needle biopsy
    MRI-guided, 588
    stereotactic-guided, 579–580
    ultrasound-guided, 566–567
  legal aspects of, 734–735
Consumer complaint mechanisms, Mammography Quality Standards Act on, 696
Contact liquid crystal thermography, 16
Contamination, and results of randomized clinical trials, 61
Contralateral breast imaging, MRI for, 198–199
Contrast, clinical image evaluation of, 123
Contrast improvement factor (CIF), 89
Contrast-enhanced dedicated breast CT (CE-DBCT), 747
Contrast-enhanced MRI, 185–187, 186*f*, 761
  agents for, 204
    reaction to, 197
  BI-RADS on, 218–219
  gadolinium compounds used in, 186, 186*t*
  history of, 18
  missed uptake of, 190
  and nephrogenic systemic fibrosis, 193
  power injector for, 187, 187*f*
  processing and uptake analysis for, 187, 187*f*
  uptake curve and washout phase for, 186, 186*f*
Cooper ligaments, 111, 224, 224*f*
  ultrasound of, 168–171, 171*f*
Cooperative Agreement for Quality Assurance Activities in Mammography, 110–111
Copeland, Murray M., 9*f*
Core needle biopsy (CNB), 612–618
  advantages of, 612–614
  benign results on, 617, 637, 638*f*
  calcifications in, 612–614, 614*f*, 615*f*
  communicating results after, 618, 642–643
  false-negative results on, 617, 637, 638*f*
  false-positive results on, 615–617
    follow-up for, 642
    myoepithelial cell markers for, 616–617, 617*f*
    due to sclerosing adenosis, 616–617, 616*f*
  limitations of, 615, 637
  management after, 635–645
    assessing for concordance in, 635–637, 636*f*, 637*f*
    with atypical ductal hyperplasia, 637–638, 639*f*
    with columnar cell lesions, 641, 642*f*
    communication responsibilities in, 642–643
    for definite benign and concordant benign cases, 637, 638*f*
    with false-negative results, 637, 638*f*
    with false-positive results, 642
    with lobular neoplasia, 640–641
    with papillary lesions, 640, 640*f*
    with radial scar, 638–640, 639*f*
    with sclerosing adenosis, 641–642, 643*f*
  MRI-guided, 210–211, 587–594
    biopsy grid for, 588–589, 589*f*
    CAD device for, 588–590, 590*f*
    contraindications to, 593–594
    dermatotomy for, 591–592
    efficacy and safety of, 587
    equipment for, 587–588
    indications for, 593
    informed consent for, 588
    introducer apparatus for, 591–592, 591*f*
    local anesthesia for, 590–591
      epinephrine with, 591
Core needle biopsy (CNB) *(Continued)*
      expected route of, 591
      injection site for, 591
      minimizing pain of, 591
    marking clip in, 591–592
    with multiple suspicious findings, 593
    number of specimens in, 591–592
    obturator placement during, 591–592, 592*f*
    positioning for, 588–589, 588*f*
    post-procedure considerations for, 592–593
    potential complications of, 594
    pre-contrast images in, 589
    pre-procedural considerations for, 588–590
    report on, 593
    with second-look ultrasound, 593
    specimen processing for, 592–593
    sterile biopsy tray for, 587–588
    sterile portion of procedure for, 590–592
    targeting of lesion for, 589–590, 590*f*
    vacuum-assisted device in, 591–592
  procedure for, 612–614
  stereotactic-guided, 564
    accuracy and cost-effectiveness of, 576
    air gap technique in, 582–583
    anesthesia for
      epinephrine with, 581
      injection tract of, 581
      local, 581
      site of, 581
      topical, 581
    coding and billing for, 723*t*
    confirming accurate needle placement for
      with prone biopsy table, 581–583, 582*f*, 583*f*
      with side-arm needle holder, 583, 584*f*
    contraindications to, 586
    dermatotomy in, 581
    description of, 577, 577*f*
    equipment for, 577–579
      add-on units as, 577–578, 578*f*, 579*f*
      dedicated prone table as, 577, 578*f*
      sterile procedure tray as, 576–587
      vacuum-assisted device as, 578–579
    indications for, 585–586
    informed consent for, 579–580
    of lesion discovered on another modality, 586
    marking clips for, 583–584
    of multiple suspicious findings, 586
    negative stroke margin in, 582–583
    positioning for, 580–581
    post-procedure considerations for, 585
    potential complications of, 586–587
    pre-procedural considerations for, 579–581
    procedure room for, 579
    record of, 585
    retargeting in, 581
    sampling in, 583–584
    scout film in, 580–581, 580*f*
    specimen processing for, 585
    specimen radiography in, 583–584, 585*f*
    sterile portion of procedure for, 581–584
    swing views in, 577, 580–581, 580*f*
    "zeroing out" in, 581
  triple test with, 615, 635–637
  ultrasound-guided, 167–168, 564–576
    advantages of, 564, 575
    air tracts in, 569–571, 571*f*
    anesthesia for
      epinephrine with, 568–569
      injection site for, 569, 569*f*
      local, 568–569
      topical, 569
    of calcifications, 170*f*
Core needle biopsy (CNB) *(Continued)*
    coaxial system for, 569, 570*f*
    coding and billing for, 723*t*
    confirmation of sampling adequacy in, 569–571, 571*f*, 572*f*
    consent form for, 566–567
    contraindications to, 576
    for cyst aspiration, 574
    of deep lesions, 569, 569*f*, 572, 573*f*
    in dense breast, 572
    dermatotomy in, 569
    description of, 564
    equipment for, 564–566
      needle and throw mechanism in, 565, 565*f*
      sterile biopsy tray in, 564–565, 564*f*
      vacuum-assisted device in, 565, 566*f*
    of fibroadenoma, 169*f*
    indications for, 575–576
    of lesion seen on another modality, 575–576
    of lymph nodes, 575
    marking clip in, 572
    of multiple suspicious findings, 575
    as one-person or two-person procedure, 568, 568*f*
    optimal needle positioning for, 569–571, 571*f*
    orientation of needle in, 568, 568*f*
    positioning for, 567, 567*f*
    post-procedure considerations for, 574–575
    potential complications of, 576
    pre-procedural considerations for, 566–568
    pre-scanning in, 567, 567*f*
    readjustment of transducer or needle position during, 569–571, 570*f*
    regional lymph node assessment with, 161–166, 162*f*, 163*f*, 164*f*, 165*f*
    report on, 575
    of small target, 573–574, 574*f*
    specimen preparation from, 575
    with steep approach angle, 569, 569*f*, 572, 573*f*
    sterile portion of procedure for, 568–574
    vacuum-assisted device for, 167–168, 565
      of calcifications, 170*f*
      confirmation of sampling adequacy with, 569–571, 572*f*
      cutting mechanism of, 565, 566*f*
      for cysts, 171–176, 176*f*
      of fibroadenoma, 169*f*
      for nipple discharge, 158–159, 159*f*
    of very superficial lesions, 569, 569*f*, 572, 573*f*
  underestimation of disease with, 615
Cortical thickening, of lymph nodes, 161–166, 162*f*, 163*f*, 164*f*
Cost-effectiveness
  of image-guided percutaneous biopsy, 563–564
    stereotactic-guided, 576
  of screening mammography, 69–70, 70*t*
Coverage, in mammography unit, 83, 83*f*
Coverslipping, of breast tissue specimens, 630–631
Cowden syndrome (CS), and breast cancer risk, 47
CP (collagenous spherulosis), cribriform DCIS *vs.*, 401–402, 403*f*
CPT (Current Procedural Terminology), 720–721, 722, 723*t*
CPT/HCFA Common Procedures Coding System, 720–721
CR (computed radiography) system, for image detection, 95–96, 96*f*

Craniocaudal (CC) view, 115, 115*f*, 116*f*
  clinical image evaluation of, 122–123, 124*f*, 125*f*
  exaggerated lateral, 117–118, 118*f*
  exaggerated medial, 122–123, 125*f*
Creams, calcifications due to, 325–326
Creatinine, and MRI, 193
Cribriform carcinoma, 453, 454*f*
Cribriform-type DCIS, 401–402, 402*f*
  vs. adenoid cystic carcinoma, 401–402, 402*f*
  case study on, 419*b*
    commentary in, 421, 421*f*
    diagnosis in, 420, 420*f*
    differential diagnosis in, 420
    findings in, 419, 419*f*, 420*f*
    history in, 419
  vs. collagenous spherulosis, 401–402, 403*f*
Criminal law, 729
Cronex LoDose I film, 10
Cryoablation, 772–773
  advantages of, 773
  confirmation of effectiveness of, 773
    histopathology for, 773, 775*f*
    imaging studies for, 773, 774*f*
  cryogen in, 773
  equipment for, 773
  history of, 773
  mechanism of action of, 772–773
CS (Cowden syndrome), and breast cancer risk, 47
CsI (cesium iodide) crystals, for image detection, 95–96, 96*f*
CT (computed tomography)
  of breast implants, 680, 680*f*
  dedicated breast, 746–747, 746*f*, 747*f*
  with PET, 748
Cumulative risk, 39–46
Curie, Marie, 13
Curie, Pierre, 13
Current Procedural Terminology (CPT), 720–721, 722, 723*t*
Cutler, Max, 15
CV (cleavage) view, 118
Cylindromatous component, in adenoid cystic carcinoma, 453–455, 455*f*
Cyst(s)
  aspiration of, in ultrasound-guided core needle biopsy, 574
  complicated, 239, 240*f*
  epidermal inclusion and sebaceous, 239–241
    case study of, 250*b*
      core needle biopsy in, 250, 253*f*
      diagnosis in, 250
      differential diagnosis in, 250
      findings in, 250, 251*f*
      fine needle aspiration in, 250, 252*f*
      impression in, 250
      patient history in, 250
    clinical presentation of, 239
    defined, 239, 240*f*
    differential diagnosis of, 240–241, 242*f*, 243*f*
    etiology and pathophysiology of, 239
    imaging indications and algorithm for, 239
    mammography of, 240, 241*f*
    MRI of, 240
    pathology of, 241, 242*f*, 243*f*
    prevalence and epidemiology of, 239
    treatment options for, 241
    ultrasonography of, 240, 241*f*, 242*f*
  galactography of, 598, 599*f*
  infundibular, 239
  lipid or oil, 283, 284*f*
    fat necrosis with, 327–329, 330*f*, 331*f*
  pilar, 239
  pseudo-, 239
Cyst(s) *(Continued)*
  retention, 239
  simple, 239, 240*f*
  trichilemmal, 239
  true, 239
  ultrasound of, 171–176
    with acute inflammation, 157, 158*f*
    containing papillomas or malignancy, 171–176, 175*f*
    with diffuse low-level internal echoes, 171–176, 174*f*
    for directional vacuum-assisted biopsy, 171–176, 176*f*
    with fat-fluid level, 171–176, 174*f*
    with fluid-debris level, 171–176, 174*f*
    mammographic correlation with, 156*f*
    with scintillating echoes, 171–176, 174*f*
Cystic hypersecretory-type DCIS, 403, 406*f*
Cystic lesion(s), benign, 239–254
  case study of, 250*b*
    core needle biopsy in, 250, 253*f*
    diagnosis in, 250
    differential diagnosis in, 250
    findings in, 250, 251*f*
    fine needle aspiration in, 250, 252*f*
    impression in, 250
    patient history in, 250
  duct ectasia as, 244–247
    classic signs of, 245
    clinical presentation of, 245
    defined, 244
    differential diagnosis of, 245–246, 247*f*
    etiology and pathophysiology of, 244
    imaging indications and algorithm for, 245
    mammography of, 245, 246*f*
    MRI of, 245
    pathology of, 245–246, 247*f*
    prevalence and epidemiology of, 244
    treatment options for, 246–247
    ultrasonography of, 245, 246*f*
  epidermal inclusion cysts and sebaceous cysts as, 239–241
    clinical presentation of, 239
    defined, 239, 240*f*
    differential diagnosis of, 240–241, 242*f*, 243*f*
    etiology and pathophysiology of, 239
    imaging indications and algorithm for, 239
    mammography of, 240, 241*f*
    MRI of, 240
    pathology of, 241, 242*f*, 243*f*
    prevalence and epidemiology of, 239
    treatment options for, 241
    ultrasonography of, 240, 241*f*, 242*f*
  fibrocystic change as, 247–249
    and breast cancer risk, 247–248, 248*b*
    clinical presentation of, 248–249
    defined, 247
    differential diagnosis of, 249
    etiology and pathophysiology of, 248
    imaging indications and algorithm for, 249
    imaging technique and findings for, 249
    pathology of, 248*f*, 249, 249*f*
    prevalence and epidemiology of, 247–248, 248*b*
    treatment options for, 249
  galactocele as, 241–244
    classic signs of, 244
    clinical presentation of, 242–244
    defined, 241
    differential diagnosis of, 244, 245*f*
    etiology and pathophysiology of, 242
    imaging indications and algorithm for, 242
    mammography of, 242–243, 243*f*
    MRI of, 244
    pathology of, 244, 245*f*
Cystic lesion(s), benign *(Continued)*
    prevalence and epidemiology of, 241
    treatment options for, 244
    ultrasonography of, 243, 244*f*
Cystosarcoma phyllodes. *See* Phyllodes tumor
Cytogenetic analysis, 229
Cytoplasmic ballooning, after neoadjuvant chemotherapy, 526*f*

D

Damadian, Raymond, 17
Damages, legal, 729
Darkroom cleanliness, quality control test of, 137*t*, 141
Darkroom fog, quality control test of, 137*t*, 142
Data, for medical audit, 703–707
  analysis of, 707–711
  collection system for, 703
  derived
    additional, 704, 705*t*
    essential, 703–704, 704*t*
  raw
    additional, 704, 705*t*
    essential, 703–704, 704*t*
  recent benchmark, 711, 712*t*
  sources of, 715
DCE-MRI. *See* Dynamic contrast enhanced magnetic resonance imaging (DCE-MRI).
DCIS. *See* Ductal carcinoma in situ (DCIS).
Dedicated breast computed tomography (DBCT), 746–747, 746*f*, 747*f*
Dedicated mammography unit, history of, 7–9, 10*f*
"Deep pockets", 735
Deficit Reduction Act (DRA), 721
Denier, Andres, 13
Depositions, 729–730
Derived data, for medical audit
  additional, 704, 705*t*
  essential, 703–704, 704*t*
Dermal calcifications, 323–325
  grid compression paddle for, 323, 326*f*
  mammography of, 323, 325*f*, 554*f*
  parenchymal *vs.*, 323–325
Dermal lymphatic invasion, in inflammatory carcinoma, 466–467, 466*f*
Dermatomyositis, calcifications in, 325, 326*f*, 327*f*
Dermatotomy, for core needle biopsy
  MRI-guided, 591–592
  stereotactic-guided, 581
  ultrasound-guided, 569
Descriptive epidemiology, 25
Desmoid tumor, extra-abdominal. *See* Fibromatosis.
Developing asymmetry, 215
  in invasive ductal carcinoma, 431–432, 433*f*, 434*f*
Development, of breast, 223–224
Diabetic mastopathy, 276–280
  classic signs of, 278
  clinical presentation of, 277
  defined, 276
  etiology and pathophysiology of, 277
  imaging indications and algorithm for, 277
  mammography of, 277–278, 277*f*
  MRI of, 278, 278*f*, 279*f*
  pathology findings in, 278, 279*f*
  prevalence and epidemiology of, 277
  treatment options for, 280
  ultrasonography of, 278, 278*f*

Diagnostic radiology, standards of care for, 731, 732
Diagnostic test, *vs.* screening, 56
Diagnost-U, 9, 79
Diaphanography, history of, 15, 16*f*
Dicta, 730
Differentiation, in invasive ductal carcinoma, 442–445, 443*f*
Diffuse large B-cell lymphoma
  case study of, 520*b*
    commentary in, 523
    diagnosis in, 522
    differential diagnosis in, 522, 523*f*
    excisional biopsy in, 521, 522*f*
    fine-needle aspiration findings in, 521, 521*f*
    history in, 520
    immunohistochemical stains in, 521
    mammography in, 520, 520*f*
    ultrasonography in, 520, 521*f*
  differential diagnosis of, 502–503, 504*f*, 523*f*
  pathology of, 502–503, 503*f*
  prevalence and epidemiology of, 502
Digital detector(s), 94–96
  computed radiography system as, 95–96, 96*f*
  flat-panel phosphor system as, 95, 95*f*
  selenium flat-panel system as, 95, 96*f*
  Slot-Scan charge-coupled device system as, 94–95, 94*f*
Digital display, for compression, 87, 88*f*
Digital image storage, 93
Digital mammography
  computer-aided detection and, 107
  full-field (*See* Full-field digital mammography (FFDM))
  history of, 12, 80, 80*t*
  for screening, 57
  stereo, 743–744, 744*f*
Digital Mammography Imaging Screening Trial (DMIST), 12
Digital tomosynthesis, 744–746, 745*f*
  with automated whole breast ultrasound, 752–753, 755*f*
Directional vacuum-assisted biopsy (DVAB), ultrasound-guided, 167–168, 565
  of calcifications, 170*f*
  confirmation of sampling adequacy with, 569–571, 572*f*
  cutting mechanism of, 565, 566*f*
  for cysts, 171–176, 176*f*
  of fibroadenoma, 169*f*
  for nipple discharge, 158–159, 159*f*
Discordance, 637
Discoverable actions, 729–730
Discovery, 729–730
Disease control programs, population trends and, 38–39
Displaced epithelial cells, *vs.* DCIS, 411–414
DMIST (Digital Mammography Imaging Screening Trial), 12
DNA amplification, as prognostic and predictive factor, 232
Dodd, Gerald, 133–134
Domingues, Carlos, 3
D'Orsi, Carl, 20
Dosimeters, history of, 20–21
Double reading
  with computer-aided detection, 104–107
  computer-aided detection *vs.*, 99
DRA (Deficit Reduction Act), 721
Drug delivery, ultrasound-activated microbubble, 759, 759*f*
Drug-related gynecomastia, 314*t*
DTPA (gadobenate dimeglumine), for contrast-enhanced MRI, 187
Duct, solitary dilated, 215
  in invasive ductal carcinoma, 435, 437*f*
Duct cut-off sign, 158, 159*f*
Duct ectasia, 244–247
  classic signs of, 245
  clinical presentation of, 245
  defined, 244
  differential diagnosis of, 245–246, 247*f*
  etiology and pathophysiology of, 244
  galactography of, 598, 598*f*
  imaging indications and algorithm for, 245
  mammography of, 245, 246*f*
  MRI of, 245
  pathology of, 245–246, 247*f*
  prevalence and epidemiology of, 244
  with secretory calcifications, 331–332
    clinical aspects of, 331
    imaging features of, 331–332, 336*f*
  treatment options for, 246–247
  ultrasonography of, 245, 246*f*
Duct extension, solid breast nodules with, 171, 172*f*
Ductal carcinoma, invasive. *See* Invasive ductal carcinoma (IDC).
Ductal carcinoma in situ (DCIS), 228, 391–422
  apocrine-type, 402, 405*f*
  architectural pattern of, 399–400
  atypical ductal hyperplasia *vs.*, 360, 361*f*, 415, 638, 639*f*
  axillary lymph node metastases of, 411–415
    vs. benign inclusion, 414*f*
    vs. dendritic cells, 413*f*
    vs. histiocyte aggregates, 412*f*
    vs. intracapsular nevus, 413*f*
    vs. nonspecific debris, 413*f*
  basal-like, 403–404
  bilateral, 393*f*
  biological factors in, 415–416
  calcifications in, 392–394
    biopsy for, 556, 557*f*
    branching, 392–394, 392*f*, 394*f*
    coarse heterogeneous, 555–556, 556*f*
    in ductal distribution, 393*f*
    in linear distribution, 392–394, 393*f*, 394*f*
    micro-, 392
    pathology of, 333–334, 343*f*
    round and punctate, 553, 554*f*
    in segmental distribution, 392–394, 392*f*, 393*f*, 394*f*
  with cancerization of lobules, 391, 400–401, 401*f*
  case study on, 419*b*
    commentary in, 421, 421*f*
    diagnosis in, 420, 420*f*
    differential diagnosis in, 420
    findings in, 419, 419*f*, 420*f*
    history in, 419
  classic signs of, 397
  classification of, 399–400
  clear cell, 403, 406*f*
  clinging- or flat-type, 403, 405*f*
  clinical presentation of, 392
  comedo-type, 392
    with cancerization of lobules, 400–401, 401*f*
    case study on, 479, 479*f*
    clinical presentation of, 392
    gross pathology of, 398–399
    microscopic findings in, 400–401, 401*f*
  cribriform-type, 401–402, 402*f*
    vs. adenoid cystic carcinoma, 401–402, 402*f*
    case study on, 419*b*
      commentary in, 421, 421*f*
      diagnosis in, 420, 420*f*
      differential diagnosis in, 420
      findings in, 419, 419*f*, 420*f*
      history in, 419
    vs. collagenous spherulosis, 401–402, 403*f*
Ductal carcinoma in situ (DCIS) *(Continued)*
  cystic hypersecretory-type, 403, 406*f*
  defined, 391–404
  detection during screening of, 67–68
  differential diagnosis of, 397–404
  dimorphic variant of, 403
  etiology and pathophysiology of, 392
  extent of, 410–411
    as prognostic and predictive factor, 232
  fine-needle aspiration findings in, 416, 416*f*, 417*f*
  galactography of, 601, 602*f*
  gross pathology of, 398–399
  imaging indications and algorithm for, 392
  incidence of, 31
  with invasive cancer
    case study on, 479, 479*f*
    with extensive intraductal component
      defined, 391
      mammography of, 394–397, 396*f*, 397*f*
  invasive potential of, 68
  LCIS *vs.*, 364–365, 365*f*
  local recurrence after breast-conserving surgery of, 411, 412*f*
  vs. lymph-vascular invasion, 446–447, 448*f*
  in male breast, 416
  mammography of, 392–394
    bilateral, 393*f*
    calcifications in, 392–394
      branching, 392–394, 392*f*, 394*f*
      in ductal distribution, 393*f*
      in linear distribution, 392–394, 393*f*, 394*f*
      micro-, 392
      in segmental distribution, 392–394, 392*f*, 393*f*, 394*f*
    extensive, 394*f*
    presenting as mass, 394, 395*f*
    with radial scar, 395*f*
    with sclerosing adenosis, 395*f*
  margin assessment for, 411
  in medical audit, 712*t*
  micropapillary, 402, 403*f*, 404*f*
  microscopic findings in, 399–403, 400*f*
  mimicking invasive carcinoma, 403–404, 407*f*, 408*f*
  MRI of, 397, 399*f*, 400*f*
  mucinous-type, 403, 407*f*
  multifocality and multicentricity of, 411
  after neoadjuvant chemotherapy, 526*f*, 527*f*
  nipple adenoma/florid papillomatosis of nipple as, 409, 409*f*
  noncomedo-type, 392
  noninvasive papillary carcinoma as, 397, 398*f*
  nuclear grade of, 409–410, 410*t*
  Paget's disease of nipple as, 404–409, 408*f*
  papillary, 456–457, 458*f*
  prevalence and epidemiology of, 67–68, 391–392
  reproducibility of diagnosis of, 415, 415*f*
  with sclerosing adenosis
    mammography of, 395*f*
    microscopic findings in, 403–404, 407*f*, 408*f*
  solid-type, 402, 404*f*
  spindle cell, 403, 406*f*
  treatment option(s) for, 416–418
    radiation therapy as, 418
    tamoxifen therapy as, 415–416, 418
  ultrasonography of, 397, 398*f*
  Van Nuys Prognostic Index for, 410–416
Ductal hyperplasia, 360, 361*f*
  atypical, 357–360
    clinical presentation of, 358
    vs. DCIS, 360, 361*f*, 415, 638, 639*f*

Ductal hyperplasia (Continued)
defined, 357
differential diagnosis of, 360
etiology and pathophysiology of, 358
imaging indications and algorithm for, 358–359
mammography of, 359, 359f
MRI of, 360
pathology findings with, 360, 361f, 362f
post-biopsy management of, 637–638, 639f
prevalence and epidemiology of, 358
treatment options for, 360
ultrasonography of, 360
benign sclerosing (See Radial scar)
calcifications with, 344f
radial scar with, 306–308, 308f
of usual type, 309–314
with central apocrine metaplasia, 312f
clinical presentation of, 309
with cribriform pattern, 313f
defined, 309
differential diagnosis of, 310–314
etiology and pathophysiology of, 309
with florid proliferation, 312f
with gynecomastia-like or micropapillary pattern, 313f
imaging indications and algorithm for, 310
mammography of, 310, 310f, 311f
MRI of, 310
normal terminal ductal lobular unit vs., 310–314, 311f, 312f
with overlapping nuclei, 313f
pathology findings with, 310–314
prevalence and epidemiology of, 309
treatment options for, 314
ultrasonography of, 310
Ductography. See Galactography.
Dussik, Karl, 13
Duty
breach of, 729
to refer, 735
DVAB. See Directional vacuum-assisted biopsy (DVAB).
Dynamic contrast enhanced magnetic resonance imaging (DCE-MRI), 185–187, 186f, 761
BI-RADS on, 218–219
gadolinium compounds used in, 186, 186t
history of, 18
missed uptake with, 190
and nephrogenic systemic fibrosis, 193
power injector for, 187, 187f
processing and uptake analysis for, 187, 187f
uptake curve and washout phase for, 186, 186f
Dynamic range, in ultrasonography, 217–218

E

E codes, 723t, 725
E-cadherin, and breast cancer risk, 47–48
Echinococcosis, mastitis due to, 380–381, 383f
Ectopic breast tissues, 223
Edinburgh trial, 57–58, 58t
and screening guidelines, 62–63
and underestimation of benefits from screening, 61
Education, in breast imaging, 19f, 20
Society of Breast Imaging on, 20
EFOV (extended field of view), in ultrasonography, 217–218
Egan, Robert, 8f, 9f
hand processing of film by, 11f
Egan, Robert (Continued)
on mammography equipment, 79
as pioneer of mammography, 5–6
standardization of technique by, 5–6, 9f
teaching aids developed by, 19f, 20
EIC. See Extensive intraductal component (EIC).
"Elapsed Time Rule", 724
Elastography, 218, 754–757
basic process of, 755
color patterns on, 755–756, 757f
defined, 754
gray scale, 755–756, 756f
rationale for, 754
shear wave, 756–757, 757f, 758f
static or compressive, 755–756, 756f
in various tissues, 754–755, 756t
Young modulus in, 754–755, 756f
Embedding, of breast tissue specimens, 630–631, 631f
Embryology, of breast, 223–224
Encapsulated papillary carcinoma, 397, 398f, 456–457, 457f, 458f
Epidemiology, of breast cancer, 25–55, 228
in African-Americans vs. whites, 34, 34f, 35–37, 36f
age standardization in, 26–29
international comparison of, 26, 26f, 27f, 28f
analytic, 25
descriptive, 25
incidence in
and age, 32–33, 32f
age-adjusted, 26, 26f, 27f, 28f
of DCIS, 31
national trends in, 30–32, 31f
and race or ethnicity, 33–34, 33f
risk factors and, 31–32
screening mammography and, 31–32, 38–39
worldwide comparison of, 26f, 27f, 28f, 29–30
international comparisons in, 29–30
age-adjusted, 26, 26f, 27f, 28f
long-term survival in, 37
mortality data in, 25–26
mortality rate in
age-adjusted, 26, 26f, 28f
national trends in, 31f, 37–38, 38f, 39f
by rate and ethnicity, 38, 39f
worldwide comparison of, 26f, 28f, 29–30
national estimates in, 25–26
national trends in, 30–33
numbers and rates in, 25–29, 26f
population trends and disease control programs in, 38–39
risk factors in, 41–45, 42t
alcohol consumption as, 42–43
body size as, 42
breastfeeding as, 41–42
exogenous hormone use as, 31–32, 43–45
and incidence, 31–32
menopausal hormones as, 44
oral contraceptives as, 43
physical activity as, 42
SERMs as, 44–45
risk in
cumulative and relative, 39–46
family history and assessment of, 45–46
histologic and mammographic markers of, 45
lifetime, 40–41, 41t
low penetrance susceptiblity genes in, 48
major genes and syndromes with increased, 46–48
worldwide comparison of, 29–30
standard population in, 29
Epidemiology, of breast cancer (Continued)
statistics in, 25–29
summary statistics in, 25–29
survival rate in
racial differences in, 35–37
screening and, 57–61
stage at diagnosis and, 35, 36f
trends in, 37, 37f
tumor size and stage at diagnosis in, 34–38, 34f, 35f, 36f
worldwide estimates in, 25–26
Epidermal inclusion cysts, 239–241
case study of, 250b
core needle biopsy in, 250, 253f
diagnosis in, 250
differential diagnosis in, 250
findings in, 250, 251f
fine needle aspiration in, 250, 252f
impression in, 250
patient history in, 250
clinical presentation of, 239
defined, 239, 240f
differential diagnosis of, 240–241, 242f, 243f
etiology and pathophysiology of, 239
imaging indications and algorithm for, 239
mammography of, 240
MRI of, 240
pathology of, 241, 242f, 243f
prevalence and epidemiology of, 239
treatment options for, 241
ultrasonography of, 240
Epinephrine, with anesthesia, for core needle biopsy
MRI-guided, 591
stereotactic-guided, 581
ultrasound-guided, 568–569
Epithelial atypia, flat, 355–357
and apocrine metaplasia, 356, 358f
with calcifications, 356, 357f
classic signs of, 356
clinical presentation of, 355
columnar cell change with, 356, 356f
columnar cell hyperplasia with, 356, 357f
cytologic atypia in, 356–357, 358f, 359f
defined, 355
differential diagnosis of, 356–357
etiology and pathophysiology of, 355
imaging indications and algorithm for, 355
mammography of, 355, 355f
MRI of, 356
pathology findings with, 356–357
prevalence and epidemiology of, 355
treatment options for, 357
ultrasonography of, 355
Epithelial hyperplasia, 309
Epitheliosis, infiltrating. See Radial scar.
Equipment, for mammography. See Mammography equipment.
Equipment changes, quality control tests required by, 139–141, 139b, 139t
Equipment-related artifacts, 126, 128f
ErbB2
expression patterns of, 229–230, 230f
as prognostic and predictive factor, 232
ESR1 gene, 230f
Estrogen excess, gynecomastia due to, 314t
Estrogen receptor(s) (ERs)
as biomarker, 626, 626f
in DCIS, 415–416
in invasive ductal carcinoma, 449, 449f
in invasive lobular carcinoma, 495
as prognostic and predictive factor, 232
Estrogen replacement therapy, and breast cancer risk, 44

Ethnicity
incidence of breast cancer and, 33–34, 33*f*
and mortality rate, 38, 39*f*
and stage at diagnosis, 35, 36*f*
and tumor size, 34, 34*f*
Evans, K.T., 14–15
Evidence, spoilation of, 729–730
Exaggerated lateral craniocaudal (XLCC) view, 117–118, 118*f*
Exaggerated medial craniocaudal (XMCC) view, 122–123, 125*f*
Excisional biopsy, 618–619, 618*f*
re-, 620–621
Excretory duct, 224*f*
Exercise, and breast cancer risk, 42
Exogenous hormone use, and breast cancer risk, 31–32, 43–45
Exposure, clinical image evaluation of, 123–124, 127*f*
Expression profiling, as prognostic and predictive factor, 232, 233*f*, 234*f*, 234*t*
Extended field of view (EFOV), in ultrasonography, 217–218
Extensive intraductal component (EIC), 446, 446*f*
case study on
moderately differentiated, 475, 475*f*
well-differentiated, 480, 480*f*
defined, 391
mammography of, 394–397, 396*f*, 397*f*
and microcalcifications, 426–427, 428*f*

F

Face-shield, 84, 84*f*
Facility physics survey, Mammography Quality Standards Act on, 693
False-negative (FN), in medical audit, 704, 706, 706*f*, 708*t*
False-positive (FP), in medical audit, 704, 706, 706*f*, 708*t*
False-positive (FP) biopsy results, 67
False-positive (FP) marks, with computer-aided detection, 102, 103*f*, 107
Familial risk, of breast cancer, 230–232
Family history, and risk assessment, 45–46
Fat distribution, and breast cancer risk, 42
Fat necrosis, 283–286
calcifications due to, 327–329
clinical features of, 327
with lipid or oil cyst, 327–329, 330*f*, 331*f*
mammographic appearance of, 327–329, 330*f*, 331*f*, 332*f*
pathology of, 345*f*
post-lumpectomy, 327–329, 332*f*, 333*f*
post-mastectomy, 332*f*
post-surgical, 327–329, 331*f*
post-traumatic, 327–329, 331*f*
ultrasound appearance of, 329, 332*f*, 333*f*
classic signs of, 286
clinical presentation of, 283
defined, 283
etiology and pathophysiology of, 283
imaging indications and algorithm for, 283
vs. invasive ductal carcinoma, 438
with lipid or oil cyst, 283, 284*f*
calcifications due to, 327–329, 330*f*, 331*f*
mammography of, 283, 283*f*, 284*f*, 285*f*
calcifications in, 327–329, 330*f*, 331*f*, 332*f*
with microcalcifications and architectural distortion, 283, 284*f*, 285*f*
MRI of, 283–286
pathology findings with, 286, 286*f*
vs. peripheral T-cell lymphoma, 504, 504*f*, 505*f*
Fat necrosis *(Continued)*
prevalence and epidemiology of, 283
after reduction mammoplasty, 686, 687*f*, 688*f*
treatment options for, 286
ultrasonography of, 283, 285*f*
calcifications in, 329, 332*f*, 333*f*
Fat saturation, in MRI, 184–185, 184*f*, 185*f*
artifacts due to errors in, 189–190, 190*f*
resolution and imaging requirements for, 183*t*
Fat suppression, in MRI, 184–185
artifacts due to errors in, 189–190, 190*f*
chemical saturation for, 184–185, 184*f*, 185*f*
inversion recovery sequence for, 185
resolution and imaging requirements for, 183*t*
Fat-fluid level, cysts with, 171–176, 174*f*
Fatty breast tissue, mammography with, 226, 227*f*
FB (from below) view, 117, 117*f*
FDA. *See* Food and Drug Administration (FDA).
FDG (2-(fluorine-18)-fluoro-2-deoxy-D-glucose), 748
FEA. *See* Flat epithelial atypia (FEA).
Federal inspection, Mammography Quality Standards Act on, 694
Feedback signal, in mammography unit, 82
Feig, Stephen, 20
FFDM. *See* Full-field digital mammography (FFDM).
FGFR1 (fibroblast growth factor receptor 1) gene, amplification of, as prognostic and predictive factor, 232
Fibroadenoma, 255–260
calcifications in involuting, 329–331
clinical aspects of, 329
mammographic appearance of, 331, 334*f*
pathology of, 346*f*
popcorn shape of, 331, 333*f*, 335*f*, 554*f*
ultrasound of, 331, 335*f*
classic signs of, 256
clinical presentation of, 255
complex, 256–259
defined, 255
with epithelial hyperplasia, 256–259, 259*f*
etiology and pathophysiology of, 255
excisional biopsy of, 618
fibrosed (old), 256–259, 258*f*, 259*f*
fine needle aspiration biopsy of, 256–259, 260*f*, 612*f*
imaging indications and algorithm for, 255
with intracanalicular growth pattern, 256–259, 258*f*
juvenile, 259–260, 261*f*
mammography of, 256, 256*f*
MRI of, 256
pathology findings with, 256–260
with pericanalicular growth pattern, 256–259, 258*f*
post-biopsy management of, 637, 638*f*
prevalence and epidemiology of, 255
treatment options for, 260
ultrasonography of, 171, 256
atypical findings in, 256, 257*f*
for short interval follow-up, 160, 160*f*
typical findings in, 171, 173*f*, 256, 257*f*
Fibroblast growth factor receptor 1 *(FGFR1)* gene, amplification of, as prognostic and predictive factor, 232
Fibrocystic change, 226–228, 247–249
and breast cancer risk, 247–248, 248*b*
clinical presentation of, 248–249
defined, 247
differential diagnosis of, 249
etiology and pathophysiology of, 248
Fibrocystic change *(Continued)*
imaging indications and algorithm for, 249
imaging technique and findings for, 249
pathology of, 248*f*, 249, 249*f*
prevalence and epidemiology of, 247–248, 248*b*
treatment options for, 249
Fibrocystic disease, 247
Fibromatosis, 270–273
clinical presentation of, 271
defined, 270
etiology and pathophysiology of, 271
imaging indications and algorithm for, 271
mammography of, 271
MRI of, 272
pathology findings with, 272, 272*f*
prevalence and epidemiology of, 270
treatment options for, 273
ultrasonography of, 271, 271*f*
Fibrosis, 273–274
classic signs of, 274
clinical presentation of, 273
defined, 273
etiology and pathophysiology of, 273
imaging indications and algorithm for, 273
mammography of, 273, 273*f*
MRI of, 274
pathology findings with, 274
prevalence and epidemiology of, 273
treatment options for, 274
ultrasonography of, 273–274
Fibrous mastopathy. *See* Fibrosis.
Fibrous tumor. *See* Fibrosis.
Field of view (FOV)
magnification and, 91
in mammography unit, 83, 83*f*, 85
in ultrasonography, 149, 151*f*, 217–218
Field strength, of MRI, 177, 179*t*
higher, 187–188
50% rule, 730
Filariasis, mammary, 386*b*
commentary on, 388
diagnosis of, 388
differential diagnosis of, 386
findings with, 386, 386*f*, 387*f*
history of, 386
Film, 93–94, 93*f*, 94*f*
Film making devices, quality control test of, 139*t*
Film processing, 80, 94
history of, 10–11, 11*f*
Film processing solutions, quality control test of, 139*t*
Film processors, 80, 94
Film-screen contact, clinical image evaluation of, 125, 128*f*
Filters, in mammography unit, 82
Fine-needle aspiration (FNA) biopsy, 611–612
advantages of, 611
of benign cystic lesions, 250, 252*f*
of DCIS, 416, 416*f*, 417*f*
diagnostic accuracy of, 612
of fibroadenoma, 256–259, 260*f*, 612*f*
history of, 611
of invasive ductal carcinoma, 613*f*
of invasive lobular carcinoma, 493–494, 494*f*, 613*f*
in case study, 497, 499*f*
limitations of, 611
procedure for, 612
stains used with, 612, 612*f*, 613*f*
triple test correlation with, 612
Fine-needle aspiration cytology (FNAC), 594–595
FISH (fluorescence in situ hybridization) testing, for *HER-2/neu*, 627–629, 629*f*
in invasive ductal carcinoma, 450, 452*f*

Fit to film, 113
Fit to viewport, 113
Fixation, for breast tissue specimens, 630–631
Fixer retention, analysis of, 137*t*, 142
Flat epithelial atypia (FEA), 355–357
 and apocrine metaplasia, 356, 358*f*
 with calcifications, 356, 357*f*
 classic signs of, 356
 clinical presentation of, 355
 columnar cell change with, 356, 356*f*
 columnar cell hyperplasia with, 356, 357*f*
 cytologic atypia in, 356–357, 358*f*, 359*f*
 defined, 355
 differential diagnosis of, 356–357
 etiology and pathophysiology of, 355
 imaging indications and algorithm for, 355
 mammography of, 355, 355*f*
 MRI of, 356
 pathology findings with, 356–357
 post-biopsy management of, 641, 642*f*
 prevalence and epidemiology of, 355
 treatment options for, 357
 ultrasonography of, 355
Flat-panel phosphor system, for image detection, 95, 95*f*
Flat-type DCIS, 403, 405*f*
Flip angle, in MRI, 177–179, 179*f*
Florid papillomatosis, of nipple. *See* Nipple adenoma.
Fluid-debris level, cysts with, 171–176, 174*f*
Fluorescence in situ hybridization (FISH) testing, for *HER-2/neu*, 627–629, 629*f*
 in invasive ductal carcinoma, 450, 452*f*
2-(fluorine-18)-fluoro-2-deoxy-D-glucose (FDG), 748
FN (false-negative), in medical audit, 704, 706, 706*f*, 708*t*
FNA biopsy. *See* Fine-needle aspiration (FNA) biopsy.
FNAC (fine-needle aspiration cytology), 594–595
Focal asymmetry(ies), 215
 on screening mammography, 546–547
  defined, 546
  diagnostic mammography for, 547
  spot compression views for, 542, 543*f*
  ultrasound-guided biopsy for, 547, 547*f*
 standards of care for, 732
Focal fibrosis. *See* Fibrosis.
Focal fibrous disease. *See* Fibrosis.
Focal spot, in mammography unit, 82, 83, 83*f*
 and patient motion, 84
 and resolution, 83–84
Focal spot selection, quality control test of, 139*t*
Focal zone setting, for ultrasound, 146, 147*f*, 217–218
Focus(i), in MRI, 218
Follow-up
 legal aspects of, 734
 short interval, ultrasound for, 159–160, 160*f*
Food and Drug Administration (FDA)
 on communicating results, 734
 for help with quality control, 144
 and Mammography Quality Standards Act, 694
 on silicone breast implants, 666
Foot pedals
 for compression, 87, 87*f*
 history of, 10
Ford, Betty, 30–31
Foreign body calcifications, 332–333
 due to bullet fragments, 332, 337*f*, 338*f*
 due to calcified sutures, 332, 340*f*
 due to gold deposits, 333, 340*f*
 parasitic, 333, 341*f*
 due to retained Hickman catheter, 332, 339*f*
 due to sewing needle or localizing wire, 332, 339*f*
Foreseeability, 730, 731
For-presentation image, 93
For-processing image, 93
Founder mutations, 47
Four-dimensional ultrasound, 149–152
FOV (field of view)
 magnification and, 91
 in mammography unit, 83, 83*f*, 85
 in ultrasonography, 149, 151*f*, 217–218
FP (false-positive), in medical audit, 704, 706, 706*f*, 708*t*
FP (false-positive) biopsy results, 67
FP (false-positive) marks, with computer-aided detection, 102, 103*f*, 107
Fraud, 736
From below (FB) view, 117, 117*f*
Frozen section, 625–626
Full resolution, 113
Full-field digital mammography (FFDM)
 accreditation for, 698–699
 acquisition workstation for, 91, 91*f*
 antiscatter grid assembly for, 88–89
 artifacts in, 125, 128*f*
 automatic exposure control for, 90
 coding and billing for, 723*t*
 compression paddles for, 86
 computer-aided detection with, 100, 100*f*
 digital detector(s) for, 94–96
  computed radiography system as, 95–96, 96*f*
  flat-panel phosphor system as, 95, 95*f*
  selenium flat-panel system as, 95, 96*f*
  Slot-Scan charge-coupled device system as, 94–95, 94*f*
 face shield for, 84
 foot pedals and digital display for compression in, 87
 history of, 80, 80*t*
 image formation in, 80, 81*f*
 laser printer for, 93
 mammography unit for, 81
 overview of equipment for, 80, 80*t*
 positioning for, legal aspects of, 731
 quality control tests for, 141
  legal aspects of, 731
 radiologist review workstation for, 91–92
 storage in, 93
 U-arm for, 85, 85*f*
 x-ray tube and filter for, 82, 83–84

G

Gadobenate dimeglumine (DTPA), for contrast-enhanced MRI, 187
Gadolinium contrast-enhanced MRI, 185–187, 186*f*
 compounds used in, 186, 186*t*
 history of, 18
 missed uptake with, 190
 power injector for, 187, 187*f*
 uptake curve and washout phase for, 186, 186*f*
Gadopentetate dimeglumine (BOPTA), for contrast-enhanced MRI, 187
Gail model, 46
Galactocele, 241–244
 classic signs of, 244
 clinical presentation of, 242–244
 defined, 241
 differential diagnosis of, 244, 245*f*
 etiology and pathophysiology of, 242
 imaging indications and algorithm for, 242
 mammography of, 242–243, 243*f*
 MRI of, 244
Galactocele *(Continued)*
 pathology of, 244, 245*f*
 prevalence and epidemiology of, 241
 treatment options for, 244
 ultrasonography of, 243, 244*f*
Galactography, 597–604
 coding and billing for, 723*t*
 contraindications and complications of, 601–604
 cysts on, 598, 599*f*
 defined, 597
 of duct ectasia, 598, 598*f*
 duct perforation in, 601, 603, 603*f*
 equipment for, 597
 indications for, 597
 interpretation of, 598–601
 of intraductal carcinoma, 601, 602*f*
 with lobular filling, 598, 599*f*
 management of lesion identified on, 604
 mastitis due to, 603
 MRI *vs.*, 601, 604*f*
 normal study in, 598, 598*f*
 vs. other modalities, 601, 603*f*, 604*f*
 of papillomas, 598–601, 599*f*, 600*f*, 601*f*
 procedure for, 597–598
 ultrasonography *vs.*, 601, 603*f*
 vasovagal reaction to, 604
Galileo, 16
Gamma imaging, breast-specific, 747–748
Gene(s)
 associated with increased breast cancer risk, 46–48
  BRCA1 and *BRCA2* as, 46–47
  CDH1 as, 47–48
  PTEN as, 47
  STK11 as, 47
  TP53 as, 47
 low penetrance breast cancer susceptibility, 48
  ATM as, 48
  BRIP1 and *PALB2* as, 48
  CHEK2 as, 48
  polymorphisms as, 48
Gene expression patterns, 229–230, 230*f*
Generalized autocalibrating partially parallel acquisition (GRAPPA), in MRI, 189
Generator, in mammography unit, 82
Genetic alterations, in breast cancer, 232, 234*f*
Genetic mutation(s), 229
 in *ATM*, 48
 in *BRCA1* and *BRCA2*, 46–47
 in *BRIP1* and *PALB2*, 48
 in *CDH1*, 47–48
 in *CHEK2*, 47, 48
 founder, 47
 gene expression patterns with, 229–230, 230*f*
 due to loss of heterozygosity, 229
 due to microsatellite instability, 229
 in *PTEN*, 47
 in *STK11*, 47
 in *TP53*, 47
 due to tumor suppressor genes, 229
Genetic susceptibility, to breast cancer, 230–232
Germline mutations
 in *BRCA1* and *BRCA2*, 46–47
 in *CDH1*, 47–48
 in *PTEN*, 47
 in *STK11*, 47
 in *TP53*, 47
Gershon-Cohen, Jacob, 4, 6*f*, 7–9
Global asymmetry, 215
GLOBOCAN, on cancer statistics, 25–26
Glomerular filtration rate (GFR), and MRI, 193
Glycogen-rich carcinoma, 462–463, 463*f*, 464*f*
Gold deposits
 calcifications due to, 333, 340*f*
 in rheumatoid arthritis, 261, 262*f*

Gothenburg Breast Screening Trial, 57–58, 58*t*
and screening guidelines, 71
on screening of women 40 to 49 years old, 71
on underestimation of benefits from screening, 61
Gould, Howard, 11
Goyanes, J, 3
Grade
in invasive ductal carcinoma, 438–445
axillary lymph node metastasis and survival in, 442–445, 445*t*
differentiation in, 442–445, 443*f*
mitotic count in, 442–445, 442*t*
Modified Scarf-Bloom and Richardson system for, 438–442
nuclear, 442–445, 444*f*
as prognostic and predictive factor, 231
Granular cell tumor, 280–283
classic signs of, 281
clinical presentation of, 280
defined, 280
etiology and pathophysiology of, 280
imaging indications and algorithm for, 280
mammography of, 280, 280*f*
MRI of, 281
pathology findings with, 281, 282*f*
prevalence and epidemiology of, 280
treatment options for, 283
ultrasonography of, 281, 281*f*
Granulocytic sarcoma, 502, 504–505, 505*f*
Granuloma, silicone
mammography of, 287*f*, 662, 663*f*, 667–668, 668*f*
MRI of, 202, 203*f*, 676*f*
due to silicone injection, 662, 663*f*
ultrasonography of, 287, 288*f*, 677–678, 679*f*
Granulomatous mastitis
mammography of, 376, 378*f*
pathology findings with, 380–381, 381*f*
GRAPPA (generalized autocalibrating partially parallel acquisition), in MRI, 189
Gray scale elastography, 755–756, 756*f*
Gray scale gain, in ultrasonography, 217–218
GRB7 gene, 229–230
Grid assembly, antiscatter, 88–89, 88*f*
Grid line artifacts, 126, 128*f*
Gros, Charles, 9*f*
on light scanning (diaphanography), 15
on mammography equipment, 79
as pioneer of mammography, 4
on Senographe, 7–9, 10*f*
Guidelines, *vs.* standards of care, 730
Guttner, W, 13
Gynecomastia, 314–318
asymmetric, 316*f*
classic signs of, 317
clinical presentation of, 315
defined, 314
dendritic pattern of, 315
differential diagnosis of, 317–318
diffuse glandular pattern of, 315
early nodular pattern of, 315, 315*f*
etiology and pathophysiology of, 314, 314*t*
imaging indications and algorithm for, 315–317
and male breast cancer, 469, 476, 476*f*
mammography of, 315, 315*f*, 316*f*
MRI of, 315–317
pathology findings with, 317–318, 317*f*, 318*f*
prevalence and epidemiology of, 314
pseudo-, 315, 316*f*
treatment options for, 318
ultrasonography of, 315, 317*f*

H

Half-value layer
in accreditation, 699
in quality control, 138*t*, 143
Hamartoma, 265–268
classic signs of, 266
clinical presentation of, 265
defined, 265
etiology and pathophysiology of, 265
imaging indications and algorithm for, 265
mammography of, 265, 266*f*
MRI of, 265, 267*f*
pathology findings with, 266, 268*f*
prevalence and epidemiology of, 265
treatment options for, 266–268
ultrasonography of, 265, 266*f*
Harm, legal, 730
Harmonic imaging, in ultrasonography, 147–148, 149*f*
HBOC (hereditary breast and ovarian cancer), 46–47
Health Care Financing Administration (HCFA), on coding and billing, 720–721
Health Insurance Plan of Greater New York (HIP) trial, 57–58, 58*t*
and screening guidelines, 62–63
and screening of women 40 to 49 years old, 59, 71
and underestimation of benefits from screening, 61
Health Maintenance Organizations (HMOs), reimbursement by, 724, 726
Heel effect, 83
Hemangioma, 288–290
cavernous, 290–291, 291*f*
clinical presentation of, 289
defined, 288
etiology and pathophysiology of, 289
imaging indications and algorithm for, 289
mammography of, 289
MRI of, 289, 290*f*
pathology findings with, 289–290, 291*f*
perilobular, 290–291, 291*f*
prevalence and epidemiology of, 288–289
treatment options for, 290
ultrasonography of, 289
Hematoma
after breast-conserving therapy, 654
due to core needle biopsy
MRI-guided, 594
stereotactic-guided, 586
ultrasound-guided, 576
Hematopoietic disease(s), 502–505
case study of, 520*b*
commentary in, 523
diagnosis in, 522
differential diagnosis in, 522, 523*f*
excisional biopsy in, 521, 522*f*
fine-needle aspiration findings in, 521, 521*f*
history in, 520
immunohistochemical stains in, 521
mammography in, 520, 520*f*
ultrasonography in, 520, 521*f*
clinical presentation of, 502
defined, 502
mammography of, 502, 503*f*
pathology of, 502–505
diffuse large B-cell lymphoma as, 502–503, 503*f*, 504*f*
granulocytic sarcoma as, 504–505, 505*f*
immunohistochemical stains in, 504
peripheral T-cell lymphoma as, 504, 504*f*, 505*f*
prevalence and epidemiology of, 502
Hendrick, R. Edward, 133–134
HER-2/neu
as biomarker, 627–629
FISH for, 627–629, 629*f*
for invasive ductal carcinoma, 450, 452*f*
immunohistochemical testing (HercepTest) for, 450, 627–629
new standard protocol and guidelines for, 450
score 0 in, 450, 450*f*, 628*f*
score 1 on, 450, 451*f*, 628*f*
score 2 on, 450, 451*f*, 628*f*
score 3 on, 450, 451*f*, 629*f*
for invasive ductal carcinoma, 449–450
FISH for, 450, 452*f*
immunohistochemical stain for, 450, 450*f*, 451*f*
rationale for, 627–629
chromosomal location of, 627–629, 627*f*
as prognostic and predictive factor, 232
HercepTest, 450, 627–629
new standard protocol and guidelines for, 450
score 0 in, 450, 450*f*, 628*f*
score 1 on, 450, 451*f*, 628*f*
score 2 on, 450, 451*f*, 628*f*
score 3 on, 450, 451*f*, 629*f*
Hereditary breast and ovarian cancer (HBOC), 46–47
Heterologous sarcomatous components, malignant phyllodes tumor with, 507*f*
Heterozygosity, loss of, 229
Hickman catheter, retained, calcifications due to, 332, 339*f*
High-intensity focused ultrasound ablation (HIFU), 775
High-risk breast disease(s), 349–372
atypical ductal hyperplasia as, 357–360
clinical presentation of, 358
defined, 357
differential diagnosis of, 360
etiology and pathophysiology of, 358
imaging indications and algorithm for, 358–359
mammography of, 359, 359*f*
MRI of, 360
pathology findings with, 360, 361*f*, 362*f*
prevalence and epidemiology of, 358
treatment options for, 360
ultrasonography of, 360
case study of, 370*b*
diagnosis in, 372, 372*f*, 373*f*
differential diagnosis in, 371
findings in, 370–371, 370*f*, 371*f*
history in, 370
flat epithelial atypia as, 355–357
and apocrine metaplasia, 356, 358*f*
with calcifications, 356, 357*f*
classic signs of, 356
clinical presentation of, 355
columnar cell change with, 356, 356*f*
columnar cell hyperplasia with, 356, 357*f*
cytologic atypia in, 356–357, 358*f*, 359*f*
defined, 355
differential diagnosis of, 356–357
etiology and pathophysiology of, 355
imaging indications and algorithm for, 355
mammography of, 355, 355*f*
MRI of, 356
pathology findings with, 356–357
prevalence and epidemiology of, 355
treatment options for, 357
ultrasonography of, 355
lobular neoplasia as, 360–366
classic signs of, 361
clinical presentation of, 360

High-risk breast disease(s) *(Continued)*
defined, 360
differential diagnosis of, 361-364
etiology and pathophysiology of, 360
mammography of, 361
MRI of, 361
pathology findings with, 362-364, 362*f*, 363*f*
prevalence and epidemiology of, 360
treatment options for, 365-366
ultrasonography of, 361
variants of, 364-365, 364*f*, 365*f*
papillary, 349-355
atypical papilloma as, 352-353, 354*f*
case study of, 370*b*
diagnosis in, 372, 372*f*, 373*f*
differential diagnosis in, 371
findings in, 370-371, 370*f*, 371*f*
history in, 370
classic signs of, 351
clinical presentation of, 349
defined, 349
differential diagnosis of, 352-353
etiology and pathophysiology of, 349
imaging indications and algorithm for, 349
intraductal papilloma as, 352, 352*f*, 353*f*
mammography of, 349-351, 350*f*, 351*f*
MRI of, 351, 352*f*
papillomatosis as, 352, 353*f*
pathology findings with, 352-353
prevalence and epidemiology of, 349
treatment options for, 353-355
ultrasonography of, 351, 351*f*
phyllodes tumor as, 366-372
classic signs of, 367
clinical presentation of, 366
defined, 366
differential diagnosis of, 367-369
etiology and pathophysiology of, 366
imaging indications and algorithm for, 366
mammography of, 366, 366*f*
MRI of, 366-367
pathology findings with, 367-369, 368*f*
prevalence and epidemiology of, 366
treatment options for, 369-372
ultrasonography of, 366
High-transmission cellular (HTC) grid, 89
HIP trial. *See* Health Insurance Plan of Greater New York (HIP) trial.
Hispanic women
incidence of breast cancer in, 33-34, 33*f*
mortality rate in, 38, 39*f*
Histologic grade
in invasive ductal carcinoma, 438-445
axillary lymph node metastasis and survival in, 442-445, 445*t*
differentiation in, 442-445, 443*f*
mitotic count in, 442-445, 442*t*
Modified Scarf-Bloom and Richardson (SBR) system for, 438-442
nuclear, 442-445, 444*f*
as prognostic and predictive factor, 231
Histologic markers, of breast cancer risk, 45
Histologic type, as prognostic and predictive factor, 231
Histology, of normal breast, 224-226, 225*f*, 226*f*
Histoplasmosis, enlarged axillary lymph nodes in, 261, 261*f*
Historical controlled studies, of computer-aided detection, 104, 105*t*
History
of breast imaging, 3-24
education and training in, 19*f*, 20
Society of Breast Imaging in, 20
era of technologic progress in, 7-12
automatic exposure timer in, 10
History *(Continued)*
Charles Gros as, 7-9, 9*f*
dedicated mammography unit in, 7-9, 10*f*
digital mammography in, 12
film processing in, 10-11, 11*f*
foot pedal in, 10
image quality in, 10
John Wolfe in, 11, 11*f*
microfocal spot x-ray tube in, 10
rare earth screens in, 10
xeromammography in, 11-12, 12*f*, 13*f*
other modality(ies) in, 12-18
light scanning (diaphanography) as, 15, 16*f*
MRI as, 17-18, 18*f*
radionuclide imaging as, 16-17, 17*f*
thermography as, 16, 16*f*
ultrasonography as, 13-15, 14*f*, 15*f*
pioneer(s) of mammography in, 3-7
Albert Salomon as, 3, 4*f*, 5*f*
Albert Strickler as, 4
Carlos Dominguez as, 3
Charles Gros as, 4
Helen Ingleby as, 4
J. Goyanes as, 3
Jacob Gershon-Cohen as, 4, 6*f*
Otto Kleinschmidt as, 3
Paul Sebold as, 3-4
R. Sigrist as, 4
Raul Leborgne as, 5, 6*f*, 7*f*, 8*f*
Robert Egan as, 5-6, 8*f*, 9*f*
Stafford Warren as, 3-4, 5*f*, 6*f*
Walter Vogel as, 3
Wendell Scott as, 6
recent challenge and accomplishments in, 22
regulation of mammography in, 20-22
screening mammography in, 18-20
legal aspects of, 732-733
HMOs (Health Maintenance Organizations), reimbursement by, 724, 726
Homer, Marc, 20
Hormone replacement therapy (HRT)
and breast cancer risk, 31-32, 44
MRI and, 204-205, 205*t*
Hospital outpatient prospective payment system (HOPPS), 721
Howry, Douglas, 13, 14*f*
HTC (high-transmission cellular) grid, 89
Hydatid disease, mastitis due to, 380-381, 383*f*

I

IARC (International Agency for Research on Cancer), on cancer statistics, 25
ICD-9-CM *(International Classification of Diseases, 9th Revision: Clinical Modifications)*, 720, 722, 722*t*
IDC. *See* Invasive ductal carcinoma (IDC).
IGF2R gene, 229
IHC testing. *See* Immunohistochemical (IHC) testing.
ILC. *See* Invasive lobular carcinoma (ILC).
Image acquisition workstation, for mammography, 91, 91*f*, 92*f*
Image formation, in MRI, 181, 181*f*, 182*f*
Image quality
in accreditation, 699
in quality control, 138*t*, 143
vs. radiation dose, 10
Image receptor(s), 82*f*, 93-96
digital detector(s) as, 94-96
computed radiography system as, 95-96, 96*f*
flat-panel phosphor system as, 95, 95*f*
Image receptor(s) *(Continued)*
selenium flat-panel system as, 95, 96*f*
Slot-Scan charge-coupled device system as, 94-95, 94*f*
film as, 93-94, 93*f*, 94*f*
processing of, 80, 94
quality control test of sizes of, 139*t*
Image sensitivity, of computer-aided detection, 102
Image storage, 93
Image-guided percutaneous biopsy, 563-596
cost-effectiveness of, 563-564
fine-needle aspiration cytology as, 594-595
MRI-guided, 210-211, 587-594
biopsy grid for, 588-589, 589*f*
CAD device for, 588-590, 590*f*
contraindications to, 593-594
dermatotomy for, 591-592
efficacy and safety of, 587
equipment for, 587-588
indications for, 593
informed consent for, 588
introducer apparatus for, 591-592, 591*f*
local anesthesia for, 590-591
epinephrine with, 591
expected route of, 591
injection site for, 591
minimizing pain of, 591
marking clip in, 591-592
with multiple suspicious findings, 593
number of specimens in, 591-592
obturator placement during, 591-592, 592*f*
positioning for, 588-589, 588*f*
post-procedure considerations for, 592-593
potential complications of, 594
pre-contrast images in, 589
pre-procedural considerations for, 588-590
report on, 593
with second-look ultrasound, 593
specimen processing for, 592-593
sterile biopsy tray for, 587-588
sterile portion of procedure for, 590-592
targeting of lesion for, 589-590, 590*f*
vacuum-assisted device in, 591-592
safety of, 563
stereotactic-guided, 576-587
accuracy and cost-effectiveness of, 576
air gap technique in, 582-583
anesthesia for
epinephrine with, 581
injection tract of, 581
local, 581
site of, 581
topical, 581
coding and billing for, 723*t*
confirming accurate needle placement for
with prone biopsy table, 581-583, 582*f*, 583*f*
with side-arm needle holder, 583, 584*f*
contraindications to, 586
dermatotomy in, 581
description of, 577, 577*f*
equipment for, 577-579
add-on units as, 577-578, 578*f*, 579*f*
dedicated prone table as, 577, 578*f*
sterile procedure tray as, 576-587
vacuum-assisted device as, 578-579
indications for, 585-586
informed consent for, 579-580
of lesion discovered on another modality, 586
marking clips for, 583-584
of multiple suspicious findings, 586
negative stroke margin in, 582-583
positioning for, 580-581

Image-guided percutaneous biopsy *(Continued)*
post-procedure considerations for, 585
potential complications of, 586-587
pre-procedural considerations for, 579-581
procedure room for, 579
record of, 585
retargeting in, 581
sampling in, 583-584
scout film in, 580-581, 580*f*
specimen processing for, 585
specimen radiography in, 583-584, 585*f*
sterile portion of procedure for, 581-584
swing views in, 577, 580-581, 580*f*
"zeroing out" in, 581
ultrasound guided, 564-576
advantages of, 564, 575
air tracts in, 569-571, 571*f*
anesthesia for
epinephrine with, 568-569
injection site for, 569, 569*f*
local, 568-569
topical, 569
coaxial system for, 569, 570*f*
coding and billing for, 723*t*
confirmation of sampling adequacy in, 569-571, 571*f*, 572*f*
consent form for, 566-567
contraindications to, 576
for cyst aspiration, 574
of deep lesions, 569, 569*f*, 572, 573*f*
in dense breast, 572
dermatotomy in, 569
description of, 564
equipment for, 564-566
needle and throw mechanism in, 565, 565*f*
sterile biopsy tray in, 564-565, 564*f*
vacuum-assisted device in, 565, 566*f*
indications for, 575-576
of lesion seen on another modality, 575-576
of lymph nodes, 575
marking clip in, 572
of multiple suspicious findings, 575
as one-person or two-person procedure, 568, 568*f*
optimal needle positioning for, 569-571, 571*f*
orientation of needle in, 568, 568*f*
positioning for, 567, 567*f*
post-procedure considerations for, 574-575
potential complications of, 576
pre-procedural considerations for, 566-568
pre-scanning in, 567, 567*f*
readjustment of transducer or needle position during, 569-571, 570*f*
regional lymph node assessment with, 161-166, 162*f*, 163*f*, 164*f*, 165*f*
report on, 575
of small target, 573-574, 574*f*
specimen preparation from, 575
with steep approach angle, 569, 569*f*, 572, 573*f*
sterile portion of procedure for, 568-574
vacuum-assisted device for, 167-168, 565
of calcifications, 170*f*
confirmation of sampling adequacy with, 569-571, 572*f*
cutting mechanism of, 565, 566*f*
for cysts, 171-176, 176*f*
of fibroadenoma, 169*f*
for nipple discharge, 158-159, 159*f*
of very superficial lesions, 569, 569*f*, 572, 573*f*
validation of, 563-564
Imaging geometry, U-arm and, 84-85, 84*f*, 85*f*
Immunohistochemical (IHC) testing, for *HER-2/neu*, 450, 627-629
new standard protocol and guidelines for, 450
score 0 in, 450, 450*f*, 628*f*
score 1 on, 450, 451*f*, 628*f*
score 2 on, 450, 451*f*, 628*f*
score 3 on, 450, 451*f*, 629*f*
Implant(s), 662-681
alternatives to, 665
comparison of imaging modalities with, 680, 680*f*
complications of, 663-665
CT of, 680, 680*f*
demographics of, 663
dual chamber (double lumen), 663, 665*f*
MRI of, 670, 670*f*
encapsulation of, 666
FDA approval of, 666
fluid on periphery of, 673, 675*f*
gel bleed from, 666
history of, 662-666
imaging indications and algorithm for, 663-666
mammography of, 667-668
with rupture, 287, 287*f*, 667-668, 668*f*
with silicone adenopathy, 667, 667*f*
with silicone granulomas, 667-668, 668*f*
Mammography Quality Standards Act on, 696
MRI of, 201-202, 668-674
in evaluation for malignancy, 201-202
with gel fracture, 674
imaging protocols for, 669-670
normal appearance in, 670-671, 670*f*
with radial folds, 671, 671*f*
rat-tail sign in, 670*f*, 673
with rupture, 288
axial and sagittal inversion recovery water saturation images in, 201, 668*f*
contour deformities in, 673
extracapsular, 673-674, 676*f*
fluid on periphery of implant in, 673, 675*f*
inconclusive signs in, 673
intracapsular, 671-673
linguine sign in, 671, 672*f*
subscapular line sign in, 671, 672*f*, 673*f*
teardrop, keyhole, or noose sign in, 673, 673*f*
water droplets in, 673, 674*f*
with silicone granulomas, 202, 203*f*, 676*f*
technical factors in, 669, 669*f*, 669*t*
multi-compartment, 671, 673*f*
pathology findings with, 287-288, 288*f*, 289*f*
prevalence and epidemiology of, 287
with radial folds
MRI of, 671, 671*f*
ultrasonography of, 674, 677*f*
rupture of, 286-288, 666
classic signs of, 287
clinical presentation of, 287
CT of, 680, 680*f*
defined, 286-287
etiology and pathophysiology of, 287
etiology of, 666
extracapsular, 666
MRI of, 673-674, 676*f*
ultrasonography of, 677-678, 678*f*, 679*f*
imaging indications and algorithm for, 287
intracapsular, 666
MRI of, 671-673
ultrasonography of, 677, 678*f*
mammography of, 287, 287*f*, 667-668, 668*f*
Implant(s) *(Continued)*
MRI of, 288
axial and sagittal inversion recovery water saturation images in, 201, 668*f*
contour deformities in, 673
extracapsular, 673-674, 676*f*
fluid on periphery of implant in, 673, 675*f*
inconclusive signs in, 673
intracapsular, 671-673
linguine sign in, 671, 672*f*
subscapular line sign in, 671, 672*f*, 673*f*
teardrop, keyhole, or noose sign in, 673, 673*f*
water droplets in, 673, 674*f*
pathology findings with, 287-288, 288*f*, 289*f*
prevalence and epidemiology of, 287
saline, 667
ultrasonography of, 674-678
extracapsular, 677-678, 678*f*, 679*f*
intracapsular, 677, 678*f*
with silicone granulomas, 287, 288*f*
saline, 663
rupture of, 667
with silicone adenopathy, 667, 667*f*
single chamber (single lumen), 663, 664*f*, 665*f*
MRI of, 670, 670*f*
stacked, 670
subglandular, 663, 664*f*
subpectoral, 663, 665*f*
ultrasonography of, 288-290, 674-679
limitations of, 678-679
normal findings in, 674, 676*f*, 677*f*
with radial folds, 674, 677*f*
with reverberation artifacts, 674, 677*f*
with rupture, 674-678
extracapsular, 677-678, 678*f*, 679*f*
intracapsular, 677, 678*f*
and silicone granulomas, 287, 287*f*
Implant views, 119
Incidence, of breast cancer
and age, 32-33, 32*f*
age-adjusted, 26, 26*f*, 27*f*, 28*f*
of DCIS, 31
national trends in, 30-32, 31*f*
and race or ethnicity, 33-34, 33*f*
risk factors and, 31-32
screening mammography and, 31-32, 38-39
worldwide comparison of, 26*f*, 27*f*, 28*f*, 29-30
Incisional biopsy, 618
Inconclusive triplets, 635-637
Independent consultants, for help with quality control, 144
"Indeterminate" category, 734
Indurative mastopathy. *See* Radial scar.
Infection, due to core needle biopsy
MRI-guided, 594
stereotactic-guided, 586
ultrasound-guided, 576
Infectious lesion(s), 375-388
abscess as, 379
mammography of, 376, 377*f*
pathology findings in, 379-380, 381*f*, 382*f*
subareolar, 377*f*, 379-380, 382*f*
ultrasonography of, 376-378, 379*f*, 380*f*, 381*f*
case study on, 386*b*
commentary in, 388
diagnosis in, 388
differential diagnosis in, 386
findings in, 386, 386*f*, 387*f*
history in, 386

Infectious lesion(s) *(Continued)*
classic signs of, 379
clinical presentation of, 375
due to coccidioidomycosis, 380-381, 384*f*
defined, 375
differential diagnosis of, 379-385
due to echinococcosis, 380-381, 383*f*
etiology and pathophysiology of, 375
due to filariasis, 386*b*
commentary on, 388
diagnosis of, 388
differential diagnosis of, 386
findings with, 386, 386*f*, 387*f*
history of, 386
granulomatous
mammography of, 376, 378*f*
pathology findings with, 380-381, 381*f*
imaging indications and algorithm for, 375-376
mammography of, 376
with abscess, 376, 377*f*
granulomatous, 376, 378*f*
with reactive lymph node, 376*f*
with skin and trabecular thickening, 376, 377*f*
with trichinosis, 376, 379*f*
MRI of, 378-379
pathology findings with, 379-385
acute inflammatory cells in, 382*f*
with breast abscess, 379
with coccidioidomycosis, 380-381, 384*f*
with echinococcosis, 380-381, 383*f*
granulomatous, 380-381, 381*f*
with subareolar abscess, 379-380, 382*f*
tuberculous, 384*f*, 385
prevalence and epidemiology of, 375
treatment options for, 385-388
due to trichinosis, 376, 379*f*
tuberculous, 384*f*, 385
ultrasonography of, 376-378, 379*f*, 380*f*, 381*f*
Inferosuperior oblique (ISO) view, 117
Infiltrating carcinoma. *See* Invasive carcinoma.
Infiltrating epitheliosis. *See* Radial scar.
Inflammatory carcinoma, 466-467
dermal lymphatic invasion in, 466-467, 466*f*
gross pathology of, 438, 438*f*
skin changes in
clinical presentation of, 425, 466-467
mammography of, 428, 430*f*
Inflammatory cell infiltrates, as prognostic and predictive factor, 231
Inflammatory lesion(s), 375-388
abscess as, 379
mammography of, 376, 377*f*
pathology findings in, 379-380, 381*f*, 382*f*
subareolar, 377*f*, 379-380, 382*f*
ultrasonography of, 376-378, 379*f*, 380*f*, 381*f*
case study on, 386*b*
commentary in, 388
diagnosis in, 388
differential diagnosis in, 386
findings in, 386, 386*f*, 387*f*
history in, 386
classic signs of, 379
clinical presentation of, 375
due to coccidioidomycosis, 380-381, 384*f*
defined, 375
differential diagnosis of, 379-385
due to echinococcosis, 380-381, 383*f*
etiology and pathophysiology of, 375
due to filariasis, 386*b*
commentary on, 388
diagnosis of, 388
differential diagnosis of, 386
findings with, 386, 386*f*, 387*f*
history of, 386

Inflammatory lesion(s) *(Continued)*
granulomatous
mammography of, 376, 378*f*
pathology findings with, 380-381, 381*f*
imaging indications and algorithm for, 375-376
mammography of, 376
with abscess, 376, 377*f*
granulomatous, 376, 378*f*
with reactive lymph node, 376*f*
with skin and trabecular thickening, 376, 377*f*
with trichinosis, 376, 379*f*
MRI of, 378-379
pathology findings with, 379-385
acute inflammatory cells in, 382*f*
with breast abscess, 379
with coccidioidomycosis, 380-381, 384*f*
with echinococcosis, 380-381, 383*f*
granulomatous, 380-381, 381*f*
with subareolar abscess, 379-380, 382*f*
tuberculous, 384*f*, 385
prevalence and epidemiology of, 375
treatment options for, 385-388
due to trichinosis, 376, 379*f*
tuberculous, 384*f*, 385
ultrasonography of, 376-378, 379*f*, 380*f*, 381*f*
Informed consent
for core needle biopsy
MRI-guided, 588
stereotactic-guided, 579-580
ultrasound-guided, 566-567
legal aspects of, 734-735
Inframammary fold, in mediolateral oblique view, 124*f*
Infundibular cyst, 239
Ingelby, Helen, 4
In-house service, for mammography equipment, 97
Inspection, Mammography Quality Standards Act on, 694
Intensifying screens, 93
quality control test of, 139*t*
Intentional torts, 735
Interlobular duct
anatomy of, 224*f*
histology of, 225*f*
Internal mammary lymph nodes
MRI of, 199
ultrasound of, 163-165, 164*f*
International Agency for Research on Cancer (IARC), on cancer statistics, 25
International Classification of Diseases, 9th Revision: Clinical Modifications (ICD-9-CM), 720, 722, 722*t*
International comparisons, of breast cancer incidence and mortality rates, 29-30
age-adjusted, 26, 26*f*, 27*f*, 28*f*
Interpreting physician, in quality control, 134-135
continuing education of, 135, 135*t*
continuing experience of, 135, 135*t*
initial qualifications of, 135, 135*t*
lead, 134, 134*t*
reestablishing qualifications of, 135
responsibilities of, 134-135, 134*t*
reviewing (audit), 134*t*
Interrogatories, 729-730
Interval cancers, 57
Interventional procedures, ultrasound-guided, 167-168, 169*f*, 170*f*
Intracystic papillary carcinoma, 397, 398*f*, 456-457, 457*f*, 458*f*
Intraductal carcinoma. *See* Ductal carcinoma in situ (DCIS).
Intraductal papillary lesions (IPLs), 158-159, 158*f*, 159*f*

Intraductal papilloma
case study of, 370*b*
diagnosis in, 372, 372*f*, 373*f*
differential diagnosis in, 371
findings in, 370-371, 370*f*, 371*f*
history in, 370
pathology findings with, 352, 352*f*, 353*f*
ultrasonography of, 351, 351*f*
Intramammary lymph node, 260-264
classic signs of, 263
clinical presentation of, 262
defined, 260
differential diagnosis of, 263-264
etiology and pathophysiology of, 261, 261*f*, 262*f*
imaging indications and algorithm for, 262
mammography of, 262-263, 262*f*, 263*f*
MRI of, 263
pathology findings with, 264, 264*f*, 265*f*
prevalence and epidemiology of, 261
reactive inflammatory, 263, 263*f*, 264*f*
treatment options for, 264
ultrasonography of, 263, 263*f*, 264*f*
Intraoperative consultation, with pathologist, 625-626
Intravenous (IV) placement, for MRI, 192
Invasive carcinoma, 228
adenoid cystic, 453-455, 454*f*, 455*f*
apocrine, 461-462, 462*f*
bilateral, 467
colloid (mucinous), 455-456, 456*f*
cribriform, 453, 454*f*
DCIS mimicking, 403-404, 407*f*, 408*f*
ductal (*See* Invasive ductal carcinoma (IDC))
with extensive intraductal component
defined, 391
mammography of, 394-397, 396*f*, 397*f*
glycogen-rich, 462-463, 463*f*, 464*f*
inflammatory, 466-467
dermal lymphatic invasion in, 466-467, 466*f*
skin changes in
clinical presentation of, 425, 466-467
mammography of, 428, 430*f*
lobular (*See* Invasive lobular carcinoma (ILC))
in male, 468-470
case study on, 476, 476*f*
clinical presentation of, 469
defined, 468
etiology and pathophysiology of, 468-469
mammography of, 469
pathology findings in, 469
prevalence and epidemiology of, 468
ultrasonography of, 469
medullary, 460-461, 461*f*
metaplastic, 463-466, 464*f*
micro-, 445-446, 445*f*
micropapillary, 459, 459*f*
vs. lymph-vascular invasion, 446-447, 448*f*
vs. ovarian metastatic carcinoma, 459, 460*f*
occult, 467, 468*t*
papillary, 456-457, 457*f*, 458*f*
secretory, 462, 463*f*
small cell, 455, 455*f*
special types of, 453-467
spindle cell, 465, 465*f*, 466*f*
tubular, 423-424, 453*f*
tubulolobular, 453, 454*f*
unusual presentations of, 467
well-differentiated, 442-445, 443*f*
case study on, 477, 477*f*
with extensive intraductal component, 480, 480*f*

Invasive ductal carcinoma (IDC), 423–482
architectural distortion in, 432–434, 434f, 435f
asymmetry in
clinical presentation of, 425
developing, 431–432, 433f, 434f
mammography of, 434–435, 436f, 437f
axillary adenopathy in, 425
axillary lymph node metastases in, 429–431, 431f, 432f
biomarker(s) for, 447–453
estrogen receptor as, 449, 449f
HER-2/neu as, 449–450
FISH for, 450, 452f
immunohistochemical stain for, 450, 450f, 451f
Ki-67 as, 453
progesterone receptor as, 453
breast pain in, 425
case study(ies) on, 471b
in male, 476, 476f
moderately differentiated, 471, 471f, 478, 478f
with DCIS, 479, 479f
with extensive intraductal component, 475, 475f
poorly differentiated, 473, 473f
well-differentiated, 477, 477f
with extensive intraductal component, 480, 480f
clinical presentation of, 424–425
asymmetry in, 425
axillary adenopathy in, 425
breast pain in, 425
in differential diagnosis, 437
mass in, 424–425
nipple discharge in, 425
nipple retraction in, 425
skin changes in, 425
with DCIS, 479, 479f
defined, 423
differential diagnosis of, 437–453
clinical presentation in, 437
vs. diffuse large B-cell lymphoma, 502–503, 504f
imaging findings in, 437
etiology and pathophysiology of, 424
with extensive intraductal component, 446, 446f
case study on
moderately differentiated, 475, 475f
well-differentiated, 480, 480f
and microcalcifications, 426–427, 428f
fine-needle aspiration findings with, 613f
histologic grade in, 438–445
axillary lymph node metastasis and survival in, 442–445, 445t
differentiation in, 442–445, 443f
mitotic count in, 442–445, 442t
Modified Scarf-Bloom and Richardson (SBR) system for, 438–442
nuclear, 442–445, 444f
intracystic, 175f
with lymph-vascular invasion, 446–447, 447f, 448f
DCIS *vs.*, 446–447, 448f
micropapillary invasive carcinoma *vs.*, 446–447, 448f
mammographic signs of
indirect, 431–435
architectural distortion as, 432–434, 434f, 435f
asymmetry as, 434–435, 436f, 437f
developing asymmetry as, 431–432, 433f, 434f
single dilated duct as, 435, 437f

Invasive ductal carcinoma (IDC) *(Continued)*
primary, 426–427
mass as, 426, 426f, 427f
microcalcifications as, 426–427, 428f, 429f
secondary, 427–431
axillary lymph node metastases as, 429–431, 431f, 432f
nipple retraction as, 428–429, 430f
skin retraction as, 428, 430f
skin thickening as, 427–428, 430f
mass in
clinical presentation of, 424–425
defined, 426
mammography of, 426
density of, 426, 426f
with irregular shape and spiculated margins, 426, 426f
with round shape and circumscribed margins, 426, 427f
spot compression in, 426, 427f
microcalcifications in, 426–427, 428f, 429f
moderately differentiated, 442–445, 443f
case study on, 471, 471f, 478, 478f
with DCIS, 479, 479f
with extensive intraductal component, 475, 475f
MRI of, 437
nipple discharge in, 425
nipple retraction in
clinical presentation of, 425
mammography of, 428–429, 430f
pathology findings in, 438–453
gross pathology in, 438, 438f
TNM staging of, 438, 439t, 440t, 442t
histologic grade in, 438–445
axillary lymph node metastasis and survival in, 442–445, 445t
differentiation in, 442–445, 443f
mitotic count in, 442–445, 442t
Modified Scarf-Bloom and Richardson (SBR) system for, 438–442
nuclear, 442–445, 444f
with perineural invasion, 446, 447f
poorly differentiated, 442–445, 443f
case study on, 473, 473f
prevalence and epidemiology of, 423–424
risk factors for, 424
single dilated duct in, 435, 437f
skin changes in, 425
skin retraction in
clinical presentation of, 425
mammography of, 428, 430f
skin thickening in
clinical presentation of, 425
mammography of, 427–428, 430f
stromal desmoplasia in, 490f
TNM staging of, 438, 439t, 440t, 442t
treatment options for, 470
ultrasonography of, 435–437
Invasive lobular carcinoma (ILC), 483–501
alveolar cell variant of, 491–493, 492f
biomarkers and prognosis for, 495
case study on, 497b
diagnosis in, 500
differential diagnosis in, 500
history in, 497
mammography in, 498f
MRI in, 499f
pathology findings in, 497–500, 497f, 498f
with core needle biopsy, 499f, 500
with excisional biopsy, 500, 500f
with fine-needle aspiration, 497, 499f
classic signs of, 488
classic type, 491–493, 491f, 492f
clinical presentation of, 483

Invasive lobular carcinoma (ILC) *(Continued)*
core needle biopsy of, 499f, 500
defined, 483
differential diagnosis of, 488–489
in case study, 500
etiology and pathophysiology of, 483
excisional biopsy of, 500, 500f
fine-needle aspiration findings with, 493–494, 494f, 613f
in case study, 497, 499f
gross pathology of, 489–491, 490f, 491f
in males, 496
mammography of, 484–485
architectural distortion in, 485, 486f
in case study, 498f
in dense breast, 484, 484f, 485f
mass with spiculated margins in, 484, 485f
microcalcifications in, 485, 486f
screening, 484, 484f
metastases of
to lymph nodes, 493f, 494–495, 495t
non-nodal, 495
microscopic pathology of, 491–493
alveolar type, 491–493, 492f
with axillary lymph node metastases, 493f
in case study, 497–500, 497f, 498f
with core needle biopsy, 499f, 500
with excisional biopsy, 500, 500f
with fine-needle aspiration, 497, 499f
classic type, 491–493, 491f, 492f
linear pattern in, 491–493, 491f, 494f
pleomorphic type, 491–493, 493f
case study of, 497b
signet ring cell type, 491–493, 492f, 494f
targetoid pattern in, 491–493, 492f
MRI of, 487–488, 489f
in case study, 499f
dynamic contrast-enhanced subtraction, 489f
fat-saturated subtraction, 490f
maximum intensity projection, 490f
after neoadjuvant chemotherapy, 528f, 529f
pleomorphic variant of, 491–493, 493f
case study of, 497b
prevalence and epidemiology of, 483–500
signet ring cell variant of, 491–493, 492f, 494f
treatment options for, 496–500
ultrasonography of, 485–487
focal shadowing in, 485–487, 488f
mass in, 485–487, 487f
Invasive micropapillary carcinoma, 459, 459f
vs. lymph-vascular invasion, 446–447, 448f
vs. ovarian metastatic carcinoma, 459, 460f
Inversion recovery sequence, in MRI, 185
Inverter circuit, in mammography unit, 82
Inverter pulsing rate, in mammography unit, 82
IPLs (intraductal papillary lesions), 158–159, 158f, 159f
ISO (inferosuperior oblique) view, 117
Isolated tumor cells (ITC), in sentinel lymph node sample, 624–625, 625f
IV (intravenous) placement, for MRI, 192

J

Jellins, Jack, 14–15, 15f
J-point-resolved spectroscopy (JPRESS), 763
Juvenile papillomatosis
clinical presentation of, 349
defined, 349
mammography of, 351
prevalence and epidemiology of, 349
treatment options for, 355

K

Karyotyping, 229
Kelly-Fry, Elizabeth, 14–15
Keyhole sign, with implant rupture, 673, 673*f*
Ki-67, as biomarker, 453
Kleinschmidt, Otto, 3
Kossoff, George, 14–15, 15*f*
K-space, in MRI, 181, 182*f*
kVp (peak kilovolt)
  accuracy and reproducibility of, quality control test of, 138*t*, 143
  clinical image evaluation of, 123

L

Labeling
  clinical image evaluation of, 126–127, 129*f*, 130*f*, 131*f*
  of imaging views, 113, 113*t*
  nonstandardized, 126–127, 129*f*, 130*f*, 131*f*
  standardized methods for, 127, 131*f*
Lactating adenoma, 274–276
  clinical presentation of, 274
  defined, 274
  etiology and pathophysiology of, 274
  imaging indications and algorithm for, 274
  mammography of, 274
  MRI of, 274
  pathology findings with, 274–276, 276*f*, 277*f*
  prevalence and epidemiology of, 274
  treatment options for, 276
  ultrasonography of, 274, 275*f*
Lactational changes in pregnancy, calcifications with, 342*f*
Lactiferous ducts
  anatomy of, 224*f*
  development of, 223
Lactiferous sinus, 224*f*
Lagios classification system, 409, 410, 410*t*
Landscape view, in ultrasonography, 149, 151*f*
Langevin, Paul, 13
"Lapsed Time Rule", 724
Laser ablation, 776
Laser printers, for mammography, 92–93
Lateromedial (LM) angled view, 115–116
Lateromedial oblique (LMO) view, 116
Latina women
  incidence of breast cancer in, 33–34, 33*f*
  mortality rate in, 38, 39*f*
Lawson, Ray, 16, 16*f*
Lawsuit, 730
LCIS. *See* Lobular carcinoma in situ (LCIS).
L-COSY. *See* Localized shift correlated spectroscopy (L-COSY).
Lead interpreting physician, in quality control, 134, 134*t*
Lead time
  and over-diagnosis, 64
  for screening, 61–62
Lead-time bias, 57
Leborgne, Raul, 6*f*
  on breast compression, 5, 7*f*, 8*f*
  on calcifications, 5, 7*f*, 8*f*
  on mammography equipment, 79
  as pioneer of mammography, 5
Legal admissions, 736
Legal harm, 730
Legal issue(s), 728–739
  administrative issues in liability as, 732–733
  agency as, 735
  communication of results as, 733–734
  consent as, 734–735
Legal issue(s) *(Continued)*
  duty to refer, negligent referral, and abandonment as, 735
  fraud as, 736
  malpractice as, 728, 729–730
  with medical audit, 717
  standards of care as, 729, 730–732
  technology development and, 736–737
Leiomyosarcoma, 511, 511*f*
Length bias, 57
Leukemia, 502, 504–505
Liability, administrative issues in, 732–733
Lidocaine, for ultrasound-guided core needle biopsy, 568–569
Lifetime risk, 39–41, 41*t*
Li-Fraumeni syndrome (LFS), and breast cancer risk, 47
Light fields, quality control test of, 139*t*
Light scanning, history of, 15, 16*f*
Lighting, quality control test of, 139*t*
Linguine sign, with implant rupture, 671, 672*f*
Lipid cyst, 283, 284*f*
  fat necrosis with, 327–329, 330*f*, 331*f*
Lipoma, 268–270
  angio-, 271*f*
  classic signs of, 268
  clinical presentation of, 268
  defined, 268
  etiology and pathophysiology of, 268
  imaging indications and algorithm for, 268
  mammography of, 268, 269*f*
  MRI of, 268
  pathology findings with, 269, 271*f*
  prevalence and epidemiology of, 268
  treatment options for, 270
  ultrasonography of, 268, 269*f*, 270*f*
Liposarcoma
  clinical presentation of, 509
  MRI of, 509
  pathology of, 510, 510*f*
Liposarcomatous heterologous element, malignant phyllodes tumor with, 507*f*
LM (lateromedial) angled view, 115–116
LMO (lateromedial oblique) view, 116
LN. *See* Lobular neoplasia (LN).
Loadability, 83, 84
Lobe, 224*f*
Lobular carcinoma, invasive. *See* Invasive lobular carcinoma (ILC).
Lobular carcinoma in situ (LCIS), 228, 360–366
  classic signs of, 361
  clinical presentation of, 360
  defined, 360
  differential diagnosis of, 361–364
    vs. DCIS, 364–365, 365*f*
  E-cadherin stain for, 364–365, 365*f*
  etiology and pathophysiology of, 360
  intermediate grade, 364–365, 365*f*
  mammography of, 361
  massive acinar distention, 364–365
  MRI of, 361
  pagetoid spread of, 405–409
  pathology findings with, 362–364, 363*f*
  pleomorphic, 364–365, 364*f*
  post-biopsy management of, 640–641
  prevalence and epidemiology of, 360
  signet ring cell type, 364–365, 364*f*
  treatment options for, 365–366
  ultrasonography of, 361
  variants of, 364–365, 364*f*, 365*f*
Lobular filling, galactography with, 598, 599*f*
Lobular hyperplasia, atypical, 360–366
  classic signs of, 361
  clinical presentation of, 360
  defined, 360
  differential diagnosis of, 361–364
Lobular hyperplasia, atypical *(Continued)*
  etiology and pathophysiology of, 360
  mammography of, 361
  MRI of, 361
  pathology findings with, 362–364, 362*f*
  post-biopsy management of, 640–641
  prevalence and epidemiology of, 360
  treatment options for, 365–366
  ultrasonography of, 361
Lobular neoplasia (LN), 360–366
  classic signs of, 361
  clinical presentation of, 360
  defined, 360
  differential diagnosis of, 361–364
  etiology and pathophysiology of, 360
  mammography of, 361
  MRI of, 361
  pathology findings with, 362–364, 362*f*, 363*f*
  post-biopsy management of, 640–641
  prevalence and epidemiology of, 360
  treatment options for, 365–366
  ultrasonography of, 361
  variants of, 364–365, 364*f*, 365*f*
Lobule(s)
  anatomy of, 224*f*
  cancerization of, 391, 400–401, 401*f*
    radiation atypia *vs.*, 531–533, 532*f*
  histology of, 225, 226*f*
Lobulitis, sclerosing lymphocytic. *See* Diabetic mastopathy.
Local anesthesia, for core needle biopsy
  MRI-guided, 590–591
    epinephrine with, 591
    expected route of, 591
    injection site for, 591
    minimizing pain of, 591
  stereotactic-guided, 581
    epinephrine with, 581
    injection tract of, 581
    site of, 581
    topical, 581
  ultrasound-guided, 568–569
    epinephrine with, 568–569
    injection site for, 569, 569*f*
    topical anesthesia with, 569
Localized shift correlated spectroscopy (L-COSY), 763
  of breast tissue, 764–766
    with benign tumor, 766*f*, 767*t*
    healthy fatty, 764*f*, 767*t*, 768*t*
    healthy glandular, 765*f*, 767*t*
    with malignant tumor, 765*f*, 767*t*, 768*t*
  choline in, 761–762
  classification and regression tree (CART) analysis for, 761–762, 766–767, 767*t*, 768*t*
  metabolites identified in, 766*t*
  phantom study using, 763–764, 764*f*
  water-to-fat ratio in, 761–762
Localizing wire, calcifications due to, 332
Long-axis focusing, in ultrasonography, 146, 147*f*
Long-term survival, with breast cancer, 37
Loss of chance doctrine, 730
Loss of heterozygosity (LOH), 229
Ludwig, George, 13
Lumpectomy. *See* Breast-conserving therapy.
Lung carcinoma, metastatic to breast, 513*f*
LVI (lymph-vascular invasion), 446–447, 447*f*, 448*f*
  DCIS *vs.*, 446–447, 448*f*
  micropapillary invasive carcinoma *vs.*, 446–447, 448*f*
Lymph node(s)
  abnormal, on screening mammography, 546, 546*f*
  axillary (*See* Axillary lymph node(s))
  complete obliteration of mediastinum of, 163

Lymph node(s) *(Continued)*
cortical thickening of, 161–166, 162*f*, 163*f*, 164*f*
intramammary, 260–264
classic signs of, 263
clinical presentation of, 262
defined, 260
differential diagnosis of, 263–264
etiology and pathophysiology of, 261, 261*f*, 262*f*
imaging indications and algorithm for, 262
mammography of, 262–263, 262*f*, 263*f*
MRI of, 263
pathology findings with, 264, 264*f*, 265*f*
prevalence and epidemiology of, 261
reactive inflammatory, 263, 263*f*, 264*f*
treatment options for, 264
ultrasonography of, 263, 263*f*, 264*f*
after neoadjuvant chemotherapy, 524, 527*f*, 528*f*, 529*f*
reactive *vs.* metastatic, 163, 163*f*
ultrasound-guided core needle biopsy of, 575
Lymph node assessment, in patients with suspicious breast lesions undergoing biopsy, ultrasound for, 161–166, 162*f*, 163*f*, 164*f*, 165*f*
Lymph node metastases
effect of neoadjuvant chemotherapy on, 524, 527*f*, 528*f*, 529*f*
of invasive lobular carcinoma, 493*f*, 494–495, 495*t*
MRI of, 199, 200*f*
Lymph node positivity, in medical audit
analysis of, 710
goals for, 710*t*
in medical literature, 708*t*
with screening and diagnostic mammography data combined, 712*t*, 713*t*
value of, 716, 716*t*
Lymph node status, as prognostic and predictive factor, 231
Lymphadenitis, silicone, 287–288, 289*f*
Lymphadenopathy
axillary
bilateral, 546
differential diagnosis of, 429–431
in invasive ductal carcinoma, 425
MRI of, 199, 200*f*
unilateral, 546
workup for, 546, 546*f*
cervical metastatic, 199, 200*f*
Lymphatic invasion, as prognostic and predictive factor, 231
Lymphoma(s), 502–505
clinical presentation of, 502
defined, 502
diffuse large B-cell
case study of, 520*b*
commentary in, 523
diagnosis in, 522
differential diagnosis in, 522, 523*f*
excisional biopsy in, 521, 522*f*
fine-needle aspiration findings in, 521, 521*f*
history in, 520
immunohistochemical stains in, 521
mammography in, 520, 520*f*
ultrasonography in, 520, 521*f*
differential diagnosis of, 502–503, 504*f*, 523*f*
pathology of, 502–503, 503*f*
prevalence and epidemiology of, 502
vs. fat necrosis, 504, 504*f*, 505*f*
vs. invasive ductal carcinoma, 502–503, 504*f*
Lymphoma(s) *(Continued)*
mammography of, 502, 503*f*
metastatic (secondary) *vs.* primary, 502–503
non-Hodgkin's, 502, 503*f*
pathology of, 502–505
peripheral T-cell, 502, 504, 504*f*, 505*f*
prevalence and epidemiology of, 502
Lymph-vascular invasion (LVI), 446–447, 447*f*, 448*f*
DCIS *vs.*, 446–447, 448*f*
micropapillary invasive carcinoma *vs.*, 446–447, 448*f*

M

M codes, 723*t*, 725
Macromastia, 682
Macrometastatic disease, in sentinel lymph node sample, 624–625
Magnetic field, in MRI, 177, 178*f*
Magnetic field strength, of MRI, 177, 179*t*
higher, 187–188
Magnetic resonance, 177–179, 179*f*, 180*f*
Magnetic resonance imaging (MRI)
acceleration factor in, 189
advantages and disadvantages of, 196–197
artifacts on, 189–192
chemical shift, 190–191
due to fat saturation errors, 189–190, 190*f*
due to magnet and coil inhomogeneities, 190, 191*f*
due to metallic clips, 191–192, 191*f*
due to missed uptake of gadolinium contrast, 190
motion and misregistration, 189, 190*f*
background enhancement on, 218
basic theory of, 177–181
image formation in, 181, 181*f*, 182*f*
magnetic resonance in, 177–179, 179*f*, 180*f*
magnetic signal in, 177, 178*f*, 179*t*
relaxation in, 17, 179–180, 180*f*
spin echo sequence in, 180–181, 180*f*
BI-RADS for, 218–219
background enhancement in, 218
dynamic contrast enhancement in, 218–219
focus or foci in, 218
of breast implants, 201–202, 668–674
in evaluation for malignancy, 201–202
with gel fracture, 674
imaging protocols for, 669–670
normal appearance in, 670–671, 670*f*
with radial folds, 671, 671*f*
rat-tail sign in, 670*f*, 673
with rupture, 288
axial and sagittal inversion recovery water saturation images in, 201, 668*f*
contour deformities in, 673
extracapsular, 673–674, 676*f*
fluid on periphery of implant in, 673, 675*f*
inconclusive signs in, 673
intracapsular, 671–673
linguine sign in, 671, 672*f*
subscapular line sign in, 671, 672*f*, 673*f*
teardrop, keyhole, or noose sign in, 673, 673*f*
water droplets in, 673, 674*f*
with silicone granulomas, 202, 203*f*, 676*f*
technical factors in, 669, 669*f*, 669*t*
with breast-conserving therapy, 198
of positive margins, 653, 653*f*
post-treatment changes in, 656
uses for, 651*t*
after chemotherapy, 205*t*
Magnetic resonance imaging (MRI) *(Continued)*
claustrophobia with, 193
coding and billing for, 723*t*
conscious sedation for, 204
contraindications to, 192–193, 192*t*, 196–197, 197*f*
contrast-enhanced, 185–187, 186*f*, 761
agents for, 204
reaction to, 197
BI-RADS on, 218–219
gadolinium compounds used in, 186, 186*t*
history of, 18
missed uptake of, 190
and nephrogenic systemic fibrosis, 193
power injector for, 187, 187*f*
processing and uptake analysis for, 187, 187*f*
uptake curve and washout phase for, 186, 186*f*
creatinine and glomerular filtration rate and, 193
dynamic contrast-enhanced, 185–187, 186*f*, 761
BI-RADS on, 218–219
gadolinium compounds used in, 186, 186*t*
history of, 18
missed uptake with, 190
and nephrogenic systemic fibrosis, 193
power injector for, 187, 187*f*
processing and uptake analysis for, 187, 187*f*
uptake curve and washout phase for, 186, 186*f*
equipment standards for, 181, 182*t*
fat suppression in, 184–185
artifacts due to errors in, 189–190, 190*f*
chemical saturation for, 184–185, 184*f*, 185*f*
inversion recovery sequence for, 185
resolution and imaging requirements for, 183*t*
field strength of, 177, 179*t*
higher, 187–188
flip angle in, 177–179, 179*f*
history of, 17–18, 18*f*, 195
and hormone replacement therapy, 204–205, 205*t*
image assessment and reporting for, 205–210
ancillary abnormalities in, 210
color-coding of contrast enhancement in, 207
findings suggesting benign lesion in, 209, 209*f*, 210*f*
focus of enhancement in, 210
history and physical examination in, 206–207
lesion classification form for, 205–206, 205*t*
lesion kinetics in, 208–209
delayed portion in, 208–209
initial portion in, 208–209
lymph nodes in, 209–210
masses in, 207, 207*f*
non-mass-like enhancement in, 207–208
clumped, 207–208, 209*f*
ductal, 207–208, 208*f*
segmental, 207–208, 208*f*
persistent enhancement pattern in, 208–209
plateau enhancement pattern in, 208–209
T2 intensity in, 207
technical review in, 207
3D MIP reformatted images in, 207
wash-out enhancement pattern in, 208–209

Magnetic resonance imaging (MRI) *(Continued)*
image formation in, 181, 181*f*, 182*f*
indication(s) for, 197-198
evaluation of difficult or equivocal mammogram, ultrasound image, or clinical findings as, 201
evaluation of known breast malignancy as, 198-199
with chest wall invasion, 198, 198*f*
contralateral breast imaging with, 198-199
after lumpectomy, 198
with lymph node metastases, 199, 200*f*
occult, 199, 199*f*
evaluation of tumor response to neoadjuvant chemotherapy as, 201
guidance for biopsy and wire localization as, 210-211
imaging of augmented breast as, 201-202, 202*f*, 203*f*
screening as, 199-201, 200*b*
of invasive ductal carcinoma, 437
IV placement for, 192
k-space in, 181, 182*f*
magnetic field in, 177, 178*f*
magnetic resonance in, 177-179, 179*f*, 180*f*
magnetic signal in, 177, 178*f*, 179*t*
magnetization of protons in, 177, 178*f*
medical audit of, 713-714
and nephrogenic systemic fibrosis, 193
parallel imaging in, 189
pathophysiology of enhancement on, 195-196
patient preparation for, 192-193
creatinine and glomerular filtration rate in, 193
IV placement in, 192
screening for contraindications in, 192-193, 192*t*
phase encode gradient in, 181, 181*f*
positioning for, 192-193, 202-204
in postmenopausal women, 204-205, 205*t*
postoperative, 205*t*
in premenopausal women, 204-205, 204*f*, 205*t*
protocols for, 181-187
dynamic contrast-enhanced scans in, 185-187, 186*f*, 186*t*, 187*f*
equipment standards in, 181, 182*t*
fat suppression in, 184-185
chemical saturation for, 184-185, 184*f*, 185*f*
inversion recovery sequence for, 185
resolution and imaging requirements for, 183*t*
resolution and imaging requirements in, 181, 183*t*
scout image in, 181-182, 183*f*
T1 weighted image in, 181, 182, 183*f*, 183*t*
T2 weighted image in, 181, 183*t*, 184, 184*f*
proton weighted sequence in, 181
after radiation therapy, 205*t*
radiofrequency coils for, 179, 179*f*, 180*f*
multi-channel bilateral, 188, 188*f*, 189*f*
radiofrequency pulse in, 177-179, 179*f*
readout gradient in, 181, 181*f*
recent hardware advancements and techniques for, 187-189
higher field strengths as, 187-188
multi-channel bilateral breast coils as, 188, 188*f*, 189*f*
parallel imaging as, 189
relaxation in, 17, 179-180, 180*f*
repetition time in, 180, 180*f*
resolution and imaging requirements for, 181, 183*t*
scanner configuration for, 177, 178*f*
scout image in, 181-182, 183*f*

Magnetic resonance imaging (MRI) *(Continued)*
screening, 57, 199-201, 200*b*
sensitivity encoding in, 189
slice select gradient in, 181
specific absorption ratio in, 188
spin echo sequence in, 180-181, 180*f*
standards of care for, 732
subtraction imaging in, 187, 187*f*
T1 weighted image in, 181, 182, 183*f*, 183*t*
T2 weighted image in, 181, 183*t*, 184, 184*f*
techniques for, 202-205, 205*t*
three-dimensional, 181
time to echo in, 180, 180*f*
time/signal-intensity curves in, 219
ultrasound correlation with, 166-167, 166*f*, 167*f*
Magnetic resonance imaging (MRI)-guided biopsy and wire localization, 210-211
Magnetic resonance imaging (MRI)-guided core needle biopsy, 210-211, 587-594
biopsy grid for, 588-589, 589*f*
CAD device for, 588-590, 590*f*
contraindications to, 593-594
dermatotomy for, 591-592
efficacy and safety of, 587
equipment for, 587-588
indications for, 593
informed consent for, 588
introducer apparatus for, 591-592, 591*f*
local anesthesia for, 590-591
epinephrine with, 591
expected route of, 591
injection site for, 591
minimizing pain of, 591
marking clip in, 591-592
with multiple suspicious findings, 593
number of specimens in, 591-592
obturator placement during, 591-592, 592*f*
positioning for, 588-589, 588*f*
post-procedure considerations for, 592-593
potential complications of, 594
pre-contrast images in, 589
pre-procedural considerations for, 588-590
report on, 593
with second-look ultrasound, 593
specimen processing for, 592-593
sterile biopsy tray for, 587-588
sterile portion of procedure for, 590-592
targeting of lesion for, 589-590, 590*f*
vacuum-assisted device in, 591-592
Magnetic resonance spectroscopy (MRS), 761-771
of breast tissue, 768
choline in, 761-762
coherence transfer based spin-echo (CABINET), 763
high field, 769, 769*f*
multidimensional, 762, 768
one-dimensional, 762-763
limitations of, 763
studies on, 761, 762
outer volume suppression (OVS) in, 762
point-resolved (PRESS), 762
J- (JPRESS), 763
principles of, 762
quantifications in, 768-769
rationale for, 761
single voxel (SV)-based, 762, 768
stimulated echo acquisition mode (STEAM) sequence in, 762
two-dimensional
acquisition schemes in, 763
benefits of, 763-766
localized J-resolved (JPRESS), 763
localized shift correlated (L-COSY), 763

Magnetic resonance spectroscopy (MRS) *(Continued)*
of benign tumor tissue, 766*f*, 767*t*
choline in, 761-762
classification and regression tree (CART) analysis for, 761-762, 766-767, 767*t*, 768*t*
of different breast tissues, 764-766, 764*f*, 765*f*, 766*f*
of healthy fatty tissue, 764*f*, 767*t*, 768*t*
of healthy glandular tissue, 765*f*, 767*t*
of malignant tumor tissue, 765*f*, 767*t*, 768*t*
metabolites identified in, 766*t*
phantom study using, 763-764, 764*f*
water-to-fat ratio in, 761-762
volume of interest (VOI) in, 762
water-to-fat ratio in, 761-762
Magnetic signal, for MRI, 177, 178*f*, 179*f*
Magnetization, of protons, in MRI, 177, 178*f*
Magnification
and mammographic views, 119
quality control test of, 139*t*
Magnification stand, in mammography unit, 90-91, 90*f*
Maintenance, of mammography equipment, 97
Male breast cancer, 468-470
case study on, 476, 476*f*
clinical presentation of, 469
colon and rectal carcinomas with, 470
DCIS as, 416
defined, 468
etiology and pathophysiology of, 468-469
gynecomastia and, 469, 476, 476*f*
invasive lobular carcinoma as, 496
mammography of, 469
metastatic spread of, 470
pathology findings in, 469
prevalence and epidemiology of, 468
survival with, 470
ultrasonography of, 469
Male-to-female transsexuals, breast cancer in, 468-469
Malignant lesions, determining extent of, ultrasound for, 160-161, 161*f*
Malignant triplets, 635-637
Malmö Mammographic Screening Trial, 57-58, 58*t*
and over-diagnosis, 64
and screening guidelines, 62
on screening of women 40 to 49 years old, 71
and service screening, 65
and underestimation of benefits from screening, 61
Malpractice, 728, 729-730
Mammary buds, primary, 223
Mammary duct ectasia, 244-247
classic signs of, 245
clinical presentation of, 245
defined, 244
differential diagnosis of, 245-246, 247*f*
etiology and pathophysiology of, 244
imaging indications and algorithm for, 245
mammography of, 245, 246*f*
MRI of, 245
pathology of, 245-246, 247*f*
prevalence and epidemiology of, 244
treatment options for, 246-247
ultrasonography of, 245, 246*f*
Mammary fat, 224*f*
Mammary zone, ultrasound of, 168-171, 170*f*
MammoDiagnost, 9, 79
Mammographic abnormalities, ultrasound of, 156-157, 156*f*, 157*f*
Mammographic image, in computer-aided detection, 100, 100*f*
Mammographic markers, of breast cancer risk, 45

- Mammographic signs, of invasive ductal carcinoma
  - indirect, 431-435
    - architectural distortion as, 432-434, 434*f*, 435*f*
    - asymmetry as, 434-435, 436*f*, 437*f*
    - developing asymmetry as, 431-432, 433*f*, 434*f*
    - single dilated duct as, 435, 437*f*
  - primary, 426-427
    - mass as, 426, 426*f*, 427*f*
    - microcalcifications as, 426-427, 428*f*, 429*f*
  - secondary, 427-431
    - axillary lymph node metastases as, 429-431, 431*f*, 432*f*
    - nipple retraction as, 428-429, 430*f*
    - skin retraction as, 428, 430*f*
    - skin thickening as, 427-428, 430*f*
- Mammographic view(s)
  - additional, 115-119
    - angled mediolateral and lateromedial, 115-116, 116*f*
    - axillary tail, 117-118, 119*f*
    - from below, 117, 117*f*
    - cleavage, 118
    - exaggerated lateral craniocaudal, 117-118, 118*f*
    - implant, 119
    - inferosuperior oblique, 117
    - lateromedial oblique, 116
    - rolled, 117
    - superoinferior oblique, 116-117
    - tangential, 119
  - labeling and soft copy display for, 113, 113*t*
  - with physical limitations or mobility impairment, 111, 112*f*
  - standard, 113-119
    - cranial caudal, 115, 115*f*, 116*f*
    - mediolateral oblique, 113-115, 114*f*
- Mammography
  - BI-RADS for, 214-217
    - assessment and management in, 216-217
    - audit in, 217
    - breast density in, 214-215
    - calcifications in, 215-216
    - masses and asymmetries in, 215
  - of breast implants, 667-668
    - with rupture, 287, 287*f*, 667-668, 668*f*
    - with silicone adenopathy, 667, 667*f*
    - with silicone granulomas, 667-668, 668*f*
  - communication of results of, 213-214
  - digital
    - computer-aided detection and, 107
    - full-field (*See* Full-field digital mammography (FFDM))
    - history of, 12, 80, 80*t*
    - for screening, 57
    - stereo, 743-744, 744*f*
  - education and training in, 19*f*, 20
    - Society of Breast Imaging on, 20
  - era of technologic progress in, 7-12
    - automatic exposure timer in, 10
    - Charles Gros as, 7-9, 9*f*
    - dedicated mammography unit in, 7-9, 10*f*
    - digital mammography in, 12
    - film processing in, 10-11, 11*f*
    - foot pedal in, 10
    - image quality in, 10
    - John Wolfe in, 11, 11*f*
    - microfocal spot x-ray tube in, 10
    - rare earth screens in, 10
    - xeromammography in, 11-12, 12*f*, 13*f*
  - with fatty breast tissue, 226, 227*f*
  - of male breast cancer, 469
  - MRI for difficult or equivocal, 201

- Mammographic view(s) *(Continued)*
  - pioneer(s) of, 3-7
    - Albert Salomon as, 3, 4*f*, 5*f*
    - Albert Strickler as, 4
    - Carlos Dominguez as, 3
    - Charles Gros as, 4
    - Helen Ingleby as, 4
    - J. Goyanes as, 3
    - Jacob Gershon-Cohen as, 4, 6*f*
    - Otto Kleinschmidt as, 3
    - Paul Sebold as, 3-4
    - R. Sigrist as, 4
    - Raul Leborgne as, 5, 6*f*, 7*f*, 8*f*
    - Robert Egan as, 5-6, 8*f*, 9*f*
    - Stafford Warren as, 3-4, 5*f*, 6*f*
    - Walter Vogel as, 3
    - Wendell Scott as, 6
  - radiation exposure from, 69, 69*t*
  - radiation risks of, 21
  - after radiation therapy, 653-656
    - calcifications in, 651-652, 652*f*, 656, 656*f*
    - diffuse changes in, 655, 655*f*
    - goals of, 653
    - indications and algorithm for, 651, 651*t*
    - parenchymal changes in, 656
    - scars in, 654-655, 655*f*
    - seromas and hematomas in, 653*f*, 654, 654*f*, 655*f*
    - skin changes in, 655
    - timing of, 653-654
    - views for, 653
  - recent challenge and accomplishments in, 22
  - regulation of, 20-22
  - screening (*See* Screening mammography)
- Mammography Accreditation Program (MAP)
  - for help with quality control, 144
  - history of, 21-22, 693
  - on positioning, 110-111
- Mammography equipment, 79-98
  - acceptance testing and annual performance audits for, 96-97
  - acquisition workstation as, 91, 91*f*, 92*f*
  - additional medical physics equipment evaluations for, 97
  - antiscatter grid assembly as, 88-89, 88*f*
  - automatic exposure control (AEC) system as, 81, 89-90, 89*f*
  - collimator as, 81, 82*f*, 85, 85*f*
  - compression devices as, 82*f*, 86-87, 86*f*, 87*f*
  - foot pedals and digital display for compression as, 87, 87*f*, 88*f*
  - generator as, 82
  - historical background of, 79, 80*t*
  - image receptor(s) as, 82*f*, 93-96
    - digital detector(s) as, 94-96
      - computed radiography system as, 95-96, 96*f*
      - flat-panel phosphor system as, 95, 95*f*
      - selenium flat-panel system as, 95, 96*f*
      - Slot-Scan charge-coupled device system as, 94-95, 94*f*
    - film as, 93-94, 93*f*, 94*f*
      - processing of, 80, 94
  - laser printers as, 92-93
  - magnification stand as, 90-91, 90*f*
  - maintenance and repair of, 97
  - Mammography Quality Standards Act on, 696
  - mammography unit as, 81-96, 82*f*
  - overview of, 80, 81*f*
  - quality control tests of (*See* Quality control (QC) tests)
  - radiation output of, 87-88
  - radiologist review workstation as, 91-92, 92*f*
  - for storage, 93

- Mammography equipment *(Continued)*
  - U-arm and imaging geometry as, 81, 84-85, 84*f*, 85*f*
  - x-ray tube and filter as, 81, 82-84, 82*f*, 83*f*
- Mammography medical audit, 702-719
  - benefits of, 702, 703
  - cancer detection rate in
    - analysis of, 710-711
    - defined, 707
    - goals for, 710*t*, 712*t*
    - in medical literature, 708*t*
    - with screening and diagnostic mammography data combined, 712*t*, 713*t*
    - value of, 715-716, 715*t*, 716*t*
  - carcinoma in situ in
    - in medical literature, 712*t*
    - with screening and diagnostic mammography data combined, 712*t*, 713*t*
    - value of, 716, 716*t*
  - categorization of results in, 704, 706*f*
  - combining screening and diagnostic outcomes in, 711-712, 712*t*, 713*t*
  - cost of, 703
  - data for, 703-707
    - analysis of, 707-711
    - collection system for, 703
    - derived
      - additional, 704, 705*t*
      - essential, 703-704, 704*t*
    - raw
      - additional, 704, 705*t*
      - essential, 703-704, 704*t*
    - recent benchmark, 711, 712*t*
    - sources of, 715
  - defined, 702
  - expanding role of, 717
  - group, 714
  - individual, 714
  - lymph node positivity in
    - analysis of, 710
    - goals for, 710*t*
    - in medical literature, 708*t*
    - with screening and diagnostic mammography data combined, 712*t*, 713*t*
    - value of, 716, 716*t*
  - medicolegal considerations with, 717
  - positive predictive value in
    - analysis of, 709-710
    - defined, 706-707
    - goals for, 710*t*
    - in medical literature, 708*t*
    - with screening and diagnostic mammography data combined, 712*t*, 713*t*
    - value of, 716, 716*t*
  - recall rate in
    - analysis of, 711
    - goals for, 710*t*
    - in medical literature, 708*t*
    - with screening and diagnostic mammography data combined, 712*t*, 713*t*
  - receiver operating characteristic curve for, 707-711, 709*f*, 710*t*
  - as required by Mammography Quality Standards Act, 703, 714-715
  - sensitivity in
    - analysis of, 709
    - defined, 706
    - goals for, 710*t*
    - in medical literature, 708*t*
  - specificity in
    - analysis of, 711
    - defined, 707
    - goals for, 710*t*
    - in medical literature, 708*t*
  - as teaching tool, 714

Mammography medical audit *(Continued)*
tumor size in
analysis of, 710
in medical literature, 708*t*
with screening and diagnostic mammography data combined, 712*t*, 713*t*
value of, 716, 716*t*
value of, 715-717, 715*t*, 716*t*
Mammography Quality Control Manual, 133-134, 144
Mammography Quality Standards Act (MQSA), 693-694
on accreditation, 693, 694
on agency, 735
on certification, 694, 695
on clinical image evaluation, 121
on communicating results, 734
on consumer complaint mechanisms, 696
on equipment, 696
on facility physics survey, 693
on federal and state inspection, 694
final rules of, 695-696
history of, 22
interim rules of, 695
key player(s) in, 694-695
accrediting body as, 694
NMQAAC as, 694, 695
state as, 694
U.S. Food and Drug Administration as, 694
on mammography reports, 214, 694, 696
on mammography units, 81
on medical audit, 703, 714-715
on medical records, 694, 696
on national advisory committee, 694
on patients with breast implants, 696
on personnel standards, 696
on positioning, 110-111
on qualification standards, 694
on quality assurance standards, 133-134, 144, 694, 696
reauthorization of, 694
requirements of, 693-694, 695
on standards of care, 731
in statutory law, 730
Mammography Quality Standards Reauthorization Act (MQSRA), 694
Mammography reports
legal aspects of, 733-734
Mammography Quality Standards Act on, 694, 696
Mammography unit, 81-96, 82*f*
Mammography unit assembly evaluation, in quality control, 138*t*, 142
Mammomat, 9, 79
Mammorex, 79
Management, BI-RADS on, 216-217
Manufacturers' representatives, for help with quality control, 143-144
MAP (Mammography Accreditation Program)
for help with quality control, 144
history of, 21-22, 693
on positioning, 110-111
Margins
close, 623
microscopic evaluation of surgical, 623, 623*f*, 624*f*
negative, 623
perpendicular, 623
positive, 623
shaved, 623, 623*f*
Marking clips, in core needle biopsy
MRI-guided, 591-592
stereotactic-guided, 583-584
ultrasound-guided, 572
Mass(es)
BI-RADS on, 215
defined, 215
in invasive ductal carcinoma
clinical presentation of, 424-425
defined, 426
mammography of, 426
density of, 426, 426*f*
with irregular shape and spiculated margins, 426, 426*f*
with round shape and circumscribed margins, 426, 427*f*
spot compression in, 426, 427*f*
palpable, 542-543, 549
mammography for, 542-543, 545*f*
MRI for, 543
ultrasonography for, 542-543, 545*f*
on screening mammography, 542-550
with benign features, 547-549
biopsy of, 547-549
fat-containing, 543, 546*b*
management algorithm for, 547, 549*f*
multiple bilateral circumscribed round or oval, 547, 548*f*
and no prior mammograms, 547
requiring no further evaluation, 543-546, 547, 548*f*
short-term imaging for, 547-549
ultrasonography for, 547, 548*f*, 549
focal asymmetries as, 546-547
defined, 546
diagnostic mammography for, 547
spot compression views for, 542, 543*f*
ultrasound-guided biopsy for, 547, 547*f*
MRI for, 542, 544*f*
spot compression views for, 542, 543*f*
suspicious and malignant, 549-550, 550*f*
ultrasonography for, 542, 543*f*
Mastectomy
fat necrosis after, 332*f*
specimen processing from, 621-622
Mastitis, 375-388
with abscess, 379
mammography of, 376, 377*f*
pathology findings in, 379-380, 381*f*, 382*f*
subareolar, 377*f*, 379-380, 382*f*
ultrasonography of, 376-378, 379*f*, 380*f*, 381*f*
case study on, 386*b*
commentary in, 388
diagnosis in, 388
differential diagnosis in, 386
findings in, 386, 386*f*, 387*f*
history in, 386
classic signs of, 379
clinical presentation of, 375
due to coccidioidomycosis, 380-381, 384*f*
comedo-, 244, 331
defined, 375
differential diagnosis of, 379-385
due to echinococcosis, 380-381, 383*f*
etiology and pathophysiology of, 375
due to filariasis, 386*b*
commentary on, 388
diagnosis of, 388
differential diagnosis of, 386
findings with, 386, 386*f*, 387*f*
history of, 386
due to galactography, 603
granulomatous
mammography of, 376, 378*f*
pathology findings with, 380-381, 381*f*
imaging indications and algorithm for, 375-376
mammography of, 376
with abscess, 376, 377*f*
Mastitis *(Continued)*
granulomatous, 376, 378*f*
with reactive lymph node, 376*f*
with skin and trabecular thickening, 376, 377*f*
with trichinosis, 376, 379*f*
MRI of, 378-379
obliterative, 244, 331
pathology findings with, 379-385
with abscess, 379
subareolar, 379-380, 382*f*
acute inflammatory cells in, 382*f*
with coccidioidomycosis, 380-381, 384*f*
with echinococcosis, 380-381, 383*f*
granulomatous, 380-381, 381*f*
tuberculous, 384*f*, 385
plasma cell, 244, 331
prevalence and epidemiology of, 375
silicone, 287-288, 288*f*
treatment options for, 385-388
due to trichinosis, 376, 379*f*
tuberculous, 384*f*, 385
ultrasonography of, 376-378, 379*f*, 380*f*, 381*f*
Mastopathy
diabetic, 276-280
classic signs of, 278
clinical presentation of, 277
defined, 276
etiology and pathophysiology of, 277
imaging indications and algorithm for, 277
mammography of, 277-278, 277*f*
MRI of, 278, 278*f*, 279*f*
pathology findings in, 278, 279*f*
prevalence and epidemiology of, 277
treatment options for, 280
ultrasonography of, 278, 278*f*
fibrous (*See* Fibrosis)
indurative (*See* Radial scar)
Medical audit, 702-719
benefits of, 702, 703
cancer detection rate in
analysis of, 710-711
defined, 707
goals for, 710*t*, 712*t*
in medical literature, 708*t*
with screening and diagnostic mammography data combined, 712*t*, 713*t*
value of, 715-716, 715*t*, 716*t*
carcinoma in situ in
in medical literature, 712*t*
with screening and diagnostic mammography data combined, 712*t*, 713*t*
value of, 716, 716*t*
categorization of results in, 704, 706*f*
combining screening and diagnostic outcomes in, 711-712, 712*t*, 713*t*
cost of, 703
data for, 703-707
analysis of, 707-711
collection system for, 703
derived
additional, 704, 705*t*
essential, 703-704, 704*t*
raw
additional, 704, 705*t*
essential, 703-704, 704*t*
recent benchmark, 711, 712*t*
sources of, 715
defined, 702
expanding role of, 717
group, 714
individual, 714

Medical audit *(Continued)*
lymph node positivity in
analysis of, 710
goals for, 710*t*
in medical literature, 708*t*
with screening and diagnostic mammography data combined, 712*t*, 713*t*
value of, 716, 716*t*
medicolegal considerations with, 717
of MRI, 713-714
positive predictive value in
analysis of, 709-710
defined, 706-707
goals for, 710*t*
in medical literature, 708*t*
with screening and diagnostic mammography data combined, 712*t*, 713*t*
value of, 716, 716*t*
recall rate in
analysis of, 711
goals for, 710*t*
in medical literature, 708*t*
with screening and diagnostic mammography data combined, 712*t*, 713*t*
receiver operating characteristic curve for, 707-711, 709*f*, 710*t*
as required by Mammography Quality Standards Act, 703, 714-715
sensitivity in
analysis of, 709
defined, 706
goals for, 710*t*
in medical literature, 708*t*
specificity in, 711
defined, 707
goals for, 710*t*
in medical literature, 708*t*
as teaching tool, 714
tumor size in
analysis of, 710
in medical literature, 708*t*
with screening and diagnostic mammography data combined, 712*t*, 713*t*
value of, 716, 716*t*
of ultrasound, 713-714
value of, 715-717, 715*t*, 716*t*
Medical Economic Index, 721
Medical physicist, in quality control, 134*t*, 135-136, 135*t*
continuing education of, 135*t*, 136
continuing experience of, 135*t*, 136
for help with questions, 143
initial qualifications of, 135*t*, 136
reestablishing qualifications of, 136
responsibilities of, 134*t*, 135-136
tests performed by, 138*t*, 142-143
on accuracy and reproducibility of peak kilovolt (kVp), 138*t*, 143
artifact evaluation as, 138*t*, 142-143
automatic exposure control system performance assessment as, 138*t*, 142
on average glandular dose, 138*t*, 143
beam quality assessment (half-value layer measurement) as, 138*t*, 143
on breast exposure, 138*t*, 143
collimation assessment as, 138*t*, 142
evaluation of system resolution as, 138*t*, 142
image quality evaluation as, 138*t*, 143
mammographic unit assembly evaluation as, 138*t*, 142
on radiation output rate, 138*t*, 143
on reproducibility of automatic exposure control, 138*t*, 143
Medical physicist, in quality control *(Continued)*
required by equipment changes, 139-141, 139*b*, 139*t*
on uniformity of screen speed, 138*t*, 142
on viewbox luminance and room illuminance, 138*t*, 143
Medical physics equipment evaluation, 97
Medical records, Mammography Quality Standards Act on, 694, 696
Medicare Fee Schedule (MFS), 721
Medicare reimbursement
acceptable codes and payment rates for, 722, 722*t*, 723*t*
background and present status of, 721-722
special rules relating to, 722-724
Mediolateral (ML) angled view, 115-116, 116*f*
Mediolateral oblique (MLO) view, 113-115, 114*f*
clinical image evaluation of, 122, 122*f*, 123*f*, 124*f*
Medullary carcinoma, 460-461, 461*f*, 462*f*
Melanoma
metastatic to breast, 513-514
desmoplastic, 514*f*
epithelioid type, 513-514, 514*f*
spindle cell, 513-514, 514*f*, 515*f*
vs. Paget's disease, 405-409
Menopausal hormones, and breast cancer risk, 31-32, 44
Menopausal status, as prognostic and predictive factor, 231
Menopause
breast histology after, 225, 226*f*
MRI after, 204-205, 205*t*
MRI prior to, 204-205, 204*f*, 205*t*
Mental distress, legal aspects of, 729
Metachronous carcinoma, 467
Metallic clip artifacts, on MRI, 191-192, 191*f*
Metaplastic carcinoma, 463-466
with chondroid element, 463-465, 464*f*
spindle cell, 465, 465*f*, 466*f*
with squamous cell carcinoma, 463-466, 465*f*
Metastasis(es)
axillary lymph node, 467
of DCIS, 411-415
vs. benign inclusion, 414*f*
vs. dendritic cells, 413*f*
vs. histiocyte aggregates, 412*f*
vs. intracapsular nevus, 413*f*
vs. nonspecific debris, 413*f*
of invasive ductal carcinoma, 429-431, 431*f*
calcified, 432*f*
and survival, 442-445, 445*t*, 467, 468*t*
tumor size and, 467, 468*t*
to breast, 511-519
of adenocarcinoma from unknown primary tumor, 513*f*
of choriocarcinoma, 516, 518*f*
clinical presentation of, 512
defined, 511
from lung carcinoma, 513*f*
mammography of, 512-513, 513*f*
of melanoma, 513-514
desmoplastic, 514*f*
epithelioid type, 513-514, 514*f*
spindle cell, 513-514, 514*f*, 515*f*
of neuroendocrine carcinoma, 514, 516*f*
of ovarian carcinoma, 514-516, 517*f*
pathology of, 513-516
prevalence and epidemiology of, 511-512
of renal cell carcinoma, 514, 515*f*
of signet cell carcinoma, 516, 518*f*
treatment options for, 516-519
of invasive lobular carcinoma
to lymph nodes, 493*f*, 494-495, 495*t*
non-nodal, 495
of male breast cancer, 470
MFS (Medicare Fee Schedule), 721
Microarray profiling, 470
Microbubble drug delivery, ultrasound-activated, 759, 759*f*
Microcalcifications
in invasive ductal carcinoma, 426-427, 428*f*, 429*f*
needle localization of, 607, 607*f*
pathology of, 333-337
with apocrine metaplasia, 342*f*, 343*f*
basophilic, 333-334, 341*f*, 342*f*
with benign terminal ductal-lobular unit, 341*f*
calcium oxalate, 333-334, 342*f*, 343*f*
calcium phosphate, 333-334, 341*f*, 342*f*
within columnar cell lesion, 346*f*
in DCIS, 333-334, 343*f*
with ductal hyperplasia, 344*f*
in involuted and hyalinized fibroadenoma, 346*f*
with lactational changes in pregnancy, 342*f*
from lumpectomy specimen, 347*f*
with radiation changes, 345*f*
with sclerosing adenosis, 344*f*
solid breast nodules with, 171, 172*f*, 173*f*
standards of care for, 731
ultrasound-guided biopsy of, 168, 170*f*
Microclips, in lumpectomy specimen, 347*f*
Microfocal spot x-ray tube, history of, 10
Microglandular adenosis, 318-319
atypical, 318-319, 320*f*, 321*f*
clinical presentation of, 318
defined, 318
etiology and pathophysiology of, 318
imaging technique and findings with, 318-319
pathology findings with, 318-319, 319*f*, 320*f*
prevalence and epidemiology of, 318
treatment options for, 319
Microinvasive carcinoma, 445-446, 445*f*
Microlobulations, solid breast nodules with, 171, 172*f*, 173*f*
Micrometastases
of DCIS, 411-414
in sentinel lymph node sample, 624-625, 625*f*
Micropapillary carcinoma
in situ, ultrasound of, 160, 161*f*, 175*f*
invasive, 459, 459*f*
vs. lymph-vascular invasion, 446-447, 448*f*
vs. ovarian metastatic carcinoma, 459, 460*f*
metastatic to breast, 514-516, 517*f*
Micropapillary DCIS, 402, 403*f*, 404*f*
Microsatellite instability (MSI), 229
Milk lines, 223
Milk of calcium, 323, 553
crescent shape (teacup sign) of, 323, 324*f*
on mammogram, 323, 324*f*, 554*f*
rounded or amorphous, 323, 324*f*, 554*f*
on ultrasound, 324*f*
Milk streaks, 223
Minimal cancer, in medical audit
in medical literature, 712*t*
with screening and diagnostic mammography data combined, 712*t*, 713*t*
value of, 716, 716*t*
Minimally invasive percutaneous breast cancer ablation, 772-776
cryoablation as, 772-773, 774*f*, 775*f*
early detection and, 772, 773*f*
high-intensity focused ultrasound ablation as, 775
historical background of, 772
laser ablation as, 776
radiofrequency ablation as, 773-775
Min-R screen, 10, 80

Misregistration artifacts, on MRI, 189, 190*f*
Missed cancers, impact of computer-aided detection on, 102-104
Mitotic count
in invasive ductal carcinoma, 442-445, 442*t*
as prognostic and predictive factor, 231
Mixed triplets, 635-637
ML (mediolateral) angled view, 115-116, 116*f*
MLH1 gene, 229
MLO (mediolateral oblique) view, 113-115, 114*f*
Mobile unit, quality control test of, 137*t*
Mobility impairment, mammographic views with, 111, 112*f*
Modified Scarf-Bloom and Richardson (SBR) grade and score, in invasive ductal carcinoma, 438-442
Mönckeberg type calcifications, 326-327, 329*f*, 345*f*
Montgomery tubercle, 224*f*
MORE (Multiple Outcomes of Raloxifene Evaluation), 44-45
Mortality data, from breast cancer, 25-26
Mortality rate
age-adjusted, 26, 26*f*, 28*f*
national trends in, 31*f*, 37-38, 38*f*
by race and ethnicity, 38, 39*f*
worldwide comparison of, 26*f*, 28*f*, 29-30
Moskowitz, Harold, 20
Moskowitz, Myron, 20
Motion artifacts, on MRI, 189, 190*f*
Motion blur, clinical image evaluation of, 125, 126*f*, 127*f*
Motion for summary judgment, 729
MQSA. *See* Mammography Quality Standards Act (MQSA).
MQSRA (Mammography Quality Standards Reauthorization Act), 694
MRI. *See* Magnetic resonance imaging (MRI).
MRS. *See* Magnetic resonance spectroscopy (MRS).
MRSI (multidimensional magnetic resonance spectroscopic imaging), 762, 768
MSH2 gene, 229
MSH6 gene, 229
MSI (microsatellite instability), 229
Mucinous carcinoma, 455-456, 456*f*
Mucinous-type DCIS, 403, 407*f*
Multi-channel bilateral breast coils, for MRI, 188, 188*f*, 189*f*
Multidimensional magnetic resonance spectroscopic imaging (MRSI), 762, 768
Multiple Outcomes of Raloxifene Evaluation (MORE), 44-45
Mutation(s), genetic. *See* Genetic mutation(s).
MYC gene, amplification of, as prognostic and predictive factor, 232
Myoepithelial cell markers, with core needle biopsy, 616-617, 617*f*
Myofibroblastoma, 293-295
clinical presentation of, 294
defined, 293
etiology and pathophysiology of, 294
imaging indications and algorithm for, 294
mammography of, 294
MRI of, 294
pathology findings with, 294-295, 294*f*, 295*f*
prevalence and epidemiology of, 294
treatment options for, 295
ultrasonography of, 294

N

NACT. *See* Neoadjuvant chemotherapy (NACT).
National advisory committee, Mammography Quality Standards Act on, 694, 695
National Alliance of Breast Cancer Organizations (NABCO), on screening, 62
National Breast Screening Study (NBSS), 57-58, 58*t*
and screening guidelines, 62
on screening of women 40 to 49 years old, 59-60, 70-71
and underestimation of benefits from screening, 61
National Cancer Institute (NCI)
on cancer statistics, 25
on screening, 62
National Health Service Breast Screening Program (NHSBSP), recall rates at, 66-67
National Mammography Quality Assurance Advisory Committee (NMQAAC), 694, 695
National Program of Cancer Registries (NPCR), on cancer statistics, 25
National Surgical Adjuvant Breast and Colorectal Project (NSABP), 44
Nationwide Evaluation of X-ray Trends (NEXT), 21-22, 693
NBSS. *See* Canadian National Breast Screening Study (NBSS); National Breast Screening Study (NBSS).
NCI (National Cancer Institute)
on cancer statistics, 25
on screening, 62
Necrosis
fat (*See* Fat necrosis)
in invasive ductal carcinoma, 438, 438*f*
as prognostic and predictive factor, 231
Needle
calcifications due to, 332, 339*f*
for ultrasound-guided core needle biopsy, 565, 565*f*
Needle localization, 605-610
challenges of, 607, 607*f*
coding and billing for, 723*t*
complications of, 607
of faint microcalcifications, 607, 607*f*
free-hand method of, 607
imaging workup prior to, 605
informed consent for, 605
local anesthesia for, 605-606
needle or hook wire system for, 605
positioning for, 605-606
procedure for, 605-609, 606*f*
scout film for, 605-606
specimen radiography with, 607-609, 608*f*, 609*f*
Negative margins, 623
Negative stroke margin, in stereotactic-guided core needle biopsy, 582-583
Negligence, law of, 729
Negligent referral, 735
Neoadjuvant chemotherapy (NACT), 524-531
advantages of, 524
DCIS after, 526*f*, 527*f*
effects on normal breast tissue of, 525
indications for, 524
invasive lobular carcinoma after, 528*f*, 529*f*
lymph nodes after, 524, 527*f*, 528*f*, 529*f*
tumor response to
Bloom and Richardson grade for, 526-529
FDG-PET and PET/CT of, 531, 531*f*
histologic changes in, 525
cytoplasmic ballooning as, 526*f*
in DCIS, 526*f*, 527*f*
degenerated tumor cells as, 525*f*
in invasive lobular carcinoma, 528*f*, 529*f*
in lymph nodes, 527*f*, 528*f*, 529*f*
and pathologic response, 525
Neoadjuvant chemotherapy (NACT) (*Continued*)
mammography of, 529-530, 529*f*
MRI of, 201, 529-530, 530*f*
predictors of, 524-525
residual tumor size in, 524, 525-526
ultrasonography of, 529-530, 530*f*
Neoangiogenesis, 185
Nephrogenic systemic fibrosis (NSF), MRI and, 193
Net magnetization, of protons, in MRI, 177, 178*f*
Neuroendocrine carcinoma, metastatic to breast, 514, 516*f*
NEXT (National Evaluation of X-ray Trends), 21-22, 693
NHSBSP (National Health Service Breast Screening Program), recall rates at, 66-67
90-degree view, 115-116, 116*f*
Nipple(s)
anatomy of, 224*f*
florid papillomatosis of (*See* Nipple adenoma)
Paget's disease of, 404-409, 408*f*
skin changes in, 425
supernumerary, 223
Nipple adenoma, 297-298, 409
classic signs of, 297
clinical presentation of, 297
defined, 297
etiology and pathophysiology of, 297
imaging indications and algorithm for, 297
mammography of, 297
MRI of, 297
pathology findings with, 297-298, 297*f*, 298*f*, 409, 409*f*
prevalence and epidemiology of, 297
treatment options for, 298
ultrasonography of, 297
Nipple discharge
bloody, 425
due to cysts, 598, 599*f*
with duct ectasia, 598, 598*f*
galactography for (*See* Galactography)
due to intraductal carcinoma, 601, 602*f*
in invasive ductal carcinoma, 425
with lobular filling, 598, 599*f*
in males, 469
MRI for, 601, 604*f*
due to papillomas, 598-601, 599*f*, 600*f*, 601*f*
trigger point for, 597
ultrasonography for, 158-159, 158*f*, 159*f*, 601, 603*f*
Nipple elevation, after reduction mammoplasty, 684, 684*f*
Nipple inversion, benign, 425
Nipple retraction
in invasive ductal carcinoma
clinical presentation of, 425
mammography of, 428-429, 430*f*
due to scarring, 429
Nipple transplantation, reduction mammoplasty with, 682, 683*f*
Nipple transposition, reduction mammoplasty with, 682, 683*f*
NMQAAC (National Mammography Quality Assurance Advisory Committee), 694, 695
Nodal metastases. *See* Lymph node metastases.
Nodal status, in medical audit
analysis of, 710
goals for, 710*t*
in medical literature, 708*t*
with screening and diagnostic mammography data combined, 712*t*, 713*t*
value of, 716, 716*t*

Nodular fasciitis, 272
Nodular fibrosis. *See* Fibrosis.
Nodular sclerosing adenosis, 302–303
Nodularity, physiologic, 425
Nodules, ultrasound of, 171
with branch pattern, 171, 172*f*
with duct extension, 171, 172*f*
due to fibroadenoma, 171, 173*f*
hard finding in, 171, 172*f*
hypoechoic, 171, 173*f*
with microcalcifications, 171, 172*f*, 173*f*
with microlobulations, 171, 172*f*, 173*f*
nonspecific findings in, 171, 173*f*
soft findings in, 171, 172*f*, 173*f*
with spiculation, 171, 172*f*
terminal duct lobular unit in, 173*f*
Noise, clinical image evaluation of, 125
Noncomedo carcinoma, 392
Noncompliance, and results of randomized clinical trials, 61
Nonencapsulated sclerosing lesion. *See* Radial scar.
Non-Hodgkin's lymphoma, 502, 503*f*
Noninvasive papillary carcinoma, 397, 398*f*, 456–457, 457*f*, 458*f*
Nonproliferative breast changes, 226–228
Noose sign, with implant rupture, 673, 673*f*
Normal breast, 223–235
anatomy of
mammographic, 224–226, 224*f*
ultrasonographic, 226, 228*f*
variations in, 226, 227*f*
embryology and development of, 223–224
histology of, 224–226, 225*f*, 226*f*
NPCR (National Program of Cancer Registries), on cancer statistics, 25
NSABP (National Surgical Adjuvant Breast and Colorectal Project), 44
NSF (nephrogenic systemic fibrosis), MRI and, 193
Nuclear grade
in DCIS, 409–410, 410*t*
in invasive ductal carcinoma, 442–445, 444*f*
Nuclear medicine breast imaging technology, 747–748
Number of deaths, from breast cancer, estimates of, 25–26
Numbers of cases, of breast cancer, estimates of, 25–26
Nurses Health Study, 44

O

Obesity, and breast cancer risk, 42
Obliterative mastitis, 244, 331
Occult breast carcinoma, 467
MRI of, 199, 199*f*
Octoson, 14–15, 15*f*
Oil cyst, 283, 284*f*
fat necrosis with, 327–329, 330*f*, 331*f*
Ointment, calcifications due to, 325–326, 328*f*
On-site surveys, in accreditation, 699–700
Oral contraceptives, and breast cancer risk, 43
Osteogenic sarcoma
mammography of, 509, 509*f*
pathology of, 510, 510*f*
Ostrum, Bernard, 10
Outer volume suppression (OVS), in magnetic resonance spectroscopy, 762
Ovarian carcinoma, metastatic to breast, 514–516, 517*f*
vs. invasive micropapillary carcinoma, 459, 460*f*
Overall cancer detection rate, in medical audit analysis of, 710–711
defined, 707
goals for, 710*t*, 712*t*
in medical literature, 708*t*
with screening and diagnostic mammography data combined, 712*t*, 713*t*
value of, 715–716, 715*t*, 716*t*
"Over-diagnosis" controversy, 39, 63–64, 71
Overexposure, 124
OVS (outer volume suppression), in magnetic resonance spectroscopy, 762

P

Pacific Islanders
incidence of breast cancer in, 33–34, 33*f*
mortality rate in, 39*f*
Paget, James, 404–405
Pagetoid spread, of LCIS, 405–409
Paget's disease, of nipple, 404–409, 408*f*
skin changes in, 425
Pain, in invasive ductal carcinoma, 425
PALB2 (partner and localizer of *BRCA2*) gene, and breast cancer risk, 48
Palpable mass, 229
workup of, 542–543, 549
mammography for, 542–543, 545*f*
MRI for, 543
ultrasonography for, 155, 155*f*, 542–543, 545*f*
Panniculitis, in peripheral T-cell lymphoma, 504, 504*f*
Panoramic imaging, in ultrasonography, 149, 151*f*
Papillary carcinoma, 456–457
intracystic (encapsulated, noninvasive), 397, 398*f*, 456–457, 457*f*, 458*f*
Papillary DCIS, 456–457, 458*f*
Papillary lesion(s), 349–355
atypical papilloma as
pathology findings with, 352–353, 354*f*
treatment options for, 353–354
case study of, 370*b*
diagnosis in, 372, 372*f*, 373*f*
differential diagnosis in, 371
findings in, 370–371, 370*f*, 371*f*
history in, 370
classic signs of, 351
clinical presentation of, 349
defined, 349
differential diagnosis of, 352–353
etiology and pathophysiology of, 349
imaging indications and algorithm for, 349
intraductal papilloma as, 352, 352*f*, 353*f*
mammography of, 349–351, 350*f*, 351*f*
MRI of, 351, 352*f*
papillomatosis as, 352, 353*f*
pathology findings with, 352–353
post-biopsy management of, 640, 640*f*
prevalence and epidemiology of, 349
treatment options for, 353–355
ultrasonography of, 351, 351*f*
Papilloma(s)
atypical
pathology findings with, 352–353, 354*f*
treatment options for, 353–354
clinical presentation of, 349
defined, 349
etiology and pathophysiology of, 349
galactography of, 598–601, 599*f*, 600*f*, 601*f*
intracystic, 171–176, 175*f*
intraductal
case study of, 370*b*
diagnosis in, 372, 372*f*, 373*f*
differential diagnosis in, 371
Papilloma(s) *(Continued)*
findings in, 370–371, 370*f*, 371*f*
history in, 370
pathology findings with, 352, 352*f*, 353*f*
ultrasonography of, 351, 351*f*
mammography of, 349, 350*f*
MRI of, 351, 352*f*
post-biopsy management of, 640, 640*f*
prevalence and epidemiology of, 349
treatment options for, 353–354
ultrasonography of, 351, 351*f*
intracystic, 171–176, 175*f*
intraductal, 351, 351*f*
Papillomatosis
clinical presentation of, 349
defined, 349
juvenile
clinical presentation of, 349
defined, 349
mammography of, 351
prevalence and epidemiology of, 349
treatment options for, 355
mammography of, 351, 351*f*
of nipple, florid (*See* Nipple adenoma)
pathology findings with, 352, 353*f*
prevalence and epidemiology of, 349
treatment options for, 354
Parallel imaging, in MRI, 189
Parasitic calcifications, 333, 341*f*
Parenchymal changes, after breast-conserving therapy, 656
Parenchymal displacement, after reduction mammoplasty, 684–685, 685*f*
Partner and localizer of *BRCA2 (PALB2)* gene, and breast cancer risk, 48
PASH. *See* Pseudoangiomatous stromal hyperplasia (PASH).
Pathologic staging, of invasive ductal carcinoma, 438, 439*t*, 440*t*, 442*t*
Patient history, legal aspects of, 732–733
Patient motion, focal spot and, 84
"Pay-for-performance" movement, 721–722
Peak kilovolt (kVp)
accuracy and reproducibility of, quality control test of, 138*t*, 143
clinical image evaluation of, 123
Peau d'orange
in inflammatory carcinoma, 466–467
in invasive ductal carcinoma, 438, 438*f*
Pectoralis muscle, in craniocaudal view, 123, 125*f*
Percutaneous biopsy, image-guided. *See* Image-guided percutaneous biopsy.
Percutaneous breast cancer ablation, 772–776
cryoablation as, 772–773, 774*f*, 775*f*
early detection and, 772, 773*f*
high-intensity focused ultrasound ablation as, 775
historical background of, 772
laser ablation as, 776
radiofrequency ablation as, 773–775
Performance audits, for mammography equipment, 96–97
Perilobular hemangioma, 290–291, 291*f*
Perineural invasion
of invasive ductal carcinoma, 446, 447*f*
as prognostic and predictive factor, 231
Peripheral T-cell lymphoma, 502, 504, 504*f*, 505*f*
Permanent sections, 630–631
Perpendicular margins, 623
Personnel standards, Mammography Quality Standards Act on, 696
PET (positron emission tomography), 748
PET/CT (positron emission tomography/computed tomography), 748

Peutz-Jeghers syndrome (PJS), and breast cancer risk, 47
Phantom dose, 96–97
Phantom image(s), in accreditation, 699, 699*t*
Phantom image quality, 96–97
Phantom image test, 137*t*, 141
Phantom study, using two-dimensional magnetic resonance spectroscopy, 763–764, 764*f*
Phase encode gradient, in MRI, 181, 181*f*
Phenotypic alterations, in breast cancer, 232, 234*f*
Phosphatase and tensin homolog *(PTEN)* gene, and breast cancer risk, 47
Phyllodes tumor, 366–372
  benign, 367
  borderline, 367
  classic signs of, 367
  clinical presentation of, 366
  defined, 366
  differential diagnosis of, 367–369
  etiology and pathophysiology of, 366
  imaging indications and algorithm for, 366
  malignant, 505–508
    clinical presentation of, 506
    defined, 505
    etiology and pathophysiology of, 505–506
    with heterologous sarcomatous components, 506–507, 507*f*
    with leaf-like projections, 506–507, 508*f*
    low-grade, 507, 508*f*
    mammography of, 506, 506*f*
    with mitotic figures, 367–369, 367*f*, 506–507, 507*f*
    pathology of, 506–508
    predicting biological behavior of, 507–508
    prevalence and epidemiology of, 505
    recurrent, 366*f*, 507–508
    with stromal overgrowth, 367–369, 368*f*, 506–507, 507*f*
    ultrasonography of, 506, 506*f*
  mammography of, 366, 366*f*
  MRI of, 366–367
  pathology findings with, 367–369, 368*f*
  prevalence and epidemiology of, 366
  treatment options for, 369–372
  ultrasonography of, 366
Physical activity, and breast cancer risk, 42
Physical limitations, mammographic views with, 111, 112*f*
Physician Insurers Association of America (PIAA), 728
Physiologic nodularity, 425
Piezoelectric effect, 13
Pilar cysts, 239
PJS (Peutz-Jeghers syndrome), and breast cancer risk, 47
Plasma cell mastitis, 244, 331
Pleomorphic variant, of invasive lobular carcinoma, 491–493, 493*f*
  case study of, 497*b*
PMF (posterior mammary fascia), ultrasound of, 168–171, 170*f*, 171*f*
PMS1 gene, 229
PMS2 gene, 229
PNL (posterior nipple line)
  in craniocaudal view, 123, 125*f*
  in mediolateral oblique view, 122, 123*f*
Point-resolved spectroscopy (PRESS), 762
  J- (JPRESS), 763
Polymorphisms, and breast cancer risk, 48
Population trends, and disease control programs, 38–39
Positioning
  for core needle biopsy
    MRI-guided, 588–589, 588*f*
    stereotactic-guided, 580–581
    ultrasound-guided, 567, 567*f*
  in mammography, 110–120
    for additional view(s), 115–119
      angled mediolateral and lateromedial, 115–116, 116*f*
      axillary tail, 117–118, 119*f*
      from below, 117, 117*f*
      cleavage, 118
      exaggerated lateral craniocaudal, 117–118, 118*f*
      implant, 119
      inferosuperior oblique, 117
      lateromedial oblique, 116
      rolled, 117
      superoinferior oblique, 116–117
      tangential, 119
    anatomy and, 111
    basic concepts of, 111–113
    breast compression and, 111–112, 112*f*
    clinical image evaluation of, 121–122
      for CC view, 122–123, 124*f*, 125*f*
      for MLO view, 122, 122*f*, 123*f*, 124*f*
    equipment and, 111
    importance of, 110–111
    labeling and soft copy display for, 113, 113*t*
    legal aspects of, 731
    with magnification, 119
    with physical limitations or mobility impairment, 111, 112*f*
    for standard view(s), 113–119
      cranial caudal, 115, 115*f*, 116*f*
      mediolateral oblique, 113–115, 114*f*
  for MRI, 192–193
  for needle localization, 605–606
Positive margins, 623
Positive predictive value (PPV), in medical audit
  analysis of, 709–710
  defined, 706–707
  goals for, 710*t*
  in medical literature, 708*t*
  with screening and diagnostic mammography data combined, 712*t*, 713*t*
  value of, 716, 716*t*
Positive predictive value-1 (PPV1), 67, 706, 709
Positive predictive value-2 (PPV2), 67, 706, 709, 710
  BI-RADS on, 217
Positive predictive value-3 (PPV3), 67, 706, 710, 712*t*
Positron emission tomography (PET), 748
Positron emission tomography/computed tomography (PET/CT), 748
Posterior acoustic shadowing, in ultrasonography, 148, 150*f*
Posterior mammary fascia (PMF), ultrasound of, 168–171, 170*f*, 171*f*
Posterior nipple line (PNL)
  in craniocaudal view, 123, 125*f*
  in mediolateral oblique view, 122, 123*f*
Postmenopausal women
  breast histology in, 225, 226*f*
  MRI in, 204–205, 205*t*
Powders, calcifications due to, 325–326
PPV. *See* Positive predictive value (PPV).
PR(s). *See* Progesterone receptor(s) (PRs).
Practice patterns, *vs.* standards of care, 730
Precessional frequency, and magnetic field strength, in MRI, 177, 179*t*
Predictive factor(s), for breast cancer, 231–232
  age as, 231
  DNA amplification as, 232
  expression profiling as, 232, 233*f*, 234*f*, 234*t*
  extent of ductal carcinoma in situ as, 232
  Her2 oncogene as, 232
  histologic grade as, 231
  histologic type as, 231
  inflammatory cell infiltrates as, 231
  lymph node status as, 231
  lymphatic and blood cell invasion as, 231
  perineural invasion as, 231
  pregnancy as, 231
  steroid hormone receptor status as, 232
  TP53 mutation as, 232
  tumor cell proliferation as, 231
  tumor necrosis as, 231
  tumor size as, 231
Predictive indicator, 626
Pregnancy
  calcifications with lactational changes in, 342*f*
  as prognostic and predictive factor, 231
Premenopausal women, MRI in, 204–205, 204*f*, 205*t*
Preoperative needle localization. *See* Needle localization.
PRESS (point-resolved spectroscopy), 762
  J- (JPRESS), 763
Presurgical needle localization. *See* Needle localization.
Price, J. L, 10
Primary mammary buds, 223
Printers, for mammography, 92–93
Problem-solving test, *vs.* screening, 56
Procedural coding, 720–727
  appropriate combination of information and, 725
  current acceptable, 722, 722*t*, 723*t*
  proper habits for, 725
  terminology for, 720–721
Processor, quality control test of, 137*t*, 141
Progesterone receptor(s) (PRs)
  as biomarker, 626, 626*f*
  in DCIS, 415–416
  in invasive ductal carcinoma, 453
  in invasive lobular carcinoma, 495
  as prognostic and predictive factor, 232
Progestins, and breast cancer risk, 44
Prognostic factor(s), for breast cancer, 231–232
  age as, 231
  DNA amplification as, 232
  expression profiling as, 232, 233*f*, 234*f*, 234*t*
  extent of DCIS as, 232
  Her2 oncogene as, 232
  histologic grade as, 231
  histologic type as, 231
  inflammatory cell infiltrates as, 231
  lymph node status as, 231
  lymphatic and blood cell invasion as, 231
  perineural invasion as, 231
  pregnancy as, 231
  steroid hormone receptor status as, 232
  TP53 mutation as, 232
  tumor cell proliferation as, 231
  tumor necrosis as, 231
  tumor size as, 231
Prognostic indicator, 626
Proliferative benign lesion(s), 300–322
  ductal hyperplasia of usual type as, 309–314
    with central apocrine metaplasia, 312*f*
    clinical presentation of, 309
    with cribriform pattern, 313*f*
    defined, 309
    differential diagnosis of, 310–314
    etiology and pathophysiology of, 309

Proliferative benign lesion(s) *(Continued)*
with florid proliferation, 312*f*
with gynecomastia-like or micropapillary pattern, 313*f*
imaging indications and algorithm for, 310
mammography of, 310, 310*f*, 311*f*
MRI of, 310
normal terminal ductal lobular unit *vs.*, 310–314, 311*f*, 312*f*
with overlapping nuclei, 313*f*
pathology findings with, 310–314
prevalence and epidemiology of, 309
treatment options for, 314
ultrasonography of, 310
gynecomastia as, 314–318
asymmetric, 316*f*
classic signs of, 317
clinical presentation of, 315
defined, 314
dendritic pattern of, 315
differential diagnosis of, 317–318
diffuse glandular pattern of, 315
early nodular pattern of, 315, 315*f*
etiology and pathophysiology of, 314, 314*t*
imaging indications and algorithm for, 315–317
mammography of, 315, 315*f*, 316*f*
MRI of, 315–317
pathology findings with, 317–318, 317*f*, 318*f*
prevalence and epidemiology of, 314
pseudo-, 315, 316*f*
treatment options for, 318
ultrasonography of, 315, 317*f*
microglandular adenosis as, 318–319
atypical, 318–319, 320*f*, 321*f*
clinical presentation of, 318
defined, 318
etiology and pathophysiology of, 318
imaging technique and findings with, 318–319
pathology findings with, 318–319, 319*f*, 320*f*
prevalence and epidemiology of, 318
treatment options for, 319
radial scar as, 304–309
clinical presentation of, 304
defined, 304
differential diagnosis of, 306–308
with ductal hyperplasia, 306–308, 308*f*
etiology and pathophysiology of, 304
imaging indications and algorithm for, 304
mammography of, 304, 304*f*, 305*f*
MRI of, 306
pathology findings with, 306–308, 306*f*, 307*f*
prevalence and epidemiology of, 304
treatment options for, 308–309
vs. tubular carcinoma, 306–308, 307*f*, 308*f*, 309*f*
ultrasonography of, 306, 306*f*
sclerosing adenosis as, 300–304
classic signs of, 302
clinical presentation of, 300
defined, 300
differential diagnosis of, 302–304
etiology and pathophysiology of, 300
imaging indications and algorithm for, 300
mammography of, 300, 301*f*, 302*f*
MRI of, 302
nodular, 302–303
pathology findings with, 302–304, 302*f*, 303*f*
prevalence and epidemiology of, 300
ultrasonography of, 302
Proliferative breast disease
with atypia, 226–228
without atypia, 226–228
Prospective, sequential read studies, of computer-aided detection, 104, 106*t*
Proton(s), magnetization of, in MRI, 177, 178*f*
Proton weighted sequence, in MRI, 181
Pseudoangiomatous stromal hyperplasia (PASH), 290–293
classic signs of, 292
clinical presentation of, 291–292
defined, 290–291
etiology and pathophysiology of, 291
imaging indications and algorithm for, 292
mammography of, 292, 292*f*
MRI of, 292
pathology findings with, 292, 293*f*
prevalence and epidemiology of, 291
treatment options for, 293
ultrasonography of, 292, 293*f*
Pseudocyst, 239
Pseudogynecomastia, 315, 316*f*
PTEN (phosphatase and tensin homolog) gene, and breast cancer risk, 47

Q

Qualification standards, Mammography Quality Standards Act on, 694
Quality assurance (QA), 133. *See also* Quality control (QC)
Quality assurance standards, Mammography Quality Standards Act on, 133–134, 144, 694, 696
Quality control (QC), 133–145
in accreditation, 699
aim of, 133
defined, 133
help with, 134–135, 143*t*
ACR Mammography Accreditation Program for, 144
independent consultants for, 144
manufacturers' representatives for, 143–144
medical physicists for, 143
U.S. Food and Drug Administration for, 144
individual(s) responsible for, 134*t*
medical physicist as, 134*t*, 135–136, 135*t*
continuing education of, 135*t*, 136
continuing experience of, 135*t*, 136
for help with questions, 143
initial qualifications of, 135*t*, 136
reestablishing qualifications of, 136
responsibilities of, 134*t*, 135–136
tests performed by, 138*t*, 139*b*, 139*t*, 142–143
radiologic technologist as, 136–137
continuing education of, 135*t*, 137
continuing experience of, 135*t*, 137
initial qualifications of, 135*t*, 136–137
reestablishing qualifications of, 137
responsibilities of, 134*t*, 136–137
tests performed by, 137*t*, 141–142
radiologist (interpreting physician) as, 134–135
continuing education of, 135, 135*t*
continuing experience of, 135, 135*t*
initial qualifications of, 135, 135*t*
reestablishing qualifications of, 135
responsibilities of, 134–135, 134*t*
reviewing (audit) interpreting physician as, 134*t*
supervising radiologist (lead interpreting physician) as, 134, 134*t*
legal aspects of, 731
with mammography, history of, 20–22, 133–134
team approach to, 134–137, 134*t*, 135*t*
Quality control (QC) tests, 137–143
due to equipment changes, 139–141, 139*b*, 139*t*
on application of compression, 139*t*
on automatic exposure, 139*t*
on beam limitation and light fields, 139*t*
on compression paddle, 139*t*
on film making devices, 139*t*
on film processing solutions, 139*t*
on focal spot selection, 139*t*
on image receptor sizes, 139*t*
on intensifying screens, 139*t*
on lighting, 139*t*
on magnification, 139*t*
on motion of tube-image receptor assembly, 139*t*
on technique factor, 139*t*
on x-ray film, 139*t*
for full-field digital mammography, 141
legal aspects of, 731
performed by medical physicists, 138*t*, 142–143
on accuracy and reproducibility of peak kilovolt (kVp), 138*t*, 143
artifact evaluation as, 138*t*, 142–143
automatic exposure control system performance assessment as, 138*t*, 142
on average glandular dose, 138*t*, 143
beam quality assessment (half-value layer measurement) as, 138*t*, 143
on breast exposure, 138*t*, 143
collimation assessment as, 138*t*, 142
evaluation of system resolution as, 138*t*, 142
image quality evaluation as, 138*t*, 143
mammographic unit assembly evaluation as, 138*t*, 142
on radiation output rate, 138*t*, 143
on reproducibility of automatic exposure control, 138*t*, 143
required by equipment changes, 139–141, 139*b*, 139*t*
on uniformity of screen speed, 138*t*, 142
on viewbox luminance and room illuminance, 138*t*, 143
performed by radiologic technologist, 137*t*, 141–142
analysis of fixer retention as, 137*t*, 142
on compression, 137*t*, 142
on darkroom cleanliness, 137*t*, 141
on darkroom fog, 137*t*, 142
on mobile unit, 137*t*
on phantom image, 137*t*, 141
on processor, 137*t*, 141
repeat analysis as, 137*t*, 142
on screen cleanliness, 137*t*, 141
on screen-film contact, 137*t*, 142
time required for, 141, 141*t*
on viewboxes and viewing conditions, 137*t*, 142
visual checklist as, 137*t*, 142
Quantum mottle, 125

R

Race
incidence of breast cancer and, 33–34, 33*f*
and mortality rate, 38, 39*f*
and stage at diagnosis, 35, 36*f*
and tumor size, 34, 34*f*
Radial folds, breast implants with
MRI of, 671, 671*f*
ultrasonography of, 674, 677*f*

Radial scar, 304-309
architectural distortion due to, 434
clinical presentation of, 304
DCIS with, 395*f*
defined, 304
differential diagnosis of, 306-308
vs. tubular carcinoma, 306-308, 307*f*, 308*f*, 309*f*
with ductal hyperplasia, 306-308, 308*f*
etiology and pathophysiology of, 304
imaging indications and algorithm for, 304
mammography of, 304, 304*f*, 305*f*
MRI of, 306
pathology findings with, 306-308, 306*f*, 307*f*
post-biopsy management of, 638-640, 639*f*
prevalence and epidemiology of, 304
treatment options for, 308-309
ultrasonography of, 306, 306*f*
Radial sclerosing lesion (RSL). *See* Radial scar
Radiation atypia
vs. cancerization of lobules, 531-533, 532*f*
vs. recurrence of DCIS, 411, 412*f*
Radiation changes, calcifications with, 345*f*
Radiation dose
in accreditation, 699
image quality *vs.*, 10
Radiation exposure
regulation of, 20-22
from screening mammography, 69, 69*t*
Radiation output, of mammography unit, 87-88
Radiation output rate, quality control test of, 138*t*, 143
Radiation risks, of mammography, 21
Radiation therapy (RT), 531-533
for DCIS, 418
histologic changes after, 531-533, 532*f*
low nuclear-to-cytoplasmic ratio after, 531-533, 532*f*
mammography after, 533*f*, 653-656
calcifications in, 651-652, 652*f*, 656, 656*f*
diffuse changes in, 655, 655*f*
goals of, 653
indications and algorithm for, 651, 651*t*
parenchymal changes in, 656
scars in, 654-655, 655*f*
seromas and hematomas in, 653*f*, 654, 654*f*, 655*f*
skin changes in, 655
timing of, 653-654
views for, 653
MRI after, 205*t*
of positive margins, 653, 653*f*
post-treatment changes in, 656
uses for, 651*t*
after positive sentinel lymph node sample, 625
recurrence after, 656-658
in axillary lymph nodes, 657-658, 658*f*
benign sequela(e) mimicking, 658-660
calcifications as, 658, 659*f*
fat necrosis as, 658, 658*f*
on mammography, 658-660, 658*f*, 659*f*
on MRI, 659-660, 660*f*
epidemiology of, 656
local, 657, 657*f*
risk factors for, 656-657
timing of, 658
skin changes after, 531-533
ultrasonography after, 533*f*
Radiofrequency ablation (RFA), 773-775
assessment of efficacy of, 775
history of, 774
mechanism of action of, 773-774
MRI-guided, 775
prior to surgical resection, 775
ultrasound-guided, 775
Radiofrequency (RF) coils, for MRI, 179, 179*f*, 180*f*
multi-channel bilateral, 188, 188*f*, 189*f*
Radiofrequency (RF) pulse, in MRI, 177-179, 179*f*
Radiographic mottle, clinical image evaluation of, 125
Radiologic technologist, in quality control, 136-137
continuing education of, 135*t*, 137
continuing experience of, 135*t*, 137
initial qualifications of, 135*t*, 136-137
reestablishing qualifications of, 137
responsibilities of, 134*t*, 136-137
tests performed by, 137*t*, 141-142
analysis of fixer retention as, 137*t*, 142
on compression, 137*t*, 142
on darkroom cleanliness, 137*t*, 141
on darkroom fog, 137*t*, 142
on mobile unit, 137*t*
on phantom image, 137*t*, 141
on processor, 137*t*, 141
repeat analysis as, 137*t*, 142
on screen cleanliness, 137*t*, 141
on screen-film contact, 137*t*, 142
time required for, 141, 141*t*
on viewboxes and viewing conditions, 137*t*, 142
visual checklist as, 137*t*, 142
Radiologist, in quality control, 134-135
continuing education of, 135, 135*t*
continuing experience of, 135, 135*t*
initial qualifications of, 135, 135*t*
reestablishing qualifications of, 135
responsibilities of, 134-135, 134*t*
reviewing (audit), 134*t*
supervising, 134, 134*t*
Radiologist review workstation, 91-92, 92*f*
Radiology benefits managers (RBMs), 540
Radionuclide imaging, 747-748
history of, 16-17, 17*f*
Raloxifene, and breast cancer risk, 44-45
Randomized clinical trials (RCTs), of screening
results of, 57-59, 58*t*
underestimation of benefit in, 60-61
Rare-earth screens, history of, 10
Rates, in epidemiology of breast cancer, 26
Rat-tail sign, with implants, 670*f*, 673
Raw data, for medical audit
additional, 704, 705*t*
essential, 703-704, 704*t*
Raw image, 93
RB1CC1 gene, 229
RBMs (radiology benefits managers), 540
RBRVS (Resource-Based Relative Value System), 721
RCTs (randomized clinical trials), of screening
results of, 57-59, 58*t*
underestimation of benefit in, 60-61
Readout gradient, in MRI, 181, 181*f*
Reasonableness, 730, 731
Recall, standards of care for, 731-732
Recall rate(s), 66-67
computer-aided detection and, 99, 105*t*, 106*t*, 107-108
defined, 66
in medical audit
analysis of, 711
goals for, 710*t*
in medical literature, 708*t*
with screening and diagnostic mammography data combined, 712*t*, 713*t*
Receiver operating characteristic (ROC) curve, in medical audit, 707-711, 709*f*, 710*t*
Rectal carcinoma, with male breast cancer, 470
Recurrence, after radiation therapy, 656-658
in axillary lymph nodes, 657-658, 658*f*
benign sequela(e) mimicking, 658-660
calcifications as, 658, 659*f*
fat necrosis as, 658, 658*f*
on mammography, 658-660, 658*f*, 659*f*
on MRI, 659-660, 660*f*
epidemiology of, 656
local, 657, 657*f*
risk factors for, 656-657
timing of, 658
Reduction mammoplasty, 682-689
appearance after, 682, 683*f*
breast cancer after, 682, 688
defined, 682
early complications of, 682
imaging indications and algorithm for, 682-688
indications for, 682
vs. liposuction, 688
mammographic change(s) after, 683-688, 683*b*
alteration of breast contour as, 684, 684*f*
architectural distortion as, 685, 685*f*, 686-688, 686*f*
asymmetric tissue as, 686-688
calcifications as, 686-688, 688*f*
displacement of breast parenchyma as, 684-685, 685*f*
disruption of subareolar ducts as, 686, 687*f*
elevation of nipple as, 684, 684*f*
fat necrosis as, 686, 687*f*, 688*f*
retroalveolar fibrotic band as, 685, 686*f*
skin thickening as, 685
with nipple transplantation, 682, 683*f*
with nipple transposition, 682, 683*f*
techniques for, 682, 683*f*
Re-excisional biopsy, after lumpectomy, 620-621
Refer, duty to, 735
Reference angle, of x-ray tube, 83*f*
Referral, negligent, 735
Regional lymph node assessment, in patient with suspicious breast lesions undergoing biopsy, 161-166, 162*f*, 163*f*, 164*f*, 165*f*
Regulation, of mammography, 20-22
Reid, John, 13, 14, 14*f*
Reimbursement, 720-727
by cash-paying customers, 724, 726
coding and billing terminology for, 720-721
by HMOs, 724, 726
Medicare
acceptable codes and payment rates for, 722, 722*t*, 723*t*
background and present status of, 721-722
special rules relating to, 722-724
by other payers, 724
by private payers, 724
strategy(ies) for successful, 724-726
appropriate combination of information and coding as, 725
challenging denials and underpayments as, 726
clinical cooperation as, 725
discounts for cash payments as, 726
facility personnel training as, 726
internal audits of data quality as, 726
knowing and applying rules as, 725
political involvement as, 726
proper coding and billing habits as, 725
using outcome data in HMO negotiations as, 726
Relative risk (RR), 39-46
Relaxation, in MRI, 17, 179-180, 180*f*

Renal cell carcinoma, metastatic to breast, 514, 515*f*
Repair, of mammography equipment, 97
Repeat analysis, in quality control, 137*t*, 142
Repetition time (TR), in MRI, 180, 180*f*
Reporting
BI-RADS for (*See* Breast Imaging, Reporting, and Data System (BI-RADS))
on breast cancer specimens, 629-631, 630*t*
on core needle biopsy
MRI-guided, 593
stereotactic-guided, 585
ultrasound-guided, 575
legal aspects of, 733-734
Mammography Quality Standards Act on, 214, 694, 696
Resolution
in MRI, 181, 183*t*
in ultrasonography, 146-147, 147*f*, 148*f*
Resolution patterns, 83-84
Resource Value System Update Committee (RUC), 721
Resource Value Unit (RVU), 721
Resource-Based Relative Value System (RBRVS), 721
Respondeat superior, 735
Restitution, 729
Retention cysts, 239
Retroalveolar fibrotic band, after reduction mammoplasty, 685, 686*f*
Retromammary fat, 224*f*
Review workstation (RW), 91-92, 92*f*
Reviewing interpreting physician, in quality control, 134*t*
RF (radiofrequency) coils, for MRI, 179, 179*f*, 180*f*
multi-channel bilateral, 188, 188*f*, 189*f*
RF (radiofrequency) pulse, in MRI, 177-179, 179*f*
RFA. *See* Radiofrequency ablation (RFA)
Rhabdomyosarcoma, 511
Rheumatoid arthritis, gold deposits in, 261, 262*f*
Risk
absolute, 39-40
cumulative and relative, 39-46
family history and assessment of, 45-46
histologic and mammographic markers of, 45
lifetime, 39-41, 41*t*
low penetrance susceptiblity genes in, 48
major genes and syndromes with increased, 46-48
worldwide comparison of, 29-30
Risk factor(s), 41-45, 42*t*
alcohol consumption as, 42-43
body size as, 42
breastfeeding as, 41-42
exogenous hormone use as, 31-32, 43-45
and incidence, 31-32
for invasive ductal carcinoma, 424
menopausal hormones as, 44
oral contraceptives as, 43
physical activity as, 42
SERMs as, 44-45
RL (rolled laterally) view, 117
RM (rolled medially) view, 117
Robbins, Lewis C., 9*f*
ROC (receiver operating characteristic) curve, in medical audit, 707-711, 709*f*, 710*t*
Rockefeller, Happy, 30-31
Roentgen, Wilhelm Conrad, 3
Rolled laterally (RL) view, 117
Rolled medially (RM) view, 117
Room illuminance, quality control test of, 138*t*, 143
Rosen's triad, columnar cell lesions in, 356-357
RR (relative risk), 39-46
RSL (radial sclerosing lesion). *See* Radial scar
RT. *See* Radiation therapy (RT)
RUC (Resource Value System Update Committee), 721
RVU (Resource Value Unit), 721
RW (review workstation), 91-92, 92*f*

S

Saline implants, 663
rupture of, 667
Salomon, Albert, 4*f*
on mammography equipment, 79
as pioneer of mammography, 3, 4*f*, 5*f*
SAR (specific absorption ratio), in MRI, 188
Sarcoma(s), 508-511
angio-
etiology of, 511
pathology of, 511, 512*f*
primary
mammography of, 509
MRI of, 509
prognosis of, 511
secondary
mammography of, 509
MRI of, 509
ultrasonography of, 509
chondro-, 510
clinical presentation of, 509
defined, 508
granulocytic, 502, 504-505, 505*f*
leiomyo-, 511, 511*f*
lipo-
clinical presentation of, 509
MRI of, 509
pathology of, 510, 510*f*
mammography of, 509, 509*f*
MRI of, 509
osteogenic
mammography of, 509, 509*f*
pathology of, 510, 510*f*
pathology of, 510-511, 510*f*, 511*f*, 512*f*
prevalence and epidemiology of, 509
rhabdomyo-, 511
ultrasonography of, 509
Sarcomatous heterologous element, malignant phyllodes tumor with, 507*f*
SBI (Society of Breast Imaging)
history of, 20
on screening, 62
Scar(s)
after breast-conserving therapy, 654-655, 655*f*
postoperative, architectural distortion due to, 434
radial *See* Radial scar
skin retraction due to, 429, 431*f*
Scarf-Bloom and Richardson (SBR) grade and score, in invasive ductal carcinoma, 438-442
Scintillating echoes, cysts with, 171-176, 174*f*
Scintimammography, 747
Scleroelastic lesion (*See* Radial scar)
Sclerosing adenosis, 300-304
calcifications with, 344*f*
classic signs of, 302
clinical presentation of, 300
DCIS with
mammography of, 395*f*
microscopic findings in, 403-404, 407*f*, 408*f*
defined, 300
differential diagnosis of, 302-304
Sclerosing adenosis *(Continued)*
etiology and pathophysiology of, 300
false positive core needle biopsy due to, 616-617, 616*f*
imaging indications and algorithm for, 300
mammography of, 300, 301*f*, 302*f*
MRI of, 302
nodular, 302-303
pathology findings with, 302-304, 302*f*, 303*f*
post-biopsy management of, 641-642, 643*f*
prevalence and epidemiology of, 300
ultrasonography of, 302
Sclerosing ductal hyperplasia, benign. *See* Radial scar.
Sclerosing lesion
nonencapsulated (*See* Radial scar)
radial (*See* Radial scar)
Sclerosing lymphocytic lobulitis. *See* Diabetic mastopathy.
Sclerosing papillary proliferation. *See* Radial scar.
SCNB. *See* Stereotactic-guided core needle biopsy (SCNB).
Scott, Wendell, 6, 20
Scout image
for MRI, 181-182, 183*f*
in stereotactic-guided core needle biopsy, 580-581, 580*f*
Screen cleanliness, quality control test of, 137*t*, 141
Screen speed uniformity, quality control test of, 138*t*, 142
Screen-film contact, quality control test of, 137*t*, 142
Screen-film mammography (SFM)
antiscatter grid assembly for, 88-89
artifacts in, 126, 129*f*
automatic exposure control for, 89, 90
compression paddles for, 86
computer-aided detection with, 100, 100*f*
face shield for, 84
film for, 93-94, 93*f*, 94*f*
processing of, 80, 94
foot pedals and digital display for compression in, 87
geometry of system for, 93, 93*f*, 94*f*
history of, 10-11, 11*f*, 79-80
image formation with, 80, 81*f*
mammography unit for, 81
overview of equipment for, 80
screen speeds for, 93-94
U-arm for, 85
x-ray tube and filter for, 82
Screening, 56-75
adverse consequences of, 65-70
breast compression with, 66
breast self-examination for, 56-57
clinical examination for, 56-57
cost-effectiveness of, 69-70, 70*t*
criteria for benefit from, 57
and DCIS, 67-68
defined, 56
vs. diagnostic (problem-solving) test, 56
digital mammography for, 57
false-positive biopsy results in, 67
and higher survival rates, 57-61
and longer survival *vs.* decreased mortality, 57
mammography for (*See* Screening mammography)
modalities of, 56-57
MRI for, 57, 199-201, 200*b*
radiation exposure due to, 69, 69*t*
randomized control trials on
results of, 57-59, 58*t*
underestimation of benefit in, 60-61

Screening *(Continued)*
  recall rates with, 66-67
  service, results of, 60, 64-65, 64*t*
  2009 U.S. Preventive Services Task Force controversy over, 70-72
  with ultrasound, 168-176
    for cysts, 171-176
      with acute inflammation, 157, 158*f*
      containing papillomas or malignancy, 171-176, 175*f*
      with diffuse low-level internal echoes, 171-176, 174*f*
      for directional vacuum-assisted biopsy, 171-176, 176*f*
      with fat-fluid level, 171-176, 174*f*
      with fluid-debris level, 171-176, 174*f*
      mammographic correlation with, 156*f*
      with scintillating echoes, 171-176, 174*f*
    goals of, 168
    identification of structures in, 168-171, 170*f*, 171*f*
    for solid breast nodules, 171, 172*f*, 173*f*
  of women 40 to 49 years old
    benefits of
      proof of, 59-60, 59*t*, 60*t*
      vs. risks, 68-69, 68*t*, 69*t*
    controversy over, 59, 70-72
    guidelines for, 62
  of women 50 to 74 years old, 71
  of women 75 years of age and older, 60, 71
Screening mammography
  vs. clinical examination, 56-57
  coding and billing for, 722-724, 723*t*
  communicating results of, 214
  cost-effectiveness of, 69-70, 70*t*
  DCIS in, 67-68
  detection rates and accuracy of, 68-69, 68*t*
  guidelines for, 61-64
    on time between screenings, 61-62
    on time to begin screening, 61
  history of, 18-20, 22
  and incidence of breast cancer, 31-32, 38-39
  mass(es) detected on, 542-550
    with benign features, 547-549
      biopsy of, 547-549
      fat-containing, 543, 546*b*
      management algorithm for, 547, 549*f*
      multiple bilateral circumscribed round or oval, 547, 548*f*
      and no prior mammograms, 547
      requiring no further evaluation, 543-546, 547, 548*f*
      short-term imaging for, 547-549
      ultrasonography for, 547, 548*f*, 549
    focal asymmetries as, 546-547
      defined, 546
      diagnostic mammography for, 547
      spot compression views for, 542, 543*f*
      ultrasound-guided biopsy for, 547, 547*f*
    MRI for, 542, 544*f*
    spot compression views for, 542, 543*f*
    suspicious and malignant, 549-550, 550*f*
    ultrasonography for, 542, 543*f*
  "over-diagnosis" controversy with, 39, 63-64, 71
  radiation exposure from, 69, 69*t*
  standards of care for, 731
Screening test, requirements for, 56
Screening trials
  results of, 57-59, 58*t*
  and screening guidelines, 61-64
  vs. therapeutic trials, 63
  underestimation of benefit in, 60-61
SDM (stereo digital mammography), 743-744, 744*f*
Seabold, Paul, 3-4
Sebaceous cysts, 239-241
  clinical presentation of, 239
  defined, 239, 240*f*
  differential diagnosis of, 240-241
  etiology and pathophysiology of, 239
  imaging indications and algorithm for, 239
  mammography of, 240, 241*f*
  MRI of, 240
  pathology of, 241
  prevalence and epidemiology of, 239
  treatment options for, 241
  ultrasonography of, 240, 241*f*, 242*f*
Sebelius, Kathleen, 70
Secretory calcifications, duct ectasia with, 331-332
  clinical aspects of, 331
  imaging features of, 331-332, 336*f*
Secretory carcinoma, 462, 463*f*
Sectioning, of breast tissue specimens, 630-631, 632*f*
SEER (Surveillance, Epidemiology, and End Results) Program, 25, 57
Selection bias, 57
Selective estrogen receptor modulators (SERMs)
  and breast cancer risk, 44-45
  for DCIS, 415-416
Selenium flat-panel system, for image detection, 95, 96*f*
Senographe, 7-9, 10*f*, 79
Sensitivity, in medical audit
  analysis of, 709
  defined, 706
  goals for, 710*t*
  in medical literature, 708*t*
Sensitivity encoding (SENSE), in MRI, 189
Sentinel lymph node sample, 623-625
  isolated tumor cells in, 624-625, 625*f*
  macrometastatic disease in, 624-625
  micrometastatic disease in, 624-625, 625*f*
  protocol for, 623-625, 624*f*
  radiation therapy after positive, 625
Serine/threonine kinase 11 *(STK11)* gene, and breast cancer risk, 47
SERMs (selective estrogen receptor modulators)
  and breast cancer risk, 44-45
  for DCIS, 415-416
Seromas, after breast-conserving therapy, 653*f*, 654, 654*f*, 655*f*
Serous papillary carcinoma, metastatic to breast, 514-516, 517*f*
Service contracts, for mammography equipment, 97
Service risk insurance, for mammography equipment, 97
Service screening, results of, 60, 64-65, 64*t*
Sestamibi scintigraphy, history of, 17
Sewing needle, calcifications due to, 332, 339*f*
SFM. *See* Screen-film mammography (SFM).
Shapiro, Sam, 18
Sharpness, clinical image evaluation of, 125, 127*f*, 128*f*
Shaved margins, 623, 623*f*
Shear wave elastography, 756-757, 757*f*, 758*f*
Short interval follow-up, ultrasound for, 159-160, 160*f*
Short-axis focusing, in ultrasonography, 147, 147*f*, 148*f*
Sickles, Edward, 9, 20
SID (source-to-image distance), in mammography unit, 83*f*, 84
Signet cell carcinoma, metastatic to breast, 516, 518*f*
Signet ring cell variant, of invasive lobular carcinoma, 491-493, 492*f*, 494*f*
Sigrist, R, 4
Silicone adenopathy, 667, 667*f*
Silicone breast implant(s), 662-681
  alternatives to, 665
  comparison of imaging modalities with, 680, 680*f*
  complications of, 663-665
  CT of, 680, 680*f*
  demographics of, 663
  dual chamber (double lumen), 663, 665*f*
    MRI of, 670, 670*f*
  encapsulation of, 666
  FDA approval of, 666
  fluid on periphery of, 673, 675*f*
  gel bleed from, 666
  history of, 662-666
  imaging indications and algorithm for, 663-666
  mammography of, 667-668
    with rupture, 287, 287*f*, 667-668, 668*f*
    with silicone adenopathy, 667, 667*f*
    with silicone granulomas, 667-668, 668*f*
  Mammography Quality Standards Act on, 696
  MRI of, 201-202, 668-674, 670*f*
    in evaluation for malignancy, 201-202
    with gel fracture, 674
    imaging protocols for, 669-670
    normal appearance in, 670-671, 670*f*
    with radial folds, 671, 671*f*
    with rupture, 288
      axial and sagittal inversion recovery water saturation images in, 201, 668*f*
      contour deformities in, 673
      extracapsular, 673-674, 676*f*
      fluid on periphery of implant in, 673, 675*f*
      inconclusive signs in, 673
      intracapsular, 671-673
      linguine sign in, 671, 672*f*
      subscapular line sign in, 671, 672*f*, 673*f*
      teardrop, keyhole, or noose sign in, 673, 673*f*
      water droplets in, 673, 674*f*
    with silicone granulomas, 202, 203*f*, 676*f*
    technical factors in, 669, 669*f*, 669*t*
  multi-compartment, 671, 673*f*
  pathology findings with, 287-288, 288*f*, 289*f*
  prevalence and epidemiology of, 287
  with radial folds
    MRI of, 671, 671*f*
    ultrasonography of, 674, 677*f*
  rupture of, 286-288, 666
    classic signs of, 287
    clinical presentation of, 287
    CT of, 680, 680*f*
    defined, 286-287
    etiology and pathophysiology of, 287
    etiology of, 666
    extracapsular, 666
      MRI of, 673-674, 676*f*
      ultrasonography of, 677-678, 678*f*, 679*f*
    imaging indications and algorithm for, 287
    intracapsular, 666
      MRI of, 671-673
      ultrasonography of, 677, 678*f*
    mammography of, 287, 287*f*, 667-668, 668*f*
    MRI of, 288
      axial and sagittal inversion recovery water saturation images in, 201, 668*f*
      contour deformities in, 673
      extracapsular, 673-674, 676*f*
      fluid on periphery of implant in, 673, 675*f*
      inconclusive signs in, 673
      intracapsular, 671-673
      linguine sign in, 671, 672*f*

Silicone breast implant(s) *(Continued)*
subscapular line sign in, 671, 672*f*, 673*f*
teardrop, keyhole, or noose sign in, 673, 673*f*
water droplets in, 673, 674*f*
pathology findings with, 287–288, 288*f*, 289*f*
prevalence and epidemiology of, 287
ultrasonography of, 674–678
extracapsular, 677–678, 678*f*, 679*f*
intracapsular, 677, 678*f*
with silicone granulomas, 287, 288*f*
with silicone adenopathy, 667, 667*f*
single chamber (single lumen), 663, 664*f*, 665*f*
MRI of, 670, 670*f*
stacked, 670
subglandular, 663, 664*f*
subpectoral, 663, 665*f*
ultrasonography of, 288–290, 674–679
limitations of, 678–679
normal findings in, 674, 676*f*, 677*f*
with radial folds, 674, 677*f*
with rupture, 674–678
extracapsular, 677–678, 678*f*, 679*f*
intracapsular, 677, 678*f*
and silicone granulomas, 287, 288*f*
Silicone granuloma(s)
mammography of, 287*f*, 662, 663*f*, 667–668, 668*f*
MRI of, 202, 203*f*, 676*f*
due to silicone injection, 662, 663*f*
ultrasonography of, 287, 288*f*, 677–678, 679*f*
Silicone injections, 662, 663*f*
Silicone lymphadenitis, 287–288, 289*f*
Silicone mastitis, 287–288, 288*f*
Simple cyst, 239, 240*f*
Single dilated duct, 215
in invasive ductal carcinoma, 435, 437*f*
Single nucleotide polymorphisms (SNPs), and breast cancer risk, 48
Single voxel (SV)-based magnetic resonance spectroscopy, 762, 768
SIO (superoinferior oblique) view, 116–117
Skin calcifications, 323–325
grid compression paddle for, 323, 326*f*
mammography of, 323, 325*f*, 554*f*
parenchymal *vs.*, 323–325
Skin changes
after breast-conserving therapy, 655
in invasive ductal carcinoma, 425
Skin dimpling, in invasive ductal carcinoma, 425
Skin flattening, in invasive ductal carcinoma, 425
Skin folds, in mediolateral oblique view, 122, 124*f*
Skin retraction
in invasive ductal carcinoma
clinical presentation of, 425
mammography of, 428, 430*f*
due to scarring, 429, 431*f*
Skin thickening
differential diagnosis of, 428
in invasive ductal carcinoma
clinical presentation of, 425
mammography of, 427–428, 430*f*
after reduction mammoplasty, 685
Skin ulceration, in invasive ductal carcinoma, 438, 438*f*
Slice select gradient, in MRI, 181
Slot-Scan charge-coupled device system, for image detection, 94–95, 94*f*
Small cell carcinoma, 455, 455*f*
SNPs (single nucleotide polymorphisms), and breast cancer risk, 48
Society of Breast Imaging (SBI)
history of, 20
on screening, 62
Soft copy display, 113
Sojourn time, 33
for screening, 61–62
Solid benign lesion(s), 255–299
adenomyoepithelioma as, 295–297
classic signs of, 295
clinical presentation of, 295
defined, 295
etiology and pathophysiology of, 295
imaging indications and algorithm for, 295
mammography of, 295
MRI of, 295
pathology findings with, 295–296, 296*f*
prevalence and epidemiology of, 295
treatment options for, 296–297
ultrasonography of, 295
adenosis as, 274–276
apocrine adenoma in, 276
clinical presentation of, 274
defined, 274
etiology and pathophysiology of, 274
imaging indications and algorithm for, 274
lactating adenoma in, 274–276, 276*f*, 277*f*
mammography of, 274
MRI of, 274
pathology findings with, 274–276
prevalence and epidemiology of, 274
treatment options for, 276
tubular adenoma in, 274, 275*f*
ultrasonography of, 274, 275*f*
diabetic mastopathy as, 276–280
classic signs of, 278
clinical presentation of, 277
defined, 276
etiology and pathophysiology of, 277
imaging indications and algorithm for, 277
mammography of, 277–278, 277*f*
MRI of, 278, 278*f*, 279*f*
pathology findings in, 278, 279*f*
prevalence and epidemiology of, 277
treatment options for, 280
ultrasonography of, 278, 278*f*
fat necrosis as, 283–286
classic signs of, 286
clinical presentation of, 283
defined, 283
etiology and pathophysiology of, 283
imaging indications and algorithm for, 283
with lipid or oil cyst, 283, 284*f*
mammography of, 283, 283*f*, 284*f*, 285*f*
with microcalcifications and architectural distortion, 283, 284*f*, 285*f*
MRI of, 283–286
pathology findings with, 286, 286*f*
prevalence and epidemiology of, 283
treatment options for, 286
ultrasonography of, 283, 285*f*
fibroadenoma as, 255–260
classic signs of, 256
clinical presentation of, 255
complex, 256–259
defined, 255
with epithelial hyperplasia, 256–259, 259*f*
etiology and pathophysiology of, 255
fibrosed (old), 256–259, 258*f*, 259*f*
fine needle aspiration biopsy of, 256–259, 260*f*
imaging indications and algorithm for, 255
with intracanalicular growth pattern, 256–259, 258*f*
Solid benign lesion(s) *(Continued)*
juvenile, 259–260, 261*f*
mammography of, 256, 256*f*
MRI of, 256
pathology findings with, 256–260
with pericanalicular growth pattern, 256–259, 258*f*
prevalence and epidemiology of, 255
treatment options for, 260
ultrasonography of, 256, 257*f*
fibromatosis as, 270–273
clinical presentation of, 271
defined, 270
etiology and pathophysiology of, 271
imaging indications and algorithm for, 271
mammography of, 271
MRI of, 272
pathology findings with, 272, 272*f*
prevalence and epidemiology of, 270
treatment options for, 273
ultrasonography of, 271, 271*f*
fibrosis as, 273–274
classic signs of, 274
clinical presentation of, 273
defined, 273
etiology and pathophysiology of, 273
imaging indications and algorithm for, 273
mammography of, 273, 273*f*
MRI of, 274
pathology findings with, 274
prevalence and epidemiology of, 273
treatment options for, 274
ultrasonography of, 273–274
granular cell tumor as, 280–283
classic signs of, 281
clinical presentation of, 280
defined, 280
etiology and pathophysiology of, 280
imaging indications and algorithm for, 280
mammography of, 280, 280*f*
MRI of, 281
pathology findings with, 281, 282*f*
prevalence and epidemiology of, 280
treatment options for, 283
ultrasonography of, 281, 281*f*
hamartoma as, 265–268
classic signs of, 266
clinical presentation of, 265
defined, 265
etiology and pathophysiology of, 265
imaging indications and algorithm for, 265
mammography of, 265, 266*f*
MRI of, 265, 267*f*
pathology findings with, 266, 268*f*
prevalence and epidemiology of, 265
treatment options for, 266–268
ultrasonography of, 265, 266*f*
hemangioma as, 288–290
cavernous, 290–291, 291*f*
clinical presentation of, 289
defined, 288
etiology and pathophysiology of, 289
imaging indications and algorithm for, 289
mammography of, 289
MRI of, 289, 290*f*
pathology findings with, 289–290, 291*f*
perilobular, 290–291, 291*f*
prevalence and epidemiology of, 288–289
treatment options for, 290
ultrasonography of, 289
intramammary lymph node as, 260–264
classic signs of, 263
clinical presentation of, 262
defined, 260
differential diagnosis of, 263–264

Solid benign lesion(s) *(Continued)*
etiology and pathophysiology of, 261, 261*f*, 262*f*
imaging indications and algorithm for, 262
mammography of, 262-263, 262*f*, 263*f*
MRI of, 263
pathology findings with, 264, 264*f*, 265*f*
prevalence and epidemiology of, 261
reactive inflammatory, 263, 263*f*, 264*f*
treatment options for, 264
ultrasonography of, 263, 263*f*, 264*f*
lipoma as, 268-270
classic signs of, 268
clinical presentation of, 268
defined, 268
etiology and pathophysiology of, 268
imaging indications and algorithm for, 268
mammography of, 268, 269*f*
MRI of, 268
pathology findings with, 269, 271*f*
prevalence and epidemiology of, 268
treatment options for, 270
ultrasonography of, 268, 269*f*, 270*f*
myofibroblastoma as, 293-295
clinical presentation of, 294
defined, 293
etiology and pathophysiology of, 294
imaging indications and algorithm for, 294
mammography of, 294
MRI of, 294
pathology findings with, 294-295, 294*f*, 295*f*
prevalence and epidemiology of, 294
treatment options for, 295
ultrasonography of, 294
nipple adenoma as, 297-298
classic signs of, 297
clinical presentation of, 297
defined, 297
etiology and pathophysiology of, 297
imaging indications and algorithm for, 297
mammography of, 297
MRI of, 297
pathology of findings with, 297-298, 297*f*, 298*f*
prevalence and epidemiology of, 297
treatment options for, 298
ultrasonography of, 297
pseudoangiomatous stromal hyperplasia as, 290-293
classic signs of, 292
clinical presentation of, 291-292
defined, 290-291
etiology and pathophysiology of, 291
imaging indications and algorithm for, 292
mammography of, 292, 292*f*
MRI of, 292
pathology findings with, 292, 293*f*
prevalence and epidemiology of, 291
treatment options for, 293
ultrasonography of, 292, 293*f*
silicone breast implant rupture as, 286-288
classic signs of, 287
clinical presentation of, 287
defined, 286-287
etiology and pathophysiology of, 287
imaging indications and algorithm for, 287
mammography of, 287, 287*f*
MRI of, 288
pathology findings with, 287-288, 288*f*, 289*f*
prevalence and epidemiology of, 287
ultrasonography of, 288-290, 288*f*
Solid breast nodules, ultrasound of, 171
with branch pattern, 171, 172*f*
with duct extension, 171, 172*f*
due to fibroadenoma, 171, 173*f*
hard finding in, 171, 172*f*
hypoechoic, 171, 173*f*
with microcalcifications, 171, 172*f*, 173*f*
with microlobulations, 171, 172*f*, 173*f*
nonspecific findings in, 171, 173*f*
soft findings in, 171, 172*f*, 173*f*
with spiculation, 171, 172*f*
terminal duct lobular unit in, 173*f*
Solid-type DCIS, 402, 404*f*
Solitary dilated duct, 215
in invasive ductal carcinoma, 435, 437*f*
SomoVu system, for automated whole breast ultrasound, 752-753, 753*f*
SonoCine system, for automated whole breast ultrasound, 752-753, 753*f*
Source-to-image distance (SID), in mammography unit, 83*f*, 84
Spatial compound imaging, in ultrasonography, 148-149, 150*f*, 151*f*, 217-218
Spatial resolution
in mammography, 83-84
in ultrasonography, 146-147, 147*f*, 148*f*
Specific absorption ratio (SAR), in MRI, 188
Specificity, in medical audit
analysis of, 711
defined, 707
goals for, 710*t*
in medical literature, 708*t*
Specimen processing, 611-634
biomarker(s) in, 626-629
Allred Score for, 626-627, 627*f*
ER and PR as, 626, 626*f*
HER-2/neu as, 627-629
chromosomal location of, 627-629, 627*f*
FISH testing for, 627-629, 629*f*
immunohistochemical testing (HercepTest) for, 450, 627-629
rationale for, 627-629
as prognostic *vs.* predictive indicators, 626
reports on, 629, 630*t*
in core needle biopsy, 612-618
calcifications in, 612-614, 614*f*, 615*f*
communicating results after, 618
false positive, 615-617
myoepithelial cell markers for, 616-617, 617*f*
due to sclerosing adenosis, 616-617, 616*f*
limitations of, 615
MRI-guided, 592-593
potential false negatives and follow-up for benign, 617
stereotactic-guided, 585
triple test with, 615
ultrasound-guided, 575
underestimation of disease with, 615
excisional biopsy for, 618-619, 618*f*
re-, 620-621
fine-needle aspiration for, 611-612, 612*f*, 613*f*
incisional biopsy for, 618
intraoperative consultation/frozen section in, 625-626
from mastectomy, 621-622
microscopic evaluation of surgical margins in, 623, 623*f*, 624*f*
reports in, 629-631, 630*t*
sentinel lymph node sample in, 623-625
isolated tumor cells in, 624-625, 625*f*
macrometastatic disease in, 624-625
micrometastatic disease in, 624-625, 625*f*
Specimen processing *(Continued)*
protocol for, 623-625, 624*f*
radiation therapy after positive, 625
tissue processing and permanent sections in, 630-631
coverslipping in, 615
embedding in paraffin in, 630-631, 631*f*
equipment for, 630-631, 631*f*
fixation in, 630-631
sectioning in, 615, 632*f*
staining in, 615, 632*f*
tumor size measurement
gross, 619-620
cassettes in, 619-620, 621*f*
initial appearance of specimen in, 619-620, 619*f*
inking of margins in, 619-620, 619*f*
recording of, 619-620, 620*f*
specimen slicing in, 619-620, 620*f*
microscopic, 620, 622*f*
Specimen radiography
in breast-conserving therapy, 651, 652*f*
with needle localization, 607-609, 608*f*, 609*f*
in stereotactic-guided core needle biopsy, 583-584, 585*f*
Speckle reduction imaging, in ultrasonography, 148-149, 151*f*
Spectroscopy, magnetic resonance. *See* Magnetic resonance spectroscopy (MRS).
S-phase fraction (SPF), as prognostic and predictive factor, 231
Spherulosis, collagenous, cribriform DCIS *vs.*, 401-402, 403*f*
Spiculation
in invasive ductal carcinoma, 426, 426*f*
in invasive lobular carcinoma, 484, 485*f*
ultrasound of, 171, 172*f*
Spin echo sequence, in MRI, 180-181, 180*f*
Spindle cell intraductal carcinoma, 403, 406*f*
Spindle cell metaplastic carcinoma, 465, 465*f*, 466*f*
vs. melanoma, 513-514, 514*f*, 515*f*
Spin-lattice relaxation time, in MRI, 17, 179-180, 180*f*
Spin-spin relaxation time, in MRI, 17, 179-180, 180*f*
Spoilation of evidence, 729-730
Spot compression views
of architectural distortion, 432, 434*f*, 435*f*
for mass, 426, 427*f*
detected on screening mammography, 542, 543*f*
Squamous cell carcinoma, 463-466, 465*f*
ST7 gene, 229
Stage at diagnosis
in epidemiology of breast cancer, 34-38, 35*f*, 36*f*
and survival rate, 35, 36*f*
Staging, of invasive ductal carcinoma, 438, 439*t*, 440*t*, 442*t*
Staining, of breast tissue specimens, 630-631, 632*f*
Stand-alone performance studies, of computer-aided detection, 102, 103*f*
Standards of care, legal aspects of, 729, 730-732
Staphylococcus aureus, mastitis due to, 375, 379
STAR (Study of Tamoxifen and Raloxifene) trial, 44-45
Stare decisis, 730
State(s), and Mammography Quality Standards Act, 694
State inspection, Mammography Quality Standards Act on, 694
Static elastography, 755-756, 756*f*

Statistics, on breast cancer, 25-29
Statute of limitations, 736
Statutory law, 730
STEAM (stimulated echo acquisition mode) sequence, in magnetic resonance spectroscopy, 762
Stereo digital mammography (SDM), 743-744, 744*f*
Stereotactic-guided core needle biopsy (SCNB), 564
  accuracy and cost-effectiveness of, 576
  air gap technique in, 582-583
  anesthesia for
    epinephrine with, 581
    injection tract of, 581
    local, 581
    site of, 581
    topical, 581
  coding and billing for, 723*t*
  confirming accurate needle placement for
    with prone biopsy table, 581-583, 582*f*, 583*f*
    with side-arm needle holder, 583, 584*f*
  contraindications to, 586
  dermatotomy in, 581
  description of, 577, 577*f*
  equipment for, 577-579
    add-on units as, 577-578, 578*f*, 579*f*
    dedicated prone table as, 577, 578*f*
    sterile procedure tray as, 576-587
    vacuum-assisted device as, 578-579
  indications for, 585-586
  informed consent for, 579-580
  of lesion discovered on another modality, 586
  marking clips for, 583-584
  of multiple suspicious findings, 586
  negative stroke margin in, 582-583
  positioning for, 580-581
  post-procedure considerations for, 585
  potential complications of, 586-587
  pre-procedural considerations for, 579-581
  procedure room for, 579
  record of, 585
  retargeting in, 581
  sampling in, 583-584
  scout film in, 580-581, 580*f*
  specimen processing for, 585
  specimen radiography in, 583-584, 585*f*
  sterile portion of procedure for, 581-584
  swing views in, 577, 580-581, 580*f*
  "zeroing out" in, 581
Sterile biopsy tray, for core needle biopsy
  MRI-guided, 587-588
  stereotactic-guided, 579
  ultrasound-guided, 564-565, 564*f*
Sternalis muscle, 226, 227*f*
Steroid hormone receptor(s)
  as biomarker, 626, 626*f*
  in DCIS, 415-416
  in invasive ductal carcinoma, 449, 449*f*
  in invasive lobular carcinoma, 495
  as prognostic and predictive factor, 232
Stewart-Treves syndrome, 511
Stimulated echo acquisition mode (STEAM) sequence, in magnetic resonance spectroscopy, 762
STK11 (serine/threonine kinase 11) gene, and breast cancer risk, 47
Stockholm trial, 57-58, 58*t*
  and underestimation of benefits from screening, 61
Storage, of mammographic images, 93
Strax, Philip, 18
Streptococcus spp, mastitis due to, 375, 379
Strickler, Albert, 4
Stroma, calcification with, 344*f*
Stromal desmoplasia, 489-491, 490*f*, 491*f*
Study of Tamoxifen and Raloxifene (STAR) trial, 44-45
Subareolar abscess, 377*f*, 379-380, 382*f*
Subareolar duct disruption, after reduction mammoplasty, 686, 687*f*
Subareolar musculature, 224*f*
Subcutaneous fat, 224*f*
Subscapular line sign, with implant rupture, 671, 672*f*, 673*f*
Subtraction imaging, in MRI, 187, 187*f*
Summary judgment, motion for, 729
Summary statistics, 26
Supernumerary nipples, 223
Superoinferior oblique (SIO) view, 116-117
Supervising radiologist, in quality control, 134, 134*t*
Surgery, fat necrosis after, 327-329, 331*f*
Surgical margins, microscopic evaluation of, 623, 623*f*, 624*f*
Surveillance, Epidemiology, and End Results (SEER) Program, 25, 57
Survival, long-term, with breast cancer, 37
Survival rate
  axillary lymph node metastases and, 442-445, 445*t*, 467, 468*t*
  with male breast cancer, 470
  racial differences in, 35-37
  screening and, 57-61
  stage at diagnosis and, 35, 36*f*
  trends in, 37, 37*f*
Susan B. Komen Foundation, on screening, 62
Susceptibility gene(s), 229
  ATM as, 48
  BRCA1 and *BRCA2* as, 46-47
  BRIP1 and *PALB2* as, 48
  CDH1 as, 47-48
  CHEK2 as, 47, 48
  founder, 47
  gene expression patterns with, 229-230, 230*f*
  due to loss of heterozygosity, 229
  low penetrance, 48
  due to microsatellite instability, 229
  PTEN as, 47
  STK11 as, 47
  TP53 as, 47
  tumor suppressor, 229
Suspicious lesions, ultrasound of
  for determining extent, 160-161, 161*f*
  for regional lymph node assessment, 161-166, 162*f*, 163*f*, 164*f*, 165*f*
Sutures, calcified, 332, 340*f*
SV (single voxel)-based magnetic resonance spectroscopy, 762, 768
Swedish Two-County Trial, 57-58, 58*t*
  and screening guidelines, 63, 71
  and underestimation of benefits from screening, 61
Swing views, in stereotactic-guided core needle biopsy, 577, 580-581, 580*f*
Synchronous carcinoma, 467
Syndrome(s), associated with increased breast cancer risk, 48
  BRCA1 and *BRCA2* in, 46-47
  Cowden syndrome as, 47
  E-cadherin in, 47-48
  Li-Fraumeni syndrome as, 47
  Peutz-Jeghers syndrome as, 47
System resolution evaluation, in quality control, 138*t*, 142

T

T1 relaxation time, in MRI, 17, 179-180, 180*f*
T1 weighted image, in MRI, 181, 182, 183*f*, 183*t*
T2 relaxation time, in MRI, 17, 179-180, 180*f*, 183*t*
T2 weighted image, in MRI, 181, 183*t*, 184, 184*f*
Tail of Spence, 111
Tamoxifen
  and breast cancer risk, 44-45
  for DCIS, 415-416, 418
Tanaka, Kenji, 13
Tangential (TAN) view, 119
Target angle, of x-ray tube, 83, 83*f*
Target materials, in mammography unit, 82
Targeted therapy, 232, 234*t*
Tattoos, calcifications due to, 325-326, 328*f*
T-cell lymphoma, peripheral, 502, 504, 504*f*, 505*f*
TDLU. *See* Terminal duct lobular unit (TDLU).
TE (time to echo), in MRI, 180, 180*f*
Tea bag, in assessing for concordance, 635
Teardrop sign, with implant rupture, 673, 673*f*
Technetium 99m (^{99m}Tc) methoxyisobutylisonitrile (sestamibi, MIBI) scintigraphy, history of, 17
Technetium 99m (^{99m}Tc) methoxyisobutylisonitrile (sestamibi, MIBI) scintimammography, 747
Technetium 99m (^{99m}Tc) pertechnetate scintigraphy, history of, 16, 17*f*
Technique factor, quality control test of, 139*t*
TechniScan system, for automated whole breast ultrasound, 752-753, 754*f*
Technology development, legal aspects of, 732, 736-737
Terminal duct
  anatomy of, 224*f*
  histology of, 226*f*
Terminal duct lobular unit (TDLU)
  anatomy of, 224-225, 225*f*
  benign calcifications with, 341*f*
  vs. ductal hyperplasia of usual type, 310-314, 311*f*, 312*f*
  histology of, 225*f*, 226*f*
  ultrasound of, 168-171, 173*f*
TFTs (thin-film transistors), for image detection
  with cesium iodide crystals, 95-96, 96*f*
  with selenium flat-panel system, 96*f*
The Joint Committee (TJC), on medical audit, 703
Thelarche, 224
Therapeutic trials, screening trials *vs.*, 63
Thermography, history of, 16, 16*f*
Thermoluminescent dosimeters (TLDs), history of, 20-21
Thin-film transistors (TFTs), for image detection
  with cesium iodide crystals, 95-96, 96*f*
  with selenium flat-panel system, 96*f*
Thomas, Louis B., 21
Three-dimensional MRI, 181
Three-dimensional ultrasound, 149-152, 152*f*
Throw mechanism, for ultrasound-guided core needle biopsy, 565, 565*f*
Thymocyte selection-associated high mobility group box member 3 *(TOX3)* gene, and breast cancer risk, 48
Time to echo (TE), in MRI, 180, 180*f*
Time/signal-intensity curves (TIC), in MRI, 219
Tissue expanders, and MRI, 196-197
Tissue processing, 630-631
  coverslipping in, 615
  embedding in paraffin in, 630-631, 631*f*
  equipment for, 630-631, 631*f*
  fixation in, 630-631
  sectioning in, 615, 632*f*
  staining in, 615, 632*f*

Tissue sections, 630-631
TJC (The Joint Committee), on medical audit, 703
TLDs (thermoluminescent dosimeters), history of, 20-21
TN (true-negative), in medical audit, 704, 706, 706*f*, 708*t*
TNM staging, of invasive ductal carcinoma, 438, 439*t*, 440*t*, 442*t*
Toker cell hyperplasia, *vs.* Paget's disease, 405-409
Tolling, of statute of limitations, 736
Tomosynthesis, 744-746, 745*f*
  digital, with automated whole breast ultrasound, 752-753, 755*f*
Topical anesthesia, for core needle biopsy
  stereotactic-guided, 581
  ultrasound-guided, 569
Torts, 729
  intentional, 735
TOX3 (thymocyte selection-associated high mobility group box member 3) gene, and breast cancer risk, 48
TP (true-positive), in medical audit, 704, 706, 706*f*, 708*t*
TP53 (tumor protein p53) gene mutation, 229
  and breast cancer risk, 47
  as prognostic and predictive factor, 232
TR (repetition time), in MRI, 180, 180*f*
Training, in breast imaging, 19*f*, 20
  Society of Breast Imaging in, 20
Tram-track appearance, of vascular calcifications, 326-327, 329*f*
Transducers, for ultrasound, 146, 147*f*, 217-218
Transillumination, history of, 15, 16*f*
Translocations, unbalanced, 229
Transsexuals, male-to-female, breast cancer in, 468-469
Trauma, fat necrosis after, 327-329, 331*f*
Trial, legal, 730
Trichilemmal cysts, 239
Trichinosis, mastitis due to, 376, 379*f*
Trigger point, for nipple discharge, 597
Triple test
  with core needle biopsy, 615, 635-637
  with fine-needle aspiration, 612
True size, 113
True-negative (TN), in medical audit, 704, 706, 706*f*, 708*t*
True-positive (TP), in medical audit, 704, 706, 706*f*, 708*t*
Tube-image receptor assembly motion, quality control test of, 139*t*
Tuberculous mastitis, 384*f*, 385
Tubular adenoma, 274-276
  clinical presentation of, 274
  defined, 274
  etiology and pathophysiology of, 274
  imaging indications and algorithm for, 274
  mammography of, 274
  MRI of, 274
  pathology findings with, 274, 275*f*
  prevalence and epidemiology of, 274
  treatment options for, 276
  ultrasonography of, 274, 275*f*
Tubular carcinoma, 453, 453*f*
  radial scar *vs.*, 306-308, 307*f*, 308*f*, 309*f*
Tubulolobular carcinoma, 424, 454*f*
Tumor cell(s), epithelial displacement of, due to core needle biopsy
  stereotactic-guided, 587
  ultrasound-guided, 576
Tumor cell proliferation, as prognostic and predictive factor, 231
Tumor necrosis, as prognostic and predictive factor, 231
Tumor protein p53 *(TP53)* gene mutation, 229
  and breast cancer risk, 47
  as prognostic and predictive factor, 232
Tumor size
  and axillary lymph node metastases, 467, 468*t*
  in epidemiology of breast cancer, 34-38, 34*f*, 36*f*
  with excisional biopsy, 618-619
  in medical audit
    analysis of, 710
    in medical literature, 708*t*
    with screening and diagnostic mammography data combined, 712*t*, 713*t*
    value of, 716, 716*t*
  as prognostic and predictive factor, 231
Tumor size measurement
  gross, 619-620
    cassettes in, 619-620, 621*f*
    initial appearance of specimen in, 619-620, 619*f*
    inking of margins in, 619-620, 619*f*
    recording of, 619-620, 620*f*
    specimen slicing in, 619-620, 620*f*
  microscopic, 620, 622*f*
Tumor suppressor genes, 229
Two-County Swedish Trial, 57-58, 58*t*
  and screening guidelines, 63, 71
  and underestimation of benefits from screening, 61

U

U-arm, of mammography unit, 81, 84-85, 84*f*, 85*f*
UK Age Trial, 57-58, 58*t*
Ulceration, in invasive ductal carcinoma, 438, 438*f*
Ultrasonography (US)
  anatomy of breast on, 226, 228*f*
  associated findings on, 218
  automated whole breast, 751-753
    ACUSON S2000 system for, 752-753, 753*f*
    digital tomosynthesis with, 752-753, 755*f*
    history of, 751-752, 752*f*
    SomoVu system for, 752-753, 753*f*
    SonoCine system for, 752-753, 753*f*
    TechniScan system for, 752-753, 754*f*
  BI-RADS for, 153-154, 154*t*, 217-218
    technical considerations in, 217-218
  of breast implants, 287, 674-679
    limitations of, 678-679
    normal findings in, 674, 676*f*
    with radial folds, 674, 677*f*
    with reverberation artifacts, 674, 677*f*
    with rupture, 674-678
      extracapsular, 677-678, 678*f*, 679*f*
      intracapsular, 677, 678*f*
    with silicone granulomas, 287, 288*f*, 677-678, 679*f*
  correlation with MRI of, 166-167, 166*f*, 167*f*
  dynamic range in, 217-218
  equipment for (*See* Ultrasound (US) equipment)
  field of view in, 149, 151*f*, 217-218
  focal zone setting in, 146, 147*f*, 217-218
  gray scale gain in, 217-218
  harmonic imaging in, 147-148, 149*f*
  history of, 13-15, 153
    A-mode and B-mode scans in, 13, 14*f*
    John Wild and John Reid in, 13, 14, 14*f*
    Octoson in, 14-15, 15*f*
    water-bath system in, 13, 14*f*
  indication(s) for, 154-176
Ultrasonography (US) *(Continued)*
    assessment of regional lymph nodes in patient with suspicious breast lesions undergoing biopsy as, 161-166, 162*f*, 163*f*, 164*f*, 165*f*
    breast pain as, 157-158, 158*f*
    correlation with MRI ("second-look") as, 166-167, 166*f*, 167*f*
    determination of extent of suspicious or malignant lesions as, 160-161, 161*f*
    guidance of interventional procedures as, 167-168, 169*f*, 170*f*
    mammographic abnormalities as, 156-157, 156*f*, 157*f*
    nipple discharge as, 158-159, 159*f*, 160*f*
    palpable abnormalities as, 155, 155*f*
    screening as, 168-176
      for cysts, 171-176, 174*f*, 175*f*, 176*f*
      goals of, 168
      identification of structures in, 168-171, 170*f*, 171*f*
      for solid breast nodules, 171, 172*f*, 173*f*
    short-interval follow-up of lesions as, 159-160, 160*f*
  of invasive ductal carcinoma, 435-437
  lexicon for, 153-154, 154*t*
  long-axis focusing in, 146, 147*f*
  of male breast cancer, 469
  medical audit of, 713-714
  MRI for difficult or equivocal, 201
  multiple focal zones in, 146, 148*f*
  posterior acoustic shadowing in, 148, 150*f*
  "second look", 166-167, 166*f*, 167*f*
    with MRI-guided core needle biopsy, 593
  short-axis focusing in, 147, 147*f*, 148*f*
  spatial compound imaging in, 148-149, 150*f*, 151*f*, 217-218
  spatial resolution in, 146-147, 147*f*, 148*f*
  speckle reduction imaging in, 148-149, 151*f*
  three-dimensional and four-dimensional, 149-152, 152*f*
  transducers for, 146, 147*f*, 217-218
Ultrasound (US) ablation, high-intensity focused, 775
Ultrasound (US) equipment, 146-152
  field of view with, 149, 151*f*
  for harmonic imaging, 147-148, 149*f*
  for spatial compound imaging, 148-149, 150*f*, 151*f*
  spatial resolution with, 146-147, 147*f*, 148*f*
  for three-dimensional and four-dimensional imaging, 149-152, 152*f*
  transducers as, 146, 147*f*
Ultrasound (US)-guided interventional procedures, 167-168, 169*f*, 170*f*
Ultrasound-activated microbubble drug delivery, 759, 759*f*
Ultrasound-guided computer-aided detection, 757-759, 758*f*
Ultrasound-guided core needle biopsy (US CNB), 167-168, 564-576
  advantages of, 564, 575
  air tracts in, 569-571, 571*f*
  anesthesia for
    epinephrine with, 568-569
    injection site for, 569, 569*f*
    local, 568-569
    topical, 569
  of calcifications, 170*f*
  coaxial system for, 569, 570*f*
  coding and billing for, 723*t*
  confirmation of sampling adequacy in, 569-571, 571*f*, 572*f*
  consent form for, 566-567
  contraindications to, 576
  for cyst aspiration, 574

Ultrasound-guided core needle biopsy (US CNB) *(Continued)*
of deep lesions, 569, 569*f*, 572, 573*f*
in dense breast, 572
dermatotomy in, 569
description of, 564
equipment for, 564-566
needle and throw mechanism in, 565, 565*f*
sterile biopsy tray in, 564-565, 564*f*
vacuum-assisted device in, 565, 566*f*
of fibroadenoma, 169*f*
indications for, 575-576
of lesion seen on another modality, 575-576
of lymph nodes, 575
marking clip in, 572
of multiple suspicious findings, 575
as one-person or two-person procedure, 568, 568*f*
optimal needle positioning for, 569-571, 571*f*
orientation of needle in, 568, 568*f*
positioning for, 567, 567*f*
post-procedure considerations for, 574-575
potential complications of, 576
pre-procedural considerations for, 566-568
pre-scanning in, 567, 567*f*
readjustment of transducer or needle position during, 569-571, 570*f*
regional lymph node assessment with, 161-166, 162*f*, 163*f*, 164*f*, 165*f*
report on, 575
of small target, 573-574, 574*f*
specimen preparation from, 575
with steep approach angle, 569, 569*f*, 572, 573*f*
sterile portion of procedure for, 568-574
vacuum-assisted device for, 167-168, 565
of calcifications, 170*f*
confirmation of sampling adequacy with, 569-571, 572*f*
cutting mechanism of, 565, 566*f*
for cysts, 171-176, 176*f*
of fibroadenoma, 169*f*
for nipple discharge, 158-159, 159*f*
of very superficial lesions, 569, 569*f*, 572, 573*f*
Unbalanced translocations, 229
Underexposure, 124, 127*f*
Unknown primary tumor, metastatic to breast, 513*f*
Up-coding, 725
Uptake curve, for contrast-enhanced MRI, 186, 186*f*
Upton, Arthur C., 21
US. *See* Ultrasonography (US).
U.S. Preventive Services Task Force (USPSTF), on screening, 62, 70-72

V

Vacuum-assisted breast (VAB) biopsy
MRI-guided, 591-592
stereotactic-guided, 578-579
ultrasound-guided, 167-168, 565
of calcifications, 170*f*
confirmation of sampling adequacy with, 569-571, 572*f*
cutting mechanism of, 565, 566*f*
of cysts, 171-176, 176*f*
of fibroadenoma, 169*f*
for nipple discharge, 158-159, 159*f*
Vagal reactions, due to core needle biopsy
MRI-guided, 594
stereotactic-guided, 586-587
ultrasound-guided, 576
Validation film checks, in accreditation, 699
Validation procedures, in accreditation, 699-700
annual updates as, 699
on-site surveys as, 699-700
validation film checks as, 699
Van Nuys Prognostic Index (VNPI), 410-416
Vascular abnormalities, in malignant lesions, 196
Vascular calcifications, 326-327
arterial, 327, 330*f*
Mönckeberg type, 326-327, 329*f*, 345*f*
tram-track appearance of, 326-327, 329*f*
Vascular endothelial growth factor (VEGF), in malignant lesions, 196
Vasovagal reaction
to galactography, 604
to needle localization, 607
Venet, Louis, 18
Vessel density, in malignant lesions, 196
View(s), mammographic. *See* Mammographic view(s).
View actual pixels, 113
Viewbox(es), quality control test of, 137*t*, 142
Viewbox luminance, quality control test of, 138*t*, 143
Viewing conditions, quality control test of, 137*t*, 142
Virtual convex view, in ultrasonography, 149, 151*f*
Visual checklist, for quality control, 137*t*, 142
VNPI (Van Nuys Prognostic Index), 410-416
Vogel, Walter, 3
Voltage divider, in mammography unit, 82
Voltage doubling circuit, in mammography unit, 82
Volume of interest (VOI), in magnetic resonance spectroscopy, 762
Volumetric ultrasound, 149-152, 152*f*

W

Wagai, Toshio, 14
Warranty, on mammography equipment, 97
Warren, Stafford, 3-4, 5*f*, 6*f*, 9
Washout phase, for contrast-enhanced MRI, 186, 186*f*
Water droplet sign, with implant rupture, 673, 674*f*
Water-to-fat ratio, in magnetic resonance spectroscopy, 761-762
Weber, William, 9
Weight, and breast cancer risk, 42
Weight gain, and breast cancer risk, 42
Wells, P. N.T., 14-15
Wheelchair, mammographic views with, 111, 112*f*
WHI (Women's Health Initiative), 44
White women
incidence of breast cancer in, 33-34, 33*f*
mortality rate in, 38, 39*f*
stage of diagnosis in, 34, 35, 35*f*, 36*f*
and survival rate, 35, 36*f*
tumor size in, 34, 34*f*
WHO (World Health Organization), on cancer statistics, 25
Wild, John, 13, 14, 14*f*, 15
Wire localization, MRI-guided, 210-211
Wolfe, John, 11, 11*f*
Women's Health Initiative (WHI), 44
Workstation
acquisition, 91, 91*f*, 92*f*
radiologist review, 91-92, 92*f*
Workup
of palpable mass, 542-543, 549
mammography for, 542-543, 545*f*
MRI for, 543
ultrasonography for, 542-543, 545*f*
of possible mass on screening mammography, 542-550
with benign features, 547-549
biopsy of, 547-549
fat-containing, 543, 546*b*
management algorithm for, 547, 549*f*
multiple bilateral circumscribed round or oval, 547, 548*f*
and no prior mammograms, 547
requiring no further evaluation, 543-546, 547, 548*f*
short-term imaging for, 547-549
ultrasonography for, 547, 548*f*, 549
focal asymmetries as, 546-547
defined, 546
diagnostic mammography for, 547
spot compression views for, 542, 543*f*
ultrasound-guided biopsy for, 547, 547*f*
MRI for, 542, 544*f*
spot compression views for, 542, 543*f*
suspicious and malignant, 549-550, 550*f*
ultrasonography for, 542, 543*f*
World Health Organization (WHO), on cancer statistics, 25
Wuchereria bancrofti, 387*f*, 388
Wunderlich, Carl, 16

X

Xeromammography, history of, 11-12, 12*f*, 13*f*, 79
XLCC (exaggerated lateral craniocaudal) view, 117-118, 118*f*
XMCC (exaggerated medial craniocaudal) view, 122-123, 125*f*
X-ray film, quality control test of, 139*t*
X-ray tube, in mammography unit, 81, 82-84, 82*f*, 83*f*

Y

Young modulus, in elastography, 754-755, 756*f*

Z

"Zeroing out" in stereotactic-guided core needle biopsy, 581
Zinc oxide-containing ointment, calcifications due to, 325-326, 328*f*

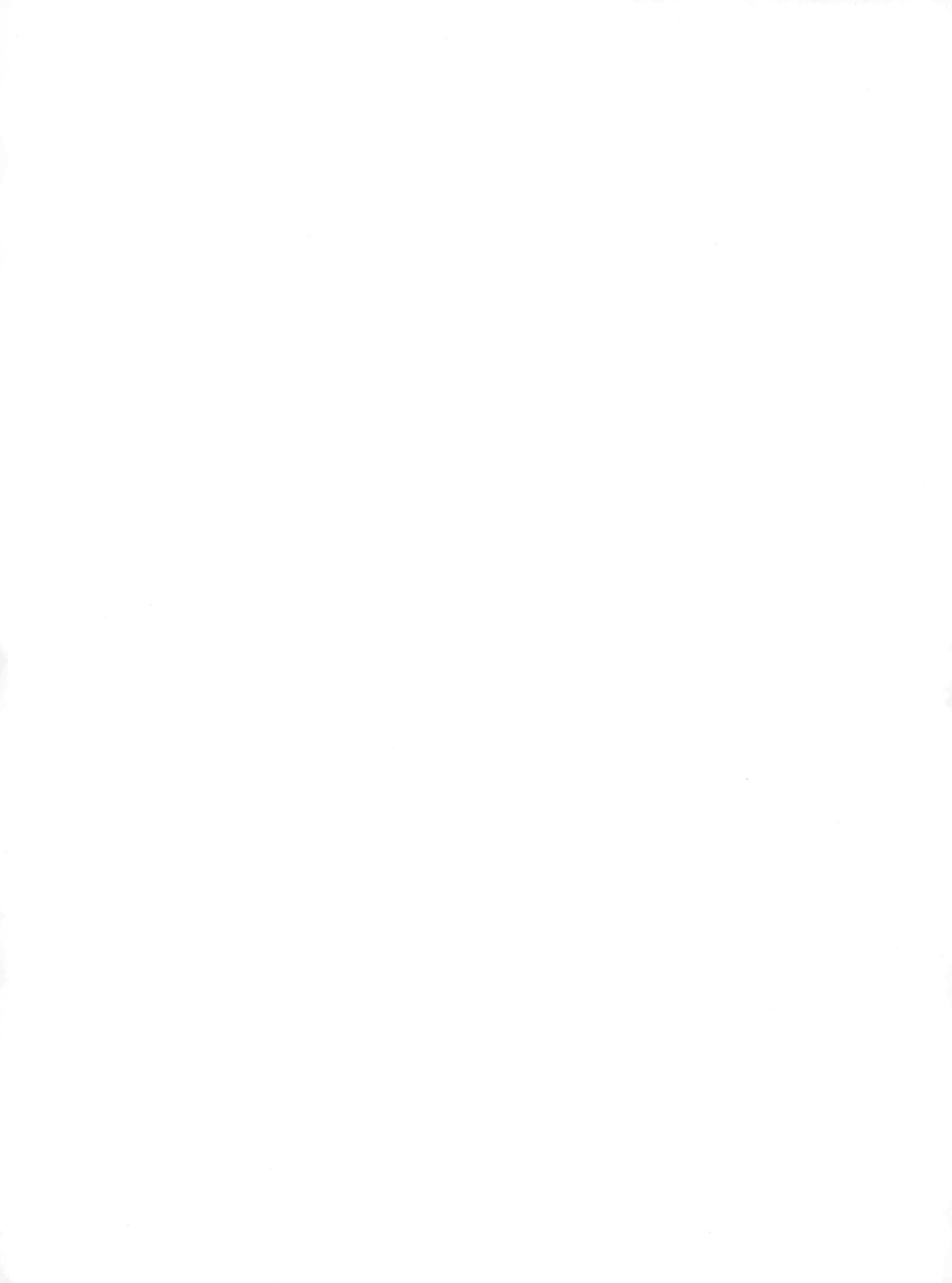